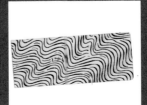

Principles and Practice of
PEDIATRIC SLEEP MEDICINE

Content Strategist: Helene Caprari
Content Development Specialist: Poppy Garraway
Content Coordinator: Humayra Rahman Khan
Project Manager: Sruthi Viswam
Design: Steven Stave
Illustration Manager: Jennifer Rose
Illustrator: Antbits
Marketing Manager (UK/USA): Nyasha Kapenzi

Principles and Practice of PEDIATRIC SLEEP MEDICINE

SECOND EDITION

Stephen H. Sheldon DO FAAP

Professor of Pediatrics
Northwestern University, Feinberg School of Medicine
Director, Sleep Medicine Center
Division of Pediatric Pulmonary Medicine
Ann & Robert H. Lurie Children's Hospital of Chicago
Chicago, IL, USA

Richard Ferber MD

Associate Professor of Neurology
Harvard Medical School
Staff Associate Emeritus
Boston Children's Hospital
Boston, MA, USA

Meir H. Kryger MD FRCPC

Professor
Department of Medicine
Section of Pulmonary, Critical Care and Sleep Medicine
Yale School of Medicine
New Haven, CT, USA

David Gozal MD

Herbert T. Abelson Professor and Chairman,
Department of Pediatrics,
Physician-in-Chief Comer Children's Hospital,
The University of Chicago
Chicago, IL, USA

ELSEVIER
SAUNDERS

London, New York, Oxford, Philadelphia, St Louis, Sydney, Toronto

ELSEVIER
SAUNDERS
an imprint of Elsevier Inc.

© 2014, Elsevier Inc. All rights reserved.

First edition 2005
Second edition 2014

Notices

Knowledge and best practice in this field are constantly changing. As new research and experience broaden our understanding, changes in research methods, professional practices, or medical treatment may become necessary.

Practitioners and researchers must always rely on their own experience and knowledge in evaluating and using any information, methods, compounds, or experiments described herein. In using such information or methods they should be mindful of their own safety and the safety of others, including parties for whom they have a professional responsibility.

With respect to any drug or pharmaceutical products identified, readers are advised to check the most current information provided (i) on procedures featured or (ii) by the manufacturer of each product to be administered, to verify the recommended dose or formula, the method and duration of administration, and contraindications. It is the responsibility of practitioners, relying on their own experience and knowledge of their patients, to make diagnoses, to determine dosages and the best treatment for each individual patient, and to take all appropriate safety precautions.

To the fullest extent of the law, neither the Publisher nor the authors, contributors, or editors, assume any liability for any injury and/or damage to persons or property as a matter of products liability, negligence or otherwise, or from any use or operation of any methods, products, instructions, or ideas contained in the material herein.

ISBN: 9781455703180
e-book ISBN: 9781455733323

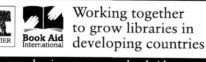

Working together
to grow libraries in
developing countries

www.elsevier.com • www.bookaid.org

Contents

Preface

Sleep medicine is a medical specialty unique in that it concentrates on events occurring during the hours of sleep to explain various aspects of a patient's health and disease. Pediatric sleep medicine is a field holding special significance because of its concern with a state that occupies over half of a child's life during the important early years of development.

The normal maturation of sleep systems is clearly among the most important neurodevelopmental milestones. The neurologic structures responsible for sleep develop rapidly during the early months and years of life and generate sleep patterns of increasing complexity and predictability. Early disruption of these vital processes can impose major cognitive and emotional consequences. Studies have confirmed the importance of sleep for the acquisition and processing of new knowledge and for maintenance of information previously gained. Recognition of both primary and secondary sleep-related disorders has also been shown as essential to the understanding and proper treatment of many other childhood disorders.

Principles and Practice of Sleep Medicine in the Child was published as a volume separate from *Principles and Practice of Sleep Medicine* for the first time in 1995. The existence of this and other texts in pediatric sleep medicine has helped move the practice of pediatric sleep medicine away from the sphere of adult medicine practitioners to one that is overseen by professionals who have dedicated their careers to the health and well-being of the pediatric patient. The preface to that 1995 volume states, in a sentence still true today, that "...*a robust scientifically based body of knowledge has emerged, and the tools to diagnose and effectively treat children with sleep disorders are now available.*" The subsequent edition, published in 2005 as *Principles and Practice of Pediatric Sleep Medicine,* along with this current edition hopefully represent additional meaningful steps in the development of pediatric sleep medicine as a distinct discipline.

Both the *American Academy of Pediatrics* and the *American Board of Pediatrics* have formally recognized and supported growth of this important discipline. In 2007, the *American Board of Pediatrics* joined several other member boards of the *American Board of Medical Specialties* in providing subspeciality certification in the field of sleep medicine. By so doing, these boards acknowledged that sleep-related disorders are not only distinctive but are also important in the evaluation and management of many disorders affecting children.

In diagnosing and managing sleep disorders in children the practitioner should be aware of various possible relationships between the disorders themselves and the effects on the child and family. Three of these very important relationships are:

1. A primary sleep-related pathology may directly cause important daytime symptoms and adverse health sequelae in the child, and only through treatment of the sleep disorder is resolution of these problems possible.
2. A sleep-related pathology may be a co-morbid condition contributing to the daytime symptoms seen in the child. In such instances, through treatment of the sleep-related pathology, the patient becomes more responsive to treatment of the co-existing disorders.
3. A child's sleep difficulties may have greater direct impact on other family members than it does on the affected child him- or herself. Thus a caretaker, for example, may be the one to become most sleep deprived and with the most medical and emotional compromise, but this compromise may include the inability to properly care for the child. Treating the child's sleep problems can improve the lives of child and family members alike.

As we continue to gain further knowledge, obtain additional evidence, and develop a better understanding of the effects of sleep and its disorders on children, major advances will be made, including insights into the often unclear area of cause and effect. Sleep disorders in infants and children reflect an interplay among many factors, including the development and maintenance of the central nervous system, the impact of environmental influences, the effects of altered patterns of parent-child interaction, and the presence of social stress and other medical conditions.

Child-care professionals must possess a comprehensive knowledge of these interactions to deliver optimal care. This book hopefully provides both the sleep medicine specialist and the primary care practitioner with resources to enable them to provide the best possible care to their pediatric patients throughout the 24-hour day and night.

Stephen H. Sheldon, Chicago
Richard Ferber, Washington
Meir H. Kryger, New Haven
David Gozal, Chicago

List of Contributors

Candice A. Alfano, PhD
Associate Professor, Department of Psychology, University of Houston; Director, Sleep and Anxiety Center for Kids (SACK), Houston, TX, USA

W. Jerome Alonso, MD
Clinical Assistant Professor, Faculty of Medicine, University of Calgary; Medical Director, Canadian Sleep Consultants, Calgary, Alberta, Canada

Raouf Amin, MD
The Hubert Dorothy Campbell Professor of Pediatric Pulmonology, Director of the Division of Pulmonary Medicine, Cincinnati Children's Hospital Medical Center, Cincinnati, OH, USA

Sarah R. Brand, PhD
Clinical Psychologist, Division of Pediatric Psychosocial Oncology, Department of Psychosocial Oncology and Palliative Care, Dana-Farber Cancer Institute/Children's Hospital of Boston, Boston, MA, USA

Chasity Brimeyer, PhD
Postdoctoral Fellow, Department of Psychology, St. Jude Children's Research Hospital, Memphis, TN, USA

Kevin L. Boyd, DDS MSc
Attending Clinical Instructor, Departments of Dentistry and Sleep Medicine, Ann & Robert H. Lurie Children's Hospital, Chicago, IL, USA

Mary A. Carskadon, PhD
Professor, E.P. Bradley Hospital Sleep Research Laboratory, Department of Psychiatry and Human Behavior, Alpert Medical School of Brown University, Providence, RI, USA; Professor, School of Psychology, Social Work and Social Policy, Director Centre for Sleep Research, University of South Australia, Adelaide, South Australia

John L. Carroll, MD
Professor, Department of Pediatrics, Division of Pediatric Pulmonary and Sleep Medicine, University of Arkansas for Medical Sciences, Arkansas Children's Hospital, Little Rock, AR, USA

Ronald D. Chervin, MD MS
Professor of Neurology, Michael S. Aldrich Collegiate Professor of Sleep Medicine; Director, University of Michigan Sleep Disorders Center, Department of Neurology, University of Michigan Health System, Ann Arbor, MI, USA

Anat Cohen Engler, MD
Resident Physician, Pediatrics Department, Meir Hospital, Kfar Saba, Israel

Jonathan Cogen, MD MPH
Department of Pediatrics, Ann & Robert H. Lurie Children's Hospital of Chicago, Northwestern University School of Medicine, Chicago, IL, USA

Valerie McLaughlin Crabtree, PhD CBSM
Director of Clinical Services and Training, Department of Psychology, St. Jude Children's Research Hospital, Memphis, TN, USA

Stephanie J. Crowley, PhD
Assistant Professor, Biological Rhythms Research Laboratory, Department of Behavioral Sciences, Rush University Medical Center, Chicago, IL, USA

Jamie A. Cvengros, PhD CBSM
Assistant Professor, Department of Behavioral Sciences, Associate Director, Behavioral Sleep Medicine Program, Sleep Disorders Service & Research Center, Rush University Medical Center, Chicago, IL, USA

Sally L. Davidson Ward MD
Associate Professor of Pediatrics, Division Chief, Pediatric Pulmonology, Keck School of Medicine of the University of Southern California; Division of Pediatric Pulmonology, Children's Hospital Los Angeles, Los Angeles, CA, USA

David F. Donnelly, PhD
Professor, Department of Pediatrics, Yale University School of Medicine, New Haven, CT, USA

Jeffrey S. Durmer, MD PhD
Adjunct Professor, Department of Health Professions, College of Health and Human Sciences; Chief Medical Officer, FusionHealth, Johns Creek, Atlanta, GA, USA

James E. Dillon, MD
Professor and Director of Residency Training, Department of Psychiatry, Central Michigan University College of Medicine, Saginaw, MI, USA

Tamar Etzioni, MD
Pediatrician and Sleep physician, Pediatrics Department and Sleep Clinic, Carmel Medical Center and Technion Faculty of Medicine, Haifa, Israel

David Gozal, MD
Herbert T. Abelson Professor and Chairman, Department of Pediatrics, Physician-in-Chief, Comer Children's Hospital, The University of Chicago, Chicago, IL, USA

Madeleine M. Grigg-Damberger, MD
Professor of Neurology, University of New Mexico School of Medicine, Department of Neurology, One University of New Mexico, Albuquerque, NM, USA

Paul Gringras, MCRPCH
Professor, Department of Children's Sleep Medicine, Evelina London Children's Hospital, Lifespan Sleep Disorder Group, Kings College London, London, UK

Guy Gut, MD
Pediatric Pulmonologist, Department of Pediatric Pulmonology, Critical Care and Sleep Medicine, Dana Children's Hospital, Tel Aviv Medical Center, Tel Aviv University Sackler Faculty of Medicine, Tel Aviv, Israel

Susan M. Harding, MD
Professor of Medicine, UAB Sleep/Wake Disorders Center, Division of Pulmonary, Allergy & Critical Care Medicine, Department of Medicine, University of Alabama at Birmingham, Birmingham, AL, USA

Mark Haupt, MD
Fellow, Division of Pulmonary Medicine, Ann & Robert H. Lurie Children's Hospital of Chicago, Northwestern University Feinberg School of Medicine, Chicago, IL, USA

John H. Herman, PhD
Professor of Psychiatry and Pediatrics, University of Texas Southwestern Medical Center at Dallas, Dallas, TX, USA

Rosemary S.C. Horne, PhD
Professor, NHMRC Senior Research Fellow and Deputy Director, The Ritchie Centre, Monash Institute of Medical Research, Monash University, Melbourne, Victoria, Australia

Anna Ivanenko, MD PhD
Associate Professor of Clinical Psychiatry and Behavioral Sciences, Feinberg School of Medicine, Northwestern University, Division of Child and Adolescent Psychiatry, Ann & Robert H. Lurie Children's Hospital of Chicago, Chicago, IL, USA

Michaela C. Johnson, BA
Department of Psychology, College of the Holy Cross, Worcester, MA, USA

Eliot Katz, MD
Assistant Professor, Harvard Medical School, Division of Respiratory Diseases, Boston Children's Hospital, Boston, MA, USA

Leila Kheirandish-Gozal, MD MSc
Associate Professor, Director of Clinical Sleep Research, Section of Pediatric Sleep Medicine, Department of Pediatrics, Pritzker School of Medicine, Biological Sciences Division, The University of Chicago, Chicago, IL, USA

Michael Kohrman, MD
Professor of Pediatrics, Neurology and Surgery, University of Chicago, Chicago, IL, USA

Suresh Kotagal, MD
Professor, Department of Neurology, Mayo Medical School; Consultant in Neurology, Pediatrics and the Center for Sleep Medicine, Mayo Clinic, Rochester, MN, USA

Harsha Kumar, MD
Assistant Professor of Pediatrics, Division of Pulmonary Medicine, University of Illinois at Chicago, Chicago, IL, USA

Jonathan Kushnir, PhD
Clinical Psychologist and Supervisor, The Child Psychiatry Unit Edmond and Lily Safra Children's Hospital, Sheba Medical Center Ramat Gan, Israel

Jyoti Krishna, MD
Assistant Professor of Pediatrics, Head, Pediatric Sleep Medicine, Sleep Disorders Center, Cleveland Clinic, Cleveland, OH, USA

Darius A. Loughmanee, MD FAAP
Assistant Professor of Pediatrics, Northwestern University Feinberg School of Medicine; Medical Director, Sleep Medicine Services at Westchester, Ann & Robert H. Lurie Children's Hospital of Chicago, Chicago, IL, USA

Carole L. Marcus, MBBCh
Professor of Pediatrics, University of Pennsylvania; Director, Sleep Center, The Children's Hospital of Philadelphia, Philadelphia, PA, USA

Susanna A. McColley, MD
Professor of Pediatrics, Northwestern University Feinberg School of Medicine; Head, Division of Pulmonary Medicine; Co-Director, Cystic Fibrosis Center; Associate Chair for Clinical Affairs, Department of Pediatrics, Ann & Robert H. Lurie Children's Hospital of Chicago, Chicago, IL, USA

Jodi A. Mindell, PhD
Professor of Psychology, Saint Joseph's University, Philadelphia; Associate Director, Sleep Center, The Children's Hospital of Philadelphia, PA, USA

Melisa Moore, PhD
Clinical Psychologist, Sleep Center, The Children's Hospital of Philadelphia, Philadelphia, PA, USA

Louise M. O'Brien, PhD MS
Associate Professor, Sleep Disorders Center, Department of Neurology; Associate Professor, Department of Obstetrics & Gynecology; Associate Research Scientist, Department of Oral & Maxillofacial Surgery, University of Michigan Health System, Ann Arbor, MI, USA

Judith A. Owens, MD MPH
Professor of Pediatrics, George Washington School of Medicine and Health Sciences; Director of Sleep Medicine, Division of Pulmonary and Sleep Medicine, Children's National Medical Center, Washington DC, USA

Pallavi P. Patwari, MD
Assistant Professor of Pediatrics, Northwestern University Feinberg School of Medicine, Ann & Robert H. Lurie Children's Hospital of Chicago, Chicago, IL, USA

Rafael Pelayo, MD
Clinical Professor, Stanford Sleep Medicine Center, Stanford University School of Medicine, Stanford, CA, USA

Iris A. Perez, MD
Assistant Professor of Pediatrics, Keck School of Medicine of the University of Southern California, Division of Pediatric Pulmonology, Children's Hospital Los Angeles, Los Angeles, CA, USA

Giora Pillar, MD, PhD
Professor and Head, Pediatrics Department and Sleep Clinic, Carmel Medical Center and Technion Faculty of Medicine, Haifa, Israel

Christian F. Poets, MD
Professor and Medical Director, Department of Neonatology, University Children's Hospital, Tuebingen, Germany

Amanda M. Roch, BA
Graduate student, Department of Psychology, University of Memphis, Memphis, TN, USA

Casey M. Rand, BS
Senior Project Coordinator, Center for Autonomic Medicine in Pediatrics (CAMP), Ann & Robert H. Lurie Children's Hospital of Chicago, Chicago, IL, USA

Gerald M. Rosen, MD
Associate Professor of Pediatrics, University of Minnesota School of Medicine, Children's Hospitals and Clinics of Minnesota, St Paul, MN, USA

Oscar Sans Capdevila, MD
Clinical Coordinator, Sleep Center, Pediatric Sleep Medicine, Division of Neurophysiology, Department of Neurology, Hospital Sant Joan de Déu, Barcelona, Spain

Abu Shamsuzzaman, MD PhD
Assistant Professor of Pediatrics, Cincinnati Children's Hospital Medical Center, University of Cincinnati, Cincinnati, OH, USA

Stephen H. Sheldon, DO FAAP
Professor of Pediatrics, Northwestern University, Feinberg School of Medicine; Director, Sleep Medicine Center, Division of Pediatric Pulmonary Medicine, Ann & Robert H. Lurie Children's Hospital of Chicago, Chicago, IL, USA

Yakov Sivan, MD
Professor and Chairman, Department of Pediatrics, Tel Aviv University Sackler, Faculty of Medicine; Director, Department of Pediatric Pulmonology, Critical Care and Sleep Medicine, Dana Children's Hospital, Tel Aviv Medical Center, Tel Aviv, Israel

Cecille G. Sulman, MD
Associate Professor, Chief, Division of Pediatric Otolaryngology, Department of Otolaryngology and Communication Sciences, Medical College of Wisconsin, Milwaukee, WI, USA

Asher Tal, MD
Professor and Head, Department of Pediatrics, Ben-Gurion University of the Negev, Beer-Sheva, Israel

Leila Tarokh, PhD
Senior Scientist, Institute of Pharmacology and Toxicology, University of Zurich, Zurich, Switzerland; Adjunct Assistant Professor, E.P. Bradley Hospital Sleep Research Laboratory, Department of Psychiatry and Human Behavior, Alpert Medical School of Brown University, Providence, RI, USA

R. Bradley Troxler, MD
Assistant Professor of Pediatric Medicine, Division of Pediatric Pulmonary and Sleep Medicine, Department of Pediatrics, University of Alabama at Birmingham, Birmingham, AL, USA

Sindhuja Vardhan, MD
Fellow in Pediatric Pulmonary Medicine, Division of Pediatric Pulmonology, The University of Chicago, Chicago, IL, USA

Merrill S. Wise, MD
Sleep Medicine Specialist, Methodist Healthcare Sleep Disorders Center, Memphis, TN, USA

Manisha Witmans, MD
Clinical Associate Professor, Faculty of Medicine and Dentistry, University of Alberta, Edmonton, Alberta, Canada; Adjunct Professor, Thompson Rivers University, Kamloops, British Columbia, Canada; Medical Director, Sound Sleep Solutions, Calgary, Alberta, Canada

Amy R. Wolfson, PhD
Professor of Psychology, Associate Dean of Faculty, College of the Holy Cross, Worcester, MA, USA

B. Tucker Woodson, MD
Professor and Chief, Division of Sleep Medicine, Department of Otolaryngology and Communication Sciences; Co-director, Froedtert Center for Sleep, Medical College of Wisconsin WN, USA

James K. Wyatt, PhD
Associate Professor of Behavioral Sciences, Rush Medical College; Director, Sleep Disorders Service and Research Center, Rush University Medical Center, Chicago, IL, USA

Rochelle Young, BA RN MN
Nurse Practitioner, Pediatric Sleep Program, Stollery Children's Hospital, Edmonton, Alberta, Canada

Acknowledgements

We would like to thank Dolores Meloni, Helene Caprari, Poppy Garraway Shereen Jameel and Sruthi Viswam for their hard work and dedication to this project.

The Editors

PRINCIPLES AND BASIC SCIENCE OF PEDIATRIC SLEEP MEDICINE

The Function, Phylogeny and Ontogeny of Sleep

Stephen H. Sheldon

Chapter 1

FUNCTION OF SLEEP

The first question asked of a biological function is an explanation of its purpose, yet the exact function of sleep still remains elusive today. Historically, physicians have, seemingly wisely, recommended sleep for the treatment of many ailments. This inexpensive prescription has been based on the assumption that sleep must have a unique restorative purpose. However, no study documents that sleep does cure anything.[1] Circadian rhythms of various biological processes, e.g., the immune system, appear to be modulated by sleep: lymphocyte functions are dramatically altered at sleep onset and during sleep.[2] Specific pokeweek mitogen response and natural killer cell activity are altered with sleep in healthy young men. Interlukin-1-like activities are followed by interlukin-2-like activities during sleep and interlukins-1 and -2 are disrupted with sleep deprivation.[3] Narcoleptic patients present disordered diurnal patterns of immune function.[4] However, what clinical effect these changes produce or how they may be therapeutically modified is unknown. The relationship between the immune system and sleep is obviously important, attractive, and possesses many clinical implications.

Theories of sleep function fall into several major categories with many overlaps. An understanding of these hypotheses provides a basis for comprehension of the varied effects disordered sleep may have on health and disease.

Restoration Theory

Sherington suggested in 1946 that sleep was a state required for enhanced tissue growth and repair.[5] This theory holds that certain somatic and/or cerebral deficits occur as a result of wakefulness and sleep either allows or promotes physiological processes to repair or restore these deficits. This will, in turn, allow normal daytime functioning.[6-8] Special focus has been placed on both restoration of somatic function and the central nervous system function. NREM sleep is thought to function in reparation of body tissue and REM sleep in restoration of brain tissue. Supporting evidence, however, is empirical and indirect. The theoretical role of NREM sleep in repair of somatic tissue comes from investigations that have shown the following:

1. Slow-wave sleep (SWS) increases following sleep deprivation.[9]
2. The percentage of SWS is increased during developmental years.[10]
3. Total sleep duration increases with body mass.[11]
4. Release of growth hormone occurs at sleep onset and peak levels occur during SWS in prepubertal children.[12]
5. The release of many endogenous anabolic steroids occurs in relation to a sleep-dependent cycle (prolactin, testosterone, and lutzinizing hormone).[13,14]
6. The nadir of catabolic steroid release, such as corticosteroids, occurs during the first hours of sleep, coincident with the largest percentage of SWS.[15]
7. Increased mitosis of lymphocytes and increased rate of bone growth occur during sleep.[16]
8. There is a gradual increase of SWS percentage of total sleep time in response to a graded increase of physical exercise.[17]

However, contrary and conflicting observations exist. For example, while peak rates of cell division occur during sleep, it appears not to be due to sleep itself. Increased mitosis is demonstrable after a night without sleep, is positively influenced by oral glucose load, and negatively influenced by cortisol secretion.[18] Similarly, in adolescents and adults, somatomedin levels are highest during waking, but not during sleep, as it is in prepubertal children.[19]

REM sleep, on the other hand, has been thought to function in restoration of central nervous system function. This state is characterized by intense CNS activation. REM sleep may have evolved in order to 'reprogram' innate behaviors and to incorporate learned behaviors and knowledge acquired during wakefulness.[20] Synthesis of CNS proteins is increased during REM sleep.[21] REM sleep also appears in significantly higher proportions in the fetus and newborn, gradually decreasing over the first few years of life. Increased protein synthesis during this sleep state may be critical in the development of the central nervous system.

Evolutionary and Adaptive Theories

Development of many physiological functions follows an orderly progression which mirrors phylogenetic development. It has been suggested that the development of sleep in the human organism also follows this same phylogenetic pattern. Evidence for this theory is scant. Animals sleep in many different ways, often more influenced by the environment and life-style than by evolution of the species.[22] SWS and REM sleep rebound are characteristic features seen after sleep deprivation in the dog, cat, rabbit, and human.[23] Definitive REM sleep, however, has never been documented in the dolphin. Dolphins do not have a pulmonary reflex to hypoxemia and have, therefore, complete voluntary control of breathing, and presumably sleep would be associated with impaired respiratory neural control. Actually, dolphins appear to exhibit hemispheric sleep. That is to say that when dolphins appear to sleep, slow-wave patterns are seen over a single hemisphere at a time, while the other hemisphere shows waking rhythm.[24] If the evolutionary theory is true, animals with highly complex central nervous system function, such as the dolphin, should follow this pattern. It stands to reason that if the dolphin sleeps in the same manner as the dog, cat, and human, survival in its aquatic environment would be impossible. Skeletal muscle atonia during REM sleep (as currently understood) would result in drowning. Therefore, the life-style and environment of the dolphin play a much more significant role in the pattern of sleep development in these species than does phylogeny.

In some species, sleep may function to enhance survival. Animals that graze for food tend to sleep in bursts over a short period of time, a behavior which may provide time needed for sufficient food-seeking while protecting the animal from predators.[25] Carnivorous animals that do not require large amounts of time for foraging and who are relatively safe from predation tend to sleep for long periods of time.

Sleep may also be an instinctive behavior, a patterned response to stimuli which conserves energy, prevents maladaptive behaviors and promotes survival.[26] According to the evolutionary theory of sleep, REM sleep cortical activation may perform additional survival functions.[27]

Energy Conservation Theory

Sleep may function to conserve energy. Mammal species exhibit a high correlation between metabolic rate and total sleep time.[28] This view states that energy reduction is greater during sleep than during periods of quiet wakefulness and sleep provides periods of enforced rest, barring the animal from activity for extended periods of time. Endothermic animals exhibit slow-wave sleep. During NREM sleep, endogenous thermoregulation continues, though functioning at levels below that of wakefulness. Poikilothermic species, on the other hand, do not exhibit clear SWS patterns. It is doubtful, however, that this theory explains the function of sleep in humans. Reduction in metabolism, which occurs during sleep, is minimal. Though the hypothesis is intriguing, energy conservation theory has been disputed and evidence exists that increase in sleep time does not correlate with increased metabolic rate.[29,30] It has been shown that there is only approximately an 8% to 10% reduction in metabolic rate during sleep when compared with relaxed wakefulness. This would be insignificant when considering an adult human's basal metabolic expenditure.

Learning Theory

A particularly interesting theory of the function of sleep centers on the role of sleep in the process of learning and memory. A significant body of knowledge exists which suggests that retention of new information depends on activation of some brain function which occurs at a critical period after the registration of this information.[31,32] Two pivotal phases appear to exist. The first is one of 'consolidation.' Medication which causes stimulation of the reticular activating system and cortical excitation during the first 90 seconds after acquisition of new information appears to enhance memory and increase retention. Though the consolidation phase of learning is important, it cannot be considered definitive for fixation of information since processing continues for a long period of time.

The second critical phase of information processing seems to occur during sleep, specifically REM sleep. Two theories have been proposed: The *passive* hypothesis (unlearning theory) and the *active* hypothesis which suggests that there are active consolidation mechanisms. An active process is supported by several facts. First, considerable brain activity occurs during this phase of sleep: brain oxygen consumption increases, there is an increase in cerebral blood flow, and there is intense activity of cortical and reticular neurons, indicating an active, functional process.

Over the past 50 years, beneficial effects of sleep on the retention of memories acquired during wakefulness have been documented.[33,34] REM sleep appears to hold special significance. Despite evidence from animal and human studies the exact function of REM sleep in childhood development and learning remains unknown. Diverse reasons have been proposed for children's learning difficulties, but no single factor appears to be consistent for all individuals. Most diagnostic and treatment protocols have empirically focused on the child's daytime capabilities.

Minor neurologic and electroencephalographic (EEG) abnormalities have been described in children with hyperactivity syndrome.[35] These abnormalities have been associated with specific or global learning difficulties and the syndrome had previously been described as 'minimal cerebral dysfunction.' Neurologic and EEG abnormalities associated with this 'hyperactivity' syndrome, however, have been shown to be non-specific and variable,[36] resulting in a change of the name of the syndrome to 'attention deficit hyperactivity disorder.'

It is noteworthy that of 15 reading-disabled (dyslexic) children studied by Levinson, 97% revealed evidence of cerebellar–vestibular (CV) dysfunction. Ninety-six percent of 22 blinded neurological examinations and 90% of 70 completed electronystagmograms indicated similar CV dysfunction.[37] Ottenbacher et al. explored the relationship between vestibular function as measured by duration of postrotatory nystagmus and human figure-drawing ability in 40 children labeled as learning-disabled.[38] Chronological age and postrotatory nystagmus durations shared significant amounts of variance with human figure-drawing. The variables of IQ and sex were non-significant. DeQuiros and Schrager have also identified vestibular dysfunction in some learning-disabled children[39] and described another related syndrome termed 'vestibular–oculomotor split,' which results in impaired ocular fixation, scanning ability, and poor eye–head coordination.

Despite the evidence that some children with learning disabilities display soft or non-focal neurologic signs[40] and low scores on tests of visual–motor integration, reading achievement, and ocular scanning,[41] contrary evidence of normal vestibular responses to rotation in dyslexic children has been published. Brown et al. measured eye movements provoked by sinusoidal rotation of the subjects at low frequencies.[42] Gain, phase, and asymmetry of the responses were calculated from the eye velocity and stimulus velocity wave forms. There were no differences between the groups in any of the measurements. These results led to the conclusion that 'there are no clinically measurable differences in this aspect of vestibular function' in their carefully selected population of dyslexic and control children. Their conclusions, however, were based on evidence obtained during the waking state. Vestibular nuclei play a major role in the control of eye movements when awake and asleep. If these nuclei are destroyed, eye movements during REM sleep are absent. In a pilot study of four reading-disabled children, a significant difference was found in the mean angular velocity of eye movements during REM sleep when compared with three normally reading controls.[43]

Correlates exist which associate the phasic events of rapid eye movements with CV control. Pompeiano et al. have shown that lesions of the medial and descending vestibular nuclei in the cat eliminated all phasic inhibition of sensory input, spinal reflexes, and all motor output associated with phasic REM bursts, including eye movements themselves.[44,45] They have also demonstrated that intense spontaneous discharges from neurons of the vestibular nuclei occur synchronous with the ocular activity of REM sleep. Nystagmus evoked by rotation can be most readily induced during sleep at the time of phasic events of REM sleep[46] and in Wernicke–Korsakoff's disease, where the vestibular nuclei are often damaged, eye movements are absent during REM sleep.[47] These observations partially confirm the influences of vestibular mechanisms of the phasic activity of REM sleep.

An age-related development of phasic inhibition of auditory evoked potentials during the ocular activity of REM sleep, and an age-related increase in the duration of the REM burst, have been described in normal subjects.[48] It seems that central vestibular influences underlie these events, and that vestibular control of phasic activity follows a developmental maturation schedule.

Considering this evidence, there may be a relationship between the CV control of REM phasic events and phasic REM sleep's importance in learning and memory. As yet, however, this relationship remains a mystery.

Significant literature exists, however, supporting a relationship between REM sleep, phasic REM activity, and learning. Sleep patterns in hyperkinetic children and normal children were studied by Busby, Firestone and Pivik.[49] Analysis of sleep pattern variables revealed a significantly longer REM onset latency and a greater absolute and relative amount of movement time for the hyperkinetic group relative to controls. No other sleep parameter differentiated the groups. Clinical observations of autistic children have suggested that fundamental symptoms of the syndrome of childhood autism involve disturbances of motility and perception. The nature of these disturbances indicates a maturational delay in the development of complex motor patterns and the modulation of sensory input.[48] Sleep studies have provided some evidence for a maturational delay in the differentiation of REM sleep patterns and the development of phasic excitatory and inhibitory mechanisms during REM sleep in these children. These findings implicate a failure of central vestibular control over sensory transmission and motor output during REM sleep. The notation that there is a dysfunction of central vestibular mechanisms underlying the delayed organization and differentiation of the REM sleep state is supported by observations of altered vestibular nystagmus in the waking state in autistic children.[48]

Studies in animals and humans support the importance of REM sleep in learning. Lucero conducted experiments which showed a significant increase in REM sleep duration with respect to controls, a non-significant increase in total sleep time, and no changes in slow-wave sleep duration in animals subjected to consecutive learning experiences.[50] Increase in REM sleep time observed after incremented learning suggests that REM sleep might be involved in the processing of information acquired during wakefulness. It has been postulated that such processing might consist of the transformation of a 'labile program' acquired in the learning session into a more 'stable program' devoid of superfluous information.

Major evidence of the importance of REM sleep in facilitating recall of complex associative information has been documented by Scrima.[51] The beneficial effect of isolated REM and isolated NREM sleep on recall was tested in 10 narcoleptic subjects. The results for complex associative tasks indicated significant differences between three conditions for free recall. Recall was significantly better after isolated REM than after isolated NREM sleep or wakefulness and was significantly better after NREM sleep than after wakefulness. It was concluded that the results were consistent with the proposed neuronal activity correlates theory of Emmons and Simon[52] that REM sleep actively consolidates and/or integrates complex associative information and that NREM sleep passively prevents retroactive interference of recently acquired complex associative information.

Newborn animals and human infants show a greater proportion of REM sleep with respect to total sleep time than adults,[53,54] and a progressive decrease in that proportion as growing continues, which is paralleled by a decrease in learning ability.[24] Fishbein has shown that REM sleep deprivation, both prior to and following learning, disrupts primarily long-term memory processes.[55] Evidence has been provided that learning induces a protracted augmentation of paradoxical sleep time, lasting for at least 24 hours.[56] This work, together with previous works, suggest that REM sleep augmentation may be a neurobiological expression of the long-term process of memory consolidation Fishbein was able to augment REM sleep using behavioral techniques of learning. Therefore, one psychobiological function of REM sleep may be to process and maintain information during wakefulness.

Results obtained from non-deprivation studies of animals provide consistent support for the hypothesis that REM sleep is functionally related to learning. Results of studies that have employed multiple training sessions may be interpreted to suggest either that prior REM sleep prepares the organism for subsequent learning, or that REM sleep facilitates consolidation and retrieval of prior learning. Given the equivocality of prior REM deprivation literature, the second interpretation seems more reasonable.[57]

Impaired cognitive functioning has been documented in studies conducted on sleep-deprived physicians. In one investigation, cognitive functioning in acutely and chronically sleep-deprived house officers was evaluated.[58] Analysis of data revealed significant deficits in primary mental tasks involving basic rote memory, language and numeric skills, as well as in tasks requiring high-order cognitive functioring and intellectual abilities.

Acquisition of many simple learning tasks in animals is followed by augmentation of REM sleep without any modification of NREM sleep.[31] Augmentation of REM sleep after learning has also been described in human infants.[59] Sleep may be particularly important for RNA and DNA synthesis linked to memory processes. There is some evidence that during sleep RNA is more actively synthesized, less rapidly degraded, or more slowly transported into the cytoplasm.[60]

As in infants, there is some evidence that REM sleep may increase following learning in older children and adults. Hartman has demonstrated an increase of REM sleep time occurring after days of increased learning, mental stress, and especially demanding events.[61] If learning does cause an increase in REM sleep, brain-damaged patients who are improving should have a higher proportion of REM sleep than patients who show no improvement. Following up a group of nine patients with severe traumatic brain damage, Ron et al. found a correlation between cognition and REM sleep improvement in seven patients.[62] Greenberg and Dewan compared the percentage of REM sleep in improving and non-improving aphasic patients and found that the latter groups did, in fact, have lower levels.[63] In 32 patients with Down syndrome, phenylketonuria, and other forms of brain damage, Feinberg found a positive relation between the amount of eye movement during REM sleep and estimates of intellectual function,[10] while in a comparison of 38 normal individuals and 15 brain-damaged subjects it was shown that mentally retarded patients had less REM sleep.[64] Linkage between REM sleep and development of the visual system has been further supported by a recent study by Oksenberg and co-workers.[65] They have reported significant anatomical changes in the microscopic anatomy of the visual cortex in REM sleep-deprived cats.

In spite of evidence from human and animal studies, the exact function of sleep in the process of learning, memory, and child development is still speculative.

Unlearning Theory

An antithetical hypothesis for the function of REM sleep in learning and memory involves a process of *unlearning*. No single memory center appears to exist in the brain.[66] Many parts of the central nervous system participate in the representation of a single event. However, localization of memory of a single event generally involves a limited number of neural pathways, and those collections of neurons within which a memory is equivalently represented probably contains a 'set' of no more than a thousand neurons. These interconnected assemblies of cells could store associations.[67,68] If the cells involved in the 'memory' of an event form mutual synapses, when part of that event is encountered again, regeneration of the activity of the entire neuronal set would occur. Crick and Mitchison proposed that the function of REM sleep, therefore, is to remove certain undesirable modes of interaction in networks of cells in the cerebral cortex.[69] This would be accomplished during REM sleep by a 'reverse learning' mechanism, so that the trace in the brain of the unconscious dream is weakened, rather than strengthened, by the activity of dreaming. A mathematical and computer model of a network of 30 to 1000 neurons has been developed by Hopfield, Fenistein, and Palmer.[70] Their model network has a content-addressable memory or 'associative memory' which allows it to learn and store many memories. A particular memory can be evoked in its entirety when the network is stimulated by an adequately sized subpart of the information of that memory. When memories are learned, spurious information is created and can also be evoked. Applying an 'unlearning' process, similar to the learning process, but with a reversed sign and starting from a noise input, enhanced the performance of the network in accessing real memories and minimizing spurious ones.

Sleep (in particular REM sleep) may then function to reduce or prevent unwanted, unnoticed, or spurious material acquired during wakefulness. Isolation of the cortex from environmental stimuli may be a necessary feature of the removal of inhibiting and/or competitive stimuli, inappropriate behavior patterns, and overloading of neuronal networks, thus permitting reprogramming and consolidation of more vital material.

Other Hypotheses

Presence of circulating hypnotoxin(s) has received some attention in the literature. This theory holds that during wakefulness, there is accumulation of sleep-producing 'toxin(s),' the presence of which stimulates or results in sleep. Once the toxin(s) have been modified by sleep, awakening occurs. Investigation of many substances claimed to be released subsequent to sleep deprivation and thalamic stimulation have failed to produce convincing evidence of the accuracy of this theory.[71] Studies of craniophagus and thoracophagus twins reveal independent sleep–wake cycles, despite the sharing of circulatory and/or nervous systems.[72]

Sleep may be required for the normal functioning of the motor system and/or skeletal musculature. Muscle aching and change in skeletal muscle enzyme activity have been reported following NREM sleep deprivation.[73] Though the ability to work is not drastically affected by sleep deprivation, physical performance follows definite circadian rhythmicity.[74] Sleep also has a profound effect on certain diseases which affect the motor system, including Parkinson's disease[75] and hereditary progressive dystonia.[76]

Though all theories of the function of sleep have had significant support, much conflicting evidence for each theory exists. The function of sleep may be explained very simply, or may be one of the more complex biological mechanisms known. A unitary explanation of the function of sleep is probably unrealistic. The exact function and purpose of sleep may prove to be a combination or a series of integrations of all proposed hypotheses.

SLEEP DEPRIVATION

Experiments conducted to unravel the meaning and function of various physiological processes have involved abolition of the function followed by observations of the consequences of its absence. For many years, research has focused on total deprivation of sleep, partial deprivation, and deprivation of various sleep stages in an attempt to identify repercussions. Unfortunately, these studies have been less fruitful in determining the function of sleep than obliteration of other physiological mechanisms.

Animal Studies

Total sleep deprivation studies in animals have shown significant deleterious effects. In early experiments, in order to keep animals awake for prolonged periods of time, constant activity was necessary, confounding the results. In 1983, Rechtschaffen and co-workers described an ingenious experimental method which controlled for the stimuli used to keep the animals awake.[77] Experimental and control rats were placed on a platform which rotated and caused awakening only when the experimental animal fell to sleep. Activity of the experimental and control animals was kept constant. Experimental animals suffered severe pathological changes from the sleep deprivation. Changes ranged from severely debilitated appearance (ungroomed and yellowed fur) to intense neurological abnormalities (ataxia and motor weakness) and death. Interestingly, there was a loss of EEG amplitude to less than half of normal waking values prior to the demise of the experimental animals. Necropsy findings included pulmonary edema, atelectasis, gastric ulcerations, gastrointestinal hemorrhage, edema of the limbs, testicular atrophy, scrotal damage, bladder enlargement, hypoplasia of the liver and spleen, and hyperplasia of the adrenal glands (indicating a significant stress response). Body weight decreased in both experimental and control animals, but was significantly greater in the experimental, sleep-deprived animals. It is also interesting to note that the animals which ate the most, lost the most weight. There was a surprisingly high correlation between the amount of paradoxical (REM) sleep obtained by the experimental animals and the survival time.

Human Studies

In comparison, effects of total sleep deprivation on human subjects have been remarkably few. Though brief psychotic episodes have been reported in some subjects, long-term psychological effects do not appear to result.[78] The only certain and reproducible effect of total sleep deprivation has been *sleepiness*.

Fatigue; decline in perceptual, cognitive, and psychomotor capabilities; and increasing transient ego disruptive episodes have been reported by Kales et al. during sleep deprivation.[79] Reality testing was impaired and regressive behavior was noted as the experiment continued. Tests for thought disorders showed shifts in thought processes to a more child-like level of cognition; however, there was no obvious evidence of schizophrenic thinking.

Performance may also be impaired by sleep deprivation. Vigilance and performance on reaction time tests have been shown to be significantly impaired by the loss of as little as one night's sleep.[80] In a study of 44 men participating in a strenuous combat course in Norway, significant impairment was observed in vigilance, reaction time, code testing, and profile of mood-state after 24 hours of sleep deprivation. Complaints of symptoms occurred first. Disturbances of senses and behavior followed. Horne et al. have reported that after 60 hours of continuous wakefulness, inherent capacity for signal detection exhibited a stepwise decline during deprivation, falling sharply during the usual sleep period time and leveling out during the daytime.[81] A clear circadian rhythm overlaid the decline due to deprivation. It was concluded that changes in inherent capacity seem to be consistent with a brain 'restitutive' role for sleep function.

Significant physiological changes after total sleep deprivation have been reported. Rebound of stage-4 sleep on the first recovery day and REM rebound on the second and third recovery days were documented by Berger and Oswald in 1962 and Williams et al. in 1964.[9,82] Kales et al. reported significant increases in stage-4 sleep and REM sleep after 205 hours of sleep deprivation, and significant decreases in stage-2 sleep.[79] On the first two recovery nights, alterations in REM sleep were noted. There was an increase in REM percentage, appearance of sleep-onset REM periods (SOREMPs), a decrease in REM latency, and a decrease in inter-REM intervals. These occurred most dramatically in those subjects who had the greatest psychological disturbances during the deprivation period.

Significant changes in performance and sleep physiology have been documented in subjects only partially deprived of sleep. In 1974, Webb and Agnew reported the results of an experiment conducted on 15 subjects restricted to a regimen of 5.5 hours of sleep a night for a period of 60 days.[83] The initial effect was an increase in the absolute volume of stage-4 sleep. By the fifth week of the experiment, the volume of stage-4 sleep returned to the baseline level. Initial effect on REM sleep was a sharp reduction when compared to the baseline. During the entire course of the experiment, there

was a reduction in REM sleep by 25%. Latency to the onset of stage-4 sleep and latency to the onset of REM sleep were also reduced. Behaviorally, only the Wilkinson Vigilance Task showed a decline in performance associated with continued sleep restriction. Initially, the subjects experienced difficulty in arousing in the morning and felt drowsy during the day. But this did not continue throughout the entire experiment. Mood scales showed no significant changes. It was concluded that the chronic loss of as much as 2.5 hours of sleep per night is not likely to result in major behavioral consequences. However, significant physiological effects were documented (especially in REM sleep) polysomnographically with partial restriction. Restricting sleep by early morning wakings generally deprives the subject of REM and stage-2 sleep, generally leaving NREM stage-4 intact. Recovery might, however, show a substantial increase in NREM stage-4 volume, suggesting that high-voltage, slow-wave sleep is (to some extent) a function of total sleep time.[84]

Sleep Deprivation in Children

Though similar to the adult, children differ in their response to acute restriction in sleep. When sleep has been restricted by 4 hours or more, there is a decrease in all stages of sleep (except slow-wave sleep); reduction in sleep-onset latency, stage-4 latency, and REM latency; and reduction of wakefulness during the sleep period. Carskadon et al. studied the effect of acute, partial restriction of sleep in children between the ages of 11 and 13.2 years.[85] Children were permitted to sleep 10 hours on baseline and recovery nights, and 4 hours on a single restricted night. No significant differences were found on any performance test. Unfortunately, the tests were brief. This may have had a significant impact on the outcome. Kleitman and Wilkinson[115] emphasized that task duration is a major factor determining a test's sensitivity to sleep loss. On the other hand, significant changes did occur on objective sleep testing. The Multiple Sleep Latency Test (MSLT) showed significant increase in daytime sleepiness which persisted into the morning following sleep restriction. This suggested that children were more severely affected by sleep restriction than adults. On polysomnography findings were comparable to adults, *but children did not show recovery rebound of slow-wave sleep and REM sleep as reported for adults*. Although children appear to be able to tolerate a single night of restricted sleep without a decrement in performance on brief tasks, perhaps more prolonged restriction and prolonged tasks similar to those required in school would show decrements. Children seem to require more time to recuperate fully from nocturnal sleep restriction than adults. The extent of daytime sleepiness that occurs is not trivial. With additional nights of partial sleep deprivation, cumulative sleepiness might rapidly become a significant problem. The importance of sleep restriction, daytime sleepiness, and performance of children in school and on their behavior may be greater than previously realized.

In 1972, Dement[86] powerfully described possible outcomes of restricted sleep on wakefulness:

After an excessively long period of wakefulness, the state of sleep becomes preemptive. When we enforce wakefulness, we are probably preventing or minimizing activity in the neural systems that subserve sleep induction and maintenance. As the potency of these systems increases during the period of their induced inactivity, they may begin to intrude upon wakefulness in an ever more aggressive manner.

The notion of total sleep deprivation could be somewhat illusory, and could result merely in a redistribution of activity in sleep and arousal systems in which NREM sleep would occur in the form of hundreds of microsleeps.

Microsleeps have been well documented in both human and animal studies.[87-89] Kales et al. have described disorientation and misperceptions during sleep deprivation that seemed to be associated with 'lapses' which become more frequent as deprivation continues.[79] Armington and Mitnick found that sleep deprivation eventually produced, in subjects who appeared to be behaviorally awake, brain wave patterns which were more or less continuously at the NREM stage-1 level.[87] The most consistent result of modest amounts of sleep loss in humans is the occurrence of these microsleep periods.[88] Microsleeps increase in frequency throughout periods of sleep deprivation. Since gross waking behavior is not affected, these lapses may have significant consequences on performance and its assessment, especially for the school-aged child whose consistent attentiveness is required for success in school. Since the perceptual shutdown can occur before EEG changes are apparent at the outset of sleep under ordinary circumstances, there may be many more such episodes in sleep-deprived subjects than EEG patterns alone would suggest.[86]

PHYLOGENETIC CONSIDERATIONS

Understanding sleep in humans requires reflection for a time on sleep in other species. Though periods of sluggish activity can be documented in reptiles, it does not appear that physiological sleep occurs.[90] Though only a relatively small number of mammalian species have been studied, it appears that most, if not all, birds and mammals sleep. Quiescent periods, intervals of reduced responsiveness to environmental stimuli, rapid reversibility of state, specific postures, and characteristic EEG changes have been observed.[91] All these criteria, however, need not be present concomitantly, and quiescence is not always equivalent to inactivity. Ritualistic pre-sleep activity and behaviors occur in many species, including humans. Timing of sleep varies; some species consolidate sleep into a single period of time and others distribute sleep throughout a 24-hour continuum.

Sleep in birds is remarkably similar to sleep in mammals. Two distinct types of sleep, with comparable electrophysiologic activity, have been documented. Major differences appear to be in the pattern of sleep and the greater number of sleep states observed in avian species.[92]

Zeplin and Rechtschaffen studied available sleep data on more than 50 mammalian species.[93] Sleeping patterns were correlated with metabolic rates, gestational periods, and brain weights. Animals with lower metabolic rates tend to sleep less than those with higher metabolic rates. Species which have longer sleep periods tend to exhibit shorter life spans and are smaller in size. Meddis replicated this study on a sample of 65 species and obtained similar results.[94]

NREM–REM cycling appears to be the basic organization of sleep in most species studied. Though the quality and quantity of NREM and REM sleep varies considerably, a regularly patterned series of state changes occurs with

demonstrable slowing of the EEG and the presence of spindling activity.[91] Paradoxical sleep has been recorded in almost all mammalian species studied. Characteristics of this sleep state include: desynchronization (activation) of central nervous system electrical activity, skeletal muscle atonia, periodic twitching, and physiological instability (especially of the cardiovascular and respiratory systems). Changes in thermoregulation and high arousal thresholds are present. Rhythmic theta activity and pontogeniculate–occipital (PGO) spikes are typically seen on EEG during mammalian paradoxical sleep.

Phylogenetic Development

Phylogenetic development of REM sleep has been studied by Allison and Van Twyver.[95] It appears to have developed approximately 130 million years ago. Allison and Cicchetti concluded that the volume of REM sleep correlated with lifestyle, risk of predation, and degree of exposure of the sleeping environment.[25]

REM sleep is the preponderant state early in life in most mammals (including humans). Though considered to be ontogenetically primitive, the role of REM sleep in the development of the central nervous system may be significant. Premature newborn humans spend approximately 90% of their total sleep time in active sleep. This falls rapidly to about 50% by term. A gradual decrease continues throughout the first few years of life to a level of about 20% to 25%. This level remains remarkably constant throughout the remainder of the life cycle.[54]

Jouvet-Mounier et al. have studied the ontogenetic development of sleep of infant cats, rats, and guinea pigs.[96] More than 70 animals underwent electrocortical, electrooocular, electromyographic, and behavioral monitoring from birth to 50 days of age. It became obvious the REM sleep was the preponderant form of sleep in these species. Each species varied significantly in the degree of development at birth, with rat pups the most immature, kittens intermediate, and guinea pigs the most mature. Degree of immaturity at birth highly correlated with the volume of paradoxical sleep recorded during the perinatal period. Rat pups exhibited 70% paradoxical sleep at birth, which decreased rapidly to near adult levels by 30 days of life. Decrease of paradoxical sleep in kittens was considerably slower. Guinea pigs showed the lowest volume of paradoxical sleep (7%); however, this was still approximately double the volume seen in the adult animal. Maturation of slow-wave sleep is late in comparison to paradoxical sleep and the time spent in paradoxical sleep and slow-wave sleep varies during the first postnatal month. These variations are different among species. Newborn kittens have a more highly developed cortex than rat pups.[97] Cortical neurons mature very rapidly and reach histological characteristics of adult cortical neurons by the twelfth postnatal day, concomitant with the appearance of slow-wave sleep. In contrast, the cortex of the newborn guinea pig appears histologically the same as that of the adult.[98]

Sleeping dolphins and porpoises are fascinating and of particular ontogenetic interest because of the complexity of the cetacean central nervous system. Mukhametov has studied the neurophysiology of sleep in the bottle-nose dolphin (*Tursiops truncatus*) and the porpoise (*Phocoena phocoena*)[99] and showed that the main characteristics of sleep in these marine mammals are unihemispheric slow-wave sleep and the apparent absence of paradoxical sleep. EEG characteristics are typical for the mammalian brain, and three distinct stages can be identified: desynchronization; intermediate synchronization with sleep spindles, theta activity, and delta waves; and maximal synchronization with slow-waves comprising more than 50% of each recording period. In all dolphins studied, unihemispheric slow-wave sleep was the main type of sleep recorded. Interestingly, this type of sleep is not found in other mammals. Synchronization of the EEG occurs in one hemisphere, while the opposite hemisphere reveals desynchronization. These cycles of synchrony and desynchrony appear to be independent. Each hemisphere exhibits different volumes of slow-wave sleep and deprivation of slow-wave sleep in one hemisphere does not result in contralateral rebound. Ipsilateral rebound is noted in the slow-wave sleep-deprived hemisphere only. Mukhametov has attempted to identify neurophysiologic and behavioral correlates of paradoxical sleeping over 30 animals of two species and concluded that paradoxical sleep does not appear to be present in the dolphin or porpoise. It is very difficult, however, to prove the complete absence of paradoxical sleep, since testing of dolphin fetuses and calves has not yet been possible. It is unknown whether these characteristics represent a phylogenetic, developmental, or adaptive phenomenon. Unraveling the mystery has fascinating teleological implications.

BEHAVIORAL AND PHYSIOLOGICAL CONSIDERATIONS

At first glance, sleep appears to be a simple process, a required part of our 24-hour life cycle. Little attention is paid to the sleeping state because human life-style focuses primarily on interactions with the environment and daily fragments of disengagement seem of secondary importance. Time spent in activities not related to goal attainment, pursuit of sustenance, fulfillment, happiness, or success appear to be intrusive, unwelcome gaps. Importance of these gaps, however, in permitting the individual to function and appropriately interact with the environment during the waking state has only recently been discovered.

Any definition of sleep is complex, both from behavioral and physiological perspectives. In simplest terms, it is a reversible disengagement with, and unresponsiveness to, the external environment, regularly alternating in a circadian manner with engagement and responsiveness. It is now known that this definition is significantly incomplete and simplistic, since sleep is a highly active and complex state.

Behavioral Correlates of Sleep

It seems easy to determine when an individual is sleeping. Behavioral correlates include a recumbent position, closure of the eyelids, quiescence, and diminished responsiveness to external stimuli. These behaviors are fairly consistent between individuals. Sleep onset, however, requires complex interactions of learned behaviors and physiological processes. Absence of sudden external stimuli; a suitable, safe, comfortable environment; relaxation of postural muscles; and learned stereotypical behaviors associated with bedtime are required.[100] There is some evidence that rhythmic, monotonous sensory stimulation helps promote sleep.[101] Whether this is behavioral, physiologic or a combination is speculative.

Physiological Correlates

Physiologically, sleep onset and maintenance are not passive processes. Isolation of the cerebrum from the brainstem and spinal cord (cerveau isole) produces a state indistinguishable from physiological sleep.[102] A series of exquisite experiments identified neurons of the reticular formation which received collateral input from somatic, visceral, and special sensory pathways, and sent ascending projections dorsally and ventrally to the basal forebrain.[103–105] These collections of neurons were termed the *reticular activating system*. Complex projections of neurons from the reticular formation to the posterior hypothalamus–subthalamus, basal forebrain, and then to the cortex are responsible for the maintenance of wakefulness.[106]

Though it was initially thought that sleep was the result of a decrease in the activity of this system, brainstem transection experiments resulting in diminished sleep suggested that sleep-inducing structures must also be present in the central nervous system.[107] This sleep-inducing structure appeared to be located in the lower brainstem, specifically the dorsal medullary reticular formation and nucleus of the solitary tract. Lesions in this area produced EEG activation in a sleeping animal.[108,109] A sleep-facilitation center appears to be present in the rostral hypothalamus[110] and cortical synchrony can be elicited by stimulation of the midline thalamus.[111] Sleep-inducing neurons are also found in the preoptic area and basal forebrain. GABA neurons located in the cortex, as well as neurons located in the hypothalamus and basal forebrain, are vital for slow-wave production.[106]

Sleep Onset

Sleep onset, therefore, results from a complex series of events involving changes in levels of somatic, visceral, and special sensory input; active inhibition of neuron networks which produce cortical desynchronization; and active stimulation of neuronal systems and pathways responsible for cortical synchrony. In addition, the rhythmic organization of these activities is extremely complex and appears to be controlled by neurons located in the suprachiasmatic nucleus.[112] Jouvet et al. described a separate system of neurons located in the upper pons which controlled the induction and manifestations of REM sleep.[113] This system was under the influence of an 'oscillator' which was separate from (though linked to) that which controlled the rhythmicity of the sleep–wake cycle.[114] A cholinergic, 'REM-on' system of neurons exists primarily located in the mesencephalic, medullary, and pontine gigantocellular tegmental fields, but may be widespread. Discharges from these neurons are responsible for REM sleep epiphenomena of cortical desynchronization, conjugate eye movements, decrease in muscle tone by active inhibition of alpha motor neurons, muscular twitching, and cardio-respiratory irregularities. It has also been shown that a self-inhibitory, aminergic, 'REM-off' system of neurons, located in the dorsal raphe nuclei, locus coeruleus, and the nucleus peribrachialis lateralis interacts with the opposing system, resulting in alternations between NREM and REM sleep.

It is clear that the behavioral, neurochemical, and neurophysiological mechanisms of the sleep–wake cycle and electrophysiological cycles during sleep itself are complex and intensely integrated. All characteristics have yet to be elucidated. Further research is needed. Answers may prove to be simple or one of the most complex physiological processes known. Implications in fetal and childhood development may be more significant than our wildest dreams.

References

1. Rechtschaffen A. The function of sleep: methodological issues. In: Drucker-Colin R, Shkurovich M, Sterman MB, editors. The functions of sleep. New York: Academic Press; 1979. p. 1.
2. Moldofsky H. Immunology and sleep. Presented at the Association of Professional Sleep Societies, First Annual Meeting. Colombus, OH: June 15–20; 1986.
3. Moldofsky H, Lue FA, Davidson JR, et al. The effect of 40 hours of wakefulness on immune functions in humans. II. Interleukins-1- & -2-like activities. Sleep Res 1988;17:34.
4. Moldofsky H, Lue FA, Davidson JR, et al. Disordered diurnal patterns of immune functions in three patients with narcolepsy-cataplexy. Sleep Res 1988;17:223.
5. Sherington CS. Man on his nature. Cambridge: Cambridge University Press; 1946. p. 413.
6. Oswald I. Sleep. Harmondsworth, Middlesex: Penguin Books; 1974.
7. Hartmann E, Orzack MH, ad Branconnier R. Deficits produced by sleep deprivation: Reversal by d- and l-amphetamine. Sleep Res 1974;3:151.
8. Adam K, Oswald I. Sleep is for tissue restoration. J Roy Col Physicians 1977;11:376.
9. Berger R, Oswald I. Effects of sleep deprivation on behavior, subsequent sleep and dreaming. J Ment Sci 1962;108:457.
10. Feinberg I. The ontogenesis of human sleep and the relationship of sleep variables to intellectual function in the aged. Comp Psychiatry 1968;9:138.
11. Adam K. Body weight correlates with REM sleep. Brit Med J 1977;1:813.
12. Sassin JF, Parker DC, Mace JW, et al. Human growth hormone release relation to slow-wave sleep and sleep-waking cycles. Science 1969;165:513.
13. Sassin JF, Frantz AG, Kapen S, et al. The nocturnal rise of human prolactin is dependent on sleep. J Clin Endocrinol Metab 1973;37:436.
14. Boyar RM, Rosenfeld RS, Kapen S, et al. Human puberty: Simultaneous augmented secretion of luteinizing hormone and testosterone during sleep. J Clin Investig 1974;54:609.
15. Weitzman ED, Hellman L. Temporal organization of the 24-hour pattern of the hypothalamic-pituitary axis. In: Ferin M, Halberg F, Richart RM, et al, editors. Biorhythms and human reproduction. New York: John Wiley; 1974. p. 371.
16. Valk IM, van der Bosch JSG. Intra-daily variation of the human ulnar length and short term growth – A longitudinal study in eleven boys. Growth 1974;42:107.
17. Griffin SJ, Trinder J. Physical fitness, exercise and human sleep. Psychophysiology 1978;15:447.
18. Fisher LB. The diurnal mitotic rhythm in the human epidermis. Brit J Dermatol 1968;80:75.
19. Finkelstein JW, Roffwarg HP, Boyar RM, et al. Age-related change in the twenty-four hour spontaneous secretion of growth hormone. J Clin Endocrinol Metab 1972;35:665.
20. Jouvet M. The function of dreaming: A neurophysiologist's point of view. In: Gazzaniga MS, Blakemore C, editors. Handbook of psychobiology. New York: Academic Press; 1975. p. 499.
21. Giuditta A, Neugebauer-Vitale A, Grassi-Zucconi G, et al. Synthesis of brain RNA and DNA during sleep. In: Borbely A, Valtax JL, editors. Sleep mechanisms. Berlin: Springer-Verlag; 1984. p. 146.
22. Bert J. Sleep in primates under natural conditions and in the laboratory. In: Koella WP, Levin P, editors. Sleep 1976: Third European Congress of Sleep Research. Basel: S Karger; 1977. p. 152.
23. Webb WB. Sleep stage responses of older and younger subjects after sleep deprivation. Electroenceph Clin Neurophysiol 1981;52:368.
24. Kovalzon VM. Brain temperature variations in ECoG in free-swimming bottle-nose dolphins. Sleep 1976: Third European Congress of Sleep Research. Basel: S Karger; 1977. p. 239.
25. Allison T, Cicchetti DV. Sleep in mammals: Ecological and constitutional correlates. Science 1976;194:732.
26. McGinty DJ, Harper TM, Fairbanks MK. Neuronal unit activity and the control of sleep states. In: Weitzman E, editor. Advances in sleep research. New York: Spectrum Publishing; 1974. p. 173.
27. Snyder F. Toward an evolutionary theory of dreaming. Am J Psychiatry 1966;123:121.
28. Zeplin H, Rechtschaffen A. Mammalian Sleep, longevity, and energy conservation. Brain Behav Evolut 1974;10:425.
29. Carpenter AC, Timiras PS. Sleep organization in hypo- and hyperthyroid rats. Neuroendocrinology 1982;34:438.
30. Eastman CI, Rechtschaffen A. Effects of thyroxin on sleep in the rat. Sleep 1979;2:215.
31. Block V, Hennevin E, Leconte P. The phenomenon of paradoxical sleep augmentation after learning: Experimental studies of its characteristics and significance. In: Fishbein W, editor. Sleep, dreams and memory. Lancaster: MTP; 1981. p. 18.
32. Smith C, d Butler S. Paradoxical sleep at selective times following training is necessary for learning. Physiol Behav 1982;29:469.
33. Jenkins J, Kallenbach K. Oblivescence during sleep and waking. Am J Psychol 1924;35:605.
34. VanOrmer EG. Retention after intervals of sleep and waking. Arch Psychol 1932;137:5.
35. Carter S, Gold A. The syndrome of minimal cerebral dysfunction. In: Barnett MH, Einhorn A, editors. Pediatrics. New York: Appleton-Century-Crofts; 1972.
36. Dykman RA, Ackerman PT, Clements S, et al. Specific learning disabilities: An attentional deficit syndrome. In: Myklebust HR, editor. Progress in learning disabilities. New York: Grune and Stratton; 1971
37. Levinson HN. Dyslexia: a solution to the riddle. New York: Springer-Verlag; 1980. p. 73.
38. Ottenbacher K, Abbott C, Haley D, et al. Human figure drawing ability and vestibular processing in learning disabled children. J Clin Psych 1984;40:1084.
39. deQuiros JB, Schrager OL. Neuropsychological fundamentals in learning disabilities. San Rafael, CA: Academic Therapy Press; 1978.
40. Steinberg M, Rendle-Short J. Vestibular dysfunction in young children with minor neurologic impairment. Dev Med Child Neurol 1977;19 639.
41. Ottenbacher K, Watson PJ, Short MA, et al. Nystagmus and ocular fixation difficulties in learning-disabled children. Am J Occupational Ther 1979;33:717.
42. Brown B, Haegerstrom-Portnoy G, Yingling CDet al. Dyslexic children have normal vestibular response to rotation. Arch Neurol 1983;40:370.
43. Sheldon SH, Spire JP, Levy HB. REM sleep eye movements in reading disabled children. Sleep Res 1990;119:34.
44. Pompeiano O. The neurophysiological mechanisms of the postural and motor events during desynchronized sleep. In: Kety SS, Evarts EV, Williams HL, editors. Sleep and altered states of consciousness. Baltimore: Williams and Wilkins; 1967. p. 351.
45. Pompeiano O. Mechanisms of sensorimotor integration during sleep. Prog Physiol Psychol 1970;3:1.
46. Reding GR, Fernandez C. Effects of vestibular stimulation during sleep. Electroencephalogr Clin Neurophysiol 1968;24:75.
47. Appenzelle O, Fisher AP. Disturbances of rapid eye movements during sleep in patients with lesions of the nervous system. Electroencephalogr Clin Neurophysiol 1968;25:29.
48. Ornitz EM. Development of sleep patterns in autistic children In: Clemente CD, Purpura DP, Mayer FE, et al, editors. Sleep and the maturing nervous system. New York: Academic Press; 1972. p. 363.
49. Busby K, Firestone P, Pivik RT. Sleep patterns in hyperkinetic and normal children. Sleep 1981;4:366.
50. Lucero MA. Lengthening of REM sleep duration consecutive to learning in the rat. Brain Res 1979;20:319.
51. Scrima L. Isolated REM sleep facilitates recall of complex associative informtion. Psychophysiology 1982;19:252.
52. Emmons W, Simon C. Response to material presented during various levels of sleep. J Exp Psychology 1956;51:89.
53. Parmelee HA, Schulz HR, Disbrow MA. Sleep patterns of the newborn. J Pediatr 1961;58:241.
54. Roffwarg HP, Dement WC, Fisher C. Preliminary observations on the sleep patterns in neonates, infants, children, and adults. In: Harms E, editor. Problems of sleep and dreams in children. London: Pergamon; 1963.
55. Fishbein W. Disruptive effects of rapid-eye-movement sleep deprivation on long-term memory. Physiol Behav 1971;6:279.
56. Fishbein W, Kastaniotis C, Chattman D. Paradoxical sleep: Prolonged augmentation following learning. Brain Res 1974;71:61.
57. McGrath MJ, Cohen DB. REM sleep facilitation of adaptive waking behavior: A review of the literature. Psychol Bull 1978;85:24.
58. Hawkins MR, Vichick DA, Silsby HD, et al. Sleep and nutritional deprivation and performance of house officers. J Med Educ 1985;60:530.
59. Paul K, Dittrichova J. Sleep patterns following learning in infants In: Levin P, Koella U, editors. Sleep: 1974. Basel: S Karger; 1975. p. 388.

60 Parkes JD. Sleep and its disorders. MPN 14, London: WB Saunders; 1985. p. 44.

61 Hartman E. The functions of sleep. New Haven: Yale University Press; 1976.

62 Ron S, Algom D, Hary D, et al. Time-related changes in the distribution of sleep stages in brain injured patients. Electroenceph Clin Neurophysiol 1980;48:432.

63 Greenberg R, Dewan EM. Aphasia and rapid-eye-movement sleep. Nature 1969;223:183.

64 Feinberg I. Eye movement activity during sleep and intellectual function in mental retardation. Science 1968;159:1256.

65 Oxsenberg A, Marks G, Farber J, et al. Effect of REM sleep deprivation during the critical period of neuroanatomical development of the cat visual system. Sleep Res 1986;15:53.

66 Squire LR. Memory and the brain. New York: Oxford University Press; 1987. p. 123.

67 Kohonen T. Associateve memory. New York: Springer-Verlag; 1977.

68 Palm G. Neural assemblies: an alternative approach to artificial intelligence, New York: Springer-Verlag; 1982.

69 Crick F, Mitchison G. The function of dream sleep. Nature 1983;304:111.

70 Hopfield JJ, Feinstein DI, Palmer RG. 'Unlearning' has a stabilizing effect in collective memories. Nature 1983;304:158.

71 Kleitman N. Sleep and wakefulness. Chicago: University of Chicago Press; 1963. p. 552.

72 Webb WB. The sleep of conjoined twins. Sleep 1978;1:205.

73 Moldofsky H, Scarisbrick P. Induction of neurasthenic musculoskeletal pain syndrome by selective sleep stage deprivation. Psychosom Med 1976;38:35.

74 Nicholson AN, Marks J. Insomnia. Lancaster: MTP; 1983. p. 22.

75 Marsden CD. 'On-off' phenomenon in Parkinson's disease. In: Rinne UK, Klinger M, Stamm G, editors. Parkinson's disease – current progress, problems and management. Amsterdam: Elsevier/North Holland; 1980 p. 241.

76 Segawa M, Hosaka A, Miyagawa F, et al. Hereditary progressive dystonia with marked diurnal fluctuation. Adv Neuro 1976;14:215.

77 Rechtschaffen A, Gilliland MA, Bergmann BM, et al. Physiological correlates of prolonged sleep deprivation in rats. Science 1983;221:182.

78 Passount P, Popoviciu L, Velok G, et al. Etude polygraphique des narcolepsies au cours du nychemere. Rev Neurol (Paris) 1968;118:431.

79 Kales A, Tan T-L, Kollar EJ, et al. Sleep patterns following 205 hours of sleep deprivation. Psychosomatic Med 1970;32:189.

80 Glenville M, Broughton R, Wing AM, et al. Effects of sleep deprivation on short duration performance measures compared to the Wilkinson Auditory Vigilance Task. Sleep 1978;1:169.

81 Horne JA, Anderson NR, Wilkinson RT. Effects of sleep deprivation on signal detection measures of vigilance: Implications for sleep function. Sleep 1983;6:347.

82 Williams HL, Hammack JT, Daly RL, et al. Response to auditory stimulation, sleep loss, and EEG stages of sleep. Electroenceph Clin Neurophysiol 1964;16:269.

83 Webb WB, Agnew HW. The effect of a chronic limitation of sleep length. Psychophysiology 1974;11:265.

84 Dement W, Greenberg S. Changes in total amount of stage 4 sleep as a function of partial sleep deprivation. Electroenceph Clin Neurophysiol 1966;20:523.

85 Carskadon MA, Harvey K, Dement WC. Acute restriction of nocturnal sleep in children. Perceptual Motor Skills 1981;53:103.

86 Dement WC. Sleep deprivation and organization of the behavioral states. In: Clemente C, Purpura D, Mayer F, editors. Sleep and the maturing nervous system. New York: Academic Press; 1972. p. 319.

87 Armington J, Mitnick L. Electroencephalogram and sleep deprivation. J Appl Physiol 1959;14:247.

88 Williams H, Lubin A, Goodnow J. Impaired performance with acute sleep loss. Psychol Monog 1959;73:1.

89 Friedman L, Bergmann BM, Rechtschaffen A. Effects of sleep deprivation on sleepiness, sleep intensity, and subsequent sleep in rats. Sleep 1979;1:369.

90 Cartwright RD. A Primer on sleep and dreaming. Reading, MA: Addison-Wesley; 1978. p. 19.

91 Zepelin H. Mammalian sleep. In: Kryger MH, Roth T, Dement WC, editors. Principles and practice of sleep medicine. Philadelphia: WB Saunders; 1989. p. 30.

92 Amlaner CJ, Ball NJ. Avian sleep. In: Kryger MH, Roth T, Dement WC, editors. Principles and practice of sleep medicine. Philadelphia: WB Saunders; 1989. p. 50.

93 Zeplin H, Rechtschaffen A. Mammalian sleep, longevity, and energy conservation. Brain, Behav Environments 1974;10:425.

94 Meddis R. The evolution of sleep. In: Mayes A, editor. Sleep mechanisms and function in humans and animals: an evolutionary perspective. Berkshire, England: Van Nostrand Reinhold (UK); 1983.

95 Allison T, Van Twyver H. The evolution of sleep. Nat Hist 1970;79:56.

96 Jouvet-Mounier D, Astic L, Lacote D. Ontogenesis of the states of sleep in rat, cat, and guinea pig during the first postnatal month. Dev Psychobiol 1970;2:216.

97 Nobak CR, Purpura DP. Postnatal ontogenesis of neurons in cat neocortex. J Comp Neurol 1961;117:291.

98 Peters HG, Bademan H. The form and growth of stellate cells in the cortex of the guinea pig. J Anat 1963;97:111.

99 Mukhametov LM. Sleep in marine mammals. Exp Brain Res 1984; 8:227.

100 Konorski J. Integrative action of the brain. Chicago: University of Chicago Press; 1967. p. 531.

101 Gastaut H, Bert B. Electroencephalographic detection of sleep induced by repetitive sensory stimuli. In: Wolstenholme GEW, O'Connor M, editors. On the nature of sleep. London: Churchill; 1961. p. 260.

102 Bremer F. Quelques proprietes de l'activite electrique du cortex cerebral 'isole.' CR SocBiol (Paris) 1935;118:1241.

103 French JD, Magoun HW. Effects of chronic lesions in central cephalic brain stem of monkeys. Arch Neurol Psychiatry 1952;69:591.

104 Lindsley DB, Bowden JW. Magoun HW. Effect upon the EEG of acute injury to the brain stem activating system. Electroencephalog Clin Neurophysiol 1949;1:475.

105 Moruzzi G. The sleep-waking cycle. Ergeb Physiol 1972;64:1.

106 Jones BE. Basic mechanisms of sleep-wake states. In: Kryger MH, Roth T, Dement WC, editors. Principles and practice of sleep medicine. Philadelphia: WB Saunders; 1989. p. 121.

107 Barini C, Moruzzi G, Palestini M, et al. Effects of complete pontine transections of the sleep-wakefulness rhythm: The midpontine pretrigeminal preparation. Arch Ital Biol 1959;97:1.

108 Freemon FR, Salinas-Garcia RF, Ward JW. Sleep patterns in a patient with a brain stem infarction involving the raphe nucleus. Electroencephalogr Clin Neurophysiol 1974;36:657.

109 Westmoreland BF, Klass DW, Sharbrough FM, et al. Alpha-coma. Arch Neurol 1975;32:713.

110 Nauta WJH. Hypothalamic regulation of sleep in rats: An experimental study. J Neurophysiol 1946 9:285.

111 Morison RS, Dempsey EW. A study of thalamo-cortical relations. J Physiol 1942;135:281.

112 Hanada Y, Kawamura H. Sleep-waking electrocorticographic rhythms in chronic cerveau isole' rats. Physiol Behav 1981;26:725.

113 Jouvet M. Paradoxical sleep: A study of its nature and mechanisms. In: Himwich WA, Schade JP, editors. Sleep mechanisms: progress in brain research. Amsterdam: Elsevier; 1965.

114 Hobson JA. The cellular basis of sleep cycle control. Adv Sleep Res 1974;1:217.

115 Wilderson RT. Sleep deprivation: Performance tests for partial and selective sleep deprivation. In: Abt LE Riess BF, editors. Progress in Clinical Psychology, vol. 3. New York: Grune and Stratton; 1968. p. 24–43.

History of Pediatric Sleep Medicine

Stephen H. Sheldon

OVERVIEW

Over the past quarter century, pediatric and adolescent sleep medicine has followed remarkable parallels with the evolution of health care for infants, children and young adults in the United States. Chronicled establishment of children's health care, as well as establishment of sleep medicine as an imperative and major medical discipline for adults provides insight into the current position of pediatric and adolescent sleep medicine and future directions for clinical practice and research. An understanding of the evolution of sleep medicine into a research and clinical field of study and branch of knowledge will create important perspective. Juxtaposition of disciplines will sensitize the reader to the need for state-of-the-art evaluation of sleep and its pathologies seen in infants, children, and adolescents.

INTRODUCTION

Over the past 25 years, the development of pediatric and adolescent sleep medicine (PASM) as an imperative child health care discipline remarkably parallels evolution of pediatric health care in the United States. Recorded evolution of health care for children as well as establishment of sleep medicine as a recognized, necessary, and vital medical discipline for adults provides lucid insight into the current position within the child health care community of pediatric and adolescent sleep medicine and future directions for research and clinical practice.

DEVELOPMENT OF PEDIATRICS AS A UNIQUE DISCIPLINE

Prior to the beginning of the twentieth century, health care for children and adolescents was virtually non-existent. Health care for children was principally provided by family members. Mortality rates for infants were high. More than one-third of infants died before their fifth birthday.[1] Despite this significant incidence of infant mortality, little was done to improve health care for children and few took particular notice of the lack of professional services. Health care for children by the medical profession was provided using adult criteria, adult standards of care, adult definitions of diseases/disorders, and utilization of therapeutic techniques developed for adult patients.[2]

Medical practitioners who limited their practice to children were few and considered 'baby feeders' since little was known of the cause of illness in children. Infectious diseases prevailed and diarrheal diseases resulting in dehydration affected many. It has been estimated that at the turn of the century there were not more than 50 medical practitioners in the United States who were particularly interested in the health care of children, and less than a dozen limited their practice exclusively to children.[3] Health care facilities for clinical evaluation and management of childhood disease, specifically designed for children's needs were non-existent.[2] Being considered the property of their parents, neither earning a living, paying taxes, nor voting, children then and now possess neither an economic nor political influence.

Childhood diseases were widespread. Prevention was the only underlying principle. Approaches to treatment of illness during childhood included tea, barley water, and protein milk. Floating hospitals and country sanatoria were occasionally utilized for management of childhood illness since sun, fresh air, and isolation were treatments of choice and standard of care. Nonetheless, because of the lack of children's clinics for diagnosis and management of pediatric diseases/disorders, care of children remained in the home.[4] Because of the lack of diagnostic methods, evaluation of childhood illness was based primarily on anecdotes, and clinical signs and symptoms. Even congenital malformations were thought by many child health care practitioners to be due to maternal influences.[5] Treatment was principally based on either adult medical interventions or was purely empiric. Climate therapy was common. Exposure to sunlight was prescribed for various illnesses including but not limited to tuberculosis, cutaneous abnormalities, anemia, and rickets. Some treatments were effective, but most were relatively ineffective. For example, treatment of pneumonia often included administration of digitalis, camphor, strichnia, and alcohol.

With the discovery and development of pasteurization of milk and immunizations for a variety of diseases, child health care practitioners were thrust into the forefront of preventive medicine. Use of antibiotics to treat infections and the development of corticosteroids were instrumental in decreasing high childhood mortality rates existing during the first half of the twentieth century.

During the second half of the twentieth century, rapid progress in pediatric medicine and surgery occurred. Practice of pediatric medicine has turned from principally treatment of infectious diseases to comprehensive preventive programs, school health, community pediatrics, developmental pediatrics, and comprehensive adolescent medicine. Extensive morbidities have been identified resulting in extensive efforts in behavioral disorders, family violence, child maltreatment, drug misuse, learning problems, school health, and developmental disabilities. Priorities have shifted and identification of many pediatric disorders requires a multi-disciplinary and inter-disciplinary approach to diagnosis and management.

DEVELOPMENT OF SLEEP MEDICINE AS A UNIQUE DISCIPLINE

Although there has been a fascination with sleep since antiquity, the scientific investigation of sleep and its disorders can be traced back to 1930 when Berger first described spontaneous EEG activity in the brains of sleeping subjects;[6] differentiation of sleep into specific and distinct states by Harvey, Loomis, and Hobart in 1937.[7] Eye movements in sleep were previously described in sleeping infants[8] and the first description of rapid eye movement (REM) sleep by Aserinsky and Kleitman at the University of Chicago in 1953.[9] Five years later, Dement and Kleitman reported the cycling of REM sleep and non-rapid eye movement (NREM) sleep throughout the sleep period, proposed a classification system of NREM sleep into four distinct stages, and the association of eye movements in REM sleep with dream mentation.[10-11]

It had become clear that these discoveries ushered in the realization that it was not enough to evaluate health and disease during only waking hours, but throughout the 24-hour continuum. A new era of medical and scientific research emerged focusing on physiology, pharmacology, pathophysiology, and even anatomy that are different during sleep than during the waking state.[12] Sleep research provided the groundwork and basis for the realization that clinical evaluation and management of patients might differ during sleep when compared to wake, resulting in the emergence of clinical sleep medicine.[13]

At first, clinical sleep medicine evolved from patient self-referrals. Most sleep complaints were related to problem insomnia. However, it became clear that the common belief that the majority of etiologies of insomnia were not purely psychiatric in origin.[13] Obstructive sleep apnea had been identified in Europe, but there had been little notice in the United States. In 1970, Lugaresi and colleagues published remarkable success of tracheostomy in the treatment of obstructive sleep apnea.[14] Nonetheless, similar evaluation and management of obstructive sleep apnea was not yet accepted. In 1972, Guilleminault demonstrated remarkable results in managing uncontrollable hypertension in a 10½-year-old boy with tracheostomy.[15] It is stunning that demonstration of the first successful treatment of sequelae of obstructive sleep apnea in the United States was in a pediatric patient.

Physiological evaluation of sleep had also progressed with adaptation of polygraphy used in monitoring EEG to evaluation of other physiological variables during sleep. Termed *polysomnography*, Holland et al.[16] changed the face of clinical assessment of sleep in adult patients. Now there were methods for both basic evaluation by history and physical examination as well as physiological assessment of sleep-related complaints in a clinical laboratory setting.

By the end of the 1970s, clinical sleep disorders medicine became an accepted area of medical inquiry, although practice of sleep disorders medicine was still couched in other disciplines of pulmonology, psychiatry, neurology, and internal medicine. In 1968, the *Manual of Standardized Terminology, Techniques, and Scoring System for Sleep Stages of Human Subjects* was published.[17] This was a significant step forward in standardizing sleep stage scoring in adults and to eliminate unreliability and inconsistencies in laboratory evaluation of sleep both between laboratories and within laboratories. It was clear at that time this standardization was not appropriate for identification of stages of sleep and evaluation of sleep in newborns, infants, and children. Anatomical and physiological variables differed markedly from the adult. Similar standardization of sleep stage identification was a daunting task due to the rapid and constantly changing biology of the maturing and developing child. Therefore, the newborn infant became

a starting point for a similar process that was started by Drs. Rechtschaffen and Kales in 1968. Drs. Anders, Emdee, and Parmelee co-chaired an ad-hoc committee to provide similar standards and the result was the publication in 1971 of *A Manual for Standardized Techniques and Criteria for Scoring of States of Sleep and Wakefulness in Newborn Infants*.[18] Strikingly, between publication of this manual and today, 42 years later, there has been no similar effort for infants and children older than 2 months of age and the beginning of puberty. Many problems precluded this task. Standardization in the pediatric age group is a formidable endeavor. First, there are rapid and dynamic changes that occur during the first two decades of life. The nervous system is constantly changing structurally and functionally during this period of life. Attempting to define cross-sectional criteria for evaluation of children both within same-age subjects and between subjects is extraordinarily difficult because of normal internal and external variability. Normal ranges can be extensive. Limitations include number of evaluations required for appropriate power. External reliability and validity can also be quite difficult to establish. Several longitudinal points are often required for appropriate comparison of polysomnographic variables. This has been suggested to be termed *developmental polysomnography*.[19] This would then take into account normal progression of maturation, rather than evaluating a single polygraphic study at a single point in time. Because of these immense difficulties, little evidence-based standardized information has been available to provide accurate and reproducible normative data, despite evidence that sleep and its normal structure and maturation has far-reaching implications on growth, development, and learning.[20,21]

Identification of effective non-invasive treatments for many sleep-related disorders developed (for example, treatment of obstructive sleep apnea in adults with nasal CPAP) and resulted in rapid development of therapeutic protocols and widespread use. Combination of high prevalence of obstructive sleep apnea in the adult population, management of the obstructive sleep-disordered breathing with a relatively innocuous procedure, and effective management of sequelae led to the rapid expansion of sleep medicine into a unique medical discipline. Sleep disorders medicine has become an accepted and distinct specialty within the medical community.

Beginning in 1978, the American Board of Sleep Medicine (ABSM) provided an examination in clinical polysomnography to assure quality of practitioners practicing sleep disorders medicine and interpreting polysomnograms. The first examination certified 21 candidates. During the next 28 years, the ABSM certified more than 3400 individuals.[22] This examination was not specialty-specific and was taken by internists, psychiatrists, psychologists, neurologists, family practitioners, and pediatricians. Successful applicants became diplomates of the ABSM. Indeed, sleep disorders medicine as a new and unique discipline became the focus of more clinical practitioners.

Pediatric and adolescent sleep medicine has become an outgrowth of this sleep disorders medicine practice. Inspiration has come from several directions: scientific and clinical interest in sudden infant death syndrome (SIDS); identification of obstructive sleep apnea and other sleep-related breathing disorders occurring with significant prevalence in the pediatric population; identification of the importance of sleep in the origin of daytime behavioral difficulties; and the influence of sleep disorders on children's daytime performance and learning.

In the early 1980s the practice of pediatrics was a highly respected medical discipline. One of the principal textbooks utilized by most students and practitioners of health care for children was entitled *Nelson's Textbook of Pediatrics*.[23] Nevertheless, the fourteenth edition of this text, published in 1992, had a total of eleven *paragraphs* uniquely devoted to sleep disorders in children.

In 1985, two seminal works were published: one for parents and the other for sleep scientists. The first was publication of Dr. Richard Ferber's book for parents entitled *Solve Your Child's Sleep Problems*.[24] Based on Dr. Ferber's work at Boston Children's Hospital, this book reviewed all aspects of sleep in childhood and provided practical information in management of many sleep-related difficulties that occur during infancy and childhood. The second publication was entitled *Sleep and Its Disorders in Children* edited by Dr. Christian Guilleminault.[25] This book was a compilation of ground-breaking scientific papers on normative data providing a basis for future direction in the scientific study of sleep and sleep–wake cycles during infancy, childhood, and adolescence.

More changes occur in anatomy, physiology, and sleep–wake patterns during the first 15 years of life than over the next four decades. Nonetheless, comparatively little evidence-based information regarding this transformation has been published. Prevalence and impact of dysfunctional sleep on the developing child requires large population-based studies. It is imperative to determine how sleep and its organization develop in infancy and early childhood, since disruption of normal progression of development during these vastly important stages in human maturation may have lifelong consequences.

Clinical pediatric sleep medicine has had to rely on nosology developed for adults.[26] Adaptations have been attempted,[27] but it is clearly apparent that adapting adult criteria to infants and children can lead to many false starts and wrong turns. Most sleep-related problems in children might carry similar nomenclature, but children are different and it would be no less inappropriate to apply adult sleep medicine anatomical, physiological, and pathological criteria to veterinary medicine.

Yet, the general pediatric community has been very slow to grasp the significance of the entirety of pediatric sleep disorders. Child health care practitioners have been resistant to absorb the importance of sleep physiology and sleep structure to human development and behavior. However, over the past 5–10 years, pediatric pulmonologists, otolaryngologists, and neurologists have increasingly recognized the importance of sleep and its disorders and have incorporated this large portion of the child's life into clinical and academic endeavors, with particular focus on sleep-related breathing abnormalities. With the 'epidemic' of obstructive sleep apnea in the adult population, this again seems to be an outgrowth of adult sleep medicine.

In 2002, the American Academy of Sleep Medicine (AASM) applied to the Accreditation Council on Graduate Medical Education (ACGME) for establishment of sleep medicine training programs under the auspices of the ACGME as part of a comprehensive plan along with the American Board of Medical Specialists (ABMS) to accept sleep medicine as an independent medical specialty. In 2003, this was approved and a consensus plan was developed for establishment of a new multi-disciplinary specialty examination in sleep medicine to be jointly offered by the ABIM, ABPN, and the ABP, ABFM, and ABO.[22] The first examination was administered in 2007. Considerations and disorders unique to childhood comprised 2% of the first examination. Although pediatrics is a required portion of a sleep medicine fellowship curriculum, it is unclear how much pediatric medicine and sleep disorders in children are afforded to internists, otolaryngologists, psychiatrists, and neurologists studying general sleep medicine in these programs. It is also unclear whether training in developmental medicine and children's health care can be translated into the practice of sleep medicine without a comprehensive underpinning of pediatric medicine.

The success of incorporating a pediatric sleep medicine objective into undergraduate, graduate, and post-graduate training curricula will depend upon outcome and cost-effectiveness. First, can the provision of comprehensive sleep medicine services to children by pediatricians specializing, and devoting full time to the practice of pediatric sleep medicine, have a significant impact on co-morbid medical illnesses such as sickle cell anemia, cystic fibrosis, neuromuscular disorders, cranio-facial malformations, or congenital/acquired cardiovascular disease? Second, what effect does early disruption of sleep and/or sleep–wake cycling have on learning, memory, and cognitive development? Finally, can understanding sleep and its disorders in childhood contribute to a better understanding of behavioral disorders, problems of attention, and learning disabilities? The mystery of establishing and integrating neural networks required for early brain development and later executive functioning may be locked within the sleeping brain.

As was true of the development of pediatrics as a unique medical discipline, further appreciation of the development of sleep and its structure, as well as the effects of disruption of its normal maturation, might lead to improved diagnosis, treatment, and prevention of a wide variety of disorders unique to both children and adults. It is evident that the present is only the beginning of the understanding of pediatric sleep and pediatric sleep medicine.

SUMMARY

Pediatric and adolescent sleep medicine has followed a similar path in its maturation to the development of pediatrics as a recognized and unique medical discipline. There has been very significant increase in evidence-based knowledge regarding sleep and its disorders in infants, children, and adolescents over the past decade. Nonetheless, what is known now about the importance of sleep in normal human development and sleep in health and disease is likely only the 'tip of the iceberg.' The future of pediatric and adolescent sleep medicine is truly before us. Many questions remain:

1. How important is the basic rest–activity cycle during gestation in growth and maturation of the central nervous system, neuronal migration, and neural network development?
2. What impact does disruption of normal sleep and/or its continuity during the first few years of life have on future human development and performance?
3. What effect does sleep deprivation during adolescence have on health and well-being as adults? How might this contribute to chronic illness affecting these individuals as adults?

Clinical Pearls

- Clinical sleep medicine is a relatively new discipline that has rapidly evolved over the past 60 years.
- Clinical sleep medicine has evolved from the scientific study of sleep in the laboratory to a unique discipline.
- Development of pediatric sleep medicine parallels the development of pediatrics as a singular profession focused on the health and well-being of infants, children, and adolescents.

References

1. Holt LE. Infant mortality ancient and modern. An historical sketch. Arch Pediatr 1943;30:885.
2. Cone TE Jr. History of American pediatrics. Boston: Little Brown; 1979. p. 99–130.
3. Smith RM. Medicine as a science: pediatrics. NEJM 1951;244:176.
4. Powers GF. Developments in pediatrics in the past quarter century. Yale J Biol Med 1939;12:1.
5. Freeman RG. Fresh air in pediatric practice. Transactions of the American Pediatric Society 1916;28:7.
6. Berger H. Uber das Elekoenkeephalogramm des Menchen. J Psychol Neurol 1930;40:160–79.
7. Harvey EN, Loomis AL, Hobart GA. Cerebral states during sleep as studied by human brain potentials. Science 1937;85:443–4.
8. de Toni G. I movimenti pendolari de bulbi ocular dei bambini durante il sonno fisiologico, ed in alcuni stati morbosi. Pediatria 1933;41:489–98.
9. Aserinsky E, Kleitman N. Regularly recurring periods of eye motility, and concomitant phenomena, during sleep. Science 1953;118:273–4.
10. Dement WC, Kleitman N. Cyclic variations in EEG during sleep and their relation to eye movements, body motility, and dreaming. Electroencephalogr Clin Neurophysiol 1957;9:673–90.
11. Dement WC, Kleitman N. The relation of eye movements during sleep to dream activity: an objective method for the study of dreaming. J Exp Psychol 1957;53:339–46.
12. Orem J, Barnes CD. Physiology in Sleep. New York: Academic Press; 1980.
13. Carskadon MA, Roth T. Normal sleep and its variations. In: Kryger M, Roth T, Dement WC, editors. Principles and practice of sleep medicine. Philadelphia: WB Saunders; 1989. p. 3–15.
14. Lugaresi E, Coccagna G, Mantovani M, et al. Effects de la tracheotomie dans les hypersomnies avec respiration periodique. Rev Neurol 1970;123: 267–8.
15. Dement WC. History of sleep physiology and medicine. In: Kryger M, Roth T, Dement WC, editors. Principles and practice of sleep medicine. 2nd ed. Philadelphia: WB Saunders, 1994. p. 3–15.
16. Holland V, Dement W, Raynal D. Polysomnography: responding to a need for improved communication. Jackson Hole, Wyoming: Presentation to the Annual Meeting of the Sleep Research Society; 1974.
17. Rechtschaffen A, Kales A. A manual of standardized terminology, techniques and scoring system for sleep stages of human subjects. Los Angeles: BIS/BRI, UCLA; 1968.
18. Anders T, Emde R, Parmelee AH, editors. A manual of standardized terminology, techniques and criteria for scoring of states of sleep and wakefulness in newborn infants. Los Angeles: UCLA Brain Information Service, NINDS Neurological Information Network; 1971.
19. Sheldon SH. Evaluating sleep in infants and children. New York: Lippincott-Raven; 1996. p. 276.
20. Karni A, Tanne D, Rubenstein BS, et al. Dependence on REM sleep of overnight improement of a perceptual skill. Science 1994;265:679–82.
21. Wilson MA, McNaughton BL. Reactivation of hippocampal ensemble memories during sleep. Science 1994:265:676–9.
22. Quan SF, Berry RB, Buyssee D, et al. Development and results of the first ABMS subspecialty certification examination in sleep medicine. J Clin Sleep Med 2008;4(5):505–8.
23. Behrman RE, editor. Nelson's textbook of pediatrics. 14th ed. Philadelphia: WB Saunders; 1992.
24. Ferber R. Solve your child's sleep problems. New York: Simon & Schuster; 1985.
25. Guilleminault C. Sleep and its disorders in children. New York: Raver Press; 1987.
26. Diagnostic Classification Steering Committee, Thorpy M chairman. International classification of sleep disorders: diagnostic and coding manual. Rochester, MN: American Sleep Disorders Association; 1990.
27. Sheldon SH, Spire JP, Levy HB. Pediatric sleep medicine. Philadelphia WB Saunders; 1992. p. 185–240.

Development of Sleep in Infants and Children

Stephen H. Sheldon

Chapter 3

SLEEP ONSET

Sleep onset is not an isolated event. Identification of an exact moment of transition from wakefulness to sleep is difficult from both a behavioral and physiological perspective. For practical purposes, sleep onset can be correlated with certain behavioral and physiological changes occurring over a period of time. This time is, nonetheless, somewhat short. Behaviors typically associated with sleep include by are not limited to closed eyes, postural change, and behavioral quiescence. Additionally, there is modulation of responsiveness to auditory and visual stimuli, decrease in the ability of performance of simple tasks, and alterations in memory of events occurring several moments prior to sleep onset. EEG activity changes commonly associated with transitional sleep (N1) are not always perceived by the individual. Conversely, individuals may believe they have slept without obvious documentable changes in the EEG from the normal waking state.[1]

Dominant posterior rhythm (DPR) varies depending upon the child's age and level of development. According to the *Manual of Scoring Sleep Stages and Other Physiological Variables of Sleep*,[1a] DPR shows only continuous slow irregular potential changes in infants less than 3 months of age. Activity attenuates with eye opening.

WAKE

During wakefulness, DPR frequency in children less than 3 months of age ranged from 3.5 to 4.5 Hz. Frequency increases as the infant matures, reaching 5–6 Hz by 5–6 months of age, and 7–9 Hz by 3 years of age.

By 3–4 months post-gestational term infants, about 75% will have an irregular 50–100 microvolt, 3–4 Hz activity over the occipital region that attenuates with eye opening. Between 5–6 months of age many infants will demonstrate 50–110 microvolt activity over the occipital region at a frequency of about 5–6 Hz. This is apparent in about 70% of infants by 1-year post-gestational term. This pattern of continued and insistent increase in DPR frequency and amplitude continues so that by 3 years of age more than 80% of children have a mean occipital frequency of more than 7.5–9.5 Hz, 65% of 9-year-old children have an average frequency of 9 Hz, and by age 15 years this increases to about 10 Hz.

EEG amplitude is generally consistently greater than 50–110 microvolts. Average amplitude of the DPR during wakefulness is 50–56 microvolts in infants and children. About 10% of children have more than 100-microvolt activity between 6 and 9 years of age. Young children rarely exhibit EEG activity in the alpha range with voltage less than 30 microvolts.

Eye blinking might be seen with conjugate vertical eye movements that occur at a frequency of about 0.5–2 Hz. Chin muscle tone is high. Sucking movements may be noted and are characterized by extended rhythmic periods of increased chin muscle tone that appears to have a waxing and waning character. There may be conjugate irregular sharply peaked eye movements with an initial deflection lasting less than 500 milliseconds.

TRANSITIONAL SLEEP (N1)

From 2 to about 8 months of age, transitional sleep (N1) is characterized by a gradual appearance of diffuse 75–200 microvolts activity at a frequency of about 3–5 Hz. This amplitude is generally greater than that seen during wakefulness, and is usually 1–2 Hz slower than the waking background rhythm.

By 8 months to 3 years of age, generalized runs or bursts of semi-rhythmic bisynchronous 75–200 microvolts activity in the range of 3–4 Hz characterize N1. This is maximal over the occipital region. There may also be higher amplitude 4–6 Hz activity noted maximally over the frontocentral or central regions.

After 3 years of age, N1 is characterized by slowing of the DPR by about 1–2 Hz. The DPR can also be gradually replaced by relatively lower-voltage mixed-frequency activity. Beginning at about 5 years of age and progressing into adolescence, rhythmic anterior theta activity (RAT) can be seen. RAT is characterized by runs of 5–7 Hz moderate-voltage activity seen best over the frontal regions.

Monophasic negative broad sharp waves seen maximally over the central regions begin to be seen during N1 (and N2) sleep at about 6 months of age. By about 16 months of age, these vertex sharp waves of about 200 milliseconds in length can occur in bursts or runs and are most often seen during transitional sleep.

A distinctive paroxysmal EEG pattern of diffuse bisynchronous 75–350 microvolts, 3–4.5 Hz activity that occurs in bursts or runs maximum over the central, frontal, or frontocentral regions during drowsiness and during N1 sleep. This activity is termed hypnogogic hypersynchrony (HH). This pattern occurs early during sleep and disappears during N3 sleep. It is present in about 30% of 3-month-old infants and almost all children by 6–8 months of age. HH decreases in prevalence as development progresses and is identified in only about 10% of normal healthy children over 10 years of age. It is rare after 12 years of age.

At sleep onset, the electromyogram may reveal a gradual fall in muscle tone; however, this is not always present and a discrete fall in tone below that of wake may not be appreciated. Sucking movements can be seen during wakefulness and can be sustained throughout transitional sleep. Spontaneous eye closure typically signals drowsiness and wake-to-sleep transition. Slow conjugate sinusoidal eye movements replace rapid conjugate movements. Blinking disappears, and sustained eye closure is noted.

STAGE N2 SLEEP

Sleep spindles typically appear between 4 and 6 weeks of age. These rudimentary spindles are noted to be maximal over the central (vertex) regions and are typically of relatively lower amplitude and slightly lower frequency, but tend to remain about 12–14 Hz. Spindles in young infants can last longer than those typically seen in adults. More than three-quarters of children less than 13 years of age show two independent locations with different frequency ranges for sleep spindles. Spindles located over the frontal regions tend to range from 10 to 12.5 Hz and those over the central or centroparietal region range from 12.5 to 14.5 Hz. Frontal sleep spindles are more prominent than centroparietal spindles in young children but are abruptly decreased in EEG power and presence beginning at about age 13 years. Centroparietal spindles persist unchanged in presence or location as development continues.

K-complexes are well-defined waves characteristic of N2 sleep. These transient events consist of an initial negative sharp wave that is immediately followed by a positive wave lasting greater than or equal to 0.5 seconds. These events begin to appear as unique identifiable waveforms at about 5–6 months post term and are maximally located over the prefrontal and frontal regions.

Electrooculogram usually shows no eye movement activity. However, there may be frontal EEG artifact noted and slow sinusoidal eye movements may continue in some children. Chin muscle EMG is of variable amplitude, is typically lower than during wakefulness, and on occasion may be as low as during REM sleep.

STAGE N3 SLEEP

Slow-wave EEG activity during N3 sleep in the pediatric patient is typically very high voltage and can range from 100 to 400 microvolts. Frequency ranged from 0.5 to 2.0 Hz activity that is maximal over the frontal region. This slow-wave activity appears as early as 2 months of age, but most often between 3 and 4.5 months of age post term. Sleep spindles may continue during N3 sleep.

Eye movements are typically absent and there is often slow-wave EEG activity artifact noted in the electrooculogram. Chin muscle EMG is of variable amplitude and is often lower than in N2 sleep. Sometimes it can be as low as during REM sleep. In infants and younger children, sucking artifact may also be noted. N3 sleep is noted when 20% or more of a given 30-second epoch consists of slow-wave activity (in otherwise normal children), regardless of age.

STAGE REM (R) SLEEP

EEG during REM sleep in infants and children resembles that of adults. Nonetheless, the dominant frequency is slower and of higher voltage the younger the infant/child. Dominant R frequency tends to increase with age with 3 Hz activity at 7–8 weeks post term, 4–5 Hz activity with bursts of saw tooth waves at about 5 months of age, 4–6 Hz at 9 months of age, and prolonged runs or bursts of notched 5–7 Hz activity at 1–5 years of age. After 5 years of age, low-voltage mixed-frequency pattern of R sleep is quite similar to that of adults, although the amplitude may be somewhat higher.

Baseline chin muscle EMG is low and no higher than other stages of sleep. It is typically the nadir of activity noted throughout the recording. Irregular brief bursts of phasic muscle activity with duration less than 0.25 seconds can be superimposed on this low chin EMG tone. This phasic activity can occur in bursts and can be concomitant with similar bursts of rapid eye movements and anterior tibialis EMG twitches. Electrooculogram reveals irregular conjugate eye movements with a rapid initial deflection of signal lasting less than 500 milliseconds.

In small infants and young children, REM sleep is sometimes difficult to differentiate from wake or other sleep states. In these cases, utilization of other recorded variables to assist in state assignation is done. Respiration during NREM sleep is classically regular and monotonous with little variation. During REM sleep, considerable respiratory instability is noted. This is characterized by variation in rate, depth, minute ventilation, brief respiratory pauses, and brief episodes of increased respiratory rate.

NORMAL COURSE OF EVOLUTION OF SLEEP ACROSS THE NIGHT

Healthy Children, Adolescents, and Young Adults
Normal, healthy pre-school-age children, school-age children, adolescents and young adults, transition into sleep through NREM sleep. This is in clear contrast to infants who normally transition to sleep through REM sleep. During transition, the posterior dominant EEG converts to an N1 pattern; theta activity appears; and eye movements become slow, rolling, and/or pendulous. EMG muscle tone changes little from waking levels. Arousal thresholds are low, but vary when meaning is assigned to a stimulus (e.g., a subject may respond to her/his name, but not to another name or a pure tone stimulus; often regardless of the amplitude which has been shown to be age-dependent). N1 sleep typically lasts briefly and is followed by transition to N2 sleep. Arousal thresholds are higher in N2 than in N1 and the same stimulus that may cause arousal or waking from N1 may cause a K-complex to appear in N2. After approximately 5 to 25 minutes of N2 sleep, there is a gradual increase in the appearance of high-voltage waves with a frequency ranging from 0.5 to 2 Hz. This is characteristic of N3 sleep, when comprising greater than 20–50% of the recording epoch. Arousal thresholds are considerably higher in N3 sleep when compared to other sleep stages. During the first cycle of the sleep period, N3 will last about 20 to 40 minutes and ends with a series of body movements and ascent to a lighter/higher NREM stage.

The first REM-sleep period of the night occurs about 70 to 110 minutes after sleep onset. The initial REM sleep period is often brief, lasting usually less than 10 minutes and is often missed during a single night of recording in the laboratory. Arousal threshold is variable during REM sleep and is generally considered to be similar to N2.

Subsequently, NREM and REM sleep cycle throughout the remainder of the sleep period at intervals of approximately

60 to 120 minutes. N3 sleep is most prominent during the early sleep period (first third to first half of the sleep period time) and propensity for N3 sleep decreases as the sleep period progresses. REM episodes, on the other hand, become longer and more intense throughout the sleep period, with the longest and most intense REM episode occurring in the early morning hours.

Though internal and external variability exists, volumes of sleep stages across sleep periods are relatively constant. N1 comprises 2–5% N2, 45–55%; N3 sleep, 13–23%; and REM, approximately 20–25%. After the age of 5 years, proportions of sleep states remain remarkably constant throughout the remainder of the life cycle. Wake after sleep onset accounts for less than 5%. There are normally four to six cycles through various stages of sleep per night.

Newborns, Infants, and Young Children

Observation of newborns, infants, and children reveals that sleep occupies a major portion of their lives. A newborn infant spends more than 70% of every 24 hours sleeping. In contrast, adults spend 25–30% of their lives sleeping. Major 'work' of the waking child has been said to be play. Because sleep occupies such a large portion of a child's life, the major 'work' of infancy and very early childhood is more likely sleep.

Behavioral and physiological characteristics of sleep in normal infants vary significantly from sleep in adults. Premature infants exhibit a lack of concordance between electrophysiological parameters and behavioral observations. This may also be true in some term infants.[7,8] In newborn infants, electrophysiological characteristics of sleep and waking states in infants are often difficult since traditional characteristics cannot be fulfilled. Solutions to these problems have been suggested by a number of investigators. Prechtl and Beintema[9] suggested state definition based on observable behaviors; Anders, Emdee and Parmelee[10] have suggested utilization of behavioral and polygraphic features; and Hoppenbrouwers[11] suggested state definition based on polygraphic features, with observational criteria used only as supplemental information. Despite differences regarding state definition, it is clear that sleep in infants and children is significantly different than in older children, adolescents, and adults. Sleep, therefore, most likely performs a different function in the developing human.

Observations in the Fetus and Premature Infants

Rhythmic cycling of periods of activity and quiescence can be identified in the human fetus between 28 and 32 weeks' gestation.[7] Neither quiet (NREM) nor active (REM) sleep can be identified in premature babies between 24 and 26 weeks' gestation.[12] By 28 to 30 weeks, active sleep can be recognized by the presence of eye movements, body movements, and irregular respiratory activity. Chin muscle hypotonia is difficult to evaluate in the fetus and premature infant since there are few periods of tonic activity before 36 weeks' gestation.[7] Quiet sleep, on the other hand, cannot be clearly identified at this time and active sleep comprises most of the sleep period. Quiet sleep does not appear to emerge significantly until approximately 36 weeks' gestation.[7] Once identifiable, this state continues to increase in proportion regularly until it becomes the dominant state at approximately 3 months of postnatal life.

Spontaneous fetal movements can be identified between 10 weeks' and 12 weeks' gestation. Rhythmic cycling of quiescence and activity can be recorded in utero by 20 weeks.[13] At 28 to 30 weeks, brief quiet periods appear, though their period is quite unstable.[14] By 32 weeks' gestational age, body movements are absent in 53% of 20-second epochs during 2- to 3-hour sleep recordings.[7] 'No movement epochs' increase to 60% at term.

Patterns of physiological EEG activity become recognizable as early as 24 weeks' gestation. Conflicting evidence exists concerning the independence of the maturation of sleep and the EEG with respect to intrauterine stage. Very young premature infants and full-term neonates have similar EEG patterns when compared at the same conceptional age. On the other hand, it has been shown that when a premature infant reaches 40 weeks' conceptional age, she or he still has not attained a degree of EEG and CNS organization of a comparable full-term newborn.[8] Premature infants show spindle development that is approximately 4 weeks in advance of that seen in full-term infants and a statistical difference between the length of quiet sleep in the term and premature infant exists, when measured at the same conceptual age.[15] Some conflicting reports, however, may be secondary to definition and calculation of gestational age and conceptional age, or may be actual differences precipitated by development in an extrauterine environment significantly different from the normal intrauterine milieu. Extrauterine development of the premature infant occurs either in a 24-hour 'light' environment or a cycled light environment, rather than in the 24-hour 'dark' conditions of the uterus. In addition, other significant medical and developmental problems often exist in the significantly preterm newborn and continuous medical interventions are often required, disrupting the natural progression of sleep–wake cycle development. The effect of constant light and medical treatment regimens on the development of the nervous system and sleep cycling has not yet been elucidated.

Term Infants: Birth to Twelve Months

By gestational term, two distinct sleep states can be identified in the term newborn: active sleep (REM), quiet sleep (NREM). Indeterminate sleep had been a state classification defined when criteria for neither REM nor NREM can be identified.[10] However, this state has recently been abandoned in the new visual classification criteria.[1a] Sucking movements are common during active sleep.[16] During this state fine twitches are almost continuous, and grimaces, smiles, vocalizations and tremors also occur. Intermittent large athetoid limb movements, stretching, can be seen. Bursts of muscle movements and irregular respiration occur concomitantly with phasic eye movements. Conversely, quiet sleep is characterized by minimal movement.[7] Chin muscle tone is increased above the level seen in active sleep. Respiration is regular and monotonous. Little, if any, phasic activity is noted.

During the first 3 months of life, striking changes occur in many physiological functions. Ten to 12 weeks of age appears to be a critical period of CNS reorganization when infantile sleep behavior and physiology shift to a more mature form. Significant changes in sleep–wake patterns occur. At birth, total sleep time in each 24-hour cycle is about 16 to 17 hours.[7] Slow decrease in total sleep time occurs, generally reaching 14 to 15 hours by 16 weeks of age, and 13 to 14 hours by 6 to 8 months.

Appearance of attentive behaviors occurs concomitantly with the development of quiet sleep and sustained sleep patterns. This evolution suggests continued development of inhibitory and controlling feedback mechanisms secondary to the increasing complexity of neural networks and neurochemical maturation.[7] By 3 months, maturation of these systems produces a relatively stable 24-hour distribution of sleep and wake. There is also a remarkably regular alternation of active and quiet sleep.[11] Prior to 3 months of age, concordance between physiological variables is remarkably high.[17] Sleep-state organization has a 'locked-in' appearance. One explanation may be a lack of maturation of essential feedback control and a lack of variability is occasionally seen in cardiac function when the conductive tissue of the heart fails to respond to regulatory input, resulting in a fixed rate, with almost equal beat-to-beat intervals. Periodic respiration, common in NREM sleep until 3 weeks of age, becomes rare after 7 weeks.[18]

During the first 6 months of life, consolidation and entrainment of sleep at night develops. Major changes seen are in the duration of single sleep periods and their placement in the 24-hour day. Coons has impressively described this progression.[19] Her study revealed that at 3 weeks of age, the mean length of the longest sleep period was 211.7 minutes, or 23.2% of the total sleep time during the 24-hour period. By 6 months of age, the longest sleep period was 358.0 minutes, or 48% of the total sleep time. Between 3 weeks and 6 weeks, sleep periods lengthen considerably, and by 6 weeks of age, the longest sleep period was no longer randomly distributed throughout the day. At 3 months, the pattern had become more consistent. Although sleep had begun to consolidate and establish its relation to the light/dark cycle by 6 weeks of age, the longest wake period was still randomly distributed at 3 months, becoming acceptably non-random at 4.5 months of age. Long 5- to 6-hour sleep periods at 6 weeks of age gradually lengthen to 8 to 9 hours and shift to nighttime, so that a diurnal pattern is relatively well established by 12 to 16 weeks of age.[7] At 6 months of age, the long sleep period immediately follows the longest wake period.[19] After 12 weeks of age, there is continuing development of the diurnal cycle and consolidation of daytime sleep into well-defined daytime naps.[20] Waking patterns change only slightly in comparison to sleep patterns. In the neonatal period, infants awaken about every 4 hours and stay awake for 1 to 2 hours. The longest period of sustained wake period increases slowly to 3 to 4 hours by 16 weeks of age.

Brief awakenings from sleep are more frequent during the first 2 months of life, than at older ages.[11] In addition, infants 1 to 2 months of age are more likely to awaken from active sleep than from quiet sleep. Bowe and Anders reported that this variable helped discriminate between infant sleep at 2 and 9 months of age.[21] Good sleepers rarely woke from quiet sleep, whereas poor sleepers typically did. Sleep-onset latencies in infants at 2 months were approximately 30 minutes. This was almost halved by 9 months of age. Anders and Keener have shown that 44% of 2-month-old infants and 78% of 9-month-old infants slept through the night.

Striking changes occur in the EEG in the immediate newborn period. _Tracé-Alternant_ EEG pattern of quiet sleep can be first identified at 32 to 34 weeks' gestation.[23] This pattern is fully developed at 37 to 38 weeks and mature neonates show this characteristic EEG pattern. _Tracé-Alternant_ pattern gradually disappears over the first month of life. Sleep spindles appear almost simultaneously with the disappearance of _tracé-Alternant_ at 4 to 6 weeks of age. Spindles are initially rudimentary, showing two spectral bands at 12 to 14 cycles per second and 18 cycles per second (cps).[18] It takes approximately 7 days for the 18-cps spindles to disappear, but the 12- to 14-cps spindles remain. The shape of these spindles changes impressively early in development. At 2 months of age, spindles contrast so slightly with background EEG activity, that no reliable measurements are possible.[24] Long spindles are seen in the 3- to 4-month-old infant (lasting 1.8 to 3.4 seconds). This duration decreases continuously to an average of 0.5 to 0.7 seconds at the end of the second year. Spindle intervals become greater with increasing age, with a mean of 9 to 11 seconds at 6 months and 19 to 28 seconds at 24 months. After this time, the spindle interval decreases with increasing age.

True continuous delta frequency activity appears at approximately 8 to 12 weeks of age[19] and quiet sleep becomes differentiated into three distinct stages, characteristic of the more mature electrophysiological pattern. At 3 months, quiet sleep is twice that of active sleep.[15] By 8 months of age, active sleep occupies approximately 30% of the total sleep time and there is a continuous but significantly slower decline until the adult proportion is reached (between 3 years and 5 years of age).[11]

Sleep onset is characteristically through REM sleep in the newborn infant (i.e., the first REM period occurs within the first 15 minutes after sleep onset). During the first 12 weeks of life, this gradually changes to sleep onset through NREM. At 3 weeks of age, an infant is likely to have 64% of sleep periods beginning with REM sleep.[19] Younger infants, less than 3 months of age, manifest REM latencies that are predominantly less than 8 minutes in length.[25] Older infants produce a mixed distribution of short and long REM latencies. By 6 months, the proportion of sleep entered through REM sleep is approximately 18%.[19] The longest sleep period is equally as likely to have sleep onset through REM at 3 weeks of age. Between 4 and 13 months, the total distribution of REM latencies appears to be bimodal with latencies either shorter than 8 minutes or longer than 16 minutes.[25] In the group of older infants, the temporal distribution of latencies constitute a diurnal rhythm, with the longest latencies appearing between 12:00 and 16:00 hours, and a tendency of short latencies to occur between 04:00 and 08:00 hours. In the older infants, REM latency also depends upon the length of prior wakefulness. Long REM latencies are significantly more often preceded by long episodes of wakefulness than are short REM latencies. By 6 months of age, the longest sleep period is only 20% more likely to be through REM.[19] The ratio of active sleep to quiet sleep is sometimes considered an indicator of maturation.[11] Active sleep time exceeds quiet sleep time during the first months of life. A reversal of this relation is noted in 60% of infants at 3 months and 90% of infants at 6 months of age.

A specific change in REM proportion occurs during this period of development. During the first 6 months of life there is a marked reduction in the total REM sleep volume. This represents a redistribution of sleep stages, since only a relatively mild decrease in the total sleep time occurs during the first year. This change is considered to be an important indicator of central nervous system maturation.[15] It is interesting to note that the reduction in the proportion of time spent in REM sleep is balanced by an increased proportion of the 24-hour day spent in wakefulness.

Two Years to Five Years

Normative data and controlled studies of children in the preschool age group and in the early school years are surprisingly few. In contrast to the dramatic changes that take place during the first year of life, transformations during this period are ongoing but gradual. Growth and all aspects of development continue in a steady manner. Sleep becomes consolidated into a long nocturnal period of approximately 10 hours.[26-29] During the first 2 to 3 years, daytime sleep continues in distinct daytime naps. The first nap is ordinarily mid morning, the second occurring early afternoon. Morning naps are slowly given up. This occurs in an irregular pattern similar to all other developmental processes. Often, this can be frustrating to parents due to the irregularity of extinction of napping. Nonetheless, by 3 to 5 years of age, sleep can be completely consolidated into a single long nocturnal period.

During the latter half of the first year of life, REM sleep averages about 30% of the total sleep time. Small and large body movements associated with REM sleep during infancy become less frequent. REM periods are of approximately uniform length, despite daytime naps, and are evenly distributed throughout the nocturnal sleep period. As the child develops, an ongoing change is seen in the uniformity and duration of these REM periods. The first REM period becomes shortened in length, while succeeding periods tend to become progressively longer and more intense as the sleep period advances. There is also a slight lengthening of the overall NREM–REM cycle length.[16] Two- to 3-year-old children still show a cycle length of about 60 minutes, with the first REM period occurring approximately 1 hour after sleep onset. By 4 to 5 years of age, cycle length increased to about 60 to 90 minutes.

Between 2 and 5 years of age, REM percentage gradually decreases from 30% of the total sleep time to near adult level of 20–25%, although the total time of each sleep state is greater than in the adult due to the longer sleep time. There appears to be a close relationship between these changes and the augmented periods of wakefulness during the daytime. Diminution of REM volume progresses until about 3 to 4.5 years, when daytime napping has ended. By this age, distinct differences between early and late portions of the sleep period have emerged.[16]

Typically, children in this age range have approximately seven cycles during each nocturnal sleep period.[29] Sleep onset latency averages about 15 minutes in the younger children, but lengthens to between 15 and 30 minutes in the older children in this developmental grouping. Slow-wave sleep predominantly occurs during the first third of the night[28] and as much as 2 hours may be spent in N3. EEG voltage is also very high during this period. N2 first appears from 3 to 4 minutes after the child falls to sleep, and N3 appears about 10 to 15 minutes after sleep onset.[29]

Distinctive characteristics of sleep occur between 2 and 5 years that may suggest stabilization and balancing of state. A relatively small number of sleep stage changes is a noticeable feature.[27] Approximately 3.5 stage shifts per hour occur, which is significantly different than that of the young adult, EEG voltage is consistently higher, and N3 is consistently longer. Another exceptional difference is the smooth progression of stages, whether moving deeper (toward N3) or moving lighter (sleep toward wake). Transition is consistent and steady in contrast to the adult pattern where there are often abrupt movements across several stages at a time with the EEG progresses toward lighter or deeper sleep.[27,28]

Five to Ten Years

Growth and development again are steady, persistent, and gradual during middle childhood. This period of development, however, is not latent. This phase is characterized by slow methodical change, searching, exploration, and increasingly sophisticated decision making. It is a time of preparation and rehearsal, trials and errors.[30]

Sleep continues to coalesce into a more mature pattern. Sleep during middle childhood resembles that of older individuals. Considerable between-subject variability exists. Nonetheless, an orderly sequence of sleep stages is preserved, spontaneously shifting from one stage to another. There is a certain within-subject stability of pattern, a fairly consistent amount of time spent in each sleep stage, and a stable number of sleep stages within nocturnal sleep periods.[28] When compared with adult sleep patterns, total sleep time in middle childhood is approximately 2.5 hours longer with equal distribution of the added time to each of the sleep stages. Stages in children of this age group tend to be longer in duration those in adults, but the sleep architecture seems to be similar.

Although quite consistent, middle childhood remains a time of regular transition. After an initially long NREM period, some children will exhibit regularly spaced REM periods of equal duration (similar to the pattern seen during infancy) while other children reveal a more mature pattern of progressively longer REM periods as sleep progresses.[16] The proportion of REM sleep approximates the adult level. But because of the decrease in total sleep time and maturation of state, there seems to be a decrease in the total number of minutes spent in REM sleep when compared to infants and younger children.

Though body movements during sleep decrease in frequency, they are generally more often seen in this age group than in adolescents and young adults. N3 sleep proportion decreases in the preschool child in the latter portion of middle childhood.[16] There does appear, however, to be a gender-related difference in the percentage of N3 sleep. Males tend to exhibit a significantly greater proportion of N3 than females of comparable age.[28,31,32]

Although naps during this period may continue, they tend to be quite irregular and sparse. Tendency to sleep during the day seems to be lowest in this age group. Consistent habitual daytime napping during middle childhood often represents an abnormal process and may be associated with unintentional daytime sleep episodes. Prepubertal children are most often significantly alert throughout the entire day. Carskadon and co-workers have shown mean daytime sleep onset latencies during MSLT testing of preadolescent (Tanner Stage 1) children to be greater than 15 minutes,[31,33] suggesting an extreme level of alertness and low homeostatic sleep pressure.

Adolescence

Persistent maturation during middle childhood gives way to a second period of rapid change during adolescence. Not since infancy are there such quantum leaps and striking changes in physical growth; hormonal alterations; and psychological, social, and cognitive development. Luxury of stability yields to the upheaval of navigating this transitional phase. These dramatic changes are important in assessing sleep and sleep disorders during this period of life.

By early adolescence, electrophysiological variables of sleep have approximated normal young adult values. For some adolescents, certain elements of less mature patterns may occasionally be observed.[16] For example, body movements during sleep are usually similar to those seen in adults, but at times may be as high as in younger children. Total REM volume is at adult levels and REM periods clearly lengthen as the sleep period progresses. Total N3 sleep time approaches adult levels of approximately 45 to 60 minutes. Total sleep requirement decreases from 9 to 10 hours during middle childhood to approximately 8.5 hours by 16 years of age.[34,35]

Sleep habits and patterns of adolescents have been extensively studies.[33,36,37] Observations have revealed interesting tendencies in the sleep of teenagers. Considerable variation can be seen in patterns between school nights and non-school nights. Where total sleep time for children 10 years of age tends to be the same on school nights and non-school nights, young adolescents sleep less on school nights than non-school nights. Bedtimes and wake times are more controlled by outside influences on school nights. Parents attempt to set bedtime limits; but homework, starting time of classes in the morning, and alarm clocks also truncate the sleep period. These influences seem to infer that sleep on non-school nights is closer to normal physiological than sleep on school nights. Increased sleep time on non-school nights may reflect recovery from partial (although cumulative) sleep restriction during the week.

Observations by Webb and Agnew[38] and Williams et al.[29] have revealed a continuous decrease in total sleep time through middle and late adolescence of approximately 2 hours. If this sleep restriction is cumulative, subjective and objective evidence of increased daytime sleepiness should appear. In fact, older adolescents report greater difficulty with daytime sleepiness and nocturnal sleep than younger adolescents.[36] Various methods have been utilized to assess sleepiness and alertness, including pupillometry,[39,40] the Stanford Sleepiness Scale (a validated seven-point Likert scale measuring subjective sleepiness),[41,42] the Epworth Sleepiness Scale,[42b] brainstem evoked potentials,[43] and the Multiple Sleep Latency Test (MSLT).[44,45] The MSLT, developed in the mid-1970s at the Stanford University Sleep Research Center, is the most widely used procedure for objective measurement of daytime sleep tendency. This test consists of a series of opportunities to sleep, administered at 2-hour intervals across a day using a standard procedure.[45] Sleepiness is measured as the speed of falling asleep (average sleep onset latency) across these nap opportunities. The presence of REM sleep during these naps is also noted. MSLT scores are related to a number of variables that range from the amount of sleep on one or several nights preceding the study[46–49] to pathological states such as narcolepsy.[50,51] An average sleep onset latency of less than 5 minutes is a range found to be associated with performance decrements and unintentional episodes of sleep.[45]

In a series of exquisite seminal experiments by Carskadon and co-workers, manifest sleepiness during adolescence was dramatically demonstrated.[46–49] Twelve girls and 15 boys were observed longitudinally over the course of 7 years to determine sleep tendency changes which may occur during puberty. When subjects were given the opportunity to sleep for 10 hours, total sleep time did not vary significantly with adolescent maturational state and all groups slept for a little more than 9 hours per night. One conclusion drawn from these data was that *there is not a reduced need for sleep as the adolescent matures*. Time spent in REM sleep also remained constant between each developmental stage in these subjects. N3 sleep, on the other hand, decreased dramatically (by approximately 35%) between Tanner Stage 1 and Tanner Stage 5. There was a concomitant fall in the mean sleep onset latency in mid adolescence, indicating reduced daytime alertness, despite a constant total sleep time. This finding also suggested that *sleep requirements do not decrease as the adolescent ages and may, in fact, increase*.

Time in bed and total sleep time decrease as the adolescent ages, resulting in a cumulative sleep debt. This sleep debt becomes significant during late adolescence and is accompanied by a continued fall in daytime alertness (as measured by the MSLT) to levels which are close to being pathological.[49] It has become clear that impact on daytime functioning may be significant. A number of normal adolescents will, therefore, have significant disturbances in daytime alertness because of normal pubertal increase in daytime sleepiness and cumulative/additive restriction of nocturnal sleep in order to meet expectations and obligations. Though there is considerable variability between individuals, many adolescents (particularly in the older age groups) have some degree of impairment.

Clinical Pearls

- Development of sleep in the pediatric and adolescent population rapidly changes and mirrors development of the biological organism.
- Structure of sleep also rapidly changes with longitudinal and cross-sectional components that are independents.
- Considerable differences occur within and between individual children. Understanding these differences begs specific expertise in evaluation, diagnosis and management of sleep-related disorders in children.
- Evaluation of management of pediatric sleep-related disorders can be best accomplished utilizing a multi-disciplinary or inter-disciplinary approach.

References

1. Agnew HW, Wegg WB. Measurement of sleep onset by EEG criteria. Am J EEG Technol 1972;12:127.
1a. Iber C, Ancoli-Israel S, Chesson A, Quan SF for the American Academy of Sleep Medicine. The AASM Manual for the Scoring of Sleep and Associated Events: Rules, Terminology and Technical Specifications. 1st ed. Westchester, Illinois: American Academy of Sleep Medicine; 2007.
2. Carskadon MA, Dement WC. Normal human sleep: An overview. In: Kryger MH, Roth T, Dement WC, editors. Principles and practice of sleep medicine. Philadelphia: WB Saunders; 1989.
3. Guilleminault C, Phillips R, Dement WC. A syndrome of hypersomnia with automatic behavior. Electroenceph Clin Neurophysiol 1975;38:403.
4. Ogilvie RD, Wilkinson RT. The detection of sleep onset: Behavioral and physiological convergence. Psychophysiology 1984;21:510.
5. Oswalk I, Taylor AM, Treisman M. Discriminative responses to stimulation during human sleep. Brain 1960;83:440.
6. Guilleminault C, Dement WC. Amnesia and disorders of excessive daytime sleepiness. In: Drucker-Colin RR, McGaugh JL, editors. Neurobiology of sleep and memory. New York: Academic Press; 1977.
7. Parmelee AH, Stern E. Development of states in infants. In: Clemente CD, Purpura DP, Mayer FE, editors. Sleep and the maturing nervous system. New York: Academic Press; 1972.

8. Dreyfus-Brisac C. Ontogenesis of sleep in human prematures after 32-weeks of conceptual age. Dev Psychobiol 1970;3:91.
9. Prechtl HFR, Beintema D. The neurological examination of the full term newborn infant. In: Clinics in Developmental Medicine, 12. London: Spastics Society and Heinemann; 1964.
10. Anders T, Emde R, Parmelee A, editors. A manual of standardized terminology, techniques and criteria for scoring of states of sleep and wakefulness in newborn infants. UCLA Brain Information Service, NINDS Neurological Information Network; 1971.
11. Hoppenbrouwers T. Sleep in infants. In: Guilleminault C, editor. Sleep and its disorders in children. New York: Raven Press; 1987.
12. Dreyfus-Brisac C. Sleep ontogenesis in early human prematurity from 24 to 27 weeks of conceptual age. Develop Psychobiol 1968;1:62.
13. Sterman MB. The basic rest-activity cycle and sleep: Developmental considerations in man and cats. In: Clemente CD, Purpura DP, Mayer FE, editors. Sleep and the Maturing Nervous System. New York: Academic Press; 1972.
14. Dreyfus-Brisac C. Ontogenese du sommeil chez le premature humain: Etude polygraphique. In: Minokowski A, editor. Regional Development of the Brain in Early Life. Oxford: Blackwell; 1967.
15. Stern E, Parmelee AH, Akiyama Y, Schultz MA, Wenner WH. Sleep cycle characteristics in infants. Pediatrics 1969;43:65.
16. Roffwarg HP, Dement WC, Fisher C. Preliminary observations of the sleep-dream pattern in neonates, infants, children, and adults. In: Harms E, editor. Problems of sleep and dreams in children. New York: Macmillian; 1964.
17. Harper RM, Leake B, Miyahara L, et al. Development of ultradian periodicity and coalescence at 1 cycle per hour in electroencephalographic activity. Exp Neurol 1981;73:127.
18. Metcalf D. The ontogenesis of sleep-awake states from birth to 3 months. Electroenceph Clin Neurophysiol 1979;28:421.
19. Coons S. Development of sleep and wakefulness during the first 6 months of life. In: Guilleminault C, editor. Sleep and its disorders in children. New York: Raven Press; 1987.
20. Parmelee A, Wenner WH, Schulz HR. Infant sleep patterns from birth to 16 weeks of age. J Pediatr 1964;65:576.
21. Bowe TR, Anders TF. The use of semi-Markof model in the study of the development of sleep-wake states in infants. Psychophysiolog 1979;16:41.
22. Anders TF, Keener M. Developmental course of nighttime sleep-wake patterns in full term and premature infants during the first years of life. Sleep 1985;8:173.
23. Nolte R, Schulte FJ, Weisse U, et al. The 'trace' alternant' of the sleeping EEG in full-term premature and hypotrophic neonates. Electroenceph Clin Neurophysiol 1969;27:625.
24. Lenard HG. The development of sleep spindles during the first two years of life. Electroenceph Clin Neurophysiol 1970;29:217.
25. Schulz H, Salzarulo P, Fagioli I, Massetani R. REM latency: Development in the first year of life. Electroenceph Clin Neurophysiol 1983;56:316.
26. Mattison RE, Handford HA, Vela-Bueno A. Sleep disorders in children. Psychiatric Medicine 1987;4:149.
27. Kohler WC, Coddington D, Agnew HW. Sleep patterns in 2-year-old children. J Pediatr 1968;72:228.
28. Ross JJ, Agnew HW Jr, Williams RL, Webb WB. Sleep patterns in pre-adolescent children: An EEG-EOG study. Pediatrics 1968;42:324.
29. Williams RL, Karacan I, Hursch CJ. Electroencephalography (EEG) of human sleep: Clinical applications. New York: John Wiley & Sons; 1975.
30. Levine ME. Middle childhood. In: Levine ME, Carey WB, Crocker AC, et al, editors. Developmental-behavioral pediatrics. Philadelphia: WB Saunders; 1983.
31. Carskadon MA, Keenan S, Dement WC. Nighttime sleep and daytime sleep tendency in preadolescents. In: Guilleminault C editor. Sleep and its disorders in children. New York: Raven Press; 1987.
32. Coble PA, Kupfer DJ, Taska LS, Kane J. EEG sleep of normal healthy children. Part I. Findings using standard measurement methods. Sleep 1984;7:289.
33. Carskadon MA, Harvey K, Duke P, et al. Pubertal changes in daytime sleepiness. Sleep 1980;2:453.
34. Ames LB. Sleep and dreams in childhood. In: Harms E, editor. Problems of sleep and dreams in children. New York: Macmillian Company; 1964.
35. Carskadon MA. The second decade. In: Guilleminault C, editor. Sleeping and waking disorders: indications and techniques. Boston: Butterworths; 1982.
36. Carskadon MA, Dement WC. Sleepiness in the normal adolescent. In: Guilleminault C, editor. Sleep and its disorders in children. New York: Raven Press; 1987.
37. Carskadon MA, Orav EJ, Dement WC. Evolution of sleep and daytime sleepiness in adolescents. In: Guilleminault C, Lugaresi E, editors. Sleep/wake disorders: natural history, epidemiology, and long-term evolution. New York: Raven Press; 1983.
38. Webb WB, Agnew HW. Sleep and dreams. Dubuque: William C Brown; 1973.
39. Lowenstein O, Loewenfeld IE. Electronic pupillography – a new instrument and some clinical applications. Arch Ophthalmol 1958;59:352.
40. Lowenstein O, Feinberg R, Loewenfeld IE. Pupullary movements during acute and chronic fatigue: A new test for the objective evaluation of tiredness. Invest Ophthalmol 1963;2:138.
41. Hoddes E, Dement W, Zarcone V. The development and use of the Stanford Sleepiness Scale (SSS). Psychophysiology 1972;9:150.
42. Herscovitch J, Broughton R. Sensitivity of the Stanford Sleepiness Scale to the effects of cumulative partial sleep deprivation and recovery oversleeping. Sleep 1981;4:83.
42b. Johns MW. A new method for measuring daytime sleepiness: the Epworth sleepiness scale. Sleep 1991;14:540–5.
43. Broughton R. Performance and evoked potential measures of various states of daytime sleepiness. Sleep 1982;5:S135.
44. Carskadon MA, Dement WC. Sleep tendency: An objective measure of sleep loss. Sleep Res 1977;6:200.
45. Carskadon MA, Dement WC, Mitler MM, et al. Guidelines for the Multiple Sleep Latency Test (MSLT): A standard measure of sleepiness. Sleep 1986;9:519.
46. Carskadon MA, Dement WC. Effects of total sleep loss on sleep tendency. Percep Mot Skills 1979;48:495.
47. Carskadon MA, Harvey K, Dement WC. Acute restriction of nocturnal sleep in children. Percept Mot Skills 1981;53:103.
48. Carskadon MA, Harvey K, Dement WC. Sleep loss in young adolescents. Sleep 1981;4:299.
49. Carskadon MA, Dement WC. Cumulative effects of sleep restriction on daytime sleepiness. Psychophysiology 1981;18:107.
50. Guilleminault C, Dement WC, Passouant P. Narcolepsy. In: Weitzman ED, editor. Advances in sleep research, vol. 3. New York: Spectrum Publications; 1976.
51. Wilson R, Raynal D, Guilleminault C, Zarcone V, Dement W. REM latencies in daytime sleep recordings of narcoleptics. Sleep Res 1972;2:166.

Chronobiology

James K. Wyatt

INTRODUCTION

The field of human chronobiology includes the study of the basic components of the circadian regulatory systems (approximately 24 hours) and their modulation of myriad biological and neurobehavioral functions. Although ultradian rhythms (shorter than 24 hours), such as those of sleep stage cycling or the basic rest activity cycle, are important if one is to fully understand sleep and alertness, the goal of this chapter is to focus exclusively on circadian rhythms chronobiology.

Some researchers see chronobiology as a discipline separate from sleep research and sleep medicine, and there are entire conferences devoted exclusively to comparative and human circadian rhythms research. According to this view, sleep and wake are merely sets of parameters that have circadian modulation. In contrast, others see all of chronobiology as a subset of sleep research. Fortunately, these distinctions are mostly artificial; and, in fact, there is growing integration of the findings of circadian rhythm basic science research with those of basic and applied sleep research, the benefit being an improved understanding of the pathophysiology of many of the disorders of sleep. This benefit is not limited merely to the so-called *circadian rhythm sleep disorders* (see Chapter 5), but also applies to all other categories of sleep disorders including insomnia. Thus, a comprehensive understanding of human chronobiology is essential to optimal evaluation and treatment of any patient with a sleep–wake complaint.

CIRCADIAN REGULATORY SYSTEM

The *circadian regulatory system* is one of the key central nervous system (CNS) processes modulating the timing and quality of sleep and wakefulness. At a global level, the circadian system affects the activity of myriad physiological processes, influencing the timing of their activity across the 24-hour day. Though the circadian system does not merely alternate between two states of activity (*on* and *off*), it is helpful to think about the *circadian night* as the range of circadian phase positions corresponding to the typical nocturnal sleep episode, and the *circadian day* as corresponding to the typical daytime wake episode.

A well-known finding in circadian physiology is that core body temperature typically rises across the circadian day and falls during the circadian night[1] independent of perturbations such as slow wave sleep deprivation.[2] Urine production falls during the circadian night.[3] A large release of cortisol precedes the beginning of the circadian day.[4] These are just a few examples of rhythmic changes in physiological processes that likely aid the consolidation of sleep at night and the level of alert functioning in the daytime. Furthermore, the circadian system also has a direct effect on sleep–wake regulation, actively driving wakefulness during the daytime and actively driving sleep at night.[5,6]

A number of different laboratory protocols have been utilized to study human circadian rhythms. Early research on the human circadian system utilized the *90-minute day*.[7,8] Here, young adults were allowed to remain awake for 60 minutes before being given a 30-minute opportunity to sleep; this 90-minute cycle was then repeated for 24 hours or more. This design allowed researchers to examine the distribution of sleep and wake episodes across the 24-hour day, learning how *sleep propensity* (the likelihood that sleep will occur) and sleep structure (e.g., the pattern of sleep stage cycling) varied across the day and night. A more recent modification of this protocol is the *ultrashort sleep–wake schedule*,[9-12] which has wake episodes of only 13 minutes alternating with sleep opportunities of only 7 minutes. Although these approaches provide interesting data on circadian modulation of sleep and wakefulness, the ability to draw meaningful conclusions about circadian modulation under normal conditions is limited since participants in these protocols never accumulate the normal 14–18 hours of continuous wakefulness or the usual 7–9 hours of sleep.

The *constant routine* protocol, as reviewed by Duffy and Dijk,[13] requires participants to remain awake while semirecumbent on bed rest – under constant illumination and temperature, and with small frequent equally spaced meals – for longer than 24 hours; the goal here is to remove or evenly distribute confounding or masking effects such as sleep–wake state, level of physical activity, light, digestion, temperature, and posture. The constant routine is the gold standard for assessing the phase of the circadian system (i.e., its timing relative to the clock) and its amplitude, but because sleep deprivation occurs during this protocol, and because the durations of the wake episodes are long and typically confounded by circadian phase, the assessment of the effects of circadian phase alone on a given function is hampered.

Free-running protocols[1,14,15] are long-duration studies (typically lasting several weeks) conducted in an environment isolated from obvious time cues; participants self-select their bed and wake-up times. The circadian system *drifts* at its intrinsic period, and the sleep–wake cycle may desynchronize from the circadian system and take on a period typically much longer than 24 hours. Unfortunately, this self-selection of light–dark cycles – in free-run studies – often allows exposure to levels of light sufficient to produce patterns of *relative coordination*, or systematic biasing of circadian phase based on light exposure, that corrupts attempts to measure variables such as intrinsic circadian period.[16]

Perhaps the most complex and labor-intensive way to investigate human circadian rhythms is with the *forced desynchrony* protocol. Pioneered by Kleitman,[17] and refined in several laboratories,[5,18,19] participants are scheduled in a multiweek protocol to a sleep–wake period (*T-cycle*) significantly different from the near-24-hour circadian period. Under this protocol, and in the absence of obvious time cues, the circadian system free runs and sleep and wake episodes appear across a wide range of circadian phases. Thus, each data point can be assigned one coordinate for circadian phase and another for, perhaps, duration of the elapsed wakefulness or duration into the scheduled sleep episode, and the data measured might be reaction time or a 30-second epoch of sleep. As reviewed later in this chapter, results from the forced desynchrony protocol have allowed a rich understanding of circadian modulation of sleep and wakefulness.

Circadian research has also demonstrated many fundamental properties of this system. The ability of the circadian system to facilitate the proper timing of physiological processes is dependent on periodic input of timing signals. The environmental light–dark cycle is the primary periodic input or *zeitgeber* (time giver) in human circadian rhythms. Without access to robust cues of bright light during daytime and darkness at night, the circadian system relies entirely on its near-24-hour intrinsic period of oscillation. As this oscillation is not exactly 24 hours in duration but is consistent in period length, absence of daily resetting from zeitgebers leads to phase drifting, typically in a later direction (though occasionally in an earlier one), relative to the 24-hour day. This type of free-running pattern is what occurs in many blind individuals; their timing system develops a progressive drift, and they complain of intermittent nighttime insomnia or daytime sleepiness. In contrast, with daily exposure to the external 24-hour light–dark cycle (with light either from the sun or from artificial light of sufficient intensity), the circadian system maintains stable alignment to the 24-hour day and produces the desired, non-drifting, sleep–wake cycle. This is known as *entrainment*. In environments free of strong zeitgebers, the period of the intrinsic circadian rhythm has been shown to be approximately 24.2 hours in healthy young and older adults.[6,20] Intrinsic periods have also been measured in adolescent children aged 10–15 and found to be approximately 24.3 hours.[18] Given that the circadian system has a non-24-hour free-running intrinsic period, it must be reset daily to maintain entrainment to the 24-hour day. Given that the average period length is (usually) slightly longer than 24 hours, the circadian phase (usually) must adjust earlier each day to remain aligned with the light–dark cycle. Larger phase shifts are required to adapt after rapid crossing of time zones (as occurs with jet travel). Hence, there is a critical reliance of the circadian system on the timing and intensity of zeitgebers (e.g., the light–dark cycle) to adjust and maintain phase.

The timing of a light stimulus affects the magnitude and direction of circadian phase shifting. An early demonstration of the relationship between the circadian phase of light exposure and the response of circadian phase shifting in a mammal was made in flying squirrels.[21] A graphical depiction of this type of response curve was developed and is known as the *phase response curve* (PRC).[21] Light exposure at certain circadian phases has minimal phase shifting effects, while light exposure at other circadian phases results in *phase delays* (shifting later) or *phase advances* (shifting earlier) of circadian rhythms with the amount and direction of shift dependent upon the timing, intensity, and duration of exposure. In humans on a normal sleep pattern (with relatively stable bedtimes and wake times, sleeping at night, and being awake during the daytime), light exposure at clock times ranging from late in the biological day to early in the biological night will produce a phase delay, whereas light exposure at times from late in the biological night to the early hours of the

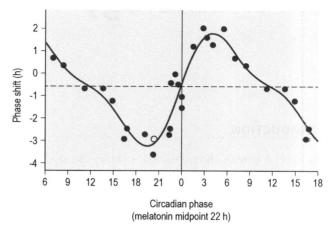

FIGURE 4-1 Type 1 Phase Response Curve for Light. The horizontal axis represents circadian phase position with hour intervals, where 0 corresponds to the trough of core body temperature, which normally occurs 1–3 hours prior to average wake time. The vertical axis represents the amount and direction of phase shifting, with the convention of phase advances being plotted as positive values and phase delays being plotted as negative values. *Figure reproduced with permission from Khalsa SB, Jewett ME, Cajochen C, Czeisler CA. A phase response curve to single bright light pulses in human subjects. J. Physiol. 6/15/2003 2003;549(Pt 3):945-952.*

biological day will produce a phase advance.[22–24] At a critical circadian phase, typically several hours prior to the morning wake time and near the trough of core body temperature, there is a *crossover zone*. Light exposure will lead to the largest phase delays when delivered just prior to the crossover zone, and the largest phase advances when delivered just after the crossover zone. Figure 4-1 illustrates the phase shifting effects of bright light.

PRCs have also been constructed to demonstrate the circadian phase shifting effects of exogenous melatonin administration. The PRCs for melatonin and light exposure are nearly opposite in their timing. Thus, melatonin administration during the period from afternoon through the early evening produces a circadian phase advance, while melatonin administration during the period from late nighttime through early morning hours produces a circadian phase delay.[25–27] Figure 4-2 illustrates the phase shifting effects of melatonin administration.

Zeitgeber intensity also affects the amount of resultant circadian phase shifting. The original PRCs[22–24] were constructed with very bright artificial indoor light (i.e., approximately 5000–10 000 lux, which is an intensity of light exposure similar to that observed outdoors at sunrise or sunset). However, the relationship between light intensity and the amount of phase shifting is nonlinear; thus, even average indoor room light intensity can produce phase shifting.[28,29]

The duration of light exposure also determines the amount of phase shifting. The original PRCs to light were constructed with multiple-hour light exposure (e.g., six consecutive hours). A 2012 study has demonstrated that even an hour of light exposure can result in significant phase shifting.[30] Similar results have been reported with intermittent light exposure[31,32] (alternating periods of bright and dim light exposure). These observations support the conclusion that a nonlinear relationship also exists between duration of light exposure and the amount of phase shift.[33]

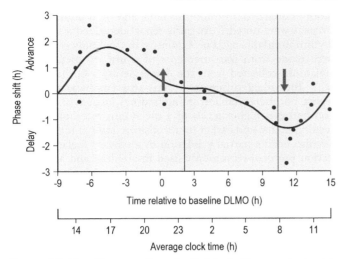

FIGURE 4-2 Phase-Response Curve for Melatonin. The upper horizontal axis represents circadian phase position with hour intervals, where 0 corresponds to the dim light melatonin onset (DLMO), which normally occurs 1–3 hours prior to average bedtime. Corresponding clock time is shown on the lower axis for clarity. The vertical axis represents the amount and direction of phase shifting, with the convention of phase advances being plotted as positive values and phase delays being plotted as negative values. *Figure reproduced with permission from Burgess HJ, Revell VL, Eastman CI. A three pulse phase response curve to three milligrams of melatonin in humans. J. Physiol. 1/15/2008 2008;586(2):639–647.*

Early research on photic circadian shifting relied upon full-spectrum artificial lighting, approximating natural sunlight. Subsequent research has found that the circadian system is maximally sensitive to visible blue light.[34] Current investigations are measuring the amount of circadian phase shifting caused by exposure to commonly encountered light-emitting devices with significant blue light spectrum, such as computer monitors, laptop monitors, and handheld computer devices. The results of these studies should improve our understanding of how some of the circadian rhythm sleep disorders develop and are maintained, explain the existence of barriers to treatment, and help us design optimal treatment protocols.

The central element of the circadian system is the *suprachiasmatic nucleus* (SCN), a bilaterally represented structure in the hypothalamus.[35,36] The SCN is sometimes referred to as the *circadian clock*. As noted above, the circadian system requires periodic input from the light–dark cycle to maintain optimal phase alignment with a nighttime sleep episode and a daytime wake episode. Environmental light is transduced to neuronal signals at the level of specialized retinal ganglion cells.[37] This circadian vision system connects to the SCN via the *retinohypothalamic tract*.[38] The SCN has many output pathways to influence other brain structures. One that has been well studied is a multi-synaptic pathway connecting the SCN to the *pineal gland*, the most important source of melatonin in the CNS.[39]

SLEEP HOMEOSTATIC SYSTEM

Although this is a chapter on chronobiology and specifically on human circadian rhythms, it would be incomplete to discuss the circadian system without discussing its equally important counterpart. The second major modulatory process affecting sleep and wakefulness is the *sleep homeostatic process*. Put simply, it is as if the CNS keeps track of each hour of continuous wakefulness, with ever-building sleepiness and sleep propensity. Though not directly measureable in humans, a proxy for the accumulation of sleep homeostatic drive can be measured via spectral composition of the waking EEG, such as spectral power in the delta band in frontal leads.[40] Similarly, the dissipation of sleep homeostatic drive during sleep episodes can be estimated from measurement of spectral power of *slow-wave activity* (SWA).[41–44] Following partial sleep restriction, there is an enhancement in SWA in recovery sleep.[42,45]

For many decades there have been *hypnotoxin* theories suggesting that across the duration of an episode of wakefulness, a substance or substances build up in the brain and/or cerebrospinal fluid (CSF) that have a negative impact on alert brain functioning, thereby increasing the likelihood of sleep. Several candidate substances have been identified to support this process, including early findings for delta sleep-inducing peptide and sleep factor S. More recent investigation has pointed to the importance of adenosine as a sleep-promoting substance that may be a key element of the sleep homeostatic process.[46,47]

THE TWO-PROCESS MODEL

The two-process model of sleep–wake regulation is a useful way of considering the simultaneous impact of the sleep homeostatic process and the circadian regulatory system on sleep and wakefulness.[48] Use of the forced desynchrony protocol over the past few decades has allowed for estimation of the independent influence of each of the two processes and, perhaps more importantly, their nonlinear interaction.[5,6] An example of this nonlinear interaction is that the amplitude of circadian modulation of alertness is quite small when measured with a concurrent low level of sleep homeostatic drive, and systematically larger with increasing extent of sleep homeostatic drive.[6,49] One of the important findings of these forced desynchrony studies has been demonstration of the difficulty knowing the extent to which certain phenomena – when they occur at a certain time of day – are caused by the homeostatic system, the circadian system, or a combination of both. For example, the depth and duration of the *midafternoon trough* of alertness is related both to the circadian and to the homeostatic systems. It is unfortunate that many published reports describing circadian rhythms of certain events or biological processes fail to measure or even estimate or consider the effects of circadian phase and sleep homeostatic pressure on the rhythms studied.

Another important outcome of forced desynchrony (and some earlier free-run) studies is the finding that circadian systems are crucial to the maintenance of sustained bouts of wakefulness during the day and sustained periods of sleep at night.[5] If the homeostatic system were the only one present, alertness would decline across the waking day, reaching critical levels of impairment in the second half of the daytime; sustained wakefulness across the daytime would be extremely difficult if not impossible. However, the circadian system actively promotes alertness across the waking day, opposing the build-up of sleep homeostatic drive. The circadian system reaches its maximal drive for alertness a few hours prior to habitual bedtime (e.g., approximately 7 p.m. for a child routinely sleeping from 9 p.m. to 6 a.m.), a period known as the *forbidden zone* for sleep[12] or as the *wake maintenance zone*.[50] Similarly, sleep homeostatic drive decreases across the nighttime sleep episode. If only a sleep homeostatic system were present, sleep would become progressively fragmented with intrusions of wakefulness in the second half of the night. Fortunately, the circadian system has a sleep-promoting function during the night, with increasingly greater sleep drive across the nocturnal sleep episode. Curiously, the circadian drive for sleep reaches its maximal level at normal wake time and for an additional 2–3 hours (e.g., approximately 6 a.m. to 9 a.m. for a child routinely sleeping from 9 p.m. to 6 a.m.). The time window of maximal sleep promotion has been called the *circadian sleep maintenance zone*.[45,51]

DEVELOPMENT OF CIRCADIAN RHYTHMS – INFANCY THROUGH ADULTHOOD

There are several limitations relevant to the discussion of the development of circadian rhythms in infants and children. First, there are only limited cross-sectional and longitudinal data addressing the ages at which the developing circadian system influences various physiological processes. Second, there are data suggesting that maternal circadian rhythms entrain those of the late-term fetus or newborn. The impact of these entraining maternal circadian rhythms persists after birth because of the infant's exposure to breastfeeding and other behavioral rhythms. Third, because of ethical and practical concerns, there are limited data to address the ability to shift the circadian rhythm of infants and children. Regardless of these caveats, there have been fascinating findings reported in this area.

It has been demonstrated that late in fetal development there is the differentiation between active and quiet sleep.[52] Confirmatory evidence comes from observations of infants born prematurely.[53] This is only to say that there is early development of sleep state regulation occurring prior to birth. Similarly, observations from nonhuman primates suggest the consolidation of circadian rhythms starts during fetal development.[54] In humans, there have been reports of variations in fetal heart rate synchronized to the mother's circadian rhythms,[55] as well as an observed 24-hour periodicity in cortisol secretion in the full-term fetus.[56] Observations such as these suggest the functioning of at least a rudimentary circadian system occurs prior to full-term birth. However, much of the animal literature on entrainment or phase shifting of fetal and/or neonatal circadian rhythms may not translate to humans and hence will not be reviewed here, given that many of the non-photic zeitgebers that can shift rhythms in animals (e.g., timing of feeding or activity) are weak or inactive as zeitgebers in humans. For a comprehensive review of the animal research findings in fetal and early-life development of the circadian system, see Sumova et al.[57]

In the human newborn, a circadian pattern of core body temperature oscillation develops by approximately 2 to 3 months of age,[58] or perhaps even earlier as suggested in a case report.[59] A circadian rhythm of salivary cortisol is established as early as the first 2 months of infancy, but different methods of data analysis produced results suggesting that this rhythm

is not established until months later, and high individual differences were noted.[60] An early report described a melatonin rhythm in infants aged 6–9 months; in this study estimations were made from measurements of a urinary metabolite of melatonin collected from the diaper across a 60-hour interval.[61] Individual differences were also emphasized in this report, but there were intriguing findings, such as of a correlation between higher levels of a melatonin metabolite in the evening hours, and earlier hours of sleep onset at night. There has also been a partial validation of a salivary melatonin collection protocol (commonly used in children and adults) for newborns, showing a reasonable correlation with blood sample melatonin levels.[62] This procedure could be utilized to sample melatonin more frequently, such as is done during the *dim light melatonin onset* (DLMO) protocol[63] in children and adults (as described below in the circadian modulation section).

Much of the literature on circadian rhythms in young children is focused on those with neurodevelopmental disorders, and hence there is a gap in knowledge for typical early childhood development of the circadian system. For example, it has been reported that 2- to 10-year-old children with autism may exhibit fragmented sleep with delayed timing relative to the sleep–wake schedule desired by the parents, and these patterns are responsive to exogenous melatonin administration.[64] A blunted or absent circadian rhythm of melatonin has also been reported in autism,[65,66] but it is unclear if this is evidence of a primary problem with the circadian pacemaker itself, with the pineal gland itself, or with the circadian regulation of pineal synthesis of melatonin. Similar sleep delay and disruption, and melatonin treatment responsiveness, has been reported for children with Angelman syndrome.[67] Other circadian research in pre-teenage children has focused on chronotype (see next section).

The most comprehensive study of circadian rhythms in children has been on youngsters in the years of pubertal development. Carskadon's research laboratories at Stanford University and Brown University have been the sites of important studies on adolescents in this age range. Much of the early studies focused on sleep and sleep deprivation, but more recent protocols have included detailed circadian assessments. A fundamental finding has been the measurement of circadian period, which is slightly longer in adolescents than in adults (approximately 24.3 hours as noted above).[18] Another well-documented finding is that of a delay of the timing of the nocturnal sleep episode during the teenage years[68] thought to result from a combination of social, behavioral, and biological factors (see Chapter 6). Implications are clear for the development of delayed sleep phase disorder (see Chapter 5), which often begins or worsens in the teenage years.

CIRCADIAN AND HOMEOSTATIC MODULATION OF NEUROBEHAVIORAL FUNCTIONS

The circadian and sleep homeostatic systems exert robust modulation of neurobehavioral functions during wakefulness. Prior to knowledge of the existence of these systems, researchers were limited to making observations of time-of-day effects or exploring the gross impact of a night of partial sleep restriction or total sleep deprivation.[69–71] Data from the constant routine protocol (described above) demonstrate relatively stable alertness, cognitive performance, and electrophysiological measures of alertness (low incidence of slow eye movements and transitions to stage 1 nonREM (NREM) sleep) during the approximately 16 hours of the normal circadian day. These measures all show impairment during the circadian night due to the combined impact of increased levels of sleep homeostatic drive and the active circadian drive for sleep. There is a minor recovery of all performance and arousal measures the following circadian day, as the circadian drive for alertness partially offsets the ever-increasing sleep homeostatic drive encountered from sleep deprivation.[72,73]

Perhaps the most comprehensive data come from the forced desynchrony protocol (as described above). Across wake episodes that are slightly shorter,[6] slightly longer,[74] or substantially longer[49] than the typical 16-hour wake episode kept by adults, the circadian system has been shown to exert approximately the same magnitude of modulation of a variety of neurobehavioral functions as the sleep homeostatic process. The implication for children (nearly all of whom sleep at night and are awake during the day) is that the build-up of sleep homeostatic pressure across daytime hours of sustained wakefulness is offset by the progressively increasing circadian drive for alertness. This results in a nearly constant level of alertness and performance across the circadian day.[75] Use of the forced desynchrony protocol has allowed for the understanding of how caffeine can attenuate certain neurobehavioral impairments encountered under conditions of sleep loss (and increased homeostatic drive) during the day, while failing to attenuate the circadian-related impairment of functioning seen during the circadian night.[49] Figure 4-3 illustrates the circadian and sleep homeostatic modulation of various neurobehavioral measures as assessed in a forced desynchrony protocol in young adults.

CHRONOTYPE

Somewhat separate from, but related to, the circadian modulation of neurobehavioral functions is the concept of chronotype, namely an individual's perception of the optimal and least favorable times of the day for mental and physical performance, alertness, and sleep. *Morning chronotypes*, also referred to as *larks* or, *early-risers*, prefer relatively early bed and wake-up times and they describe their optimal mental and physical performance to be in the early part of the wake episode. *Evening chronotypes*, sometimes referred to as *owls* or *late sleepers*, prefer relatively late bed and wake-up times and they describe their period of optimal mental and physical performance to be late in the wake episode. Two commonly reported questionnaires of chronotype are the *Morningness Eveningness Questionnaire*[76] and the *Munich Chronotype Questionnaire.*[77] A recent development is the creation of a subjective chronotype scale for young children, which has been validated in a sample of 4–11-year-olds.[78] This study showed a relatively even distribution of the number of children in each chronotype category, from *definitely morning type* through *definitely evening type*. Use of chronotype questionnaires validated in children should allow for measurement of the age at which these patterns emerge and how they may change across development.

While not perfectly correlated with biologic or physiologic study, subjective chronotype classification does show important correlations with certain circadian parameters. For example, compared to evening types, healthy young adult morning types have been noted to have not only an earlier circadian phase (relative to clock time), but also an even earlier phase of the circadian rhythms of melatonin and core body temperature (relative to their sleep schedule).[79] Baehr et al. reported a similar finding of the impact of chronotype on the relationship between core body temperature and the sleep episode, also noting that the circadian phase was later in men than in women.[80] A relationship between chronotype and circadian period has also been reported, with longer circadian period length associated with higher eveningness ratings.[81]

CIRCADIAN MODULATION OF ENDOCRINE SYSTEMS AND OTHER PHYSIOLOGY

The circadian system modulates the timing of the release of a number of endocrine components. Under normal conditions (e.g., sleep at night, wake during the day, and relatively consistent bedtimes and wake times) the primary release of cortisol begins just prior to wake time and drops to its lowest levels prior to bedtime.[1,82] In contrast, thyroid stimulating hormone (TSH) release begins shortly before bedtime, but sleep itself has an inhibitory effect.[83] Early studies reported that prolactin levels are enhanced by sleep.[84] But, under constant routine conditions where sleep is prohibited, a daily rhythm of this hormone has been observed, suggesting that the nocturnal release may be predominantly due to circadian modulation. Substantial gender differences were also found, as would be expected (with higher circadian amplitude of prolactin levels in women).[85] Growth hormone release, in contrast, appears to be directly related to sleep itself and not the circadian system, with release of growth hormone in the early night tied to slow-wave sleep.[4]

Perhaps the most well-studied hormone with a prominent circadian pattern of release is melatonin. In people on a regular sleep schedule, the nocturnal release of melatonin begins shortly before bedtime. This is commonly studied using the DLMO protocol.[63] Frequent episodic sampling (e.g., every 30 or 60 minutes) of blood or, more recently, of saliva is sufficient to capture this typically nocturnal rise in melatonin levels, and the onset is defined as that point when levels rise about a certain threshold (e.g., 10 pg/mL in blood and 3 or 4 pg/mL in saliva). Since light exposure suppresses melatonin levels, sampling must be conducted under conditions of very dim lighting.[86]

There are myriad findings of time-of-day changes in various physiological parameters and the incidence of medical events, not all of which can fully separate confounding factors of time-of-day, duration of prior wake or sleep, circadian phase itself, or other variables. Only a few examples will be provided here. There is a well-known morning increase in the onset of symptoms of myocardial infarction.[87] Perhaps related is the finding of increased platelet aggregability in the 6–9 a.m. window,[88] though much of this may have to do with posture changes from supine to upright at the end of a nocturnal sleep episode.[89] Data obtained during the constant routine protocol have shown a circadian variation in respiratory control, with lowest values of several parameters of respiratory functioning occurring toward the end of the circadian day with maximal values occurring during the early circadian day.[90]

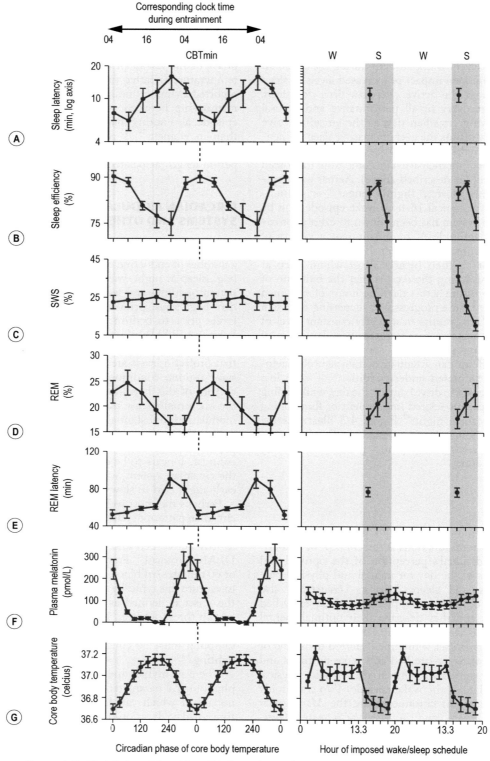

FIGURE 4-3 Circadian vs. Homeostatic Modulation of Cognition. This figure depicts the circadian (left panels) and sleep homeostatic (right panels) modulation of various neurobehavioral measures during forced desynchrony, relative to average baseline performance (0 on each y-axis). Circadian phase is double-plotted relative to the minimum of core body temperature (CBTmin, dotted vertical line spanning Rows A–F). Sleep homeostatic depicts the 13.33 h wake episodes and the 6.67 h sleep episodes (highlighted by the vertical stippled rectangle spanning Rows A–F). Rows A and B: an addition task and the digit symbol substitution task, two measures of cognitive throughput. Row C: the Probed Recall Memory task, assessing free-recall memory after a 10-minute delay with distraction. Rows D and E: median reaction time and the number of response lapses on the Psychomotor Vigilance Task, a test of visual attention and simple reaction time. Row F: KSS = Karolinska Sleepiness Scale, a report of subjective sleepiness. *Figure reproduced with permission of author from Wyatt JK, Ritz-De Cecco A, Czeisler CA, Dijk DJ. Circadian temperature and melatonin rhythms, sleep, and neurobehavioral function in humans living on a 20-h day. Am. J. Physiol. 10/1999 1999;277(4 Pt 2):R1152–R1163.*

CIRCADIAN AND HOMEOSTATIC MODULATION OF SLEEP

Experiments using the forced desynchrony and the free-run protocols have revealed important details of the independent and shared modulation of sleep by the sleep homeostatic and circadian systems. Sleep propensity, as assessed by simply measuring the time from lights out to sleep onset, has a strong circadian modulation. Sleep onset occurs most rapidly when trials are initiated at the circadian phase at or just following the average morning wake-up time, i.e., near the trough of core body temperature[5,91] and several hours after the time of maximal endogenous melatonin levels,[6] during the circadian sleep maintenance zone. Rapid eye movement (REM) sleep has a similar circadian pattern, with the amount of REM sleep occurring (during a given period of sleep) showing the same relationship to circadian phase as does sleep propensity.[6,44,92–94] Latency to REM sleep is also shortest in the circadian sleep maintenance zone.[6] This is an important observation relevant to the practice of sleep medicine, as there may be a false-positive sleep onset REM period (SOREMP) observed in the first nap of a multiple sleep latency test (MSLT), as this first nap is scheduled near the peak time of circadian propensity for REM sleep. REM sleep also occurs in increasing amounts across a major sleep episode, a process that has been referred to as *sleep-dependent disinhibition* of REM sleep.[44] Interestingly, during free-running conditions, a similar propensity for REM sleep that is linked to the circadian phase is observed, but REM sleep density (e.g., the number of rapid eye movements per epoch of REM sleep) does not show circadian modulation.[95] There is very little circadian modulation of slow-wave sleep (NREM stage 3).[6,44] Slow-wave sleep is predominantly modulated by the sleep homeostatic process, showing decreased prevalence across successive NREM–REM cycles in a major sleep episode.[6,44] Figure 4-4 illustrates the circadian and sleep homeostatic modulation of various polysomnographic measures as assessed in a forced desynchrony protocol in young adults.

The microstructure of sleep has also been assessed in forced desynchrony protocols via spectral analysis of the sleep EEG, predominantly in young adults, revealing the sleep homeostatic and circadian modulation of slow-wave activity and sleep spindles.[4] The circadian propensity for sleep spindles peaks at the circadian phase normally occurring at the beginning of the nocturnal sleep episode. Slow-wave activity shows much lower amplitude of circadian modulation. In contrast, the homeostatic system shows strong modulation of slow-wave activity, with high levels in the first NREM episode and declining levels in subsequent NREM episodes of the sleep episode. Homeostatic influence on sleep spindle activity progressively increases across the length of the sleep episodes, independent of circadian phase. The decline in slow-wave activity across sleep cycles independent of circadian phase has also been reported in children and teenagers.[96]

Unique information about the circadian modulation of sleep and wake comes from exogenous melatonin studies. Melatonin administration increases the duration of sleep in naps and in sleep episodes during the circadian day, and it may shorten sleep latency.[97–99] However, melatonin administration does not increase sleep duration for sleep episodes scheduled during the circadian night (e.g., a nocturnal sleep episode) in either normal sleepers or patients with insomnia.[100,101] In a forced desynchrony protocol with melatonin administration given prior to sleep episodes scheduled at a full range of circadian phases, a sleep-promoting effect of melatonin was found only in sleep episodes occurring during the circadian day,[102] supporting the hypothesis that melatonin administration during the circadian day could suppress the circadian system's drive for alertness that normally occurs at that time.[103–106]

CONCLUSION

Understanding both the intrinsic circadian timekeeping system and the complimentary sleep homeostatic process is fundamental to understanding daily changes in multiple behavioral and physiological measures. The circadian system modulates sleep and alertness, core body temperature, pineal melatonin, cortisol, and numerous other physiological processes. Its phase alignment is controlled by exposure to light via a special class of retinal ganglion cells that project to the suprachiasmatic nucleus in the hypothalamus. The resultant shift in circadian phase is dependent on timing, intensity, duration and spectral characteristics of the light. Exogenous melatonin ingestion has circadian phase-shifting properties as well.

The circadian system actively drives wakefulness in increasing amounts across the normal waking day, counteracting the impairment in neurobehavioral performance that would otherwise result from the build-up of sleep homeostatic drive. Similarly, the circadian system maintains consolidated sleep in the second half of the night, counteracting the dissipation of the homeostatic pressure that occurs across the night during sleep. These findings have been demonstrated in adolescents, young adults, and older adults using a forced desynchrony protocol. Given the demands and the nearly 1-month duration of this protocol, it is unlikely ever to be employed to study circadian and sleep homeostatic modulation in infants or young children. Similarly, the requirements necessary to directly assess the circadian modulation of many physiological parameters are difficult to adapt to safely and ethically study the rhythms in infants and young children; however, novel approaches – such as urinary sampling of a melatonin metabolite – have been applied and show promise.

Clinical Pearls

- The circadian timing system and the sleep homeostatic system are the two major modulatory processes that work together to permit consolidated periods of sleep and wakefulness.
- Light is the major zeitgeber ('time giver') affecting the alignment and entrainment of circadian rhythms in children and adults.
- Assessment of circadian phase can be approximated by history and determined with greater certainty by measurement of melatonin levels (in saliva or blood), of melatonin metabolite levels (in urine), or of core body temperature.
- Chronotype refers to the perceived time of day (morning, evening, or neither) of optimal mental and physical performance.

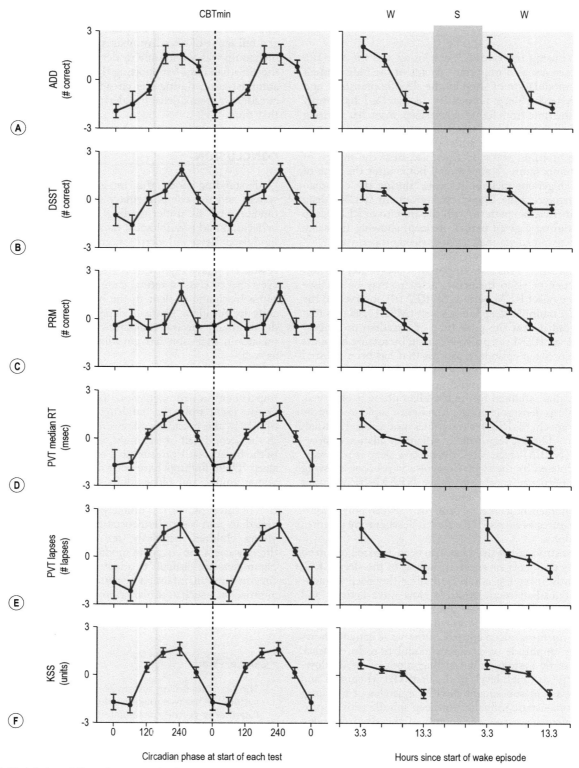

FIGURE 4-4 Modulation of Sleep Structure. This figure depicts the circadian (left panels) and sleep homeostatic (right panels) modulation of various sleep measures during forced desynchrony. Circadian phase is double-plotted relative to the minimum of core body temperature (CBTmin, dotted vertical line spanning Rows A–G). Sleep homeostatic modulation is double-plotted depicting the 13.33 h wake episodes and the 6.67 h sleep episodes (highlighted by the vertical stippled rectangle spanning Rows A–G). Plasma melatonin and core body temperature measures are presented in Rows F and G, to allow visualization of circadian phase (left panels), and the variation on body temperature based on sleep–wake state (right panel G). *Figure reproduced with permission of author from Wyatt JK, Ritz-De Cecco A, Czeisler CA, Dijk DJ. Circadian temperature and melatonin rhythms, sleep, and neurobehavioral function in humans living on a 20-h day. Am. J. Physiol. 10/1999 1999;277(4 Pt 2):R1152–R1163.*

References

1. Weitzman ED, Czeisler CA, Moore-Ede MC. Sleep-wake, neuroendocrine and body temperature circadian rhythms under entrained and non-entrained (free-running) conditions in man. In: Suda M, Hayaishi O, Nakagawa H, editors. Bioilogical rhythms and their central mechanisms. Elsevier/North-Holland Biomedical Press; 1979. p. 199–227.
2. Beersma DG, Dijk DJ. Selective SWS suppression does not affect the time course of core body temperature in men. J Sleep Res 1992;1(3):201–4.
3. Shanahan TL, Czeisler CA. Light exposure induces equivalent phase shifts of the endogenous circadian rhythms of circulating plasma melatonin and core body temperature in men. J Clin Endocrinol Metab 1991;73(2):227–35.
4. Weitzman ED, Czeisler CA, Zimmerman JC, Moore-Ede MC. Biological rhythms in man: relationship of sleep-wake, cortisol, growth hormone, and temperature during temporal isolation. Adv Biochem Psychopharmacol 1981;28:475–99.
5. Dijk DJ, Czeisler CA. Paradoxical timing of the circadian rhythm of sleep propensity serves to consolidate sleep and wakefulness in humans. Neurosci Lett 1994;166(1):63–8.
6. Wyatt JK, Ritz-De Cecco A, Czeisler CA, et al. Circadian temperature and melatonin rhythms, sleep, and neurobehavioral function in humans living on a 20-h day. Am J Physiol 1999;277(4 Pt 2):R1152–63.
7. Carskadon MA, Dement WC. Sleep studies on a 90-minute day. Electroencephalogr Clin Neurophysiol 1975;39(2):145–55.
8. Carskadon MA, Dement WC. Sleepiness and sleep state on a 90-min schedule. Psychophysiology 1977;14(2):127–33.
9. Lavie P, Scherson A. Ultrashort sleep-walking schedule. I. Evidence of ultradian rhythmicity in 'sleepability'. Electroencephalogr Clin Neurophysiol 1981;52(2):163–74.
10. Lavie P, Zomer J. Ultrashort sleep-waking schedule. II. Relationship between ultradian rhythms in sleepability and the REM-non-REM cycles and effects of the circadian phase. Electroencephalogr Clin Neurophysiol 1984;57(1):35–42.
11. Lavie P. Ultradian cycles in wakefulness – possible implications for work-rest schedules. In: Folkard S, Monk TH, editors. Hours of work: temporal factors in work-scheduling. New York: John Wiley and Sons Ltd.; 1985. p. 97–106.
12. Lavie P. Ultrashort sleep-waking schedule. III. 'Gates' and 'forbidden zones' for sleep. Electroencephalogr Clin Neurophysiol 1986;63(5):414–25.
13. Duffy JF, Dijk DJ. Getting through to circadian oscillators: why use constant routines? J Biol Rhythms 2002;17(1):4–13.
14. Monk TH, Weitzman ED, Fookson JE, et al. Circadian rhythms in human performance efficiency under free-running conditions. Chronobiologia 1984;11(4):343–54.
15. Monk TH, Moline ML. The timing of bedtime and waketime decisions in free-running subjects. Psychophysiology 1989;26(3):304–10.
16. Klerman EB, Dijk DJ, Kronauer RE, et al. Simulations of light effects on the human circadian pacemaker: implications for assessment of intrinsic period. Am J Physiol 1996;270(1 Pt 2):R271–2.
17. Kleitman N. Sleep and Wakefulness. Chicago: University of Chicago Press; 1939.
18. Carskadon MA, Labyak SE, Acebo C, et al. Intrinsic circadian period of adolescent humans measured in conditions of forced desynchrony. Neurosci Lett 1999;260(2):129–32.
19. Hiddinga AE, Beersma DG, Van den Hoofdakker RH. Endogenous and exogenous components in the circadian variation of core body temperature in humans. J Sleep Res 1997;6(3):156–63.
20. Czeisler CA, Duffy JF, Shanahan TL, et al. Stability, precision, and near-24-hour period of the human circadian pacemaker [see comments]. Science 1999;284(5423):2177–81.
21. De Coursey PJ. Daily light sensitivity rhythm in a rodent. Science 1960;131(3392):33–5.
22. Honma K, Honma S. A human phase response curve for bright light pulses. Jap J Psychiatr Neurol 1988;42(1):167–8.
23. Minors DS, Waterhouse JM, Wirz-Justice A. A human phase-response curve to light. Neurosci Lett 11/25/1991 1991;133(1):36–40.
24. Khalsa SB, Jewett ME, Cajochen C, et al. A phase response curve to single bright light pulses in human subjects. J Physiol 2003;549(Pt 3):945–52.
25. Lewy AJ, Ahmed S, Jackson JML, et al. Melatonin shifts human circadian rhythms according to a phase-response curve. Chronobiol Int 1992;9(5):380–92.
26. Burgess HJ, Revell VL, Molina TA, et al. Human phase response curves to three days of daily melatonin: 0.5 mg versus 3.0 mg. Clin Endocrinol Metab 2010;95(7):3325–31.
27. Burgess HJ, Revell VL, Eastman CI. A three pulse phase response curve to three milligrams of melatonin in humans. J Physiol 2008;586(2):639–47.
28. Boivin DB, Duffy JF, Kronauer RE, et al. Sensitivity of the human circadian pacemaker to moderately bright light. J Biol Rhythms 1994;9(3-4):315–31.
29. Boivin DB, Duffy JF, Kronauer RE, et al. Dose-response relationships for resetting of human circadian clock by light. Nature 1996;379(6565):540–2.
30. St Hilaire MA, Gooley JJ, Khalsa SB, et al. Human phase response curve to a 1 h pulse of bright white light. J Physiol 2012;590(Pt 13):3035–45.
31. Burgess HJ, Crowley SJ, Gazda CJ, et al. Preflight adjustment to eastward travel: 3 days of advancing sleep with and without morning bright light. J Biol Rhythms 2003;18(4):318–28.
32. Revell VL, Burgess HJ, Gazda CJ, et al. Advancing human circadian rhythms with afternoon melatonin and morning intermittent bright light. J Clin Endocrinol Metab 2006;91(1):54–9.
33. Nelson DE, Takahashi JS. Sensitivity and integration in a visual pathway for circadian entrainment in the hamster (Mesocricetus auratus). J Physiol 1991;439:115–45.
34. Lockley SW, Brainard GC, Czeisler CA. High sensitivity of the human circadian melatonin rhythm to resetting by short wavelength light. J Clin Endocrinol Metab 2003;88(9):4502–5.
35. Moore RY, Eichler VB. Loss of a circadian adrenal corticosterone rhythm following suprachiasmatic lesions in the rat. Brain Res 1972;42:201–6.
36. Stephan FK, Zucker I. Circadian rhythms in drinking behavior and locomotor activity of rats are eliminated by hypothalamic lesions. Proc Natl Acad Sci USA 1972;69(6):1583–6.
37. Berson DM, Dunn FA, Takao M. Phototransduction by retinal ganglion cells that set the circadian clock. Science 2002;295(5557):1070–3.
38. Moore RY, Lenn NJ. A retinohypothalamic projection in the rat. J Comparative Neurol 1972;146(1):1–14.
39. Cassone VM. Melatonin's role in vertebrate circadian rhythms. Chronobiol Int 1998;15(5):457–73
40. Cajochen C, Wyatt JK, Czeisler CA, et al. Separation of circadian and wake duration-dependent modulation of EEG activation during wakefulness. Neuroscience 2002 114(4):1047–60.
41. Borbely AA, Baumann F, Brandeis D, et al. Sleep deprivation: effect on sleep stages and EEG power density in man. Electroencephalogr Clin Neurophysiol 1981;51(5):483–95.
42. Brunner DP, Dijk DJ, Tobler I, et al. Effect of partial sleep deprivation on sleep stages and EEG power spectra: evidence for non-REM and REM sleep homeostasis. Electroencephalogr Clin Neurophysiol 1990;75(6):492–9.
43. Dijk DJ, Brunner DP, Beersma DG, et al. Electroencephalogram power density and slow wave sleep as a function of prior waking and circadian phase. Sleep 1990;13(5):430–40.
44. Dijk DJ, Czeisler CA. Contribution of the circadian pacemaker and the sleep homeostat to sleep propensity, sleep structure, electroencephalographic slow waves, and sleep spindle activity in humans. J Neurosci 1995;15(5 Pt 1):3526–38.
45. Brunner DP, Dijk DJ, Borbély AA. Repeated partial sleep deprivation progressively changes in EEG during sleep and wakefulness. Sleep 1993;16(2):100–13.
46. Porkka-Heiskanen T, Strecker RE, Thakkar M, et al. Adenosine: a mediator of the sleep-inducing effects of prolonged wakefulness. Science 1997;276(5316):1265–8.
47. Strecker RE, Morairty S, Thakkar MM, et al. Adenosinergic modulation of basal forebrain and preoptic/anterior hypothalamic neuronal activity in the control of behavioral state. Behav Brain Res 2000;115(2):183–204.
48. Borbély AA. A two process model of sleep regulation. Hum Neurobiol 1982;1(3):195–204.
49. Wyatt JK, Cajochen C, Ritz-De CA, et al. Low-dose repeated caffeine administration for circadian-phase-dependent performance degradation during extended wakefulness. Sleep 2004;27(3):374–81.
50. Strogatz SH, Kronauer RE, Czeisler CA. Circadian pacemaker interferes with sleep onset at specific times each day: role in insomnia. Am J Physiol 1987;253(1 Pt 2):R172–8.
51. Stepanski EJ, Wyatt JK. Use of sleep hygiene in the treatment of insomnia. Sleep Med Rev 2003;7(3):215–25.
52. Nijhuis JG, Prechtl HF, Martin CB, Jr., et al. Are there behavioural states in the human fetus? Early Hum Dev 1982;6(2):177–95.

53. Curzi-Dascalova L, Figueroa JM, Eiselt M, et al. Sleep state organization in premature infants of less than 35 weeks' gestational age. Pediatr Res 1993;34(5):624–8.

54. Reppert SM, Schwartz WJ. Functional activity of the suprachiasmatic nuclei in the fetal primate. Neurosci Lett 1984;46(2):145–9.

55. Lunshof S, Boer K, Wolf H, et al. Fetal and maternal diurnal rhythms during the third trimester of normal pregnancy: outcomes of computerized analysis of continuous twenty-four-hour fetal heart rate recordings. Am J Obstetr Gynecol 1998;178(2):247–54.

56. Seron-Ferre M, Riffo R, Valenzuela GJ, et al. Twenty-four-hour pattern of cortisol in the human fetus at term. Am J Obsteetr Gynacol 2001;184(6):1278–83.

57. Sumova A, Sladek M, Polidarova L, et al. Circadian system from conception till adulthood. Progress Brain Res 2012;199:83–103.

58. Petersen SA, Anderson ES, Lodemore M, et al. Sleeping position and rectal temperature. Arch Dis Child 1991;66(8):976–9.

59. McGraw K, Hoffmann R, Harker C, et al. The development of circadian rhythms in a human infant. Sleep 1999;22(3):303–10.

60. de Weerth C, Zijl RH, Buitelaar JK. Development of cortisol circadian rhythm in infancy. Early Hum Dev 2003;73(1–2):39–52.

61. Sadeh A. Sleep and melatonin in infants: a preliminary study. Sleep 1997;20(3):185–91.

62. Bagci S, Mueller A, Reinsberg J, et al. Saliva as a valid alternative in monitoring melatonin concentrations in newborn infants. Early Hum Dev 2009;85(9):595–8.

63. Lewy AJ, Sack RL. The dim light melatonin onset as a marker for circadian phase position. Chronobiol Int 1989;6(1):93–102.

64. Giannotti F, Cortesi F, Cerquiglini A, et al. An open-label study of controlled-release melatonin in treatment of sleep disorders in children with autism. J Autism Dev Disord 2006;36(6):741–52.

65. Tordjman S, Anderson GM, Pichard N, et al. Nocturnal excretion of 6-sulphatoxymelatonin in children and adolescents with autistic disorder. Biol Psychiatry 2005;57(2):134–8.

66. Kulman G, Lissoni P, Rovelli F, et al. Evidence of pineal endocrine hypofunction in autistic children. Neuro Endocrinol Lett 2000;21(1):31–4.

67. Zhdanova IV, Wurtman RJ, Wagstaff J. Effects of a low dose of melatonin on sleep in children with Angelman syndrome. J Pediatr Endocrinol Metab 1999;12(1):57–67.

68. Carskadon MA, Vieira C, Acebo C. Association between puberty and delayed phase preference. Sleep 1993;16(3):258–62.

69. Wilkinson RT, Edwards RS, Haines E. Performance following a night of reduced sleep. Psychonom Sci 1966;5(12):471–2.

70. Patrick GTW, Gilbert JA. Studies from the Psychological Laboratory of the University of Iowa. The Psychological Review 1896;3(5):468–83.

71. Gates AI. Diurnal variations in memory and association. University of California Publications in Psychology 1916;1(5):323–44.

72. Johnson MP, Duffy JF, Dijk DJ, et al. Short-term memory, alertness and performance: a reappraisal of their relationship to body temperature. J Sleep Res 1992;1(1):24–9.

73. Cajochen C, Khalsa SB, Wyatt JK, et al. EEG and ocular correlates of circadian melatonin phase and human performance decrements during sleep loss. Am J Physiol 1999;277(3 Pt 2):R640–9.

74. Dijk DJ, Duffy JF, Czeisler CA. Circadian and sleep/wake dependent aspects of subjective alertness and cognitive performance. J Sleep Res 1992;1(2):112–17.

75. Czeisler CA, Dijk DJ, Duffy JF. Entrained phase of the circadian pacemaker serves to stabilize alertness and performance throughout the habitual waking day. In: Ogilvie RD, Harsh JR, editors. Sleep onset: normal and abnormal processes. Washington, D.C.: American Psychological Association; 1994. p. 89–110.

76. Horne JA, Ostberg O. A self-assessment questionnaire to determine morningness-eveningness in human circadian rhythms. Int J Chronobiol 1976;4(2):97–110.

77. Roenneberg T, Wirz-Justice A, Merrow M. Life between clocks: daily temporal patterns of human chronotypes. J Biol Rhythms 2003;18(1):80–90.

78. Werner H, Lebourgeois MK, Geiger A, et al. Assessment of chronotype in four- to eleven-year-old children: reliability and validity of the Children's Chronotype Questionnaire (CCTQ). Chronobiology Internat 2009;26(5):992–1014.

79. Duffy JF, Dijk DJ, Hall EF, et al. Relationship of endogenous circadian melatonin and temperature rhythms to self-reported preference for morning or evening activity in young and older people. J Investig Med 1999;47(3):141–50.

80. Baehr EK, Revelle W, Eastman CI. Individual differences in the phase and amplitude of the human circadian temperature rhythm: with an emphasis on morningness- eveningness. J Sleep Res 2000;9(2):117–27.

81. Duffy JF, Rimmer DW, Czeisler CA. Association of intrinsic circadian period with morningness-eveningness, usual wake time, and circadian phase. Behavioral Neurosci 2001;115(4):895–9.

82. Hellman L, Nakada F, Curti J, et al. Cortisol is secreted episodically by normal man. J Clin Endocrinol Metab 1970;30(4):411–22.

83. Allan JS, Czeisler CA. Persistence of the circadian thyrotropin rhythm under constant conditions and after light-induced shifts of circadian phase. J Clin Endocrinol Metab 1994;79(2):508–12.

84. Sassin JF, Frantz AG, Weitzman ED, et al. Human prolactin: 24-hour pattern with increased release during sleep. Science 1972;177(4055):1205–7.

85. Waldstreicher J, Duffy JF, Brown EN, et al. Gender differences in the temporal organization of proclactin (PRL) secretion: evidence for a sleep-independent circadian rhythm of circulating PRL levels- a clinical research center study. J Clin Endocrinol Metab 1996;81(4):1483–7.

86. Lewy AJ, Wehr TA, Goodwin FK, et al. Light suppresses melatonin secretion in humans. Science 1980;210:1267–9.

87. Muller JE, Stone PH, Turi ZG, et al. Circadian variation in the frequency of onset of acute myocardial infarction. N Engl J Med 1985;313(21):1315–22.

88. Tofler GH, Brezinski D, Schafer AI, et al. Concurrent morning increase in platelet aggregability and the risk of myocardial infarction and sudden cardiac death. N Engl J Med 1987;316(24):1514–18.

89. Brezinski DA, Tofler GH, Muller JE, et al. Morning increase in platelet aggregability. Association with assumption of the upright posture. Circulation 1988;78(1):35–40.

90. Spengler CM, Czeisler CA, Shea SA. An endogenous circadian rhythm of respiratory control in humans. J Physiol 2000;526(Pt 3):683–94.

91. Czeisler CA, Weitzman E, Moore-Ede MC, et al. Human sleep: its duration and organization depend on its circadian phase. Science 1980;210(4475):1264–7.

92. Czeisler CA, Zimmerman JC, Ronda JM, et al. Timing of REM sleep is coupled to the circadian rhythm of body temperature in man. Sleep 1980;2(3):329–46.

93. Weitzman ED, Czeisler CA, Zimmerman JC, et al. Timing of REM and stages 3 + 4 sleep during temporal isolation in man. Sleep 1980;2(4):391–407.

94. Carskadon MA, Dement WC. Distribution of REM sleep on a 90 minute sleep-wake schedule. Sleep 1980;2(3):309–17.

95. Zimmerman JC, Czeisler CA, Laxminarayan S, et al. REM density is dissociated from REM sleep timing during free-running sleep episodes. Sleep 1980;2(4):409–15.

96. Tarokh L, Carskadon MA, Achermann P. Dissipation of sleep pressure is stable across adolescence. Neuroscience 2012;216:167–77.

97. Dollins AB, Zhdanova IV, Wurtman RJ, et al. Effect of inducing nocturnal serum melatonin concentrations in daytime on sleep, mood, body temperature, and performance. Proc Natl Acad Sci USA 1994;91(5):1824–8.

98. Hughes R, Badia P, French J, et al. The effects of exogenous melatonin on body temperature and daytime sleep. J Sleep Res 1994;3(Supp 1):111.

99. Tzischinsky O, Lavie P. Melatonin possesses time-dependent hypnotic effects. Sleep 1994;17(7):638–45.

100. James SP, Mendelson WB, Sack DA, et al. The effect of melatonin on normal sleep. Neuropsychopharmacology 1987;1(1):41–4.

101. James SP, Sack DA, Rosenthal NE, et al. Melatonin administration in insomnia. Neuropsychopharmacology 1990;3(1):19–23.

102. Wyatt JK, Dijk DJ, Ritz-de Cecco A, et al. Sleep-facilitating effect of exogenous melatonin in healthy young men and women is circadian phase dependent. Sleep 2006;29(5):609–18.

103. Shochat T, Luboshitzky R, Lavie P. Nocturnal melatonin onset is phase locked to the primary sleep gate. Am J Physiol 1997;273(1 Pt 2):R364–70.

104. Cajochen C, Krauchi K, Wirz-Justice A. Role of melatonin in the regulation of human circadian rhythms and sleep. J Neuroendocrinol 2003;15(4):432–7.

105. Sack RL, Hughes RJ, Edgar DM, et al. Sleep-promoting effect of melatonin: at what dose, in whom, under what conditions, and by what mechanisms? Sleep 1997;20(10):908–15.

106. Dijk DJ, Cajochen C. Melatonin and the circadian regulation of sleep initiation, consolidation, structure, and the sleep EEG. J Biol Rhythms 1997;12(6):627–35.

Circadian Rhythm Disorders: Diagnosis and Treatment

John H. Herman

INTRODUCTION

Normal sleep quantity and sleep quality at an undesirable hour is the hallmark of a circadian rhythm sleep disorder. Work, school, or family demands dictate normal sleep hours. Circadian rhythm disorders are not disorders of sleep quality; instead, they are disorders in the timing of sleep.

Unlike insomnia or obstructive sleep apnea, sleep is normal in circadian rhythm disorders, only its timing is abnormal. Sleep architecture is normal, the distribution of sleep stages is normal, and sleep is normally refreshing. Circadian rhythm disorders are persistent. They emerge as early as when a child begins attending school and as late as adolescence. Before a child attends school, circadian rhythm disorders may be present but might not be problematic. Only with the introduction of a school start-time do these behaviors create a conflict between a child's hours of sleep and school requirements.

In some children, circadian rhythm disorders emerge with the start of a school year after the child slept abnormal hours throughout the summer. We do not know why some children easily transition back to a school sleep schedule and others are locked into the summer's aberrant hours.

The emergence of a circadian rhythm disorder in a child may result from a genetic polymorphism,[1] as a parent frequently suffers from the same symptoms or propensity. Parents perceive their child as sleep-deprived on school days. As a result, they allow the child to sleep as late as he or she wishes on weekends and holidays. Therefore, the child is unable to initiate sleep on Sunday night or awaken Monday for school.

SOME CONSEQUENCES OF CIRCADIAN RHYTHM DISORDERS

Circadian rhythm disorders' major consequences are daytime sleepiness, inattention, combativeness, irritability, and hyperactivity. Children who are sleep-deprived secondary to delayed sleep phase disorder (DSPD) frequently have symptoms similar to attention deficit hyperactivity disorder. DSPD may result in problems with school attendance and school performance. Some children with delayed sleep phase disorder may become school dropouts. A study of adolescents found that those with a tendency towards phase delay have more sleep problems, more daytime sleepiness and more emotional difficulties than do those without morning or evening preference or those with a morning chronotype.[2]

BIOLOGICAL CLOCKS AND CIRCADIAN RHYTHMS

All individuals possess inherent circadian rhythms greater or less than 24 hours, the vast majority longer than 24 hours

(Figure 5-1). The Horne and Ostberg Morningness/Eveningness Questionnaire (MEQ)[3] is a widely used scale that measures an individual's preference to engage in various activities at an early or late hour. It is used to define an individual's chronotype, or 'lark' versus 'owl' preferences. Fourth-grade children are mostly morning chronotypes. By adolescence, the majority are evening chronotypes.[4] Chronotype shifts from preference to a disorder when the individual cannot sleep or wake at desired hours and suffers consequential academic or work-related difficulties.

PREVALENCE

Circadian rhythm disorders appear in approximately 10–18% of children and adolescents. Delayed sleep phase disorder alone effects up to 16% of adolescents but may appear in children as early as the start of school. It appears much less frequently in working adults. About 0.15% of adults, or 3 in 2000, have DSPD. Using the strict International Classification of Sleep Disorders diagnostic criteria, a random study in 1993 of 7700 adults (aged 18–67) in Norway estimated the prevalence of DSPD at 0.17%.[5] Advanced sleep phase disorder children are seen much less frequently. This disorder also appears at the age of starting school. Before school age, waking at an early hour is normal. Normal infants and young children who wake at an early hour will nap during the day. Irregular sleep–wake disorder is extremely rare in children but typically emerges in adolescence. Non-24-hour circadian rhythm is relatively rare and appears in blind individuals, including children.

DIFFERENTIAL DIAGNOSIS OF CIRCADIAN RHYTHM DISORDERS

A careful history is essential to distinguish circadian rhythm disorders from other sleep disorders. The hallmark of circadian rhythm disorders is that when the child is allowed to sleep at his or her desired schedule, sleep is normal and daytime sleepiness rapidly subsides. Children with DSPD have no daytime sleepiness when allowed to sleep late on weekends. Children with sleep onset insomnia differ from children with DSPD as they are unable to sleep late on weekends and sleep is chronically non-restorative. Children with early morning awakening insomnia differ from children with advanced sleep phase disorder (ASPD) as they are unable to initiate sleep at an early hour and as a result are chronically fatigued. Circadian rhythm sleep disorders should also be distinguished from settling disorders, generalized anxiety disorder, mood disorders, ADD/ADHD, restless legs/periodic limb movements, and obstructive sleep apnea syndrome. School avoidance/refusal may be confused with DSPD.

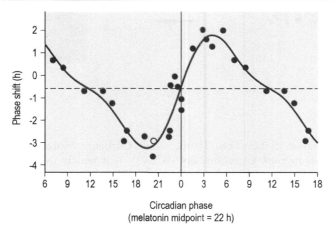

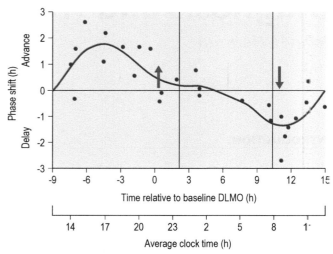

FIGURE 5-1   The PRC to the Bright Light Stimulus Using Melatonin Midpoints as the Circadian Phase Marker. Phase advances (positive values) and delays (negative values) are plotted against the timing of the center of the light exposure relative to the melatonin midpoint on the pre-stimulus CR (defined to be 22 h), with the core body temperature minimum assumed to occur 2 h later at 0 h. Data points from circadian phases 6–18 are double plotted. The filled circles represent data from plasma melatonin, and the open circle represents data from salivary melatonin in subject 18K8 from whom blood samples were not acquired. The solid curve is a dual harmonic function fitted through all of the data points. The horizontal dashed line represents the anticipated 0.54 h average delay drift of the pacemaker between the pre- and post-stimulus phase assessments. (*The figure legend is from the original text.*) Sat Bir S Khalsa, SB, Jewett, ME, Cajochen, C and Czeisler, C, A phase response curve to single bright light pulses in human subjects, J Physiol June 15, 2003 vol. 549 no. 3 945–952.

FIGURE 5-2   The Three Pulse Phase Response Curve (PRC) to 3 mg of Exogenous Melatonin Generated from Subjects Free-Running during an Ultradian LD Cycle. Phase shifts of the DLMO are plotted against the time of administration of the melatonin pill relative to the baseline DLMO (top x-axis). The average baseline DLMO is represented by the upward arrow, the average baseline DLMOff by the downward arrow, and the average assigned baseline sleep times from before the laboratory sessions are enclosed by the vertical lines. Each dot represents the phase shift of an individual subject, calculated by subtracting the phase shift during the placebo session (free-run) from the phase shift during the melatonin session. The curved line illustrates the dual harmonic curve fit. The average clock time axis (bottom x-axis) corresponds to the average baseline sleep times. This PRC can be applied to people with different sleep schedules by moving the average clock time axis until the vertical lines align with the individual's sleep schedule. (*The figure legend is from the original text.*) Burgess, HJ, Revel, VL, and Eastman, CI, A three pulse phase response curve to three milligrams of melatonin in humans, January 15, 2008 The Journal of Physiology, 586, 639–647.

DELAYED SLEEP PHASE DISORDER

In DSPD, the major sleep episode is delayed by one or more hours of the desired bedtime, resulting in significant academic, work, or family issues. In general, children appear to be less tolerant of sleep deprivation than adults and an hour delay in sleep onset may result in pathological symptoms. DSPD is likely much more frequent than ASPD because the cycle length of the biological clock exceeds 24 hours in the overwhelming majority of individuals (Figure 5-2).

Presenting Complaints
- Bedtime struggles or difficulty awakening at the desired time
- Complaint of insomnia at bedtime and/or excessive sleepiness in the morning
- Falling asleep at school or being too sleepy in the morning to participate in normal activities
- Symptoms consistent with behavioral hyperactivity, ADHD, or depression
- The child prefers not to eat breakfast and is hungry at or close to bedtime.

Diagnostic Criteria
The criteria below are similar to those described in the International Classification of Sleep Disorders, revised: diagnostic and coding manual. Diagnosis requires that:
- the sleep pattern is significantly delayed, typically by more than one hour,
- there is an inability to fall asleep at the desired clock time and an inability to awaken spontaneously at the desired time of awakening,

- this sleep pattern has been present for at least 1 month,
- normal quality and quantity sleep are observed when the child can sleep on his or her desired schedule,
- children with DSPD sleep later on weekends and holidays,
- they report less daytime sleepiness on weekends when they awaken spontaneously at a later hour,
- no other sleep or psychiatric disorder is present that could explain the patient's symptoms,
- the delayed phase is not the result of social preference or an overloaded school, social activity, or work schedule.

Coexistence with Psychiatric/Behavioral Symptoms
Attention deficit hyperactivity disorder (ADHD), oppositional symptoms, conduct disorder, aggressive symptoms, and symptoms of depression appear frequently in many but not all children with DSPD.[6] In some instances, DSPD leads to chronic sleep deprivation which may aggravate underlying psychopathological tendencies in a child.[7] When psychiatric symptoms and DSPD are present conjointly, it is important to establish if the psychiatric symptoms are present independent of the DSPD or only occur with it.[8] For example, on weekends or holidays, when the child sleeps until spontaneous awakening, do psychiatric symptoms lessen? If the psychiatric symptoms and DSPD coexist temporarily, it is best to treat the DSPD before addressing the psychiatric symptoms. If the

psychiatric symptoms are present regardless of prior sleep, it is best to treat both the psychiatric symptoms and the DSPD concurrently.

Evaluation

Children with DSPD:

- usually have one parent with DSPD symptoms or 'night owl' preference,
- typically feel their best and best accomplish tasks such as homework at a later hour,
- 'feel best' at or near bedtime,
- encounter academic, emotional, and behavioral problems during morning hours,
- might require a urinary toxicology screen in some adolescents,
- in certain cases should be evaluated for depression, ADHD, school refusal, conduct disorder, oppositional defiant disorder, and anxiety disorders,
- in some cases it is helpful for the family to maintain a diary of bedtime, time of sleep onset, and wake up time for a minimum of two weeks and as long as one month to establish a pattern,
- may give a significantly different description of their sleep habits then do their parents,
- tend to cover windows to black out sunlight,
- watch TV or are in front of computer monitors near or after their desired bedtime.

The Singular Significance of Sunday Night

Sunday night bedtime frequently is the major flash point for school-age children. Many children with DSPD awaken and retire at a considerably later hour on weekends, effectively 'moving' to a more westward time zone. This is also called social jet lag.[9] Parents and child expect to return to a weekday schedule Sunday night (or move east) and the child finds it impossible.

In adolescents, failure to cooperate with a plan to reschedule their sleep may be a sign of clinical depression or oppositional defiant symptoms. Adolescence is a particularly vulnerable life stage for the development of this syndrome: in some children, the concept of adolescence with its increased autonomy and noncompliance becomes synonymous with delayed sleep phase disorder.

Treatment of DSPD
Treatment of DSPD with Optimally Timed Light Exposure

There is a phase response curve to bright light (Figure 5-1) describing the amplitude or phase advance or delay when an individual is exposed to bright light at various times. Light advances or delays circadian rhythms in humans more than any other zeitgeber.

Light exposure at dawn signals to the brain that awakening has occurred too late. It resets the suprachiasmatic nuclei to advance gene expression to an earlier hour. Consequently, light exposure at the time of awakening is a powerful tool in shifting the circadian rhythm to an earlier hour, resulting in an individual becoming sleepy earlier. This is a phase advance.

Light exposure close to bedtime shifts the circadian rhythm later, causing the individual to initiate sleep later and wake up later. This is a phase delay. Both are discussed below as a treatment for DSPS and ASPD.

Light Switches from Causing a Phase Delay to Causing a Phase Advance during Sleep

Light exposure during the first half of an individual's normal sleeping hours likewise has a phase-delaying effect. Light exposure during the individual's last two or three normal sleeping hours has a phase-advancing effect. The nadir of core body temperature, or the minimum temperature in the circadian cycle, typically occurs about two-thirds of the way through the sleep cycle. A child who begins sleep at 9:00 p.m. and spontaneously awakens at 7:00 a.m. on weekends typically has a temperature minimum approximately 3–4:00 a.m.

A child with DSPD who begins sleep at 3:00 a.m. on weekends and awakens at 1:00 p.m. will have a temperature minimum about 9–10:00 a.m. Light administered *before* the minimum causes a *phase delay*, or results in sleep occurring later, and light administered *after* the minimum causes a *phase advance*, or results in sleep occurring earlier (Figure 5-3).

The timing of the temperature nadir is established by a careful history of when the child or adolescent prefers to begin sleep and to awaken. This sometimes requires a sleep diary or actigraphy for a week. In children or adolescents with phase delay, it is best to expose them to sunlight, bright light, or blue light about the time they normally awaken and prevent them from being exposed to morning light before their estimated temperature minimum. A child who awakens at noon weekends should wear sunglasses after sunrise to the estimated time of their temperature minimum on school days.

Between the vernal and autumnal equinoxes, when day is longer than night, morning sunlight alone is extremely helpful in advancing phase. As soon as a child awakens, have him or her play in sunlight, preferably outdoors, but possibly indoors, in an area illuminated by sunlight. It also has a mood-elevating and antidepressant effect, as morning exposure to bright light boxes is a recognized treatment for seasonal affective disorder (SAD) and other mild depressive disorders.[10]

Blue Light Therapy

Rods and cones were the only known photoreceptors that transduce light into a neural signal until the recent discovery of a third retinal photoreceptor called melanopsin.[11] Neural signals from melanopsin-containing cells are transmitted from the retina to the suprachiasmatic nucleus (SCN). These cells are most sensitive to light of a blue wavelength.[12]

Bright light boxes have been replaced to a great extent by iPad-sized, blue, LED boxes. These are lightweight, run on rechargeable batteries, and are sufficiently portable to fit in a purse or compact briefcase. They have demonstrated efficacy in a number of studies.[13] The patient uses blue light or daylight exposure for 20 minutes to an hour soon after wake-up and avoids bright light after approximately 5–6:00 p.m. as much as possible.[14] The light of dawn is extremely important in entraining circadian rhythms,[15] in children as well as adults.[16] Phase shifting with blue or white light is more effective when it is associated with active play or exercise (a running wheel in rats[17]).

Treatment of DSPD with Optimally Timed Melatonin Administration

Melatonin is a greatly misunderstood compound. Many believe it is a sedative hypnotic. Although it has sedating effects in a minority of individuals (approximately 20%), it has no sedating effect in most. In population-based studies, melatonin does not

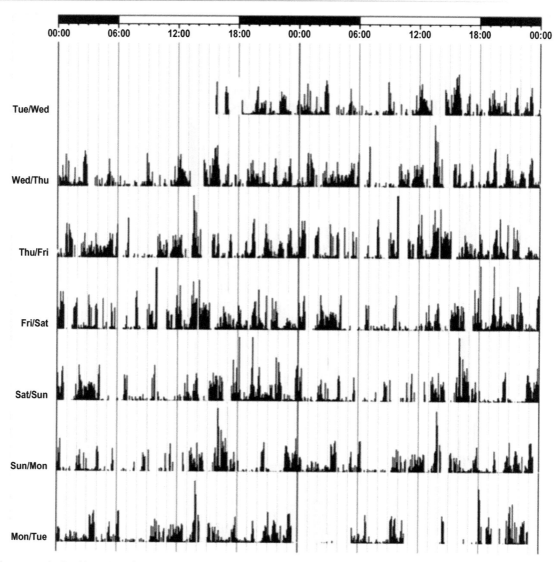

FIGURE 5-3 Actogram obtained by actigraphy over a 7-day period from an older adult patient who has ISWRD. The yellow bars indicate timing and level of ambient light exposure, and the black bars indicate activity levels recorded at the non-dominant wrist. Note the lack of a discernible circadian sleep–wake rhythm. Sleep is characterized by nocturnal fragmentation and multiple short periods of sleeping and waking across the entire 24-hour day. (*Legend from original text.*) *Zee PC, Vitiello MV. Circadian Rhythm Sleep Disorder: Irregular Sleep Wake Rhythm Type. Sleep Med Clin. 2009 Jun 1;4(2):213–218.*

have sedative hypnotic effects.[18] It is more accurately regarded as a chronobiotic or a chemical agent that advances or delays circadian rhythms.[19] In fact, it is the only non-prescription substance with demonstrated phase shifting properties.

The pineal gland secretes approximately 300 picograms of melatonin each night or 0.3 milligrams.[20] Over-the-counter melatonin typically is sold in quantities far exceeding this amount. Melatonin has powerful phase-shifting properties when administered in low doses. Doses exceeding 1 mg remain in blood long enough to cancel their desired effect, as they are present in blood during both the phase advance and phase delay portion of the circadian rhythm.

Melatonin has a relatively small ability to shift circadian rhythms when the pineal normally secretes it, beginning 2 hours before normal sleep onset. It has its most powerful effect in advancing circadian rhythms when administered approximately 4–6 hours before its normal secretion. For an individual with DSPD, who normally initiates sleep at 2:00 a.m., DLMO would occur at approximately midnight. To phase advance such an individual, melatonin would be administered at 6–8:00 p.m.

The Phase Response Curve for Melatonin and Light

The phase response curve describes when either light or melatonin has various degrees of phase-advancing or phase-delaying effects or has no effect at all. Light's maximum phase-advancing effect occurs about the time of normal awakening and its maximal delaying effect occurs around normal bedtime, or later (Figure 5-1). Melatonin's maximal phase-advancing effect occurs approximately 4–6 hours before normal DLMO and its maximal delaying effect occurs about the time of normal awakening (Figure 5-2).

Phase Shifting in a Family Systems Approach

Behavioral issues frequently overlay circadian rhythm disorders. Treatment is most effective if parents understand the basic principles underlying their child's inability to initiate sleep and awaken. Effective treatment of DSPD by a sleep specialist requires that he or she convinces the parents of the nature of the disorder and the necessity of each proposed intervention. Expectations and possible resistance to treatment are best brought into the open and discussed.

If the child is sufficiently mature, he or she should be encouraged to 'own' the problem, or to take responsibility for it. The sleep specialist should offer a list of fun activities for parent and child to enjoy after early awakenings on weekends, such as playing outdoors, going to a neighborhood park, or going out for breakfast. Older children should be encouraged to set their own alarms and wake up on their own as they might soon leave their parent's household, such as when they leave for college.

Sleep Hygiene

Treatment of DSPD should begin with ensuring that optional sleep hygiene is adhered to, or manipulations with light and melatonin might not be effective.

- Expose the child to dim light, or light dim enough to make reading somewhat difficult, for 2 hours preceding bedtime. Dim light permits the expression of melatonin. Normal room illumination, televisions, and computer screens suppress melatonin secretion, interfering with any attempt to help the child initiate sleep earlier.
- Parents should establish a set bedtime that is consistent across weekdays, weekends, and vacations. Every child deserves a bedtime. As much as a child might protest, a set bedtime, similar to a home-cooked meal, is a basic component of good parenting.
- Precede the bedtime with bedtime rituals. Children thrive on rituals and repetition of enjoyable behavioral sequences prepares a child for sleep. These might include reading to the child, quiet games, prayers, or storytelling. Having a set time for bathing and pajamas helps a child prepare for sleep.
- Minimize the child's naps to optimize an earlier bedtime. Naps reduce homeostatic sleep pressure, which is problematic if the child has sleep onset difficulties. If a child with DSPD requires a nap, allow as little sleep as possible.
- For children with DSPD, it is best if they have approximately the same wake-up time 7 days a week. Other children might be able to sleep late on weekends and still fall asleep earlier on Sunday night, but the hallmark of children with DSPD is that they can't. Children with the same wake-up time every morning do better in school[21] and have fewer behavioral and emotional problems.
- Avoid all foods or beverages with caffeine.
- Make sure your child's bedroom is quiet, dark, and comfortable. Darkness and quiet have been coupled with sleep since prehistoric times. There are no published data to support claims that sound machines enhance sleep quality or quantity.
- There should be no screens (phones, computers, video) in any child's bedroom.

Melatonin and Circadian Rhythms

Melatonin onset, when its blood levels rise to exceed 5 picograms/mL, is called dim light melatonin onset (DLMO).

DLMO is the marker of the beginning of biological night and dim light melatonin offset is the end of biological night. The clock hour of DLMO determines if an individual is normal, phase advanced, or phase delayed. The phase response curve to exogenous melatonin shows its phase advance or phase delay properties (Figure 5-2).[22]

In attempting to correct an individual's phase advance or phase delay, the biomarker employed is the shift in DLMO to an earlier or later hour, as measured by saliva melatonin concentration. Advancing DLMO not only advances the time of sleep onset, but also the time of the body's core temperature minimum and the time of dim light melatonin offset, allowing the individual to awaken at an earlier hour. DLMO accurately predicts wake-up time.[23] The phase response curve to melatonin is the opposite of the phase response curve to light. The phase response curve shows a maximal phase advance to melatonin when it is administered 6 hours before DLMO, or 8 hours before sleep onset.

Chronotherapy

Chronotherapy is a behavioral technique in which bedtime is systematically delayed, which follows the natural tendency of human biology.[24] Bedtime is delayed by 3-hour increments each day, establishing a 27-hour day. The procedure is maintained until the desired bedtime is reached (say 10 p.m.), when the normal 24-hour day is then established. This approach is favored by adolescents who are extreme night owls. It is difficult to administer, as a parent typically must be present to oversee unusual sleep and wake-up times, such as noon to 8:00 p.m.

Successful Phase Advance Therapy

The first sign that the light and/or melatonin are having their desired effect is an earlier hour of sleep onset and less struggles with morning awakening. This is followed by the parents reporting the child's morning appetite to be increased.

Maintenance Phase

A strategy must be determined in advance for counteracting the natural tendency of an adolescent to slip back into a later bedtime and awakening hour on weekends. The adolescent should agree that he or she may remain awake late on occasion but must arise and be in sunlight early. Parents need to be vigilant that weekends, school holidays, or summer vacations do not result in a return of phase delay.

ADVANCED SLEEP PHASE DISORDER

Presenting Complaints

Advanced sleep phase disorder is a disorder in which the major sleep episode is advanced in relation to the desired clock time. It results in compelling early sleepiness, an early sleep onset, and an awakening that is earlier than desired.

Diagnostic Criteria

- Inability to stay awake until the desired bedtime or inability to remain asleep until the desired time of awakening. Children or adolescents with ASPD fall asleep doing homework, at social events, immediately after dinner, or before dinner if it is at a late hour.
- There is a phase advance of the major sleep episode in relation to the desired time for sleep. Children with advanced

sleep phase disorder also awaken before the desired time of awakening.
- Symptoms are present for at least 3 months.
- When not required to remain awake until the later bedtime, patients will:
  - have a habitual sleep period that is of normal quality and duration, with a sleep onset earlier than desired,
  - awaken spontaneously earlier than desired,
  - maintain stable entrainment to a 24-hour sleep–wake pattern.

Unlike other sleep maintenance disorders, the early morning awakening occurs after a normal amount of undisturbed sleep. Unlike other causes of excessive sleepiness, daytime school or activities early in the day are not affected by sleepiness. This problem becomes apparent in children and adolescents when social and academic activities stretch into evening hours.

Sleep onset times may be as early as 5–6 p.m. and wake times may be 3 a.m. to 5 a.m. These sleep-onset and wake times occur despite the family's best efforts to delay sleep to later hours.

Attempts to delay sleep onset to a time later than usual may result in embarrassment due to falling asleep during social gatherings. If chronically forced to stay up later for social or vocational reasons, the early awakening aspect of the syndrome could lead to chronic sleep deprivation and daytime sleepiness or napping.

In one subtype of ASPD, called familial ASPD, at least one parent will carry the ASPD gene and exhibit a phenotype similar to the child. As with narcolepsy, the gene and gene product responsible for ASPD have been identified.[25] The genetic mechanism of ASPD has been identified in an extended family, in which it is called familial advanced sleep phase disorder.[26]

Interpersonal Dynamics
The child with ASPD often views his or her symptoms as a positive character attribute. These children are frequently in a good mood following early morning awakening. The child needs to mature sufficiently to allow caretakers to sleep to a later hour when he or she is old enough to be awake alone. ASPD becomes more problematic in middle school or high school. These children ask to go to bed and wish their family would comply with their need for an early bedtime.

Coexistence with Psychiatric/Behavioral Symptoms
Unlike DSPD, which coexists with a host of psychiatric and behavioral disorders, ASPD has not been associated with a psychiatric or behavioral disorder. This must speak to the vastly different genetics of delayed and advanced phases. Advancing the phase of an individual's circadian rhythm is a treatment for some forms of depression, especially seasonal affective disorder. It is possible that advanced sleep phase is *protective* against psychiatric disorders such as depression.

Age of Onset
Symptoms of ASPD appear as early as infancy and become apparent when the infant grows into a child with the same early hour of awakening. It may be problematic with an infant who requires supervision but not so with a child who can entertain him- or herself with a television, books, or other electronic device, such as an iPad.

Epidemiology
It is more likely to appear in children who have one parent or grandparent with ASPD tendencies, which may not be sufficiently severe to be syndromic.

Evaluation
Advanced sleep phase disorder is differentiated from other disorders producing early evening sleepiness, such as obstructive sleep apnea, disrupted nocturnal sleep, chronic sleep deprivation, or narcolepsy. Like DSPD patients, ASPD patients have no intrinsic sleep abnormalities; they report that sleep itself is restful and restorative.

Treatment
Advanced sleep phase disorder is treated with light or melatonin. Use either a bright light box emitting white light or a blue light panel. Greatest efficacy for creating a phase delaying effect is obtained by exposing the child to the light source at or near bedtime. Outdoor light exposure in months with daylight saving is equally effective to a bright light box.

The phase response curve to melatonin shows that administering melatonin when the child wakes up has the maximal efficacy in achieving a phase delay. If the melatonin has a sedating effect, it might also help the child to return to sleep. More than 1 milligram will reduce efficacy.

The child with ASPD should be kept out of bright light as much as possible before noon. Dark shades on windows may be necessary. Children with ASPD should wear sunglasses with blue-light-blocking properties riding in the car to school in the morning. Begin exposing the child with ASPD to bright light in the afternoon and continue until bedtime.

IRREGULAR SLEEP–WAKE RHYTHM DISORDER

Irregular sleep–wake rhythm disorder (ISWRD) differs from other circadian rhythm disorders in that it appears to be the result of an impaired circadian pacemaker, as opposed to a normal pacemaker out of phase or not entrained.

Presenting Complaints
Contrary to normal circadian rhythms in which individuals have one main sleeping period and one main period of wakefulness during a typical 24-hour stretch, individuals with irregular sleep–wake rhythms have more than one sleep and wake episode during a typical 24-hour day. Sleep might occur in several blocks somewhat randomly during the 24-hour period, and none might be long enough to be considered the major sleep period (Figure 5-3).

This sleeping pattern is normal in newborn infants who sleep about 12 hours broken up into chunks spread around the clock. This pattern is uncommon by 6 months of age by which time most infants have a major sleep period at night and one or more naps during the day.

Unlike DSPD or ASPD, individuals with ISWRD are extremely impaired and unable to engage in most normal activities such as normal school and work at a normal hour. The unpredictable timing of sleep episodes can have a crippling effect.

Diagnostic Criteria

Irregular sleep–wake rhythm disorder presents with a complaint of insomnia, excessive daytime sleepiness, or both. If the patient keeps a sleep log or is monitored by actigraphy for a week or longer, it shows at least three sleep episodes in most 24-hour periods. Nevertheless, total sleep time per 24 hours is essentially normal (Figure 5-3).

Family Dynamics

The burden on a family to care for a child with IRSWD is that a caretaker needs to be present continually. In such cases, the adolescent experiences insomnia for much of the night, sleeps from 2 to 6:00 a.m., then is awake for several hours before napping for 1–2 hours 2–3 times during the day.

Coexistence with Psychiatric/Behavioral Symptoms

This disorder appears mostly in adults with dementia but may be seen in a child with traumatic brain injury or a psychiatric syndrome.

Age of Onset

Irregular sleep–wake rhythm disorder increases in frequency with age, because it is brought about by medical and psychiatric conditions associated with aging.[27]

Evaluation

There are children who nap for an extended period after school and are then unable to initiate sleep until 2:00 a.m. They arise for school about 6:00 a.m. and exhibit daytime sleepiness until they return home for their extended nap. This is not ISWRD, as it consists of two major sleep episodes at approximately the same time each day. Unlike ISWRD, this two-sleep episode resolves gradually with nap restriction and introduction of an outdoor activity after school.

Treatment

Irregular sleep–wake rhythm disorder is treated with as much bright light and outdoor activity during daylight hours as possible. Total darkness during a window of time beginning at bedtime is recommended. A constant routine of a light–dark schedule 7 days a week is indicated. Melatonin can be given prior to the sleep period to take advantage of its body-temperature-lowering properties.[28,29] A sedative hypnotic might be considered in some patients without co-morbid medical conditions.

NON-24-HOUR SLEEP–WAKE DISORDER

Presenting Complaints

Non-24-hour sleep–wake disorder goes by many names. It is often called free-running or non-entrained circadian rhythm disorder. It occurs when the intrinsic period of the circadian pacemaker 'free-runs' with respect to the 24-h day: typically, the patient has sleep onset 30 minutes to 1.5 hours later each day. Affected children are not able to maintain a stable phase relationship with the 24-h day. Parents initially report that their child's sleep pattern is completely random and has no pattern. A careful history, sleep log over several weeks, and 2 weeks or more of actigraphy reveal a delay in the onset of sleep of 30 minutes to 2 hours each night (Figure 5-4).

When the child's endogenous rhythms are out of phase with the family and school, both insomnia and excessive daytime sleepiness are present. Conversely, when the child's endogenous rhythm is in phase with home and school, symptoms remit. The intervals between symptomatic periods may last several weeks to several months. Non-24-h sleep disorder patients typically sleep 8 hours or longer; approximately two-thirds sleep 9–11 hours.[30] Approximately 50% of blind individuals are unentrained and free-run, most with a phase delay pattern.[31,32] Reviewing the literature, there are about 90 cases described, with 57 being published in one 10-year Japanese study.[22]

Diagnostic Criteria

The ICSD requires a chronic complaint of insomnia, excessive sleepiness or both, based upon a lack of synchronization between the 24-hour clock and the patient's non-24-hour sleep–wake cycle. Diagnosis is established by maintaining a sleep log and/or actigraphy for at least 14 days showing a greater than 24-hour period length for the sleep–wake schedule.

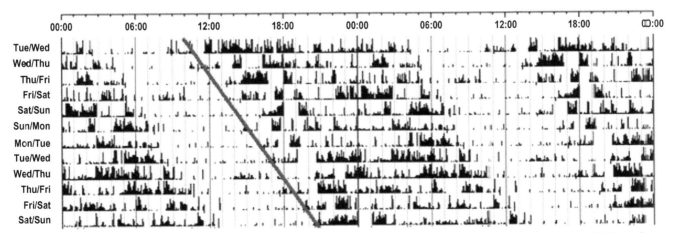

FIGURE 5-4 Illustration of 12 days of actigraphy from a patient with non-24-hour circadian rhythm disorder showing a cumulative delay of 10 hours for a 24.83 hour free-running sleep–wake cycle. Data are double plotted. The patient begins monitoring beginning sleep at about 10 a.m. and ends beginning sleep at 8 p.m. *Barion A, Zee PC, A clinical approach to circadian rhythm sleep disorders, Sleep Medicine, 8, 6, September 2007, Pages 566–577.*

Family Dynamics

This disorder is frequently of great consternation to the patient's family, as the child is unable to attend school or work at a designated hour.

Interpersonal Dynamics

Individuals with this disorder frequently lack normal social relationships[22] and do not attend school or work a normal job. In the above study of 57 individuals carefully diagnosed with non-24-hour CR disorder, 56 did not attend school or work normal hours.[22]

Coexistence with Psychiatric/Behavioral Symptoms

There are about 15 published single-case reports and two published series of cases of non-24 CRD for a total of about 90 patients. About 25–30% have a pre-existing psychiatric disorder, the most frequent being social adjustment disorder and major depressive disorder. The non-24 CRD emerges concurrently with the emergence of the psychiatric symptoms.

Age of Onset

Symptoms emerge in the second decade of life in the majority of cases. In only one of the 90 cases did the disorder emerge before age 10 and the remainder became symptomatic as adults. A sizeable proportion of the non-24-hour CR disorder patients had pre-existing delayed sleep phase disorder, suggesting a genetic link between these two disorders.

Evaluation

Diagnosis is established by a 2-week or longer diary completed daily and by concurrent actigraphy. When plotting the 24-hour logs.

Treatment

Melatonin administration has been reported to improve the timing of sleep in non-24-hour sleep–wake disorder, especially in the blind. Begin at 3 mg 1 h before the desired hour of sleep onset. Once a patient is entrained, melatonin may be lowered to 0.5 mg.[24] The patient should be in as much light and as active as possible during the intended wake period and in conditions of dark, quiet, and bed rest during the intended sleep period. In non-blind individuals, exposure to the light of dawn or a bright light box at the time of dawn may be essential to maintain entrainment.

CONCLUSION

Circadian rhythm disorders are fairly common in children and frequently masquerade as other sleep disorders, most notably insomnia and daytime sleepiness. Many children have been evaluated extensively from a medical perspective before they are referred to a sleep specialist. For the most part, an in-depth interview including the child and caretakers is sufficient to establish circadian rhythm disorder diagnoses. In many cases, a 1-week to 1-month diary is absolutely essential to make the diagnosis, especially when the family describes the child's sleep as 'chaotic' and not following any pattern. In almost every case, a sleep diary that is collected over a sufficient period of time will reveal an underlying pattern for when sleep occurs.

Frequently a second disorder coexists along with the circadian rhythm disorder, such as depression, an anxiety disorder, obstructive sleep apnea, or RLS/PLMD. In some instances polysomnography is required to establish the severity of a coexisting disorder and it should be treated before the circadian rhythm disorder can be addressed. Treating obstructive sleep apnea first will make it much easier for a child to comply with changing his or her sleep schedule. If a psychiatric disorder coexists with a circadian rhythm disorder, treating the circadian rhythm disorder first may alleviate depression or anxiety. It is known that early morning bright light has an antidepressant effect in some individuals and is the preferred treatment for seasonal affective disorder. Children with phase delay syndrome and anxiety symptoms frequently become most anxious with regard to their inability to initiate sleep. The correction of the delayed sleep phase disorder may exert an anxiolytic effect in such children.

Discussions with children and their families about circadian rhythm disorders are frequently profound, as the sleep disorders specialist is informing the child about symptoms that may continue throughout his or her life and offering treatment strategies for addressing the disorder. It is extremely rewarding when diagnosing and treating a circadian rhythm disorder in a child with only bright light, and sometimes melatonin, results in an enormous improvement in the child's quality of life.

Clinical Pearls

- Circadian rhythm disorders are not sleep disorders: they are normal sleep at an abnormal time.
- Delayed sleep phase disorder (DSPD) is especially prevalent in adolescents, most of whom sleep late weekends.
- Late-night light, including room light, screens, and cell phones, worsens DSPD.
- New blue-light LED small-screens are mobile, a novel treatment for circadian rhythm disorders.
- Melatonin is largely ineffective as a treatment if it is given in the 2 hours before normal bedtime.

References

1. Barclay NL, Eley TC, Mill J, et al. Sleep quality and diurnal preference in a sample of young adults: associations with 5HTTLPR, PER3, and CLOCK 3111. Am J Med Genet B Neuropsychiatr Genet 2011;156B(6): 681–90.
2. Gelbmann G, Kuhn-Natriashvili S, Pazhedath, et al. Morningness: protective factor for sleep-related and emotional problems in childhood and adolescence? Chronobiol Int 2012;29(7):898–910.
3. Horne JA, Ostberg O. Individual differences in human circadian rhythms. Biol Psychol 1977;5(3):179–90.
4. Kanevoshi I, Yukako H, Susumu M. Investigation of the children's version of the morningness-eveningness questionnaire with primary and junior high school pupils in Japan. Percept Mot Skills 1990;71: 1353–4.
5. Schrader H, Bovim G, Sand T. The prevalence of delayed and advanced sleep phase syndromes. J Sleep Res 1993;2(1):51–5.
6. Cardinali DP. The human body circadian: How the biologic clock influences sleep and emotion. Neuroendocrinol Lett 2000;21(1):9–15.
7. Dahl RE, Lewin DS. Pathways to adolescent health sleep regulation and behavior. J Adolesc Health 2002;31(6 Suppl):175–84.
8. Kayumov L, Zhdanova IV, Shapiro CM. Melatonin, sleep, and circadian rhythm disorders. Semin Clin Neuropsychiatry 2000;5(1):44–55.
9. Roenneberg T, Allebrandt KV, Merrow M, et al. Social jetlag and obesity. Curr Biol 2012;22(10):939–43.

10. Niederhofer H, von Klitzing K. Bright light treatment as mono-therapy of non-seasonal depression for 28 adolescents. Int J Psychiatry Clin Pract 2012;16(3):233–7.

11. Provencio I, Jiang G, De Grip WJ, et al. Melanopsin: an opsin in melanophores, brain, and eye. Proc Natl Acad Sci USA 1998;95(1):340–5.

12. Enezi J, Revell V, Brown T, et al. A "melanopic" spectral efficiency function predicts the sensitivity of melanopsin photoreceptors to polychromatic lights. J Biol Rhythms 2011;26(4):314–23.

13. Revell VL, Molina TA, Eastman CI. Human phase response curve to intermittent blue light using a commercially available device. J Physiol 2012. [Epub ahead of print]

14. Lafrance C, Dumont M, Lesperance P, et al. Daytime vigilance after morning bright light exposure in volunteers subjected to sleep restriction. Physiol Behav 1998;63(5):803–10.

15. Danilenko KV, Wirz-Justice A, Krauchi K, et al. The human circadian pacemaker can see by the dawn's early light. J Biol Rhythms 2000;15(5): 437–46.

16. Clodore M, Foret J, Benoit O, et al. Psychophysiological effects of early morning bright light exposure in young adults. Psychoneuroendocrinology 1990;15(3):193–205.

17. Baehr EK, Fogg LF, Eastman CI. Intermittent bright light and exercise to entrain human circadian rhythms to night work. Am J Physiol 1999;277(6 Pt 2):R1598–604.

18. Buscemi N, Vandermeer B, Hooton N, et al. The efficacy and safety of exogenous melatonin for primary sleep disorders. A meta-analysis. J Gen Intern Med 2005;20(12):1151–8.

19. Dawson D, Armstrong SM. Chronobiotics – drugs that shift rhythms. Pharmacol Ther 1996;69(1):15–36.

20. Fourtillan JB, Brisson AM, Fourtillan M, et al. Melatonin secretion occurs at a constant rate in both young and older men and women. Am J Physiol Endocrinol Metab 2001;280(1):E11–22.

21. Kim SJ, Lee YJ, Cho SJ, et al. Relationship between weekend catch-up sleep and poor performance on attention tasks in Korean adolescents. Arch Pediatr Adolesc Med 2011;165(9):806–12.

22. Burgess HJ, Revel VL, Eastman CI. A three pulse phase response curve to three milligrams of melatonin in humans. J Physiol 2008;586: 639–47.

23. Crowley SJ, Acebo C, Fallone G, et al. Estimating dim light melatonin onset (DLMO) phase in adolescents using summer or school-year sleep/wake schedules. Sleep 2006;29(12):1632–41.

24. Czeisler CA, Richardson GS, Coleman RM, et al. Chronotherapy: resetting the circadian clocks of patients with delayed sleep phase insomnia. Sleep 1981;4(1):1–21.

25. Reid KJ, Chang AM, Dubocovich ML, et al. Familial advanced sleep phase disorder. Arch Neurol 2001;58(7):1089–94.

26. Jones CR, Campbell SS, Zone SE, et al. Familial advanced sleep-phase syndrome: A short-period circadian rhythm variant in humans. Nat Med 1999;5(9):1062–5.

27. Zee PC, Vitiello MV. Circadian rhythm sleep disorder: irregular sleep wake rhythm type. Sleep Med Clin 2009;4(2):213–18.

28. Arendt J. Complex effects of melatonin. Therapie 1998;53(5):479–88.

29. Dawson D, Gibbon S, Singh P. The hypothermic effect of melatonin on core body temperature: is more better? J Pineal Res 1996;20(4):192–7.

30. Hayakawa T, Uchiyama M, Kamei Y, et al. Clinical analyses of sighted patients with non–24-hour sleep-wake syndrome: a study of 57 consecutively diagnosed cases. Sleep 2005;28(8):945–52.

31. Sack RL, Brandes R, Kendall AR, et al. Entrainment of free-running circadian rhythms by melatonin in blind people. N Engl J Med 2000; 343:1070–7.

32. Emens J, Lewy AJ, Laurie AL, Songer JB. Rest-activity cycle and melatonin rhythm in blind free-runners have similar periods. J Biol Rhythms 2010;25:381–4.

Sleep during Adolescence

Stephanie J. Crowley, Leila Tarokh, and Mary A. Carskadon

INTRODUCTION

Sleep–wake behavior changes across adolescence are the product of changing intrinsic regulatory sleep mechanisms and an evolving psychosocial milieu.[1] Often, these changing biological processes regulating sleep are in direct conflict with social demands, creating a state of chronically restricted and ill-timed sleep. A description of these sleep–wake patterns begins the chapter. To understand how these patterns emerge, the intrinsic regulatory mechanisms of sleep and wake – the homeostatic sleep system and the circadian timing system – and our current understanding of how they change across adolescent development are reviewed next. The chapter then identifies some of the salient psychosocial factors that likely contribute to adolescent sleep–wake behavior and how they interact with maturational changes in sleep-regulatory processes to modify sleep patterns.

For the purpose of this chapter, adolescence is defined as the second decade of human life. Puberty, the process of sexual maturation and reproductive competence, usually occurs during adolescence, but is not assumed to be synonymous with adolescence. When possible, the distinction is made between these development terms.

SLEEP–WAKE PATTERNS

A hallmark behavioral change of adolescence is the tendency for sleep timing to become later. This delay of sleep patterns has been reported across the globe in pre-industrial and industrial countries.[2] To start, many adolescents report going to bed later as they get older, especially on weekend and vacation nights. Self-reported school-night bedtimes in the US range from about 9:30 p.m. to 11:30 p.m.,[3] and reported bedtimes are as late as midnight or 1:00 a.m. in European and Asian samples.[4] Older adolescents (ages 14–19 years) typically report later bedtimes than their younger peers (ages 11–13 years).[3,4] Wake-up times on school days remain relatively stable or get earlier across these age groups because they are dictated by school start times. The majority of US schools begin before 8:15 a.m., and many start before 7:30 a.m.[5] School-day wake times range from about 6:00 a.m. to 7:00 a.m.,[3,4] with some reports noting a tendency for older adolescent girls to wake earlier than boys.[e.g.,6]

Late bedtimes and early wake times on school nights reduce sleep opportunity time for the average teen. The range of self-reported time in bed is about 6.5 to 8.5 or 9 hours, with older adolescents usually reporting less time in bed than younger adolescents.[4,7] The majority of high-school-aged adolescents (≈14–18 years) report 8 h of sleep or less, and Korean adolescents average closer to 5.5 to 6.5 hours of time in bed on school nights.[8,9] Using actigraphy and self-reported pubertal status in a longitudinal design, Sadeh and colleagues[10] reported that delayed sleep onset and a shortening in sleep duration emerges before the manifestation of secondary sexual characteristics associated with puberty. Later sleep onset and shorter total sleep time also predicted a faster progression of self-rated puberty status. Thus, the onset of puberty in this study was linked to the behavioral sleep changes observed during adolescence.

Despite this decreased time devoted to sleep on school nights, however, laboratory studies reveal that more mature adolescents may 'need' the same amount of sleep, and perhaps more compared to their younger and less mature peers. Carskadon and colleagues[11] studied youngsters aged 10 to 12 years old longitudinally across three consecutive summers. Participants were given 10-hour nocturnal sleep opportunities (10 p.m.–8 a.m.) for 1 week before and then while in the laboratory for three consecutive nights. Polysomnographic (PSG) recordings revealed that the amount of time spent asleep during these 10 hours remained constant across puberty stages (Tanner stages[a] 1 through 5), and averaged 9.2 hours. Furthermore, the mature adolescents were often awakened at the end of the 10-hour sleep opportunity, suggesting that these teenagers may have slept longer if permitted. The disparity between this estimate of sleep 'need' and reported school-night sleep duration suggests that most adolescents, especially older and more mature adolescents, are severely sleep-restricted, and are likely carrying residual sleep pressure during the school week.

It remains unclear whether the sleep loss accumulated over the school week can be 'recovered' on weekends. Many teenagers, however, exhibit behavior similar to a 'behavioral sleep rebound' on weekend nights which may indicate that adolescents try to compensate for insufficient school-week sleep by sleeping more on non-school nights. Weekend time in bed averages about 1 to 1.5 hours more on weekend nights compared to school nights, and this disparity in sleep duration increases with age.[4,13] Indeed, preteens and younger adolescents may show no weekend rebound. Furthermore, a majority of mid to older adolescents typically go to sleep about 1 to 2 hours later on weekends compared to school-nights and extend their sleep by waking 1 to as many as 4 hours later on weekend mornings.[3] Self-reported average bedtime typically ranges from about 10:00 p.m. to as late as 2:00 a.m. on weekend nights, and weekend wake times typically range between 8:30 a.m. and 10 a.m. Standard deviations of an hour or more in some studies suggest that many teens sleep later than this average on weekend mornings. Again, older adolescents report later weekend bedtimes and wake times than their younger adolescent peers, on average.[3,4] Changes to sleep–wake timing on weekends compared to school-nights results in sleep irregularity for many adolescents.

---

[a]*Tanner stage, an index of pubertal development, is based on secondary sexual characteristics, including pubic hair growth and distribution, stage of genital development for boys, and stage of breast development for girls.[12]*

SLEEP–WAKE REGULATION

Borbély[14] was the first to describe a model clearly identifying the interaction between sleep–wake homeostasis and the circadian timing system. In his 'Two-Process Model of Sleep Regulation,' he designated the homeostatic sleep–wake component as Process S and the circadian component as Process C. Since its original description, this model has been refined and variations have been developed,[15–20] and these models now guide our understanding of developmental changes to sleep timing and duration across adolescence.

Homeostatic Sleep–Wake System

A simple way to characterize the homeostatic sleep–wake process is that the 'pressure' to sleep increases the longer an individual is awake and dissipates as the individual sleeps. Physiological correlates of this process have been quantified using the sleep EEG. For example, EEG slow-wave activity, or SWA (power in the 0.75–4.5 Hz range) is a useful marker of 'sleep pressure.' SWA predominates at the beginning of the nocturnal sleep episode when sleep pressure is greatest and shows a decline across the night as sleep pressure dissipates.[14,18,21,22] The SWA decline over the course of the night can be fit with an exponential decaying function, from which the time constant of the decline gives a metric of the rate of dissipation of sleep pressure. If the system is challenged by extending wakefulness, SWA increases during subsequent sleep episodes, and this increase is proportional to the time spent awake.[21] The build-up of SWA is modeled using an exponential increasing function. The specific neuroanatomical and neurochemical factors involved in sleep–wake homeostasis are not fully understood.

Circadian Timing System

In contrast to the homeostatic sleep/wake system, the circadian system does not depend on prior sleep and wake duration, but is rather a self-sustaining system that intrinsically regulates a multitude of 24-hour rhythms, including sleep propensity. The 'master clock' that organizes the timing of these rhythms in mammals has been localized to the suprachiasmatic nuclei (SCN) of the hypothalamus.[23]

Physiological or behavioral outputs of systems regulated by the SCN can be measured over extended periods of time (hours to days), and events associated with these approximate 24-hour rhythms (e.g., when a hormone 'turns on' or 'turns off') are used to infer circadian time or phase. For example, melatonin, a hormone secreted by the human pineal gland, is regulated by the SCN and therefore oscillates with a circadian rhythm. Levels of the hormone are nearly absent during the day, rise in the evening, stay relatively constant during the night, and decline close to habitual wake-up time. The onset of melatonin secretion, also called the dim light[b] melatonin onset (DLMO),[24] is the most common and reliable marker of the human circadian timing system.[25–27] The decline of melatonin, also called the dim light melatonin offset (DLMOff) phase is another phase marker of the circadian timing system derived from the melatonin rhythm (see also Chapter 5).

Circadian rhythms oscillate with an intrinsic period slightly different from 24 hours. In adults, this period ranges from 23.5 to 24.9 hours,[28,29] and one analysis of over 150 adults reported an average period of 24.15 ± 0.2 hours.[28] The majority of people have an endogenous period longer than 24 hours; only an estimated 21% have an intrinsic period of less than 24 hours.[30] Sex[30] and race[29] differences in endogenous period have also been reported in adults. The circadian timing system is capable of entrainment, the process by which the endogenous period is synchronized to the environmental 24-hour day using external time-givers, or *zeitgebers*. The primary entraining stimulus to the system is light and dark,[31,32] and the system shows some sensitivity to short-wavelength ($\approx$460 nm) light.[33,34] A small subset of intrinsically photosensitive retinal ganglion cells (ipRGCs) containing melanopsin and projecting to the SCN have been described in rodents.[35–37] The small percentage of ipRGCs that contain melanopsin are photosensitive,[38] are modulated by synaptic input from rods and cones,[39] and are necessary for circadian entrainment by light.[40] Light–dark cues come from the daily cycles of daylight and darkness and can also be artificially imposed in modern environments by switching an electric light on and off or by drawing a window shade.

One proposed entrainment mechanism ('discrete entrainment'[41]) describes the process as a daily phase shift in response to photic cues that corrects the difference between the endogenous period and the external solar day length. This entrainment mechanism is predicted by a phase response curve (PRC) to light. Light PRCs are experimentally derived and describe how light shifts circadian rhythms to an earlier or later time when light is presented at various times across the circadian cycle. In general, the human system responds in a systematic and predictable manner: light just before habitual bedtime or in the first half of habitual sleep shifts circadian rhythms later (phase delay), while light during the second half of habitual sleep or just after waking shifts circadian rhythms earlier (phase advance).[42–47] According to these general properties of the adult light PRC, morning light exposure facilitates entrainment in those with an intrinsic period greater than 24 hours, whereas evening light exposure entrains individuals with a period shorter than 24 hours. In adults, endogenous circadian period also predicts differences in how the system aligns to sleep,[48] and those with a long period have a later entrained phase (clock time) than those with a short period.[49]

Two-Process Model of Sleep Regulation

Figure 6-1 is a schematic representation of how Process S and Process C may interact as opponent processes, and is based on the models proposed by others.[19,20,50] The broad concept of 'sleep pressure' is on the y-axis as a function of time on the x-axis. Sleep pressure varies across the 24-hour day (Process C, red line), and also depends on the amount of time awake and asleep (Process S, blue line). In this schematic example, sleep occurs from 10 p.m. to 7 a.m. The onset of melatonin production (DLMO phase) usually occurs before habitual bedtime and is illustrated by the upward-facing arrow at 9 p.m. Process S is anchored to the onset of sleep and the onset of wake. The homeostatically driven pressure to sleep decreases as sleep progresses across a night of sleep and increases with hours of wakefulness across the day. Sleep pressure dictated by the circadian timing system is greatest about 7 hours after DLMO phase, near the end of habitual sleep and is lowest just before DLMO phase near to habitual bedtime. According

---

[b]*Melatonin synthesis is blocked by light; hence, measures are taken in the presence of a dimly lit environment.*

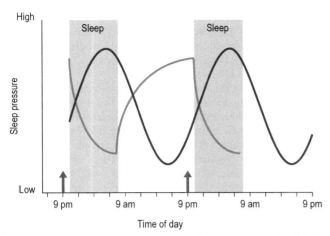

FIGURE 6-1 A schematic representation of the Two Process Model of Sleep Regulation. The broad concept of 'sleep pressure' is illustrated on the y-axis as a function of time spanning over 2 days. An ideal sleep duration of 9 hours per night from 10 p.m. to 7 a.m. is illustrated by shaded gray rectangles. The upward-facing arrow at 9 p.m. illustrates the time of melatonin onset (DLMO phase), which usually occurs 1 to 2 hours before bedtime. Process C (red curve) shows sleep pressure changing with a cycle length of 24 hours. The pressure to sleep is highest approximately 7 hours after DLMO phase and sleep pressure is lowest just before DLMO phase, and thus just before bedtime. Process S is illustrated by the blue curve, and is dependent on the timing and duration of sleep and wake. At sleep onset, sleep pressure is highest and dissipates over the course of sleep, whereas sleep pressure is lowest at the beginning of the waking day and accumulates over the course of wakefulness. Ideally, these two processes interact with one another to maintain sleep at night and maintain alertness during the day (see text). *This figure was published in S.J. Crowley, C.N. Kyriakos, and A.R. Wolfson. Sleep Patterns and Challenges. In: Encyclopedia of Adolescence. B.B. Brown and M. Prinstein (eds.). Copyright Elsevier (2011).*

to this two-process model, the alerting signal of the circadian process opposes a wake-dependent sleep-promoting process to maintain wakefulness across the day.[19] Similarly, homeostatic sleep pressure dissipating across a night of sleep is countered by the circadian timing system as it reaches its maximal levels of sleep propensity during the second half of the habitual sleep period, thus maintaining or 'protecting' the second half of nocturnal sleep.[20] Theoretically, the alignment of these two processes predicts maintenance of wakefulness and alertness during the daytime and maintenance of sleep at night. This ideal balance between the systems is challenged during adolescence as both processes show developmental changes and as behavioral demands and choices alter the balance.

CHANGES TO SLEEP–WAKE REGULATION ACROSS ADOLESCENCE

Puberty, or the process of sexual maturation and reproductive competence, usually occurs during adolescence and is initiated with a re-activation of the hypothalamic–pituitary–gonadal axis after a dormant period during childhood. The brain also undergoes major structural reorganization during this time. One of the most prominent structural changes during development is a sharp decline of cortical synapses ('pruning') in the second decade of life. This change is further illustrated by cortical gray matter volume declining throughout the teen years. These changes to brain structure influence sleep physiology.

One of the most readily observed and striking changes to the sleep EEG is a progressive developmental decline in the amplitude of the signal across adolescence. This decline typically begins around ages 9 or 10 and continues until the early 20s, though the precise timing of the beginning and termination of this decline varies across individuals and is debated.[51,52] This decline likely reflects the pruning of synapses that occurs in the healthy adolescent cortex[53,54] and is not state-specific. As a result, EEG power is diminished during waking[55–57] and sleep.[58–63]

One sleep-specific change to the EEG is a redistribution of sleep-stage variables. Minutes of slow-wave sleep (SWS; sleep characterized by high-amplitude, low-frequency waves) declines by approximately 40%.[60,61,64–67] At the same time, an approximate 20% increase in stage 2 sleep is observed in both longitudinal[60] and cross-sectional[61] samples. Whether these changes are also a reflection of adolescent cortical restructuring or are of functional significance to sleep-dependent processes remains unknown. Finally, young adolescents tend to 'skip' their first REM episode.[60,66] The 'skipped REM' episodes are characterized by the emergence from 'deep' sleep stages 3 and 4 (SWS) into 'lighter' stages such as stages 1 and 2 for a duration of at least 12 minutes.[61] In adults, 'skipped REM' episodes often accompany sleep deprivation protocols; therefore, some have speculated that the skipped REM episodes in young individuals may reflect increased sleep drive observed in younger individuals.[68]

The dynamics of the homeostatic system are also altered during puberty, though not involving the dissipation of Process S with sleep. One cross-sectional and two longitudinal studies which modeled the dissipation of sleep pressure across nights of sleep found that the time constant of the decay does not change across adolescent development.[69–71] This finding lends further support to the notion that the recovery process occurring during sleep, from which some infer sleep 'need,' does not change across adolescent development. One cross-sectional study modeled the build-up of SWA using sleep before and after 36 hours of sleep deprivation and found an increase in the time constant of the build-up in post-pubertal versus pre-pubertal teens.[70] In other words, mature adolescents accumulated sleep pressure at a slower rate across a waking period compared to their younger pre-pubertal peers. Longer sleep onset latency near bedtime in Tanner 5 adolescents compared to Tanner 1 adolescents provides further support for this developmental difference in sleep pressure at the end of the waking day.[72] Figure 6-2 illustrates this relative change across adolescence. Process S of the mature adolescent (blue dashed line) increases across the waking day at a slower rate than the immature, young adolescent (blue solid line), and thus at a 10 p.m. bedtime has not reached the same level of sleep pressure as the immature adolescent. This slower accumulation of sleep pressure is thought to explain, in part, why mature adolescents are able to stay awake longer into the evening or night, whereas younger pre-pubertal adolescents are able to, and often do, fall asleep more rapidly and earlier in the evening.

The circadian timing system is also altered during adolescence. Changes to chronotype – whether an individual is a morning/early type or an evening/late type – provided the first indication of this circadian change. Chronotype can be measured via questionnaires[73–75] that ask what time of day one would choose to engage in different activities, such as when

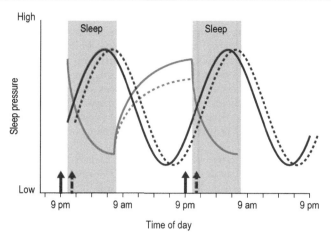

FIGURE 6-2 A Schematic Representation Illustrating the Relative Change to Process C and Process S with Maturation. Illustration symbols are the same as in Figure 6.1. Young, immature adolescents are shown in solid lines and mature, older adolescents are shown in dashed lines. The dissipation of Process S is shown as a solid blue line for both immature and mature adolescents since this recovery process shows little change across adolescence. A delayed Process C and a slower accumulation of Process S are permissive of later sleep times with maturation (see text).

they prefer to wake up, go to bed, take a test, exercise, and so forth. More recently, the midpoint of sleep on weekend or vacation days ('free days') has also been used to assess whether an individual is a late or early chronotype.[76] Carskadon and colleagues[75] noted an association between 'eveningness' and a more mature self-assessed puberty rating. This study was particularly informative because these data were sampled from a group with similar psychosocial contexts (6th grade students), thus reducing the potential impact of social factors driving this association between puberty and time-of-day preference. In a longitudinal study of 14-year-old Brazilian adolescents, Andrade and colleagues[77] reported sleep midpoint on weekend nights delayed in adolescents who matured from one Tanner stage to another, whereas weekend mid-sleep time did not change in those who remained at the same Tanner stage during the study. Others have since confirmed this change across puberty[78] and with age.[79–82] This 'evening' tendency, which appears to be most pronounced during late adolescence (≈20 years),[81] suggests that underlying properties of the adolescent circadian timing system are altered compared to children and adults. Indeed, laboratory studies show that a more mature stage is associated with later onset and offset of melatonin secretion even when sleep (dark) is fixed in young humans.[83,84] Hagenauer and colleagues[85] reviewed similar findings of a circadian phase delay shift from pre- to post-pubertal development in other mammalian species. Pubertal humans and several other non-human mammalian species are also phase-delayed compared to later during adulthood.

Similar to Process S, Process C also undergoes developmental changes that allow mature adolescents to stay awake later into the evening or night compared to younger adolescents. Figure 6-2 shows this relative delay of the circadian system. The dashed red curve and the dashed red arrow representing DLMO phase of the older adolescent is shifted later compared to the young adolescent (red solid curve and red solid

upward-facing arrow). Thus, the time of greatest pressure for sleep dictated by the circadian system in older adolescents is now closer to wake-up time, and the time when the circadian process promotes alertness (low sleep pressure) at the end of the day becomes later into the evening.

Specific factors that contribute to the developmental circadian delay during adolescence are an active area of investigation. One hypothesized mechanism includes a lengthening of the endogenous circadian period during adolescence since a longer intrinsic period length is associated with a later entrained phase in adults.[49] In a preliminary study,[86] average period in 27 adolescents aged 9–15 years was 24.27 h. In this cross-sectional study, the sample size was too small to observe a difference among pubertal groups classified by Tanner stage; however, period measured in this group of adolescents was significantly longer than in a group of adults measured by others.[87,88] Pubertal changes to intrinsic period are also observed in laboratory animals; however, the change appears to be sex-dependent and does not necessarily predict the concomitant change in phase.[89]

An alternative or additional hypothesized mechanism that may explain the adolescent delay in circadian timing is a developmental difference in the phase response to light. Because most humans have an intrinsic circadian period longer than 24 hours, most entrainment occurs with discrete phase advances in response to light occurring shortly after habitual wake-up time. One suggestion is that older adolescents have an attenuated response to this phase-advancing light. Alternatively, adolescents may develop a heightened sensitivity to delaying light in the evening. Either or both of these hypothesized differences in light sensitivity would favor a delayed circadian phase. Preliminary data[90] suggest that light sensitivity measured via melatonin suppression does not differ between pre- to early-pubertal adolescents and mid- to late-pubertal adolescents. The less mature group, however, showed melatonin suppression in response to low light levels (≈15 lux) at a time that would advance the system, whereas the more mature adolescents did not. Two additional studies report older adolescents showing minimal phase advances in response to 2[91] or 6[92] days of short-wavelength light exposure after waking. Collectively, these studies may lend some preliminary support to an attenuated phase advance response to light in more mature adolescents. Preliminary animal data[93] also support the hypothesized exaggerated response to delaying light in juvenile female mice compared to adults. Ongoing studies are testing these hypotheses in humans.

PSYCHOSOCIAL CONTEXT

In addition to the sleep-regulatory changes reviewed above, a number of psychosocial factors evolve as youngsters pass through adolescence. First, parent-set bedtimes become less common.[6,13,94,95] With less restriction over bedtime and greater evening alertness permitted by changes to sleep-regulatory systems, many older adolescents stay awake later to study,[95,96] watch television or play video games,[97] and socialize.[95,98] In recent years, social interactions increasingly occur through use of technology (e.g., text messaging, Facebook®, Twitter®, and so forth).[99] Recent reports indicate that 70–88% of teens living in industrialized countries spend time on social network sites daily,[100–102] and this estimate will likely increase over the coming years. Access to media screens, such as TV, video games, cell phones, and computers contributes to late bedtimes on school nights,[97] and more access to these screens is associated with fewer hours of sleep[13] and more disturbed sleep[103] on school nights. Recent studies indicate that light from media screens in the evening before bedtime may delay the circadian system and increase alertness,[104,105] though further work is needed. If so, such effects likely exacerbate the delayed circadian phase and heightened evening alertness that older adolescents already experience due to altered sleep regulation. Data also indicate that staying awake later on weekends to socialize or engage in other leisure activities and sleeping in on weekends may also exacerbate the already-delayed circadian system of teens.[91]

The combination of these biological and psychosocial factors that favor (and perhaps exacerbate) late bedtimes are in direct conflict with the school schedule, particularly in communities with early school start times. As a consequence, school-night sleep is chronically restricted and many teens wake at an inappropriate time with respect to the circadian timing system. The negative consequences of short and ill-timed sleep are numerous, including sleepiness, depressed mood, immune and metabolic dysfunction, poor school performance, substance use, and driving accidents (see Chapters 5 and 9). Education of school administrators, teachers, parents, and students about adolescent sleep needs remains critical, and targeted sleep interventions are needed to attenuate the risk of such poor outcomes.

Clinical Pearls

- Encourage parents to set a bedtime for their teenager.
- Encourage teens to avoid bright light, bright 'screens,' and other stimulating activities in the evening before bedtime and to seek bright light (sunlight if possible) in the morning.
- Encourage teens to keep a consistent sleep–wake schedule across the week, including on weekends.
- As part of the medical community and a local community, be part of the discussion with school administrators, teachers, parents, and students about adolescent sleep needs and consequences of insufficient sleep in this age group.

ACKNOWLEDGMENTS

We thank the National Institutes of Health for support of our research summarized in this chapter: MH52415, MH01358, MH45945, MH58879, HL71120, MH076969, MH079179, AA13252, and MH078662. We also acknowledge our colleagues, fellows, students, staff, and participants who make important contributions to our research.

References

1. Carskadon MA. Sleep in adolescents: the perfect storm. Pediatr Clin North Am 2011;58(3):637–47.
2. Carskadon MA. Maturation of processes regulating sleep in adolescents. In: Marcus CL, Carroll JL, Donnelly DF, et al, editors. Sleep in children: developmental changes in sleep patterns. 2nd ed. New York, NY: Informa Healthcare USA, Inc.; 2008. p. 95–114.
3. Crowley SJ, Acebo C, Carskadon MA. Sleep, circadian rhythms, and delayed phase in adolescence. Sleep Med 2007;8(6):602–12.
4. Gradisar M, Gardner G, Dohnt H. Recent worldwide sleep patterns and problems during adolescence: a review and meta-analysis of age, region, and sleep. Sleep Med 2011;12(2):110–18.
5. Wolfson AR, Carskadon MA. A survey of factors influencing high school start times. NASSP Bulletin 2005;89(642):47–66.
6. Wolfson AR, Carskadon MA. Sleep schedules and daytime functioning in adolescents. Child Dev 1998;69(4):875–87.
7. Olds T, Blunden S, Petkov J, et al. The relationships between sex, age, geography and time in bed in adolescents: a meta-analysis of data from 23 countries. Sleep Med Rev 2010;14(6):371–8.
8. Yang CK, Kim JK, Patel SR, Lee JH. Age-related changes in sleep/wake patterns among Korean teenagers. Pediatrics 2005;115 (Suppl. 1):250–6.
9. Kim SJ, Lee YJ, Cho SJ, et al. Relationship between weekend catch-up sleep and poor performance on attention tasks in Korean adolescents. Arch Pediatr Adolesc Med 2011;165(9):806–12.
10. Sadeh A, Dahl D, Shahar G, et al. Sleep and the transition to adolescence: a longitudinal study. sleep 2009;32(12):1602–9.
11. Carskadon MA, Harvey K, Duke P, et al. Pubertal changes in daytime sleepiness. Sleep 1980;2(4):453–60.
12. Tanner J. Growth at adolescence. Oxford: Blackwell; 1962.
13. National Sleep Foundation. Sleep in America poll. A National Sleep Foundation Poll www.sleepfoundation.org/. 2006;1–76.
14. Borbely AA. A two process model of sleep regulation. Hum Neurobiol 1982;1:195–204.
15. Achermann P, Dijk DJ, Brunner DP, et al. A model of human sleep homeostasis based on EEG slow-wave activity: quantitative comparison of data and simulations. Brain Res Bull 1993;31(1–2):97–113.
16. Borbely AA, Achermann P. Sleep homeostasis and models of sleep regulation. J Biol Rhythms 1999;14(6):557–68.
17. Borbely AA, Achermann P, Trachsel L, et al. Sleep initiation and initial sleep intensity: interactions of homeostatic and circadian mechanisms. J Biol Rhythms 1989;4(2):149–60.
18. Daan S, Beersma DG, Borbely AA. Timing of human sleep: recovery process gated by a circadian pacemaker. Am J Physio 1984;246(2 Pt 2):R161–83.
19. Edgar DM, Dement WC, Fuller CA. Effect of SCN lesions on sleep in squirrel monkeys: evidence for opponent processes in sleep-wake regulation. J Neurosci 1993;13(3):1065–79.
20. Dijk DJ, Czeisler CA. Contribution of the circadian pacemaker and the sleep homeostat to sleep propensity, sleep structure, electroencephalographic slow waves, and sleep spindle activity in humans. J Neurosci 1995;15(5 Pt 1):3526–38.
21. Borbely AA, Baumann F, Brandeis D, et al. Sleep deprivation: Effect on sleep stages and EEG power density in man. Electroencephalogr Clin Neurophysiol 1981;51:483–93.
22. Dijk DJ, Brunner DP, Beersma DG, et al. Electroencephalogram power density and slow wave sleep as a function of prior waking and circadian phase. Sleep 1990;13(5):430–40.
23. Moore RY. Circadian rhythms: Basic neurobiology and clinical applications. Ann Rev Med 1997;48 253–66.
24. Lewy AJ, Sack RL. The dim light melatonin onset as a marker for circadian phase position. Chronobiol Int 1989;6(1):93–102.
25. Klerman H, St Hilaire MA, Kronauer RE, et al. Analysis method and experimental conditions affect computed circadian phase from melatonin data. PLoS One 2012;7(4):e33836.
26. Klerman EB, Gershengorn HB, Duffy JF, et al. Comparisons of the variability of three markers of the human circadian pacemaker. J Biol Rhythms 2002;17(2):181–93.
27. Benloucif S, Guico MJ, Reid KJ, et al. Stability of circadian phase markers under regular sleep schedules. Sleep 2003;25:A106.
28. Duffy JF, Cain SW, Chang A, et al. Sex difference in the near-24-hour intrinsic period of the human circadian timing system. PNAS 2011;108(supplement 3):15602–8.
29. Eastman CI, Molina TA, Dziepak ME, et al. Blacks (African Americans) have shorter free-running circadian periods than whites (Caucasian Americans). Chronobiol Int 2012;29(8):1072–7.
30. Duffy JF, Wright KP. Entrainment of the human circadian system by light. J Biol Rhythms 2005;20(4):326–38.
31. Aschoff J, Hoffmann K, Pohl H, et al. Re-entrainment of circadian rhythms after phase shifts of the zeitgeber. Chronobiologia 1975;2: 23–78.
32. Czeisler CA, Richardson GS, Zimmerman JC, et al. Entrainment of human circadian rhythms by light-dark cycles: A reassessment. Photochem Photobiol 1981;34:239–47.

33. Brainard GC, Hanifin JP, Greeson JM, et al. Action spectrum for melatonin regulation in humans: evidence for a novel circadian photoreceptor. J Neurosci 2001;21:6405–12.

34. Thapan K, Arendt J, Skene DJ. An action spectrum for melatonin suppression: evidence for a novel non-rod, non-cone photoreceptor system in humans. J Physiol 2001;535:261–7.

35. Hannibal J, Hindersson P, Knudsen SM, et al. The photopigment melanopsin is exclusively present in pituitary adenylate cyclase-activating polypeptide-containing retinal ganglion cells of the retinohypothalamic tract. J Neurosci 2002;22:RC191

36. Provencio I, Rodriguez IR, Jiang G, et al. A novel human opsin in the inner retina. J Neurosci 2000;20(2):600–5.

37. Gooley JJ, Lu J, Chou TC, et al. Melanopsin in cells of origin of the retinohypothalamic tract. Nat Neurosci 2001;4(12):1165.

38. Berson DM, Dunn FA, Takao M. Phototransduction by retinal ganglion cells that set the circadian clock. Science 2002;295(5557):1070–3.

39. Wong KY, Dunn FA, Graham DM, et al. Synaptic influences on rat ganglion-cell photoreceptors. J Physiol 2007;582(Pt 1):279–96.

40. Guler AD, Ecker JL, Lall GS, et al. Melanopsin cells are the principal conduits for rod-cone input to non-image-forming vision. Nature 2008;453(7191):102–5.

41. Moore-Ede MC, Sulzman FM, Fuller CA. The clocks that time us. Physiology of the circadian timing system. Cambridge, London: Harvard University Press; 1982.

42. Minors DS, Waterhouse JM, Wirz-Justice A. A human phase-response curve to light. Neurosci Lett 1991;133:36–40.

43. Revell VL, Eastman CI. How to trick Mother Nature into letting you fly around or stay up all night. J Biol Rhythms 2005;20(4):353–65.

44. Khalsa SBS, Jewett ME, Cajochen C, et al. A phase response curve to single bright light pulses in human subjects. J Physiol 2003;549(3):945–52.

45. Czeisler CA, Kronauer RE, Allan JS, et al. Bright light induction of strong (type 0) resetting of the human circadian pacemaker. Science 1989;244:1328–33.

46. Kripke DF, Elliott JA, Youngstedt SD, et al. Circadian phase response curves to light in older and young women and men. J Circadian Rhythms 2007;5(1):4.

47. Revell VL, Molina TA, Eastman CI. Human phase response curve to intermittent blue light using a commercially available device. J Physiol 2012;590(19):4859–68.

48. Wright KP, Gronfier C, Duffy JF, et al. Intrinsic period and light intensity determine the phase relationship between melatonin and sleep in humans. J Biol Rhythms 2005;20:168–77.

49. Duffy JF, Rimmer DW, Czeisler CA. Association of intrinsic circadian period with morningness-eveningness, usual wake time, and circadian phase. Behavioral Neurosci 2001;115:895–9.

50. Carskadon MA, Acebo C. Regulation of sleepiness in adolescents: Update, insights, and speculation. Sleep 2002;25(6):606–14.

51. Tarokh L, Carskadon MA. EEG delta power decline can begin before age 11: A reply to Campbell and Feinberg. Sleep 2010;33(6):738.

52. Feinberg I, Campbell IG. The onset of the adolescent delta power decline occurs after age 11 years: a comment on Tarokh and Carskadon. Sleep 2010;33(6):737; author reply 8.

53. Feinberg I. Schizophrenia: caused by a fault in programmed synaptic elimination during adolescence? J Psychiatr Res 1982;17(4):319–34.

54. Feinberg I, Thode HC Jr., Chugani HT, et al. Gamma distribution model describes maturational curves for delta wave amplitude, cortical metabolic rate and synaptic density. J Theor Biol 1990;142(2):149–61.

55. Matousek M, Petersen I. Automatic evaluation of EEG background activity by means of age-dependent EEG quotients. Electroencephalogr Clin Neurophysiol 1973;35(6):603–12.

56. Gasser T, Jennen-Steinmetz C, Sroka L, et al. Development of the EEG of school-age children and adolescents. II. Topography. Electroencephalogr Clin Neurophysiol 1988;69(2):100–9.

57. Dustman RE, Shearer DE, Emmerson RY. Life-span changes in EEG spectral amplitude, amplitude variability and mean frequency. Clin Neurophysiol 1999;110(8):1399–409.

58. Campbell IG, Darchia N, Khaw WY, et al. Sleep EEG evidence of sex differences in adolescent brain maturation. Sleep 2005;28(5):637–43.

59. Tarokh L, Van Reen E, Lebourgeois M, et al. Sleep EEG provides evidence that cortical changes persist into late adolescence. Sleep 2011;34(10):1385–93.

60. Tarokh L, Carskadon MA. Developmental changes in the human sleep EEG during early adolescence. Sleep 2010;33(6):801–9.

61. Jenni OG, Carskadon MA. Spectral analysis of the sleep electroencephalogram during adolescence. Sleep 2004;27(4):774–83.

62. Gaudreau H, Carrier J, Montplaisir J. Age-related modifications of NREM sleep EEG: from childhood to middle age. J Sleep Res 2001;10:165–72.

63. Feinberg I, Higgins LM, Khaw WY, et al. The adolescent decline of NREM delta, an indicator of brain maturation, is linked to age and sex but not to pubertal stage. Am J Physiol Regul Integr Comp Physiol 2006;291(6):R1724–9.

64. Williams RL, Karacan I, Hursch CJ, et al. Sleep patterns of pubertal males. Pediatr Res 1972;6(8):643–8.

65. Feinberg I, Koresko RL, Heller N. EEG sleep patterns as a function of normal and pathological aging in man. J Psychiatr Res 1967;5(2):107–44.

66. Carskadon MA. The second decade. In: Guilleminault C, editor. Sleep and waking disorders: indications and techniques. Menlo Park: Addison Wesley; 1982. p. 99–125.

67. Karacan I, Anch M, Thornby JI, et al. Longitudinal sleep patterns during pubertal growth: four-year follow up. Pediatr Res 1975;9(12):842–6.

68. Kupfer DJ, Ulrich RF, Coble PA, et al. Application of automated REM and slow wave sleep analysis:II. Testing the assumptions of the two-process model of sleep regulation in normal and depressed subjects. Psychiatr Res 1984;13:335–43.

69. Tarokh L, Carskadon MA, Achermann P. Dissipation of sleep pressure is stable across adolescence. Neuroscience 2012;216:167–77.

70. Jenni OG, Achermann P, Carskadon MA. Homeostatic sleep regulation in adolescents. Sleep 2005;28(11):1446–54.

71. Campbell IG, Darchia N, Higgins LM, et al. Adolescent changes in homeostatic regulation of EEG activity in the delta and theta frequency bands during NREM sleep. Sleep 2011;34(1):83–91.

72. Taylor DJ, Jenni OG, Acebo C, et al. Sleep tendency during extended wakefulness: insights into adolescent sleep regulation and behavior J Sleep Res 2005;14(3):239–44.

73. Horne JA, Ostberg O. A self-assessment questionnaire to determine morningness-eveningness in human circadian rhythms. Int J Chronobiol 1976;4:97–110.

74. Smith CS, Reilly C, Midkiff K. Evaluation of three circadian rhythm questionnaires with suggestions for an improved measure of morningness. J Appl Psychol 1989;74(5):728–38.

75. Carskadon MA, Vieira C, Acebo C. Association between puberty and delayed phase preference. Sleep 1993;16(3):258–62.

76. Roenneberg T, Wirz-Justice A, Merrow M. Life between clocks: daily temporal patterns of humans chronotypes. J Biol Rhythms 2003;18(1):80–90.

77. Andrade MMM, Menna-Barreto L, Benedito-Silvo AA, et al. Sleep characteristics following change in adolescent maturity status. Sleep Res 1993;22:521.

78. Randler C, Bilger S. Associations among sleep, chronotype, parental monitoring, and pubertal development among German adolescents. J Psychol 2009;143(5):509–20.

79. Giannotti F, Cortesi F, Sebastiani T, et al. Circadian preference, sleep and daytime behaviour in adolescence. J Sleep Res 2002;11(3):191–9.

80. Kim S, Dueker GL, Hasher L, et al. Children's time of day preference: age, gender and ethnic differences. Pers Individ Dif 2002;33(7):1083–90.

81. Roenneberg T, Kuehnle T, Pramstaller PP, et al. A marker for the end of adolescence. Curr Biol 2004;14(24):R1038–9.

82. Roenneberg T, Kuehnle T, Juda M, et al. Epidemiology of the human circadian clock. Sleep Med Rev 2007;11(6):429–38.

83. Carskadon MA, Acebo C, Jenni OG. Regulation of adolescent sleep: Implications for behavior. Ann NY Acad Sci 2004;1021:276–91.

84. Carskadon MA, Acebo C, Richardson GS, et al. An approach to studying circadian rhythms of adolescent humans. J Biol Rhythms 1997;12(3):278–89.

85. Hagenauer MH, Perryman JI, Lee TM, et al. Adolescent changes in the homeostatic and circadian regulation of sleep. Dev Neurosci 2009;31(4):276–84.

86. Carskadon MA, Acebo C. Intrinsic circadian period in adolescents versus adults from forced desynchrony. Sleep 2005;28(Abstract Supplement):A71.

87. Czeisler CA, Duffy JF, Shanahan TL, et al. Stability, precision, and near-24-hour period of the human circadian pacemaker. Science 1999;284:2177–81.

88. Wright KP, Hughes RJ, Kronauer RE, et al. Intrinsic near-24-h pacemaker period determines limits of circadian entrainment to a weak synchronizer in humans. Proc Nat Acad Sci USA 2001;98(24):14027–32.

89. Hagenauer MH, Lee TM. The neuroendocrine control of the circadian system: Adolescent chronotype. Front Neuroendocrinol 2012;33(3): 211–29.

90. Carskadon MA, Acebo C, Arnedt JT. Failure to identify pubertally-mediated melatonin sensitivity to light in adolescents. Sleep 2002;25 (Suppl.):A191.

91. Crowley SJ, Carskadon MA. Modifications to weekend recovery sleep delay circadian phase in older adolescents. Chronobiol Int 2010;27(7): 1469–92.

92. Sharkey KM, Carskadon MA, Figueiro MG, et al. Effects of an advanced sleep schedule and morning short wavelength light exposure on circadian phase in young adults with late sleep schedules. Sleep Med 2011;12(7):685–92.

93. Weinert D, Kompauerova V. Light-induced phase and period reponses of circadian activity rhythms in laboratory mice of different age. Zoology 1998;101:45–52.

94. Carskadon MA. Patterns of sleep and sleepiness in adolescents. Pediatrician 1990;17(1):5–12.

95. Loessl B, Valerius G, Kopasz M, et al. Are adolescents chronically sleep-deprived? An investigation of sleep habits of adolescents in the Southwest of Germany. Child Care Health Dev 2008;34(5):549–56.

96. Carskadon MA. Adolescent sleepiness: increased risk in a high-risk population. Alcohol, Drugs Driving 1989–1990;5/6(4/1):317–28.

97. Van den Bulck J. Television viewing, computer game playing, and Internet use and self-reported time to bed and time out of bed in secondary-school children. Sleep 2004;27(1):101–4.

98. Knutson KL, Lauderdale DS. Sociodemographic and behavioral predictors of bed time and wake time among US adolescents aged 15 to 17 years. J Pediatr 2009;154(3):426–30, e1.

99. Valkenburg PM, Peter J. Online communication among adolescents: an integrated model of its attraction, opportunities, and risks. J Adolesc Health 2011;48(2):121–7.

100. Center on Addiction and Substance Use at Columbia University. National Survey of American Attitudes on Substance Abuse XVI: Teens and Parents. New York, NY: Columbia University, 2011.

101. O'Dea B, Campbell A. Online social networking amongst teens: friend or foe? Stud Health Technol Inform 2011;167:133–8.

102. Dowdell EB, Burgess AW, Flores JR. Original research: online social networking patterns among adolescents, young adults, and sexual offenders. Am J Nurs 2011;111(7):28–36.

103. Munezawa T, Kaneita Y, Osaki Y, et al. The association between use of mobile phones after lights out and sleep disturbances among japanese adolescents: a nationwide cross-sectional survey. Sleep 2011;34(8): 1013–20.

104. Cajochen C, Frey S, Anders D, et al. Evening exposure to a light-emitting diodes (LED)-backlit computer screen affects circadian physiology and cognitive performance. J Appl Physiol 2011;110(5): 1432–8.

105. Chang A, Aeschbach D, Duffy JF, et al. Impact of evening use of light-emitting electronic readers on circadian timing and sleep latency. Sleep 2012;35(Suppl.):A205.

Pharmacology of Sleep

Judith A. Owens

INTRODUCTION

This chapter will cover general principles of medication use for sleep disorders in children with a focus on sedative/hypnotic medications for insomnia in children and adolescents.[1,2] Specific pharmacologic interventions for other sleep disorders (such as narcolepsy or restless legs syndrome) are discussed in those respective chapters. General recommendations will be described first, followed by a discussion of specific features of those sleep medications that have been identified as commonly used in pediatric settings.

It should be noted that – other than for the treatment of enuresis – the only medication currently approved by the US Food and Drug Administration (FDA) for use in treating any sleep disorders in children under 18 years old is chloral hydrate (due to an old indication for its use in treating insomnia in children). In general, empirical data are limited regarding the efficacy, safety, and tolerability of pharmacologic interventions for sleep problems in the pediatric population. Most of the information available regarding use of these medications is taken from adult data or from case reports or small case series in pediatric populations. Only a few published studies have specifically examined the effectiveness of hypnotic/sedative use in children and adolescents in randomized placebo-controlled clinical trials. Despite this lack of evidence, a number of studies, in both the United States and Europe, suggest that prescribing, or recommending over-the-counter (OTC) use of, sedatives or hypnotics for sleep complaints is a relatively common practice among pediatricians, general practitioners, and child psychiatrists.[3] Thus, while empirical data will be included whenever possible, recommendation for the rational use of these medications in clinical practice in this chapter will be largely based on recently developed consensus statements[1,2] rather than on empirically based guidelines.

GENERAL RECOMMENDATIONS

Clinical Considerations
Treatment Strategies
Treatment strategies should always be diagnostically driven and based on systematic evaluation of possible etiologic factors.

Combination of Treatment Modalities
Medication should rarely be the first choice or sole treatment. In almost all cases, medication should be used in combination with non-pharmacologic behavioral management strategies. Although pharmacologic interventions are likely to have a more rapid and potent effect, non-pharmacologic treatments have been shown to result in more sustained improvement (persisting after medication has been discontinued).[4] Combining therapies also helps to minimize side effects.

Sleep Hygiene
When working with children with sleep difficulties, existing unhealthy sleep practices should always be uncovered and addressed, and treatment recommendations must include institution of more appropriate sleep behaviors. Healthy sleep practices, commonly referred to as good *sleep hygiene*, include modifying daytime, bedtime, and within-sleep practices that positively impact wake-to-sleep transitions, for example by decreasing psychophysiological arousal and improving the sleep environment. Specific recommendations are usually made across a wide range of activities and typically include such suggestions as adoption of a nightly pleasant bedtime routine, maintenance of a consistent bedtime and wake time, use of a quiet, dark and cool bedroom, avoidance of caffeinated products, and assurance of appropriate levels of daily physical activity.

Sleep Education
Psycho-education regarding the basics of sleep and sleep regulation is a critical component of responsible medication management. For example, families should understand medication effects in relationship to homeostatic sleep regulation. Thus, they should know that a late-day nap might reduce the sleep drive such that even large doses of medication may be ineffective in facilitating sleep initiation at the desired bedtime. Clinicians can help parents to understand the appropriate role of pharmacotherapy by explaining that sleep is a biological function that is influenced by multiple internal and external facilitating and inhibiting factors and that medication acts to facilitate but does not 'cause' sleep.

Treatment Goals
Clear, well-defined treatment goals must be established with the patient and family. Treatment outcomes should be realistic, clearly defined, and measurable (with goals for example, for sleep onset to be consistently less than 30 minutes, for improvement in mood and attentiveness, and for a decrease in subjective distress about the insomnia in caregiver and patient). Caregiver expectations regarding the potential impact of pharmacotherapy must be explicitly stated and appropriate; hence, the immediate goal of treatment will usually be to *alleviate* or *improve*, rather than to completely *eliminate*, sleep problems.

Exit Strategy
It is important at the outset of treatment to have a defined *exit strategy* regarding expectations of treatment and its duration (ideally less than 1 month). In fact, the duration of therapy should be discussed and clarified with the family at the outset; and, the clinician should begin planning for discontinuation of medication at the time of initiation. In most situations, medications should be used for the shortest possible duration.

Dosing

Dosing should be initiated at the lowest level likely to be effective and increased only as necessary. There should be clearly defined criteria for dose escalation with simultaneous monitoring for side effects. Close communication with the family, including during frequent follow-up visits, is a key component of successful and safe management.

Discontinuation

Abrupt discontinuation of medications – especially ones used on a nightly basis over an extended period of time – should generally be avoided. Drugs should be tapered gradually to reduce the possibility of rebound insomnia, an occurrence that is especially common when treatment is with high doses or with drugs having short or intermediate half-lives.

Dose Modification

Potential modifications in dosage and timing should be reviewed ahead of time with the family. For example, it should be clear if the medication is to be given on a nightly, or on an intermittent as needed basis. If the latter, then the criteria for administering the medication on any given night should be made completely clear (e.g., if still awake after 45 minutes of trying). If middle-of-the-night dosing for night wakings is to be employed, then the specific indications for such usage must be understood (e.g., only if there is at least 4 hours of remaining sleep opportunity).

Hazardous Activities

Patients, especially adolescents, should be cautioned to avoid hazardous activities – such as driving or using power tools – after taking a hypnotic medication.

Non-accidental Overdose

Any hypnotics, particularly those with high toxicity at overdose levels, should be used with extreme caution in patients with a history of depression due to the risk of non-accidental overdose.

Drug Screening

Adolescents should be screened for alcohol and drug use prior to initiation of sleep medication, as many recreational substances may have additive effects when combined with sedatives and hypnotics.

Use in Pregnancy

Because some sleep medications are contraindicated in pregnancy, pregnancy screening should be carefully considered in sexually active girls before initiating therapy, and the importance of contraception use during the course treatment should be discussed. This concern warrants checking for pregnancy in adolescent girls.

Pharmacologic Considerations
Patient and Drug Selection

Selection of patients to be treated should be based on the clinician's judgment of the best possible match between the clinical circumstances (e.g., type of sleep problem and patient characteristics) and the properties of currently available drugs (including onset of action, safety, and tolerability). Medications selected should have pharmacologic characteristics (particularly onset and duration of action) appropriate for the presenting complaint. For children with sleep-onset problems, a shorter-acting medication is generally desirable, whereas longer-acting medications should be considered for sleep maintenance problems. Medications and time of administration should be chosen to minimize morning hangover or persistent grogginess. Usually, this means choosing an agent with the shortest possible half-life.

Timing

Consideration should be given to the timing of drug administration relative to the targeted time of sleep onset (e.g., 'within 30 minutes of lights out'). There should be awareness of the wakeful period that precedes sleep readiness. This is the circadian-mediated period of alertness that occurs in adults and children, (usually) in the evening hours, just before sleep onset during a 1- or 2-hour window in which it becomes difficult or almost impossible to fall asleep. This is the so-called second-wind or wake maintenance zone (see Chapter 4). Most hypnotic medications have their onset of action within 30 minutes of administration and peak within 1–2 hours. Thus, giving the medication too early (e.g., 2 hours before sleep onset) is not only less likely to be effective than dosing closer to bedtime but – when administered during this window of increased circadian alertness – may induce dissociative phenomenon (i.e., disinhibition and hallucinations).[5]

Drug–drug Interaction

Medication should be used with caution when there is a potential for pharmacodynamic drug–drug interaction with concurrent medications (e.g., opiates) or pharmacokinetic drug–drug interaction (e.g., between fluoxetine, a CYP2D6 and -2C19 inhibitor, and diphenhydramine).[6]

Metabolic Considerations

Based on the meager pediatric pharmacokinetic/ pharmacodynamic data that exist for hypnotic drugs, it appears that some medications (such as zolpidem (Ambien®)) are metabolized differently in younger children (see below). These data suggest that children may require higher doses than adults.[7] Additionally, a dose that is not adequate to induce sleep could result in a paradoxical reaction in which the child becomes groggy, and subsequently agitated and disinhibited.[7]

Concurrent use of OTC Agents

Caregivers and patients should be questioned regarding concurrent use of parent- or self-initiated non-prescription sleep medications (Tylenol PM®, melatonin, herbals), as well as other OTC medications. In some cases, OTC sleep medications may interact with other prescription or OTC drugs, or they may exacerbate an underlying medical condition. Some of these medications have similar ingredients (e.g., diphenhydramine is the soporific ingredient in many OTC allergy/cold preparations and sleep aids). Although most complementary alternative therapies (e.g., herbal preparations such as chamomile or synthetic melatonin) are generally viewed by parents as safe, the potential drug–drug interactions between these agents and sedatives, hypnotics, and other medications are largely unknown. Such use should be approached with caution.

Tolerability
Adverse Effects
All medications prescribed for sleep problems should be closely monitored for the emergence of adverse effects. Some medications may even precipitate new, or exacerbate co-existing, sleep-related problems such as sleepwalking and daytime sleepiness. Discontinuation of these agents may also result in increased sleep problems. For example, when REM-suppressing medications are abruptly withdrawn, an increase in nightmares may be seen as a result of a subsequent *rebound* in REM sleep.[8]

Co-existing Sleep Problems
Insomnia in children commonly occurs in conjunction with other primary sleep disorders (e.g., obstructive sleep apnea, restless legs syndrome). Thus, the possibility of simultaneous occurrence of both medically based and behaviorally based sleep disorders warrants attention. In addition, pharmacologic treatment of insomnia could exacerbate the symptoms of co-existing sleep problems. For example, sedative/hypnotics with respiratory depressant properties (such as the benzodiazepines (BZDs)), and medications that may cause significant weight gain (e.g., mirtazapine), should be avoided if the insomnia occurs in the presence of obstructive sleep apnea, and sedating selective serotonin reuptake inhibitors (SSRIs) should be used with caution in the presence of insomnia as they may increase symptoms of restless legs syndrome (RLS).

SPECIFIC MEDICATIONS COMMONLY USED FOR PEDIATRIC INSOMNIA

Summaries of pharmacologic and clinical properties of sedatives/hypnotics frequently used in pediatric clinical settings are presented in Tables 7.1 and 7.2. The following discussion describes drug properties and specific cautions regarding use in the pediatric population. OTC drugs are discussed first; then there follows a description of prescription medications that are currently FDA-approved for treatment of insomnia in adults (BZD receptor agonists, melatonin receptor agonists, low-dose doxepin).[9] Prescription medications commonly used *off-label* for childhood insomnia are discussed below, but the order of presentation should not be interpreted as implying any preference (given that the currently available empirical evidence regarding safety and efficacy of pharmacological insomnia treatment in children is inadequate to rank recommendations). Of the OTC medications discussed, most do not have pediatric dosing listed by the manufacturer, and dosing in clinical practice is often determined by choosing a proportion of the adult dose.

Nonprescription Medications
Antihistamines
Antihistamines – both OTC (e.g., diphenhydramine) and prescription (e.g., hydroxyzine) – are the most commonly prescribed or recommended sedatives in pediatric practice.[3] Because of their widespread use and familiarity, many families and providers view antihistamines an acceptable choice for the treatment of childhood insomnia. Clinical experience suggests that these medications are generally well tolerated in children. First-generation drugs (diphenhydramine, hydroxyzine, chlorpheniramine) cross the blood–brain barrier and bind to H_1 receptors in the central nervous system (CNS).[10]

By contrast, second- and third-generation antihistamines, such as terfenadine and loratadine, are significantly less sedating.[10] Antihistamines are generally rapidly absorbed, and effects on sleep architecture appear to be minimal.[10] Most OTC sleep aids (such as Tylenol PM®) contain diphenhydramine or doxylamine. A double-blind placebo-controlled study in 50 children with diphenhydramine HCL (1 mg/kg) showed significant subjective improvement in sleep latency and night waking.[11] However, a more recent study in 6- to 15-month-old children found that diphenhydramine was no better than placebo in reducing night wakings.[12]

Potential adverse effects of antihistamine usage include anticholinergic effects (e.g., dry mouth, blurred vision, urinary retention), morning hangover with daytime drowsiness, and paradoxical excitation. Tolerance to antihistamines may develop, necessitating increasing doses.

Melatonin
Melatonin is a hormone secreted by the pineal gland that binds to receptors in the suprachiasmatic nucleus in the hypothalamus. Melatonin is a key biomarker of circadian sleep–wake cycles; its release is suppressed by exposure of the retina to light. The goal of treatment with commercially available (synthetic) melatonin is (theoretically) to supplement the endogenous pineal hormone. Depending upon the dose and timing of administration, melatonin has both chronobiotic (i.e., shifting of the circadian sleep–wake cycle) and mild hypnotic (i.e., sedating) effects.[13] Because plasma levels of exogenous melatonin peak within 1 hour of administration, reduction in sleep latency in insomnia appears to be maximal when melatonin is taken in doses of 3–5 mg close to bedtime.[13] However, studies of melatonin in adults with delayed sleep phase disorder have reported that smaller doses (e.g., 0.5 mg) 5–6 hours before the usual time of sleep onset may be of some corrective value in treating sleep onset delay caused by the existence of the phase delay.[14]

In general, there is more empirical support confirming the safety and efficacy of melatonin use than there is for other sedative/hypnotic drugs frequently used in clinical practice in the pediatric population. For example, studies have demonstrated efficacy in reducing sleep-onset latency both in healthy children[15] and in children with ADHD,[16–19] based on the premise that some children with ADHD have a circadian-mediated phase delay (i.e., delayed sleep onset and offset compared to developmental norms). Additional clinical uses for melatonin include in normal children with chronic or acute circadian rhythm disturbances (e.g., delayed sleep phase syndrome, jet lag) and in children with special needs or neurodevelopmental disorders (e.g., blindness, Rett syndrome, autism).[20,21]

Although generally regarded as safe even under conditions of long-term use,[22] potential adverse effects of melatonin include suppression of the hypothalamic–gonadal axis, potentially triggering precocious puberty on discontinuation,[23] and anti-inflammatory effects.[24] Since melatonin is not regulated by the FDA, the commercially available formulations tend to vary in strength and purity; therefore, consideration may be given to use of pharmaceutical-grade melatonin (available on the Internet). Commonly used doses of melatonin are 1 mg in infants, 2.5–3 mg in older children, and 5 mg in adolescents;[25] in children with special need's doses ranging from 0.5 to 10 mg have been reported[26] irrespective of age. As noted above, delay in sleep-onset initiation due to a circadian-based

TABLE 7.1	Pharmacology of Selected Medications Used For Pediatric Insomnia						
DRUG	CLASS	MECHANISM OF ACTION	ELIMINATION HALF-LIFE	METABOLIC PATHWAYS	TIME TO MAX PLASMA CONCENTRATION	DRUG-DRUG INTERACTIONS (PHARMACOKINETIC/ DYNAMIC)	SLEEP ARCHITECTURE EFFECTS
Diphenhydramine (Benadryl®) Brompheniramine Chlorpheniramine Hydroxyzine (Atarax®)	Antihistamines	H₁ subtype receptor agonists. First-generation drugs cross blood–brain barrier	4–6 h 4–6 h 4–6 h 6–24 h	Hepatic	Rapid absorption and onset of action; Peak levels 2–4 h	ETOH and CNS depressants (barbiturates, opiates)	Decrease SOL; may impair sleep quality
Melatonin	Hormone analogue	Main effect is at suprachiasmatic nucleus; weak hypnotic (may have GABA-receptor effects)	30–50 min; returns to baseline levels in 4–8 h Biphasic elimination: 3 min and 45 min 90% excreted in 4 h	Hepatic	30–60 min; (sustained release peak level 4 h)	Largely unknown; NSAIDs, ETOH, caffeine, BZDs may interfere with normal melatonin production	Decrease SOL; main effect on circadian rhythms
Clonazepam (Klonopin®)*	Benzodiazepine receptor agonists (BzDRA): Benzodiazepines	Bind to central GABA (γ-aminobutyric acid) receptors	19–60 h	Hepatic	Rapid absorption; slowed by food 20–60 min	CYP4503A inhibitors (fluoxetine/grapefruit juice) increase levels; ETOH/barbiturates increase CNS depression	Suppress SWS; reduce frequency of nocturnal arousals
Zolpidem (Ambien®/ Ambien CR®)* Zaleplon (Sonata®)* Eszopiclone (Lunesta®)*	Benzodiazepine receptor agonists (BzDRA): nonbenzo- diazepines	BZD-like	2.5–3 h 1 h 5–6 h	CYP450 oxidation; aldehyde oxidation	90 min 60 min 60 min	ETOH, CNS depressants may potentiate effects	Decrease SOL; little effect on sleep architecture
Ramelteon (Rozerem®)*	Synthetic melatonin receptor agonist	Selective affinity MT₁, MT₂ receptors	1–2.6 h	CYP1A2 (CYP3A4/ CYP2A9)	45 min	Avoid use with P1A2 inhibitors (fluvoxamine)	Decrease SOL; no effect on NW
Clonidine (Catapres®) Guanfacine (Tenex®)	α agonists	α adrenergic receptor agonists; (guanfacine more selective) decrease NE release	6–24 h 17 h	50–80% of dose excreted unchanged in urine	Rapid absorption; bioavailability 100%; onset action within 1 h; peak effects 2–4 h		Decrease SOL; reduce REM, SWS
Trazodone (Desyrel®)	Atypical antidepressant	5-HT, serotonin agonist	Biphasic; first T ½ 3–6 h; second T ½ 5–9 h	CYP450/ CYP2D6	30–120 min	Potentiate effects of ETOH, CNS depressants, digoxin, phenytoin, antihypertensives	Decrease SOL, improve sleep continuity, decrease REM, increase SWS

SWS, slow-wave sleep (stage 3–4); SOL, sleep-onset latency; NW, night wakings; BZD, benzodiazepine; NSAID, nonsteroidal anti-inflammatory drug; ETOH, alcohol.
*FDA-approved as hypnotic in adults.

Reprinted by permission of Oxford University Press, USA. From Owens, J. Insomnia in Children and Adolescents. Pediatric Psychopharmacology. 2003;2660.

TABLE 7.2   Clinical Properties of Selected Medications Used for Pediatric Insomnia

DRUG	ADULT DOSING RANGE (MG/DOSE)	FORMULATION	SIDE EFFECTS	DEVELOPMENT TOLERANCE/ WITHDRAWAL EFFECTS	SAFETY PROFILE/ (OVERDOSE)	COMMENTS
Diphenhydramine Brompheniramine Chlorpheniramine Hydroxyzine	25–50 (should not exceed daily dose 300mg) 4 4 25–100 0.6mg/kg (children)	Tablet, capsule, syrup, injectable	Daytime drowsiness, GI (appetite loss, nausea/vomiting, constipation, dry mouth), paradoxical excitation		OD: hallucinations, seizures, excessive stimulation	Weak soporifics; high level parental/ practioner acceptance
Melatonin	2.5–5 (0.3–25)	Tablet; various strengths	Largely unknown; reported hypotension, bradycardia, nausea, headache. Possible exacerbation of co-morbid autoimmune diseases		unknown	Used in children with developmental disabilities, MR, autism, PDD, neurologic impairment, blindness; jet lag
Clonazepam*	0.5–2.0	Tablets	Residual daytime sedation, rebound insomnia on discontinuation, psychomotor/cognitive impairment, anterograde amnesia (dose dependent); impairment in respiratory function	Yes, especially with shorter acting BZD; withdrawal effects include seizures	Marked abuse potential	Also used to control partial arousal parasomnias (night terrors, sleepwalking); use short half-life BZD for sleep onset; longer half-life for sleep maintenance
Zolpidem* Zaleplon*	5–10 5–10	Tablet, oral spray, sublingual tablet	Headache, retrograde amnesia; few residual next-day effects	May develop tolerance/ adaptation with extended use; may develop rebound insomnia on discontinuation	Well-tolerated in adults; OD: CNS depression; hypotension	Little clinical experience in children
Ramelteon*	8	Tablet	Dizziness, nausea; nipple discharge (increased prolactin?)	No withdrawal; low abuse potential; not a controlled substance	Anaphylaxis; abnormal cognitions	Avoid co-administration with fluvoxamine
Clonidine	0.025–0.3 (increase by 0.05 increments)	Tablet, transdermal patch	Dry mouth, bradycardia, hypotension, rebound hypertension on discontinuation		Narrow therapeutic index; OD: bradycardia, decreased consciousness hypotension	Also used in daytime treatment of ADHD
Trazodone	20–50	Tablets	Dizziness, CNS overstimulation. Cardiac arrhythmias, hypotension, priapism		OD: hypotension, cardiac effects	May be used with co-morbid depression

*FDA-approved as hypnotic in adults.

Reprinted by permission of Oxford University Press, USA. From Owens, J. Insomnia in Children and Adolescents. Pediatric Psychopharmacology, 2003;2:660.

phase delay may respond better to a small dose (0.5 mg) 5–6 hours before the desired bedtime.[14]

Herbal Preparations

Most herbal preparations are generally considered safe; however, these products remain largely untested in children. Valerian root, St. John's wort, and *Humulus lupulus* (hops) have some evidence for efficacy in adult and/or pediatric studies.[27,28] Valerian root, which has BZD-like properties, has been shown in several studies in adults to have sleep-promoting effects without the hangover effects seen with the BZDs, although effects may not be seen until after several weeks of treatment.[28] Data on the efficacy of lemon balm, chamomile, and passionflower are limited; chamomile is reported anecdotally to have mild sedating effects. Kava-kava and tryptophan have been associated with significant safety concerns (e.g., hepatotoxicity and eosinophilic myalgia syndrome, respectively).[27,28] Aromatherapy with the volatilized oil of lavender has been reported in several small studies to improve sleep quality in both adults and children.[29,30]

FDA-Approved Prescription Insomnia Drugs
Benzodiazepine Receptor Agonists; Benzodiazepines
Gamma-aminobutyric acid (GABA) is the major inhibitory neurotransmitter in the brain. The hypnotic effect of the BZDs is mediated by their action at GABA type A receptors ($GABA_A$).[31] These medications shorten sleep-onset latency, increase total sleep time (TST), and improve non-REM sleep maintenance; however, most disrupt slow-wave sleep. The BZDs also have muscle-relaxant, anxiolytic, and anticonvulsant properties. The shorter onset of action of some BZDs has led to their use in treating sleep-onset insomnia; agents with a longer duration of action have been more commonly used to address sleep maintenance. However, use of longer-acting BZDs may lead to morning hangover, daytime sleepiness, and compromised daytime functioning. Anterograde amnesia and disinhibition may also occur. In general, this class of medication should only be used for short-term or transient insomnia, or in clinical situations in which their other properties (e.g., anxiolytic) are advantageous. BZDs are occasionally used to treat severe partial arousal parasomnias (e.g., sleep terrors, sleepwalking) in children, with their efficacy possibly related to their slow-wave sleep suppressant effects. There is a risk of habituation or addiction with these medications, as well as withdrawal phenomena, all of which limits their use in children and adolescents.

Nonbenzodiazepine Receptor Agonists
The nonbenzodiazepine receptor agonists (NBzRAs) bind preferentially to $GABA_A$ receptor complexes containing α_1 subunits.[32] Effects on sleep architecture appear minimal, although they may increase slow-wave sleep.[10] There are two short-acting NBzRAs approved for use in adults, zaleplon (Sonata®) and zolpidem. Zaleplon has a very short half-life, making it potentially useful for middle-of-the-night administration (if at least 5 hours remain before the desired wake time), as well as for sleep-onset insomnia.[33] Side effects include dizziness, anterograde amnesia, confusion, and hallucinations. The most common adverse event reported in adults is headaches. Zolpidem has a half-life of 2–3 hours and is available in oral tablets as well oral spray and sublingual formulations; the low-dose sublingual form has recently been approved for middle-of-the-night insomnia in adults. Longer-duration trials in adults suggest continued hypnotic benefit at 6 months without the development of tolerance.

There are several studies that have reported on the use of zolpidem in pediatric patients.[7,34,35] While an open-label dose-escalation study suggested that children may require higher doses compared to adults, a randomized clinical trial in 200 children with ADHD-associated insomnia found that zolpidem doses up to 10 mg were ineffective and were associated with significant adverse events (hallucinations).[7]

Two NBzRAs with longer half-lives are also approved for sleep maintenance as well as sleep initiation insomnia

in adults: zolpidem-CR (Ambien-CR®) and eszopiclone (Lunesta®). Peak drug concentration of eszopiclone occurs at 60 minutes; half-life and clinical effect are approximately 6 hours. Fatty foods tend to delay the absorption. Side effects include unpleasant taste and headache. Abrupt withdrawal with prolonged use (over 2 weeks) may be associated with rebound insomnia. Studies in adults have shown no development of tolerance effects at 6 months, and this medication has been approved for longer-term use.[36]

As noted above, disinhibition with any of the NBzRAs may occur in the period immediately after ingesting the medication, and hallucinations have been reported.[37] Recent reports of rare sleep-related events (sleep-eating, sleep-driving) in adults taking zolpidem[38] have raised additional concerns about its use in children. Although rebound insomnia may occur with either of these compounds, studies in adults suggest non-nightly administration can be effective.[38]

Melatonin Receptor Agonists
Melatonin receptor agonists act selectively at the MT_1 and MT_2 receptors, and have been reported to be potentially useful in the pediatric population.[39] Ramelteon (Rozerem®) is the only drug in this class that has FDA approval for the treatment of insomnia in adults; it does not appear to have abuse potential and is not a scheduled drug. The sleep-promoting effect of ramelteon is postulated to be related both to a circadian-advancing effect and to reduction of the circadian-based surge in alertness level (wake maintenance zone) just prior to sleep onset.[40] While it has shown moderate efficacy in clinical trials in reducing sleep-onset latency, subjective improvements in sleep-onset latency are typically less consistently reported than are objective ones (i.e., those that are polysomnographically determined).[40] Side effects include dizziness and fatigue; co-administration with fluvoxamine should be avoided.

Low-dose Doxepin
The antidepressant doxepin (Silenor®) acts as a selective histamine receptor antagonist in low doses. It has a long half-life and was approved for sleep maintenance insomnia in adults in 2010. It appears to have no abuse potential and is not a scheduled drug

Off-label Insomnia Drugs Used in Pediatrics
Alpha Agonists
Central α_2 agonists, which decrease adrenergic tone, are used to treat both symptoms of attention deficit hyperactivity disorder during the day and ADHD-associated sleep-onset delay at bedtime in children.[41] Despite their widespread use,[3,42] particularly of clonidine, data regarding safety and efficacy in children are limited. Although several descriptive studies have reported adequate clinical response and a relatively low adverse effect profile,[43] clonidine has a narrow therapeutic index, and there have been reports of overdose with this medication.[44] The drug is rapidly absorbed, with an onset of action within 1 hour and peak effects at 2–4 hours. Tolerance to the sedating effects may develop with sedative effects tending to decrease over time, thus necessitating gradual increases in dose and associated increased potential for adverse effects. In general, the maximum bedtime dose is 0.3 mg; the failure to respond at this level suggests that an alternative hypnotic should be considered. Night awakening may also occur as blood levels drop.

Effects on sleep architecture appear fairly minimal but may include decreases in both REM and slow-wave sleep.[45] Discontinuation can lead to rebound in these sleep stages (thus causing vivid dreams or increased sleepwalking and sleep terrors).[46] Potential adverse effects include hypotension and bradycardia, anticholinergic effects, irritability, and dysphoria. Rebound hypertension may occur on abrupt discontinuation.

Antidepressants

Sedating atypical antidepressants, SSRIs, and tricyclic antidepressants (TCAs) are frequently used in clinical practice to treat insomnia in both adult and pediatric populations.[47,48] Antidepressants most likely mediate sleep promotion by influencing activity of non-GABA sleep–wake regulating neurotransmitters (e.g., histamine, acetylcholine, serotonin).[47] The majority of these antidepressants, especially those with anticholinergic effects, suppress REM and increase latency to REM sleep; thus, abrupt withdrawal may lead to REM rebound and increased nightmares.

Despite their widespread use, especially in mental health settings, overall there is a lack of methodologically rigorous research that supports the use of any of the antidepressants for insomnia in either adults or children. Thus, the use of antidepressants for insomnia should generally be limited to clinical situations in which there are concurrent mood issues, since treating the underlying mood disorder will often result in improvements in sleep, and vice versa. However, it should be kept in mind that if hypersomnia is part of the clinical picture of depression, the use of an antidepressant with sedative effects may further increase daytime sleepiness. Furthermore, the dose of antidepressants for insomnia is typically less than the dose used to treat mood disorders.

Atypical antidepressants that are sedating, such as mirtazapine (Remeron®), nefazodone (Serzone®), and trazodone (Desyrel®), are used in mental health settings to treat both adult and childhood insomnia. Mirtazapine is an α_2-adrenergic, 5-HT antagonist with a high degree of sedation at low doses (e.g., 7.5 mg HS); this may result in residual daytime sleepiness.[49] It has been shown to decrease sleep-onset latency, increase sleep duration, and reduce wake after sleep onset (WASO) in both healthy adults and in those with major depression, with relatively little effect on REM.[50] Nefazodone is a 5-HT antagonist and norepinephrine reuptake inhibitor that is also associated with significant sedation. Trazodone, a 5-HT$_{2A/C}$ antagonist, is one of the most sedating antidepressants and appears to inhibit postsynaptic binding of serotonin and block histamine receptors.[50] Despite its widespread use in psychiatry practice, the empirical evidence supporting the efficacy of trazodone is modest at best and generally limited to clinical trials in adults with psychiatric disorders.[51] Trazodone is an REM suppressant and may increase slow-wave sleep; morning hangover is a common side effect. Trazodone has been associated with hypotension, arrhythmias, and serotonin syndrome; in the 50–150-mg dose range, it has been associated with reports of priapism in adults.[52]

Serotonin antagonists and SSRIs are believed to promote sleep primarily by inhibiting uptake of the wake-promoting neurotransmitter serotonin.[53] These drugs vary widely in their propensity to cause sedation (and better sleep) or activation (with resulting sleep-onset delay and sleep disruption). Use of the more activating SSRIs (e.g., fluoxetine) is often associated with reports of insomnia in adults.[49] Newer-generation SSRI medications, such as citalopram (Celexa®) and escitalopram (Lexapro®), appear to have fewer sleep-disrupting effects and may be useful in the management of insomnia associated with depression. The SSRIs tend to suppress slow-wave sleep; they also suppress REM sleep, often prolong REM latency, and may increase the number of rapid eye movements, resulting in the characteristic polysomnographic finding of so-called *Prozac eyes*.[49] SSRIs may also exacerbate symptoms of restless legs and periodic limb movements.

The TCAs are largely sedating, although they vary in degree. Amitriptyline, doxepin, and trimipramine are the most sedating and are the TCAs most frequently used for insomnia (in adults).[49] Most TCAs are potent REM suppressants, thus rapid withdrawal may lead to REM rebound and increased nightmares. The TCAs also tend to suppress slow-wave sleep and have been used clinically to treat severe partial arousal parasomnias because of these direct effects on delta sleep.[54] Conversely, anecdotal reports suggest that abrupt withdrawal after chronic use may lead to slow-wave sleep rebound and an increase in partial arousal parasomnias (sleepwalking, sleep terrors).[54]

The most commonly reported side effects of tricyclics are anxiety, agitation, and anticholinergic effects (blurred vision, dry mouth, urinary retention, and orthostatic hypotension). TCAs are associated with an increased risk of cardiotoxicity, especially with desipramine and in prepubertal children, and should be used with extreme caution in clinical situations in which there is a risk of accidental or intentional overdose. TCAs may also exacerbate RLS symptoms.

ADDITIONAL MEDICATIONS

Other classes of medications that are not indicated for insomnia but which have been reportedly used in pediatric clinical practice include anticonvulsants (carbamazepine, valproic acid, topiramate, gabapentin), atypical antipsychotics (risperidone, olanzapine, quetiapine), and (at least when taking into account current knowledge) chloral hydrate. Antipsychotics in general interfere with neurotransmitters regulating sleep and wakefulness, including dopamine, norepinephrine, serotonin, acetylcholine, and histamine.[55] *Traditional* antipsychotics (e.g., thioridazine and, to a lesser extent, haloperidol) are often associated with significant daytime somnolence. Newer atypical agents tend to be less sedating, but there is some variability among individual agents (clozapine is more sedating than olanzapine or quetiapine which in turn are more sedating than risperidone). Most antipsychotics decrease sleep-onset latency, increase sleep continuity, and suppress REM sleep (in higher doses). They also may promote sleep by attenuating psychiatric symptoms that interfere with sleep.

In most instances, these medications are being prescribed for alternative indications (e.g., bipolar disorder, mood dysregulation, aggression), and the associated side effect of sedation is used to advantage in an attempt to reduce sleep-onset latency and night wakings. In general, these medications should be used with caution, if at all, for insomnia in children. There are no or limited data on safety and tolerability for this indication in either adults or children. Tolerance to the hypnotic effects may develop, necessitating dose increases. Furthermore, the sedating effects may interfere with daytime functioning and learning. These medications can also have negative effects on coexisting sleep disorders. For example, many of the newer atypical antipsychotics have significant associated weight gain and thus can worsen obstructive sleep apnea.

Anticonvulsants typically cause dose-dependent sedation, although tolerance to this effect may develop.[56] Carbamazepine, phenobarbital, and valproic acid are all associated with increased daytime somnolence; conversely, phenytoin may cause relatively less daytime sleepiness than other anticonvulsants. Newer anticonvulsants have varying degrees of daytime sedation. Gabapentin, which has effects on dopamine, serotonin, and norepinephrine, also appears to increase slow-wave sleep and has been shown to decrease restless legs syndrome symptoms.[57] Direct effects of these medications on sleep are largely unknown. Finally, since 1993, the American Academy of Pediatrics has recommended against the use of chloral hydrate in children except for short-term sedation, because of the risk of hepatotoxicity.[58]

In summary, sedative and hypnotic medications should be used with caution to treat insomnia in children and adolescents, as little empirical data exist regarding safety, efficacy, and tolerability in the pediatric population. Every effort should be made by the clinician to evaluate potential etiologic and exacerbating factors for the insomnia symptoms before prescribing medication, and hypnotics should always be combined with behavioral treatment strategies. Selection of medication, when determined to be appropriate, should be based on pharmacokinetic and pharmacodynamic profiles of the individual drugs and the specific clinical circumstances (such as age, presence of comorbid medical or psychiatric conditions, concomitant medications, and abuse potential). Potential drug–drug interactions and sleep-related effects of medications commonly prescribed in pediatric practice should also be taken into consideration.

Clinical Pearls

- Medication should rarely be the first or sole choice for the treatment of insomnia in children.
- Use of sedative/hypnotic medication in children should always be combined with behavioral interventions and education regarding healthy sleep practices.
- Selection of medication should be based on assessment of relative risks and benefits, type of sleep problem, patient characteristics, and pharmacologic properties of individual agents.
- Clinicians should approach the use of these drugs with caution in pediatric practice (since, in contrast to adults, there are very limited data in children demonstrating safety and efficacy).

References

1. Owens JA, Babcock D, Blumer J, et al. The use of pharmacotherapy in the treatment of pediatric insomnia in primary care: rational approaches. A consensus meeting summary. J Clin Sleep Med 2005;1(1):49–59.
2. Mindell JA, Emslie G, Blumer J, et al. Pharmacologic management of insomnia in children and adolescents: consensus statement. Pediatrics 2006;117(6):e1223–32.
3. Owens JA, Rosen CL, Mindell JA. Medication use in the treatment of pediatric insomnia: results of a survey of community-based pediatricians. Pediatrics 2003;111(5 Pt 1):e628–35.
4. Mindell JA, Kuhn B, Lewin DS, et al. Behavioral treatment of bedtime problems and night wakings in infants and young children. Sleep 2006;29(10):1263–76.
5. Pelayo R, Dubik M. Pediatric sleep pharmacology. Semin in Pediatr Neurol 2008;15:79–90.
6. Lee JY, Lee SY, Oh SJ, et al. Assessment of drug-drug interactions caused by metabolism-dependent cytochrome P450 inhibition. Chem Biol Interact 2012;198(1–3):49–56.
7. Blumer JL, Findling RL, Shih WJ, et al. Controlled clinical trial of zolpidem for the treatment of insomnia associated with attention-deficit/hyperactivity disorder in children 6 to 17 years of age. Pediatrics 2009;123(5):e770–6.
8. Nielsen TA, Paquette T, Solomonova E, et al. REM sleep characteristics of nightmare sufferers before and after REM sleep deprivation. Sleep Med 2010;11(2):172–9.
9. Feren S, Katyal A, Walsh J. Efficacy of hypnotic medications and other medications used for insomnia. Sleep Med Clin 2006;1:387–97.
10. Zisapel N. Drugs for insomnia. Expert Opin Emerg Drugs 2012;17(3):299–317.
11. Russo RM, Gururaj VJ, Allen JE. The effectiveness of diphenhydramine HCI in pediatric sleep disorders. J Clin Pharmacol 1976;16(5–6):284–8.
12. Merenstein D, Diener-West M, Halbower AC, et al. The trial of infant response to diphenhydramine: the TIRED study–a randomized, controlled, patient-oriented trial. Arch Pediatr Adolesc Med 2006;160(7):707–12.
13. Ioachimescu OC, El-Solh AA. Pharmacotherapy of insomnia. Expert Opin Pharmacother 2012;13(9):1243–60.
14. Coogan AN, Thome J. Chronotherapeutics and psychiatry: setting the clock to relieve the symptoms. World J Biol Psychiatry 2011 12(1):40–3.
15. Van Geijlswijk IM, Korzilius HP, Smits MG. The use of exogenous melatonin in delayed sleep phase disorder: a meta-analysis. Sleep 2010;33(12):1605–14.
16. Bendz LM, Scates AC. Melatonin treatment for insomnia in pediatric patients with attention-deficit/hyperactivity disorder. Ann Pharmacother 2010;44(1):185–91.
17. Van der Heijden KB, Smits MG, Van Someren EJ, et al. Prediction of melatonin efficacy by pretreatment dim light melatonin onset in children with idiopathic chronic sleep onset insomnia. J Sleep Res 2005;14(2):187–94.
18. Van der Heijden KB, Smits MG, Van Someren EJ, et al. Effect of melatonin on sleep, behavior, and cognition in ADHD and chronic sleep-onset insomnia. J Am Acad Child Adolesc Psychiatr 2007;46(2):233–41.
19. Weiss MD, Wasdell MB, Bomben MM, et al. Sleep hygiene and melatonin treatment for children and adolescents with ADHD and initial insomnia. J Am Acad Child Adolesc Psychiatr 2006;45(5):509–12.
20. Jan J, Wasdell M, Reiter R, et al. Melatonin therapy of pediatric sleep disorders: recent advances, why it works, who are the candidates, and how to treat. Curr Pediatr Rev 2007;3:214–24.
21. Malow B, Johnson K. Sleep in children with autism spectrum disorders. J Child Neurol 2008;10:350–9.
22. Carr R, Wasdell MB, Hamilton D, et al. Long-term effectiveness outcome of melatonin therapy in children with treatment-resistant circadian rhythm sleep disorders. J Pineal Res 2007;43(4):351–9.
23. Luboshitzky R, Lavi S, Thuma I, et al. Increased nocturnal melatonin secretion in male patients with hypogonadotropic hypogonadism and delayed puberty. J Clin Endocrinol Metab 1995;80(7):2144–8.
24. Mauriz JL, Collado PS, Veneroso C, et al. A review of molecular aspects of melatonin's anti-inflammatory actions: recent insights and new perspectives. J Pineal Res 2012;Epub ahead of print.
25. Sánchez-Barceló EJ, Mediavilla MD, Reiter RJ. Clinical uses of melatonin in pediatrics. Int J Pediatr 2011; Epub ahead of print.
26. Guénolé F, Godbout R, Nicolas A, et al. Melatonin for disordered sleep in individuals with autism spectrum disorders: systematic review and discussion. Sleep Med Rev 2011;15(6):379–87.
27. Gyllenhaal C, Merritt SL, Peterson SD, et al. Efficacy and safety of herbal stimulants and sedatives in sleep disorders. Sleep Med Rev 2000;4(3):229–51.
28. Meolie AL, Rosen C, Kristo D, et al. Oral nonprescription treatment for insomnia: an evaluation of products with limited evidence. J Clin Sleep Med 2005;1(2):173–87.
29. Lewith GT, Godfrey AD, Prescott P. A single-blinded, randomized pilot study evaluating the aroma of Lavandula augustifolia as a treatment for mild insomnia. J Altern Complement Med 2005;11(4):631–7.

30. Hirokawa K, Nishimoto T, Taniguchi T. Effects of lavender aroma on sleep quality in healthy Japanese students. Percept Mot Skills 2012; 111–22.
31. Witek MW, Rojas V, Alonso C, et al. Review of benzodiazepine use in children and adolescents. Psychiatr Q 2005;76(3):283–96.
32. Mohler H, Fritschy JM, Rudolph U. A new benzodiazepine pharmacology. J Pharmacol Exp Ther 2002;300(1):2–8.
33. Zammit GK, Corser B, Doghramji K, et al. Sleep and residual sedation after administration of zaleplon, zolpidem, and placebo during experimental middle-of-the-night awakening. J Clin Sleep Med 2006;2(4): 417–23.
34. Blumer JL, Reed MD, Steinberg F, et al. Potential pharmacokinetic basis for zolpidem dosing in children with sleep difficulties. Clin Pharmacol Ther 2008;83(4):551–8.
35. Colle M, Rosenzweig P, Bianchetti G, et al. Nocturnal profile of growth hormone secretion during sleep induced by zolpidem: a double-blind study in young adults and children. Horm Res 1991;35(1):30–4.
36. Walsh JK, Krystal AD, Amato DA, et al. Nightly treatment of primary insomnia with eszopiclone for six months: effect on sleep, quality of life, and work limitations. Sleep 2007;30(8):959–68.
37. Liskow B, Pikalov A. Zaleplon overdose associated with sleepwalking and complex behavior. J Am Acad Child Adolesc Psychiatr 2004;43(8): 927–8.
38. Zammit G. Comparative tolerability of newer agents for insomnia. Drug Saf 2009;32(9):735–48.
39. Stigler KA, Posey DJ, McDougle CJ. Ramelteon for insomnia in two youths with autistic disorder. J Child Adolesc Psychopharmacol 2006;16(5):631–6.
40. Liu J, Wang LN. Ramelteon in the treatment of chronic insomnia: systematic review and meta-analysis. Int J Clin Pract 2012;66(9):867–73.
41. Prince JB, Wilens TE, Biederman J, et al. Clonidine for sleep disturbances associated with attention-deficit hyperactivity disorder: a systematic chart review of 62 cases. J Am Acad Child Adolesc Psychiatr 1996;35(5):599–605.
42. Owens JA, Rosen CL, Mindell JA, et al. Use of pharmacotherapy for insomnia in child psychiatry practice: A national survey. Sleep Medicine 2010;11(7):692–700.
43. Ingrassia A, Turk J. The use of clonidine for severe and intractable sleep problems in children with neurodevelopmental disorders – a case series. Eur Child Adolesc Psychiatry 2005;14(1):34–40.
44. Kappagoda C, Schell DN, Hanson RM, et al. Clonidine overdose in childhood: implications of increased prescribing. J Paediatr Child Health 1998;34(6):508–12.
45. Danchin N, Genton P, Atlas P, et al. Comparative effects of atenolol and clonidine on polygraphically recorded sleep in hypertensive men: a randomized, double-blind, crossover study. Int J Clin Pharmacol Ther 1995;52–5.
46. Ghanizadeh A. Insomnia, night terror and depression related to clonidine in attention-deficit/hyperactivity disorder. J Clin Psychopharmacol 2008;28(6):725–6.
47. Buysee D, Schweitzer P, Moul D. Clinical pharmacology of other drugs used as hypnotics. In: Kryger M, Roth T, Dement B, editors. Principles and practices of sleep medicine. 4th ed. Philadelphia: Elsevier Saunders; 2005. p. 452–67.
48. Walsh JK, Erman M, Erwin CW, et al. Subjective hypnotic efficacy of trazodone and zolpidem in DSM III-R primary insomnia. Hum Psychopharm Clin 1998;13(3):191–8.
49. Wichniak A, Wierzbicka A, Jernajczyk W. Sleep and antidepressant treatment. Curr Pharm Des 2012; Epub ahead of print.
50. Younus M, Labellarte MJ. Insomnia in children: when are hypnotics indicated? Paediatr Drugs 2002;4(6):391–403.
51. Carrey N, Baath S. Trazodone for sleep in children. Child Adolesc Psychopharmacol News 1996;1:10–11.
52. Mendelson WB. A review of the evidence for the efficacy and safety of trazodone in insomnia. J Clin Psychiatry 2005;66(4):469–76.
53. Satterlee W, Faries D. The effects of fluoxetine on symptoms of insomnia in depressed patients. Psychopharmacol Bull 1995;31:227–37.
54. Kierlin L, Littner MR. Parasomnias and antidepressant therapy: a review of the literature. Front Psychiatry 2011;2:71.
55. Keshavan M, Prasad K, Montrose D, et al. Sleep quality and architecture in quetiapine, risperidone, or never-treated schizophrenia patients. J Clin Psychopharm 2007;27(6):703–5.
56. Bourgeois B. The relationship between sleep and epilepsy in children. Semin Pediatr Neurol 1996;3(1):29–35.
57. Aurora RN, Kristo DA, Bista SR. The treatment of restless legs syndrome and periodic limb movement disorder in adults-an update for 2012: practice parameters with an evidence-based systematic review and meta-analyses: an American Academy of Sleep Medicine Clinical Practice Guideline. Sleep 2012;35(8):1039–62.
58. Hoffman GM, Nowakowski R, Troshynski TJ, et al. Risk reduction in pediatric procedural sedation by application of an American Academy of Pediatrics/American Society of Anesthesiologists process model. Pediatrics 2002;109(2):236–43.

Promoting Healthy Sleep Practices

Darius A. Loghmanee and Jamie A. Cvengros

INTRODUCTION

Of the myriad pediatric sleep disorders children in our society face, inadequate total sleep time provides perhaps the greatest challenge. Families tend to underestimate children's sleep need and lack understanding of the relationship between inadequate sleep and behavioral, health, and neurocognitive problems. Developments in technology have given increasing numbers of stimulation-seeking children access to movies, video games, and social media 24 hours a day, 7 days a week. Advertising and media have normalized consumption of wake-promoting agents such as caffeine, guarana, ginseng, and taurine in the form of energy drinks, increasingly utilized by children and adolescents to fend off sleep in order to have enough time to complete homework assignments, study for tests, or participate in extracurricular activities. Early school start times for adolescents, a population with a physiologic delay in sleep phase, also contributes to insufficient sleep. In this context, the importance of the role of health care providers, parents, and family members in helping children and adolescents recognize the importance of adequate sleep and assisting them as they develop healthy sleep habits comes into focus. This chapter will review guidelines for total sleep need over the lifetime, identify some of the sequelae associated with inadequate total sleep time, and provide an overview of concepts essential to establishing healthy sleep habits, often referred to as good sleep hygiene.

ALLOWING FOR ADEQUATE SLEEP TIME

From a clinical perspective, there is no magic number of hours that a child or adolescent must sleep. The adequacy of the quality and quantity of a child's sleep can be determined based on descriptions of sleep continuity, time spent in bed awake after bedtime, and signs of sleepiness during the day. It is clear, however, that children and adolescents need more sleep than adults, and accommodations must be made to enable children to achieve the amount of sleep they require. These accommodations may include limiting after-school and evening activities to allow for an adequately early bedtime, preparation for the next day (e.g., packing backpack, laying out clothes) to allow for later waketimes, and the establishment of a consistent timeframe for daytime napping. As children grow, new accommodations such as monitoring of nighttime socialization (e.g., talking on telephone, texting, and computer use) or media consumption may also be required to assure that adolescents are able to achieve their ideal total sleep time.

Although it is known that individual sleep requirements can vary significantly, there are reliable guidelines to help establish target total sleep times by age. Sleep need varies throughout the life span with infants sleeping 14–15 hours per day, toddlers sleeping 12–14 hours per day, preschoolers sleeping 11–13 hours, school-aged children sleeping 10–11

hours, and teenagers needing 8.5–9 hours per day.[1] Epidemiological research suggests that children and adolescents are frequently getting less sleep than needed. The 2004 Sleep in American Poll found that 54% of school-aged children are getting less than 10 hours of sleep per day; the median hours of total sleep time among children aged 6–10 year was 9.5 hours.[2] Eighty percent of parents reported that their children are getting 'just the right amount of sleep,' suggesting that parents are aware of the increased sleep need among children and adolescents as compared to adults. In addition, 27% of school-aged children were getting *more* sleep on the weekends, suggesting that these children are building up a sleep debt throughout the week and have significant variability in their sleep–wake schedule between school days and weekends.[6]

CONSEQUENCES ASSOCIATED WITH INSUFFICIENT SLEEP

Insufficient total sleep time among children and adolescents has been associated with significant health consequences. A recent meta-analysis which included 12 studies (with data for over 30 000 children) found that short sleep duration was significantly associated with increased weight defined as a body weight greater than 85th percentile for age.[3] Furthermore, short sleep time is associated with metabolic changes (e.g., insulin resistance, increased fasting plasma glucose) among overweight and obese children.[4] In a longitudinal study of 200 children from birth to 5 years, normal-weight and overweight children did not differ in terms of nighttime sleep duration; however, overweight children demonstrated significantly less daytime napping, and thus shorter total sleep times.[5] While these studies highlight the importance of adequate total sleep time, a potential moderating factor of the relationship between sleep duration and weight may be timing of sleep. In the Spruyt et al. study of 2011, variability in total sleep time was associated with metabolic changes, as was total sleep time itself. Similarly, a recent study found that adolescents with later bedtimes and rise times were significantly more likely to be overweight as compared to adolescents with earlier bed- and rise-times, despite similar total sleep times between the two groups.[6]

DEVELOPING HEALTHY SLEEP HABITS

Traditionally, the term 'sleep hygiene'[7] has been used to include a wide variety of behaviors aimed at creating an environment conducive to sleep and avoiding activities that are disruptive to sleep. Although education about good sleep hygiene is frequently used as part of treatment for insomnia in adult populations, there is no standard definition of sleep hygiene.[8] For example, good sleep hygiene in adults is commonly presented as: (1) maintaining a cool, quiet, and dark sleep environment, (2) avoiding caffeine and alcohol near bedtime, and (3) not watching television or reading in bed, representing a conceptual overlap with stimulus control treatment for insomnia.[9] Given the non-standard definition of sleep hygiene, the present chapter instead presents recommendations to promote 'healthy sleep practices' among children and adolescents. Specifically, the chapter will review the importance of allowing for adequate time for sleep, maintaining a consistent sleep–wake pattern, creating a comfortable sleep environment, avoiding physiological barriers to sleep, and establishing effective bedtime routines. This chapter will not focus on specific treatments for childhood insomnia, as this is presented elsewhere (see Chapters 16 and 17).

MAINTAINING A CONSISTENT SLEEP–WAKE PATTERN

As currently understood, the sleep–wake cycle depends on the interactions between two processes: process C, the circadian wakefulness drive, and process S, the homeostatic sleep drive. These processes are presented in Figure 8-1.[10]

Process C has a period of about 24 hours established primarily through melatonin secretion mediated by light exposure, although other *zeitgebers*, or time markers, such as physical activity, social activity, or food intake also play a role. Process S, the drive to sleep, begins to accumulate gradually during wakefulness and drops off after sleep onset more quickly than it accumulates. Sleep onset occurs as the increasing sleep pressure due to Process S intersects with the decreasing circadian wakefulness drive of Process C. Sleep offset occurs when the increasing circadian wakefulness drive intersects with the decreasing sleep drive. Trying to stay awake or asleep out of sync with these processes can lead to sleepiness or difficulty initiating sleep. For example, if a child were to be put to bed prior to the intersection of these two processes, or if the two processes were not aligned, the circumstances would not be optimal for the child to fall asleep.

Establishing a consistent sleep–wake cycle requires that the child avoid activities that would shift either process. Process

C can be delayed through light exposure at the beginning of the night from activities such as watching television, playing in brightly lit rooms, or playing video games. Other *zeitgebers* such as playing with siblings, eating a meal, or exercising close to bedtime can also delay Process C, though they tend to have a lesser effect. Delaying Process C moves the height of the wakefulness drive closer to bedtime, making it less likely that the child will fall asleep. Napping and sleeping-in will also significantly reduce the power of the sleep drive (Process S) and will delay the intersection with Process C, thereby delaying sleep onset. Key recommendations to establish conditions for a consistent sleep–wake pattern are presented in Box 8-1.

CREATING A SUITABLE SLEEP ENVIRONMENT

A suitable sleep environment plays a significant role in helping children fall asleep at the beginning of the night and stay asleep for the duration of the night. Above all, it is important that a child's sleep environment remain consistent. If the environment changes after sleep onset, whether due to a parent leaving the room or due to a change in ambient noise, the child is more likely to awaken during the night. Ideal sleep environments will vary from child to child, but the following elements are generally important:

- It is important to maintain a cool, dark room for sleeping. Bedroom temperature should be less than 75 degrees Fahrenheit.
- Any music or white noise that is present at sleep onset should continue throughout the night. This can mask regular household noises, preventing associated arousals by means of competitive noise inhibition.
- If the child is noted to have nasal congestion that seems worse at night, the sleep environment should be evaluated for potential allergens (e.g., dust from old pillows or stuffed animals).
- Items that are associated with wakefulness (e.g., homework, mobile phones) should be kept outside of the sleep environment. This will prevent the association between these activities and the sleep environment. Isolating the bed for sleep will strengthen the association between the sleep environment and drowsiness at sleep onset.[9]
- Televisions, video games, and computers should also be kept out of the sleep environment. Use of these items in the bedroom and near bedtime are associated with variability in sleep and wake times, shorter sleep times, and poorer sleep quality.[11,12]

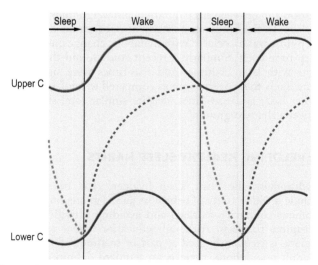

FIGURE 8-1 The two-process model of sleep regulation.[17]

Box 8-1   Tips for Maintaining a Consistent Sleep-wake Pattern

- Limit light exposure in the evening, including light from television, video games, and computer screens.
- Avoid physical activity, large meals, and social activity for at least 3 hours prior to bedtime.
- Bedtime and wake time should remain as consistent as possible.
- Naps should be timed early enough in the afternoon so as to allow for adequate sleep pressure to accumulate by bedtime.

REDUCING PHYSIOLOGIC BARRIERS TO SLEEP

Identifying physiologic barriers can be a complex process because an activity that excites one child can sometimes help another child relax. For example, in some children a bath can be very calming, making it an effective part of their bedtime routine. For other children, however, bath time is a time for playing, and it can take them quite a while to wind down afterwards. In general, activities that excite the child, such as vigorous play, conflicts with family members, or video games, should be avoided close to bedtime. Physical exertion should be avoided at least 3 hours prior to bedtime to allow enough time for the child to settle down and get into bed at a reasonable level of activation.[13]

Attention must also be given to potentially stimulating medications, drinks, and food that a child might take prior to bedtime. In children who are on extended-release stimulants or are given short-acting stimulants after school, problems with increased sleep-onset latency may be associated with prolonged medication effect. Chocolate, energy drinks, or caffeinated beverages can also provide a powerful barrier to successfully achieving sleep onset. A good general rule is that no caffeine should be ingested for at least 4 hours prior to sleep.[13] Children with high sensitivity to the effect of sugar and caffeine should avoid them any time after lunch.

Hunger itself can provide a barrier to sleep, and incorporating a snack into the bedtime routine can be an effective way of addressing issues with sleep onset. While the data are not very strong, there is a suggestion that tryptophan[14] or carbohydrates can be particularly helpful.

For some children, fear of the dark, separation anxiety, or other issues can increase activation at bedtime. For these children, use of graduated extinction or 'fading out' techniques which allow for the presence of a caregiver as the child develops the confidence to rest in bed alone can be applied.

ESTABLISHING A RELAXING BEDTIME ROUTINE

Establishing a consistent, progressively less stimulating bedtime routine prior to bedtime has been demonstrated to significantly improve sleep quality.[15] The reasons for this are not fully understood, but are likely to be associated with a combination of factors. Children value routine, and being able to rely on a predictable sequence of activities can have a significant calming effect. The gradual reduction of stimulation as the routine progresses allows a child to transition smoothly from days full of new experiences to a relaxed state conducive to sleep. Also, receiving positive attention from a caregiver just prior to bed can help make bedtime a highlight of the day rather than a dreaded obligation.

There are no bedtime routines that are guaranteed to work for every child, and routines change as children grow and develop. There are, however, consistent features of successful bedtime routines. As a sequence of activities is consistently repeated prior to bedtime, those activities begin to serve as 'sleep cues.' Initially the child may require the involvement of a caregiver as the routine is being established, but gradually responsibility for moving through the sequence can be given to the child. A sticker chart can be useful in reinforcing compliance with the steps of the routine. Listing the steps in the routine and positively reinforcing each one helps the child

start to enjoy participating and, since both the child and the parent are referring to the same chart, interpersonal conflicts can be avoided. Regardless of the specific steps, the ultimate goal remains the same: by the end of the routine the child ends up relaxed, sleepy, and resting comfortably in bed.

CONCLUSION

Healthy sleep habits can play a significant role in helping children and adolescents meet their total sleep need. The recommendations about such habits should not be applied formulaically. A recent review of data from the National Sleep Foundation Poll found there may be developmental changes in 'good sleep hygiene,' and different aspects of sleep hygiene (consistent sleep–wake pattern, consistent bedtime routine, etc.) may differentially affect sleep quality across childhood.[16] With this in mind, the recommendations in this chapter should be seen as guidelines and illustrative examples intended to draw attention to the impact that maintaining a consistent sleep–wake pattern, creating a comfortable sleep environment, avoiding physiological barriers to sleep, and establishing appropriate bedtime routines can have on a child's ability to fall asleep and stay asleep. Parents, children, and adolescents should be invited into regular discussions about what they are learning from the application of these concepts and principles, and consultations should be focused on advancing the process of developing healthy sleep habits. In this way, health care practitioners and families will see a significant increase in their capacity to help their children achieve adequate sleep.

Clinical Pearls

- There is no magic number of hours of sleep needed; total sleep need should be individually assessed based on nighttime sleep quality and daytime functioning.
- Insufficient total sleep time is associated with significant behavioral, health, and neurocognitive problems.
- Children and adolescents should maintain a regular sleep–wake schedule, with particular attention paid to maintaining consistency between schooldays and weekends.
- A suitable sleep environment is one that is comfortable, cool, dark, quiet, and free from media such as televisions, computers, video games, and mobile phones.
- Physiologic barriers to sleep such as physical exercise, hunger, and separation anxiety should be addressed prior to bedtime.
- Parents should help children and adolescents develop an individualized bedtime routine.

References

1. Children and sleep [Internet]. Available from: http://www.sleep foundation.org/article/sleep-topics/children-and-sleep.
2. National Sleep Foundation. 2004 Sleep in America Poll: Children and sleep. http://www.sleepfoundation.org/sites/default/files/FINAL%20 SOF%202004.pdf; 2004.
3. Cappuccio FP, Taggart FM, Kandala NB, et al. Meta-analysis of short sleep duration and obesity in children and adults. Sleep 2008;31 (5):619–26.

4. Spruyt K, Molfese DL, Gozal D. Sleep duration, sleep regularity, body weight, and metabolic homeostasis in school-aged children. Pediatrics 2011;127(2):e345–52.

5. Agras WS, Hammer LD, McNicholas F, et al. Risk factors for childhood overweight: A prospective study from birth to 9.5 years. J Pediatr 2004;145(1):20–5.

6. Olds TS, Maher CA, Matricciani L. Sleep duration or bedtime? Exploring the relationship between sleep habits and weight status and activity patterns. Sleep 2011 1;34(10):1299–307.

7. Hauri PJ. Sleep hygiene, relaxation therapy, and cognitive interventions. In: Hauri PJ, editor. Case studies in insomnia. New York: Plenum; 1991. p. 65–84.

8. Stepanski EJ, Wyatt JK. Use of sleep hygiene in the treatment of insomnia. Sleep Med Rev 2003;7(3):215–25.

9. Bootzin RR, Epstien D, Wood JM. Stimulus control instruction. In: Hauri PJ, editor. Case studies in insomnia. New York: Plenum; 1991. p. 19–28.

10. Borbely AA. A two process model of sleep regulation. Hum Neurobiol 1982;1(3):195–204.

11. Munezawa T, Kaneita Y, Osaki Y, et al. The association between use of mobile phones after lights out and sleep disturbances among Japanese adolescents: A nationwide cross-sectional survey. Sleep 2011;34(8):1013–20.

12. Van den Bulck J. Television viewing, computer game playing, and internet use and self-reported time to bed and time out of bed in secondary-school children. Sleep 2004 1;27(1):101–4.

13. Morin CM, Hauri PJ, Espie CA, et al. Nonpharmacologic treatment of chronic insomnia. An American Academy of Sleep Medicine Review. Sleep 1999;22(8):1134–56.

14. Hartmann E. Effects of L-tryptophan on sleepiness and on sleep. J Psychiatr Res 1982–1983;17(2):107–13.

15. Mindell JA, Telofski LS, Wiegand B, et al. A nightly bedtime routine: Impact on sleep in young children and maternal mood. Sleep 2009;32(5):599–606.

16. Mindell JA, Meltzer LJ, Carskadon MA, et al. Developmental aspects of sleep hygiene: Findings from the 2004 National Sleep Foundation Sleep in America poll. Sleep Med 2009;10(7):771–9.

17. Waterhouse J, Fukuda Y, Morita T. Daily rhythms of the sleep-wake cycle. J Physiol Anthropol 2012;31(1):5.

Sleep History and Differential Diagnosis

Stephen H. Sheldon

Chapter 9

INTRODUCTION

Clinical evaluation is the most important part of the process of assessment and diagnosis of sleep and its disorders in the pediatric and adolescent patient. Next in importance comes the physical examination. Laboratory assessment may be valuable as well, though it is not always necessary.

DEVELOPING A DIFFERENTIAL DIAGNOSIS: PROCESS OF SOLVING CLINICAL PROBLEMS

Hypotheses form the basis of inquiry into patients' presenting problems. They are generated very early in the assessment, and they are then refined by completing the clinical history and by performing a physical examination. The set of hypotheses is then further refined into an actual diagnosis or a list of possible (differential) diagnoses.[1] Laboratory testing may be needed when the history and physical examination alone do not lead to a final diagnosis.

Evaluation of the Clinical History

The abilities for establishing an appropriate initial hypothesis set and to subsequently test it by clinical inquiry require a wide knowledge base. Understanding of the pathophysiology, natural history, clinical manifestations, and patterns of symptom presentation for the various disorders is essential if one is to make an accurate diagnosis.

Sleep disturbances in children are common. When a sleepless child frequently disturbs parents during the night, parents will generally be quick to seek medical attention (especially when the child's sleep problems lead to symptoms of sleep deprivation in the parents themselves). Similarly, profoundly sleepy children may reach the sleep professional early on (particularly if the child is falling asleep at inappropriate times such as during meals, while talking on the phone, or when opening presents at a birthday party). On the other hand, the child who is only mildly sleepy may not reach appropriate professional care until late in the course of the disorder because the symptoms of less than profound sleepiness are easy to miss. A youngster in a state of hypo-arousal may have symptoms considerably different than those of a sleepy adult. Thus, instead of overt sleepiness, sleepy children may present with hyperactivity, distractibility, attention difficulties, mood swings, increased frustration, and learning problems. These symptoms are too often inadequately addressed, usually with behavioral interventions with only limited consideration of the possibility of a sleep disorder. This is unfortunate, since screening for sleep problems generally does not take very long to do.

In one study of 202 children who presented consecutively to a developmental and behavioral pediatric practice, parents and other primary caretakers were found to only infrequently report that the child under their care had a sleep problem, even when symptoms suggesting a sleep disorder were present.[2] Simply asking the parent the single question, 'Does your child have a sleep problem?' is inadequate to determine the presence or absence of problematic sleep.

A sleep history obtained from a frustrated, sleepy parent can be vague and inaccurate, with the parent focusing, at times, on the wrong details. For example, parents often describe the child's sleep pattern only for the most severe or most recent night or period. A more accurate depiction of the sleep patterns across time can be obtained from a sleep diary, log, or chart. For this reason, the parent can be asked to maintain a sleep chart or log for a period of 2 to 4 weeks prior to the first visit (and then again during treatment). This item then becomes very helpful in identifying habitual sleep–wake cycle patterns and provides documentation of abnormalities occurring from night to night.[2] Maintaining a sleep log seems to improve observational skills of the child's care-taker, increases validity of observational data, and can be indirectly therapeutic. Parents might see on paper what actually happened most nights. Sleep disorder professionals might find review of such documents useful to clarify the actual pattern of what is happening and such review might well be the most accurate way of documenting progress.

It is important to begin with a screening process that might provide insight or cues to the practitioner that a problem requiring further consideration might be present. A structured approach to screening the history has been tested and validated.[3] An important first step is obtaining information regarding the typical/habitual sleep patterns and difficulties. A number of screening tools have been developed to assist the child health care practitioner in assessing for sleep-related disorders and have been comprehensively reviewed by Spruyt and Gozal.[4] These authors, however, conclude that very few of these tools fulfill all the necessary properties required, and only a few are standardized. None of the tools had any diagnostic power in and of itself – thus, making the diagnosis remains in the domain of the clinician. One questionnaire, the *BEARS* Screening Tool developed by Owens and Dalzell, had particular usefulness in the primary care setting as well as in the sleep medicine center.[5] It has questions regarding **B**edtime, **E**xcessive daytime sleepiness, **A**wakenings at night, **R**egularity/duration, and **S**noring, the answers to which suggest a series of possible diagnoses (see Figures 9-1 to 9-5).

HISTORICAL DETAILS

Bedtime

Knowledge of what parents believe is an appropriate bedtime and length of expected sleep can provide insight into the reasons for the problem sleep. For example, a 5-year-old child whose bedtime is 7:30 p.m. and whose scheduled waking is

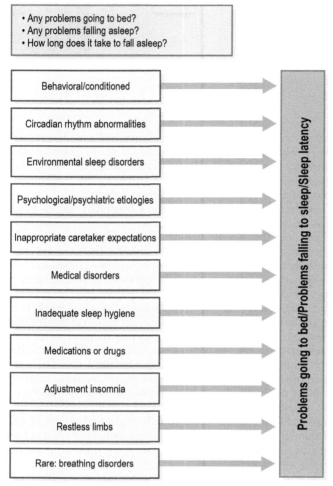

- Any problems going to bed?
- Any problems falling asleep?
- How long does it take to fall asleep?

Behavioral/conditioned

Circadian rhythm abnormalities

Environmental sleep disorders

Psychological/psychiatric etiologies

Inappropriate caretaker expectations

Medical disorders

Inadequate sleep hygiene

Medications or drugs

Adjustment insomnia

Restless limbs

Rare: breathing disorders

Problems going to bed/Problems falling to sleep/Sleep latency

FIGURE 9-1 Bedtime. *Adapted from: Owens JA, Dalzell V. Use of the 'BEARS' sleep screening tool in a pediatric residents' continuity clinic: a pilot study.* Sleep Medicine 2005:6:63–69. With permission.

- Any difficulty waking in the morning?
- Feels sleepy during the day?
- Has difficulty paying attention?
- Has difficulty sitting still?

Circadian rhythm disorder

Sleep-related movement disorder

Sleep-related arousal disorder

Partial arousal disorder

Sleep-related breathing disorder

Narcolepsy with or without cataplexy

Idiopathic hypersomnia with or without long sleep time

Medical conditions

Medication

Insufficient sleep syndrome

Recurrent hypersomnia

Excessive daytime sleepiness

FIGURE 9-2 Excessive daytime sleepiness. *Adapted from: Owens JA, Dalzell V. Use of the 'BEARS' sleep screening tool in a pediatric residents' continuity clinic: a pilot study.* Sleep Medicine 2005: 6: 63–69. With permission.

7:00 a.m. most likely will be in bed too early (at a time when his or her circadian rhythm may not permit easy settling) and in bed too long (*inappropriate caretaker expectation*). On the other hand, knowledge that a child both falls asleep and wakes early (7:30 p.m. and 5:00 a.m.) suggests a circadian rhythm disorder might be present (*advanced sleep phase*). Similarly, a 2-year-old child whose bedtime is at 01:00 a.m. (because of the parents' work schedules) and who then wakes at 11:00 a.m. (and is difficult to wake earlier) may have a *delayed sleep phase* that, at least on weekdays when earlier wakings are necessary, can lead to a syndrome of *insufficient sleep* and profound daytime problems.

Sleep Latency

Sleep latency can provide information regarding the ease and speed of settling at night. This information, combined with the knowledge of habitual bedtime, can help in determination of the presence of behavioral, circadian, psychological, and medical sleep-onset difficulties (*behavioral insomnia of childhood, sleep onset association disorder, limit-setting sleep disorder,*

delayed or advanced sleep phase, anxiety-related sleep disorders, and *restless limb syndrome*).

The history that the youngster can fall asleep easily and without difficulty when at the grandparent's house, or in the parents' bed, or on the sofa, or in front of the television strongly suggests a behavioral/conditioned etiology or anxiety rather than an organic cause for the sleeplessness since, when the cause of a child's sleeplessness is medically based, a child typically has difficulty falling asleep anywhere and under any circumstances. And, when the cause is anxiety, the child usually has difficulty falling asleep in a room alone. Prolongation of the sleep latency must be assessed in conjunction with knowledge of bedtime for accurate interpretation. For example, a 4-hour sleep latency in a 9-year-old child has different meaning when the bedtime is 7:00 p.m. (which may be too early) than when it is 10:00 p.m.

Habitual Time of Morning Waking

Time of habitual morning waking helps determine total nocturnal sleep time and provides information as to circadian

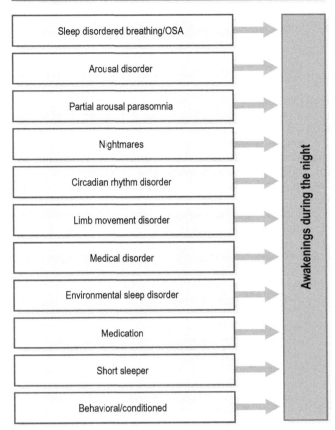

- Awakening frequently during the night?
- Sleepwalk or sleep talk?
- Any trouble falling back to sleep after waking up in the middle of the night?

Sleep disordered breathing/OSA

Arousal disorder

Partial arousal parasomnia

Nightmares

Circadian rhythm disorder

Limb movement disorder

Medical disorder

Environmental sleep disorder

Medication

Short sleeper

Behavioral/conditioned

Awakenings during the night

FIGURE 9-3 Awakenings. *Adapted from: Owens JA, Dalzell V. Use of the 'BEARS' sleep screening tool in a pediatric residents' continuity clinic: a pilot study.* Sleep Medicine 2005: 6: 63–69. *With permission.*

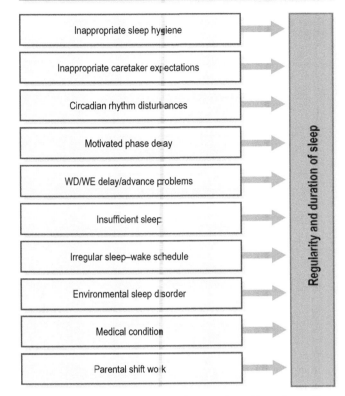

- Has a regular sleep schedule been established?
- When does the patient get into bed?
- What time does the patient wake in the morning?
- Any significant differences in bedtime and wake time between weekdays and weekends?

Inappropriate sleep hygiene

Inappropriate caretaker expectations

Circadian rhythm disturbances

Motivated phase delay

WD/WE delay/advance problems

Insufficient sleep

Irregular sleep–wake schedule

Environmental sleep disorder

Medical condition

Parental shift work

Regularity and duration of sleep

FIGURE 9-4 Regularity and duration of sleep. *Adapted from: Owens JA, Dalzell V. Use of the 'BEARS' sleep screening tool in a pediatric residents' continuity clinic: a pilot study.* Sleep Medicine 2005: 6: 63–69. *With permission.*

phase. Determination of whether morning waking is spontaneous or induced is also important. The times of morning waking are also powerful contributors to circadian rhythm entrainment; if the times are inconsistent, *sleep–wake schedule abnormality* might be suggested.

It is important to determine the times of waking on weekends and holidays in addition to on weekdays (school days). Late sleep offset on weekends and holidays might suggest a *delayed sleep phase*. When wake-up times are variable, a *non-24-hour sleep–wake schedule* might be suspected, especially in a youngster with severe neurological abnormalities.

Sleep Continuity

Sleep continuity problems may occur as isolated symptoms or in association with sleep-onset difficulties. Determination of timing, frequency, length, and characteristics of, and parental responses to, nocturnal wakings provides information regarding possible behavioral, circadian/schedule-related, and physiological (medical) causes. Sleep-onset difficulties accompanied by sleep continuity problems in the absence of physiological abnormalities suggest the presence of *behavioral, schedule-related*, or *psychological* etiologies that should be pursued by

careful history. *Limit-setting problems* and insufficient parental tolerance are sometimes easy to detect when similar findings exist during the day. A history of wakings that are short only and whenever specific parental interventions are initiated (rocking, pacifier, feeding) may suggest (if not diagnose) the actual problem (*sleep onset association disorders* or *excessive nocturnal feedings*).

Excessive Daytime Sleepiness

Determination of the presence of daytime sleepiness is vitally important. It can be difficult to determine the presence of excessive sleepiness in young infants, toddlers, and young children in whom daytime sleep is normal as expected. Total sleep times range from about 16–18 hours in the newborn to about 9–10 hours by late childhood. There is a gradual decline in total sleep time as the child matures.

By about 12 weeks of age (if not before) circadian rhythmicity of the sleep–wake cycle begins to be clear, with the longest sleep period occurring at night and the longest wake period occurring during the day. At this age, daytime sleep occurs in about 3–4 discrete daytime naps. Naps consolidate at around 6 months into two briefer daytime sleep periods

- Does the patient snore more than three nights per week?
- Are there pauses, snorts, gasps, or choking?
- Does the child breathe through her/his mouth?
- Does the child wake with headaches?
- Does the child wet the bed?
- Are there reported witnessed apneas?
- Is there sleep-related diaphoresis?
- Is/are there daytime sleepiness/hyperactivity/attention problems?
- Does the child wake with a dry mouth?

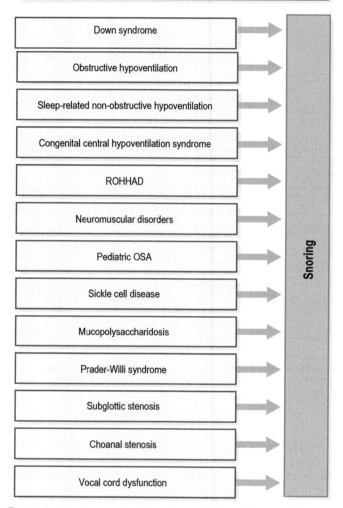

FIGURE 9-5 Snoring. *Adapted from: Owens JA, Dalzell V. Use of the 'BEARS' sleep screening tool in a pediatric residents' continuity clinic: a pilot study. Sleep Medicine 2005: 6: 63–69. With permission.*

and, into the second year of life, into a single early afternoon sleep period. Daytime naps are typically given up by 3–5 years of age. There is a wide variation of normal, but youngsters habitually still napping at 6–7 years of age might be exhibiting symptoms of daytime sleepiness.

THE PHYSICAL EXAMINATION

The physical examination needed depends on the medical history, the specifics of the sleep complaint, and the hypotheses generated during assessment. A healthy toddler who simply needs help giving up the pacifier at night may not need

TABLE 9.1 Modified Mallampati Scoring Criteria[11]
Modified Mallampati Scoring:

- Class I: Soft palate, uvula, fauces, pillars visible.
- Class II: Soft palate, uvula, fauces visible.
- Class III: Soft palate, base of uvula visible.
- Class IV: Only hard palate visible.

Adapted from Samsoon GL, Young JR. Difficult tracheal intubation: a retrospective study. Anaesthesia 1987;42:487–90.

a full examination. A child with enuresis may require examination of the genitals, perineum, and spine. And a child with possible seizures or known neurologic abnormalities will require a more comprehensive and extensive neurodevelopmental evaluation. A complete discussion of the physical and developmental evaluation of children at various developmental levels may be found in several excellent resources.[6,7]

The most common areas requiring evaluation in children presenting with sleep complaints are those related to the airway since airway-related problems are often part of the differential diagnosis regardless of presenting complaint.[3–10]

These areas include:

- Habitus: For abnormal height, weight, and body mass index (obesity or failure to thrive);
- HEENT:
  1. For abnormal skull or facial features (craniosynostosis, facial asymmetry, midface hypoplasia, retrognathia, macroglossia, dental overjet);
  2. For adenotonsillar and uvular enlargement and oropharyngeal crowding (modified Mallampati scale,[11] see Table 9.1);
  3. For nasal obstruction (septal deviation, polyps, enlarged turbinates);
  4. For palatal abnormalities (high arching, presence of cleft); and
  5. For thyroid enlargement;
- Chest and back: For chest or spine abnormalities (pectus excavatum, barrel-shaped, scoliosis);
- Neurologic: For abnormal tone (hypertonia, spasticity, hypotonia).

Clinical Pearls

- Clinical history is the most important part of the process of solving clinical problems.
- The ability to establish an initial hypothesis set and subsequent testing of these hypotheses requires a wide knowledge base.
- A structured approach to obtaining pertinent clinical information is essential to the diagnosis and management of sleep disorders in infants, children, and adolescents.

References

1. Barrows HS, Tamblyn RM. Problem-based learning: an approach to medical education. New York: Springer; 1980.
2. Ferber R. Solve your child's sleep problems. New York: Simon & Schuster; 2006.
3. Sheldon SH, Ahart S, Levy HB. Sleep patterns in abused and neglected children. Sleep Res 1991;20:333.
4. Spruyt K, Gozal D. Pediatric sleep questionnaires as diagnostic or epidemiological tools: a review of currently available instruments. Sleep Med Rev 2011;15(1):19–32.

5. Owens JA, Dalzell V. Use of the 'BEARS' sleep screening tool in a pediatric residents' continuity clinic: a pilot study. Sleep Med 2005;6:63–9.

6. Frankenberg WK, Thornton SM, Cohrs ME. Pediatric developmental diagnosis. New York: Thieme-Stratton, Inc.; 1981.

7. Behrman RE, Kliegman RM, Nelson WE, et al, editors. Nelson: textbook of pediatrics. 14th ed. Philadelphia: WB Saunders; 1992.

8. Epstein LJ, Kristo D, Strollo PJ, et al. Clinical guideline for the evaluation, management and long-term care of obstructive sleep apnea in adults. J Clin Sleep Med 2009;5(3):263–76.

9. Cataletto ME, Lipton AJ, Murphy TD. Childhood sleep apnea clinical presentation. http://emedicine.medscape.com/article/1004104, update 5/14/2012.

10. Chan J, Edman JC, Koltai PJ. Obstructive sleep apnea in children. Am Fam Physician 2004;69(5):1147–55.

11. Samsoon GL, Young JR. Difficult tracheal intubation: a retrospective study. Anaesthesia 1987;42:487–90.

PRACTICE AND CLINICAL SCIENCE OF PEDIATRIC SLEEP MEDICINE

PART

II

THE INSOMNIAS (SLEEP ONSET AND MAINTENANCE DIFFICULTIES)

Sleep and Colic

Anat Cohen Engler, Tamar Etzioni, and Giora Pillar

TERMINOLOGY AND DEFINITIONS

The most distinctive feature of infantile colic is excessive crying. Crying, especially in the evening, is a normal behavior of infants.[1] Recognizing which crying behavior should be considered excessive and requires further evaluation is a challenge for the clinician.

There is an extensive variety of definitions for excessive crying and colic. The most widely used is the one defined by Wessel at 1954, also known as 'the rule of three:' crying for more than 3 hours per day, for more than 3 days per week, and for longer than 3 weeks in an infant who is well-fed and is otherwise healthy.[2–5]

Other definitions of a 'fussy/colicky infant' can be grossly divided into two large groups. One group uses different time limits, while the other group relies on the different subjective estimation of the parents.[5,6] When using definitions from the latter group, one has to keep in mind that there could be disconcordance between parental expectations and a 'normal for age' behavior. As of now, there is still no consensus on which definition is the most accurate or appropriate to be used. Despite relatively many studies in this field, more research needs to be done to elucidate this issue and lead to more commonly accepted terms and definitions.

Regarding the duration of symptoms, there are also various opinions. Reijneveld et al. demonstrated that when applying a different time frame to the same definition there is a change in the prevalence of excessive crying. When applying a time frame of '3 preceding weeks or longer' in comparison with 'during the preceding week' the prevalence substantially declines.[6] The most commonly used and the most validated is the original Wessel definition for 'seriously fussy children' with the requirement of 'over 3 preceding weeks.' For the purpose of research it is highly important to adhere to a unified definition in order for results to be comparable and for meta-analysis to be carried out. In practice, that may not be applicable, as many parents will not be willing to wait for that long. Nevertheless, acute crying might be an obvious sign of a serious illness or even a life-threatening one, and must clearly not be ignored.

PROPERTIES AND 'NATURAL COURSE'

The typical colicky crying episodes are prolonged, practically unsoothable and associated with a high-pitched cry.[7,8] The episodes are sometimes accompanied by posture changes such as drawing up of the legs or clenched fists, flushing, and passing gas.[8,9] Episodes are more common during evening and night hours.[3,7,10,11]

Besides differences in crying duration and intensity, it seems that the crying curve of the colicky infant resembles the one of the 'average' infant. The overall duration of crying increases gradually until it peaks at about the age of 6–8 weeks, then declines until it reaches a plateau around the age of 3–4 months.[4,10,11]

PREVALENCE

The prevalence of infantile colic in the community is estimated to be 10–40%, depending on the definition used. Since there is a large variety of definitions and different considerations to babies' cries, it is hard to determine the exact prevalence rates.[5,6]

PATHOGENESIS

While infantile colic is a well-known syndrome of excessive cry, the etiology and pathogenesis remains an enigma. Many theories exist, yet none is adequately evidence-based.

Most of the theories argue that a gastrointestinal disturbance causes the crying paroxysms. That belief is somewhat supported by clinical evidence and the infant's behavior during the bouts as described above. Some parents' report of alleviation of symptoms with gas absorbers also supports this theory. Other theories suggest that the crying bouts may be related to temperament and regulation. This section will describe the most accepted proposed causes of infantile colic.

Excessive Air Load in the Gastrointestinal Tract

Based on clinical observations that infants with colic tend to pass relatively large amounts of gas,[2,7] it is a common belief that excessive gas in the gastrointestinal tract causes painful abdominal distention and subsequently crying bouts. Possible sources for excessive gas may be aerophagia and colonic bacterial fermentation of malabsorbed carbohydrates.[12] Though very common and accepted by clinicians and parents, this theory has never been successfully proven.[3,9,12,13] Nevertheless, clinical trials with Simethicone (gas absorber) failed to prove symptomatic relieve in comparison with placebo, when treating colicky infants.[14]

Dysmotility

Another common belief is that the origin of infants' crying is gut hyperperistalsis and intestinal smooth muscle spasm.[9,13] This theory is supported by evidence that antispasmodic agents, such as Dicyclomine hydrochloride and Cimetropium bromide, alleviate colic symptoms.[14,15] Transient dysregulation of the central nervous system was suggested as the reason for dysmotility, though no difference was found in the balance of autonomic nervous system between colicky and other infants.[16]

Gut Hormones

The gastrointestinal tract activity is highly regulated by different hormones. Some of them were suggested to play a role in the pathogenesis of infantile colic. Different studies found higher levels of motilin in colicky infants.[17–19] Motilin is speculated to promote gastric emptying, which increases small bowel peristalsis and decreases transient time. This can also relate to the dysmotility theory. Higher levels of ghrelin were also found in colicky infants, though only in one small study.[19]

A recent study showed that colicky infants had higher urinary levels of 5-hydroxy indoleacetic acid, a metabolite of serotonin.[20] This supported the hypothesis that some features of colic might be caused by a serotonin–melatonin counter-balancing system involving the gastrointestinal smooth muscles. Serotonin and melatonin have opposite effects on intestinal smooth muscle: serotonin causes contraction while melatonin causes relaxation.[21] It was hypothesized that in some infants, the balance between circulating serotonin concentrations and intestinal smooth muscle sensitivity to serotonin might lead to painful gastrointestinal cramps in the evening when serotonin concentrations are highest.

Lack of melatonin in the first months of life may explain the lack of its needed relaxing effect.[22] However, some researchers believe there is no solid scientific evidence to support this hypothesis.[23]

Gastroesophageal Reflux

This was suggested to be related to the pathogenesis of infantile colic, though no convincing evidence exists. Apparently, this is a distinctive common GI pathology that may coexist with infantile colic.[9,13,24]

Food Allergy

Food allergy was also suggested to have a role in infantile colic. Infantile colic is sometimes related to a food allergy and may represent, particularly when severe, the first clinical manifestation of atopic disease.[25,26] Like gastroesophageal reflux, food allergy may also be a distinctive pathology that might mimic or co-exist with infantile colic.

Psychosocial Factors

Over the years, it was widely argued that excessive infant crying is an early manifestation of a difficult temperament, and the colicky infant is often considered to be irritable and hypersensitive.[3,9] In the literature, there is only weak evidence to support this theory, as it is almost impossible to examine it in an unbiased longitudinal manner. One study attempted to explore the theory using objective physiologic tools and found no support for this theory.[27] Other theories suggested that the excessive crying originates in an inadequate parent–infant interaction, though there is no clear evidence to support this theory either.[3,4,9]

Parental Smoking

Recent studies indicated that exposure of the child to tobacco smoking by the mother during pregnancy and after delivery, and smoking by the father, were associated with excessive crying. Moreover, it was suggested that smoking is linked to increased plasma and intestinal motilin levels, and higher-than-average intestinal motilin and ghrelin levels seem to be related to elevated risk of infantile coli.[28,29]

OUTCOME AND PROGNOSIS

Infantile colic is a transient, self-limiting condition considered to have a favorable outcome, usually resolving by the age of 4–6 months.[9]

On psychological grounds, several studies suggested that infants with colic are more emotional and are somewhat prone to negative moods and temper tantrums.[30,31]

DIAGNOSIS

Excessive infant crying is a very common situation and the differential diagnosis is extremely broad. When excessive crying is prolonged, an organic disease is estimated to account for less than 5% of the cases.[32] Nevertheless, before making the diagnosis of infantile colic, an organic cause must be ruled out.

When faced with a crying infant, the importance of a thorough history and physical examination cannot be over-emphasized. Situations that may cause similar symptoms such as gastroesophageal reflux, constipation and cow milk protein allergy must be considered, as well as an acute illness or a neurologic or developmental problem. Any history suggestive of a specific pathology should be considered appropriately. Box 10-1 lists potential causes for prolonged, excessive infantile crying.

Parents should be asked about characteristics of the crying episodes such as duration, time of the day and accompanying behavior.

Physical examination should be completed in a systematic head-to-toe manner with emphasis on the gastrointestinal and neurologic systems. Signs of abuse or trauma must be sought as well.

The infant's weight percentile should be considered.

If the history and physical examination reveal no pathological condition in an infant that gains weight properly, laboratory or radiographic examinations are usually not necessary.[5]

Box 10-1   Potential Causes for Prolonged Excessive Infantile Crying

Gastrointestinal:
  Infantile colic
  Gastroesophageal reflux
  Rumination
  Feeding problems
  Constipation
  Milk protein allergy
Neurological:
  Psychomotor retardation
  Communication problems
Difficulty breathing:
  Choanal atresia
  Laryngomalacia
  Congenital lung disease
Infection:
  Urinary tract infection
  Otitis media
Pain:
  Fracture
  Hernia
  Corneal abrasion
  Atopic dermatitis
Social problems:
  Neglect
  Abuse
  Inadequate relation with care giver
  Limit-setting sleep disorders

A recent retrospective cohort study found that the only useful laboratory examination when evaluating a crying infant with a normal history and physical examination is urine evaluation.[32] If there is a pathology suspected in the history and physical examination, evaluation should be followed accordingly.

TREATMENT

Once the diagnosis of infantile colic is made, the first step of management is reassuring of the parents, explaining that colic is a self-limiting condition and that the excessive crying does not reflect an underlying disease or bad parenting.[9] In addition, parents should be reassured that there is no negative prognosis for infantile colic.

As for interventional therapies, over the years many remedies have been proposed and studied as possible treatments for infantile colic. The main groups are pharmacological, dietary and behavioral interventions based on the different possible etiologies/mechanisms. Unfortunately, due to lack of a standard definition and methodological weaknesses in many of the clinical trials, the data do not deliver convincing evidence to support a specific treatment. Currently, it is still not clear which is the optimal treatment, and watchful waiting might just be the best medicine.

Dietary Interventions

Some trials examined the efficacy of elimination of potentially allergenic agents from the infant's diet. Data regarding utilizing of hypoallergenic diets by breastfeeding mothers are inconclusive, but suggest that there may be some therapeutic benefits.[33] The use of hypoallergenic formula for bottle-fed infants also appears to have a beneficial effect on colic symptoms. The benefit of using a soy-based formula is less conclusive.[35,34] Further validated studies are needed to evaluate these dietary interventions.

High-fiber formulas were also tested. While the enriched formula did have a significant effect on stool characteristics, it did not influence crying duration.[34,35]

Two randomized-controlled trials studied the effect of lactase on infantile colic. Neither of them found a beneficial effect.[33]

Some researchers recommend at least one attempt of dietary modification in the management of infantile colic.

Pharmacologic Interventions

Several pharmacologic agents were suggested and tested as treatment of infantile colic.

Simethicone, a commonly used drug aimed to relieve gas-related symptoms, was tested in three different validated trials. The results did not demonstrate conclusive benefit as a treatment for infantile colic.[33,34]

Anticholinergic drugs were tested as possible therapies due to their anti-spasmodic effect.

Dicyclomine has been proved to be an effective treatment for infantile colic; however, due to life-threatening side effects such as apnea, seizures and coma, the manufacturer has contraindicated the use of the drug in infants younger than 6 months and does not consider infantile colic as an indication for using the drug.[33,36]

One study found cimetropium bromide to be effective but that it had side effects of sleepiness.[37] Another trial found methylscopolamine to be ineffective.[33]

Lactobacillus

The role of intestinal microflora has been growing in importance, and lower counts of intestinal lactobacilli were observed in colicky infants, in comparison with healthy infants. *Lactobacillus reuteri*, one of the few endogenous *Lactobacillus* species in the human gastrointestinal tract, has been used safely for many years as a probiotic dietary supplement in adults, and recent data demonstrated safety after long-term dietary supplementation for newborn infant. One study, which included 90 breastfed colicky infants, demonstrated that supplementation with *L. reuteri* improved colicky symptoms significantly in breastfed infants, compared with the standard therapy with simethicone, within 7 days of treatment (response rate of 95% and 7%, respectively). No adverse effects were reported.[38]

Behavioral Interventions

Clinical trials examining the efficacy of behavioral interventions are problematic in nature. First, it is impossible to conduct a double-blind study, and bias may affect the results. Second, many of the examined interventions can cause overstimulation and therefore influence the results.

Increased carrying of the child was found useful in reducing the amount of crying.[39]

Parkin et al. found that specific management techniques such as early response to the crying, gentle soothing motion, avoidance of overstimulation, use of pacifier and car-ride simulators were not more helpful than support and reassurance alone in reducing infant crying.[40]

Any combination of these approaches can be tried and individualized to each infant. If the diagnosis of infantile colic is correct, the most important approaches are parental reassurance and gaining time. As stated, the natural history is spontaneous alleviation by 6 months of age.

INFANTILE COLIC AND SLEEP PROBLEMS

An association between infantile colic and sleep problems later on in life has previously been suggested by subjective parental testimonies.[41–43] This association was further explored, supported by some research and confounded by others.

Such association is very difficult to explore for several reasons. First, as described above, there is a lack of a globally acceptable definition of colic. Results of different studies are incomparable, as different colic definitions were used. Second, most of the research used questionnaires to evaluate infants' sleep. This method was found unreliable,[44] especially as mothers of 'quiet' infants tend to overestimate their child's sleeping time,[8] while mothers of colicky infants tend to consider their child to be more difficult.[43]

Currently, no consensus is established. The two phenomena may influence each other, and both may be affected by many factors, some of which may overlap. As the base of both phenomena is very complex and may be attributed to physiologic as well as psychological factors, empiric isolation of each factor and a full understanding of the nature and relation of those behaviors may never be accomplished.

Infantile Colic and Sleep Problems before the Age of Three Months

Some subjective studies supported the hypothesis that infants with colic tend to sleep less. This was ratified by subjective studies, but not corroborated by objective researches.

A very large population-based study was conducted by Crowcroft et al. Their results showed that colicky babies had significantly shorter periods of 'longest continuous time asleep' and longer periods of 'longest time awake' than other infants.[45] St. James-Roberts et al. found that colicky infants slept on average 77 minutes less than non-colicky infants at the age of 6 weeks; the clearest group differences were in the daytime.[46] White et al. found that colicky infants slept about 1.5–2 hours less in a course of the day when compared to infants without colic.[27] On the other hand, a recent longitudinal study found that most infants with prolonged colic at 5–6 weeks of age were settled at night at 12 weeks of age, and they 'slept through the night' as soon as other infants.[47]

Those studies, while very important and informative, were based on parental reports alone.

Objective studies, which used polysomnography to evaluate sleep, found that colicky infants have a similar total and nocturnal sleeping time and structure as other infants, and shed new light on the validity of observational diaries.

One study found that during late evening and night sleep, excessively and non-excessively crying infants had an equal total sleeping time, a normal nocturnal sleep structure and similar sleep onset time.[48]

A more recent study used a 24-hour polysomnography (PSG) to compare between two groups, colicky and non-colicky infants, according to modified Wessel criteria. The study found that colicky infants had the same total sleep time as non-colicky infants, though sleep structure was somewhat different. The total REM sleep time in a 24-hour period was equal between the two groups, but the excessively crying infants had relatively less REM sleep during the evening, and they 'catch up' during the long night sleep, when they had a longer REM sleep compared to the control group.[49]

The studies described above used both PSG and diaries to assess infants' sleep time and compared the results. A clear discrepancy between diary reports and PSG results was revealed, as reported sleep time in the diary data for the control group was longer than the objectively observed sleep time. These findings suggest that research based on diary reports alone may be biased, and more objective studies are needed.

Infantile Colic and Sleep after the Age of Three Months

Another aspect studied is whether colicky infants have sleeping problems later on in life, after colic symptoms had subsided.

Some studies argued that formerly colicky infants had more night awakenings.[41,42] Others have found no significant differences in reported sleeping patterns.[50]

Canivet et al. approached mothers of ex-colicky infants and infants who did not have colic when the children were 4 years old and interrogated them about their children's sleep-related behaviors in several ways: (1) whether they went to sleep easily, (2) whether they talked and cried in sleep, (3) whether they did not mind going to bed, (4) frequency of nightmares,

and (5) being overtired. No differences were found in the two groups in any aspect.[31]

Again, these are all subjective reports. Kirjavainen et al. in the same research described above, examined also 6-month-old babies. There was no difference in reported sleeping time. Polysomnography showed more short awakenings (shorter than five minutes) in the control group, but other than that, the sleep was practically similar between the two groups.[48]

Explanations for a Possible Direct Relation

Few theories attempted to explain a possible direct relation between infantile colic and sleeping problems.

As crying and sleeping are mutually exclusive in nature, it is reasonable to think that crying bouts during sleeping hours may come at the expense of sleep itself. White et al. found that, in a group of colicky infants, there is an inverse relation between time spent crying and duration of sleep, though in non-colicky infants such a relationship did not exist. However, they also showed that when controlling for crying statistically, colicky infants still have a shorter nocturnal sleep time, though less dramatic than the original differences.[27]

The theory of excessive crying as a result of sleep deprivation was not supported by the aforementioned studies which used PSG. The proportion of sleep stages, the number of stage shifts, the total sleep time and number of sleep apneas of excessively crying infants were similar to the known structure of normal sleep for their age.[48,49]

As described above, there is a difference between the sleeping time as reported by parents and the actual sleeping time that was objectively measured, meaning that at least part of the real difference may not be in the sleeping habits of the infants but rather at their behavior during waking hours or how they are perceived by their parents. It is possible that while awake, 'non-colicky' infants stay quiet and soothe themselves back to sleep, making it hard to recognize their night wakening, in contrast to colicky infants who tend to cry or fuss. This ties in with the hypothesis that infant sleep–waking problems usually involve maintenance of signaling behaviors rather than a generalized disturbance.[47]

Another possible explanation is that parents of colicky infants are more stressed and more sensitive to their infant's night wakening and tend to describe their child as more difficult than it actually is.

Common Causes

The two nocturnal behaviors may not be dependent on each other, but may have common escalating factors. There are several potential such factors, which may influence both sleep and behavior and, when disturbed, result in both fragmented sleep and excessive crying/colic. The following is a brief discussion of such potential factors.

Circadian Disturbance

The circadian production of hormones such as cortisol and melatonin begins around the age of 6–8 weeks and a mature day–night-related secretion pattern is established by the age of 3–4 months,[51] the same age that nocturnal crying bouts and fragmented nocturnal sleep resolves. A difference in the nature of both behaviors in some infants may, in part, be attributed to a difference in day–night rhythmicity development.

Colicky and non-colicky infants were found to have similar average salivary cortisol levels during a 24-hour period, though infants with colic had a less clearly defined daily rhythm of cortisol secretion.[27]

Melatonin, 'the dark hormone,' has well-known sleep-promoting effects[52–54] as well as a relaxing effect on intestinal smooth muscle.[21,23] Therefore, it is possible that an earlier maturation of circadian melatonin secretion might play a role in the resolution of infantile colic and the consolidation of nocturnal sleep.

Feeding Method

The influence of feeding method on excessive crying and nocturnal sleep has been sparsely studied and the database in this matter is slim. Different studies which investigated the influence of breastfeeding on infantile colic had contradictory results.[45,55,56] As for the relation between feeding method and sleep–wake patterns of the infant, there are consistent findings suggesting that breastfed infants are more easily aroused and have a more fragmented nocturnal sleep.[22,57] There are not enough supporting data about the differences in the overall length of nocturnal sleep in order to make a solid conclusion.[55]

In our recent research, we found that exclusively breastfed infants had significantly fewer colic attacks and a decreased attack intensity when compared to exclusively formula-fed infants. We found that the breastfed infants, while waking up more often, tend to have an overall longer nocturnal sleep than formula-fed ones, though these results were not statistically significant.[22]

We also confirmed, as had been previously described, that breast milk contains melatonin while artificial formulas do not. Considering the aforementioned properties of melatonin, this provides a possible explanation to a common factor affecting both crying and nocturnal infantile sleep, as breastfed infants enjoy an extrinsic melatonin supplementation. More research in this area might be beneficial.

Cow Milk Protein Allergy

In the late 1980s, cow milk protein allergy was found to cause sleeping problems.[59–61] It is also believed to elicit colic symptoms, as described above. However, cow milk allergy is rare in comparison to both infant sleeping problems and infantile colic and therefore cannot indicate a common pathology.

Temperament

Infants with colic, using Wessel's criteria, are significantly more likely to have a difficult temperament than non-colicky babies, when the temperament assessment is performed at 4 months of age. Nonetheless, colic does not appear to be an expression of a permanently difficult temperament. Temperament assessments performed at a mean age of 3.6 months showed an association between problems of sleep–wake organization, difficult temperament, and extreme crying.[62]

In a study that assessed 105 infants at 4–5 months of age, those with difficult temperaments slept 12.8 hours and those with easy temperaments slept 14.9 hours.[63] It thus appears that infants who have a difficult temperament have briefer total sleep durations.

Group differences in sleep duration between colicky and non-colicky infants, and between easy and difficult infants, were observed to generally decrease over time.

Clinical Pearls

- Infantile colic is a common syndrome characterized by excessive crying. The most widely used definition is the one defined by Wessel in 1954: crying for more than 3 hours per day, for more than 3 days per week, and for longer than 3 weeks in an infant who is well fed and is otherwise healthy.
- Infantile colic is a transient, self-limiting condition, considered to have a favorable outcome, which resolves spontaneously by the age of 6 month.
- The etiology and pathogenesis remain an enigma. Many theories exist; most of them argue that a gastrointestinal disturbance causes the crying paroxysms. Other theories suggest that the crying bouts may be related to temperament and regulation.
- An organic disease is estimated to account for less than 5% of the cases; nevertheless, before making the diagnosis of infantile colic an organic cause must be ruled out.
- The differential diagnosis of excessive crying is wide, consisting of gastrointestinal, neurological, social, behavioral, respiratory and other factors.
- The main groups of interventional therapies are pharmacological, dietary and behavioral, based on the different possible etiologies/mechanisms. It is still not clear which is the optimal treatment and watchful waiting might just be the best approach, in addition to parental reassurance.
- There is an association between infantile colic and sleep problems, according to subjective parental testimonies. Some subjective studies supported the hypothesis that infants with colic tend to sleep less. This was confronted by objective studies using a PSG, showing no substantial differences compared to the known structure of normal sleep for their age.
- At least part of this discrepancy may not be in the sleeping habits of the infants but rather their behavior during waking hours or how they are perceived by their parents.
- The two nocturnal behaviors may not be dependent on each other, but rather have common escalating factors such as circadian disturbance, feeding method, cow milk protein allergy, temperament, etc.
- Melatonin has both sleep-promoting effects and a relaxing effect on the GI tract.
- Low levels of melatonin in early infancy may lead to both fragmented sleep and colic.

References

1. St James-Roberts I, Halil T. Infant crying patterns in the first year: normal community and clinical findings. J Child Psychol Psychiatry 1991;32(6):951–68.
2. Wessel MA, Cobb JC, Jackson EB, et al. Paroxysmal fussing in infancy, sometimes called colic. Pediatrics 1954;14(5):421–35.
3. Roberts DM, Ostapchuk M O'Brien JG. Infantile colic. Am Fam Phys 2004;70(4):735–40.
4. Herman M, Le A. The crying infant. Emerg Med Clin North Am 2007;25(4):1137–59, vii.
5. Lucassen PL, Assendelft W, van Eijk JT, et al. Systematic review of the occurrence of infantile colic in the community. Arch Dis Child 2001;84(5):398–403. Review.
6. Reijneveld SA, Brugman E, Hirasing RA. Excessive infant crying: the impact of varying definitions. Pediatrics 2001;108(4):893–7.
7. Barr RG. Colic and crying syndromes in infants. Pediatrics 1998;102(5 Suppl. E):1282–6.
8. Current diagnosis and treatment: Pediatrics 20e chapter 2, Child Development & Behavior. Edward Goldson, Ann Reynolds
9. Savino F. Focus on infantile colic. ActaPaediatr 2007;96(9):1259–64.
10. Brazelton TB. Crying in infancy. Pediatrics 1962;29 579–88.
11. St James-Roberts I. Persistent infant crying. Arch Dis Child 1991;66(5):653–5.

12. Sferra TJ, Heitlinger LA. Gastrointestinal gas formation and infantile colic. Pediatr Clin North Am 1996;43(2):489–510. Review.

13. Gupta SK. Is colic a gastrointestinal disorder? Curr Opin Pediatr 2002;14(5):588–92.

14. Garrison MM, Christakis DA. A systematic review of treatments for infant colic. Pediatrics 2000;106(1 Pt 2):184–90.

15. Savino F, Brondello C, Cresi F, et al. Cimetropium bromide in the treatment of crisis in infantile colic. J Pediatr Gastroenterol Nutr 2002;34(4):417–19.

16. Kirjavainen J, Jahnukainen T, Huhtala V, et al. The balance of the autonomic nervous system is normal in colicky infants. Acta Paediatr 2001;90(3):250–4.

17. Lothe L, Ivarsson SA, Ekman R, et al. Motilin and infantile colic. A prospective study. Acta Paediatr Scand 1990;79(4):410–16.

18. Ivarsson SA, Lindberg T. Motilin, vasoactive intestinal peptide and gastrin in infantile colic. Acta Paediatr Scand 1987;76(2):316–20.

19. Savino F, Grassino EC, Guidi C, et al. Gherlin and motilin concentration in colicky infants. Acta Paediatr 2006;95(6):738–41.

20. Kurtoglu S, Uzum K, Hallac IK, et al. 5 Hydroxy-3-indole acetic acid levels in infantile colic: Is serotoninergic tonus responsible for this problem? Acta Paediatr 1997;86:764–5.

21. Bubenik GA. Thirty four years since the discovery of gastrointestinal melatonin. J Physiol Pharmacol 2008;59(Suppl. 2):33–51.

22. Cohen-Engler A, Hadash A, Shehadeh N, et al. Breastfeeding may improve nocturnal sleep and reduce infantile colic: potential role of breast milk melatonin. Eur J Pediatr 2012;171(4):729–32.

23. Bubenik GA. Gastrointestinal melatonin: localization, function, and clinical relevance. Dig Dis Sci 2002;47(10):2336–48.

24. Douglas P, Hill P. Managing infants who cry excessively in the first few months of life. BMJ 2011;343:d7772.

25. Hill DJ, Hosking CS. Infantile colic and food hypersensitivity. J Pediatr Gastroenterol Nutr 2000;30(Suppl):67–76.

26. Iacono G, Carroccio A, Montaldo G. Severe infantile colic and food intolerance: a long-term prospective study. J Pediatr Gastroenterol Nutr 1991;12:332–5.

27. White BP, Gunnar MR, Larson MC, et al. Behavioral and physiological responsivity, sleep, and patterns of daily cortisol production in infants with and without colic. Child Dev 2000;71(4):862–77.

28. Reijneveld SA, Lanting CI, Crone MR, et al. Exposure to tobacco smoke and infant crying. Acta Paediatr 2005;94:217–21.

29. Shenassa ED, Brown MJ. Maternal smoking and infantile gastrointestinal dysregulation: the case of colic. Pediatrics 2004;114:497–505.

30. Rautava P, Lehtonen L, Helenius H, et al. Infantile colic: child and family three years later. Pediatrics 1995;96(1 Pt 1):43–7.

31. Canivet C, Jakobsson I, Hagander B. Infantile colic. Follow-up at four years of age: still more "emotional". Acta Paediatr 2000;89(1):13–17.

32. Freedman SB, Al-Harthy N, Thull-Freedman J. The crying infant: Diagnosis testing and frequency of serious underlying disease. Pediatrics 2009;123(3):841–8.

33. Garrison MM, Christakis DA. A systematic review of treatments for infant colic. Pediatrics 2000;106(1 Pt 2):184–90.

34. Lucassen PL, Assendelft WJ, Gubbels JW, et al. Effectiveness of treatments for infantile colic: systematic review. BMJ 1998;316(7144):1563–9.

35. Treem WR, Hyams JS, Blankschen E, et al. Evaluation of the effect of a fiber-enriched formula on infant colic. J Pediatr 1991;119(5):695–701.

36. Williams J, Watkins-Jones R. Dicyclomine: worrying symptoms associated with its use in some small babies. Br Med J (Clin Res Ed) 1984;288(6421):901.

37. Savino F, Brondello C, Cresi F, et al. Cimetropium bromide in the treatment of crisis in infantile colic. J Pediatr Gastroenterol Nutr 2002;34(4):417–19.

38. Savino F, Pelle E, Palumeri E, et al. *Lactobacillus reuteri* (American type culture collection strain 55730) versus simethicone in the treatment of infantile colic: a prospective randomized study. Pediatrics 2007;119:e124.

39. Hunziker UA, Barr RG. Increased carrying reduces infant crying: a randomized controlled trial. Pediatrics 1986;77(5):641–8.

40. Parkin PC, Schwartz CJ, Manuel BA. Randomized controlled trial of three interventions in the management of persistent crying of infancy. Pediatrics 1993;92(2):197–201.

41. Weissbluth M, Davis AT, Poncher J. Night waking in 4- to 8-month-old infants. J Pediatr 1984;104(3):477–80.

42. Ståhlberg MR. Infantile colic: occurrence and risk factors. Eur J Pediatr 1984;143(2):108–11.

43. Rautava P, Lehtonen L, Helenius H, et al. Infantile colic: child and family three years later. Pediatrics 1995;96(1 Pt 1):43–7.

44. Sadeh A. Assessment of intervention for infant night waking: parental reports and activity-based home monitoring. J Consult Clin Psychol 1994;62:63–8.

45. Crowcroft NS, Strachan DP. The social origins of infantile colic: questionnaire study covering 76,747 infants. BMJ 1997;314(7090):1325–8.

46. St James-Roberts I, Conroy S, Hurry J. Links between infant crying and sleep-waking at six weeks of age. Early Hum Dev 1997;48(1–2):143–52.

47. St James-Roberts I, Peachey E. Distinguishing infant prolonged crying from sleep-waking problems. Arch Dis Child 2011;96(4):340–4.

48. Kirjavainen J, Kirjavainen T, Huhtala V, et al. Infants with colic have a normal sleep structure at 2 and 7 months of age. J Pediatr 2001;138(2):218–23.

49. Kirjavainen J, Lehtonen L, Kirjavainen T, et al. Sleep of excessively crying infants: a 24-hour ambulatory sleep polygraphy study. Pediatrics 2004;114(3):592–600.

50. Lehtonen L, Korhonen T, Korvenranta H. Temperament and sleeping patterns in colicky infants during the first year of life. J Dev Behav Pediatr 1994;15(6):416–20.

51. Larson MC, White BP, Cochran A, et al. Dampening of the cortisol response to handling at 3 months in human infants and its relation to sleep, circadian cortisol activity, and behavioral distress. Dev Psychobiol 1998;33(4):327–37.

52. Doghramji K. Melatonin and its receptors: a new class of sleep-promoting agents. J Clin Sleep Med 2007;3(Suppl. 5):S17–23.

53. Lavie P. Sleep-wake as a biological rhythm. Annu Rev Psychol 2001;52:277–303.

54. Cajochen C, Kräuchi K, Wirz-Justice A. Role of melatonin in the regulation of human circadian rhythms and sleep. J Neuroendocrinol 2003;15(4):432–7.

55. Saavedra MA, da Costa JS, Garcias G, et al. Infantile colic incidence and associated risk factors: a cohort study. J Pediatr (Rio J) 2003;79(2):115–22.

56. Lucassen PL, Assendelft WJ, van Eijk JT, et al. Systematic review of the occurrence of infantile colic in the community. Arch Dis Child 2001;84(5):398–403.

57. Eaton-Evans J, Dugdale AE. Sleep patterns of infants in the first year of life. Arch Dis Child 1988;63(6):647–9.

58. Rosen LA. Infant sleep and feeding. J Obstet Gynecol Neonatal Nurs 2008;37(6):706–14.

59. Kahn A, François G, Sottiaux M, et al. Sleep characteristics in milk-intolerant infants. Sleep 1988;11(3):291–7. abstract.

60. Kahn A, Mozin MJ, Rebuffat E, et al. Milk intolerance in children with persistent sleeplessness: a prospective double-blind crossover evaluation. Pediatrics 1989;84(4):595–603.

61. Kahn A, Rebuffat E, Blum D, et al. Difficulty in initiating and maintaining sleep associated with cow's milk allergy in infants. Sleep 1987;10(2):116–21.

62. Papousek M, von Hofacker N. Persistent crying in early infancy: a non-trivial condition of risk for the developing mother-infant relationship. Child Care Health Dev 1998;24(5):395–424.

63. Weissbluth M, Liu K. Sleep patterns, attention span, and infant temperament. J Dev Behav Pediatr 1983;4(1):34–6.

Sleep and Gastroesophageal Reflux

R. Bradley Troxler and Susan M. Harding

Chapter 11

INTRODUCTION

Gastroesophageal reflux disease (GERD) is common in children of all ages and can impact sleep. In infants, it is the most common GI problem presenting to the pediatrician's office.[1] Despite its high prevalence, minimal research is available examining the impact of GERD on sleep in children.

Gastroesophageal reflux (GER) is the retrograde passage of gastric contents into the esophagus and it is normally seen post-prandially. Regurgitation is a symptom of GER and is common in infants.[2] The refluxate is acidic and contains digestive enzymes that can injure the mucosal lining of the esophagus and upper airway. Intrinsic protective mechanisms exist to prevent or minimize this damage. Reflux becomes pathologic GERD when GER episodes are more frequent and produce symptoms including heartburn, esophagitis, failure to thrive, or respiratory symptoms such as cough and wheeze.[2]

We will discuss esophageal physiology during wakefulness and sleep, along with the epidemiology and clinical manifestations of GERD, and its impact on sleep in pediatric populations. The diagnosis and treatment of GERD in pediatric populations and future directions in sleep-related GERD research will be discussed.

ESOPHAGEAL PHYSIOLOGY

The esophagus develops initially during the fourth week of gestation as a small outgrowth of the endoderm and later includes all three germ layers: the endoderm, mesoderm, and ectoderm. These layers give rise, respectively, to the epithelial lining; muscular layers, angioblast, and mesenchyme; and the neural components.[3]

The esophagus slowly increases its length so that at 20 weeks of gestation, esophageal length approximates 11 cm.[4] Esophageal length doubles during the first year of life.[3] Ultimately, the esophageal body in adults has a length of 18–22 cm, with the lower esophageal sphincter (LES) representing the distal 2–4 cm of the esophagus.[5] The LES grows from a few millimeters in newborns and reaches its adult length during adolescence. In older children, the proximal 1.5–2 cm of the LES is encircled by the crural diaphragm and sits in the thoracic cavity, and the lower 2 cm resides in the abdominal cavity.[5]

The esophagus consists of three functionally distinct zones, including the upper esophageal sphincter (UES), the esophageal body, and the lower esophageal sphincter (LES).[3]

The UES is an intraluminal high-pressure zone located between the pharynx and the cervical esophagus. The anterior wall includes the posterior surface of the cricoid cartilage, the arytenoid cartilage, and the interarytenoid muscles. The posterior wall includes the cricopharyngeus and thyropharyngeus muscles. The UES prevents refluxate from getting into the

upper airway, and it prevents air from entering the esophagus during inspiration. The UES opens during belching, rumination, deglutition, regurgitation, and vomiting.[5]

The esophageal body begins at the edge of the cricopharyngeal muscle and, in adults, is comprised of striated skeletal muscle for the first 4–5 cm, followed by a transitional zone that contains both skeletal muscle and smooth muscle cells. The distal 10–14 cm comprises smooth muscle cells.[3]

The LES is a high-pressure zone controlling the flow of materials between the esophagus and the stomach. The LES comprises an intrinsic muscular layer (intrinsic LES) and the extrinsic LES, which is the crural diaphragm.[5] These two components of the LES are superimposed and linked together by the phrenoesophageal ligament. Both the intrinsic and extrinsic components of the LES contribute to LES competence. The LES is tonically contracted at rest and relaxes with esophageal distention and deglutination. The crural diaphragm portion of the LES creates spike-like increases in LES pressure during inspiration and relaxes with esophageal distention and vomiting.[5]

The esophagus accomplishes its role as a conduit to move food from the mouth to the stomach through peristalsis. The esophagus exhibits three different forms of peristalsis: primary peristalsis, secondary peristalsis, and deglutitive inhibition.[6]

Primary peristalsis is a reflex esophageal contraction that is initiated by swallowing and a contraction wave that moves from the pharynx to the stomach. This propulsive force is caused by the sequential contraction of the esophageal muscle layers. In children, the typical amplitude of the contraction ranges between 40 and 89 mmHg, has a duration of 2.5–5 seconds, and a propagation velocity of 3.0 cm/second.[7,3]

Secondary peristalsis occurs with esophageal luminal distention and is not associated with a swallow. It helps remove refluxate that was not cleared with primary peristalsis.[6]

Deglutitive inhibition results when a second swallow is initiated while a prior peristalsis is still occurring. This results in complete inhibition of the peristaltic contraction caused by the first swallow. With successive swallows, the esophagus remains in stasis until a final swallow produces a large 'clearing wave' that sweeps the esophagus of its contents.[6]

The LES is constantly adapting to the changing pressure gradients between the stomach and the esophagus in order to maintain competency. During inspiration, the pressure gradient between the stomach and esophagus is 4–6 mmHg and is countered by an LES pressure between 10 and 35 mmHg. During the migrating motor complex of esophageal contractions, the LES vigorously contracts to prevent reflux of stomach contents into the esophagus. During inspiration, there is an increasingly negative intra-esophageal pressure, while abdominal muscle contractions augment gastric pressure. Both of these situations increase the pressure gradient, predisposing to GER events. However, the contraction of the crural diaphragm during abdominal muscle contraction, vomiting, or straining helps to prevent reflux.[5] In addition to

TABLE 11.1 Factors that Influence Lower Esophageal (LES) Pressure and Transient Lower Esophageal Sphincter Relaxation (TLESR) Frequency.[9]

	INCREASES LES PRESSURE	DECREASES LES PRESSURE	INCREASES TLESR FREQUENCY	DECREASES TLESR FREQUENCY
Food(s)	Protein	Fat, chocolate, ethanol, peppermint	Fat	
Hormone(s)	Gastrin, motilin, substance P	Secretin, cholecystokinin, glucagon, gastric inhibitory polypeptide, vasoactive intestinal polypeptide, progesterone	Cholecystokinin	
Neural agent(s)	α-Adrenergic agonists, β-adrenergic antagonists, cholinergic agonists	α-Adrenergic antagonists, β-adrenergic agonists, cholinergic antagonists, serotonin	L-Arginine	Baclofen, metabotropic glutamate receptor antagonists, cannaboid receptor agonists, L-NAME, serotonin
Medication(s)	Metoclopramide, domperidone, prostaglandin F2α, cisapride	Nitrates, calcium chanel blockers, theophylline, morphine, meperidinem, diazepam, barbituates	Sumatriptan	Atropine, morphine, loxiglumide

L-NAME, N(G)-nitro-L-arginine methyl ester.

Reprinted with permission from Wiley-Blackwell, publisher: From Kahrilas P, Pandolfino J. Esophageal Motor Function. In: Yamada, T, editor. Textbook of Gastroenterology. Hoboken NJ: Wiley-Blackwell; 2009. p. 187–206.[9]

abdominal and intrathoracic pressures, the LES pressure is influenced by many other factors, as listed in Table 11.1.[9]

During swallowing, the LES relaxes within 1–2 seconds of the primary peristaltic contraction and this relaxation lasts approximately 5–10 seconds. When the bolus arrives at the LES, the LES pressure declines to gastric pressure, and the sphincter remains closed. Then, the intrabolus pressure forces the LES to open and the bolus enters the stomach. After 5–7 seconds, the LES rebounds to its original pressure and the LES undergoes an after-contraction, which ends the peristaltic contraction wave.[6]

Gas is vented from the stomach by belching, where there is a transient relaxation of the LES (TLESR). TLESRs are abrupt declines in the LES pressure to gastric pressure that are not related to primary peristalsis, secondary peristalsis, or swallowing. There is also inhibition of the crural diaphragm with TLESRs.[10] TLESRs have a typical duration of 10–45 seconds. TLESRs occur up to six times per hour in normal adults and are more frequent immediately post-prandially. They occur during arousals but not during stable sleep.[11]

TLESRs can be triggered by gastric distention or vagal stimulation that occurs with endotracheal intubation. Gamma-amino-butyric acid (GABA) serves as an inhibitor of TLESRs.[5] Table 11.1 also reviews factors influencing TLESRs.[9]

LES pressures in children range between 10 and 40 mmHg. LES pressures that are 5 mmHg above the intragastric pressure are usually sufficient to prevent GER.[5,12] LES motor patterns in infants and children are similar to those observed in adults.[5]

MECHANISMS OF GASTROESOPHAGEAL REFLUX

Gastroesophageal reflux occurs when intra-abdominal pressure exceeds intrathoracic pressure and the LES barrier. GER is prevented by normal LES function. The intra-abdominal

portion of the esophagus is squeezed closed by abdominal pressure. In addition, the acuity of the angle where the esophagus enters the stomach (angle of His) serves as a component of the barrier at the gastroesophageal junction. A compromise in this region, as seen in hiatal hernia, predisposes to GER.[5]

The majority (81% to 100%) of GER episodes in infants, children, and adults are caused by TLESRs.[13] Omari et al noted that 82% of GER episodes in premature infants and 91% of GER episodes in term infants occurred in association with TLESRs.[14,15] Kawahara et al. noted TLESRs in association with 58% to 69% of GER episodes in children being evaluated for GERD.[13]

Protective mechanisms limit damage to the esophagus and airway. Immediately after the refluxate enters the lower esophagus, the UES contracts to prevent entry into the pharynx. Secondary peristalsis also occurs, which helps clear the refluxate. Saliva, which contains bicarbonate, is then swallowed, neutralizing any adherent acidic remnants. Finally, mucosal glands in the esophagus produce mucus and bicarbonate, limiting esophageal mucosal damage.[6]

Airway protective mechanisms include the UES reflex, whose function depends on refluxate volume. Small refluxate volumes result in UES contraction, while large volumes stimulate a vagally mediated relaxation of the UES, allowing the refluxate to enter the pharynx. Simultaneously, this vagal response evokes a centrally mediated apnea with laryngeal closure to prevent aspiration. In older children, apnea is not provoked, but a coughing spell occurs in this situation.[16]

ESOPHAGEAL PHYSIOLOGY DURING SLEEP

Sleep and the circadian rhythm alter upper gastroesophageal function. Gastric acid secretion peaks between 8 p.m. and 1 a.m.[11] Gastric myoelectric function is disrupted by sleep, resulting in delayed gastric emptying.[11] There is also delayed esophageal acid clearance during sleep. These factors predispose to GER during sleep.

The UES pressure decreases with sleep onset. Kahrilas et al. reported that UES pressure decreases from 40 ± 17 mmHg during wakefulness to 20 ± 17 mmHg during N1 sleep, and was lowest (8 ± 3 mmHg) during N3 sleep.[17] The UES contractile reflex is also altered during sleep. The UES contractile reflex is triggered by smaller volumes of refluxate during REM sleep, and does not occur during N3 sleep.[18] The UES reflex is preempted by coughing and/or arousal. Basal LES pressure does not change during sleep. The frequency of TLESRs declines during sleep time. Almost all TLESRs occur during wakefulness or during brief arousals from sleep.[18]

In addition, swallowing frequency decreases by 50% to 80% during sleep time compared to wakefulness.[11] Similar to TLESRs, swallowing occurs during arousals and is almost nonexistent during stable sleep.[19] Salivary secretion is not detectable during stable sleep.[11] Esophageal acid clearance is also delayed during sleep. Orr et al. observed that 15 mL of 0.1 N HCl was cleared from the distal esophagus within 25 minutes during sleep, whereas it took only 6 minutes to clear when awake.[19] Sleep prolongs the latency to the first swallow if esophageal acid is present. Finally, during sleep, 40% of the refluxate reaches the proximal esophagus near the UES compared to <1% during wakefulness.[20] This, in addition to the lower UES pressure during sleep, might predispose to microaspiration of refluxate into the pharynx.

Despite the lack of some GERD-protective mechanisms during sleep, individual GER events are much less frequent during sleep than during wake. However, if GER occurs, the events are of a longer duration, and are more likely to result in esophagitis and Barrett's esophagus.[11]

GASTROESOPHAGEAL REFLUX DISEASE (GERD)

Gastroesophageal reflux disease is a common pediatric illness and has protean manifestations.[21] GERD can present with recurrent vomiting (regurgitation), poor weight gain, heartburn, chest pain, esophagitis, vomiting, Sandifer syndrome, hematemesis, anemia, Barrett's esophagus, esophageal adenocarcinoma, asthma exacerbation, chronic cough, acute life-threatening events (ALTEs), recurrent pneumonia, sleep apnea, and dental erosions.[2,22] A prospective Italian study documents that 12% of infants had regurgitation and 1% of children met criteria for GERD.[23] Among US adolescents, aged 10 to 17 years, 5.2% reported heartburn and 8.2% reported acid regurgitation during the previous week.[24] GERD is also more frequent during early childhood when large fluid boluses are used for feeding.[2]

Adolescents and older children experience similar clinical presentations as adults with GERD. Typical complaints include heartburn, dyspepsia, and regurgitation. Gupta et al. described the presenting symptoms of GERD in pediatric patients.[22] The most common symptoms included abdominal pain (70%), regurgitation (69%), and cough (69%). In patients between 1 and 36 months of age, symptoms of GERD included regurgitation (98%), irritability (41%), feeding problems (10%), failure to thrive (7%) and respiratory problems (18.6%).[22] Toddlers and younger children (less than 6 years) more likely reported cough, anorexia/food refusal, and vomiting.[22] In a Finnish study examining children with GERD

(mean age 6.7 years), the presenting symptoms included abdominal pain (63%), heartburn (34%), regurgitation (22%), vomiting (16%), retrosternal pain (18%), and respiratory symptoms (29%).[25] Adolescents with GERD reported esophageal symptoms (22.4%), regurgitation (21.4%), dysphagia (14.5%), shortness of breath (24.4%), wheezing (1.7%), and cough (17.9%).[26]

Extra-esophageal manifestations of GERD are also present in children.[27] El-Serag et al. compared 1980 children with GERD (mean age 9.2 years) to a control group without GERD, examining the association of GERD with upper and lower respiratory disorders.[27] They demonstrated that children with GERD were more likely to have sinusitis (4.2% vs. 1.4%), laryngitis (0.7% vs. 0.2%), asthma (13.2% vs. 6.8%), pneumonia (6.3% vs. 2.3%), and bronchiectasis (1.0% vs. 0.1%). After adjusting for age, gender, and ethnicity, GERD remained associated with all of these conditions.[27]

SLEEP-RELATED GERD

Sleep-related GERD

Sleep-related GERD may present with nocturnal awakenings with a sour taste in the mouth, burning discomfort in the chest, or nocturnal arousals. These arousals may disrupt sleep, leading to daytime sleepiness or insomnia.[11]

Few studies examine the epidemiology, severity, or range of clinical impact that is associated with sleep-related GERD in children. In children, GERD during sleep is associated with increased sleep arousals, sleep fragmentation, and other sleep disturbances.[21] Kahn et al. evaluated 50 infants with occasional regurgitation and noted that 41 of the 50 infants had proximal GER events, with 97 episodes occurring during sleep time. Reflux during sleep time occurred commonly during wakefulness (41%) or was associated with arousals.[28] This study did not determine whether arousals led to the reflux or if the reflux led to the arousal from sleep.[28] Ghaem et al. examined 72 children with GERD and 3102 controls, with a questionnaire, finding that children with GERD (aged 3 to 12 months) were less likely to have ever slept through the night by 12 months of age (20%) compared to the controls.[29] Fifty percent of GERD children awakened and required parental attention more than three times nightly. These findings continued in children with GERD aged 12–24 months and 24–36 months, with only 8% and 4% sleeping through the night compared to 45% and 56% of controls. Sixty percent of 12–24-month-olds and 50% of 24–36-month-olds with GERD woke up more than three times nightly. Children with GERD had more awakenings and were less likely to sleep through the night.[29]

A prospective randomized, controlled study in adolescents with GERD (ages 12 to 17 years) assessed the impact of 8 weeks of a proton pump inhibitor (esomeprazole) on quality of life (QOL) using the Quality of Life in Reflux and Dyspepsia Questionnaire.[30] After 8 weeks of PPI, there was an improvement in the sleep dysfunction domains of the QOL instrument in the PPI-treated group. These findings suggest that GERD treatment may improve sleep in adolescents.[30]

Obstructive Sleep Apnea

Both GERD and obstructive sleep apnea (OSA) share confounding variables and risk factors, including obesity.[11] The relationship between sleep-related GERD and OSA was assessed by Wasilewska and Kaczmarski with simultaneous esophageal pH monitoring and polysomnography in 24 children (ages 2 to 36 months) with sleep disturbances indicative of GERD and possible sleep-disordered breathing.[31] Children with sleep-related GERD had a higher REM apnea–hypopnea index (AHI) (23.4 events per hour) compared to children without sleep-related GERD (AHI: 4.9 events per hour). These observations suggest that GERD is associated with more severe OSA during early childhood.[31]

The impact of sleep-related GERD among children aged 6 to 12 years was assessed by Noronha et al.[32] Eighteen children with OSAS and tonsilar hypertrophy were evaluated with polysomnography with concomitant esophageal pH monitoring and the OSA-18 Questionnaire. The AHI was greater than 1.0 for all patients and 41.1% of patients had esophageal pH values below 4 for more than 10% of sleep time. The esophageal pH values correlated with emotional distress and daytime problems on the OSA-18. A temporal correlation between individual GER events and apnea–hypopnea events was not apparent.[32]

A second study, by Wasilewska et al., assessed 57 children with OSA, 19 of whom had residual OSA after prior adenotonsillectomy, using pH monitoring and polysomnography to determine the risks for residual OSA. Compared to newly diagnosed patients, children with residual OSA had more severe OSA (AHI 20.61 versus 8.57, $p=0.03$), lower mean intraluminal esophageal pH (5.36 versus 5.86, $p=0.007$), higher reflux index (9.67% versus 4.35%, $p=0.006$), and a lower minimum esophageal pH during sleep (1.53 versus 2.15, $p=0.04$). The minimal value of esophageal pH was noted to correlate with respiratory indices on the polysomnography, a particularly interesting finding as this value is often not reported and is not required to diagnose GER.[33]

Asthma, Laryngospasm, Hoarseness

Sleep-related GERD can trigger asthma and/or laryngospasm during sleep. There is an association between GERD and asthma but the direction of causality is not known, and may be bi-directional. Proposed mechanisms of interaction include microaspiration and a vagally mediated reflex bronchoconstriction.[11] A systematic review assessed the association of pediatric asthma and GERD.[34] Twenty articles met the *a priori* inclusion criteria. Estimates of GERD prevalence in children with asthma ranged from 19.3% to 80.0%. Five studies compared 1314 asthma patients to 2434 controls. Based on these data, the average GERD prevalence in pediatric asthmatics was 22.0% compared to 4.8% in the controls. The pooled odds ratio (OR) for having GERD in the asthma group was 5.6 (95% confidence interval (CI) of 4.3–6.9).[34]

A prospective cohort of 1037 New Zealanders was examined for GER symptoms and airway responsiveness at ages 11 years and 26 years.[35] GER symptoms that were at least 'moderately bothersome' were associated with asthma (OR 3.2, 95% CI 1.7–7.2), wheeze (OR 4.3, 95% CI 2.1–8.7), and nocturnal cough (OR 4.3, 95% CI 2.1–8.7) independent of body mass index. Women with GER symptoms were more likely to have airflow obstruction. The direction of causality is not clear since patients with airway hyper-responsiveness at age 11 were more likely to report GER symptoms at age 26.[35]

The effect of GERD therapy on asthma outcomes shows conflicting data in children.[36,37] Khoshoo and Haydel described

44 pediatric asthmatics with GERD who were treated with omeprazole and metoclopramide, ranitidine, or fundoplication.[36] Patients treated with omeprazole/metoclopramide or fundoplication had significantly fewer asthma exacerbations (0.33 and 0.66) over 6 months compared to patients on ranitidine (2.2).[36] Antithetically, Størdal et al. performed a randomized trial utilizing omeprazole or placebo for 12 weeks in 38 children with asthma and GERD (mean age 10.8 years).[37] After 12 weeks, esophageal acid contact times decreased in the omeprazole group, but there were no differences in the asthma symptom score, lung function, or number of rescue beta-agonist uses between groups.[37] More information regarding the association between GERD and asthma in children is needed.

Sleep-related GERD may be associated with laryngeal findings as the acidic refluxate migrates into the larynx. Block and Brodsky reported a retrospective review of 337 children (mean age 7.2 years) with hoarseness.[38] Eighty-eight percent had laryngeal reflux and 30% had cough. Among the patients with cough and hoarseness (99 patients), 66% were found to have GERD. Also, 50% of patients who were treated for GERD utilizing a variety of behavioral and medical therapies had improvement or resolution of their hoarseness at 3 months, and 68% had resolution by 4.5 months.[37]

Acute Life-Threatening Events (ALTEs)

Acute life-threatening events are episodes occurring in infants that are frightening to the observer. Findings include apnea, color change, sudden limpness, and/or choking and gagging. Many disorders are implicated in ALTEs including seizures, infections, arrhythmias, and GERD.[39] In a systematic review of 2912 publications including 643 infants with ALTEs, GERD was diagnosed in 227 (35%) infants, seizures in 83 (13%), lower respiratory tract infection in 58 (9%), and in 169 (26%) infants, no diagnosis was made.[39] Despite the high prevalence of GERD, there are few data to support the role of GERD in ALTEs.[39] Molloy et al. noted that there is rarely a temporal relationship between GERD events and apnea in premature infants.[40] Finally, Semeniuk et al. evaluated 264 patients aged 4 to 102 months with GERD and found 8 patients with symptoms of ALTEs. They describe GERD as a causative factor of ALTEs in only 4.8% of their cohort.[41]

GERD DIAGNOSIS

For patients presenting with stereotypical features of sleep-related GERD, a thorough history and physical examination are sufficient to make the diagnosis.[2] Questions directed at the frequency of nighttime awakenings, substernal chest pain, indigestion, heartburn, nocturnal cough or choking, or chronic vomiting should lead to the diagnosis in most older children or adolescents.[2] Other patients may have only extra-esophageal symptoms and present with excessive daytime sleepiness without an obvious historical cause, or waking up with laryngospasm, wheeze, or cough. Additionally, patients may note refluxate on their pillows.[11] However, historical findings do not discriminate patients with esophagitis.[2]

Esophageal pH monitoring identifies acid GER episodes, and can be used in patients without typical GER symptoms. Esophageal pH monitoring is performed by placing a pH probe at a level corresponding to 87% of the nares–LES distance, based on published regression equations, by fluoroscopy or through manometric measurement of the LES location. Interpretation of the results involves calculating the reflux index, which is the percentage of the recording time when esophageal pH falls below 4.0. The mean upper limit of normal is 12% in children up to 11 months, and 6% in children and adults.[2] The test is performed over 24 hours to increase the test's sensitivity and specificity, which approximates 90%.[42] The reproducibility of the test ranges between 69–85%.[42] Additionally, esophageal pH monitoring can be integrated with polysomnography to allow unified visualization of the patient's sleep and esophageal pH.[11]

Esophageal electrical impedance monitoring allows for the detection of liquid and gas in the esophagus, regardless of pH.[11] It is commonly combined with pH monitoring. Since a large number of GER events, especially post-prandial GER, are non-acidic, this technology allows for detection of more GER episodes. This technology is expensive, however, and requires a high degree of skill to interpret and has not been widely available to date. In addition, the clinical importance of non-acidic GER on sleep is unclear.[11]

GERD TREATMENT

Management options for GERD include non-pharmacologic behavioral interventions, medical therapy, and surgical therapy. Appropriate treatment requires a thorough knowledge of chrono-therapeutic principles in order to obtain optimal control of GERD.[2] Figure 11-1 reviews behavioral and medical therapy of GERD in children.[2]

Behavioral Interventions

Behavioral interventions during early childhood include formula thickening, positioning changes, nasogastric/nasojejunal feeds, and elevation of the head of the bed by 30 degrees during sleep.[2] Milk thickening agents decrease regurgitation that aids in weight gain. However, these agents did not improve esophageal acid contact times, number of reflux episodes lasting greater than 5 minutes, or number of reflux episodes per hour.[43] Positioning may also prevent GER episodes in infants. Tobin et al. studied 24 infants with GERD less than 5 months old with esophageal pH monitoring while being placed in different positions.[44] Esophageal acid contact times were greatest in the supine position (15.3%) and lowest in the prone position (6.7%). There are conflicting data regarding the benefit of elevating the head of the bed by 30 degrees. The authors note that the left decubitis position (esophageal acid contact time 7.7%) is a suitable alternative to prone positioning for the postural management of infants with symptomatic GERD.[44] Note that this recommendation is in contrast to the American Academy of Pediatrics recommendation that infants should sleep in the supine position.[45] Supine positioning confers the lowest risk of SIDS and is the preferred sleeping position for infants. Prone positioning should only be considered in unusual cases where the risk of complications from GERD outweighs the potential of SIDS.[2]

The efficacy of non-pharmacological therapy in infant GERD was recently evaluated by Orenstein and McGowan.[46] Caregivers of infants implemented a program utilizing GER feeding modifications, positioning, and tobacco smoke avoidance. Outcomes included the Infant Gastroesophageal Reflux Questionnaire-Revised. Among the 37 infants followed, GER scores improved in 59%, and 24% of patients no longer met diagnostic criteria for GERD after 2 weeks.[46]

Behavioral interventions during childhood and adolescence include weight management, dietary changes, sleep positional therapy, and smoking cessation.[11] There are minimal data examining behavioral therapy in children. Medications that can decrease LES pressure or increase the likelihood of GERD include theophylline, anticholinergics, prostaglandins, calcium channel blockers, and alendronate.[11] Avoidance of these medications should be considered; however, there are no data in children examining the impact of these medications on GERD.

Pharmacological Therapy

Pharmacological treatment of GERD includes gastric acid secretion inhibitors and prokinetic agents. Antacids have major side effects and toxicities in children and are not recommended.[2] Furthermore, H_2 receptor antagonists are associated with side effects and are not recommended for long-term treatment in children.[2] Also, currently available prokinetic agents should not be used in children.[2] Proton pump inhibitors are used and are well tolerated in children.

Histamine-2 Receptor Antagonists

Histamine-2 receptor antagonists (H_2RAs) inhibit the histamine-2 receptor of the gastric parietal cell and decrease gastric acid secretion. H_2RAs have a relatively quick onset of action and are useful for episodic symptom relief. A systematic evaluation of the side effects of H_2RAs in children has not been performed. Commonly used H_2RAs include famotidine, cimetidine, nizatidine, and ranitidine. Famotidine, the most commonly studied H_2RA, has been shown to cause agitation and signs concerning for headaches in infants.[47] Other side effects include dizziness, constipation, anemia, and urticaria. Cimetidine has been associated with gynecomastia, neutropenia, thrombocytopenia, and reduces the hepatic metabolism of medications such as theophylline.[2] Tolerance to the H_2RA class of medications does develop in both children and adults. Thus, H_2RAs are not ideal for chronic therapy for GERD in pediatric populations.

Proton Pump Inhibitors

Proton pump inhibitors (PPIs) inhibit the hydrogen–potassium ATPase channels that are the final step in gastric acid secretion. PPIs bind covalently with the cysteine residues of the hydrogen–potassium ATPase pump. PPIs are more effective at suppression of acidic secretions than the H_2RAs.[11] Commonly used PPIs include omeprazole, lansoprazole, pantoprazole, rabeprazole, and esomeprazole. There is some variation in the rates of activation and plasma half-life with the different PPIs; however, average half-life approximates 1–2 hours. Due to covalent bonding to the ATPase pump, the duration of action ranges from 15 hours for lansoprazole to 28 hours for omeprazole, and 46 hours for pantoprazole. PPIs are slow to achieve steady-state inhibition and generally require 3 days to achieve maximum impact. Children, ages 1 to 10 years, metabolize PPIs faster than adults and require a higher per kilogram dose compared to adults.[48] PPIs should be tapered and not discontinued abruptly as this would result in gastric acid hypersecretion.

	Infants (Less than 12 months old)	Children (1–12 years old)	Adolescents (12–18 years old)
Behavioral interventions **Medical Interventions**	Hydrolyzed protein formula for 2–4 weeks Thickening formula decreases number of regurgitation episodes Prone positioning is best for GERD, but supine position recommended due to risk of SIDS	No evidence to support dietary restriction in children or adolescents Adult studies support limiting late night eating Weight loss if obese Avoid foods that decrease LES tone (peppermint, caffeine, chocolate, alcohol, high-fat meals)	

Gastric Anti-secretory Therapy (Histamine-2 Receptor Antagonists)

Cimetidine	10–20 mg/kg/day PO div Q8–12 hours	20–40 mg/kg/day PO div Q6H	1600 mg/day PO div Q6-12 hours
Famotidine	<3 mos: 0.5 mg/kg/day PO 3–12 mos: 1 mg/kg/day PO div BID	1–2 mg/kg/day div BID max 40 mg/day	20–40 mg PO BID
Nizatidine	>6 mos: 5–10 mg/kg/day PO div BID	5–10 mg/kg/day PO div BID	150 mg PO BID, max 300 mg per day
Ranitidine	5–10 mg/kg/day PO div BID; max 300 mg/day	5–10 mg/kg/day PO div BID; max 300 mg/day	150 mg po BID

Gastric Anti-secretory Therapy (Proton-Pump Inhibitors)*

Esomeprazole	Not approved	1–11 yr: 10 mg PO QD	20–40 mg PO QD
Lansoprazole	Not approved	<30 kg: 15 mg PO QD >30 kg: 30 mg PO QD	15–30 mg PO QD
Omeprazole	Not approved	10–20 kg: 10 mg PO QD or 1 mg/kg/day PO div BID >20 kg: 20 mg PO QD	20 mg PO QD
Pantoprazole	Not approved	>5 yrs: 15–40 kg: 20 mg PO QD >40 kg: 40 mg PO QD	20–40 mg PO QD
Rabeprazole	Not approved	Not approved	20–40 mg PO QD

Gastric Acid Buffers/Barriers (Antacids, Alginate, Sucralfate)
Not recommended in chronic therapy as safe and convenient alternatives exist (H_2RAs and PPIs)

Prokinetic therapies (Cisapride, bethanachol, baclofen, metoclopramide)
Currently insufficient evidence to justify the use of these agents in the treatment of GERD

FIGURE 11-1 Summary of behavioral and medical therapies for pediatric GERD. *Preferred therapy. *Adapted from Vandenplas Y, Rudolph CD, Di Lorenzo C, et al. Pediatric gastroesophageal reflux clinical practice guidelines: joint recommendations of the North American Society for Pediatric Gastroenterology, Hepatology, and Nutrition (NASPGHAN) and the European Society for Pediatric Gastroenterology, Hepatology, and Nutrition (ESPGHAN). J Pediatr Gastroenterol Nutr 2009;49(4):498–547.*[2]

Minor side effects occur in 1–3% of patients on PPIs and include headache, diarrhea, abdominal pain, nausea, and rash. Major side effects are rare and include interstitial nephritis with omeprazole, hepatitis with omeprazole or lansoprazole, and visual disturbances with pantoprazole and omeprazole.[49]

There is a high frequency of nocturnal acid breakthrough among children on PPIs. Pfefferkorn et al. studied 18 children with esophagitis (mean age of 10.3 years) treated with 1.4 mg/kg of PPI divided twice daily and underwent esophageal pH testing after 3 weeks of therapy.[50] They demonstrated

that 89% of the patients had nocturnal acid breakthrough on the PPI.[50]

Finally, PPIs are most effective if they are administered as a single daily dose, 30 minutes before breakfast. This dosing corresponds with the timing of activation of stomach proton-potassium pumps after the overnight fast.[11]

Risks of Chronic Acid Suppression
Children taking H_2RAs or PPIs long term are at an increased risk of developing community-acquired pneumonia, acute

gastroenteritis., and *Clostridium difficile* infection. These risks are thought to be conferred due to the medications limiting the gastric acid's ability to kill possible pathogenic microorganisms.[51]

Referral to a Pediatric Gastroenterologist

In general, medical therapy with a PPI should be continued for 3 months. If GERD-related symptoms resolve, then the PFI should be stopped with plans for patient follow-up for evaluation of any recurrent symptoms. However, if the patient continues to have persistent GERD symptoms after 3 months of PPI therapy, then evaluation by a pediatric gastroenterologist should be considered. Other indications for a pediatric gastroenterologist referral include 'alarming' symptoms such as upper gastrointestinal bleeding, persistence of failure to thrive, acute worsening of weight loss or having difficulty swallowing or controlling secretions.[2]

Positive Airway Pressure

Continuous positive airway pressure (CPAP) is used for successful OSA treatment in children.[52] Despite this, there are scant data examining the effect of CPAP on sleep-related GERD in children. In adults, CPAP controls OSA and decreases sleep-related GERD symptoms and esophageal acid contact times.[11] CPAP increases esophageal, LES, and gastric pressures.[53] The differential pressure between the esophagus and stomach (the so-called barrier pressure) increases with CPAP. Finally, CPAP causes a disproportionate increase in LES pressure compared to esophageal and gastric pressures. This increase may be due to reflex activation of the LES, or by the transmission of the CPAP pressure to the LES.[53]

Surgical Therapy

Surgical fundoplication involves wrapping a portion of the stomach around the LES to strengthen or tighten the LES. Published reports vary widely in the success of surgical interventions for GERD in children, with success rates ranging from 40% to 95%. Complication rates from open and laparoscopic reflux surgery are similar.[54] Complications of GERD surgery include splenectomy (0.2%), esophageal laceration (0.2%), infection, recurrent GERD (2.5–40%), small bowel obstruction, gastroparesis, and dumping syndrome. Long-term outcome studies of fundoplication show that 14% of children have GERD recurrence after Nissen fundoplications, and 20% have GERD recurrence in loose wrap procedures (i.e., <360 degree wrap).[2] Optimally, prior to considering surgical therapy, the child should be evaluated carefully by a pediatric gastroenterologist.

FUTURE DIRECTIONS

Minimal data exist evaluating sleep-related GERD in children. There is also a need for well-designed randomized trials evaluating the efficacy of GERD therapy in sleep-related GERD in children. Data emerging from adults cannot be extrapolated to children. Furthermore, pediatricians need to be educated that GERD does occur during sleep time and can adversely affect sleep and daytime functioning as well as potentially contribute to other comorbid disease states.

CONCLUSION

During sleep, there is significant alteration in the physiology of the gastroesophageal system that increases the likelihood of GER. Sleep-related GERD is associated with GER symptoms and alters sleep architecture. Sleep-related GERD can impact sleep, contribute to excessive daytime sleepiness, impair quality of life, impact asthma severity, impact laryngitis, and is associated with OSA. There is still much research needed to assess the exact impact of sleep-related GERD on pediatric health and disease. Hopefully, future research will provide better methods of GERD identification, treatment, and prevention.

Clinical Pearls

- Transient relaxations of the lower esophageal sphincter are responsible for most gastroesophageal reflux (GER) episodes that commonly occur during arousals from sleep.
- Weekly heartburn is reported in 5.2% and/or regurgitation is reported in 8.2% of US adolescents.
- Sleep-related GER is associated with GER symptoms during sleep, arousals, obstructive sleep apnea, asthma, laryngospasm, hoarseness, and acute life-threatening events.
- Diagnosis of sleep-related GER includes symptoms and esophageal pH and impedance monitoring.
- Treatment includes behavioral interventions, pharmacologic therapy (primarily proton pump inhibitors) and, in carefully evaluated children, surgical fundoplication.

References

1. Suwandhi E, Ton MN, Schwarz SM. Gastroesophageal reflux in infancy and childhood. Pediatr Ann 2006;35(4):259–66.
2. Vandeplas Y, Rudolph CD, and committee members. Pediatric gastroesophageal reflux clinical practice guidelines: Joint recommendation of the North American Society for Pediatric Gastroenterology, Hepatology, and Nutrition (NASPGHAN) and the European Society for Pediatric Gastroenterology, Hepatology, and Nutrition (ESPGHAN). J Pediatr Gastroenterol Nutr 2009;49(4):498–547.
3. Skandalakis JE, Ellis H. Embryologic and anatomic basis of esophageal surgery. Surg Clin North Am 2000;80(1):85–155.
4. Gupta A, Jadcherla SR. The relationship between somatic growth and *in vivo* esophageal segmental and sphincteric growth in human neonates. J Pediatr Gastroenterol Nutr 2006;43(1):35–41.
5. Mittal RK, Balaban DH. The esophagogastric junction. N Engl J Med 1997;336(13):924–32.
6. Diamant NE. Functional anatomy and physiology of swallowing and esophageal motility. In: Richter JE, Castell DO, editors. The esophagus. West Sussex, UK: Wiley-Blackwell; 2012. p. 65–96.
7. Hillemeier AC, Grill BB, McCallum R, et al. Esophageal and gastric motor abnormalities in gastroesophageal reflux during infancy. Gastroenterology 1983;84(4):741–6.
8. Mahony MJ, Migliavacca M, Spitz L, et al. Motor disorders of the oesophagus in gastro-oesophageal reflux. Arch Dis Child 1988;63(11):1333–8.
9. Kahrilas P, Pandolfino J. Esophageal motor function. In: Yamada Y, editor. Textbook of gastroenterology. Hoboken, NJ: Wiley-Blackwell; 2009. p. 187–206.
10. Mittal RK, Holloway RH, Penagini R, et al. Transient lower esophageal sphincter relaxation. Gastroenterology 1995;109(2):601–10.
11. Harding SM. Gastroesophageal reflux during sleep. Sleep Med Clin 2007;2(1):41–50.
12. Cucchiara S, Staiano A, Di Lorenzo C, et al. Esophageal motor abnormalities in children with gastroesophageal reflux and peptic esophagitis. J Pediatr 1986;108(6):907–10.

13. Kawahara H, Dent J, Davidson G. Mechanisms responsible for gastroesophageal reflux in children. Gastroenterology 1997;113(2):399–408.

14. Omari TI, Barnett C, Snel A, et al. Mechanisms of gastroesophageal reflux in healthy premature infants. J Pediatr 1998;133(5):650–4.

15. Omari TI, Barnett CP, Benninga MA, et al. Mechanisms of gastro-oesophageal reflux in preterm and term infants with reflux disease. Gut 2002;51(4):475–9.

16. Jadcherla SR, Hogan WJ, Shaker R. Physiology and pathophysiology of glottis reflexes and pulmonary aspiration: from neonates to adults. Semin Resp Care Med 2010;31(5);554–60.

17. Kahrilas PJ, Dodds WJ, Dent J, et al. Effect of sleep, spontaneous gastroesophageal reflux, and a meal on upper esophageal sphincter pressure in normal human volunteers. Gastroenterology 1987;92(2):466–71.

18. Bajaj JS, Bajaj S, Dua KS, et al. Influence of sleep stages on esophago-upper esophageal sphincter contractile reflex and secondary esophageal peristalsis. Gastroenterology 2006;130(1):17–25.

19. Orr WC, Johnson LF, Robinson MG. Effect of sleep on swallowing, esophageal peristalsis, and acid clearance. Gastroenterology 1984;86(5 Pt 1):814–19.

20. Orr WC, Elsenbruch S, Harnish MJ, et al. Proximal migration of esophageal acid perfusions during waking and sleep. Am J Gastroenterology 2000;95(1);37–42.

21. Sherman PM, Hassall E, Fagundes-Neto U, et al. A global, evidence-based consensus on the definition of gastroesophageal reflux disease in the pediatric population. Am J Gastroenterol 2009;104(5):1278–95.

22. Gupta SK, Hassall E, Chiu Y-L, et al. Presenting symptoms of nonerosive and erosive esophagitis in pediatric patients. Dig Dis Sci 2006;51(5):858–63.

23. Campanozzi A, Boccia G, Pensabene L, et al. Prevalence and natural history of gastroesophageal reflux: Pediatric prospective survey. Pediatrics 2009;123(3):779–83.

24. Nelson SP, Chen EH, Syniar GM, et al. Prevalence of symptoms of gastroesophageal reflux during childhood: a pediatric practice-based survey. Pediatric Practice Research Group. Arch Pediatr Adolesc Med 2000;154(2):150–4.

25. Ashorn M, Ruuska T, Karikoski R, et al. The natural course of gastroesophageal reflux disease in children. Scand J Gastroenterol 2002;37(6):638–41.

26. Gunasekaran TS, Dahlberg M, Ramesh P, et al. Prevalence and associated features of gastroesophageal reflux symptoms in a Caucasian-predominant adolescent school population. Dig Dis Sci 2008;53(9):2373–9.

27. El-Serag HB, Gilger M, Kuebeler M, et al. Extraesophageal associations of gastroesophageal reflux disease in children without neurologic defects. Gastroenterology 2001;121(6):1294–9.

28. Kahn A, Rebuffat E, Sottiaux M, et al. Arousals induced by proximal esophageal reflux in infants. Sleep 1991;14(1):39–42.

29. Ghaem M, Armstrong KL, Trocki O, et al. The sleep patterns of infants and young children with gastro-oesophageal reflux. J Paediatr Child Health1998;34(2):160–3.

30. Gunasekaran T, Tolia V, Colletti RB, et al. Effects of esomeprazole treatment for gastroesophageal reflux disease on quality of life in 12- to 17-year-old adolescents: an international health outcomes study. BMC Gastroenterol 2009;9:84.

31. Wasilewska J, Kaczmarski M. Sleep-related breathing disorders in small children with nocturnal acid gastro-oesophageal reflux. Rocz Akad Med Bialymst 2004;49:98–102.

32. Noronha AC, de Bruin VMS, Nobre e Souza MA, et al. Gastroesophageal reflux and obstructive sleep apnea in childhood. Int J Pediatr Otorhinolaryngol 2009;73(3):383–9.

33. Wasilweska J, Kaczmarski M, Debkowska D. Obstructive hypopnea and gastroesophageal reflux as factors associated with residual obstructive sleep apnea syndrome. Int J Pediatr Otorhinolaryng 2011;75:657–63.

34. Thakkar K, Boatright RO, Gilger MA, et al. Gastroesophageal reflux and asthma in children: a systematic review. Pediatrics 2010;125(4):e925–30.

35. Hancox RJ, Poulton R, Taylor DR, et al. Associations between respiratory symptoms, lung function and gastro-oesophageal reflux symptoms in a population-based birth cohort. Respir Res 2006;7:142.

36. Khoshoo V, Haydel R. Effect of antireflux treatment on asthma exacerbations in nonatopic children. J Pediatr Gastroenterol Nutr 2007;44(3):331–5.

37. Størdal K, Johannesdottir GB, Bentsen BS, et al. Acid suppression does not change respiratory symptoms in children with asthma and gastro-oesophageal reflux disease. Arch Dis Child 2005;90(9):956–60.

38. Block BB, Brodsky L. Hoarseness in children: the role of laryngopharyngeal reflux. Int J Pediatr Otorhinolaryngol 2007;71(9):1361–9.

39. McGovern MC, Smith MB. Causes of apparent life threatening events in infants: a systematic review. Arch Dis Child 2004;89(11):1043–8.

40. Molloy EJ, Di Fiore JM, Martin RJ. Does gastroesophageal reflux cause apnea in preterm infants? Biol Neonate 2005;87(4):254–61.

41. Semeniuk J, Kaczmarski M, Wasilewska J, et al. Is acid gastroesophageal reflux in children with ALTE etiopathogenetic factor of life threatening symptoms? Adv Med Sci 2007;52:213–21.

42. Michail S. Gastroesophageal reflux. Pediatr Rev 2007;28(3):101–10.

43. Horvath A, Dziechciarz P, Szajewska H. The effect of thickened-feed interventions on gastroesophageal reflux in infants: Systematic review and meta-analysis of randomized, controlled trials. Pediatrics 2008;122(6):e1268–77.

44. Tobin JM, McCloud P, Cameron DJ. Posture and gastro-oesophageal reflux: a case for left lateral positioning. Arch Dis Child 1997;76(3):254–8.

45. American Academy of Pediatrics. Task Force on Infant Sleep Position and Sudden Infant Death Syndrome. Changing concepts of sudden infant death syndrome: implications for infant sleeping environment and sleep position. Pediatrics 2000;105(3 Pt 1):650–6.

46. Orenstein SR, McGowan JD. Efficacy of conservative therapy as taught in the primary care setting for symptoms suggesting infant gastroesophageal reflux. J Pediatr 2008;152(3):310–14.

47. Orenstein SR, Shalaby TM, Davandry SN, et al. Famotidine for infant gastro-oesophageal reflux: a multicentre, randomized, placebo-controlled, withdrawal trial. Aliment Pharmacol Ther 2003;17(9):1097–107.

48. Sachs G, Shin JM, Howden CW. Review article: the clinical pharmacology of proton pump inhibitors. Aliment Pharmacol Ther 2006;23(Supp 2):2–8.

49. Thomson ABR, Sauve MD, Kassam N, et al. Safety of the long-term use of proton pump inhibitors. World J Gastroenterol 2010;16(19):2323–30.

50. Pfefferkorn MD, Croffie JM, Gupta SK, et al. Nocturnal acid breakthrough in children with reflux esophagitis taking proton pump inhibitors. J Pediatr Gastroenterol Nutr 2006;42(2):160–5.

51. Canani RB, Cirillo P, Roggero P, et al. Therapy with gastric acidity inhibitors increases the risk of acute gastroenteritis and community-acquired pneumonia in children. Pediatrics 2006;117(5):e817–20.

52. Waters KA, Everett FM, Bruderer JW, et al. Obstructive sleep apnea the use of nasal CPAP in 80 children. Am J Respir Crit Care Med 1995;152(2):780–5.

53. Shepherd KL, Holloway RH, Hillman DR, et al. The impact of continuous positive airway pressure on the lower esophageal sphincter. Am J Physiol Gastrointest Liver Physio 2007;292(5):G1200–5.

54. Hassall E. Outcomes of fundoplication: causes for concern, newer options. Arch Dis Child 2005;90(10):1047–52.

Sleep and Pain

Valerie McLaughlin Crabtree, Amanda M. Rach, and Merrill S. Wise

INTRODUCTION

Chronic pain, described as pain occurring for 3 months or longer, is a relatively common condition and is reported to affect up to 44% of children and adolescents, with higher rates of chronic pain reported in girls beginning at age 4.[1] Many chronic pain conditions – including fibromyalgia, rheumatologic disorders, and other causes of musculoskeletal pain, functional abdominal pain, headaches and migraine, cancer, and spasticity-related pain in cerebral palsy – have been linked to both disturbed sleep and daytime fatigue in children and adolescents. In fact, approximately half of all pediatric pain patients report disturbed sleep.[2-7] In a sample of adolescent patients with chronic pain, reports of insomnia were six times higher than in the healthy adolescent population.[6] Poor sleep is also associated with episodic acute pain, as is commonly seen in many conditions including sickle cell disease.[8,9] A disturbance of sleep in children and adolescents with pain has been demonstrated convincingly through the use of self- and parent-reports, diary methodology, and actigraphy; far fewer studies have utilized polysomnography (PSG). It is likely that chronic pain and related sleep disturbances in children also have a strong negative impact on the sleep and quality of life of parents and caregivers, although this has not been carefully investigated.

This chapter will explore the consistent finding that sleep is disrupted in children and adolescents with pain, and it will examine it from the perspective that a bi-directional relationship exists between pain and sleep.[10] Additionally, we will review more recent investigations that examine the mediating and moderating impact of mood on the relationship between pain and sleep and on the functional impact of this relationship on children and adolescents. Not only is sleep disrupted in children and adolescents with chronic pain, but daytime fatigue and reduced health-related quality of life are present in this population as well. Finally, there will be a discussion of pharmacologic and non-pharmacologic interventions designed to ameliorate sleep disturbances and, when possible, to diminish pain.

Chronic Pain

The most frequent sleep-related complaints in youth with chronic pain are: difficulty initiating and maintaining sleep, difficulty awakening in the morning, daytime sleepiness, napping, snoring, and nightmares.[4-6,11] Poor sleep in children with chronic pain has a significant negative impact on health-related quality of life through such pathways as activity limitation and functional disability.[5,12] Adolescents, for example, with poor sleep quality, poor sleep efficiency, and difficulty initiating and maintaining sleep have more limited daytime activities than do adolescents with chronic pain who do not have poor sleep – even when controlling for pain and mood disturbances.[12] These observations highlight the importance of understanding the role of disturbed sleep in pediatric pain patients instead of solely attributing daytime activity limitations and poor quality of life to chronic pain. Furthermore, levels of pre-sleep cognitive arousal and sleep-related anxiety are reported to be higher in youth with chronic pain and are predictive of reports of insomnia.[4,6] This anxiety – likely reflecting intrusions of worry or anxiety related to pain and functional limitations – also interferes with sleep onset and lends itself to implementation of cognitive-behavioral interventions for insomnia.

Acute Pain

Although the majority of reports in the literature on sleep and pain focus on the relationship between sleep disturbance and chronic pain, acute pain is also known to disrupt sleep. Post-surgical pain, acute injury, or dental pain, for example, may negatively impact sleep, and such painful occurrences are typically part of all children's lives on occasion. Acute pain may disrupt sleep directly, or it may do so indirectly through efforts to reposition or mobilize during sleep. In some cases the psychological impact of a traumatic event that caused the acute pain may contribute to sleep disturbance as well.[10]

METHODS OF SLEEP ASSESSMENT

Evaluation of the child with pain and sleep issues begins with a thorough history. The healthcare provider should try to understand and characterize the child's pain and other medical issues as well as taking a careful sleep history. Ideally, the clinician should possess a thorough understanding of normal sleep physiology in children and must be willing to devote time to eliciting the history directly from the child, whenever possible, as well as from the parent or caregiver. In addition to typical details, such as bedtime routines, habitual bed and rise times, and sleep continuity, the clinician should ask about sleep quality during the night, the degree of restoration after the major sleep period, possible sleep-related breathing problems, symptoms of restless legs syndrome and periodic limb movements, and parasomnias (sleepwalking, sleep talking, sleep terrors, and sleep bruxism). Obtaining a history of nap frequency is important, as is other evaluation of alertness or sleepiness during the day. Parents should be asked their perceptions about the associations among nocturnal pain, sleep quality, and daytime function. A thorough medication history is also important, especially since children with chronic or acute pain are likely to be taking several. Questions about mood, emotional regulation, and anxiety should not be forgotten and lead further toward a comprehensive understanding of the child's sleep.

Both subjective and objective means of assessment are helpful in children with chronic pain. Subjective measures range from single time point self-report questionnaires to daily diary methods filled out over weeks or months. Depending on the age and ability of the child, measures can be completed by the child, the parent, or (ideally) by both. Within pediatric sleep research, parents are often the primary source of information; however, results of Valrie et al. suggest retrospective and concurrent reports by child and parent show adequate correspondence.[8]

Because interviews, questionnaires, and diaries are subjective, they are more appropriate to assess perception and awareness of sleep behaviors (night wakings, resistance to sleeping alone, sleepwalking, night terrors, snoring, restless and disrupted sleep, and apneic pauses) than are objective measures of sleep.[13] Objective data are also critical to obtain, for obvious reasons. The most commonly used objective methods are actigraphy and polysomnography (PSG), with videography growing in usage. Objective measurement periods can last from 1 day (PSG) to up to several weeks (actigraphy) and are best used to assess amount and timing of sleep (PSG or actigraphy) and stages of sleep, sleep quality, and causes of disrupted sleep (such as sleep apnea, periodic leg movements, parasomnias, or seizures) (PSG).[14] Since methods vary in terms of duration, effort, cost, and reliability, the use of multiple measures is helpful when feasible.

Self-Report Questionnaires

The multifaceted nature of sleep has led to the development of questionnaires assessing sleep patterns and habits, symptoms of disrupted sleep, and thoughts or beliefs about sleep (Tables 12.1a, 12.1b). Although most questionnaires assess sleep retrospectively (typically over the preceding 1–4 weeks),

some inquire about current sleep on a night-to-night basis;[15] thus, care should be taken when selecting a measure for a particular purpose and population.

Despite the inherent limitations associated with self-report questionnaires, their low cost and ease of implementation make them the most commonly used method in research with pediatric pain patients. Studies comparing the accuracy of self-reports to objective measures have found acceptable levels of agreement on certain sleep markers (total sleep time, sleep quality); however, parents sometimes tend to underreport the prevalence of night awakenings.[16,17]

Self-Report Daily Diaries

Prior to the development of actigraphy and PSG, daily diaries were considered the gold standard for sleep assessment in both adults and children.[18] More recently, studies found acceptable reliability and validity when child-completed daily sleep logs were compared against objective measures (actigraphy).[19,20] Sleep diaries are completed upon awakening and may capture much information including: bedtime, wake time, planned wake time, elements of sleep quality, number of perceived night wakings, time from lights out to sleep onset (sleep latency), time awake between sleep onset at night and time of rising in the morning (wake after sleep onset (WASO)), and other relevant information such as where the child slept, medications taken prior to bed, and bedtime difficulties.[21,22] Daily diaries have provided a unique methodology for elucidating the bi-directional relationship between

TABLE 12.1a   Parent Report Measures of Sleep Used in Chronic Pain Populations

Children's Sleep Hygiene Scale; CSHS[79]	17 item; 2–8 years	Activities surrounding sleep such as bedtime routines, stable bedtime and wake times over the past month
Children's Sleep Habits Questionnaire; CSHQ[75,81]	35 item; 4–10 years	Behavioral and medical-based sleep problems over the last week
Children's Sleep Wake Scale; CSWS[80]	40 item; 2–8 years	Child's sleep over the last month in the areas of going to bed, falling asleep, awakening, reinitiating sleep, and wakefulness
Sleep Disturbance Scale for Children; SDSC[82]	26 item; 5–15 years	Sleep initiation and maintenance, daytime sleepiness, sleep-disordered breathing, and sleep arousal
Epworth Sleepiness Scale; ESS[85]	8 item; 2–18 years	Assess daytime sleepiness, falling asleep during daytime activities

TABLE 12.1b   Child Self-Report Measures of Sleep Used in Chronic Pain Populations

Sleep Habits Survey; SHS[59]	36 item; 10–19 years	Usual sleeping and waking on school and weekend nights, school performance, daytime sleepiness, and sleep–wake behavior problems past 2 weeks
Sleep Self Report; SSR[75]	18 item; 7–12 years	Sleep habits, problems falling asleep, sleep duration, night waking, and daytime sleepiness past week
Adolescent Sleep Hygiene Scale; ASHS[83]	28 item; 12–18 years	Sleep-facilitating and sleep-inhibiting practices on 9 domains over the last month
Adolescent Sleep Wake Scale; ASWS[83]	28 item; 12–18	Assesses sleep initiation, maintenance, and quality across five dimensions in the past month
Pre-sleep Arousal Scale; PSAS[84]	16 items; 12–18 years	Cognitive and somatic arousal prior to sleep onset
Epworth Sleepiness Scale; ESS[85,86]	8 item; 2–18 years	Assess daytime sleepiness, falling asleep during daytime activities

pain and sleep in pediatric patients, which will be discussed later in this chapter.[9,23]

Actigraphy

An actigraph is a wristwatch-sized instrument usually worn on the non-dominant hand or ankle that measures movement over time and uses this as an indirect measure of sleep and wakefulness.[15] Some models include an event button that can be pressed to signal bedtime and morning waking. The actigraph can be worn 24 hours a day for many days, and it captures data while the child sleeps in his or her normal environment.[24-28] Actigraphy records sleep parameters such as total sleep duration (from sleep onset to final waking), sleep onset latency (minutes from bedtime to the first 20-minute period of sleep), total time in bed (from *lights out* to *got out of bed* events), and sleep efficiency (ratio of total sleep duration to total time spent in bed).[21] Actigraphy has been deemed useful for characterizing and monitoring circadian rhythms and sleep disturbances in children by the Standards of Practice Committee of the American Academy of Sleep Medicine (AASM),[29] and it has been successfully used to measure the sleep patterns of children and adolescents experiencing a range of chronic pain conditions including migraine,[21] recurrent abdominal pain (RAP),[30] and chronic musculoskeletal pain.[31]

The majority of actigraphy studies suggest that children and adolescents with chronic pain have sleep patterns similar to their peers without pain. Children and adolescents with RAP, as well as those with migraines, demonstrated no group differences in sleep duration, WASO, and sleep efficiency compared to control groups.[21,30] However, adolescents recruited from a multidisciplinary pain clinic had similar total sleep times but lower sleep efficiencies and more night wakings compared to a pain-free control group.[32] Further, a 2008 study of 17 females with chronic musculoskeletal pain found that the majority of participants experienced disturbed sleep with reduced nighttime sleep, increased nighttime wakefulness, and decreased sleep efficiency.[31]

A 2010 study by Lewandowski et al.,[15] investigating the relationship between pain and sleep, reported results similar to the 2004 studies by Haim et al.[30] and by Bruni et al.[21] Adolescents receiving treatment for chronic pain did not differ from a sample of peers with intermittent pain complaints on measures of average sleep duration, sleep efficiency, or WASO. Across both groups, longer sleep durations were associated with increased next-day pain in both chronic and occasional pain sufferers. Interestingly, increased sleep duration was not associated with self-reported higher levels of sleep quality, sleep efficiency, or restorative sleep.[15]

Nocturnal Polysomnography

The clinical utility of PSG in children with chronic pain has not been systematically evaluated; however, by taking a thorough sleep history, the clinician can identify sleep concerns that may indicate the need for PSG. For example, children with habitual snoring or witnessed apnea require PSG for characterization of breathing during sleep as part of the evaluation for obstructive sleep apnea (OSA) or other forms of sleep-related breathing disorders. Children on chronic steroids (as may be prescribed for some forms of cancer or other painful conditions) may experience significant weight gain and (thus) an increased risk for OSA. There are limited data

that suggest an association between chronic opioid treatment and central or obstructive sleep apnea.[33-35] Evidence-based practice parameters for respiratory indications for PSG in children, by the AASM, provide clinical guidance regarding which children may benefit from PSG.[36]

Non-respiratory indications for PSG in this population include atypical or potentially injurious parasomnias and suspected periodic limb movement disorder (PLMD). PSG may be indicated when nocturnal seizures are being considered, particularly when there is uncertainty about whether seizures, respiratory disturbances during sleep, or parasomnias are occurring. Evidence-based practice parameters for non-respiratory indications for PSG in children provide additional guidance.[37]

Nocturnal PSG is a valid and reliable method for assessing sleep stage distribution and sleep architecture in children but, in the absence of clinical indications for respiratory or non-respiratory sleep disorders, use of PSG to characterize sleep architecture in children with chronic pain is not likely to alter management or be cost-effective. From a research perspective, PSG (either in-laboratory or portable testing) may provide a useful method to investigate the important relationships between sleep and chronic pain in children. For example, PSG evaluations of sleep in children with juvenile fibromyalgia[38] and juvenile rheumatoid arthritis (JRA),[39] document significant sleep fragmentation.

Comparing Subjective and Objective Measures

Studies suggest subjective and objective measures capture unique and complementary aspects of the sleep experience and, thus, both methods have a place in pediatric sleep assessment.[24,40,41] These different dimensions of sleep and sleep problems captured by subjective and objective measures also provide an explanation for discrepant research findings. Subjective reports reflect the child's or parents' actual perceptions of sleep. Objective measures, however, may be insensitive to the subtle causes of these perceived changes in sleep quality that contribute to the subjective experiences.[42] Because the perception of both sleep quality and pain are subjective, the role of subjective reports in studying the sleep of pediatric chronic pain patients is essential.

MOOD AND SLEEP

The relationship between mood disorders and sleep disruptions is best characterized as bi-directional and mutually interacting. Investigations show that emotional disturbances can contribute to sleep difficulties,[43,44] and insufficient sleep can lead to significant disturbances in mood.[45,45-50] Disturbed sleep (including too much or too little sleep) is a commonly reported symptom in both depressive and anxiety disorders.[51,52] A 2002 study found that of adolescents who met criteria for major depressive disorder (MDD), 88.6% described sleep disturbances as a contributing symptom.[51]

The relationship between mood and sleep is not straightforward, however, as mood is known to influence sleep differentially depending on whether the child has an anxiety or a depressive disorder.[53] Children experiencing symptoms of depression (anhedonia, psychomotor retardation, social withdrawal, fatigue, decreased appetite and weight, and hopelessness/helplessness) are more likely to suffer from hypersomnia, whereas children with anxiety symptoms (separation anxiety, somatic complaints, brooding/worry, and psychomotor agitation) are more likely to suffer from insomnia.[54] This suggests early mood disorders may influence the development of sleep disturbances and may be used to assist with differential diagnosis.[43]

The relationship between mood and sleep may be more a function of subjective complaints than objectively captured sleep disturbances.[14] A number of objective studies have failed to find a difference in sleep between children with mood disorders and age-matched controls.[52,55,56] However, by subjective report, youth with anxiety disorders have been found to underestimate or underreport sleep difficulties compared to those with depression who perceive their sleep as disturbed despite normal objective results.[42] That being said, some studies have found objective differences in sleep quality,[57] damped circadian amplitude, and lower activity levels[58] in children with depression.

Although the presence of *subjectively* reported disrupted sleep in children and adolescents with mood disorders is well established, inconsistencies within the literature do exist. Many of the discrepancies can likely be attributed to age and cultural differences across study populations, to expected changes associated with normal development, and to the assessment methods used to capture the sleep experience.[5,24,59] However, it is important to consider that once both sleep disturbance complaints and a mood disorder have developed it becomes essential to intervene to disrupt the cycle and re-establish developmentally appropriate mood and sleeping patterns.

For additional discussion of mood and sleep, see Chapter 46.

MOOD AND PAIN

Depressive and emotional symptoms are consistently associated with increased pain in studies of children with and without chronic disease.[60–65] One study found depression alone explained 25.4% of the variance in pain scores,[66] and children who reported increased emotional distress were more likely to report pain in multiple areas of the body compared to children with low levels of distress.[67] In a manner similar to that reported in the literature on sleep and pain, daily vacillations of depressed mood and stress have been found to affect reports of pain in children; thus, daily increases of depressed mood or stress are highly predictive of increased pain.[68,69] Furthermore, depressive symptoms are associated with increased functional disability scores; however, this may be due to the overlapping characteristics of fatigue, diminished interest in activities, and psychomotor retardation.[62] Finally, as anxiety and depression increase, negative emotions and chronic pain can trigger both negative thinking[66] and increased somatic sensitivity. When both negative mood and pain are present, a negative feedback loop can occur, with each symptom exacerbating the other.[70]

BI-DIRECTIONAL RELATIONSHIP OF PAIN AND SLEEP

Lewin and Dahl posited a theory whereby sleep and pain have a bi-directional relationship.[10] As such, pain may directly

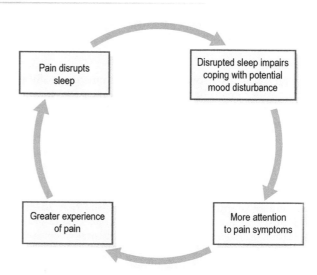

FIGURE 12-1 Cyclic Nature of Pain and Sleep. *(Adapted from Lewin DS, Dahl RE. Importance of sleep in the management of pediatric pain. Journal of Developmental and Behavioral Pediatrics 1999;20(4):244–252.)*[10]

interfere with sleep whereby it inhibits sleep onset, induces nocturnal awakenings, and interferes with return to sleep. Conversely, a poor night's sleep is hypothesized to lead to increased experience of pain and decreased pain tolerance the following day. The role of potential mood dysregulation resulting from poor sleep is essential in Lewin & Dahl's model (see Figure 12-1).

Because of the importance of coping in the context of managing chronic pain on a daily basis, the impact of adequate sleep is crucial for assisting children and adolescents in managing daily pain through improved coping mechanisms. Lewin and Dahl describe specific benefits of sufficient sleep in children and adolescents with chronic pain, including the role of deep nonREM (N3) sleep in inhibiting pain signals and promoting the release of growth hormone (thereby assisting healing), and the role of sleep in modulating the relation between stress and immune function.

Daily Diary Methodology

In an attempt to elucidate the bi-directional theory, daily diaries provide a methodology to assist with the determination of directionality in the pain–sleep relationship. Through daily diary methodology, poor sleep has been demonstrated to be predictive of reports of pain the following day. Mood has been identified as a moderator variable in this relationship, whereby with increasingly positive mood, the impact of poor sleep on reports of pain decreases.[9,15,23] Furthermore, while daily variations in sleep predicted pain, typical sleep quality had a greater influence on reports of pain.[23] Interestingly, while pain has been reported to be predictive of poor sleep quality the following evening in children with sickle cell disease,[9] this was not found in a sample of children with juvenile polyarticular arthritis,[23] or in youth from a multidisciplinary pain clinic.[15] Thus, while evidence is increasing for the impact of poor sleep on the experience of pain in children with chronic and episodic pain (particularly when negative mood is present), the reverse, i.e., the impact of pain on sleep in this population, is less clear.

PSYCHOLOGICAL INTERVENTIONS/TREATMENTS

Currently, no formalized psychological interventions exist which are designed to treat comorbid sleep disturbances and pain in children. However, a number of studies implementing a cognitive-behavioral treatment for insomnia (CBT-I) in adults experiencing chronic pain due to injury or medical conditions show promise.

Heavily based on Morin's treatment for insomnia,[71] CBT-I primarily focuses on stimulus control, sleep restriction (limited time in bed with strict bed and rise times), and cognitive restructuring (to change unrealistic beliefs and irrational fears regarding sleep), but it also incorporates relaxation training (deep breathing, progressive muscle relaxation, autogenic training, and imagery). Compared to a control group, participants with osteoarthritis receiving CBT-I achieved a shorter sleep-onset latency, decreased WASO, and increased sleep efficiency, and there were reduced self-reports of pain, all of which were maintained at 1-year follow-up.[72] Importantly, the CBT-I intervention made no reference to pain management techniques, whereas the treatment provided to the control group contained several treatment components that have previously been included in effective multi-component interventions for chronic pain management.[72] As the CBT-I group reported reduced immediate and long-term pain, this suggests the importance of healthy sleep in the treatment of chronic pain.

When measuring pain outcomes, it is important not only to assess pain severity but also pain interference, which captures how the pain sensation interferes with a person's ability to engage in daily tasks. It is possible that improvements in sleep quality may not influence pain severity directly but rather improves pain interference and other pain-related outcomes indirectly by bolstering coping resources.[22]

A pilot study investigating treatment for children with JRA reported that eight children treated with CBT described significant improvements in sleep quality, pain control, and physical functioning compared to a control group.[73] A second pilot study using the same intervention reported improved sleep (defined as decreased sleep latency and more restorative sleep) associated with decreased levels of pain.[74]

Results from these pilot studies – specifically their demonstration of a link between improved sleep and pain reduction – led researchers to specifically introduce sleep as the first module within an 8-week multimodal, outpatient, cognitive-behavioral intervention for youth with fibromyalgia.[75] The sleep module assists with making changes in sleep hygiene and identifying maladaptive sleep cognitions, and it uses stimulus control, sleep restriction, relaxation, and deep breathing instruction. Children also maintain daily sleep logs to identify problematic patterns of behavior and track changes in sleep quality. Additional modules in the intervention focus on psycho-education, pain management techniques, and skills to manage activities of daily living.[73] The pain management protocol includes exploring maladaptive cognitions regarding pain and the teaching of cognitive reframing, thought stopping, distraction techniques, the use of visual imagery, and self-hypnosis.

To date, this study has found that children receiving the CBT intervention report decreased pain and fatigue and increased sleep quality.[73] Furthermore, there was an increase from 1% to 24% of children who reported experiencing no current pain at all. Although the pain, fatigue, sleep disturbance, sleep latency, and physical symptoms (headaches and gastric disturbances) did not remit completely, the authors suggested the treatment instilled optimism in the children and empowered them to assume control over symptom management.[73]

PHARMACOLOGICAL INTERVENTIONS

Interventions directed at controlling pain during the major sleep period are likely to improve sleep quality and quantity. However, it is important that the clinician monitor closely for side effects including those that have an adverse impact on sleep or daytime alertness.

There are few prospective studies designed to systematically evaluate pharmacological interventions that address both chronic pain and sleep issues in children. The effect of pregabalin on sleep and pain in adult participants with fibromyalgia was investigated in two studies, and findings were generally positive and associated with meaningful improvement in sleep and pain.[76,77] Generalization of these findings is limited by the disease model (fibromyalgia) and the age group (adults). Nevertheless, it appears likely that certain medications have efficacy for controlling some forms of pain and improving sleep fragmentation.

Tricyclic antidepressants, such as amitriptyline, have been used at bedtime for chronic pain and to help consolidation of sleep. Children with chronic pain plus restless legs syndrome or PLMD may benefit from gabapentin or pregabalin, or from other anticonvulsant medications such as carbamazepine or lamotrigene. Duloxetine (Cymbalta™) is a newer selective serotonin and norepinephrine reuptake inhibitor with US Food and Drug Administration (FDA) approval in adults for treatment of diabetic peripheral neuropathic pain, fibromyalgia, chronic musculoskeletal pain, major depressive disorder, and generalized anxiety disorder.[78] However, use of duloxetine in children is *off label* (not approved by the FDA) and the increased risk of suicidal thinking and behavior in children, adolescents, and young adults taking antidepressants for major depressive disorder and other psychiatric disorders limits use of this medication. Given the paucity of FDA-approved options in this area, it is clear that much work is needed to develop and evaluate pharmacological treatment options for children with chronic pain and sleep issues.

CONCLUSION

A bi-directional relationship between disrupted sleep and pain exists in children and adolescents with acute, episodic, and chronic pain. This relationship appears to be moderated to some degree by mood and has an impact on daytime function including health-related quality of life. This chapter addresses the importance of fully assessing mood and sleep in pediatric patients with chronic pain as well as the utility of non-pharmacologic and pharmacologic methods of intervention in this patient population.

Clinical Pearls

- Evaluation of the child with pain and sleep issues begins with a thorough history of the child's pain, other medical and psychological issues, and sleep.
- A bi-directional relationship between sleep and chronic pain is postulated: pain may inhibit sleep onset, induce nocturnal awakenings, and interfere with return to sleep; poor sleep may lead to increased experience of pain.
- Because the perception of sleep quality and pain is subjective, it is essential to assess subjective reports of both.
- Improvements in sleep quality may influence pain perception indirectly by bolstering coping resources, thus limiting the degree that pain sensations interfere with the ability to engage in daily activities.
- The relationship between sleep and pain is moderated by mood: with increasingly positive mood, the negative impact of poor sleep on reports of pain decreases.
- Children with chronic pain receiving non-pharmacologic interventions such as CBT-I report decreased pain and fatigue and improved sleep quality.
- Research is needed to develop and evaluate pharmacological treatment options for children with chronic pain and sleep issues.

References

1. Perquin CW, Hazebroek-Kampschreur AAJM, Hunfeld JAM, et al. Pain in children and adolescents: A common experience. Pain 2000;87(1):51–8.
2. Berrin SJ, Malcarne VL, Varni JW, et al. Pain, fatigue, and school functioning in children with cerebral palsy: A path-analytic model. J Pediatr Psychol 2007;32(3):330–7.
3. Hinds PS, Hockenberry M, Rai SN, et al. Clinical field testing of an enhanced-activity intervention in hospitalized children with cancer. J Pain Sympt Manag 2007;33(6):686–97.
4. Huntley ED, Campo JV, Dahl RE, et al. Sleep characteristics of youth with functional abdominal pain and a healthy comparison group. J Pediatr Psychol 2007;32(8):938–49.
5. Long AC, Krishnamurthy V, Palermo TM. Sleep disturbances in school-age children with chronic pain. Jf Pediatr Psychol 2008;33(3):258–68.
6. P alermo TM, Wilson AC, Lewandowski AS, et al. Behavioral and psychosocial factors associated with insomnia in adolescents with chronic pain. Pain 2011;152(1):89–94.
7. Varni JW, Seid M, Kurtin PS. The PedsQL in pediatric cancer: reliability and validity of the Pediatric Quality of Life Inventory Generic Core Scales, Multidimensional Fatigue Scale, and Cancer Module. Med Care 2001;39(8):800–12.
8. Valrie CR, Gil KM, Redding-Lallinger R, et al. The influence of pain and stress on sleep in children with sickle cell disease. Childr Health Care 2007;36(4):335–53.
9. Valrie CR, Gil KM, Redding-Lallinger R, et al. Brief Report: Daily mood as a mediator or moderator of the pain–sleep relationship in children with sickle cell disease. J Pediatr Psychol 2008;33(3):317–22.
10. Lewin DS, Dahl RE. Importance of sleep in the management of pediatric pain. J Dev Behavior Pediatr 1999;20(4):244–52.
11. Law EF, Dufton L, Palermo TM. Daytime and nighttime sleep patterns in adolescents with and without chronic pain. Health Psychol 2011. Dec 12. [Epub ahead of print]
12. Palermo TM, Fonareva I, Janosy NR. Sleep quality and efficiency in adolescents with chronic pa1in: Relationship with activity limitations and health-related quality of life. Behavior Sleep Med 2008;6(4):234–50.
13. Sadeh A. Commentary: Comparing actigraphy and parental report as measures of children's sleep. J Pediatr Psychol 2008;33(4):406–7.
14. Gregory AM, Sadeh A. Sleep, emotional and behavioral difficulties in children and adolescents. Sleep Med Rev 2012;16(2):129–36.
15. Lewandowski AS, Palermo TM, Motte SDl, et al. Temporal daily associations between pain and sleep in adolescents with chronic pain versus healthy adolescents. Pain 2010;151(1):220–25.
16. Werner H, Molinari L, Guyer C, et al. Agreement rates between actigraphy, diary, and questionnaire for children's sleep patterns. Arch Pediatr Adolesc Med 2008;162(4):350–8.
17. Sadeh A. Evaluating night wakings in sleep-disturbed infants: A methodological study of parental reports and actigraphy. Sleep 1996;19(10):757–62.
18. Knab B, Engel-Sittenfeld P. The many facets of poor sleep. Neuropsychobiology 1983;10:141–7.
19. Gaina A, Sekine M, Chen X, et al. Validity of child sleep diary questionnaire among junior high school children. J Epidemiol 2004;14(1):1–4.
20. Sadeh A, Raviv A, Gruber R. Sleep patterns and sleep disruptions in school-age children. Dev Psychol 2000;36(3):291–301.
21. Bruni O, Russo PM, Violani C, et al. Sleep and migraine: An actigraphic study. Cephalalgia 2004;24(2):134–9.
22. Jungquist CR, O'Brien C, Matteson-Rusby S, et al. The efficacy of cognitive-behavioral therapy for insomnia in patients with chronic pair. Sleep Med 2010;11(3):302–9.
23. Bromberg MH, Gil KM, Schanberg LE. Daily sleep quality and mood as predictors of pain in children with juvenile polyarticular arthritis. Health Psychol 2011;31(2):202–9.
24. Holley S, Hill CM, Stevenson J. A comparison of actigraphy and parental report of sleep habits in typically developing children aged 6 to 11 years. Behavior Sleep Med 2009;8(1):16–27.
25. Meltzer LJ, Westin AML. A comparison of actigraphy scoring rules used in pediatric research. Sleep 2011;12(8):793–6.
26. Sadeh A, Lavie P, Scher A, et al. Actigraphic home-monitoring sleep-disturbed and control infants and young children: A new method for pediatric assessment of sleep-wake patterns. Pediatrics 1991;87(4):494–9.
27. Sadeh A, Sharkey K, Carskadon MA. Activity-based sleep-wake identification: An empirical test of methodological issues. Sleep 1994;17(3):201–7.
28. Sitnick SL, Goodlin-Jones BL, Anders TF. The use of actigraphy to study sleep disorders in preschoolers: Some concerns about detection of nighttime awakenings. Sleep 2008;31(3):395–401.
29. Littner M, Kushida CA, Anderson MW, et al. Practice parameters for the role of actigraphy in the study of sleep and circadian rhythms: An update for 2002. Am Acad Sleep Med 2003;26:754–60.
30. Haim A, Pillar G, Pecht A, et al. Sleep patterns in children and adolescents with functional recurrent abdominal pain: Objective versus subjective assessment. Acta Paediatrica 2004;93(5):677–80.
31. Tsai S-Y, Labyak SE, Richardson LP, et al. Brief Report: Actigraphic sleep and daytime naps in adolescent girls with chronic musculoskeletal pain. J Pediatr Psychol 2008;33(3):307–11.
32. Palermo TM, Toliver-Sokol M, Fonareva I, et al. Objective and subjective assessment of sleep in adolescents with chronic pain compared to healthy adolescents. Clin J Pain 2007;23(9):812–20.
33. Amos LB, D'Andrea LA. Severe central sleep apnea in a child with leukemia on chronic methadone therapy. Pediatr Pulmonol 2013;48(1):85–7.
34. Jungquist CR, Flannery M, Perlis ML, et al. Relationship of chronic pain and opioid use with respiratory disturbance during sleep. Pain Management Nursing 2012;13(2):70–9.
35. Farney RJ, Walker JM, Cloward TV, et al. Sleep-disordered breathing associated with long-term opioid therapy. Chest J 2003;123(2):632–9.
36. Aurora NR, Zak RS, Karippot A, et al. Practice parameters for the respiratory indications for PSG in children. Sleep 2011;34(3):379–88.
37. Kotagal S, Nichols CD, Grigg-Damberger MM, et al. Non-respiratory indications for polysomnography and related procedures in children: An evidence-based review. Sleep 2012;35(11):1451–66.
38. Roizenblatt S, Tufik S, Goldenberg J, et al. Juvenile fibromyalgia: Clinical and polysomnographic aspects. The J Rheumatol 1997;24(3):579–35.
39. Passarelli CM, Roizenblatt S, Len CA, et al. A case-control sleep study in children with polyarticular juvenile rheumatoid arthritis. J Rheumatol 2006;33(4):796–802.
40. Short MA, Gradisar M, Lack LC, et al. The discrepancy between actigraphic and sleep diary measures of sleep in adolescents. Sleep Med 2012;13(4):378–84.
41. Wiggs L, Montgomery P, Stores G. Actigraphic and parent reports of sleep patterns and sleep disorders in children with subtypes of attention-deficit hyperactivity disorder. Sleep 2005;28(11):1437–45.
42. Forbes EE, Bertocci MA, Gregory AM, et al. Objective sleep in pediatric anxiety disorders and major depressive disorder. J Am Acad Child Adolesc Psychiatr 2008;47(2):148–55.
43. Ivanenko A, McLaughlin Crabtree V, Gozal D. Sleep and depression in children and adolescents. Sleep Med Rev 2005;9(2):115–29.
44. Patten CA, Choi WS, Gillin JC, et al. Depressive symptoms and cigarette smoking predict development and persistence of sleep problems in US

adolescents. Pediatrics 2000;106(2):1–9. http://pediatrics.aappublications. org/content/106/2/e23.abstract. Accessed August 1, 2000.

45. Carskadon MA, Acebo C. Regulation of sleepiness in adolescents: Update, insights, and speculation. Sleep 2002;25(6):606–14.

46. Dahl RE. The consequences of insufficient sleep for adolescents: Links between sleep and emotional regulation. Phi Delta Kappan 1999;80(5): 354–9.

47. Dahl RE, Harvey AG. Sleep in children and adolescents with behavioral and emotional disorders. Sleep Med Clin 2007;2(3):501–11.

48. Gregory AM, O'Connor TG. Sleep problems in childhood: A longitudinal study of developmental change and association with behavioral problems. J Am Acad Child Adolesc Psychiatr 2002;41(8):964–71.

49. Johnson EO, Roth T, Breslau N. The association of insomnia with anxiety disorders and depression: Exploration of the direction of risk. J Psychiatr Res 2006;40(8):700–8.

50. Roberts RE, Ramsay Roberts C, Ger Chen I. Impact of insomnia on future functioning of adolescents. J Psychosomatic Res 2002;53(1): 561–9.

51. Moldofsky H. Sleep and pain. Sleep Med Rev 2001;5(5):385–96.

52. Puig-Antich J, Goetz R, Hanlon C, et al. Sleep architecture and REM sleep measures in prepubertal children with major depression: A controlled study. Arch Gen Psychiatr 1982;39(8):932–9.

53. Cousins JC, Whalen DJ, Dahl RE, et al. The bidirectional association between daytime affect and nighttime sleep in youth with anxiety and depression. J Pediatr Psychol 2011;36(9):969–79.

54. Ryan ND, Puig-Antich J, Ambrosini P, et al. The clinical picture of major depression in children and adolescents. Arch Gen Psychiatr 1987;44(10):854–61.

55. Benca RM, Obermeyer WH, Thisted RA, et al. Sleep and psychiatric disorders. Arch Gen Psychiatr 1992;49(8):651–68.

56. Dahl RE, Puig-Antich J, Ryan ND, et al. EEG sleep in adolescents with major depression: the role of suicidality and inpatient status. J Affective Disorders 1990;19(1):63–75.

57. Dahl RE, Ryan ND, Matty MK, et al. Sleep onset abnormalities in depressed adolescents. Biological Psychiatry 1996;39(6):400–10.

58. Armitage R, Hoffmann R, Emslie G, et al. Rest-activity cycles in childhood and adolescent depression. J Am Acad Child Adolesc Psychiatr 2004;43(6):761–9.

59. Wolfson AR, Carskadon MA, Acebo C, et al. Evidence for the validity of a Sleep Habits Survey for adolescents. Sleep 1998;26(2):213–16.

60. Gil KM, Carson JW, Porter LS, et al. Daily stress and mood and their association with pain, health-care use, and school activity in adolescents with sickle cell disease. J Pediatr Psychol 2003;28(5):363–73.

61. Hoff AL, Palermo TM, Schluchter M, et al. Longitudinal relationships of depressive symptoms to pain intensity and functional disability among children with disease-related pain. J Pediatr Psychol 2006;31(10):1046–56.

62. Kashikar-Zuck S, Vaught MH, Goldschneider KR, et al. Depression, coping, and functional disability in juvenile primary fibromyalgia syndrome. J Pain 2002;3(5):412–19.

63. Packham JC, Hall MA. Long-term follow-up of 246 adults with juvenile idiopathic arthritis: functional outcome. Rheumatology 2002;41(12): 1428–35.

64. Sandstrom MJ, Schanberg LE. Brief report: Peer rejection, social behavior, and psychological adjustment in children with juvenile rheumatic disease. J Pediatr Psychol J 2004;29(1):29–34.

65. Timko C, Stovel K, Moos RH, et al. Adaptation to juvenile rheumatic disease: A controlled evaluation of functional disability with a one-year follow-up. Health Psychol 1992;11(1):67–76.

66. Margetic B, Aukst-Margetić B, Bilić E, et al. Depression, anxiety and pain in children with juvenile idiopathic arthritis (JIA). Eur Psychiat 2005;20(3):274–6.

67. Bruusgaard D, Smedbråten BK, Natvig B. Bodily pain, sleep problems and mental distress in schoolchildren. Acta Pædiatrica 2000;89(5): 598–600.

68. Schanberg LE, Gil KM, Anthony KK, et al. Pain, stiffness, and fatigue in juvenile polyarticular arthritis: Contemporaneous stressful events and mood as predictors. Arthritis & Rheumatis 2005;52(4):1196–204.

69. Varni JW, Rapoff MA, Walcron SA, et al. Chronic pain and emotional distress in children and adolescents. J Dev Behavioral Pediatr 1996; 17(3):154–61.

70. Keefe FJ, Lumley M, Anderson T, et al. Pain and emotion: New research directions. J Clin Psychol 2001;57(4):587–607.

71. Morin C. Insomnia: Psychological assessment and management. New York, NY: Guilford Press; 1993.

72. Vitiello MV, Rybarczyk B, Von Korff M, et al. Cognitive behavioral therapy for insomnia improves sleep and decreases pain in older adults with comorbid insomnia and osteoarthritis. J Clin Sleep Med 2009;5(4):355–62.

73. Degotardi PJ, Klass ES, Rosenberg BS, et al. Development and evaluation of a cognitive-behavioral intervention for juvenile fibromyalgia. J Pediatr Psychol 2006;31(7):714–23.

74. Fox DG, Degotardi PJ, Klass ES, et al. Sleep in children with fibromyalgia [Abstract]. Arthritis Care Res 1999;12(S14).

75. Goodlin-Jones BL, Sitnick SL, Tang K, et al. The Children's Sleep Habits Questionnaire in toddlers and preschool children. J Dev Behavioral Pediatr 2008;29(2):82–3 10.1097/DBP.1090b1013e318163c318139a.

76. Pauer L, Winkelmann A, Arsenault P, et al. An international, randomized, double-blind, placebo-controlled, phase III trial of pregabalin monotherapy in treatment of patients with fibromyalgia. J Rheumatol 2011;38(12):2643–52.

77. Roth T, Lankford DA, Bhadra P, et al. Effect of pregabalin on sleep in patients with fibromyalgia and sleep maintenance disturbance: A randomized, placebo-controlled, 2-way crossover polysomnography study. Arthritis Care Res 2012;64(4):597–606.

78. Eli Lilly and Company. Prescribing information. Indianapolis, IN. 2011.

79. LeBourgeois MK, Harsh J. A new research instrument for measuring children's sleep. Sleep 2001;24:A213.

80. LeBourgeois MK, Harsh J, Hancock M. Validation of the children's sleep-wake scale. Sleep 2001;24:A14.

81. Owens JA, Spirito A, McGuinn M. The Children's Sleep Habits Questionnaire (CSHQ): psychometric properties of a survey instrument for school-aged children. Sleep 2000;23(8):1043–51.

82. Bruni O, Ottaviano S, Guidetti V, et al. The Sleep Disturbance Scale for Children (SDSC): Construction and validation of an instrument to evaluate sleep disturbances in childhood and adolescence. J Sleep Res 1996;5(4):251–61.

83. LeBourgeois MK, Giannotti F, Cortesi F, et al. The relationship between reported sleep quality and sleep hygiene in Italian and American adolescents. Pediatrics 2005;115(Suppl. 1):257–65.

84. Nicassio PM, Mendlowitz DR, Fussell JJ, et al. The phenomenology of the pre-sleep state: The development of the pre-sleep arousal scale. Behaviour Res Ther 1985;23(3):263–71.

85. Melendres CS, Lutz JM, Rubin ED, et al. Daytime sleepiness and hyperactivity in children with suspected sleep-disordered breathing. Pediatrics 2004;114(3):768–75.

86. Moore M, Kirchner HL, Drotar D, et al. Relationships among sleepiness, sleep time, and psychological functioning in adolescents. J Pediatr Psychol 2009;34(10):1175–83.

Sleep Related Enuresis

Oscar Sans Capdevila

INTRODUCTION

The symptom of involuntary urine loss is termed urinary incontinence. Urinary incontinence during the night (the terms bedwetting, enuresis, enuresis nocturna and sleep-related enuresis (SRE) are used synonymously) is the commonest urinary symptom in children and adolescents, and can lead to major distress for the affected child and parents. SRE is estimated to affect 5 to 7 million children in the United States alone, occurring much more often in boys than in girls, with a 3:1 reported ratio in most cohorts.

Up to the fifth year of life, urinary incontinence is regarded as a physiological phenomenon, even if many children develop complete continence well before this age.[1] According to the International Children's Continence Society, enuresis is classified as either primary – when the child has never achieved nighttime dryness, or secondary – when nocturnal enuresis occurs after a period of dryness of at least 6 months.

Among the known risk factors for the occurrence of nocturnal enuresis, significant associations between sleep-disordered breathing and SRE have emerged both in children and in adults over the last decade.[2–6] It has become apparent that increased upper airway resistance during sleep manifesting either as habitual snoring (HS) or as documented obstructive sleep apnea syndrome (OSAS) leads to increases in the risk of SRE. Most importantly, after successful treatment of the respiratory disorder during sleep, SRE can be reduced in frequency or severity, and even eliminated. Thus, careful evaluation of sleep-disordered breathing in enuretic patients is important, especially in those children with concomitant daytime incontinence.[6]

EPIDEMIOLOGY

The epidemiology of bedwetting is complicated by the variety of definitions used in studies (Box 13-1).

Children develop stable bladder control in the third to sixth year of life – initially during the day and later also during the night. At age 7 years, approximately 10% still have nocturnal enuresis, and 2–9% are affected during the day.[8] Similar results were reported by the Avon Longitudinal Study, a prospective and large longitudinal cohort from birth that examined a variety of developmental trajectories specifically assessing growth and pediatric milestones. Another epidemiological study in Hong Kong, which defined bedwetting as the occurrence of one wet night over a 3-month period, reported a prevalence of 16.1% at age 5 years, 10.1% at 7 years and 2.2% at 19 years.[9] In all studies, the prevalence is markedly greater for boys than for girls at all ages, with an average ratio of 3:1.[9–12] Children tend to outgrow SRE, with a spontaneous remission rate of about 14–15% annually among bedwetters, with 3% remaining enuretic into adulthood.[8,10,11] Male gender and age younger than 9 years are considered major contributors to sleep-related enuresis in children.[12]

Interestingly, in a recent population-based study made in 6147 children by Su and collaborators, the prevalence of nocturnal enuresis (NE) was not greater in children with OSA, but was increased with increasing severity of OSA in girls only, demonstrating, for the first time, a sex-associated prevalence of NE in relation to increasing OSA severity.[13]

ETIOLOGY

Important risk factors for SRE include family history, nocturnal polyuria, impaired sleep arousal and nocturnal bladder dysfunction. Nocturnal enuresis has been linked to chromosomes 13, 12, 8 and 22, with a predominantly autosomal dominant inheritance.[14]

In two-thirds of children with SRE, disturbed circadian rhythms in ADH release and nocturnal polyuria have been reported.[15] Defects in sleep arousal have also been associated with SRE.[16] As many as a third of children with SRE may have nocturnal detrusor overactivity along with reduced functional bladder capacity. Interestingly, these children have normal detrusor activity and a normal functional bladder capacity when they are awake, but a reduced functional bladder capacity with detrusor hyperactivity when asleep.[7]

Other risk factors for sleep-related enuresis include constipation,[17] developmental delay and other neurological dysfunction,[18] attention deficit hyperactivity disorder (ADHD),[19] upper airway resistance,[20,21] and sleep-disordered breathing.[2–6,22]

PATHOPHYSIOLOGY

Urinary incontinence is a heterogeneous entity with multifactorial contributors, which is also affected by coexisting morbidities. Two major entities are reported.

Physiological Urinary Incontinence

This term clarifies urinary incontinence as a symptom that is regarded as a normal feature during the first few years of life, and is considered as pathological only after the fifth year of life. The range of normal continence development is, however, very wide, such that one can assume that many children experience 'physiological' urinary incontinence beyond the completed fifth year of life ('late developers'). The clinical and diagnostic test findings in such children are negative and reveal the absence of any pathological features.[7]

Organic Urinary Incontinence

This form of urinary incontinence is rare. However, special efforts have to go into the detection of possible organic causes, particularly among treatment-refractory cases. The

---

Box 13-1 Definitions[7]

- *Enuresis*: Intermittent incontinence while asleep in a child over 5 years of age.
- *Monosymptomatic enuresis*: Enuresis with no other lower urinary tract symptoms.
- *Expected bladder capacity* (EBC): Calculated as [30 + (age in years × 30)] in milliliters.
- *Nocturnal polyuria* (NP): Overproduction of urine at night, defined as nocturnal urine output exceeding 130% of EBC for age.
- *Non-monosymptomatic enuresis*: Enuresis with other, mainly daytime, lower urinary tract symptoms.
- *Overactive bladder* (OAB): All children with complaints of urgency and frequency with or without incontinence.

---

permanent leaking of small amounts of urine during the day and at night is typical for girls with duplex kidney and ectopic ureter implantation. Malformations of the urethra may also be the cause of organic urinary incontinence. Polyuric renal disease – such as tubulopathies, chronic renal failure, or diabetes insipidus – can also manifest as treatment-refractory enuresis.

Neurogenic Disorders

In congenital diseases (e.g., myelomeningocele/spina bifida) or acquired neoplastic or inflammatory disorders of the nervous system, the innervation of the bladder is often affected. Occult spinal dysraphisms (for example, spina bifida occulta, tethered cord syndrome, sacral agenesis) often remain undetected for a long time and can manifest as treatment-resistant SRE.[1]

MANIFESTATIONS OF THE SYMPTOMS OF FUNCTIONAL URINARY INCONTINENCE

Monosymptomatic Enuresis Nocturna (MEN)

The causes underlying many of the enuretic cases remain frequently only partially explained. It may be assumed that a combination of developmental delays in neurological bladder control and the regulation of urine production play the major crucial roles in the causation of enuresis.

There are children who present nocturnal polyuria, with or without vasopressin deficiency. These children usually have no associated daytime bladder dysfunction,[23] and wet their beds because nocturnal urine output exceeds the amount of urine that the bladder can accommodate. In general, they sleep too deeply to wake up when the bladder is full – high arousal thresholds. Experts have chosen to call this subtype of MEN as *diuresis-dependent enuresis*.[24]

There is a second group of children with SRE and MEN who suffer from detrusor overactivity.[23,24] Many of these children have daytime symptoms such as urgency and/or incontinence, or are constipated,[10] and they wet their beds because of uninhibited detrusor contractions that fail to awaken the child from sleep. The term *detrusor-dependent enuresis* is commonly used to define this MEN subgroup.[24] There are also children who exhibit signs of both diuresis-dependent and detrusor-dependent SRE.[25]

Since neither nocturnal polyuria nor diminished functional bladder capacity adequately explain why children with SRE do not wake up to void, the primary mechanisms in patients with enuresis are believed to represent *multifactorial pathways*, with several different pathophysiologic mechanisms being proposed.

Nocturnal Polyuria

The findings by Nørgaard et al. showing that many enuretic children have nocturnal polyuria (due to the lack of the physiological nocturnal peak of vasopressin secretion) causing nocturnal urine production and exceeding their functional bladder capacity[26] have been replicated[27,28] and contradicted.[29] The possibility has also been put forward that polyuria is not necessarily always caused by vasopressin deficiency.[16]

Detrusor Overactivity

Support for the *detrusor overactivity* hypothesis is provided by the finding that children with enuresis go to the toilet more often than dry children, that they void smaller volumes, and that urgency symptoms are more common in this group.[17,23] However, the European Bladder Dysfunction Study (EBDS) did not find any correlation between clinical urge symptoms and cystomanometric detrusor overactivity.[24] It is likely that the overactive bladder in children is not pathophysiologically identical to the better-understood overactive bladder in adults. The cardinal symptom of overactive bladder is an imperative urinary urge. By intentionally restricting fluid intake and paying frequent visits to the toilet many children remain continent during the day, but once these control mechanisms are absent, for example, during sleep, such children manifest enuresis, a very different situation from that seen in adults.[1]

Sleep-Disordered Breathing

Over the last decade, a significant correlation between SRE and sleep-disordered breathing (SDB) has been firmly established. Habitual snoring is the most common clinical manifestation of SDB in children, a condition that ranges from primary snoring to severe OSAS.[30] Studies on the epidemiology and symptoms of sleep-disordered breathing have reported an increased frequency of enuresis in children with habitual snoring. Wang and colleagues reported that 46% of children with OSAS diagnosed by polysomnography had nocturnal enuresis.[31]

In a European population questionnaire-based study, Kaditis and colleagues showed that 23.3% of children with SRE were habitual snorers.[32] In a recent questionnaire-based survey of a community sample of children in Greece by the same authors, children with HS reported more often the concurrent presence of SRE than those children without HS.[21] Similar results were reported by a North American population-based study, in which 26.9% of habitual snorers presented with enuresis.[33] The existence of a significant association between enuresis and SDB has been further supported by the decreases in frequency of SRE or even complete resolution of nocturnal enuresis after successful treatment of the breathing disorder during sleep.

As a general recommendation, mouth breathing and nasal congestion during sleep should be more carefully evaluated in cases of children with NE who do not respond to standard treatment and present with SDB.[4]

Deep Sleep with Reduced Arousabilty

A great deal of controversy has existed for many years about whether enuresis reflects a sleep disorder or not. In fact, some studies based on surveys have found that children with nocturnal enuresis are more subject to parasomnias (such as night terrors or sleepwalking) than children who do not wet the bed.[14] Considering that most patients with sleep apnea frequently complain about their more frequent awakenings to urinate, some of them may not fully awaken to urinate, and thus have SRE. Accordingly, it is reasonable to assume that there may be something abnormal with the arousal response when SRE is present. To explore this issue, several studies examined whether sleep characteristics might differ among children with and without SRE, and have analyzed the 'arousability' of these patients.[3,20,34–36] In most of the children with SRE, normal polysomnographic findings were reported, failing to identify a specific 'deep-sleep phenotype' that may explain the occurrence of enuresis. However, when surveyed, parents consistently indicate that their children with SRE are 'deep sleepers,' compared with their siblings who are not bedwetters.[14] Furthermore, when assessing the timing of SRE within the sleep cycle, it becomes apparent that the involuntary and accidental voiding events might occur during any sleep stage,[31] even if children with severe, therapy-resistant enuresis preferably void during non-REM sleep, particularly stages 3–4.[32]

Increased Glomerular Filtration

It has been described that in obese adult patients glomerular filtration rate is increased. Krieger and colleagues found in obese subjects with sleep apnea, higher fractional urinary flows, increased fractional sodium and chloride excretion, and a lower percentage of filtered sodium reabsorption, compared to normal subjects.[37] Interestingly, treatment with CPAP tended to normalize renal function in patients with OSAS and was associated with reduced urinary output and sodium reabsorption. No studies in children with SRE have been made in order to corroborate this hypothesis. However, a recent study by Kaditis and colleagues suggested that increased natriuresis is indeed present in children with OSAS and is probably related to increased systemic blood pressure.[38]

Natriuretic Peptides

One of the potential mechanisms accounting for the increased prevalence of SRE in the context of SDB may be related to the release of both atrial and brain natriuretic peptides from cardiac myocytes following cardiac wall distension, as induced by the increased negative intrathoracic pressure swings that accompany the increased upper airway resistance associated with SDB. Increased respiratory effort against a closed or partially closed airway elicits a rise in the negative intrathoracic pressures with a subsequent increase in the venous return and cardiac distension, the latter leading to the release of atrial wall diuretic peptides. In addition, the hypoxia associated with an apneic event may induce pulmonary vasoconstriction, causing right ventricular overload and additional atrial distension. All these mechanisms may explain the increases in atrial natriuretic peptide (ANP) release, which would then enhance urinary excretion. To test these assumptions, Krieger and collaborators examined and confirmed the presence of a correlation between ANP levels and the degree of negative intrathoracic pressures associated with apneic events and hypoxemia.[37] However, the role of ANP and that of brain natriuretic peptide (BNP) remains controversial. Patwardhan and colleagues showed the absence of any association between natriuretic peptides and OSAS in a community-based sample, suggesting that undiagnosed OSAS may not be associated with major alterations in left ventricular function, as reflected by changes in morning natriuretic peptide levels.[39]

In a study on children, Kaditis and colleagues showed that children with an apnea hypopnea index (AHI) ≥5 events/hour of total sleep time had fourfold higher risk of nocturnal increase in BNP levels when compared to subjects with AHI ≤5. These investigators concluded that BNP levels were higher among snoring children, and appeared to correlate with the severity of respiratory disturbance during sleep.[32] Based on the cumulative evidence presented heretofore, SDB may increase the frequency of enuresis in children though BNP-dependent mechanisms. In further exploration of this hypothesis, Sans and colleagues found that habitual snoring (HS) was associated with increased prevalence of SRE in a young school-aged community-based sample, and that morning BNP levels were increased in enuretic children. However, the prevalence of enuresis did not appear to be modified by the severity of respiratory disturbance during sleep. Taken together, even mild increases in sleep pressure due to HS may raise the arousal threshold and promote enuresis, particularly among prone children, and more so among those with elevated BNP levels. Thus, in children with a genetic propensity for enuresis, BNP levels may tend to be enhanced by both HS and OSAS, thereby tipping the balance in favor of a more pronounced propensity to develop SRE.[33]

To summarize the role of BNP in enuretic children with sleep-disordered breathing we could use increased plasma levels of BNP as an indicator of increased prevalence of enuresis in the context of SDB.[40]

Comorbidities in Functional Urinary Incontinence

Risk factors associated with a greater prevalence or severity of SRE include urinary tract infections (which may cause temporary detrusor and/or urethral instability), diabetes mellitus and diabetes insipidus, stress, sexual abuse and other psychopathological conditions, as well as some of the risk factors for sleep-related enuresis, such as constipation and upper airway obstruction.[1,4,7]

THERAPEUTIC OPTIONS IN CHILDREN WITH SLEEP-RELATED ENURESIS

Given the pathophysiological processes potentially underlying SRE, it should come as no surprise that therapies of enuresis that have aimed to address either sleep and urine production or detrusor function have not achieved increased success than when compared to placebo. Only three therapies have withstood the test of proper randomized, placebo-controlled trials: the enuresis alarm, desmopressin, and imipramine treatment. Among those, only the enuresis alarm and treatment with desmopressin can presently be recommended for routine treatment of SRE.[24]

The Enuresis Alarm

The alarm is triggered when a sensor in the sheets or night clothing becomes wet, setting off an auditory signal causing the child to wake up, cease voiding, and go to the bathroom to complete the voiding. Parents are advised to wake their child up when the alarm is activated, since otherwise SRE children are prone to turn it off and go back to sleep.[7] The alarm should be worn every night. Response is not immediate and treatment should be continued for 2–3 months or until the child is dry for 14 consecutive nights.[7] The success rate is reported to be around 60–70%. Relapse after successful treatment occurs in 5–30% of children.[41]

Treatment with Desmopressin

Desmopressin is a synthetic analog of arginine vasopressin, the naturally occurring antidiuretic hormone. One of its major actions is to reduce the volume of urine produced overnight to within normal limits. Medication should be taken 1 hour before the last void and before bedtime to allow timely enhanced concentration of urine to occur. Fluid intake should be reduced from 1 hour before desmopressin administration and for 8 h subsequently to encourage optimal concentrating capacity and treatment response, as well as to reduce the risk of hyponatremia/water intoxication. Desmopressin is only effective on the night of administration; therefore, it must be taken on a daily basis. Full adherence is required to avoid wet nights. Based on a recent international consensus guideline for the treatment of enuresis, the initial duration of treatment should be 2–6 weeks, to ascertain its antienuretic effect.[7]

Side effects are rare and treatment is generally considered safe, if the patient does not consume large amounts of liquids while taking the drug.[42] Reported success rates have varied between 40% and 80%, but most children relapse after treatment, so the curative effect is low.[42,43]

TREATING COMORBIDITIES

Children with urinary incontinence and clinically relevant comorbidities need a comprehensive therapeutic strategy that considers the patient and the families' individual situation.

Here, the author would like to make a special mention for SRE in the context of SDB.

Effect of Appropriate Treatment of Sleep-Disordered Breathing on Sleep-Related Enuresis

Overall, the available data are scant. Weider and Hauri reported resolution or decreased frequency of sleep-related enuresis and diurnal incontinence after relief of upper airway obstruction following adenotonsillectomy.[20] Basha et al.[44] and Firoozi et al.[45] reported similar results.

A lower response rate to adenotonsillectomy seemed to be associated with prematurity, obesity, family history of nocturnal enuresis (NE), presence of non-monosymptomatic NE, severe NE preoperatively, and arousal difficulties.[46]

Interestingly, resolution of enuresis has also been reported in children with habitual snoring and nasal obstruction who received treatment with intranasal corticosteroids.[47]

Appropriate treatment for sleep-disordered breathing is extensively described in other chapters of this book.

CONCLUSION: CLINICAL IMPLICATIONS AND FUTURE RESEARCH

Nocturnal enuresis refers to the involuntary loss of urine after the age of 5 years, an age at which children are expected to

have achieved full bladder control at night. It is classified as primary when the child has never achieved nighttime dryness and secondary when bedwetting occurs after being dry for at least 6 months. The condition is considered primary in a child who has never been consistently dry during sleep for 6 months. Primary sleep enuresis is more common in boys than in girls with a 3:1 ratio.

As discussed earlier, enuresis is clinically and pathogenetically a heterogeneous disorder and, in this chapter, we have emphasized the role of sleep-disordered breathing in the disease. A link between habitual snoring and SRE has been established in children and adults. Several pathophysiological mechanisms have been proposed to explain this association but, in the end, genetic predisposition to enuresis seems to be the most important factor, even when compared to OSAS severity. Effective treatment of upper way resistance, even habitual snoring, may improve or resolve enuresis in affected children.

Given all these considerations, careful evaluation of the presence of sleep-disordered breathing (from habitual snoring to OSAS) in enuretic patients is most significant. Proper treatment can lead to resolution of the problem, improving patient's self-esteem and quality of life.

Clinical Pearls

- Male sex and age younger than 9 years are considered major contributors to sleep-related enuresis in children.
- Urinary incontinence is a heterogeneous entity that has multifactorial causes and is affected by comorbidities.
- Children with urinary incontinence and clinically relevant comorbidities need a comprehensive therapeutic strategy that considers the patient's and their families' individual situation.
- Upper airway resistance during sleep manifested either as habitual snoring (HS) or a documented obstructive sleep apnea (OSA) syndrome increases the risk of enuresis.
- Only the enuresis alarm and treatment with desmopressin can presently be recommended for routine use.

References

1. Schultz-Lampel D, Steuber C, Hoyer PF, et al. Urinary incontinence in children. Dtsch Arztebl Int 2011;108(37):613–20. doi: 10.3238/arztebl.2011.0613.
2. Barone JG, Hanson C, DaJusta DG, et al. Nocturnal enuresis and overweight are associated with obstructive sleep apnea. Pediatrics 2009;124(1):e53–9.
3. Brooks LJ. Enuresis and sleep apnea. Pediatrics 2005;116:799–800.
4. Sakellaropoulou AV, Hatzistilianou MN, Emporiadou MN, et al. Association between primary nocturnal enuresis and habitual snoring in children with obstructive sleep apnoea-hypopnoea syndrome. Arch Med Sci. 2012;8(3):521–7. doi: 10.5114/aoms.2012.28809. PubMed PMID: 22852010; PubMed Central PMCID: PMC3400898.
5. Jeyakumar A, Rahman SI, Armbrecht ES, et al. The association between sleep-disordered breathing and enuresis in children. Laryngoscope 2012;122(8):1873–7. doi: 10.1002/lary.23323. Epub 2012 May 1. Review. PubMed PMID:22549900.
6. Bascom A, Penney T, Metcalfe M, et al. High risk of sleep disordered breathing in the enuresis population. J Urol 2011;186(Suppl. 4):1710–13. doi: 10.1016/j.juro.2011.04.017. PubMed PMID: 21862067.
7. Vande Walle J, Rittig S, Bauer S, et al. American Academy of Pediatrics; European Society for Paediatric Urology; European Society for Paediatric Nephrology; International Children's Continence Society. Practical consensus guidelines for the management of enuresis. Eur J Pediatr 2012;171(6):971–83. doi: 10.1007/s00431-012-1687-7. Epub 2012 Feb 24. Erratum in: Eur J Pediatr. 2012;171(6):1005.

8. Butler R, Heron J. The prevalence of infrequent bedwetting and nocturnal enuresis in childhood. A large British cohort. Scand J Urol Nephrol 2008;2:257–64.

9. Yeung CK, Sreedhar B, Sihoe JD, et al. Differences in characteristics of nocturnal enuresis between children and adolescents: a critical appraisal from a large epidemiological study. BJU Int 2006;97(5):1069–73.

10. Heilenkötter K, Bachmann C, Janhsen E, et al. Prospective evaluation of inpatient and outpatient bladder training in children with functional urinary incontinence. Urology 2006;67:176–80.

11. Bower WF, Moore KH, Shepherd RB, et al. The epidemiology of childhood enuresis in Australia. Br J Urol 1996;78(4):602–6.

12. Wille S. Nocturnal enuresis: sleep disturbance and behavioural patterns. Acta Paediatr 1994;83:772–4.

13. Su MS, Li AM, So HK, et al. Nocturnal enuresis in children: prevalence, correlates, and relationship with obstructive sleep apnea. J Pediatr 2011;159(2):238–42.e1. doi: 10.1016/j.jpeds.2011.01.036. Epub 2011 Mar 12.PubMed PMID: 21397910.

14. Hunskaar S, Burgio K, Diokno A, et al. Epidemiology and natural history of urinary incontinence in women. Urology 2003;62(4 Suppl. 1):16–23.

15. Rittig S, Knudsen UB, Nørgaard JP, et al. Abnormal diurnal rhythm of plasma vasopressin and urinary output in patients with enuresis. Am J Physiol 1989;56(4 Pt 2):F664–71.

16. Kawauchi A, Imada N, Tanaka Y, et al. Changes in the structure of sleep spindles and delta waves on electroencephalography in patients with nocturnal enuresis. Br J Urol 1998;81(Suppl. 3):72–5.

17. Yazbeck S, Schick E, O'Regan S. Relevance of constipation to enuresis, urinary tract infection and reflux. A review. Eur Urol 1987;13(5):318–21. Review. PubMed PMID: 3315689.

18. Järvelin MR. Developmental history and neurological findings in enuretic children. Dev Med Child Neurol 1989;31(6):728–36.

19. Duel BP, Steinberg-Epstein R, Hill M, et al. A survey of voiding dysfunction in children with attention deficit-hyperactivity disorder. J Urol 2003;170(4 Pt 2):1521–3; discussion 1523–4.

20. Weider DJ, Hauri PJ. Nocturnal enuresis in children with upper airway obstruction. Int J Pediatr Otorhinolaryngol 1985; 9(2):173–82.

21. Alexopoulos EI, Kostadima E, Pagonari I, et al. Association between primary nocturnal enuresis and habitual snoring in children. Urology 2006;68(2):406–9.

22. Brooks LJ, Topol HI. Enuresis in children with sleep apnea. J Pediatr 2003;142:515–18.

23. Nevéus T, Hetta J, Cnattingius S, et al. Depth of sleep and sleep habits among enuretic and incontinent children. Acta Paediatr 1999;88:748–52.

24. Nevéus T. Sleep enuresis. Handb Clin Neurol 2011;8:363–9. Review.

25. Nijman RJ. Role of antimuscarinics in the treatment of nonneurogenic daytime urinary incontinence in children. J Urol 2004;63(3 Suppl. 1):45–50.

26. Nørgaard JP, Pedersen EB, Djurhuus JC. Diurnal antidiuretic hormone levels in enuretics. J Urol 1985;134:1029–31.

27 Hunsballe JM, Hansen TK, Rittig S, et al. The efficacy of DDAVP is related to the circadian rhythm of urine output in patients with persisting nocturnal enuresis. Clin Endocrinol (Oxf) 1998;49(6):793–801. PubMed PMID: 10209568.

28. Vurgun N, Yiditodlu MR, Ypcan A, et al. Hypernatriuria and kaliuresis in enuretic children and the diurnal variation. J Urol 1998;159(4):1333–7. PubMed PMID: 9507879.

29. Läckgren G, Nevéus T, Stenberg A. Diurnal plasma vasopressin and urinary output in adolescents with monosymptomatic nocturnal enuresis. Acta Paediatr 1997;86(4):385–90. PubMed PMID: 917.

30. Gozal D, O'Brien LM. Snoring and obstructive sleep apnoea in children: why should we treat? Pediatr Respir Rev 2004;5:S371–6.

31. Wang RC, Elkins TP, Keech D, et al. Accuracy of clinical evaluation in pediatric obstructive sleep apnea. Otolaryngol Head Neck Surg 1998;118:69–73.

32. Kaditis AG, Alexopoulos EI, Hatzi F, et al. Overnight change in brain natriuretic peptide levels in children with sleep disordered breathing. Chest 2006;130:1377–384.

33. Sans Capdevila O, McLaughlin Crabtree V, Kheirandish-Gozal L, et al. Increased morning brain natriuretic peptide levels in children with nocturnal enuresis and sleep-disordered breathing: A community-based study. Pediatrics 2008;121:e1208–14.

34. Umlauf MG, Chasens ER. Sleep disordered breathing and nocturnal polyuria: nocturia and enuresis. Sleep Med Rev 2003;7(5):373–6.

35. Mikkelsen EJ, Rapoport JL. Enuresis: psychopathology, sleep stage, and drug response. Urol Clin North Am 1980;7(2):361–77. PubMed PMID: 6996271.

36. Nevéus T, Stenberg A, Läckgren G, et al. Sleep of children with enuresis: a polysomnographic study. Pediatrics 1999;106(6 Pt 1):1193–7.

37. Krieger J, Petiau C, Sforza E, et al. Nocturnal pollakiuria is a symptom of obstructive sleep apnea. Urol Int 1993;50(2):93–7.

38. Kaditis AG, Alexopoulos EI, Evangelopoulos K, et al. Correlation of urinary excretion of sodium with severity of sleep-disordered breathing in children: a preliminary study. Pediatr Pulmonol 2010;45(10):999–1004.

39. Patwardhan AA, Larson MG, Levy D, et al. Obstructive sleep apnea and plasma natriuretic peptide levels in a community-based sample. Sleep 2006;29(10):1301–6.

40. Waleed FE, Samia AF, Samar MF. Impact of sleep-disordered breathing and its treatment on children with primary nocturnal enuresis. Swiss Med Wkly 2011;141:w13216. doi: 10.4414/smw.2011.13216. PubMed PMID: 21720969.

41. Glazener CM, Evans JH. Desmopressin for nocturnal enuresis in children. Cochrane Database Syst Rev 2002;(3):CD002112. Review. PubMed PMID: 12137645.

42. Monda JM, Husmann DA. Primary nocturnal enuresis: a comparison among observation, imipramine, desmopressin acetate and bed-wetting alarm systems. J Urol 1995;154(2 Pt 2):745–8.

43. Robson WL, Leung AK. Side effects and complications of treatment with desmopressin for enuresis. J Natl Med Assoc 1994;86(10):775–8.

44. Basha S, Bialowas C, Ende K, et al. Effectiveness of adenotonsillectomy in the resolution of nocturnal enuresis secondary to obstructive sleep apnea. Laryngoscope 2005;115(6):1101–3.

45. Firoozi F, Batniji R, Aslan AR, et al. Resolution of diurnal incontinence and nocturnal enuresis after adenotonsillectomy in children. J Urol 2006;175(5):1885–8; discussion 1888. PubMed PMID: 16600788.

46. Kovacevic L, Jurewicz M, Dabaja A, et al. Enuretic children with obstructive sleep apnea syndrome: Should they see otolaryngology first? J Pediatr Urol 2012. [Epub ahead of print] PubMed PMID: 22285485.

47. Alexopoulos EI, Kaditis AG, Kostadima E, et al. Resolution of nocturnal enuresis in snoring children after treatment with nasal budesonide. Urology 2005;66(1):194. PubMed PMID: 15961142.

Bedtime Problems and Night Wakings

Jodi A. Mindell and Melisa Moore

INTRODUCTION

In young children, bedtime difficulties and frequent night wakings are both common and persistent. It is estimated that 20–30% of children under the age of 3 years experience these sleep problems.[1,2] Furthermore, 84% of children with a sleep problem at age 1–2 still have the same problem at age 3.[3] Studies have provided solid evidence that sleep problems affect emotional, cognitive, behavioral, and academic functioning in children[4–6] and also are associated with important health concerns such as obesity.[7] The sleep and daytime functioning of parents is affected as well.[8]

Bedtime Problems

Bedtime problems occur in about 10–30% of preschoolers and toddlers.[9] Typical symptoms include avoidance of bedtime (such as refusal to get into bed, stay in bed, or participate in the bedtime routine) and frequent requests after lights out (such as for food, drinks, or stories). Bedtime problems often begin as part of the emerging independence of toddlers, but they can continue or develop in preschoolers and school-aged children as well. Often, children will test limits in order to determine boundaries and gain independence, both at night and during the day. In most cases these behaviors are developmentally appropriate; however, at bedtime these behaviors may be more difficult for parents to address, and they can result in inconsistent bedtime routines or parental limits that change with the child's requests. When nighttime routines and appropriate rules are absent, inconsistent, or dependent upon the child's requests, bedtime problems may emerge.

Night Wakings

Frequent night wakings of children are reported by 25–50% of parents[10–12] and are found to be most problematic in infants and toddlers aged 6 months to 3 years. The conditions under which the child learns to fall asleep (i.e., sleep associations) may have a direct impact on the frequency of night wakings, as may other behavioral factors and circadian issues; however, medical causes, such as reflux and obstructive sleep apnea, should be considered. When sleep associations involve another person (typically a caregiver), it is more difficult for the child to return to sleep independently following normative night wakings. Parental presence (e.g., rocking, feeding, or lying down with the child) has been shown to be one of the most common predictors of frequent night waking.[10] Although parents often perceive that their children with night wakings have more frequent arousals than do other children, in fact such wakings are a normal part of sleep architecture and are experienced equally by children with and without reported night waking.[13] It is the child's signaling at times of waking – by crying, calling, or getting out of bed (because of difficulty returning to sleep independently) – that makes the parents aware of, and thus report as frequent, the night wakings.

Children often have frequent night wakings and bedtime problems as coexisting symptoms. When bedtime problems lead to a long bedtime routine and increased time to sleep onset, caregivers may eventually do whatever it takes for everyone to get to sleep. Furthermore, inconsistent limit setting may facilitate the development of negative sleep associations. For example, a child may repeatedly prolong bedtime with demands (typically by calling out, crying, or having tantrums). If the caregiver eventually gives in to these demands, perhaps by lying down with the child or bringing him or her into the parental bed, these behaviors are reinforced. Thus, the sleep problem is related to both the negative sleep onset associations and to the lack of appropriate limit setting.

INTERVENTIONS

Interventions for bedtime problems and frequent night wakings have been supported by a broad foundation of research.[14] The review by Mindell et al.[1] found that 94% of 52 treatment studies for bedtime problems and frequent night wakings were efficacious, with over 80% of children demonstrating improvement; and, these improvements were maintained for 3 to 6 months. Behavioral approaches for the treatment of bedtime problems and night waking are discussed below and include: sleep hygiene, extinction, graduated extinction, positive routines and bedtime fading, scheduled awakenings, and parent education/prevention. More recently, internet-based interventions incorporating these treatment modalities have been developed.

Sleep Hygiene

Sleep hygiene is typically a component of treatments for bedtime problems and frequent night wakings. Any intervention to address childhood sleep problems should begin with an assessment and, if necessary, recommendations for improving sleep hygiene. Positive sleep habits include having a consistent sleep schedule on weekdays and weekends (that provides the opportunity for adequate sleep duration), a regular bedtime routine, and conditions that are conducive to falling asleep. Several large-scale studies have found that absence of these sleep practices has a significant negative impact on bedtime and nighttime sleep behaviors.[2,15]

The evidence as to whether sleep hygiene itself directly results in improvements in sleep is mixed. For example, one study[16] found that sleep hygiene alone significantly improved sleep in almost 20% of children with ADHD and insomnia. In contrast, another study found that although combined behavioral–educational intervention for new mothers resulted in significant improvement in maternal and infant sleep, just teaching maternal sleep hygiene and providing basic information about infant sleep did not.[17] (Also see section on Education/Prevention below.)

Although inclusion of a bedtime routine is often recommended to caregivers as part of well child care or as a component of behavioral sleep interventions, the importance of the bedtime routine itself may be underappreciated. For example, a 2009 study found that, compared to controls, a bedtime routine alone resulted in improvements in sleep onset latency, number of night wakings, sleep continuity, problematic sleep behaviors, and maternal mood.[18] Other important aspects of good sleep hygiene (besides having an appropriate bedtime routine) include avoiding letting the child fall asleep while feeding and moving the feeding to the beginning of the routine, eliminating caffeine, and avoiding use of electronics 30–60 minutes before bedtime.

Extinction

Standard extinction involves putting the child in the crib or bed at a consistent time and ignoring the child's negative behaviors (such as crying, yelling, tantrums), while monitoring for safety, until a specified wake time. Extinction is one of the earliest behavioral interventions developed and tested for bedtime problems and frequent night wakings, and it has been well validated.[1] At least three randomized-controlled trials (RCTs)[19–21] provide empirical support for standard extinction. One RCT compared extinction to scheduled awakenings and to a control group. Based on parental reports it was found that the extinction group had fewer night wakings than controls, and that the improvements seen occurred more quickly than in the scheduled awakenings group.[19] Extinction alone has also been compared with extinction combined with a medication (trimeprazine) or placebo.[21] Extinction was effective in all three groups – with improvements maintained at both 6 and 30 months – but the fastest response was in the extinction plus medication group.

Consistency is the key to success with extinction, yet most caregivers find their child's prolonged crying to be extremely stressful; thus the standard approach to extinction may be difficult for some parents. If parents respond to their child's yelling and crying after a period of time, the child's negative behavior is reinforced with attention and reward, increasing the likelihood of the behavior continuing. Parents should also be advised about the possibility of an initial or delayed *extinction burst* or brief worsening of negative behaviors. While this is a normative part of the extinction process, parents may perceive this as evidence that the intervention is not working.

Graduated Extinction

Graduated extinction, like standard extinction, involves ignoring negative behaviors, but only for a specified duration, before checking on the child and providing only brief reassurance and limited attention. These regular checks continue until the child falls asleep. The overall goal is to extinguish negative behaviors, thereby increasing the independence of the child (e.g., by moving them into their bed/crib/room and allowing them to develop their own soothing skills and positive sleep associations) and decreasing the child's reliance on a caregiver to help fall asleep at bedtime and return to sleep following normative night wakings. This treatment can be implemented in a number of ways including gradually moving the parent out of the room (e.g., first sitting beside the bed, then in the doorway), checking at fixed intervals (e.g., 3 minutes between checks), or checking at increasing intervals (3 minutes, then 5 minutes, then 10 minutes). Studies have found all such approaches to be efficacious.[1,22,23] In a clinical situation, the decision regarding the time between checks is usually based on parental comfort and acceptability, as well as on child temperament and the length of time the child will stay in bed (for toddlers).

A number of RCTs support the use of graduated extinction as an effective intervention for bedtime problems and frequent wakings. Hiscock et al.[24] compared graduated extinction, instituted at an 8-month well-child visit, to a control group. The intervention group demonstrated fewer sleep problems at 10 and 12 months. Adams and Rickert[25] compared graduated extinction (ignoring the child for a set amount of time determined by the child's age and parent input) with positive bedtime routines. Both intervention groups were effective at reducing negative bedtime behaviors when compared with controls.

An RCT of 3–6-year-olds found the use of a *bedtime pass* to be an effective modification of graduated extinction. In this study, children were given a card (the bedtime pass), which could be traded in for a reasonable request (such as a visit from a caregiver or a drink of water).[26] After the bedtime pass was used, caregivers were instructed to ignore negative, attention-seeking behaviors from the child. Results demonstrated less frequent calling and crying out and shorter time to quieting in the intervention group compared to controls, and these improvements were maintained at 3 months. High parental satisfaction was noted.

Despite evidence that both graduated and standard extinction are effective, of the two approaches, graduated extinction is almost always the one recommended, as it is often perceived by parents and providers to be a 'gentler' approach. Overall, graduated extinction interventions are typically the most widely utilized behavioral treatment for bedtime problems and night wakings.

Positive Routines with Faded Bedtime

Positive routines with faded bedtime involves developing a short, enjoyable bedtime routine to be implemented at a later than desired bedtime (closer to the time the child is currently falling asleep). The goal is for the child to develop an association between the positive bedtime routine and falling asleep quickly. Once this association is established, the child's bedtime is moved earlier in 15-minute increments. Unlike extinction, where the goal is to reduce negative behaviors the goal of positive routines and faded bedtime is to reduce the physiological and emotional arousal that accompanies bedtime conflict and for the child to develop or increase appropriate bedtime behaviors.[1]

At least three studies have found positive routines with faded bedtime to be effective in the treatment of bedtime problems and night waking.[25,27,28] The only study of positive routines with faded bedtime to include a control group also had a group treated with graduated extinction. Prior to the later bedtime (in the positive routine group), the parent and child would complete 4–7 calm, pleasurable activities together; if the child began to tantrum, the parent was to end the activities and tell the child that it was time for bed; finally, the child's bedtime was gradually moved earlier until the desired time was reached. In this study, the positive routines with faded bedtime and the graduated extinction treatments were both significantly more effective than was no treatment (the control group) but were not significantly different from each other.

Scheduled Awakenings

Though used much less frequently than other approaches discussed in this chapter, scheduled awakenings are an alternative treatment for frequent wakings if the child wakes at consistent, predictable times during the night. Parents first track the number and times of night wakings to determine a baseline.[29,30] Then, they wake the child at a specified time (typically 15–20 minutes before a usual waking) and provide their usual response to the night waking (e.g., feeding, rocking) until the child returns to sleep. The interval between scheduled wakings is then gradually increased with the intention of increasing the duration of sleep between wakings. Several studies have found scheduled awakenings to be successful,[19,29–31] although this procedure may take longer than extinction (e.g., several weeks) and may be difficult for parents to implement (as they need to wake their child throughout the night). Additionally, this approach is not applicable to children with bedtime struggles.

Education/Prevention

Parent education and prevention focuses on providing written or in-person information during the prenatal or newborn period in order to prevent the development of bedtime problems and frequent night wakings. Education typically involves provision of information about helping children develop self-soothing skills (including positive associations) and recommending positive sleep hygiene practices (including a consistent sleep schedule and a bedtime routine). Many educational programs advise putting infants to bed awake and allowing them to return to sleep independently following normative night waking.[17] Multiple studies have been conducted showing that short interventions (1–4 sessions) greatly impact infant sleep,[32–36] although longer-term outcomes are unknown. St. James-Roberts et al.[35] and Adair et al.[32] incorporated written sleep information into two routine well-child visits and found benefits in infant sleep. Wolfson et al.[36] randomly assigned first-time parents in child birthing classes to a sleep education group (2 classes before and 2 classes after childbirth) or to a control group. According to parent diary, 72% of 3-week-old infants 'slept through the night' compared with 48% in the control group. A study by Pinilla and Birch[34] found that by 8 weeks, 100% of infants in a parent education intervention slept through the night compared with 23% of controls.

An emerging area in prevention is the intersection of sleep and obesity. As early as the first 6 months of life, a link has been found between sleep duration and weight-for-length measures,[37] and it has been shown that total daily sleep duration of less than 12 hours during infancy is associated with overweight status in preschool-aged children.[38] Thus, there has been a call for clinicians and researchers to include sleep interventions in obesity-prevention efforts.[39] One pilot study from 2001[40] found that a behavioral intervention targeting feeding as well as sleep resulted in lower weight-for-length percentiles at 1 year of age.

Internet Interventions

Though behavioral interventions have typically been conducted face-to-face, at least one study has demonstrated efficacy using an internet-based intervention for young children.[41] Based on responses to an expanded version of the Brief Infant Sleep Questionnaire (BISQ),[42] parents were given information about how their child's sleep compared to a normative sample of same-aged children (*excellent*, *good*, or *disrupted*) along with customized, behaviorally based advice for how to improve their child's sleep. One week following the internet intervention, improvements were seen in latency to sleep onset, number and duration of night wakings, and sleep continuity. Maternal confidence in managing their child's sleep, maternal sleep, and maternal mood were also significantly improved. These improvements were maintained at 1 year post intervention.[43]

TREATMENT CHALLENGES AND IMPLICATIONS

While research clearly demonstrates that behavioral treatments for bedtime problems and night wakings are effective at improving children's sleep, there are many who are resistant to behavioral interventions because of worries about harmful effects on other aspects of child development, such as the quality of the parent–child relationship. Concerns have been raised about the impact of behavioral sleep interventions on attachment, security, and mental health.[44,45] A recent review of secondary outcomes of behavioral sleep interventions did not find evidence to support iatrogenic effects.[46] Of 35 treatment studies that included a secondary outcome measure, no systematic negative effects were found on any measured child variable. Conversely, improvements were demonstrated in child mood,[47] daytime behavior,[48–56] and temperament.[24,34] Several studies that focused on the impact of behavioral sleep interventions on the parent–child relationship were also reviewed.[52–54,57–59] Again, rather than demonstrating harmful effects, these studies found just the opposite. Young children with sleep disturbances initially scored lower on measures of attachment, security, and maternal bonding compared to good sleepers, and treatment actually improved security, attachment, and parent–child interactions.

BEDTIME PROBLEMS, NIGHT WAKINGS, AND SPECIAL POPULATIONS

While bedtime problems and frequent night wakings are common in typically developing children, children in special populations such as autism spectrum disorders (ASDs) and attention deficit hyperactivity disorder (ADHD) are at increased risk for problems with sleep (see Chapters 15 and 16).

Autism Spectrum Disorders

Children with developmental conditions such as autism spectrum disorders (ASDs) may be at increased risk for bedtime problems and night wakings compared to typically developing children, with 44–83% of children diagnosed with ASDs having a sleep problem based on actigraphy or parent report.[60–62] Sleep problems and shorter sleep duration in children with ASDs have been shown to relate to more energetic, excited, and problematic daytime behaviors[62] as well as to decreased social skills and increased stereotypic behaviors.[63]

Though behavioral interventions may be more difficult to implement and, therefore, are offered less frequently than medications, parents of children with ASDs prefer behavioral interventions to sleep medications.[64] One study evaluated the efficacy of faded bedtime with response cost (that is, negative consequences for inappropriate behaviors) combined with positive reinforcement in three children with ASD.[65] Sleep onset latency improved in all three during treatment and was still present 12 weeks later. Daytime behavior, as measured by the Child Behavior Checklist (CBCL),[66] a commonly used screening tool for externalizing and internalizing behaviors, improved, with scores moving from the borderline clinical range to the average range in two of the three children. Another study[67] of 20 children with ASDs (ages 3–10 years), whose parents attended a 3-part workshop on the treatment of sleep issues, found significant improvements in hyperactivity, self-stimulatory behaviors, and repetitive behaviors in addition to significant improvements in sleep.

For a more complete discussion of this topic, see Chapter 16.

ATTENTION DEFICIT HYPERACTIVITY DISORDER

Children with attention deficit hyperactivity disorder (ADHD) have been reported to have more bedtime problems (e.g., longer time to sleep onset and bedtime resistance) than do children without ADHD. This remains a controversial issue, as reviews of objective evidence have not confirmed findings from parent report studies.[68,69] Regardless, behavioral interventions for bedtime problems and night wakings in children with ADHD are promising, with at least one case series[70] and one small study[16] showing feasibility and parent satisfaction. There has also been one recent RCT of a behavioral intervention for 27 children (aged 5–14 years) that found small changes in ADHD symptom scores from baseline to 5 months post treatment following either a brief or extended treatment of sleep issues.[71] Early implementation of behavioral treatment may be critical as sleep disturbances can exacerbate symptoms of ADHD.[72,73]

For a more complete discussion of this topic, see Chapter 15.

CONCLUSION

Studies have found that bedtime problems and nighttime wakings are highly prevalent sleep disturbances in typically developing children as well as in children with ASDs and ADHD. Behavioral interventions and preventive educational approaches have been shown to be highly effective, and internet-based interventions appear to be quite promising. Not only do these behavioral interventions improve sleep, but they also appear to have a positive impact on secondary outcomes in such areas as daytime behavior, parent–child relationship, and parental well-being.

Clinical Pearls

- Bedtime problems and problematic nighttime wakings occur in 20–30% of children.
- Most such problems can be effectively treated using behavioral approaches.
- Nighttime arousals are a normal part of sleep architecture.
- Helping children learn to fall asleep independently at bedtime also helps them to learn to return to sleep independently after waking during the night.
- An appropriate bedtime routine and consistent sleep schedule are essential to develop and maintain normal sleep patterns at night.
- Feedings that are part of the bedtime routine should happen before bed and before sleep.
- Infants and children should be put to bed wide awake.

References

1. Mindell JA, Kuhn B, Lewin DS, et al. Behavioral treatment of bedtime problems and night wakings in infants and young children. Sleep 2006;29:1263–76.
2. Sadeh A, Mindell JA, Luedtke K, et al. Sleep and sleep ecology in the first 3 years: a web-based study. J Sleep Res 2009;18:60–73.
3. Kataria S, Swanson MS, Trevathan GE. Persistence of sleep disturbances in preschool children. J Pediatr 1987;110:642–6.
4. Sadeh A, Gruber R, Raviv A. Sleep, neurobehavioral functioning, and behavior problems in school-age children. Child Dev 2002;73:405–17.
5. Sadeh A, Gruber R, Raviv A. The effects of sleep restriction and extension on school-age children: What a difference an hour makes. Child Dev 2003;74:444–55.
6. Fallone G, Acebo C, Seifer R, et al. Experimental restriction of sleep opportunity in children: Effects on teacher ratings. Sleep 2005; 28:1279–85.
7. Hart CN, Cairns A, Jelalian E. Sleep and obesity in children and adolescents. Pediatr Clins N Am 2011;58:715–33.
8. Meltzer LJ, Mindell JA. Relationship between child sleep disturbances and maternal sleep, mood, and parenting stress: A pilot study. J Family Psychol 2007;21:67–73.
9. Liu X, Liu L, Owens JA, et al. Sleep patterns and sleep problems among schoolchildren in the United States and China. Pediatrics 2005;115:241–9.
10. Sadeh A, Mindell JA, Luedtke K, et al. Sleep and sleep ecology in the first 3 years: a web-based study. J Sleep Res 2009;18(1):60–73.
11. Burnham MM, Goodlin-Jones BL, Gaylor EE, et al. Nighttime sleep-wake patterns and self-soothing from birth to one year of age: a longitudinal intervention study. J Child Psychol Psychiatry 2002;43:713–25.
12. Gaylor EE, Burnham MM, Goodlin-Jones BL, et al. A longitudinal follow-up study of young children's sleep patterns using a developmental classification system. Behav Sleep Med 2005;3:44–61.
13. Sadeh A. Assessment of intervention for infant night waking: parental reports and activity-based home monitoring. J Consult Clin Psychol 1994;62:63–8.
14. Morgenthaler TI, Owens J, Alessi C, et al. Practice parameters for behavioral treatment of bedtime problems and night wakings in infants and young children. Sleep 2006;29:1277–81.
15. Mindell JA, Meltzer LJ, Carskadon MA, et al. Developmental aspects of sleep hygiene: findings from the 2004 National Sleep Foundation Sleep in America Poll. Sleep Med 2009;10:771–9.
16. Weiss MD, Wasdell MB, Bomben MM, et al. Sleep hygiene and melatonin treatment for children and adolescents with ADHD and initial insomnia. J Am Acad Child Adolesc Psychiatry 2006;45:512–19.
17. Stremler R, Hodnett E, Lee K, et al. A behavioral-educational intervention to promote maternal and infant sleep: a pilot randomized, controlled trial. Sleep 2006;29:1609–15.
18. Mindell JA, Telofski LS, Wiegand B, et al. A nightly bedtime routine: Impact on sleep problems in young children and maternal mood. Sleep 2009;32:599–606.
19. Rickert VI, Johnson CM. Reducing nocturnal awakening and crying episodes in infants and young children: A comparison between scheduled awakenings and systematic ignoring. Pediatrics 1988;81:203–12.
20. Seymour FW, Brock P, During M, et al. Reducing sleep disruptions in young children: evaluation of therapist-guided and written information approaches: a brief report. J Child Psychol Psychiatry 1989;30:913–18.
21. France KG, Blampied NM, Wilkinson P. Treatment of infant sleep disturbance by trimeprazine in combination with extinction. J Dev Behav Pediatr 1991;12:308–14.
22. Sadeh A. Assessment of intervention for infant night waking: Parental reports and activity-based home monitoring. J Consult Clin Psychol 1994;62:63–8.
23. Blunden S. Behavioural treatments to encourage solo sleeping in preschool children: an alternative to controlled crying. J Child Health Care 2011;15:107–17.
24. Hiscock H, Bayer J, Gold L, et al. Improving infant sleep and maternal mental health: a cluster randomised trial. Arch Dis Child 2007; 92:952–8.
25. Adams LA, Rickert VI. Reducing bedtime tantrums: Comparison between positive routines and graduated extinction. Pediatrics 1989;84:756–61.
26. Moore BA, Friman PC, Fruzzetti AE, et al. Brief report: evaluating the Bedtime Pass Program for child resistance to bedtime – a randomized, controlled trial. J Pediatr Psychol 2007;32:283–7.
27. Milan ZP, Berger MI, Pierson DF. Positive routines: A rapid alternative to extinction for elimination of bedtime tantrum behavior. Child Behav Ther 1981;3:13–25.

28. Galbraith L, Hewitt KE. Behavioural treatment for sleep disturbance. Health Visit 1993;66:169–71.
29. Johnson CM, Lerner M. Amerlioration of infant sleep disturbances II: Effects of scheduled awakenings by compliant parents. Infant Mental Health J 1985;6:21–30.
30. Johnson CM, Bradley-Johnson S, Stack JM. Decreasing the frequency of infants' nocturnal crying with the use of scheduled awakenings. Fam Practice Res 1981;1:98–104.
31. McGarr RJH. In search of the sand man: Shaping an infant to sleep. Educ Treat Child 1980;3:173–82.
32. Adair R, Bauchner H, Philipp B, et al. Night waking during infancy: role of parental presence at bedtime. Pediatrics 1991;87:500–4.
33. Kerr S, Jowett SA, Smith LN. Preventing sleep problems in infants: A randomized controlled trial. J Adv Nursing 1996;24:938–42.
34. Pinilla T, Birch LL. Help me make it through the night: behavioral entrainment of breast-fed infants' sleep patterns. Pediatrics 1993;91:436–44.
35. St. James-Roberts I, Sleep J, Morris S, et al. Use of a behavioural programme in the first 3 months to prevent infant crying and sleeping problems. J Paediatr Child Health 2001;37:289–97.
36. Wolfson A, Lacks P, Futterman A. Effects of parent training on infant sleeping patterns, parents' stress, and perceived parental competence. J Consult Clin Psychol 1992;60:41–8.
37. Sadeh A, Tikotzky L, Scher A. Parenting and infant sleep. Sleep Med Rev 2010;14:89–96.
38. Taveras EM, Rifas-Shiman SL, Oken E, et al. Short sleep duration in infancy and risk of childhood overweight. Arch Pediatr Adolesc Med 2008;162:305–11.
39. Paul IM, Bartok CJ, Downs DS, et al. Opportunities for the primary prevention of obesity during infancy. Adv Pediatr 2009;56:107–33.
40. Paul IM, Savage JS, Anzman SL, et al. Preventing obesity during infancy: a pilot study. Obesity (Silver Spring) 2011;19:353–61.
41. Mindell JA, Du Mond CE, Sadeh A, et al. Efficacy of an internet-based intervention for infant and toddler sleep disturbances. Sleep 2011; 34:451–8.
42. Sadeh A. A brief screening questionnaire for infant sleep problems: Validation and findings for an Internet sample. Pediatrics 2004;113:e570–7.
43. Mindell JA, Du Mond CE, Sadeh A, et al. Long-term efficacy of an internet-based intervention for infant and toddler sleep disturbances: one year follow-up. J Clin Sleep Med: JCSM: official publication of the American Academy of Sleep Medicine 2011;7:507–11.
44. Blunden SL, Thompson KR, Dawson D. Behavioural sleep treatments and night time crying in infants: challenging the status quo. Sleep Med Rev 2011;15:327–34.
45. Narvaez D. Dangers of 'crying it out': Damaging children and their relationships for the longterm. (December 11, 2011) Available at: http://www.psychologytoday.com/blog/moral-landscapes/201112/dangers-crying-it-out. Accessed 15 August 2013.
46. Mindell JA, Moore M. The impact of behavioral interventions for sleep problems on secondary outcomes in young children and their families. In: Montgomery-Downs H, Wolfson A, editors. Oxford handbook of infant, child, and adolescent sleep: development and problems. Oxford University Press; in press.
47. Skuladottir A, Thome M. Changes in infant sleep problems after a family-centered intervention. Pediatr Nurs 2003;29:375–8.
48. Burke RV, Kuhn BR, Peterson JL. Brief report: A 'storybook' ending to children's bedtime problems—the use of a rewarding social story to reduce bedtime resistance and frequent night waking. J Pediatr Psychol 2004;29:389–96.
49. Richman N, Douglas J, Hunt H, et al. Behavioural methods in the treatment of sleep disorders – a pilot study. J Child Psychol Psychiatry, and Allied Disciplines 1985;26:581–90.
50. Sanders MR, Bor B, Dadds M. Modifying bedtime disruptions in children using stimulus control and contingency management techniques. Behavl Psychother 1984;12:130–41.
51. Seymour FW, Bayfield G, Brock P, et al. Management of night-waking in young children. Austr J Family Ther 1983;4:217–23.
52. France KG. Behavior characteristics and security in sleep-disturbed infants treated with extinction. J Pediatr Psychol 1992;17:467–75.
53. Hiscock H, Bayer JK, Hampton A, et al. Long-term mother and child mental health effects of a population-based infant sleep intervention: cluster-randomized, controlled trial. Pediatrics 2008;122:e621–7.
54. Minde K, Faucon A, Falkner S. Sleep problems in toddlers: Effects of treatment on their daytime behavior. J Am Acad Child Adolesc Psychiatry 1994;33:1114–21.
55. Keech A, Collins R, MacMahon S, et al. Three-year follow-up of the Oxford Cholesterol Study: assessment of the efficacy and safety of simvastatin in preparation for a large mortality study. Eur Heart J 1994;15:255–69.
56. Reid MJ, Walter AL, O'Leary SG. Treatment of young children's bedtime refusal and nighttime wakings: A comparison of 'standard' and graduated ignoring procedures. Jo Abnormal Child Psychol 1999;27:5–16.
57. Eckerberg B. Treatment of sleep problems in families with young children: Effects of treatment on family well-being. Acta Paediatrica 2004;93:126–34.
58. France KG, Blampied NM, Wilkinson P. Treatment of infant sleep disturbance by trimeprazine in combination with extinction. J Dev Behav Pediatr: JDBP 1991;12:308–14.
59. Matthey S, Speyer J. Changes in unsettled infant sleep and maternal mood following admission to a parentcraft residential unit. Early Hum Dev 2008;84:623–9.
60. Wiggs L, Stores G. Sleep patterns and sleep disorders in children with autistic spectrum disorders: Insights using parent report and actigraphy. Devl Med Child Neurol 2004;46:372–80.
61. Richdale AL. Sleep problems in autism: Prevalence, cause, and intervention. Dev Med Child Neurol 1999;41:60–6.
62. Richdale AL, Prior MR. The sleep/wake rhythm in children with autism. Eur Child Adolesc Psychiatry 1995;4:175–86.
63. Schreck KA, Mulick JA, Smith AF. Sleep problems as possible predictors of intensified symptoms of autism. Res Dev Disabilities 2004;25:57–66.
64. Wiggs L, Stores G. Behavioural treatment for sleep problems in children with severe learning disabilities and challenging daytime behaviour: effect on daytime behaviour. J Child Psychol Psychiatry, and Allied Disciplines 1999;40:627–35.
65. Moon EC, Corkum P, Smith IM. Case study: A case-series evaluation of a behavioral sleep intervention for three children with autism and primary insomnia. J Pediatr Psychol 2011;36:47–54
66. Achenbach TM. Integrative guide to the 1991 CBCL/4-18, YSR, and TRF profiles. Burlington, VT: University of Vermont, Department of Psychology; 1991.
67. Reed HE, McGrew SG, Artbee K, et al. Parent-based sleep education workshops in autism. J Child Neurol 2009;24:936–45.
68. Cortese S, Lecendreux M, Mouren MC, et al. ADHD and insomnia. J Am Acad Child Adolesc Psychiatry 2006;45:384–5.
69. Sadeh A, Pergamin L, Bar-Haim Y. Sleep in children with attention-deficit hyperactivity disorder: a meta-analysis of polysomnographic studies. Sleep Med Rev 2006;10:381–98.
70. Mullane J, Corkum P. Case series: evaluation of a behavioral sleep intervention for three children with attention-deficit/hyperactivity disorder and dyssomnia. J Attention Dis 2006;10:217–27.
71. Sciberras E, Fulton M, Efron D, et al. Managing sleep problems in school aged children with ADHD: a pilot randomised controlled trial. Sleep Med 2011;12:932–5.
72. Dahl RE, Pelham WE, Wierson M. The role of sleep disturbances in attention deficit disorder symptoms: a case study. J Pediatr Psychol 1991;16:229–39.
73. O'Brien LM, Ivanenko A, Crabtree VM, et al. Sleep disturbances in children with attention deficit hyperactivity disorder. Pediatr Res 2003;54:237–43.

Attention Deficit, Hyperactivity, and Sleep Disorders

James E. Dillon and Ronald D. Chervin

INTRODUCTION

Two decades of burgeoning research in pediatric sleep disorders have produced compelling evidence, with broad consequences for public health, that complex relationships among sleep, behavior, and cognition account for serious and common neurobehavioral morbidity in children.[1,2] The evidence linking sleep pathology to symptoms of hyperactivity, inattention, and other neurobehavioral deficits is robust and convincing yet replete with contradictions. Seldom is there so much agreement on the scope and significance of a problem with so little consensus on its meaning and mechanism. Here we summarize this work, rationalize it within a multidimensional model, and suggest directions for investigation in the next decade. Several very competent reviews have been published recently that simplify our task considerably and allow us to emphasize a few key concepts.[1,3–14]

SLEEP DISORDER AND NEUROBEHAVIORAL PATHOLOGY AS COMORBID PROBLEMS

Parents report sleep problems in 25–50% of their children with attention deficit/hyperactivity disorder (ADHD), according to a widely quoted estimate,[15] and depending upon how sleep problems are defined, they may occur in as many as 80%.[16] Typical complaints include difficulties falling asleep or returning to sleep, bedtime anxiety or resistance, snoring, restless sleep, enuresis, nightmares, shortened sleep, and daytime sleepiness. A wide range of objective sleep findings, such as reduced sleep efficiency, sleep fragmentation, and elevated apnea–hypopnea index (AHI), have been detected with polysomnography (PSG) and actigraphy. Among children presenting with primary sleep complaints, behavioral symptoms (such as hyperactivity, defiance, and aggression), neuropsychiatric diagnoses (such as ADHD and oppositional defiant disorder (ODD)), and significant neuropsychological deficits (such as impaired attention and memory, impulsive responding, dull general intelligence, and delayed academic skill development) are common. Parent ratings, sometimes referred to as *subjective* measurements, are more likely than are objective measures (such as PSG, actigraphy, and multiple sleep latency tests (MSLT)) to produce substantial correlations with behavioral measures. This is especially true in clinical populations. Community samples of ostensibly normal children assessed by objective means are less likely to generate robust correlations.[17]

Inconsistencies between subjective and objective measures may reflect differential sensitivities to specific sleep phenomena.[18] Parents observe behavior continually over periods of years, whereas the PSG detects behavioral events for a single night, usually in a laboratory setting (and typically one bearing only superficial resemblance to home). An important though seldom appreciated phenomenon affecting parent ratings is the *halo* effect[19] (and its reverse, the infelicitously dubbed *devil* effect[20]). These effects occur when high ratings on one desirable (or undesirable) trait are accompanied by unwarranted elevations on other desirable (or undesirable) traits, producing strong but not necessarily true correlations. Abikoff et al.[21] showed that teachers observing children with oppositional defiant behaviors, for example, tended to document ADHD symptoms that were not present. Whether this devil effect contributes to the consistently high correlations between daytime behavioral problems and nighttime sleep difficulties in studies based upon parent ratings has not been investigated.

Because ADHD so commonly presents with comorbid psychiatric conditions it has not always been clear whether associated sleep findings are attributable to ADHD or to other psychopathology. Some associations may vanish when children with comorbid disorders such as depression and anxiety are eliminated from subject pools. This possibility was recently examined (2012) by Accardo et al.[22] who used a structured interview to diagnose ADHD in 317 children among whom 60 had comorbid anxiety and 62 had comorbid depression. On the *Children's Sleep Habits Questionnaire* (CSHQ)[23] only the anxious children showed modestly higher total scores relative to the ADHD group without comorbid conditions. Subscale scores, however, revealed sleep onset delay in both comorbid groups, high bedtime resistance and night wakings in the anxious children, and higher sleep duration scores for the depressed group. Comorbidities did not affect ratings on symptoms related to sleep-disordered breathing. Although this study suggested that psychiatric comorbidity is a relevant factor contributing to the frequency of sleep problems in persons with ADHD, it could also be interpreted to indicate that the magnitude of that contribution may be modest and, with respect to symptoms of sleep-disordered breathing (SDB), inconsequential.

Other confounds may account for conflicting findings in the literature. Patterns of sleep and psychiatric morbidity may also depend upon age, sex, obesity and body mass index. Treatment status (i.e., medication in the recent past) introduces the complexity of both direct and rebound effects.[24] Difficulties interpreting the literature are further magnified by inconsistencies among experts on important diagnostic thresholds in both sleep and psychiatric symptom criteria. For example, there is at best uneasy agreement on the AHI threshold that should define obstructive sleep apnea.[25,26] To some extent, the reconciliation of views depends upon the outcome of research establishing the AHI levels strongly associated with neurobehavioral morbidity. Similarly, the optimal threshold for determining clinical significance of periodic leg movements (PLMs) and associated arousals is not well studied.

Diagnostic inconsistencies in sleep have their counterparts in psychiatric conditions as well. In 1980 the DSM-III – the third edition of the American Psychiatric Association's Diagnostic and Statistical Manual of Mental Disorders (DSM)[26] – established a radically categorical (and medical) model to define childhood psychopathology. In this system, attributes widely and continuously distributed in the population, such as attention and activity level, are defined as deviant mainly on the basis of quantity or severity rather than quality or nature. Disorders defined in this way have boundaries that are somewhat arbitrary and indistinct, particularly to the extent that the measures of defining traits may be subjective or depend upon judgments of developmental norms.

Given these limitations in defining and measuring sleep and behavioral attributes, it is not surprising that conflicting reports on many key sleep-behavior findings make the literature as a whole rather difficult to digest. Two meta-analyses of particular note are discussed below; they offer complementary summaries of dependable findings gleaned from existing evidence, though most conclusions are based on only a few studies.

Sadeh and colleagues[12] reviewed reports that used PSGs to compare ADHD children with controls. Multiple confounds were examined including age, sex, rigor of psychiatric diagnosis, recruitment source, medication status, and use of an adaptation night prior to PSG. Studies with manifest recruitment bias were eliminated, but presence of comorbidity was not an exclusion criterion. Twelve samples were analyzed including data from 333 children with ADHD and 231 controls. After sleep time, sleep efficiency, sleep latency, sleep architecture, AHI and respiratory distress indices (RDI), arousals, and PLMs were examined, only PLMs statistically separated ADHD from control children, though the effect size of 0.26 was quite modest. Studies with older subjects and using more rigorous psychiatric diagnostic protocols contributed most to this result. Only seven studies contributed to the PLMs analysis, and a handful of additional subjects negative for PLMs would have moved the results into the statistically non-significant range. In a subset of studies analyzed by Sadeh in which psychiatric comorbidities had been excluded, ADHD children had longer sleep latencies than controls.

Cortese and colleagues[8] subsequently conducted a meta-analysis that involved a broader array of variables (such as PSG, actigraphy, MSLT, and subjective measures), and they included several published studies that had been unavailable a few years earlier. They excluded studies that lacked explicit diagnostic criteria and studies with subjects who were medicated or who had comorbid anxiety or depressive disorders. This left 722 ADHD children and 638 controls in 16 reports. The PLMs were not analyzed. Table 15.1 shows 11 significant effects distinguishing ADHD from control children in these analyses, along with the small number of studies (only three to four on average) upon which each conclusion was based (an indication of the slender thread upon which we can base current opinion). The ADHD children displayed longer sleep onset latency when measured by actigraphy but not by PSG. Sleep efficiency, stage shifts per hour, and true sleep time also differed between groups, but sleep onset latency measured by PSG, and percentage of time in stages 1, 2, slow-wave, and

TABLE 15.1   Positive Sleep Findings in Attention-Deficit/Hyperactivity Disorder

FINDING	SUBJECTIVE VS OBJECTIVE MEASURE	STANDARDIZED MEAN DIFFERENCE (95% CI)	NUMBER OF COMPONENT STUDIES WITH INDIVIDUALLY SIGNIFICANT OR NON-SIGNIFICANT RESULTS	
			Significant	Non-Significant Same/Opposite Direction
Bedtime resistance	Subjective	−0.86 (−1.10, -0.62)	3	1/0
Sleep onset difficulties	Subjective	−0.73 (−0.88, −0.58)	4	1/0
Night awakenings	Subjective	−0.21 (−0.39, −0.02)	2	1/0
Difficulty with morning wakenings	Subjective	−0.83 (−1.14, −0.51)	2	0/0
Daytime sleepiness	Subjective	−0.19 (-0.37, −0.00)	1	2/0
Sleep disordered breathing	Subjective	−0.37 (−0.72, −0.02)	0	2/0
Sleep onset latency (actigraphy)	Objective	−0.36 (−0.56, −0.15)	1	1/2
Stage shifts per hour	Objective	−0.59 (−1.06, −0.11)	1	1/0
True sleep (actigraphy)	Objective	0.36 (0.11, 0.60)	1	2/0
Sleep efficiency (PSG)	Objective	0.25 (0.03, 0.47)	1	4/1
MSLT	Objective	−1.43 (−1.87, −0.99)	1	1/0
Apnea-hypopnea index	Objective	−0.52 (−0.81, −0.23)	2	1/0

Standardized mean differences are determined by subtracting ADHD scores from controls; thus, a negative score means that the mean score for the ADHD group was higher than that of controls.
  The fourth column shows the number of studies that independently yielded statistically significant findings. For these variables statistically significant findings in the component studies were in the same direction as that of the meta-analytic finding.
  The fifth column shows the number of studies with non-significant findings. To the left of the 'slash' is the number of studies in which the mean scores were in the same direction as that of the meta-analytic finding; to the right is the number with findings in the opposite direction.

This table, which is based on Cortese S, Faraone SV, Konofal E, Lecendreux M. Sleep in children with attention-deficit/hyperactivity disorder: Meta-analysis of subjective and objective studies. Journal of the American Academy of Child & Adolescent Psychiatry. 2009;48:894–908,[8] shows positive findings extracted from figure 2 in that paper.

rapid eye movement (REM) sleep, did not. The AHI was higher in ADHD subjects and was in accord with subjective parent-reported measures for SDB.

ATTENTION-DEFICIT/HYPERACTIVITY DISORDER: HETEROGENEITY, SYMPTOMS, AND DISORDERS

Attention deficit disorder with and without hyperactivity (ADD w/ H and ADD w/o H) was introduced in the DSM-III largely on the expectation that the core symptom was inattention and that the ADD w/o H phenotype would prove to be an alternative expression, perhaps more common in girls, of the same presumably familial condition. Numerous studies spanning nearly 30 years have consistently highlighted the distinctiveness of ADHD that is characterized by inattention alone from the combined and hyperactive–impulsive types. The inattentive type tends to be sluggish, anxious, shy, socially withdrawn, unpopular, and poor in sports and academics. Compared to hyperactive children, they have fewer externalizing problems and cause less family stress.[27–30] Impressions drawn from descriptive psychopathology have more recently been buttressed by sophisticated imaging methodologies – such as magnetic resonance spectroscopy[31] and functional magnetic resonance imaging (fMRI)[32] – that have been able to discriminate between central physiological correlates of inattentive and combined types of ADHD.

Sleep characteristics also differ in the two major ADHD types. Chiang et al.[33] interviewed youth aged 10–17 in whom they established diagnoses of ADHD-combined in 174, ADHD-inattentive in 130, and ADHD-hyperactive-impulsive in 21. Compared to 257 non-ADHD controls, combined and inattentive ADHD groups were more prone to daytime napping and to sleep disorders generally, but the combined type alone displayed circadian rhythm problems and sleep talking, whereas the inattentive type had more symptoms of hypersomnia. The distinction between ADHD types associated with movement may prove especially relevant to understanding the connection between ADHD and disorders such as restless legs syndrome for which the urge to move is a defining feature.

The problem of heterogeneity in ADHD does not end with the types specified in the DSM.[34] Within the combined ADHD phenotype multiple genetic and non-genetic variants may well be discovered.[35] There is no need for a single grand hypothesis that explains ADHD or each of its relationships to diverse sleep disorders through a single mechanism. There is room for multiple hypotheses to guide different aspects of future investigation. Comorbidities with sleep disorders may be an important pathway for discriminating homogeneous ADHD phenotypes that would improve the specificity and biological relevance of psychiatry's classification system.

NATURE OF INTERACTIONS BETWEEN SLEEP AND NEUROBEHAVIORAL PATHOLOGY

In general, the association between two correlated disorders may be causal in either direction or it may arise from a third condition. A cause need not be an exclusive or sole cause but may be a contributing one. The sleep problems most characteristic of ADHD have been hypothetically associated with each of these pathways. Despite limited evidence that may change with time, organizing relationships in this way is worthwhile if it sheds new light on what ADHD is (or, rather, what the different forms of ADHD are) and if it offers a rational way to simplify a complex subject.

Figure 15-1 diagrams a few of the multiple pathways proposed as explanations for the comorbidity of sleep disorders and neurobehavioral pathology. The potential for these mechanisms to interact can be easily appreciated from a glance at this picture, though our understanding of these complex interactions is quite limited.

ADHD AND STIMULANTS AS A CAUSE OF SLEEP DYSFUNCTION

Bedtime has long been a minefield for parent–child conflict in otherwise healthy families and, even more likely, in chaotic homes with parents struggling to rear overactive and defiant children. Irregular execution of good sleep hygiene by parents, abetted by the ubiquitous lure of increasingly available electronic devices, fosters resistance to bedtime, especially among temperamentally irritable youngsters whose instinct for fight-or-flight tilts decidedly in favor of the former. Bedtime thus becomes a predictable source of conflict, its mere anticipation a potent source of arousal in its own right. Behavioral impediments to settling or falling asleep in children with ADHD may be compounded by the effects of stimulant medications, including both the direct alerting effects and the *rebound* hyperactivity associated with withdrawal.

It is not surprising, therefore, that difficulties initiating or maintaining sleep represent the most common sleep complaints related to ADHD. These complaints often fall diagnostically into the International Classification of Sleep Disorders-Second Edition (ICSD-2)[36] grouping of behavioral insomnias of childhood (BIC), especially the limit-setting type which develops when the caretaker rewards avoidance behaviors by allowing the child to delay bedtime.

The dynamics of BICs are well understood in terms of behavioral theory, the validity of which is supported by the effectiveness of behavioral interventions such as extinction (which usually means ignoring protests or other entreaties for attention), graduated extinction, positive bedtime routines with fading in of a target bedtime, scheduled awakenings, and parent education. A committee of the American Academy of Sleep Medicine (AASM) reviewed the literature and adapted the most effective techniques in a practice parameter to guide treatment interventions for preschool children, though nothing comparable exists specifically for ADHD.[37,38] Surprisingly, no trials have been published with appropriate controls proving the efficacy of a systematic behavioral approach to BIC in children with ADHD. Preliminary, unpublished results for a manualized 5-week intervention suggest that children with ADHD respond as well as others.[16] Another trial that compared two versions of an intervention geared to ADHD did not include an untreated control group.[39]

Although sleep initiation problems in most children with ADHD have been understood and treated largely on the basis of learned behavior, family conflict, and medication effects, the extent to which endogenous cycles contribute to bedtime resistance in some children with ADHD may deserve closer attention than it has previously received. Delayed sleep phase

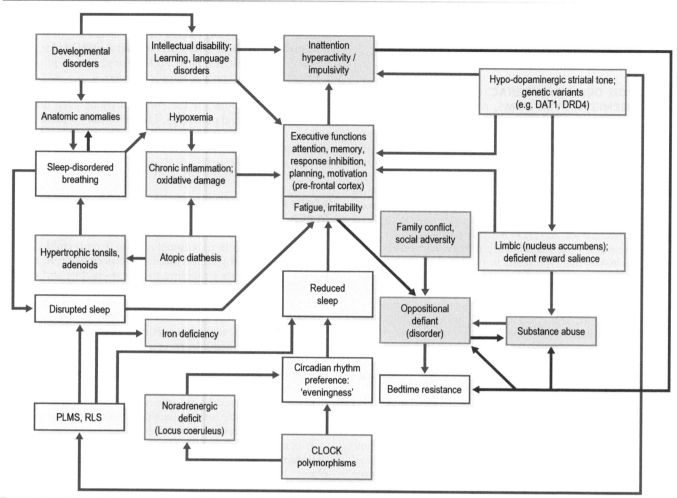

FIGURE 15-1 Model of Hypothetical Causal Pathways Linking Sleep Disorders with Inattention and Hyperactivity. PLMS, periodic limb movements in sleep; RLS, restless legs syndrome; DAT1, dopamine transporter 1; DRD4, dopamine receptor D4; *CLOCK, Circadian Locomotor Output Cycles Kaput* gene. Blue boxes, sleep disorders; yellow boxes, behavioral pathology; green boxes, biological cognitive dysfunction and biological factors. Blue arrows show possible functional or causal sequences; red arrows show positive feedback loops. Deeper green colored boxes (near the center of the diagram) show executive functions as the common pathway of several causal chains, with fatigue and irritability as closely allied subjective experiences.

disorder typically becomes most severe in or after adolescence, but similar tendencies also can be identified in younger children.[40,41] Interestingly, in a sample of 5- to 14-year-old ADHD children with common sleep disorders who had been recruited for a pilot trial of a simple behavioral intervention, 56% were diagnosed with delayed sleep phase while only 28% were diagnosed with limit-setting disorders.[39]

Medications for ADHD have varying impacts on bedtime compliance. Atomoxetine, clonidine, and guanfacine all promote sleep, and the latter two are sometimes administered primarily for that purpose. Stimulants may affect sleep directly by promotion of alertness and reduction of sleepiness – even after the major therapeutic effects have disappeared – by aggravation of symptoms during a period of rebound hyperactivity that extends into the child's bedtime.[42] Or, somewhat paradoxically, they may facilitate sleep through a direct therapeutic effect on the hyperactivity. For some children the impact of stimulants is tantamount to a chemically induced phase delay. When medication underlies a serious sleep problem, simple behavioral interventions such as educating

parents and improving sleep hygiene, though potentially of benefit, may be inadequate without changes in the medication regimen. Some evidence exists that the longer-acting stimulants are less likely to trigger problems in sleep initiation.[24]

AN INTRINSIC SLEEP DISORDER AS THE HYPOTHETICAL ETIOLOGY OF INATTENTION, HYPERACTIVITY, AND OTHER NEUROCOGNITIVE IMPAIRMENT: SLEEP-DISORDERED BREATHING

Even brief experimental restrictions of sleep can affect attention and cognition in healthy children. Thus, a single night's experimental reduction in sleep produced inattentive behaviors[43] and impairment in higher cognitive functions such as verbal fluency and flexibility and acquisition of abstract concepts.[44] Similarly, during a week of restricted sleep, normal children displayed decrements in teacher-rated academic and attention scores, though without changes in hyperactivity or oppositional behavior.[45] Gruber et al.[46] reported that parent ratings of alertness, and teacher ratings of emotional regulation and restless-impulsive behavior, improved among children aged 7–11 who had extended their sleep time by an average 27.36 minutes during an experimental trial lasting a week. In contrast, children who restricted sleep by an average of 54.04 minutes deteriorated with respect to these measures.

Sleepiness due to either sleep disruption or reduced sleep duration is a common problem among children with ADHD symptoms. A survey of parents of more than 800 children at general pediatric clinics, for example, found a substantial association between sleepiness and behaviors that characterize ADHD,[2] while MSLT has objectively confirmed this observation in three studies employing this measure.[47–49] Actigraphic studies of sleep onset latency and sleep duration have produced mixed findings[50] but at least two reports, not confounded by medication effects, have shown sleep latency to be greater,[51] and sleep duration to be shorter,[52] in ADHD children than in controls.

Behavior is largely the product and manifestation of high-level cognitive functions, collectively referred to as executive functions, that influence self-control, reasoning, and judgment. One formulation of these functions defines six major domains that include inhibition, set shifting, self-regulation of affect and arousal, working memory, analysis/synthesis, and contextual memory.[53] In some measure, impaired executive function is present in all persons with ADHD, at least to the extent that the defining features of ADHD can be said to be executive functions *per se* (namely the capacities to control attention and to regulate behavior, including modulation of activity and impulse). A more granular dissection of cognition usually will identify additional features of executive dysfunction among children with the ADHD diagnosis, but at its core it can be said that ADHD *is* executive dysfunction.

Impaired executive function can result from disordered sleep or daytime sleepiness. In a model posited by Beebe and Gozal,[53] the disrupted sleep and intermittent hypoxia and hypercarbia resulting from obstructive sleep apnea impair restorative sleep and cellular homeostasis. These effects, in turn, cause prefrontal cortical dysfunction manifested in executive dysfunction. A neurobehavioral phenotype emerges with difficulty manipulating information, poor planning and execution, disorganization, poor judgment, rigid thinking, poorly maintained attention and motivation, emotional lability, and overactivity/impulsivity. This description is generally consistent with a diagnosis of ADHD, and many cases of ADHD would neatly fit such a description.

The prefrontal cortex, the brain region thought to be most responsible for executive functions, is particularly vulnerable to sleep deprivation. Thus, sleep-deprived adults have paradoxical prefrontal activation demonstrable on fMRI during a verbal learning task.[54] In contrast, subjects with OSA have shown reduced prefrontal activation in a brief visual delayed matching-to-sample task.[55] Even where neuropsychological deficits are mild, adults with OSA may show widespread functional changes in cerebral cortex, including in prefrontal regions.[56] Functional and anatomic imaging of children and adults with ADHD has shown prefrontal cortical abnormalities consistent with the neuropsychological models of executive function.[57–60]

Gozal[61] has extended the executive function model of sleep and ADHD to emphasize the role of inflammation and oxidative stress as potential mechanisms for cellular changes underlying neurocognitive deficits in children with OSA. This perspective is supported by experimental rodent studies showing that intermittent hypoxia leads to cellular damage, including changes in gene expression,[62,63] and to behavioral outcomes similar to those observed in OSA. Furthermore, in children with OSA, and especially those with snoring and with neurocognitive deficits, levels of C-reactive protein, found in high-sensitivity testing, are elevated.[64] In addition, in non-obese children with OSA, levels of soluble CD40 ligand – an indicator of endothelial inflammation – are also high.[65] Insulin-like growth factor 1 (IGF-1), a neuroprotective hormone, is also elevated in children with OSA, more so in children with less neurocognitive dysfunction who are presumably benefitting from greater neuroprotection provided by higher hormone levels.[66] Among children with ADHD but without reported sleep problems, a role for oxidative stress and cellular immunity has been suggested as well. Thus, 35 children and adolescents with ADHD were found to have high nitric oxide synthetase, xanthine oxidase, and adenosine deaminase activities but low glutathione S-transferase and paraoxonase-1 activity.[67] The importance of inflammation may be related to the apparent excess of atopic disorders and food sensitivities among children with ADHD.[68–73] Although *fad* diets – such as the Feingold diet[74,75] – have rarely survived rigorous clinical trials, elimination diets have consistently identified children with behavioral sensitivities to specific foods or ingredients that can be demonstrated on repeat food challenges.[76,77] Practicability, perhaps more than noteworthy weaknesses in the evidence, has prevented these approaches from entering mainstream practice or attracting a large body of research.[78]

There is little doubt that the severest forms of pediatric obstructive sleep apnea can cause a characteristic daytime syndrome comprising irritability, languor, and cognitive dulling with prominently impaired attention and memory. Osler[79] vividly described the impact of adenoid hypertrophy in his classic text:

At night the child's sleep is greatly disturbed; the respirations are loud and snorting, and there are sometimes prolonged pauses, followed by deep, noisy inspirations. The child may wake up in a paroxysm of shortness of breath. … In long-standing cases the child is very stupid-looking, responds slowly to questions, and may be sullen and cross. …
The influence upon the mental development is striking. Mouth-breathers are usually dull, stupid, and backward. It is impossible for them to fix the attention for long. … Headaches, forgetfulness, inability to study without discomfort, are frequent symptoms of this condition in students. Among other symptoms … general listlessness, and an indisposition for physical or mental exertion

Osler's patient was sluggish, rather than hyperactive, and would likely meet DSM-IV criteria for the inattentive type of ADHD, though the prominence of the sleep disturbance and the associated mental dullness and listlessness, of which inattention is but one feature, would immediately draw clinical interest to the physical cause rather than to the comparatively abstract psychiatric construct. Current debate, however, focuses upon whether less pronounced sleep-associated disturbances in breathing, presenting without the obvious physical and mental stigmata described by Osler, can also cause clinically significant neurobehavioral pathology, including the ADHD syndrome.

Many publications suggest that PSG measures such as the AHI, usually considered to be valid indices of the presence and severity of nocturnal respiratory disturbance, may fail to detect labored nocturnal respiration that is relevant for neurobehavioral pathology. A German study, for example, has challenged the assumption that primary snoring – which by definition is not associated with significant apnea, hypopnea, or associated arousals – is benign.[80] Of 92 habitual snorers studied (from a community population of 1114 school-age children) 69 had primary snoring and the remaining 23 had either upper airway resistance syndrome (UARS) or OSA. All three of these objectively diagnosed forms of SDB were associated with significant neurobehavioral morbidity – including both hyperactivity and inattention – to about the same extent. Primary snoring was an important risk factor for hyperactivity (OR=2.8), inattentive behavior (OR=4.4), daytime sleepiness (OR=10.7), and diminished performance in mathematics, science, and spelling.

Like Osler's case, most prepubertal children with significant SDB have enlarged adenoids and tonsils for which adenotonsillectomy is often recommended. Several groups have systematically examined the consequences of adenotonsillectomy in children with putative SDB. Huang et al.[80A] offered children with ADHD and mild OSA, defined by an AHI between one and five events/hour, the choice of adenotonsillectomy, conventional stimulant treatment for ADHD, or no treatment. The group choosing surgery had the best outcome on the ADHD rating scale and on a continuous performance test, leading the authors to conclude that mild SDB warranted surgical treatment. Chervin and colleagues[81] studied children selected to undergo adenotonsillectomy on surgical grounds before formal psychiatric and sleep assessment had been performed. Comprehensive diagnostics including PSG with esophageal pressure monitoring, MSLT, neuropsychological testing, and structured psychiatric interviews, took place immediately before surgery and about 1 year later. In most instances clinician-diagnosed SDB had been an indication for surgery, though only about half the children were subsequently diagnosed with OSA (even when only requiring an obstructive apnea index of 1). Both neurobehavioral measures and DSM-IV diagnoses improved substantially after surgery. At baseline, 37% of 79 subjects compared to 11% of 27 controls were assigned diagnoses of attention or disruptive behavior disorders, whereas a year later only 23% of post-surgical cases still met criteria for at least one of these diagnoses.[82] Figure 15-2 summarizes diagnostic changes before and after surgery. ODD, a disorder that is characterized by traits of irritability and proneness to protests and tantrums, was particularly amenable to improvement through surgery. These findings were replicated in a second cohort.[83]

As in other studies of the impact of adenotonsillectomy, sleep parameters improved along with measures of behavior and cognition. The most curious finding of the Chervin study was that changes in psychiatric diagnosis and neurobehavioral functioning were unrelated to pre-surgical diagnoses of OSA. Huang's conclusion that mild SDB was an important source of neurobehavioral morbidity implicitly assumed that children without SDB, who were excluded from the study, would not similarly benefit.[80A] Among 81 children from the second cohort studied by Chervin's group, however, it was possible to show that respiratory findings not recorded routinely with

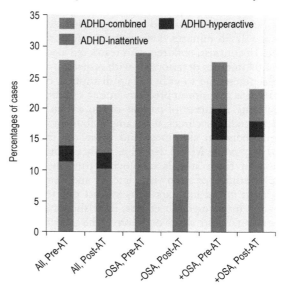

ADHD diagnoses before and after adenotonsillectomy

(A)

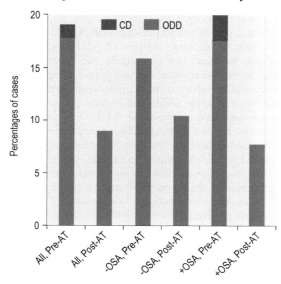

Oppositional defiant disorder and conduct disorder diagnoses before and after adenotonsillectomy

(B)

FIGURE 15-2 Figures show changes in DSM-IV diagnostic rates of disorders of attention and disruptive behavior before and about 1 year after adenotonsillectomy in 79 children aged 5 to 12. The bars show stacked rates for ADHD types (2a), and for disruptive behavior disorders (2b), both in cases without polysomnographic evidence of OSA, and in those with such evidence (obstructive apnea index of 1 or more). ADHD, attention-deficit/hyperactivity disorder; ADHD-hyperactive, predominantly hyperactive/impulsive type; ADHD-inattentive, predominantly inattentive type; CD, conduct disorder; ODD, oppositional defiant disorder; OSA, obstructive sleep apnea; –OSA, no OSA present on polysomnography; +OSA, OSA present. AT, adenotonsillectomy. 'All' refers to 79 subjects undergoing AT, whereas the –OSA group comprised 38 subjects and the +OSA group 40. * p < .05 (McNemar's test). *Data for this figure have been adapted from Dillon JE, Blunden S, Ruzicka DL, Guire KE, Champine D, Weatherly RA, et al. DSM-IV diagnoses and obstructive sleep apnea in children before and 1 year after adenotonsillectomy. Journal of the American Academy of Child & Adolescent Psychiatry 2007;46:1425–36.[82]*

PSG could predict diagnosis and outcome. Thus, the AHI – counted with or without respiratory effort-related arousals – failed to predict the presence of DSM-IV attention and disruptive behavior disorders. However, esophageal manometry – specifically, the lowest pressure recorded and the proportion of sleep time during which pressure was more negative than -10 cm H_2O – did predict the presence and resolution of these psychiatric conditions.[84] Esophageal manometry did not, however, predict composite measures of inattentive and hyperactive behavior or cognitive and executive function, nor did it predict their improvement after surgery. Chervin's study raises the possibility that even with sensitive accommodations for children's sleep studies – use of nasal pressure monitoring and pediatric definitions for scoring short apneic events and respiratory effort-related arousals – measures of intrathoracic pressure may (in some circumstances) be better indicators of mild but significant SDB than the respiratory measurements that are routinely part of traditional PSG. Although Calhoun et al.[17] were unable to detect relationships between mild SDB (or PSG) and multiple neuropsychological measures in a general population sample of 571 school-aged children, it is possible that a more sensitive measure (such as intrathoracic pressure) would have been a better indicator for subtle but outcome-relevant SDB. In a subsequent analysis of the *Penn State Cohort*,[85] a more complex relationship between PSG and neurobehavioral findings did emerge: parent-rated daytime sleepiness, adjusted for AHI, was associated with parent-rated learning, attention/hyperactivity levels, and conduct problems, a relationship mediated by objective measures of working memory and processing speed.

Longitudinal studies have pointed to the importance of early symptoms of SDB for subsequent behavior. In a 2-year follow-up of 506 children initially assessed at ages 4–5, Ali and colleagues[86] found that among persistent habitual snorers, hyperactivity, sleepiness, and restless sleep increased during the 2-year interval. Chervin et al.[87] followed a cohort of children aged 2 to 13 for four years and found that ratings for snoring and other indicators of SDB at baseline were strong predictors of later elevations on the hyperactivity index of the *Conners Parent Rating Scale*,[88,89] even after adjusting for stimulant use and for baseline hyperactivity. The *Avon Longitudinal Study of Parents and Children*, an epidemiologic examination of health from early life, included questions concerning snoring, mouth-breathing, and witnessed apnea in sequential surveys obtained from 6 through 69 months of age.[90] Development of SDB symptoms followed four distinct trajectories that variously predicted hyperactivity, conduct problems, peer difficulties, and emotional problems at ages four and seven, even after controlling for 15 possible confounders. The evolution of substantial behavioral effects from early respiratory symptoms suggests that early interdiction of SDB may be necessary to prevent emergence of important behavioral sequelae. Population rates of SDB – estimated by Lumeng and Chervin[91] as 1.5–6% for 'always' snoring (i.e., habitual snoring), 0.2–4% for parent-reported apnea, and 4–11% for SDB defined in various ways – emphasize the potential public health significance of these phenomena. Although common, these disorders may not be recognized before they become entrenched. One retrospective study from an allergy service found that over half of children experienced symptoms more than 2 years before undergoing adenotonsillectomy.[92]

SDB judged to be mild on traditional PSG testing might have significant ramifications for behavior and treatment planning in individual patients. O'Brien et al.[93] observed that among children aged 5–7 who underwent polysomnography after screening of a large public school sample, SDB was present in 26% of those with mild hyperactivity but in only 5% with severe symptoms of OSA or no symptoms at all. This is consistent with observations that more extreme cases of OSA present with lethargy and sluggishness rather than overactivity. It may be that mild cases increase activity as compensation for sleepiness, but that as fatigue becomes overwhelming, the compensatory response breaks down and is superseded by lassitude and sleepiness. Analogous compensatory responses can be observed in the imaging of some brain regions that activate in response to sleep loss.[54] The same regions may be hypoactive after prolonged disturbance damages them. More severe hyperactivity persisting after adenotonsillectomy might be understood to reflect either a more advanced and less reversible process or an alternative pathophysiology altogether.

ARE THERE COMMON ETIOLOGIES OR MECHANISMS THAT EXPLAIN THE COMORBIDITY OF SLEEP DISORDERS AND NEUROBEHAVIORAL DYSFUNCTION?

Because of the sensitivity of behavior to sleep deprivation and disruption, any sleep disturbance might be a cause of neurobehavioral problems. Some sleep disturbances, however, may also be linked to behavior problems on a deeper level, through neurochemical or genetic mechanisms common to both.

Circadian Rhythm Disturbances
Evidence for circadian rhythm variations in ADHD has given new life to the hypo-arousal/noradrenergic-deficit hypothesis of hyperactivity.[94] More than 70 years ago Bradley and Bowen observed that stimulants rather than sedatives provide effective treatment for hyperactivity.[95,96] Electrophysiological studies of skin conductance, electroencephalogram, and auditory- and sensory-evoked responses suggested that children with ADHD show hypo- rather than hyperarousal.[45] Weinberg and Brumback[97] attempted to define a primary disorder of vigilance that described many ADHD children.

The comorbidity of ADHD with delayed sleep phase syndrome (DSPS) in children was first reported in a 10-year-old child[98] whose chronic behavioral and sleep symptoms resolved with chronotherapy. Systematic research addressing variations in circadian rhythms in ADHD has focused upon chronotypes and apparent phase delays associated with sleep initiation difficulties rather than upon rigorously diagnosed DSPS. Van der Heijden et al.[99] compared children diagnosed with both ADHD and sleep-onset insomnia (SOI) with children diagnosed with ADHD who did not have SOI. The ADHD + SOI group displayed late dim light melatonin onset (DLMO) which was interpreted as strong evidence that the sleep disturbance arose from a delayed sleep phase. Treatment with melatonin produced improvement in sleep initiation and normalization of DLMO, but it did not lead to change in behavioral symptoms – findings suggesting that ADHD symptoms were not simply the result of poor sleep or of phase delay as such.[100,101] Susman and colleagues[102] assessed chronotypes in a community sample aged 8–13 and found that children with elevations of the attention and rule-breaking behavior scales on the Child Behavior Checklist (CBCL)[103,104] were likely to display an eveningness profile. Several studies have found that children with ADHD were significantly more hyperactive relative to controls during the afternoon compared to morning.[105–107]

As is the case in children, adults with ADHD often complain of sleep problems. Rybak et al.[108,109] found that among 29 adults with ADHD, over 40% exhibited an evening chronotype. Eveningness was associated with impulsive responding and difficulty sustaining mental effort. Noting that adults with ADHD may be sensitive to seasonal mood changes, these investigators administered bright light therapy to ADHD subjects between November and February (fall–winter). They found that circadian preference changes, interpreted as phase advances, predicted improvement in core ADHD symptoms, whereas mood as such did not influence these symptoms.

Examining the evidence for disturbances in circadian rhythms in ADHD, Imeraj et al.[110] have reasoned that dysfunction of the *locus coeruleus*, which regulates noradrenergic activity and arousal through widespread projections to the cortex, including to prefrontal structures, implicates noradrenergic dysfunction in executive processes that interact with reward systems. They propose that the locus coeruleus is integrated within a circuit that includes the suprachiasmatic nucleus, which is associated with the circadian clock, and the dorsomedial hypothalamic nucleus, which is involved in circadian regulation of corticosteroid secretion and other endocrine functions. These structures hypothetically would impose a circadian influence upon widespread central and autonomic processes promoting vigilance, motivation, memory, information processing, motor behavior, metabolism, and cardiovascular function. Imeraj and colleagues also suggest that persons with ADHD may exhibit elevated tonic, and reduced phasic, locus coeruleus discharges that together cause distractibility and performance deficits.

Whether or not the noradrenergic hypothesis ultimately prevails, a compelling line of research developing in the next few years concerns the identification and function of genetic variations associated both with ADHD and the sleep–wake cycle. The *CLOCK* (for 'Circadian Locomotor Output Cycles Kaput') gene, which codes a transcription factor that is critical for circadian rhythms, has been associated both with chronotype and with ADHD. The gene's role in dopamine metabolism and the brain's reward system[111] makes *CLOCK* an attractive place to look for mechanisms linking biological rhythms to ADHD. One single-nucleotide polymorphism (SNP), referred to either as the 'rs180126' polymorphism or by its location '3111' on the gene, has been examined with respect to both circadian preferences and ADHD. Katzenberg and colleagues[112] reported that subjects who possessed the 'C' allele (most of whom were heterozygotes, as the number of 'C' homozygotes was small) had lower chronotype scores, indicating a skew toward eveningness. This finding was contradicted by a second study finding no such association,[113] but was supported by a third[114] reporting greater eveningness in 'C' homozygotes than among subjects manifesting the 'T' allele. A fourth study suggested a weak association between the 'T' allele and DSPS.[115] Kissling et al.[116] then reported that the 'T' allele was associated with measures of ADHD in adults, but the finding was difficult to interpret because the sample, comprising subjects referred to a forensic psychiatry

institute, included an unspecified number of cases that had been diagnosed as having ADHD. Xu et al.[117] studied within-family transmission disequilibrium in distinct samples of children and their families from the UK and from Taiwan. The 'T' allele was preferentially transferred in the Taiwanese families and in the combined samples, though not in the UK families when analyzed separately. Cao et al.[118] more recently compared prevalence of these alleles in ADHD children (n = 162) and controls (n = 150) and found that the 'C' allele appeared more frequently in the ADHD sample than it did in the controls; and, among those with ADHD, it was found more often in those with sleep-onset difficulties.

Two other genes contributing to the circadian pacemaker, BMAL1 and PER2, were examined in a study of adults with ADHD.[119] This study measured the daily rhythms of certain hormones (salivary cortisol and melatonin), gene expression (BMAL1 and PER2), and movement (actigraphically recorded) among 13 adults with, and 19 without, ADHD. The circadian rhythmicity of gene expression observed in controls was absent in ADHD subjects, and hormone secretion exhibited a phase delay in subjects with ADHD.

Other functional components of the sleep–wake cycle, such as the melatonin synthetic pathway, may also be implicated in ADHD.[120] While the genetic studies as a whole do not lead to any firm conclusions, they point to interesting directions for further exploration.

Restless Legs Syndrome, Periodic Leg Movements

The dopamine-deficit hypothesis of ADHD, which has generated much of the basic and clinical neuroscience in ADHD, is predicated upon several well-established observations. First, the prominence of motor activity *per se* implicates some role for dopamine function in the expression of ADHD. Second, the historical epidemic of *encephalitis lethargica* that caused profound and persistent parkinsonism in some afflicted adults produced in children a paradoxical syndrome of hyperkinesis, emotional lability, and antisocial behavior.[121] Third, the stimulant medications, which bring about prompt and dramatic behavioral changes in many children with ADHD, are distinguished from less effective treatments, such as tricyclic antidepressants, by their impact upon dopamine reuptake.[122] Fourth, novelty seeking and reward salience, traits strongly associated with ADHD, are closely linked to dopamine function.[123–127] Fifth, animal models of ADHD can be produced by destruction of dopamine pathways through fetal hydroxydopamine exposure or by creating knock-outs of the dopamine transporter gene.[128] Sixth, human imaging studies show anatomical and functional brain differences in persons with ADHD that implicate dopamine involvement. These include, for example, reduced volume of the caudate and globus pallidus and reduced D2/D3 receptor density in the nucleus accumbens and midbrain.[129] Finally, though sometimes contradictory and difficult to interpret, genetic studies generally support the role of genes that are linked to dopamine function and metabolism as having a role in ADHD.[130–134]

In searching for a common underlying pathophysiology between ADHD and sleep dysfunction, recent discoveries concerning RLS and PLMs are extremely promising. First, the presence of both RLS and PLMs in children is now well established.[135–139] RLS, diagnosed by narrow criteria, occurs in about 2% of children and adolescents.[140] Second, RLS/PLMs appears to be mediated, at least in part, by dopaminergic hypofunction. Indeed, the experience of RLS resembles the experience of akathisia associated with dopamine blockade in individuals receiving antipsychotic drugs, and the most effective pharmacological treatments for RLS are dopamine agonists. Third, children with RLS and low ferritin levels – an abnormality hypothetically affecting dopamine function – often benefit from iron supplementation.[141–143] Fourth, some children with ADHD have lower than expected ferritin levels.[144] Early reports claim that the behavior of such children is ameliorated by iron supplementation, though the long history of discarded cures for ADHD makes this at best a preliminary finding.[145] Fifth, rates of RLS and PLMs are elevated in ADHD, and vice versa.[9,146,147] And sixth, in children with comorbid ADHD and RLS/PLMs who have low ferritin levels, iron supplementation seems to improve both behavior and sleep movements.[145,148] Such findings point to the possibility that ADHD and RLS/PLMs have a common underlying etiology that has some connection to iron metabolism and dopamine function.[149]

The hypothesis that ADHD and RLS/PLMs share mechanisms or causes should probably be modified by a working assumption that, because ADHD is heterogeneous, we expect the comorbidity of ADHD and RLS/PLMs to include a subtype of ADHD that has not hitherto been distinguished from the broadly inclusive ADHD syndrome. If that were the case, then the diurnal behavioral phenotype of the relevant ADHD subtype might well have observable features that differentiate it from other ADHD syndromes. Like ADHD, RLS is probably heterogeneous etiologically.[150] This is suggested by a bimodal distribution in age of onset, the earlier-onset cases exhibiting especially high familial loading, greater severity, and more prominent polysomnographic findings such as PLMs and microarousals. One would expect an imperfect overlap between two syndromes, RLS and ADHD, each of which is etiologically diverse and, indeed, the magnitude of comorbidity in children is around 25% in either direction.[140] Ferritin levels as correlates of both symptom severity and reversibility by iron supplementation in RLS and ADHD may point to genetic mechanisms that produce diurnal and nocturnal phenotypes with different thresholds for penetrance based upon exogenous factors such as nutrition.

CONCLUSION: SIGNIFICANCE AND FUTURE DIRECTIONS

Both the DSM-IV-TR[151] and its successor, the DSM-5,[152] share with ICSD-2 a criterion-based approach to diagnosis that emphasizes clinical features that can be ascertained using conventional medical approaches with little emphasis upon how comorbid conditions may be interrelated. A deeper view of clinical assessment benefits immensely from perspectives on sleep and behavioral pathology that broadly take both night and day into account. Thus, a young child presenting with sleeplessness and ADHD may be diagnosed with a BIC for which parental education in sleep, sleep hygiene, and a few straightforward behavioral techniques is likely to be adequate intervention. The presence of ADHD, however, raises the specter of a much broader differential diagnosis including medication effects (for which changes in dosing, schedules, or agents may be needed), nocturnal movement disorders (for which ferritin levels, iron supplementation, or dopamine

agonists may be indicated), and circadian rhythm disorders (which require a systematic and sometimes extended diagnostic approach that may ultimately suggest the need for adaptations in sleep schedule, phototherapy, or oral melatonin administration). Conversely, children who present for treatment of ADHD, ODD, or intellectual and learning problems may have primary or contributory sleep disorders such as OSA. Because behavioral disorders and sleep are so often intimately linked, the clinician is obliged to consider how a given treatment affects both daytime and nighttime behavior. Usually, the improvement of one is paralleled by improvement of the other; but, at times, just the opposite is true, especially with stimulant therapy.

The complexity of associations between different disorders cautions the clinician against an overly simplistic formulation of cause and effect. Thus, while adenotonsillectomy sometimes produces dramatic improvement in daytime behavior, there are many cases in which changes are more modest, leaving residual symptoms of the same kind, chronic symptoms that are not readily reversed, or a separate problem aggravated by SDB but not caused by it. Put in the simplest possible way, non-sleep-specialist practitioners ought to think routinely in etiological terms about even the most ordinary presentations of behavior and learning disorders, attending in particular to the possibility that sleep plays an etiologic role in daytime behavior complaints. Thoughtful diagnosis will suggest novel treatment strategies that are not yet well integrated into the behavioral specialist's technical arsenal. Likewise, sleep specialists using conventional approaches to diagnosis may not detect mild respiratory disturbances during sleep, yet in an individual case that cannot be well formulated in any other way, mild SDB might be the best explanation for significant behavioral and cognitive disturbance. The relative contributions of conditioning and intrinsic biological rhythms to sleep problems in ADHD youngsters are not always easily dissected, and both may contribute in varying degrees to insomnia that does not respond to simple educational and behavioral measures.

Molecular genetics, neuroimaging, and animal models are now making critical contributions to understanding the relationships between sleep and behavior. Genetic techniques that employ family pedigrees by their nature address disorder variants that are relatively homogeneous, unlike methods using subjects from general populations. There is already reason to distinguish predominantly inattentive ADHD from the combined and hyperactive–impulsive types, and it is hard to see how it can be useful to unify these distinctive presentations of inattentiveness in conceptualizing their respective interactions with sleep. Both groups may be of interest for understanding behavior arising from a presumed primary sleep disorder such as OSA, as the manifestations of OSA in behavior and cognition are probably varied and diagnostically diverse. Efforts to find the best ways to divide the ADHD population into more homogeneous subgroups may help to clarify fundamental links with sleep pathology.

We have examined the sleep disorders associated with neurobehavioral problems in children from the perspective of hypothetical causal relationships. Attention, hyperactivity, ADHD, and other behavioral problems have been repeatedly and robustly associated with sleep disorders in numerous studies employing both parent questionnaires and objective findings from PSG, actigraphy, and MSLT. The literature as a whole has been criticized, however, for confounding comorbidity, referral bias, and other factors with the primary contribution of ADHD to these associations. Conservative analyses, including meta-analyses of research meeting exacting specifications, have been helpful in separating the noise – a tendency for most variables measured to correlate with something of apparent significance – from the signal, namely, the associations that hold up well when confounds are eliminated by design or statistical methods. These include PLMs and a handful of sleep findings summarized in Table 15.1. The significance of SDB has been especially controversial, but newer evidence suggests that early symptoms of SDB are associated with later neurobehavioral morbidity and that PSG may not always detect mild but clinically important sleep breathing abnormalities. The role of circadian rhythms in ADHD is a promising area of research that will be further elucidated by study of how the behavioral rhythms of psychiatrically disordered children correspond to biological cycles and circadian pathology.

It has been suggested that the diagnosis of ADHD be reserved for cases in which the syndrome persists after treatment of a coexisting sleep disorder. Owens has advised, 'A prudent approach would then be to treat any documented sleep disorder (i.e., adenotonsillectomy for OSA) before confirming (or rejecting) the diagnosis of ADHD and initiating treatment.'[153] If the treatment targeting a sleep disorder resolves ADHD symptoms, according to this reasoning, then there was no ADHD in the first place. What, then, is *true* ADHD, and how does it differ from look-alikes?

The view proposed in this chapter, that ADHD is a heterogeneous syndrome with multiple causes, is inconsistent with the notion of a unique or *real* ADHD that implicitly has a distinct but unknown pathophysiology. For clinical purposes, it may be prudent to treat a sleep disorder before prescribing stimulants for an associated behavior problem; but, for several reasons, it does not follow that the treatment outcome should decide the diagnosis. First, while several follow-up reports of adenotonsillectomy have documented remission of ADHD, no randomized, controlled trials have been published to prove this claim. Data from the *Child Adenotonsillectomy Trial* (CHAT)[154] are currently being analyzed and may help to resolve this issue. Second, the ADHD syndrome associated with SDB satisfies DSM criteria that are unmodified in any respect. ADHD that is cured by adenotonsillectomy looks and behaves like any other ADHD. Third, the failure of surgery to cure ADHD in a given case does not tell us whether SDB was the cause, especially where long-standing sleep difficulties may have caused irreversible damage. Fourth, the presence of strictly defined OSA apparently does not predict which children will have ADHD, even in a population referred for adenotonsillectomy. Among those who do have ADHD, children without OSA may benefit from surgery as much as those without it.[81-84] Fifth, a treatment's efficacy is at best weak proof for the mechanism of illness. Gold salts were introduced for rheumatoid arthritis on the theory that the disease was a form of tuberculosis; yet the success of the intervention did not prove that rheumatoid arthritis was a mycobacterial disease.[155] Similarly, children with RLS and iron deficiency do not shed the RLS diagnosis when iron supplementation successfully mitigates symptoms of the disorder. Finally, mild SDB is quite common in the pediatric population and theoretically could account for a substantial proportion of children

diagnosed with ADHD. If this is true, then the entire literature on the nature and treatment of ADHD may be predicated upon populations in which the SDB pathway to ADHD is among the most common. If there is a *real* ADHD, then the one associated with SDB is as good a candidate as any for that designation.

Controversy illuminates gaps in knowledge and theory and helps to shape the research agenda. In this chapter we have emphasized the importance of comorbidity as a clue to hypothetical ADHD subtypes having unique mechanistic and etiologic characteristics. Although the presence of comorbid conditions is usually presumed to confound the interpretation of research data, here just the opposite may be true. If it is true that some cases of ADHD are generated by mechanisms that also underlie RLS/PLMs, for example, then a group of children who have been diagnosed with both may include relatively few with unrelated causes or mechanisms. Even greater homogeneity may be achieved by selecting cases on the basis of other features closely related to the putative pathophysiology, such as the presence of iron deficiency or response to iron supplementation in ADHD-RLS/PLMs. At least in principle this is a straightforward approach, not yet widely exploited, for creating more homogeneous subject populations and analytic subgroups. The same principle might be used in examining ADHD chronotypes. Thus, rather than ask whether ADHD as a whole is characterized by a specific chronotype, it may be more fruitful to ask whether ADHD children with an evening preference differ in other relevant ways from ADHD children reporting a morning preference.

The study of pediatric OSA has already taken multiple directions. Perhaps the most fundamental of these addresses the definition and measurement of the syndrome, since traditional PSG measures and disease thresholds may not capture some children with clinically relevant SDB. Better understanding of the extent and characteristics of neurobehavioral morbidity in milder presentations of OSA will help to define the boundaries of the syndrome and the indications for treatment. Examination of inflammatory changes in SDB is a promising area of research that may ultimately be relevant to understanding the familiality of the condition[156] and the nature of atopic influences long alleged to underlie some cases of ADHD. Tonsils removed from children with OSA exhibit more proinflammatory cytokines, higher levels of thioredoxin, and higher rates of T-cell proliferation than do tonsils recovered from children with recurrent tonsillitis.[157] Is it possible that these or other substances produced in the lymphoid tissues have a direct effect on behavior? Such a finding might explain the dissociation between diagnoses of OSA and resolution of behavior problems following adenotonsillectomy reported in follow-up studies.[81,82,84]

If it is true that ADHD is a syndrome providing an umbrella for many distinct variants, then research will increasingly recognize a diversity of behavioral conditions related to many different forms of sleep disturbance. Answers to key questions may come from genetic and functional imaging studies, especially as these techniques become more accessible; but the power of these methodologies depends upon study populations that are relatively uniform with respect to the characteristics being examined. The clues provided by close examination of the relationships between psychiatric and sleep pathology can help to inform the search for etiologies and mechanisms while guiding the development of novel approaches to treatment.

Clinical Pearls

- Heterogeneity of ADHD syndromes helps to explain its myriad associations with pediatric sleep disorders.
- Standard PSG procedures and scoring may be inadequate to exclude treatable SDB when presentation is of both distressed nocturnal breathing and neurobehavioral morbidity.
- Children with complaints related to attention, behavior, and learning should be screened for major sleep disorders, especially SDB, RLS, and circadian rhythm disturbances.
- The developmental origin of ADHD usually can be traced to the preschool years; when onset is later, careful evaluation for underlying sleep disorders is warranted.
- Recognition of mechanistic relationships between sleep and behavioral symptoms helps inform the choice and sequence of treatments for comorbid conditions; ideally, a single intervention will be effective for both.

References

1. Owens JA. Neurocognitive and behavioral impact of sleep disordered breathing in children. Pediatr Pulmonol 2009;44:417–22.
2. Chervin RD, Archbold KH, Dillon JE, et al. Inattention, hyperactivity, and symptoms of sleep-disordered breathing. Pediatrics 2002;109:449–56.
3. Yoon SYR, Jain U, Shapiro C. Sleep in attention-deficit/hyperactivity disorder in children and adults: Past, present, and future. Sleep Med Rev 2012;16:371–88.
4. Gregory AM, Sadeh A. Sleep, emotional and behavioral difficulties in children and adolescents. Sleep Med Rev 2012;16:129–36.
5. Spruyt K, Gozal D. Sleep disturbances in children with attention-deficit/hyperactivity disorder. Exp Rev Neurotherapeut 2011;11:565–77.
6. Konofal E, Lecendreux M, Cortese S. Sleep and ADHD. Sleep Med 2010;11:652–8.
7. O'Brien LM. The neurocognitive effects of sleep disruption in children and adolescents. Child Adolesc Psychiatr Clin N Am 2009;18:813–23.
8. Cortese S, Faraone SV, Konofal E, et al. Sleep in children with attention-deficit/hyperactivity disorder: Meta-analysis of subjective and objective studies. J Am Acad Child Adolesc Psychiatry 2009;48:894–908.
9. Walters AS, Silvestri R, Zucconi M, et al. Review of the possible relationship and hypothetical links between attention deficit hyperactivity disorder (ADHD) and the simple sleep related movement disorders, parasomnias, hypersomnias, and circadian rhythm disorders. J Clin Sleep Med 2008;4:591–600.
10. Owens JA. Sleep disorders and attention-deficit/hyperactivity disorder. Curr Psychiatr Rep 2008;10:439–44.
11. Gozal D, Kheirandish-Gozal L. Neurocognitive and behavioral morbidity in children with sleep disorders. Curr Opin Pulm Med 2007;13:505–9.
12. Sadeh A, Pergamin L, Bar-Haim Y. Sleep in children with attention-deficit hyperactivity disorder: A meta-analysis of polysomnographic studies. Sleep Med Rev 2006;10:381–98.
13. Kheirandish L, Gozal D. Neurocognitive dysfunction in children with sleep disorders. Dev Sci 2006;9:388–99.
14. Cortese S, Konofal E, Yateman N, et al. Sleep and alertness in children with attention-deficit/hyperactivity disorder: a systematic review of the literature. Sleep 2006;29:504–11.
15. Corkum P, Tannock R, Moldofsky H. Sleep disturbances in children with attention-deficit/hyperactivity disorder. J Am Acad Child Adolesct Psychiatry 1998;37:637–46.
16. Corkum P, Davidson F, Macpherson M. A framework for the assessment and treatment of sleep problems in children with attention-deficit/hyperactivity disorder. Pediatr Clin N Am 2011;58:667–83.
17. Calhoun SL, Mayes SD, Vgontzas AN, et al. No relationship between neurocognitive functioning and mild sleep disordered breathing in a community sample of children. J Clin Sleep Med 2009;5:228–34.
18. Wiggs L, Montgomery P, Stores G. Actigraphic and parent reports of sleep patterns and sleep disorders in children with subtypes of attention-deficit hyperactivity disorder. Sleep 2005;28:1437–45.
19. Thorndike EL. A constant error in psychological ratings. J Appl Psychol 1920;4:25–9.
20. Koenig MA. Characterizing children's expectations about expertise and incompetence: Halo or pitchfork effects? Child Dev 2011;82:1634–47.
21. Abikoff H, Courtney M, Pelham WE Jr, et al. Teachers' ratings of disruptive behaviors: the influence of halo effects. J Abnorm Child Psychol 1993;21:519–33.
22. Accardo JA, Marcus CL, Leonard MB, et al. Associations between psychiatric comorbidities and sleep disturbances in children with attention-deficit/hyperactivity disorder. J Dev Behav Pediatr 2012;33:97–105.
23. Owens JA, Spirito A, McGuinn M. The Children's Sleep Habits Questionnaire (CSHQ): Psychometric properties of a survey instrument for school-aged children. Sleep 2000;23:1–9.
24. Cox DJ, Moore M, Burket R, et al. Rebound effects with long-acting amphetamine or methylphenidate stimulant medication preparations among adolescent male drivers with attention-deficit/hyperactivity disorder. J Child Adolesc Psychopharmacol 2008;18:1–10.
25. Chervin RD, Aldrich MS. Effects of esophageal pressure monitoring on sleep architecture. Am J Resp Crit Care Med 1997;156:881–5.
26. Claman DM, Votteri BA. Effects of esophageal pressure monitoring on sleep architecture. Am J Resp Crit Care Med 1998;157:1697–8.
27. Lahey BB, Schaughency EA, Strauss CC, et al. Are attention deficit disorders with and without hyperactivity similar or dissimilar disorders? J Am Acad Child Psychiatry 1984;23:302–9.
28. Lahey BB, Schaughency EA, Hynd GW, et al. Attention deficit disorder with and without hyperactivity: comparison of behavioral characteristics of clinic-referred children. J Am Acad Child Adolesc Psychiatry 1987;26:718–23.
29. Milich R, Balentine AC, Lynam DR. ADHD combined type and ADHD predominantly inattentive type are distinct and unrelated disorders. Clin Psychol: Sci Pract 2001;8:463–88.
30. Bauermeister JJ, Matos M, Reina G, et al. Comparison of the DSM-IV combined and inattentive types of ADHD in a school-based sample of Latino/Hispanic children. J Child Psychol Psychiatry 2005;46:166–79.
31. Ferreira PEMS, Palmini A, Bau CHD, et al. Differentiating attention-deficit/hyperactivity disorder inattentive and combined types: a (1) H-magnetic resonance spectroscopy study of fronto-striato-thalamic regions. J Neural Transm 2009;116:623–9.
32. Solanto MV, Schulz KP, Fan J, et al. Event-related FMRI of inhibitory control in the predominantly inattentive and combined subtypes of ADHD. J Neuroimag 2009;19:205–12.
33. Chiang H-L, Gau SS-F, Ni H-C, et al. Association between symptoms and subtypes of attention-deficit hyperactivity disorder and sleep problems/disorders. J Sleep Res 2010;19:535–45.
34. Steinhausen HC. The heterogeneity of causes and courses of attention-deficit/hyperactivity disorder. Acta Psychiatr Scand 2009;120:392–9.
35. Zhou K, Chen W, Buitelaar J, et al. Genetic heterogeneity in ADHD: DAT1 gene only affects probands without CD. Am J Med Genet Part B, Neuropsychiat Genet: the Official Publication of the International Society of Psychiatric Genetics 2008;147B:1481–7.
36. American Academy of Sleep Medicine. International Classification of Sleep Disorders – Second Edition (ICSD-2): Diagnostic and coding manual. Westchester, Illinois: American Academy of Sleep Medicine, 2005.
37. Mindell JA, Kuhn B, Lewin DS, et al. Behavioral treatment of bedtime problems and night wakings in infants and young children. Sleep 2006;29:1263–76.
38. Morgenthaler TI, Owens J, Alessi C, et al. Practice parameters for behavioral treatment of bedtime problems and night wakings in infants and young children. Sleep 2006;29:1277–81.
39. Sciberras E, Fulton M, Efron D, et al. Managing sleep problems in school aged children with ADHD: a pilot randomized controlled trial. Sleep Med 2011;12:932–5.
40. Werner H, LeBourgeois MK, Geiger A, et al. Assessment of chronotype in four- to eleven-year-old children: reliability and validity of the Children's Chronotype Questionnaire (CCTQ). Chronobiol Int 2009;26:992–1014.
41. Russo PM, Bruni O, Lucidi F, et al. Sleep habits and circadian preference in Italian children and adolescents. J Sleep Res 2007;16:163–9.

42. Johnston C, Pelham WE, Hoza J, et al. Psychostimulant rebound in attention deficit disordered boys. J Am Acad Child Adolesc Psychiatry 1988;27:806–10.

43. Fallone G, Acebo C, Arnedt JT, et al. Effects of acute sleep restriction on behavior, sustained attention, and response inhibition in children. Percept Mot Skills 2001;93:213–29.

44. Randazzo AC, Muehlbach MJ, Schweitzer PK, et al. Cognitive function following acute sleep restriction in children ages 10–14. Sleep 1998;21:861–8.

45. Fallone G, Acebo C, Seifer R, et al. Experimental restriction of sleep opportunity in children: effects on teacher ratings. Sleep 2005;28:1561–7.

46. Gruber R, Cassoff J, Frenette S, et al. Impact of sleep extension and restriction on children's emotional lability and impulsivity. Pediatrics 2012;130(5):e1155–61.

47. Golan N, Shahar E, Ravid S, et al. Sleep disorders and daytime sleepiness in children with attention-deficit/hyperactive disorder. Sleep 2004;27:261–6.

48. Lecendreux M, Konofal E, Bouvard M, et al. Sleep and alertness in children with ADHD. J Child Psychol Psychiatry 2000;41:803–12.

49. Wiebe S, Carrier J, Frenette S, et al. Sleep and sleepiness in children with attention deficit/hyperactivity disorder and controls. J Sleep Res 2013;22(1):41–9.

50. Corkum P, Tannock R, Moldofsky H, et al. Actigraphy and parental ratings of sleep in children with attention-deficit/hyperactivity disorder (ADHD). Sleep 2001;24:303–12.

51. Hvolby A, Jorgensen J, Bilenberg N. [Sleep and sleep difficulties in Danish children aged 6–11 years]. Ugeskr Laeger 2008;170:448–51.

52. Owens J, Sangal RB, Sutton VK, et al. Subjective and objective measures of sleep in children with attention-deficit/hyperactivity disorder. Sleep Med 2009;10:446–56.

53. Beebe DW, Gozal D. Obstructive sleep apnea and the prefrontal cortex: towards a comprehensive model linking nocturnal upper airway obstruction to daytime cognitive and behavioral deficits. J Sleep Res 2002;11:1–16.

54. Drummond SPA, Brown GG, Gillin JC, et al. Altered brain response to verbal learning following sleep deprivation. Nature 2000;403:655–7.

55. Zhang X, Ma L, Li S, et al. A functional MRI evaluation of frontal dysfunction in patients with severe obstructive sleep apnea. Sleep Med 2011;12:335–40.

56. Yaouhi K, Bertran F, Clochon P, et al. A combined neuropsychological and brain imaging study of obstructive sleep apnea. J Sleep Res 2009;18:36–48.

57. Bush G, Valera EM, Seidman LJ. Functional neuroimaging of attention-deficit/hyperactivity disorder: a review and suggested future directions. Biol Psychiatry 2005;57:1273–84.

58. Schneider M, Retz W, Coogan A, et al. Anatomical and functional brain imaging in adult attention-deficit/hyperactivity disorder (ADHD) – a neurological view. Eur Arch Psychiatry Clin Neurosci 2006;256(Suppl 1):i32–41.

59. Seidman LJ, Valera EM, Makris N. Structural brain imaging of attention-deficit/hyperactivity disorder. Biol Psychiatry 2005;57:1263–72.

60. Shaw P, Rabin C. New insights into attention-deficit/hyperactivity disorder using structural neuroimaging. Curr Psychiatry Rep 2009;11:393–8.

61. Gozal D. Sleep, sleep disorders and inflammation in children. Sleep Med 2009;10(Suppl 1):S121–6.

62. Zhou Y-H, Cai X-H, Zhang C-X, et al. [The effect of chronic intermittent hypoxia on p38MAPK in cerebral tissues of weanling rats]. Chung-Kuo Ying Yung Sheng Li Hsueh Tsa Chih. Chin J Appl Physiol 2009;25:45–8.

63. Hambrecht VS, Vlisides PE, Row BW, et al. G proteins in rat prefrontal cortex (PFC) are differentially activated as a function of oxygen status and PFC region. J Chem Neuroanat 2009;37:112–17.

64. Gozal D, Crabtree VM, Sans Capdevila O, et al. C-reactive protein, obstructive sleep apnea, and cognitive dysfunction in school-aged children. Am J Resp Crit Care Med 2007;176:188–93.

65. Gozal D, Kheirandish-Gozal L, Serpero LD, et al. Obstructive sleep apnea and endothelial function in school-aged nonobese children: effect of adenotonsillectomy. Circulation 2007;116:2307–14.

66. Gozal D, Sans Capdevila O, McLaughlin Crabtree V, et al. Plasma IGF-1 levels and cognitive dysfunction in children with obstructive sleep apnea. Sleep Med 2009;10:167–73.

67. Ceylan MF, Sener S, Bayraktar AC, et al. Changes in oxidative stress and cellular immunity serum markers in attention-deficit/hyperactivity disorder. Psychiatr Clinl Neurosci 2012;66:220–6.

68. Tsai M-C, Lin H-K, Lin C-H, et al. Prevalence of attention deficit/hyperactivity disorder in pediatric allergic rhinitis: a nationwide population-based study. Allergy Asthma Proc 2011;32:41–6.

69. Saricoban HE, Ozen A, Harmanci K, et al. Common behavioral problems among children with asthma: is there a role of asthma treatment? Ann Allergy Asthma Immunol 2011;106:200–4.

70. Romanos M, Buske-Kirschbaum A, Folster-Holst R, et al. Itches and scratches – is there a link between eczema, ADHD, sleep disruption and food hypersensitivity? Allergy 2011;66:1407–9.

71. Fasmer OB, Riise T, Eagan TM, et al. Comorbidity of asthma with ADHD. J Atten Disord 2011;15:564–71.

72. Schmitt J, Buske-Kirschbaum A, Roessner V. Is atopic disease a risk factor for attention-deficit/hyperactivity disorder? A systematic review. Allergy 2010;65:1506–24.

73. Romanos M, Gerlach M, Warnke A, et al. Association of attention-deficit/hyperactivity disorder and atopic eczema modified by sleep disturbance in a large population-based sample. J Epidemiol Commun Health 2010;64:269–73.

74. Feingold BE. Feingold diet. Aust Fam Phys 1980;9:60–1.

75. Mattes JA, Gittelman R. Effects of artificial food colorings in children with hyperactive symptoms. A critical review and results of a controlled study. Arch Gen Psychiatry 1981;38:714–18.

76. Egger J, Stolla A, McEwen LM. Controlled trial of hyposensitisation in children with food-induced hyperkinetic syndrome. Lancet 1992 339:1150–3.

77. Pelsser LM, Frankena K, Toorman J, et al. Effects of a restricted elimination diet on the behaviour of children with attention-deficit hyperactivity disorder (INCA study): a randomised controlled trial. Lancet 2011;377:494–503.

78. Millichap JG, Yee MM. The diet factor in attention-deficit/hyperactivity disorder. Pediatrics 2012;129:330–7.

79. Osler W. The principles and practice of medicine. Edinburgh: Young J. Pentland; 1892.

80. Brockmann PE, Urschitz MS, Schlaud M, et al. Primary snoring in school children: prevalence and neurocognitive impairments. Sleep Breath 2012;16:23–9.

80A. Huang YS, Guilleminault C, Li HY, et al. Attention-deficit/hyperactivity disorder with obstructive sleep apnea: a treatment outcome study. Sleep Med 2007;8:18–30.

81. Chervin RD, Ruzicka DL, Giordani BJ, et al. Sleep-disordered breathing, behavior, and cognition in children before and after adenotonsillectomy. Pediatrics 2006;117:e769–78.

82. Dillon JE, Blunden S, Ruzicka DL, et al. DSM-IV diagnoses and obstructive sleep apnea in children before and 1 year after adenotonsillectomy. J Am Acad Child Adolesc Psychiatry 2007;46:1425–36.

83. Dillon JE, Hodges EK, Felt B, et al. DSM-IV diagnoses in children before and six months after adenotonsillectomy. Sleep 2010;33:A241.

84. Chervin RD, Ruzicka DL, Hoban TF, et al. Esophageal pressures, polysomnography, and neurobehavioral outcomes of adenotonsillectomy in children. Chest 2012;142:101–10.

85. Calhoun SL, Fernandez-Mendoza J, Vgontzas AN, et al. Learning, attention/hyperactivity, and conduct problems as sequelae of excessive daytime sleepiness in a general population study of young children. Sleep 2012;35:627–32.

86. Ali NJ, Pitson D, Stradling JR. Natural history of snoring and related behaviour problems between the ages of 4 and 7 years. Arch Dis Child 1994;71:74–6.

87. Chervin RD, Ruzicka DL, Archbold KH, et al. Snoring predicts hyperactivity four years later. Sleep 2005;28:885–90.

88. Conners CK, Barkley RA. Rating scales and checklists for child psychopharmacology. Psychopharmacol Bull 1985;21:809–68.

89. Conners CK, Sitarenios G, Parker JDA, et al. The Revised Conners' Parent Rating Scale (CPRS-R): Factor structure, reliability, and criterion validity. J Abnorm Child Pscyhol 1998;26:257–68.

90. Bonuck K, Freeman K, Chervin RD, et al. Sleep-disordered breathing in a population-based cohort: behavioral outcomes at 4 and 7 years. Pediatrics 2012;129:e857–65.

91. Lumeng JC, Chervin RD. Epidemiology of pediatric obstructive sleep apnea. Proc Am Thoracic Soc 2008;5:242–52.

92. Richards W, Ferdman RM. Prolonged morbidity due to delays in the diagnosis and treatment of obstructive sleep apnea in children. Clin Pediatr 2000;39:103–8.

93. O'Brien LM, Holbrook CR, Mervis CB, et al. Sleep and neurobehavioral characteristics of 5- to 7-year-old children with parentally reported

symptoms of attention-deficit/hyperactivity disorder. Pediatrics 2003; 111:554–63.

94. Pliszka SRMD, McCracken JTMD, Maas JWMD. Catecholamines in attention-deficit hyperactivity disorder: current perspectives. J Am Acad Child Adolesc Psychiatry 1996;35:264–72.

95. Bradley C. The behavior of children receiving Benzedrine. Am J Psychiatry 1937;94:577–85.

96. Bradley C, Bowen M. Amphetamine (Benzedrine) therapy of children's behavior disorders. Am J Orthopsychiatry 1941;11:92–103.

97. Weinberg WA, Brumback RA. Primary disorder of vigilance: a novel explanation of inattentiveness, daydreaming, boredom, restlessness, and sleepiness. J Pediatr 1990;116:720–5.

98. Dahl RE, Pelham WE, Wierson M. The role of sleep disturbances in attention deficit disorder symptoms: a case study. J Pediatr Psychol 1991;16:229–39.

99. Van der Heijden KB, Smits MG, Van Someren EJW, et al. Idiopathic chronic sleep onset insomnia in attention-deficit/hyperactivity disorder: a circadian rhythm sleep disorder. Chronobiol Int 2005;22:559–70.

100. Hoebert M, van der Heijden KB, van Geijlswijk IM, et al. Long-term follow-up of melatonin treatment in children with ADHD and chronic sleep onset insomnia. J Pineal Res 2009;47:1–7.

101. Van der Heijden KBPD, Smits MGMDPD, Van Someren EUSJWPD, et al. Effect of melatonin on sleep, behavior, and cognition in ADHD and chronic sleep-onset insomnia. J Am Acad Child Adolesc Psychiatry 2007;46:233–41.

102. Susman EJ, Dockray S, Schiefelbein VL, et al. Morningness/eveningness, morning-to-afternoon cortisol ratio, and antisocial behavior problems during puberty. Dev Psychol 2007;43:811–22.

103. Achenback TM, Edelbrock C. Manual for the child behavior checklist and revised child behavior profile. Burlington: University of Vermont, Department of Psychiatry; 1983.

104. Achenback T. ASEBA, Child behavior checklist for ages 4–18 (CBCL/4-18). Burlington: University of Vermont; 2001.

105. Antrop I, Buysse A, Roeyers H, et al. Activity in children with ADHD during waiting situations in the classroom: a pilot study. Br J Educ Psychol 2005;75:51–69.

106. Tsujii N, Okada A, Kaku R, et al. Association between activity level and situational factors in children with attention deficit/hyperactivity disorder in elementary school. Psychiatr Clin Neurosci 2007;61:181–5.

107. Imeraj L, Antrop I, Roeyers H, et al. Diurnal variations in arousal: a naturalistic heart rate study in children with ADHD. Eur Child Adolesc Psychiatry 2011;20:381–92.

108. Rybak YE, McNeely HE, Mackenzie BE, et al. An open trial of light therapy in adult attention-deficit/hyperactivity disorder. J Clin Psychiatry 2006;67:1527–35.

109. Rybak YE, McNeely HE, Mackenzie BE, et al. Seasonality and circadian preference in adult attention-deficit/hyperactivity disorder: clinical and neuropsychological correlates. Compr Psychiatry 2007;48:562–71.

110. Imeraj L, Sonuga-Barke E, Antrop I, et al. Altered circadian profiles in attention-deficit/hyperactivity disorder: an integrative review and theoretical framework for future studies. Neurosci Biobehav Rev 2012; 36:1897–919.

111. McClung CA, Sidiropoulou K, Vitaterna M, et al. Regulation of dopaminergic transmission and cocaine reward by the Clock gene. Proc Natl Acad Sci USA 2005;102:9377–81.

112. Katzenberg D, Young T, Finn L, et al. A CLOCK polymorphism associated with human diurnal preference. Sleep 1998;21:569–76.

113. Robilliard DL, Archer SN, Arendt J, et al. The 3111 Clock gene polymorphism is not associated with sleep and circadian rhythmicity in phenotypically characterized human subjects. J Sleep Res 2002;11:305–12.

114. Mishima K, Tozawa T, Satoh K. The 3111T/C polymorphism of hClock is associated with evening preference and delayed sleep timing in a Japanese population sample. Am J Med Genet Part B, Neuropsychiatr Genet: the Official Publication of the International Society of Psychiatric Genetics 2005;133B:101–4.

115. Iwase T, Kajimura N, Uchiyama M, et al. Mutation screening of the human Clock gene in circadian rhythm sleep disorders. Psychiatry Res 2002;109:121–8.

116. Kissling C, Retz W, Wiemann S, et al. A polymorphism at the 3'-untranslated region of the CLOCK gene is associated with adult attention-deficit hyperactivity disorder. Am J Med Genet Part B, Neuropsychiatr Genet 2008;147:333–8.

117. Xu X, Breen G, Chen C-K, et al. Association study between a polymorphism at the 3'-untranslated region of CLOCK gene and attention deficit hyperactivity disorder Behav Brain Funct [Electronic Resource]: BBF 2010;6:48.

118. Cao Y-L, Cui Q-T, Tang C-H, et al. [Association of CLOCK gene T3111C polymorphism with attention deficit hyperactivity disorder and related sleep disturbances in children]. Zhongguo Dangdai Erke Zazhi 2012;14:285–8.

119. Baird AL, Coogan AN, Siddiqui A, et al. Adult attention-deficit hyperactivity disorder is associated with alterations in circadian rhythms at the behavioural, endocrine and molecular levels. Mol Psychiatry 2012;17:988–95.

120. Chaste P, Clement N, Botros HG, et al. Genetic variations of the melatonin pathway in patients with attention-deficit and hyperactivity disorders. J Pineal Res 2011;51:394–9.

121. Krusz JC, Koller WC, Ziegler DK. Historical review: abnormal movements associated with epidemic encephalitis lethargica. Movement Disord 1987;2:137–41.

122. Wilens TE. Mechanism of action of agents used in attention-deficit/hyperactivity disorder. J Clin Psychiatry 2006;67(Suppl 8):32–8.

123. Anckarsater H, Stahlberg O, Larson T, et al. The impact of ADHD and autism spectrum disorders on temperament, character, and personality development. Am J Psychiatry 2006;163:1239–44.

124. Huang HY, Lee IH, Chen KC, et al. Association of novelty seeking scores and striatal dopamine D2/D3 receptor availability of healthy volunteers: single photon emission computed tomography with 123i-iodobenzamide. J Formos Med Assoc 2010;109:736–9.

125. Munafo MR, Yalcin B, Willis-Owen SA, et al. Association of the dopamine D4 receptor (DRD4) gene and approach-related personality traits: meta-analysis and new data. Biol Psychiatry 2008;63:197–206.

126. Nemoda Z, Szekely A, Sasvari-Szekely M. Psychopathological aspects of dopaminergic gene polymorphisms in adolescence and young adulthood. Neurosci Biobehav Rev 2011;35:1665–86.

127. Nyman ES, Loukola A, Varilo T, et al. Impact of the dopamine receptor gene family on temperament traits in a population-based birth cohort. Am J Med Genet Part B, Neuropsychiatr Genet: the Official Publication of the International Society of Psychiatric Genetics 2009; 150B:854–65.

128. Russell VA. Overview of animal models of attention deficit hyperactivity disorder (ADHD). Curr Protocols Neurosci 2011;Chapter 9:Unit9.35.

129. Volkow ND, Kollins SH, et al. Evaluating dopamine reward pathway in ADHD: clinical implications. JAMA 2009;302:1084–91.

130. Coghill D, Banaschewski T. The genetics of attention-deficit/hyperactivity disorder. Exp Rev Neurotherapeut 2009;9:1547–65.

131. Gainetdinov RR. Strengths and limitations of genetic models of ADHD. Attent Deficit Hyperactiv Disord 2010;2:21–30.

132. Gizer IR, Ficks C, Waldman ID. Candidate gene studies of ADHD: a meta-analytic review. Hum Genet 2009;126:51–90.

133. Nikolaidis A, Gray JR. ADHD and the DRD4 exon III 7-repeat polymorphism: an international meta-analysis. Social Cognit Affect Neurosci 2010;5:188–93.

134. Sharp SI, McQuillin A, Gurling HMD. Genetics of attention-deficit hyperactivity disorder (ADHD). Neuropharmacology 2009;57:590–600.

135. Muhle H, Neumann A, Lohmann-Hedrich K, et al. Childhood-onset restless legs syndrome: clinical and genetic features of 22 families. Movement Disord 2008;23:1113–21; quiz 1203.

136. Picchietti DL, Stevens HE. Early manifestations of restless legs syndrome in childhood and adolescence. Sleep Med 2008;9:770–81.

137. Rajaram S-S, Walters AS, England SJ, et al. Some children with growing pains may actually have restless legs syndrome. Sleep 2004; 27:767–73.

138. Turkdogan D, Bekiroglu N, Zaimoglu S. A prevalence study of restless legs syndrome in Turkish children and adolescents. Sleep Med 2011;12:315–21.

139. Walters AS, Picchietti DL, Ehrenberg BL, et al. Restless legs syndrome in childhood and adolescence. Pediatr Neurol 1994;11:241–5.

140. Picchietti D, Allen RP, Walters AS, et al. Restless legs syndrome: prevalence and impact in children and adolescents–the Peds REST study. Pediatrics 2007;120:253–66.

141. Oner P, Dirik EB, Taner Y, et al. Association between low serum ferritin and restless legs syndrome in patients with attention deficit hyperactivity disorder. Tohoku J Experiment Med 2007;213:269–76.

142. Patrick LR. Restless legs syndrome: pathophysiology and the role of iron and folate. Altern Med Rev 2007;12:101–12.

143. Trotti LM, Bhadriraju S, Becker LA. Iron for restless legs syndrome. Cochrane Database Syst Rev 2009.

144. Konofal E, Lecendreux M, Arnulf I, et al. Iron deficiency in children with attention-deficit/hyperactivity disorder. Arch Pediatr Adolesc Med 2004;158:1113–15.

145. Konofal E, Lecendreux M, Deron J, et al. Effects of iron supplementation on attention deficit hyperactivity disorder in children. Pediatr Neurol 2008;38:20–6.

146. Chervin RD, Archbold KH, Dillon JE, et al. Associations between symptoms of inattention, hyperactivity, restless legs, and periodic leg movements. Sleep 2002;25:213–18.

147. Picchietti DL, Underwood DJ, Farris WA, et al. Further studies on periodic limb movement disorder and restless legs syndrome in children with attention-deficit hyperactivity disorder. Movement Disord 1999; 14:1000–7.

148. Picchietti D. Is iron deficiency an underlying cause of pediatric restless legs syndrome and of attention-deficit/hyperactivity disorder? Sleep Med 2007;8:693–4.

149. Picchietti MA, Picchietti DL. Advances in pediatric restless legs syndrome: Iron, genetics, diagnosis and treatment. Sleep Med 2010;11: 643–51.

150. Whittom S, Davuvilliers Y, Pennestri MH, et al. Age-at-onset in restless legs syndrome: a clinical and poolysomnographic study. Sleep Med 2007;9:54–9.

151. American Psychiatric Association. Diagnostic and Statistical Manual of Mental Disorders (Fourth Edition, text revision). Washington, D.C.: American Psychiatric Association; 2000.

152. American Psychiatric Association. Diagnostic and Statistical Manual of Mental Disorders. 5th ed. Arlington, VA: American Psychiatric Association; 2013.

153. Owens JA. A clinical overview of sleep and attention-deficit/hyperactivity disorder in children and adolescents. J Can Acad Child Adolesc Psychiatry 2009;18:92–102.

154. Redline S, Amin RS, Beebe DW, et al. Childhood Adenotonsillectomy Trial (CHAT): rationale, design, and challenges of a randomized controlled trial evaluating a standard surgical procedure in a pediatric population. Sleep 2011;34:1509–17.

155. Cecil RL, Kammerer WH, DePrume FJ. Gold salts in the treatment of rheumatoid arthritis: a study of 245 cases. Ann Intern Med 1942;16: 811–27.

156. Friberg D, Sundquist J, Li X, et al. Sibling risk of pediatric obstructive sleep apnea syndrome and adenotonsillar hypertrophy. Sleep 2009;32:1077–83.

157. Kim J, Bhattacharjee R, Dayyat E, et al. Increased cellular proliferation and inflammatory cytokines in tonsils derived from children with obstructive sleep apnea. Pediatr Res 2009;66:423–8.

Sleep and Its Disturbances in Autism Spectrum Disorder

Paul Gringras

INTRODUCTION

Families of young people with autism spectrum disorders (ASD) often report that their children have problems falling asleep or staying asleep and that they don't seem to need as much sleep as their peers. These difficulties can arise in infancy, even before the child has a formal autism spectrum diagnosis. Although every day brings behavioral and learning challenges, for these families sleep is often the final straw.

Epidemiological studies in children with ASD now lend support to the suggestion that their sleep difficulties start at a very young age and tend to persist.[1,2] Even when children with learning difficulties and medical comorbidities are excluded, an excess of sleep problems are still found in children with ASD.[2]

Given that the causes of ASD themselves are poorly understood, it comes as no surprise that the origins of sleep disorders in ASD are still unclear. Despite efforts by diagnostic systems to classify ASD as a single entity, the evidence is to the contrary. Indeed, the symptoms of ASD cluster in dimensions rather than into clear categories, and such an interpretation is likely to provide an easier framework for exploring some of the associated sleep problems.[3]

A combination of epidemiological and biological studies is required to explore potential causal links and answer important questions such as: do sleep problems appear as a secondary consequence of having an ASD; do early and persistent sleep problems cause, or contribute to, the emergence of ASD; or, do ASD and its associated sleep problems both share a common underlying pathophysiological basis?

Autism is rarely the discrete entity described in many research studies. Comorbidity is the rule rather than the exception, and it is necessary to appreciate the often additive contributions of common comorbidities such as attention deficit hyperactivity disorder (ADHD), learning difficulties, tics, and seizures, all of which have their own independent effects on sleep.

After discussing the prevalence and possible causes of sleep problems in ASD, an attempt will be made to review the various intervention modalities that are used in treating these sleep problems in children. This is an exciting and rapidly developing area that challenges researchers and clinicians, not just to establish what interventions can work, but also to determine how best to deliver them to the large numbers of patients. Finally, we will look briefly beyond childhood at what is known about the long-term prognosis.

EPIDEMIOLOGY

In general, solid epidemiological studies of sleep patterns, sleep behaviors, and sleep quality in patients with ASD are lacking. Studies have been small, lacked controls, and have often used non-validated diagnostic tools.[4]

Two complementary research protocols that can be helpful are longitudinal cohort studies and controlled cross-sectional ones. The former have all the strengths of studying the temporal sequence of sleep problems in young people with ASD, and they can shed more light on possible directions of causality. However, they are often costly, retaining a cohort for years is difficult, and parameters studied are usually subjective. The latter are less expensive, they allow for the teasing out of possible confounders and, if subjects are carefully matched, they permit the combination of objective and subjective measures.

Evidence from one of the longitudinal protocols comes from the Avon Longitudinal Study of Parents and Children (ALSPAC), a prospective study of a cohort of over 14 000 children born in 1991–2 in southwest England.[5] Parental reports of sleep duration were collected by questionnaires at eight time points from 6 months to 11 years, including from 86 children with an ASD diagnosis (determined at age 11 from health and education records).[1] Children with ASD slept for 15 to 45 minutes less each day compared to contemporary controls aged 30 months to 11 years old (Figure 16-1). The difference remained significant after adjusting for gender, epilepsy, high parity, and ethnicity. The difference in sleep duration mostly reflected changes in nighttime rather than daytime sleep duration. Nighttime sleep duration was shortened because of both later bedtimes and earlier waking times. Frequent wakings, defined as three or more times a night, were significantly more common in children with ASD from 30 months of age.

Another population-based cohort study assessed sleep problems at two age ranges (7–9 and 11–13 years).[2] A screening questionnaire was used to define autism spectrum problems and, in this group, the prevalence of chronic insomnia was more than ten times that seen in controls; and, in the ASD children, the sleep problems were more persistent over time.

Evidence from a cross-sectional study comes from a study of children between 4 and 10 years of age randomly selected from a regional autism center.[4] This descriptive cross-sectional study compared both subjective and objective measures of sleep in an ASD cohort with those of typically developing (TD) controls. In this study more than half of the families of the children with ASD (57.6%) voiced concerns about sleep problems, including the presence of long sleep latencies despite a bedtime routine, frequent night wakings, sleep terrors, and early risings. Only 12.5% of families of the TD cohort reported sleep concerns. Objective actigraphy measurements showed children with ASD took longer to fall asleep, were more active during the night, and had the longest nighttime duration of a wake episode. However, sleep efficiency, total sleep time, and the number of long wake episodes,

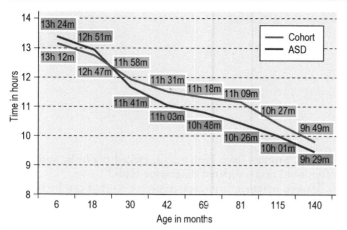

FIGURE 16-1 Total mean sleep duration in ASD children compared to total cohort. Adapted from Humphreys J et al.[1]

as determined by actigraphy, were not statistically different between the ASD and TD cohorts.

Sleep Profiles and Sleep Architecture

Wiggs and Stores[6] used sleep questionnaires, parental diaries, and actigraphy to describe the profile of sleep disturbance in children with ASD. They found that the sleep disorders underlying the sleeplessness were most commonly behavioral, although sleep–wake cycle disorders and anxiety-related problems were also seen. They did not find that sleep patterns measured with actigraphy differed between those ASD children with or without reported sleeplessness. Similar findings were reported in studies by Malow et al.[7] and Souders et al.[4] They used International Classification of Sleep Disorders-2 (ICSD-2)[8] nomenclature and found the commonest sleep diagnoses were behavioral insomnia of childhood – sleep-onset type and insomnia due to PDD.

Importantly, Wiggs and Stores observed that some children with ASD woke at night without alerting their parents, which they termed 'contented sleeplessness.' This contented behavior contrasts with TD children with sleep association disorder who signal or come into their parents' bedrooms. These important differences have contributed to the design of many of the current or proposed behavioral interventions discussed later in this chapter.

Sleep Architecture and Dreaming in ASD

A small controlled study found that young adults with ASD have fewer recollections of dreaming than controls.[9] Their dream content narratives following REM sleep awakenings were shorter with fewer social and emotional experiences. Spectral analysis of the same group showed distinctive slower alpha EEG patterns and asymmetries in the ASD group.[10]

Objective support for REM differences is still in the early stages and is inconsistent. A recent controlled single-night PSG study found rapid eye movement (REM) sleep percentage was lower in children with ASD compared with both children with typical development and children with other developmental disorders.[11] Although interesting, the numbers of children were small and some of the differences found might relate to differences in mean age of the different groups

of children. Additionally, a *first night effect* might account for part of this finding and, in fact, one two-night study did find that REM sleep percentage was lower on night 1 but not night 2.[12]

If REM differences in ASD are real, the potential implications are intriguing. REM sleep is greatest in the developing brain and may represent a protected time for neuroplasticity.[13] REM sleep is involved in memory consolidation and, according to several studies, normal cognitive function and processing of emotional memory.[14,15] In the autism research field where rat and mouse models of autism are being developed, it has been shown that REM deprivation in the neonatal rat induces social deficiencies in the adult animal.[16] The hypothesis elaborated most recently by Buckley et al.[11] goes so far as to suggest that 'a primary cholinergic deficiency may simultaneously produce deficits in REM sleep in autism and contribute to the socio-emotional deficits at the core of the autistic phenotype ...' There is enough belief in this hypothesis to support a recent open-label study, discussed later in this chapter,[17] designed to pharmacologically increase REM percentage in children.

CAUSES OF SLEEP PROBLEMS IN CHILDREN WITH ASD

Learning Difficulty

Children with ASD may present with varied language and cognitive phenotypes. Young people with high-functioning autism and Asperger's syndrome might have average or above-average cognitive abilities, in contrast to non-verbal children with profound learning difficulties. This level of cognitive impairment, although normally a strong predictor for sleep problems, seems less so in ASD where children across a wide range of cognitive abilities have been reported as having sleep problems at an equally high rate. It is tempting to speculate that, although sleep problems in general may be equally common among these groups, the specific nature of these problems is group-dependent. A high rate of anxiety in many of the young people with Asperger's syndrome is often encountered that exacerbates bedtime insomnia[18] with perseverative rituals that further increase sleep latency.[19]

Sensory Issues

Hypersensitivities are well described in people with ASD.[20] Parents attest to the challenges of trimming nails, cutting hair, and even getting their children to wear clothes. The environmental nuances occurring at bedtime, with demands or needs around room and bed (e.g., special sheets, particular sounds, favorite pajamas) are often marked and problematic for families of children with ASD. The theory underlying the reasons for using weighted blankets and other weighted items for calming purposes on these youngsters is based on the idea of sensory integration, a concept initially developed by the occupational therapist Jean Ayres[21] and further developed by occupational therapists and other professionals.[22] It has been hypothesized that the deep pressure provided by weighted items provides proprioceptive input to the body resulting in an inhibitory response that reduces the body's physiological level of arousal and stress.[23] The safety and efficacy of this intervention is not known although a large controlled study in the UK is underway (L. Wiggs and P. Gringras, personal communication).

Genes, Neurobiological Factors, and Melatonin

Although there have been many attempts to use putative genetic and biochemical findings from ASD studies to explain the sleep difficulties seen in children with ASD,[24] these attempts suffer from two fundamental problems: first, there is no evidence that ASD exists as a single disorder with a single cause, and second, the actual causal pathways that lead to ASD are poorly understood.

Although ASD was once thought to be caused by environmental factors, genetic factors are now considered to be more contributory to its pathogenesis. These include, for example, mutations in certain clock-related genes and in other genes that encode synaptic molecules associated with neuronal communication.[25] However, epigenetic mechanisms are also likely to be important; and, these mechanisms are affected by environmental factors (such as nutrition, drugs and mental stress), and they control gene expression without changing DNA sequence.[26] For a more complete review of autism neurobiology, the reader is directed to a comprehensive summary by Silver and Rapin.[27]

Perhaps the greatest efforts have centered on the hormone melatonin because of its known importance in sleep neurobiology and relevance also to ASD research. Abnormal platelet serotonin level remains one of the few consistent biochemical findings in children with autism.[28] Serotonin is a biochemical precursor to melatonin, and there has been considerable research into the components of this pathway. Genetic abnormalities have been reported in the two melatonin receptors,[29] and a variety of mutations have been described in acetylserotonin-o-methyltransferase (ASMT), one of the enzymes responsible for the synthesis of melatonin from serotonin.[29,30] However, the overall numbers of children in these studies whose ASD and sleep problems were associated with these specific ASMT mutations are very small and the findings have not been replicated in all genetic studies.[31]

Although the genetic findings still only explain a few case findings, there is other evidence that melatonin physiology is important in ASD. In one study by Malow and colleagues, the level of a melatonin metabolite was directly related to the amount of deep sleep in children with ASD.[32] The role of exogenous melatonin in treating the sleep of children with ASD is discussed later in the treatment section of this chapter.

Seizures

When a child (and particularly a very young child) presents initially with seizures, the focus of caretakers and clinicians is reducing the frequency and intensity of the seizures and investigating their causes. It is usually only later, when the seizures are under control, that a range of language, cognitive, social, behavioral, and sleep problems emerge or become recognized.[33] About 30% of children with autism also have epilepsy,[34] but it is still not known how often a shared underlying cause accounts for both disorders. However, seizures are often activated in sleep. So, when evaluating a child with autism who experiences unusual repetitive sleep-associated behaviors (or possible parasomnias), one should maintain a high index of suspicion of a possible underlying seizure disorder. Despite the technical challenges of studying these children (who may well be aversive to the investigations

required), full EEG and polysomnography are often essential. For additional information on epilepsy and sleep, also see Chapter 44.

Co-morbidities in ASD

Unfortunately, much of the sleep and ASD research has sought to study *pure* groups of children with ASD. While this approach has certain advantages, it also reduces the generalizability to the real clinical situation where comorbidity of both medical and psychiatric conditions is the rule.[35]

When the prevalence of current comorbid DSM-IV disorders was carefully assessed in children and adolescents with ASD, 72% were diagnosed with at least one comorbid disorder.[35] Anxiety disorders (41%) and ADHD (31%) were the most common, but higher rates of obsessive–compulsive disorder, oppositional defiant disorder, and tic disorders were also present. Many of these disorders are themselves associated with sleep problems (see Chapters 15 and 46), and their frequency in children with ASD suggests they should not be ignored. Clinically, we have observed that there is often an additive effect, where the prolonged sleep latency and bedtime resistance commonly seen in children with ADHD[36] is exacerbated in ASD by an additional degree of cognitive rigidity and by a lack of empathy regarding the sleep of other family members.

Diagnostic Overshadowing – Diagnosing Other Sleep Disorders

Diagnostic overshadowing[37] – in the context of ASD with sleep problems – is the phenomenon of inadvertently over-focusing on the child's ASD (and assuming that the ASD itself is the cause of the child's insomnia), instead of remaining vigilant to other potential causes of the sleep disorders.

Obstructive sleep apnea syndrome (OSAS) is common in the general pediatric population, and its peak incidence in preschool-aged children[38] occurs at a similar age to that when ASD is often first diagnosed.[39] However, there is no convincing epidemiological evidence to suggest that OSAS is more common in ASD, at least once one adjusts for confounders such as low muscle tone.[40]

Parents report an increased frequency of non-rapid eye movement (NREM) arousal disorders in children with ASD,[41] although robust studies are still lacking. Much of the time, simple clinical history combined with home video is sufficient to rule out much rarer nocturnal seizure disorders.[42]

In ASD, rhythmic movement disorder (RMD), such as head banging, can be severe; and, it can also be seen during the day – unrelated to sleep – as well as at night. The movements can persist to adulthood.[43] There is very little research on causes or treatments specific to ASD.

The diagnosis of restless leg syndrome (RLS) in children with ASD is difficult because of the child's cognitive and language limitations. In some cases the finding of frequent arousing PLMs on PSG can be very suggestive. Low long-term stores of iron (usually determined by low serum ferritin levels) can worsen such a disorder, and iron supplementation was shown to improve restless sleep in children with ASD in an open-label pilot study.[44]

REM sleep behavior disorder (RBD) has been reported in one case series of children with ASD who were studied with PSG[12] although a larger polysomnographic study that excluded children on psychotropic medication did not document RBD or even periods of REM sleep without atonia.[7]

TREATMENT OF SLEEP PROBLEMS IN ASD

Size of the Problem

Autism is certainly more common than was previously thought, and current estimates are of over 1 in 100 children being affected.[45] As already discussed, over half of these children will have significant sleep problems. Although complex face-to-face multidisciplinary interventions may be effective, they are time-consuming and will fail to reach many youngsters suffering from a disorder this common. It is for this reason that booklet or web interventions are being proposed, and perhaps this is why behavioral interventions are often neglected in favor of perceived quicker pharmacological options.

What and Who are We Trying to Treat?

We need to differentiate those interventions designed to improve the sleep and quality of life of family members and other caretakers from those that demonstrably improve sleep quantity and quality for the child. Often, there is an assumption that, because parents report an improvement on a subjective sleep questionnaire, there is an actual improvement in the child's objective sleep parameters. In fact, this is rarely the case and, with the exception of sleep latency, parental questionnaires in interventional studies do not agree with objective findings on PSG or actigraphy.[46] This is, of course, not surprising as they are looking at different outcome measures, although both are clinically important.

Sleep disturbances in typically developing children are known to impact maternal sleep and daytime functioning with the extent of sleep disturbance significantly predicting maternal mood, stress and fatigue. There has not been enough research on health-related quality of life outcomes for parents and siblings in specific ASD groups. In part, this is because there is still debate about the best *disease-specific* quality of life measure for caretakers of children with autism.[47] Support groups have been shown to help the mental health and quality of life of mothers of children with ASD, but these have not focused on sleep issues alone.[48,49]

Sleep Behavioral Interventions in ASD

The basic principles of behavioral interventions for children and young people with ASD do not differ greatly from general principles of sleep environment normalization and appropriate *sleep hygiene* as discussed in Chapters 8 and 14. Systematic reviews highlight the lack of robust studies.[50] An often unwritten aspect of all such interventions is to anticipate the important behavioral extinction burst that often occurs on about the third night of the intervention and provide enough support for the emotionally drained and physically exhausted parents to help them be as consistent and persistent as required during that period.

Specific *parent training workshops* for sleep difficulties in children with autism have potential to be helpful, and in one non-controlled pilot study improvements were found both in objective measures (such as sleep latency) and in subjective ones (such as ratings of daytime behavior).[51] Future studies of parenting education interventions will need to be performed using controlled studies measuring both subjective and objective sleep outcomes.

Montgomery et al. showed the effectiveness of a booklet-delivered intervention[51] that has recently been used in the Melatonin in Children with Neurodevelopmental Disorders and Impaired Sleep (MENDS) study.[52] This booklet was designed for children with neurodevelopmental delay as well as ASD, and it is freely available on the web.[53] Interestingly, there was no evidence of any differential response between children with and without ASD.

In the US, the Autism Treatment Network (ATN) has developed an algorithm and a behavioral sleep medicine toolkit for the evaluation and treatment of insomnia in children with ASD.[54] The algorithm emphasizes screening for sleep problems in children with ASD, followed by identification and treatment of associated medical comorbidities that may affect sleep.

Sensory Interventions in ASD

There is very limited evidence available to support the effectiveness of use of weighted blankets and similar items in the treatment of children with presumed sensory integration (SI) issues. There is one controlled study using such sensory blankets in children with ADHD that showed a small reduction in sleep latency.[55] There is no evidence for the efficacy of weighted blankets in children with ASD, and – although case reports exist – there are safety concerns about their use, and the cost of weighted blankets is considerable. Controlled studies are now underway in the UK (Wiggs L., personal communication), but given that the sensory profile of young people with ASD is as varied as are other aspects of their phenotype, it will be interesting to see if specific profiles (obtained using standardized questionnaires) predict treatment response.

Melatonin and other Pharmacological Interventions in ASD

This section will primarily focus on melatonin, as there is so little robust evidence for the use of any other medications for sleep problems in ASD.

A number of systematic reviews have aimed to determine the effect of melatonin on sleep parameters in children with autism and other developmental problems (see Table 16.1). The trials included within each meta-analysis are heterogeneous in terms of patient populations studied, the doses used, and the time and durations of treatment. Of methodological concern are the number of small trials, suspicions of outcome reporting bias within the trials, and the use of a crossover design (the suitability of which has been questioned due to the impact on the circadian timing system outlasting drug washout periods).

Perhaps the main difficulty with meta-analyses is that the included studies ignored behavioral interventions that could have taken place before or alongside treatment with melatonin. There is good clinical rationale and growing evidence that behavioral and psychopharmacological interventions are complimentary, and any behavioral intervention should either precede, or take place alongside, a pharmacological one.[52,56]

There are two well-powered studies that shed more light on the effects of behavioral interventions and melatonin. The MENDS study was a randomized clinical trial (RCT) specifically designed and powered to assess impact of a systematic dose escalation of melatonin on total sleep time over a 3-month period using subjective and objective assessments of sleep.[52] Of the 146 children randomized, 63 had autism and learning difficulties, and the rest other non-specific causes of

TABLE 16.1   Results of Systematic Reviews of Melatonin vs Placebo[52]

SYSTEMATIC REVIEW	POPULATION	TOTAL SLEEP TIME			SLEEP ONSET LATENCY			AUTHOR CONCLUSION
		TRIALS[1]	NO. OF CHILDREN	ESTIMATE (95% CI)	TRIALS	NO. OF CHILDREN	ESTIMATE (95% CI)	
Buscemi et al.[66] 12 trials, 7 cross over	Secondary sleep disorders; heterogeneous population	9	382	WMD[2]: 15.6 (7.2 to 24.0)	6	163	WMD: −13.2 (−27.3 to 0.9)	No significant effect on SOL and a small and clinically unimportant effect on sleep efficiency
Braam et al.[67] 9 trials, 7 crossover	Intellectual disability; adults and children	7	257	WMD: 49.8 (34.2 to 64.8)	7	273	WMD: −33.8 (−42.97 to −24.70)	Decreases SOL and increases TST
Rossignol and Frye[68] 5 controlled trials- 5 crossover, 57 patients	Autism spectrum disorders	5	57	Hedge's g: 1.07 (0.49 to 1.65)	5	57	Hedge's g: 2.46 (1.96 to 2.98)	Improved sleep parameters and minimal side effects. Call for a large RCT. ≤4 min longer TST and 39 min shorter SOL with melatonin.
		5	57	Glass's Δ: 0.93 (0.33 to 1.53)	5	57	Glass's Δ: 1.28 (0.67 to 1.89)	
Philips and Appleton[69] 3 cross over studies, 35 children	Children with neurodevelopmental disabilities	No meta-analysis			No meta-analysis			May be effective in reducing SOL. No evidence of an effect on TST. Call for a large RCT

[1] Trials = number of trials relating to either Total Sleep Time (TST) outcomes, or Sleep Onset Latency (SOL) Trials. Depending on variables captured by each study these will be less, or the same as the total number of trials in the systematic review.

[2] WMD = weighted mean difference.

Adapted from Gringras P, Gamble C, Jones A, et al. Melatonin for sleep problems in children with neurodevelopmental disorders: randomised double masked placebo controlled trial. BMJ 2012;345:e6664.

learning difficulty. One of the standardized parental sleep behavioral interventions already discussed[51] was used for a month prior to any melatonin treatment during which a routine bedtime was established. Over half of the subjects on this trial improved during this run-in, to the extent their sleep problems were no longer severe enough to qualify for the pharmacological RCT.

The pharmacological placebo-controlled intervention administered 0.5–12 mg immediate-release melatonin in a stepwise fashion. The results only showed a small increase of 23 minutes in total sleep time (TST) but a larger 38-minute reduction of sleep latency. For some children these effects were seen at the lowest dose (0.5 mg). Melatonin had no demonstrable effect on night wakings. There was no evidence that exogenous melatonin was differentially more effective in children with learning disability and ASD than in children with other non-specific causes of learning difficulty. Melatonin was well tolerated and there were no excess adverse effects in the treatment group such as, in particular, any increase in, or new onset of, epileptic seizures.

The effect of melatonin on sleep latency was consistent with other reports of the use of melatonin in typically developing children (35 minute reduction),[57] in children with intellectual disabilities (34 minutes)[58] and in children with autism (39 minutes).[59] In keeping with another study on typically developing children,[57] the MENDS study found melatonin was most effective for those children with the longest sleep latency. The study also found that children on melatonin woke

earlier than controls by the end of the 3-month period; this finding has not been previously reported in children with neurodevelopmental disorders. It is consistent with melatonin's effect in laboratory-controlled studies,[60,61] and suggests that evening exogenous fast-release melatonin advances sleep phase over time – therefore causing children to both fall asleep and wake earlier – and explaining the smaller effect on TST. Levels of salivary melatonin in some children in the study remained high, even when melatonin had not been taken the previous evening. It is likely that these children are the well-described *slow metabolizers*, those children who seem to initially respond well to melatonin but then need to have their dose lowered.[62]

Cortesi et al.[56] employed a different design where 160 children with ASD, aged 4–10 years, suffering from sleep onset and sleep maintenance insomnia, were assigned in equal numbers randomly to one of four groups: (1) combination of controlled-release melatonin and cognitive–behavioral therapy; (2) controlled-release melatonin; (3) four sessions of cognitive–behavioral therapy; or (4) placebo drug treatment condition. Children were studied at baseline and after 12 weeks of treatment. Treatment response was assessed by actigraphy, sleep diary, and sleep questionnaire. Melatonin treatment was mainly effective in reducing insomnia symptoms, while cognitive–behavioral therapy had a small positive impact mainly on sleep latency, suggesting that some behavioral aspects might play a role in determining initial insomnia. The combination treatment group showed a trend to outperform the other active treatments. This study demonstrated that adding a behavioral intervention to melatonin treatment seems to result in a better treatment response, at least in the short term.

The use of clonidine, trazodone, and occasionally atypical antipsychotic medications has been reported in case series and open-label studies as improving sleep of children with ASD.[63,64] Such medications are often prescribed to also address behavioral and mood comorbidities in ASD, and carefully designed studies will be required to isolate which effects are specific to sleep.

A different approach has been to focus on the limited evidence that REM sleep is decreased in children with ASD, and, therefore, to use pharmacological means to try to *normalize* REM sleep. An open-label trial of donepezil has recently shown that REM percentage can indeed be increased pharmacologically.[17] The design of the study, and its duration, raise unanswered questions about whether such an intervention may result in clinical benefit or, indeed, cause long-term harm.

DO CHILDREN WITH ASD GROW OUT OF THEIR SLEEP PROBLEMS?

Well-meaning family members, friends, and professionals will often try to reassure an exhausted family that their sleepless child with ASD 'will grow out of it.' Unfortunately, there is no empirical evidence to suggest this is true. Anecdotally, parents whose children with ASD had reached young adulthood have told us that they simply gave up mentioning it, as 'there seemed to be nothing more we could do.' In addition, some young children with ASD eventually enter sheltered accommodation, where caretakers are awake at night anyway (so without having their own sleep disturbed), and the sleep problems of the youngsters under their care are less likely to be reported.

In the only adult study with a clear control group, 20 adults with Asperger's syndrome (without medication) were compared with 10 healthy controls.[18] On subjective questionnaires and sleep diaries, the Asperger's subjects had more frequent difficulties falling asleep, longer sleep latencies, and more frequent early morning wakings than did the controls. In another non-controlled study, objective and subjective measures were used to investigate sleep in adolescents and young adults, aged 15 to 25 years, with autism and Asperger's syndrome.[65] This study found that although the sleep questionnaires completed by parents and caretakers revealed only a moderate degree of sleep problem, greater sleep disturbance was recorded with actigraphy.

This finding suggests that even though subjective complaints of sleep disturbances are less common in adolescents and young adults with autism (than they are in younger children), this may be due to the caretakers adapting to the sleep patterns rather than to an actual reduction in sleep disturbances. The adult studies discussed above focus on adults who would not have not been exposed to many of the newer behavioral and pharmacological interventions discussed in this chapter. Although the hope is that long-term improvements in sleep for people with ASD will be possible with current treatment options, this will require evidence from controlled trials with much longer follow-up periods than those used to date.

Clinical Pearls

- Sleep difficulties may emerge in infancy and precede a formal diagnosis of ASD.
- Behavioral interventions are often effective and should precede pharmacological treatments.
- Melatonin treatment is most effective when accompanied by a behavioral intervention.
- Melatonin primarily improves sleep-onset difficulties; it has less impact on total sleep duration and is unlikely to improve nighttime waking.
- Doses of melatonin as low as 0.5 mg will be helpful for some children.
- Although high doses of melatonin may promote its sedative action in some children, this may not be the case for slow metabolizers.

References

1. Humphreys J, Gringras P, Blair P, et al. Sleep patterns in children with autistic spectrum disorders: a prospective cohort study. Arch Dis Child 2013; online first doi:10.1136/arcdischild.
2. Sivertsen B, Posserud MB, Gillberg C, et al. Sleep problems in children with autism spectrum problems: a longitudinal population-based study. Autism 2012;16(2):139–50.
3. Happé F, Ronald A. The 'fractionable autism triad': a review of evidence from behavioural, genetic, cognitive and neural research. Neuropsychol Rev 2008;18(4):287–304.
4. Souders MC, Mason TBA, Valladares O, et al. Sleep behaviors and sleep quality in children with autism spectrum disorders. Sleep 2009;32(12):1566–78.
5. Blair PS, Humphreys JS, Gringras P, et al. Childhood sleep duration and associated demographic characteristics in an English cohort. Sleep 2012;35(3):353–60.
6. Wiggs L, Stores G. Sleep patterns and sleep disorders in children with autistic spectrum disorders: insights using parent report and actigraphy. Dev Med Child Neurol 2004;46(6):372–80.
7. Malow BA, Marzec ML, McGrew SG, et al. Characterizing sleep in children with autism spectrum disorders: a multidimensional approach. Sleep 2006;29(12):1563–71.
8. American Academy of Sleep Medicine. International classification of sleep disorders. 2nd ed. Diagnostic and coding manual. Westchester, Illinois: American Academy of Sleep Medicine; 2005.
9. Daoust AM, Lusignan FA, Braun CMJ, et al. Dream content analysis in persons with an autism spectrum disorder. J Autism Dev Disord 2008;38(4):634–43.
10. Daoust AM, Limoges E, Bolduc C, et al. EEG spectral analysis of wakefulness and REM sleep in high functioning autistic spectrum disorders. Clin Neurophysiol 2004;115(6):1368–73.
11. Buckley AW, Rodriguez AJ, Jennison K, et al. Rapid eye movement sleep percentage in children with autism compared with children with developmental delay and typical development. Arch Pediatr Adolesc Med 2010;164(11):1032–7.
12. Thirumalai SS, Shubin RA, Robinson R. Rapid eye movement sleep behavior disorder in children with autism. J Child Neurol 2002;17(3):173–8.
13. Hobson JA. REM sleep and dreaming: towards a theory of protoconsciousness. Nat Rev Neurosci 2009;10(11):803–13.
14. Stickgold R. Sleep-dependent memory consolidation. Nature 2005;437(7063):1272–8.
15. Maquet P. The role of sleep in learning and memory. Science 2001;294(5544):1048–52.
16. Vogel G, Hagler M. Effects of neonatally administered iprindole on adult behaviors of rats. Pharmacol Biochem Behav 1996;55(1):157–61.
17. Buckley AW, Sassower K, Rodriguez AJ, et al. An open label trial of donepezil for enhancement of rapid eye movement sleep in young children with autism spectrum disorders. J Child Adolesc Psychopharmacol 2011;21(4):353–7.
18. Tani P, Lindberg N, Nieminen-von Wendt T, et al. Sleep in young adults with Asperger syndrome. Neuropsychobiology 2004;50(2):147–52.
19. Gabriels RL, Cuccaro ML, Hill DE, et al. Repetitive behaviors in autism: relationships with associated clinical features. Res Dev Disabil 2005;26(2):169–81.

20. Lane AE, Dennis SJ, Geraghty ME. Brief report: Further evidence of sensory subtypes in autism. J Autism Dev Disord 2011;41(6):826–31.
21. Ayres AJ, Heskett WM. Sensory integrative dysfunction in a young schizophrenic girl. J Autism Child Schizophr 1972;2(2):174–81.
22. Champagne T, Stromberg N. Sensory approaches in inpatient psychiatric settings: innovative alternatives to seclusion and restraint. J Psychosoc Nurs Ment Health Serv 2004;42(9):34–44.
23. Mullen B, Champagne T, Krishnamurty S, et al. Exploring the safety and therapeutic effects of deep pressure stimulation using a weighted blanket. Occupational Therapy in Mental Health 2008;24(1):65–89.
24. Kotagal S, Broomall E. Sleep in children with autism spectrum disorder. Pediatr Neurol 2012;47(4):242–51.
25. Bourgeron T. The possible interplay of synaptic and clock genes in autism spectrum disorders. Cold Spring Harb Symp Quant Biol 2007;72:645–54.
26. Miyake K, Hirasawa T, Koide T, Kubota T. Epigenetics in autism and other neurodevelopmental diseases. Adv Exp Med Biol 2012;724:91–8.
27. Silver WG, Rapin I. Neurobiological basis of autism. Pediatr Clin North Am 2012;59(1):45–61, x.
28. Zafeiriou DI, Ververi A, Vargiami E. The serotonergic system: its role in pathogenesis and early developmental treatment of autism. Curr Neuropharmacol 2009;7(2):150–7.
29. Jonsson L, Ljunggren E, Bremer A, et al. Mutation screening of melatonin-related genes in patients with autism spectrum disorders. BMC Med Genomics 2010;3:10.
30. Melke J, Goubran Botros H, Chaste P, et al. Abnormal melatonin synthesis in autism spectrum disorders. Mol Psychiatry 2008;13(1):90–8.
31. Toma C, Rossi M, Sousa I, et al. Is ASMT a susceptibility gene for autism spectrum disorders? A replication study in European populations. Mol Psychiatry 2007;12(11):977–9.
32. Leu RM, Beyderman L, Botzolakis EJ, et al. Relation of melatonin to sleep architecture in children with autism. J Autism Dev Disord 2011;41(4):427–33.
33. Baca CB, Vickrey BG, Caplan R, et al. Psychiatric and medical comorbidity and quality of life outcomes in childhood-onset epilepsy. Pediatrics 2011;128(6):e1532–43.
34. Tuchman R, Cuccaro M. Epilepsy and autism: neurodevelopmental perspective. Curr Neurol Neurosci Rep 2011;11(4):428–34.
35. Abdallah MW, Greaves-Lord K, Grove J, et al. Psychiatric comorbidities in autism spectrum disorders: findings from a Danish historic birth cohort. Eur Child Adolesc Psychiatry 2011;20(11–12):599–601.
36. Konofal E, Lecendreux M, Cortese S. Sleep and ADHD. Sleep Med 2010;11(7):652–8.
37. Jopp DA, Keys CB. Diagnostic overshadowing reviewed and reconsidered. Am J Ment Retard 2001;106(5):416–33.
38. Tauman R, Gozal D. Obstructive sleep apnea syndrome in children. Expert Rev Resp Med 2011;5(3):425–40.
39. Fountain C, King MD, Bearman PS. Age of diagnosis for autism: individual and community factors across ten birth cohorts. J Epidemiol Community Health 2011;65(6):503–10.
40. Cortesi F, Giannotti F, Ivanenko A, et al. Sleep in children with autistic spectrum disorder. Sleep Med 2010;11(7):659–64.
41. Goldman SE, Richdale AL, Clemons T, et al. Parental sleep concerns in autism spectrum disorders: variations from childhood to adolescence. J Autism Dev Disord 2012;42(4):531–8.
42. Kotagal S. Parasomnias in childhood. Sleep Med Rev 2009;13(2):157–68.
43. Chisholm T, Morehouse RL. Adult headbanging: sleep studies and treatment. Sleep 1996;19(4):343–6.
44. Dosman CF, Brian JA, Drmic IE, et al. Children with autism: effect of iron supplementation on sleep and ferritin. Pediatr Neurol 2007;36(3):152–8.
45. Autism and Developmental Disabilities Monitoring Network Surveillance Year 2008 Principal Investigators. Prevalence of Autism Spectrum Disorders – Autism and Developmental Disabilities Monitoring Network, 14 Sites, United States, 2008-Surveillance Summaries. Morb Mort Weekly Rep 2012;61(SS03):1–19, CDC.
46. Sadeh A. The role and validity of actigraphy in sleep medicine: an update. Sleep Med Rev 2011;15(4):259–67.

47. Tavernor L, Barron E, Rodgers J, et al. Finding out what matters: validity of quality of life measurement in young people with ASD. Child Care Health Dev 2013;39(4):592–601.
48. Shu BC, Lung FW. The effect of support group on the mental health and quality of life for mothers with autistic children. J Intellect Disabil Res 2005;49(Pt 1):47–53.
49. Hall HR. Families of children with autism: behaviors of children, community support and coping. Issues Compr Pediatr Nurs 2012;35(2):111–32.
50. Montgomery P, Dunne D. Sleep disorders in children. Clin Evid 2007;2007:pii.
51. Montgomery P, Stores G, Wiggs L. The relative efficacy of two brief treatments for sleep problems in young learning disabled (mentally retarded) children: a randomised controlled trial. Arch Dis Child 2004;89(2):125–30.
52. Gringras P, Gamble C, Jones A, et al. Melatonin for sleep problems in children with neurodevelopmental disorders: randomised double masked placebo controlled trial. BMJ 2012;345:e6664.
53. Montgomery P. Encouraging good sleep habits in children with learning disabilities [Internet]. 2007. Available from: http://www.research autism.net/pages/research_autism_projects_studies/research_autism_project_016.
54. Autism Treatment Network. ATN/AIR-P Sleep Tool Kit for Children with ASD [Internet]. 2012 Available from: http://www.autismspeaks.org/science/resources-programs/autism-treatment-network/tools-you-can-use/sleep-tool-kit.
55. Hvolby A, Bilenberg N. Use of Ball Blanket in attention-deficit/hyperactivity disorder sleeping problems. Nord J Psychiatry 2011;65(2):89–94.
56. Cortesi F, Giannotti F, Sebastiani T, et al. Controlled-release melatonin, singly and combined with cognitive behavioural therapy, for persistent insomnia in children with autism spectrum disorders: a randomized placebo-controlled trial. J Sleep Res 2012 May 22. doi: 10.1111/j.1365-2869.2012.01021.x. [Epub ahead of print].
57. van Geijlswijk IM, van der Heijden KB, Egberts ACG, et al. Dose finding of melatonin for chronic idiopathic childhood sleep onset insomnia: an RCT. Psychopharmacology (Berl) 2010;212(3):379–91.
58. Braam W, Smits MG, Didden R, et al. Exogenous melatonin for sleep problems in individuals with intellectual disability: a meta-analysis. Dev Med Child Neurol 2009;51(5):340–9.
59. Rossignol DA, Frye RE. Melatonin in autism spectrum disorders: a systematic review and meta-analysis. Dev Med Child Neurol 2011;53(9):783–92.
60. Czeisler CA. Commentary: evidence for melatonin as a circadian phase-shifting agent. J Biol Rhythms 1997;12(6):618–23.
61. Lewy AJ, Sack RL. Exogenous melatonin's phase-shifting effects on the endogenous melatonin profile in sighted humans: a brief review and critique of the literature. J Biol Rhythms 1997;12(6):588–94.
62. Braam W, van Geijlswijk I, Keijzer H, et al. Loss of response to melatonin treatment is associated with slow melatonin metabolism. J Intellect Disabil Res 2010;54(6):547–55.
63. Ming X, Gordon E, Kang N, et al. Use of clonidine in children with autism spectrum disorders. Brain Dev 2008;30(7):454–60.
64. Gringras P. When to use drugs to help sleep. Arch Dis Child 2008;93(11):976–81.
65. Oyane NMF, Bjorvatn B. Sleep disturbances in adolescents and young adults with autism and Asperger syndrome. Autism 2005;9(1):83–94.
66. Buscemi N, Vandermeer B, Hooton N, et al. The efficacy and safety of exogenous melatonin for primary sleep disorders. A meta-analysis. J Gen Intern Med 2005;20(12):1151–8.
67. Braam W, Smits MG, Didden R, et al. Exogenous melatonin for sleep problems in individuals with intellectual disability: a meta-analysis. Dev Med Child Neurol 2009;51(5):340–9.
68. Rossignol DA, Frye RE. Melatonin in autism spectrum disorders: a systematic review and meta-analysis. Dev Med Child Neurol 2011;53(9):783–92.
69. Phillips L, Appleton RE. Systematic review of melatonin treatment in children with neurodevelopmental disabilities and sleep impairment. Dev Med Child Neurol 2004;46(11):771–5.

Metabolic Syndrome and Obesity

Jerome Alonso

METABOLIC SYNDROME

The metabolic syndrome (MetS) was originally described in the adult population, with the observance of the tendency for the aggregation of a number of cardiovascular risk factors that are associated with increased risk for atherosclerotic cardiovascular disease (ASCVD)[1-3] and type 2 diabetes (T2DM).[4] A central, albeit not exclusive, factor in the pathogenesis of MetS is insulin resistance.[5,6] Other mechanisms that have been thought to play a role include the effect of obesity, increased inflammatory mediators, aggravated oxidative stress, endothelial dysfunction, and elevated cortisol levels. However, the exact definition of MetS has continued to be a center of debate. Only recently has there been harmonization of the definition in the adult population to include cut-off points for fasting glucose, HDL cholesterol, triglycerides, waist circumference, and blood pressure.[7] Defining the condition in the pediatric population is a greater challenge, since it needs to incorporate considerations such as criteria across ages, take into account physiologic changes in metabolism throughout the life-cycle, and the requirement to define morphologic scores for truncal obesity. The International Diabetes Federation published its definition of MetS in 2007 as listed in Table 17.1 with the following parameters: (1) waist circumference, (2) triglyceride level, (3) blood pressure, and (4) fasting glucose. Other proposed criteria for MetS are listed on Table 17.1. A further hindrance to unified criteria is that prevalence rates vary greatly from 6% to 39% of the general population.[8] The diagnosis of MetS also appears to be unstable as children age.[9,10] Nonetheless, there is significant evidence that the presence of MetS and its attendant cardiovascular risk factors in childhood and adolescence are associated with markers for early and subclinical atherosclerosis[11-14] and increased risk for the development of T2DM and ASCVD.[15,16]

SLEEP AND THE COMPONENTS OF THE METABOLIC SYNDROME (see also Chapter 31)

Sleep deprivation and sleep disruption have been observed to have associations with many of the parameters of MetS. In fact, the inclusion of obstructive sleep apnea (OSA) as a component of MetS in the form of syndrome Z has been proposed, because of the strength of the association and evidence of increased risk for ASCVD and DM.[17] In the pediatric population, Redline et al. found a sixfold increase in risk for MetS in adolescents who were obese and had sleep-disordered breathing (SDB).[18] Both sleep fragmentation[19] and obstructive sleep apnea[20] have been observed to be associated with insulin resistance. Dysregulation of lipid metabolism and its subsequent improvement have been shown with obstructive sleep apnea. A bidirectional relationship between obesity and disrupted sleep has also been demonstrated in models of artificial sleep disturbance and clinical OSA, as described in later sections.

Insulin Resistance

Insulin resistance has been considered a central mechanism in the increased risk for diabetes and ACVD in MetS. Early studies on sleep deprivation demonstrated a reduction in glucose utilization and insulin sensitivity with acute sleep deprivation.[21] Epidemiologic data from cross-sectional studies have also demonstrated an association between short sleep and diabetes;[22,23] while prospective studies have supported an increase in incident diabetes with baseline short sleep.[24,25] Sleep stage deprivation and fragmentation have been observed to present a similar phenomenon. In one particular SWS deprivation trial that utilized acoustic stimuli, a 90% reduction of SWS over a 3-day period produced approximately a 25% reduction in insulin sensitivity without the expected compensatory rises in insulin secretion.[19] The fragmentation and SWS curtailment that was produced during this study can be thought to correspond to what can typically be seen in the context of OSA.

OSA in the adult population has been demonstrated in the Sleep Heart Health Study, a large multicenter population-based study, to be associated with derangement in various aspects of glucose metabolism.[26,27] The cross-sectional analysis employed data from fasting serum glucose samples and 2-hour oral glucose tolerance tests to evaluate utilization and responsiveness to a glucose challenge. The study revealed that insulin resistance and glucose intolerance were independently associated with SDB after controlling for age, sex, race, BMI, and waist circumference.[27] In a separate sub-analysis involving obese/overweight individuals with a sleep-related breathing disorder (SDB) and non-obese subjects with SDB, those with a SDB had a higher prevalence rate and adjusted odds of having impaired fasting glucose (IFG), impaired glucose tolerance (IGT), IFG and IGT and occult diabetes, after controlling for the same factors.[26] Another large cross-sectional study involving over 1000 subjects showed that there was an independent association between OSA and incident diabetes with increasing severity of OSA linked to higher risk of developing diabetes.[28] As summarized by Tesali and Ip,[29] the majority of adult cross-sectional investigations have shown similar findings with only a few small studies showing contradictory results. Unfortunately, pediatric data has not been as consistent and is plagued by small population sizes. An observational study from de la Eva et al. demonstrated a significant correlation between the apnea-hypopnea index (AHI) and fasting glucose, independent of BMI in an population of obese subjects.[30] Unfortunately, other studies failed to show similar associations between SDB and impairment in glucose metabolism.[31-33] In a study involving non-obese children, Kaditis et al. found no significant correlation between SDB and insulin resistance, fasting glucose levels or fasting insulin after controlling for BMI.[32] In an investigation with both obese and non-obese children, Tauman et al. failed to show significant correlations between AHI, SpO₂ nadir, arousal index, and parameters of insulin resistance such as the insulin/fasting glucose ratio (I/G ratio) and the homeostasis model

TABLE 17.1   Proposed Criteria for the Metabolic Syndrome in Children

	OBESITY	GLUCOSE DYSREGULATION	TRIGLYCERIDES	HDL	BLOOD PRESSURE
IDF Consensus 2007	Ages 10 – <16 yrs, 90th percentile WC. Age ≥16, WC ≥94 cm for men and ≥80 cm for women	Fasting glucose = 100 mg/dL (5.6 mmol/L) or known T2DM	≥150 mg/dL (1.7 mmol/L)	≤40 mg/dL (1.03 mmol/L)	Systolic ≥130 / Diastolic ≥85 mmHg
Ford et al. (2005)[149]	WC ≥90th percentile for age	Fasting glucose ≥110 mg/dL (6.1 mmol/L)	≥110 mg/dL	≤40 mg/dL (1.03 mmol/L)	≥90th percentile for age
De Ferranti et al. (2004)[150]	WC ≥75th percentile for age	Fasting glucose ≥110 mg/dL (6.1 mmol/L)	≥100 mg/dL (1.1 mmol/L)	<50 mg/dL (1.3 mmol/L)	≥90th percentile for age
Cruz et al. (2004)[151]	WC ≥90th percentile for age	Impaired glucose tolerance	≥90th percentile for age	≤10th percentile for age	≥90th percentile for age
Weiss et al. (2004)[152]	BMI Z-score ≥2.0	Impaired glucose tolerance	≥95th percentile for age	≤5th percentile for age	≥95th percentile for age
Cook et al. (2003)[153]	WC ≥90th percentile for age	Fasting glucose ≥110 mg/dL (6.1 mmol/L)	≥110 mg/dl	≤40 mg/dL (1.03 mmol/L)	≥90th percentile for age

WC, waist circumference; T2DM, type 2 diabetes; BMI, body mass index.

assessment equation (HOMA).[33] On the contrary, the same group later published an interventional study with 62 children (37 obese and 25 non-obese) with SDB who underwent adenotonsillectomy that did show an association between parameters of SDB and the I/G ratio, and found a significant improvement in insulin resistance after treatment.[34]

Dyslipidemia
The current evidence surrounding the relationship between sleep disturbance and dysregulation of lipid metabolism is primarily based on SDB and its accompanying hypoxemia. Much of it is founded on animal model data and theoretical mechanisms, with sparse clinical data partially supportive of a direct relationship. Mechanistically, there is evidence that intermittent hypoxemia stimulates the production of hypoxia-inducible factor-1 in the liver, which in turn activates sterol regulatory element-binding protein-1(SREBP-1) and stearoyl-CoA desaturase-1 (SCD).[35] SCD is an important enzyme controlled by SRBEP-1 that is instrumental in triglyceride and phospholipid biosynthesis. In the above-cited study, in was demonstrated in lean mice that there was an increase in total cholesterol, high-density lipoprotein (HDL), triglycerides and phospholipids with intermittent hypoxemia for 5 days. This was not observed in the opposite arm of the study that involved obese mice. In another study involving 4 weeks of intermittent hypoxemia, there was an observed increase in low-density lipoprotein (LDL) levels.[36]

Cross-sectional data from larger adult studies have demonstrated a tendency for a decrease in HDL cholesterol and an increased in triglycerides with the presence of SDB.[37–40] However, this is inconsistent, with a similar studies showing no significant association.[41–44] In the pediatric population, Tauman et al.[33] examined a convenience sample of 135 children (64 moderate to severe OSA, 56 mild OSA and 16 controls) with the complaint of snoring. In their study, they failed to demonstrate a difference in those with mild sleep apnea, moderate to severe sleep apnea, and matched controls, in terms of total cholesterol, triglycerides, HDL and LDL cholesterol. There have also been a number of interventional studies in adults and children examining the effect of the

treatment of obstructive sleep apnea on profiles of cholesterol metabolism. Gozal et al.[34] examined the response on the lipid profile of children with OSA after having an adenotonsillectomy. The study involved 62 individuals (35 obese and 27 non-obese) and demonstrated a significant reduction in total cholesterol and LDL with a reciprocal increase in HDL cholesterol after a 6–12-month follow-up in both obese and non-obese children. Similar findings were also seen in two adult population studies from Japan that utilized nasal CPAP as the primary treatment for SDB. Chin et al.[45] observed a reduction in LDL and reciprocal increase in HDL with 6 months of CPAP therapy for OSA in two groups – a group with significant body weight reduction and a group with no significant reduction in body weight. This was accompanied with a reduction in visceral fat accumulation. In a subsequent study from the same group,[46] CPAP therapy for 1 month demonstrated a statistically significant rise in HDL with a reduction in LDL. In a study of 32 individuals in Slovakia, nasal CPAP was associated with a reduction in total cholesterol and triglycerides without evident improvement in HDL.[47] In terms of randomized control trials, Robinson et al.[48] evaluated the response of the lipid profiles of 220 obese adults with severe sleep apnea, of which 108 individuals were placed on CPAP therapy and 112 were started on sham CPAP. The study demonstrated a significant reduction in total cholesterol as compared to baseline in those subjects on therapeutic CPAP; this difference was not observed with sham CPAP. In comparing CPAP and sham CPAP, the difference between the two groups only closely approached statistical significance (mean difference in change 0.2 mmol/L, 95% CI 20.12 to 0.41, p=0.06). However, smaller randomized, controlled trials have failed to show significant changes to the lipid profile with therapy.[49–51]

Hypertension
Elevated blood pressure (BP) has been demonstrated to have contributions from both insulin resistance[52] and obesity.[53] Hypertension has a strong association with SDB in adulthood, with the condition being present in up to 50% of subjects.[54] In children, there are a number of studies that have

also reported an association between SDB and elevated systolic and diastolic blood pressure.[55–63] However, evidence of the relationship is not extensive, and the magnitude of the blood pressure effect appears smaller.

The development of hypertension in the context of MetS is predominantly described as arising from the collaboration between increased sympathetic nervous system (SNS) tone, insulin resistance and derangement in vascular structure or function. As a parallel, SDB is also associated with a sympathetic predominance[64] and has shown an association with insulin resistance, with subsequent reversibility with the treatment of SDB.[20,65] Hypoxemia, which is commonly seen in SDB, has been postulated to trigger vascular remodeling and an increase in inflammatory markers as seen in atherosclerosis.[56] Affectation of the renin–angiotensin–aldosterone system by hypoxemia in OSA has also been postulated, with animal trials supporting this model.[67] Sleep deprivation and/or fragmentation separate from SDB may also play a role in the development of hypertension.

The physiologic profile of BP over a 24-hour period is characterized by a nighttime reduction described as the 'nocturnal dipping' phenomenon. This reduction in blood pressure has been associated with an overall increase in markers of vagal tone, and a decrease in sympathetic tone – even with the elimination of the effect of physical activity.[68] In comparison, wakefulness is characterized by BP variation being primarily reactive to the physical activity and posture,[69] while BP during sleep is controlled by posture and the transition into the stages of sleep.[68] Non-rapid eye movement (NREM) sleep is associated with an overall reduction in blood pressure with an accompanying reduction in sympathetic tone, while rapid eye movement (REM) sleep is associated with bursts of sympathetic activation and an overall BP similar to wakefulness.[70] With partial sleep deprivation, there is an increase in mean BP during 24-hour BP monitoring, with the finding being more pronounced during nighttime sleep – this normalizes with subsequent sleep. There is also an increase in early morning BP surge with sleep deprivations.[71,72] In examining the effects of sleep fragmentation and SWS deprivation, there is evidence of attenuation in nocturnal arterial blood pressure dipping. However, subsequent day ambulatory blood pressure is not significantly elevated.[73] The effect of poor sleep efficiency and short sleep on blood pressure has also been investigated in the adolescent population. Javaheri et al. performed a cross-sectional analysis of 238 individuals without obstructive sleep apnea to evaluate the odds of prehypertension (≥90th percentile for age, sex and height) for both short sleep (≤6.5 hours or sleep) and low efficiency sleep (≤85%). After adjusting for sex, body mass index percentile, and socioeconomic status, the odds of prehypertension increased 3.5-fold (95% CI, 1.5–8.0) for low sleep efficiency subjects, and 2.5-fold (95% CI, 0.9–6.9) for short sleepers. In those with a low sleep efficiency, there was an average increase in systolic blood pressure of 4.0±2.1 mmHg.[74] Naturally, short sleep and low sleep efficiency can be seen as a surrogate for primary sleep disorders such as obstructive sleep apnea.

As described earlier, obstructive sleep apnea in childhood is associated with the presence of elevated BP.[55–63] In a multicenter community-based study including 306 subjects between the ages of 6 and 13 years, children diagnosed with obstructive sleep apnea had significantly higher nocturnal systolic (95% CI, 1.4–10.5) and diastolic (95% CI, 1.4–8.1) BP – this

elevation was also noted to be present during wakefulness. There was no significant difference in nocturnal dipping.[59] In comparing children referred to a specialty sleep clinic for snoring, Marcus et al. observed that children with obstructive sleep apnea had a higher diastolic BP index than those with primary snoring alone. There was no significant difference in systolic blood pressure index or the magnitude of nocturnal BP dipping.[56] In a similar study using 24-hour blood pressure monitoring examining 19 children between the ages of 8 to 12 years who referred to a sleep clinic for suspected OSA, there was a significant increase in diastolic BP and mean BP, and a significant reduction in the degree of BP nocturnal dipping, among those with OSA versus primary snorers. In addition, the odds of non-dipping in nocturnal blood pressure was 6.66 times higher in children with OSA.[58] A similar investigation evaluating data from consecutive patients between the ages of 6 and 15 years who were also referred for suspected OSA divided patients into two groups, high-AHI (>5 events/hour) and low-AHI (≤5 events/hour), and demonstrated elevated sleep-related diastolic and systolic blood pressures. In their sub-analysis of obese children, those with a high-AHI had a higher prevalence of hypertension (OR=6.667; 95% CI, 1.004–44.284). However, the BMI characteristics for the two groups were not described.[61] In 90 children between the ages of 4.4 and 18.8 years (mean =10.7), Reade et al. noted a statistically significant elevation in office-recorded systolic and diastolic BP in the obese. However, they noted that children with obesity and hypertension had significantly higher hypopnea indexes, AHIs, and incidence of OSA, as compared to normotensive obese subjects. The BMI score (ratio of BMI to 95th percentile BMI for age, sex and race) was not significantly different between their hypertensive and normotensive obese subjects.[62] The two latter studies suggest that obesity and OSA may have a synergistic effect in causing elevations in diurnal blood pressure. In supporting the hypothesis that OSA has a causal relationship in the development of hypertension, studies have demonstrated a significant reduction in blood pressure in subjects with OSA.[75–77] Apostolidou et al. evaluated the effect of adenotonsillectomy (AT) on blood pressure in 58 subjects with OSA and 17 controls who underwent AT for recurrent tonsillitis or otitis media. In subjects who were able to attain an AHI ≤1 event per hour, there was a significant improvement in diastolic BP (p=0.002).[75] In a retrospective study involving 44 children with OSA who had undergone AT, 24-hour BP monitoring demonstrated a significant reduction in diastolic BP load (percentage of blood pressure readings above the 95th percentile for age, sex and height) in the overall analysis. In sub-analysis of 10 subjects who were noted to be hypertensive, there was a significant reduction in nocturnal systolic and diastolic BP.[76] Unfortunately, a recent meta-analysis from Friedman et al. has demonstrated only a 59.8% success rate in the treatment of OSA with AT.[78] Furthermore, AT is not as effective in the treatment of OSA in obese children and therefore likely to be less effective in the context of MetS.[34,79,80]

Obesity in the Context of the Metabolic Syndrome

Obesity has been associated with elevations in blood pressure,[81] insulin resistance and impaired glucose tolerance,[82–84] inflammatory markers,[85–87] elevated triglycerides and low HDL,[83] and arterial wall stiffness and endothelial dysfunction.[88] Childhood obesity also confers an increased risk of future obesity and insulin resistance,[89] further weight gain over expected growth, and risk for development of cardiovascular risk factors as young adults.[90] In particular, visceral fat has more adverse health outcomes in comparison to BMI or subcutaneous fat and offers an increase in the odds of developing MetS.[91] Although obesity has been demonstrated to have a larger role in the development of insulin resistance in comparison to OSA,[33,34] there is evidence that OSA in the context of obesity may amplify the risk for insulin resistance and dyslipidemia.[30,34] Gozal et al. demonstrated an improvement in insulin resistance with AT in the context of obesity, and not in their non-obese subjects, which supports additive interactions between OSA and obesity.[34] Figure 17-1 describes a mechanistic model of the contribution of OSA and obesity to the MetS. Unfortunately, the potential advantages conferred by treating OSA might be limited by parallel evidence suggesting that the treatment of OSA is associated with weight gain even in overweight populations.[92]

OBESITY

The significance of obesity in modern-day society cannot be overstated, with recent evidence demonstrating 31.7% of US children between the ages of 2 and 19 were at or above the 85th percentile for weight between 2007 and 2008.[93] The consequences of obesity are broad and far-reaching, with implications on physical health and psychosocial well-being. As described earlier, there are associations with hypertension,[81] insulin resistance and glucose dysregulation,[82–84] inflammatory markers,[85–87] elevated triglycerides and low HDL,[83] and vascular dysfunction.[88] There is also evidence of body image dissatisfaction, reduced quality of life and lower self-esteem.[94] Recent interest has also been placed in the relationship between sleep fragmentation and deprivation, including a wealth of epidemiologic data supporting an association between short sleep and being overweight or obese.[95] Experimental studies demonstrated an association between sleep deprivation and decreased leptin[96,97] and elevated ghrelin;[98] these findings correlate with increased appetite and

food intake.[99–101] Buxton and colleagues presented findings in adult subjects showing a reduction in resting metabolic rate with an extended sleep restriction coupled with a circadian disruption.[102] The odds of have an elevated BMI in a short sleeper have also been demonstrated to increase in the context of genetic heritability of elevated BMI, suggesting less environmental control of weight with a plausible increase in obesity potential with short sleep.[103] Behavioral obesogenic correlates of insufficient sleep include maladaptive habits such as increased snacking[104] and general food intake.[105] Among sleep disorders, obstructive sleep apnea has naturally been front and center, with evidence supporting a phenotypic subtype with obesity. Other disorders with significant relationships with obesity include narcolepsy and nocturnal eating disorders.

Hart et al.[95] recently completed a systematic review of 30 studies from 16 countries examining the epidemiologic evidence of association between sleep duration and obesity. There was significant agreement across the studies, demonstrating the presence of an inverse relationship between sleep duration and obesity risk. There were also six prospective studies that helped clarify temporal characteristics of short sleepers versus longer sleepers. In a particular study involving 2281 children between the ages of 3 and 12 years, BMI at follow-up was lower by 0.75 kg/m² for each hour of additional sleep during baseline recording.[106] In a separate study involving 1138 children between the ages of 2.5 and 6 years, those who were persistent short sleepers (<10 hours a night throughout follow-up) were 4.2 times more likely to become overweight or obese (OR=4.2; 95% CI 1.6–11.1, p=0.003).[107]

Among sleep disorders, obstructive sleep apnea is most affected by significantly elevated BMI. Epidemiologic characteristics in the general population suggest that 2% of school-aged children,[108] and 13% of preschool children are afflicted by the condition.[109] In contrast, 46% to 59% of obese children have obstructive sleep apnea.[110–112] Contributing anatomic factors include adenotonsillar hypertrophy[113] and fat deposition in the lateral fat pads,[114] uvula[115] and tongue.[116] There is also increased collapsibility of the upper airway with obesity

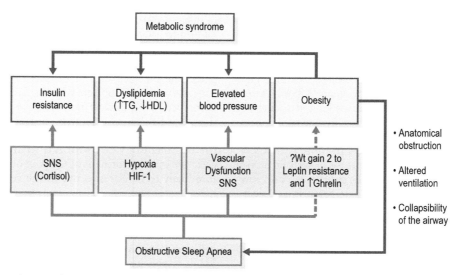

FIGURE 17-1 Potential contributions of obstructive sleep apnea to the metabolic syndrome. TG, triglycerides; HDL, high-density lipoprotein; BP, blood pressure; SNS, sympathetic nervous system; HIF-1, hypoxia-inducible factor-1; OSA, obstructive sleep apnea.

in terms of the pharyngeal critical pressure of collapse (Pcrit).[117] Pcrit improves significantly with weight loss.[118] There is also increased work of breathing and lower oxygen reserves with truncal obesity.[119] With the reverse relationship, observational data suggest that obstructive sleep apnea may predispose individuals to gain weight by derangement in adipocyte hormone functioning. Levels of the satiety hormone leptin are elevated in adults with obesity and OSA – this has been postulated to be secondary to leptin resistance.[120–122] This relationship has also been demonstrated in children, with further elevations in leptin with increases in severity of hypoxemia independent of BMI Z scores.[123] In support of a causal relationship between OSA and elevations of leptin, a fall in leptin has been observed in children with MetS and OSA with initiation of CPAP therapy.[31] Unfortunately, treatment of OSA is complicated and less successful in this population. In a recent meta-analysis by Friedman et al., 59.8% of children undergoing AT were cured of the condition when cure was defined as a residual AHI < 1 event per hour.[78] This is compared to a 12% cure rate (AHI < 1) demonstrated in a meta-analysis of AT in obesity-related OSA.[124] Therefore, the American Academy of Sleep Medicine supports the implementation of a repeat polysomnographic study after AT in the context of obesity.[125] CPAP is the commonly acceptable secondary treatment modality for residual OSA and has been demonstrated to be effective in pediatric OSA.[126–129] The use of nasal steroids and leukotriene inhibitors is also associated with significant improvements in reducing SDB events.[130,131] Their combination also increases the likelihood of resolution of residual OSA after AT.[132] However, evidence of their benefit in the context of obesity needs further clarification. Rapid maxillary expansion (RME) is another therapy that may be effective in the treatment of OSA[133,134] but it will need further studies to examine its effectiveness in the context of obesity. Guilleminault et al. published a pilot study with a randomized cross-over design utilizing RME and AT that showed great promise for the use of RME with AT for residual OSA.[135] Naturally, weight loss should be addressed in weight-related OSA to impact SDB, secondary metabolic consequences, and cardiovascular risk – but the current body of evidence does not yet elucidate the effectiveness of this strategy in treating OSA in the pediatric population. A case series of six young adolescents with morbid obesity demonstrated reductions in their apnea index from 14.1 events per hour to 1.6 events per hour with an average weight reduction of 18.7 kg.[136] Bariatric surgery in morbidly obese children has cautiously been investigated with the inherent concern about possible adverse effects on physiologic growth and bone maturity. However, evidence from Kalra et al. showed resolution of OSA in a population of 10 morbidly obese adolescents (mean BMI=60.8±11.07) who underwent laparoscopic Roux en Y gastric bypass that resulted in a mean weight loss of 58 kg (mean AHI at baseline versus follow-up, 9.1 versus 0.65).[110]

Narcolepsy has also been associated with obesity, particularly with rapid onset of weight gain in a number of case series.[137–139A] Indeed, rapid weight gain and ultimately obesity appear to be a relatively consistent feature of many children with narcolepsy, and have been described as far back as in the 1930s.[140] The tendency for obesity has been further demonstrated in mouse models of the disease in which hypocretin (orexin) neurons were genetically ablated. The association

with obesity occurred despite decreased food consumption in comparison to non-ablated mice.[141] The exact mechanism has yet to be ascertained, with evidence leading towards a complex set of relationships that entail the involvement of neurotransmitters in diurnal activity, feeding and metabolism. In rats, the neuropeptide dynorphin is co-localized with hypocretin neurons and the loss of these specific neurons is associated with hypophagia and obesity in comparison to rodents with only a loss of the hypocretin peptide.[142] In regards to sleep distribution, total sleep has been observed to be similar between narcoleptic and non-narcoleptic human subjects, with a tendency for more disrupted nocturnal sleep in narcoleptics, as well as increased daytime sleep and an earlier peak in propensity for daytime sleep as compared to habitual nappers.[143]

Nocturnal eating disorder (NED) and sleep-related eating disorder (SRED) are other conditions that have been described in the context of obesity. NED involves excessive eating during the habitual sleep period while SRED entails recurrent episodes of nocturnal awakenings with associated eating, with or without recollection. NED is the more common of these two conditions and is self-reported in 15.7% of adults enrolled in a weight-loss program,[144] and in up to 27% of subjects having completed bariatric surgery.[145] These elevated figures are clearly different from the 1.5% prevalence in the general population that was recorded through a survey sample.[145] SRED is a less prevalent condition in the general population, but has a high propensity in individuals with eating disorders. In a study by Winkelman et al. examining a population of psychiatric and non-psychiatric subjects, 16.7% of in-patients and 8.7% of out-patients with eating disorders were noted to have the condition in comparison to 4.6% of a student population and 1% of obese controls.[146] The condition can be quite severe in those afflicted, with up to half of subjects described in one study as having daily eating,[147] and another citing a mean duration period of affliction spanning 15.8 years.[148]

Clinical Pearls

- The metabolic syndrome in children has been associated with the development of diabetes and cardiovascular disease.
- The components of the condition include impaired glucose metabolism, lipid dysregulation, elevated blood pressure and excessive weight and/or visceral obesity.
- Parameters of glucose metabolism have shown inconsistent associations with SDB in children; however, there is evidence of improvement in some interventional studies involving OSA.
- There also appears to be some degree of variability in the association between SDB and low HDL and elevated triglycerides.
- Interventional studies have demonstrated improvement in total cholesterol, HDL and LDL.
- SDB has consistent associations with diastolic hypertension, which has been observed to respond to adenotonsillectomy and CPAP.
- In regards to obesity, epidemiologic data support an association between sleep curtailment and obesity.
- Prospective data support a dose–response relationship between sleep and the degree of potential weight excess.
- Obesity also increases the risk of OSA and reduces the success rate of adenotonsillectomy.

References

1. Ford ES. Risks for all-cause mortality, cardiovascular disease, and diabetes associated with the metabolic syndrome: a summary of the evidence. Diabetes Care 2005;28(7):1769–78.
2. Galassi A, Reynolds K, He J. Metabolic syndrome and risk of cardiovascular disease: a meta-analysis. Am J Med 2006;119(10):812–19.
3. Gami AS, Witt BJ, Howard DE, et al. Metabolic syndrome and risk of incident cardiovascular events and death: a systematic review and meta-analysis of longitudinal studies. J Am Coll Cardiol 2007;49(4):403–14.
4. Ford ES, Li C, Sattar N. Metabolic syndrome and incident diabetes: current state of the evidence. Diabetes Care 2008;31(9):1898–904.
5. Pladevall M, Singal B, Williams LK, et al. A single factor underlies the metabolic syndrome: a confirmatory factor analysis. Diabetes Care 2006;29(1):113–22.
6. Park YW, Zhu S, Palaniappan L, et al. The metabolic syndrome: prevalence and associated risk factor findings in the US population from the Third National Health and Nutrition Examination Survey, 1988–1994. Arch Intern Med 2003;163(4):427–36.
7. Alberti KG, Eckel RH, Grundy SM, et al. Harmonizing the metabolic syndrome: a joint interim statement of the International Diabetes Federation Task Force on Epidemiology and Prevention; National Heart, Lung, and Blood Institute; American Heart Association; World Heart Federation; International Atherosclerosis Society; and International Association for the Study of Obesity. Circulation 2009;120(16):1640–5.
8. Reinehr T, Wunsch R, de Sousa G, et al. Comparison of metabolic syndrome prevalence using eight different definitions: a critical approach. Arch Dis Child 2007;92(12):1067–72.
9. Goodman E, Daniels SR, Meigs JB, et al. Instability in the diagnosis of metabolic syndrome in adolescents. Circulation 2007;115(17):2316–22.
10. Gustafson JK, Yanoff LB, Easter BD, et al. The stability of metabolic syndrome in children and adolescents. J Clin Endocrinol Metab 2009;94(12):4828–34.
11. Berenson GS, Srinivasan SR, Bao W, et al. Association between multiple cardiovascular risk factors and atherosclerosis in children and young adults. The Bogalusa Heart Study. N Engl J Med 1998;338(23):1650–6.
12. Juonala M, Jarvisalo MJ, Maki-Torkko N, et al. Risk factors identified in childhood and decreased carotid artery elasticity in adulthood: the Cardiovascular Risk in Young Finns Study. Circulation 2005;112(10):1486–93.
13. Chinali M, de Simone G, Roman MJ, et al. Cardiac markers of preclinical disease in adolescents with the metabolic syndrome: the Strong Heart Study. J Am Coll Cardiol 2008;52(11):932–8.
14. Toledo-Corral CM, Ventura EE, Hodis HN, et al. Persistence of the metabolic syndrome and its influence on carotid artery intima media thickness in overweight Latino children. Atherosclerosis 2009;206(2):594–8.
15. Morrison JA, Friedman LA, Gray-McGuire C. Metabolic syndrome in childhood predicts adult cardiovascular disease 25 years later: the Princeton Lipid Research Clinics Follow-up Study. Pediatrics 2007;120(2):340–5.
16. Morrison JA, Friedman LA, Wang P, Glueck CJ. Metabolic syndrome in childhood predicts adult metabolic syndrome and type 2 diabetes mellitus 25 to 30 years later. J Pediatr 2008;152(2):201–6.
17. Wilcox I, McNamara SG, Collins FL, et al. "Syndrome Z": the interaction of sleep apnoea, vascular risk factors and heart disease. Thorax 1998;53(Suppl 3):S25–8.
18. Redline S, Storfer-Isser A, Rosen CL, et al. Association between metabolic syndrome and sleep-disordered breathing in adolescents. Am J Respir Crit Care Med 2007;176(4):401–8.
19. Tasali E, Leproult R, Ehrmann DA, et al. Slow-wave sleep and the risk of type 2 diabetes in humans. Proc Natl Acad Sci USA 2008;105(3):1044–9.
20. Harsch IA, Pour Schahin S, Radespiel-Troger M, et al. Continuous positive airway pressure treatment rapidly improves insulin sensitivity in patients with obstructive sleep apnea syndrome. Am J Respir Crit Care Med 2004;169(2):156–62.
21. Spiegel K, Leproult R, Van Cauter E. Impact of sleep debt on metabolic and endocrine function. Lancet 1999;354(9188):1435–9.
22. Gottlieb DJ, Punjabi NM, Newman AB, et al. Association of sleep time with diabetes mellitus and impaired glucose tolerance. Arch Intern Med 2005;165(8):863–7.
23. Knutson K., Spiegel K, Penev P, et al. Role of sleep duration and quality in the risk and severity of type 2 diabetes mellitus. Arch Intern Med 2006;166(16):1768–74.
24. Mallon L, Broman JE, Hetta J. High incidence of diabetes in men with sleep complaints or short sleep duration: a 12-year follow-up study of a middle-aged population. Diabetes Care 2005;8(11):2762–7.
25. Ayas NT, White DP, Al-Delaimy WK, et al. A prospective study of self-reported sleep duration and incident diabetes in women. Diabetes Care 2003;26(2):380–4.
26. Seicean S, Kirchner HL, Gottlieb DJ, et al. Sleep-disordered breathing and impaired glucose metabolism in normal-weight and overweight/obese individuals: the Sleep Heart Health Study. Diabetes Care 2008;31(5):1001–6.
27. Punjabi NM, Shahar E, Redline S, et al. Sleep-disordered breathing, glucose intolerance, and insulin resistance: the Sleep Heart Health Study. Am J Epidemiol 2004;160(6):521–30.
28. Botros N, Concato J, Mohsenin V, et al. Obstructive sleep apnea as a risk factor for type 2 diabetes. Am J Med 2009;122(12):1122–7.
29. Tasali E, Ip MS. Obstructive sleep apnea and metabolic syndrome: alterations in glucose metabolism and inflammation. Proc Am Thorac Soc 2008;5(2):207–17.
30. de la Eva RC, Baur LA, Donaghue KC, et al. Metabolic correlates with obstructive sleep apnea in obese subjects. J Pediatr 2002;140(6):654–9.
31. Nakra N, Bhargava S, Dzuira J, et al. Sleep-disordered breathing in children with metabolic syndrome: the role of leptin and sympathetic nervous system activity and the effect of continuous positive airway pressure. Pediatrics 2008;122(3):e634–42.
32. Kaditis AG, Alexopoulos EI, Damani E, et al. Obstructive sleep-disordered breathing and fasting insulin levels in nonobese children. Pediatr Pulmonol 2005;40(6):515–23.
33. Tauman R, O'Brien LM, Ivanenko A, et al. Obesity rather than severity of sleep-disordered breathing as the major determinant of insulin resistance and altered lipidemia in snoring children. Pediatrics 2005;116(1):e66–73.
34. Gozal D, Capdevila OS, Kheirandish-Gozal L. Metabolic alterations and systemic inflammation in obstructive sleep apnea among nonobese and obese prepubertal children. Am J Respir Crit Care Med 2008;177(10):142–9.
35. Li J, Thorne LN, Punjabi NM, et al. Intermittent hypoxia induces hyperlipidemia in lean mice. Circ Res 2005;97(7):698–706.
36. Li J, Savransky V, Nanayakkara A, et al. Hyperlipidemia and lipid peroxidation are dependent on the severity of chronic intermittent hypoxia. J Appl Physiol 2007;102(2):557–63.
37. Newman AB, Nieto FJ, Guidry U, et al. Relation of sleep-disordered breathing to cardiovascular disease risk factors: the Sleep Heart Health Study. Am J Epidemiol 2001;154(1):50–9.
38. Roche F, Sforza E, Pichot V, et al. Obstructive sleep apnoea/hypopnea influences high-density lipoprotein cholesterol in the elderly. Sleep Med 2009;10(8):882–6.
39. Coughlin SR, Mawdsley L, Mugarza JA, et al. Obstructive sleep apnoea is independently associated with an increased prevalence of metabolic syndrome. Eur Heart J 2004;25(9):735–41.
40. Czerniawska J, Bieleń P, Pływaczewski R, et al. [Metabolic abnormalities in obstructive sleep apnea patients]. Pneumonol Alergol Pol 2008;76(5):340–7.
41. Tan KC, Chow WS, Lam JC, et al. HDL dysfunction in obstructive sleep apnea. Atherosclerosis 2006;184(2):377–82.
42. Drager LF, Bortolotto LA, Lorenzi MC, et al. Early signs of atherosclerosis in obstructive sleep apnea. Am J Respir Crit Care Med 2005;172(5):613–18.
43. Drager LF, Bortolotto LA, Maki-Nunes C, et al. The incremental role of obstructive sleep apnoea on markers of atherosclerosis in patients with metabolic syndrome. Atherosclerosis 2010;208(2):490–5.
44. Kono M, Tatsumi K, Saibara T, et al. Obstructive sleep apnea syndrome is associated with some components of metabolic syndrome. Chest 2007;131(5):1387–92.
45. Chin K, Shimizu K, Nakamura T, et al. Changes in intra-abdominal visceral fat and serum leptin levels in patients with obstructive sleep apnea syndrome following nasal continuous positive airway pressure therapy. Circulation 1999;100(7):706–12.
46. Chin K, Nakamura T, Shimizu K, et al. Effects of nasal continuous positive airway pressure on soluble cell adhesion molecules in patients with obstructive sleep apnea syndrome. Am J Med 2000;109(7):562–7.
47. Dorkova Z, Petrasova D, Molcanyiova A, et al. Effects of continuous positive airway pressure on cardiovascular risk profile in patients with severe obstructive sleep apnea and metabolic syndrome. Chest 2008;134(4):686–92.
48. Robinson GV, Pepperell JC, Segal HC, et al. Circulating cardiovascular risk factors in obstructive sleep apnoea: data from randomised controlled trials. Thorax 2004;59(9):777–82.

49. Comondore VR, Cheema R, Fox J, et al. The impact of CPAP on cardiovascular biomarkers in minimally symptomatic patients with obstructive sleep apnea: a pilot feasibility randomized crossover trial. Lung 2009;187(1):17–22.

50. Coughlin SR, Mawdsley L, Mugarza JA, et al. Cardiovascular and metabolic effects of CPAP in obese males with OSA. Eur Respir J 2007;29(4):720–7.

51. Drager LF, Bortolotto LA, Figueiredo AC, et al. Effects of continuous positive airway pressure on early signs of atherosclerosis in obstructive sleep apnea. Am J Respir Crit Care Med 2007;176(7):706–12.

52. Landsberg L. Hyperinsulinemia: possible role in obesity-induced hypertension. Hypertension 1992;19(1 Suppl):161–6.

53. Sorof J, Daniels S. Obesity hypertension in children: a problem of epidemic proportions. Hypertension 2002;40(4):441–7.

54. Shepard JW Jr. Hypertension, cardiac arrhythmias, myocardial infarction, and stroke in relation to obstructive sleep apnea. Clin Chest Med 1992;13(3):437–58.

55. Kohyama J, Ohinata JS, Hasegawa T. Blood pressure in sleep disordered breathing. Arch Dis Child 2003;88(2):139–42.

56. Marcus CL, Greene MG, Carroll JL. Blood pressure in children with obstructive sleep apnea. Am J Respir Crit Care Med, 1998;157(4 Pt 1):1098–103.

57. Serratto M, Harris VJ, Carr I. Upper airways obstruction. Presentation with systemic hypertension. Arch Dis Child 1981;56(2):153–5.

58. Weber SA, Santos VJ, Semenzati Gde O, et al. Ambulatory blood pressure monitoring in children with obstructive sleep apnea and primary snoring. Int J Pediatr Otorhinolaryngol 2012;76(6):787–90.

59. Li AM, Au CT, Sung RY, et al. Ambulatory blood pressure in children with obstructive sleep apnoea: a community based study. Thorax 2008; 63(9):803–9.

60. Enright PL, Goodwin JL, Sherrill DL, et al. Blood pressure elevation associated with sleep-related breathing disorder in a community sample of white and Hispanic children: the Tucson Children's Assessment of Sleep Apnea study. Arch Pediatr Adolesc Med 2003;157(9):901–4.

61. Leung LC, Ng DK, Lau MW, et al. Twenty-four-hour ambulatory BP in snoring children with obstructive sleep apnea syndrome. Chest 2006;130(4):1009–17.

62. Reade EP, Whaley C, Lin JJ, et al. Hypopnea in pediatric patients with obesity hypertension. Pediatr Nephrol 2004;19(9):1014–20.

63. Guilleminault C, Eldridge FL, Simmons FB, et al. Sleep apnea in eight children. Pediatrics 1976;58(1):23–30.

64. Narkiewicz K, Somers VK. Cardiovascular variability characteristics in obstructive sleep apnea. Auton Neurosci 2001;90(1–2):89–94.

65. Harsch IA, Schahin SP, Brückner K, et al. The effect of continuous positive airway pressure treatment on insulin sensitivity in patients with obstructive sleep apnoea syndrome and type 2 diabetes. Respiration 2004;71(3):252–9.

66. Lavie L. Obstructive sleep apnoea syndrome – an oxidative stress disorder. Sleep Med Rev 2003;7(1):35–51.

67. Raff H, Roarty TP. Renin, ACTH, and aldosterone during acute hypercapnia and hypoxia in conscious rats. Am J Physiol 1988;254(3 Pt 2):R431–5.

68. Van de Borne P, Nguyen H, Biston P, et al. Effects of wake and sleep stages on the 24-h autonomic control of blood pressure and heart rate in recumbent men. Am J Physiol 1994;266(2 Pt 2):H548–54.

69. Kario K, Schwartz JE, Pickering TG. Ambulatory physical activity as a determinant of diurnal blood pressure variation. Hypertension 1999;34(4 Pt 1):685–91.

70. Somers VK, Dyken ME, Mark AL, et al. Sympathetic-nerve activity during sleep in normal subjects. N Engl J Med 1993;328(5):303–7.

71. Lusardi P, Zoppi A, Preti P, et al. Effects of insufficient sleep on blood pressure in hypertensive patients: a 24-h study. Am J Hypertens 1999;12(1 Pt 1):63–8.

72. Tochikubo O, Ikeda A, Miyajima E, et al. Effects of insufficient sleep on blood pressure monitored by a new multibiomedical recorder. Hypertension 1996;27(6):1318–24.

73. Sayk F, Teckentrup C, Becker C, et al. Effects of selective slow-wave sleep deprivation on nocturnal blood pressure dipping and daytime blood pressure regulation. Am J Physiol Regul Integr Comp Physiol 2010;298(1):R191–7.

74. Javaheri S, Storfer-Isser A, Rosen CL, et al. Sleep quality and elevated blood pressure in adolescents. Circulation 2008;118(10):1034–40.

75. Apostolidou MT, Alexopoulos EI, Damani E, et al. Absence of blood pressure, metabolic, and inflammatory marker changes after adenotonsillectomy for sleep apnea in Greek children. Pediatr Pulmonol 2008; 43(6):550–60.

76. Ng DK, Wong JC, Chan CH, et al. Ambulatory blood pressure before and after adenotonsillectomy in children with obstructive sleep apnea. Sleep Med 2010;11:721–5.

77. Amin R, Anthony L, Somers V, et al. Growth velocity predicts recurrence of sleep-disordered breathing 1 year after adenotonsillectomy. Am J Respir Crit Care Med, 2008;177(6):654–9.

78. Friedman M, Wilson M, Lin HC, et al. Updated systematic review of tonsillectomy and adenoidectomy for treatment of pediatric obstructive sleep apnea/hypopnea syndrome. Otolaryngol Head Neck Surg 2009; 140(6):800–8.

79. Tauman R, Gulliver TE, Krishna J, et al. Persistence of obstructive sleep apnea syndrome in children after adenotonsillectomy. J Pediatr 2006;149(6):803–8.

80. Mitchell RB, Kelly J. Outcome of adenotonsillectomy for obstructive sleep apnea in obese and normal-weight children. Otolaryngol Head Neck Surg 2007;137(1):43–8.

81. Sorof JM, Lai D, Turner J, et al. Overweight, ethnicity, and the prevalence of hypertension in school-aged children. Pediatrics 2004;113(3 Pt 1):475–82.

82. Sinha R, Fisch G, Teague B, et al. Prevalence of impaired glucose tolerance among children and adolescents with marked obesity. N Engl J Med 2002;346(11):802–10.

83. Steinberger J, Moorehead C, Katch V, et al. Relationship between insulin resistance and abnormal lipid profile in obese adolescents. J Pediatr 1995;126(5 Pt 1):690–5.

84. Arslanian S, Suprasongsin C. Insulin sensitivity, lipids, and body composition in childhood: is "syndrome X" present? J Clin Endocrinol Metab 1996;81(3):1058–62.

85. Cook DG, Mendall MA, Whincup PH, et al. C-reactive protein concentration in children: relationship to adiposity and other cardiovascular risk factors. Atherosclerosis 2000;149(1):139–50.

86. Ford ES. National health and nutrition examination, C-reactive protein concentration and cardiovascular disease risk factors in children: findings from the National Health and Nutrition Examination Survey 1999–2000. Circulation 2003;108(9):1053–8.

87. Visser M, Bouter LM, McQuillan GM, et al. Low-grade systemic inflammation in overweight children. Pediatrics 2001;107(1):E13.

88. Tounian P, Aggoun Y, Dubern B, et al. Presence of increased stiffness of the common carotid artery and endothelial dysfunction in severely obese children: a prospective study. Lancet 2001;358(9291):1400–4.

89. Steinberger J, Moran A, Hong CP, et al. Adiposity in childhood predicts obesity and insulin resistance in young adulthood. J Pediatr 2001; 138(4):469–73.

90. Sinaiko AR, Donahue RP, Jacobs DR Jr, et al. Relation of weight and rate of increase in weight during childhood and adolescence to body size, blood pressure, fasting insulin, and lipids in young adults. The Minneapolis Children's Blood Pressure Study. Circulation 1999;99(11):1471–6.

91. Taksali SE, Caprio S, Dziura J, et al. High visceral and low abdominal subcutaneous fat stores in the obese adolescent: a determinant of an adverse metabolic phenotype. Diabetes 2008;57(2):367–71.

92. Soultan Z, Wadowski S, Rao M, et al. Effect of treating obstructive sleep apnea by tonsillectomy and/or adenoidectomy on obesity in children. Arch Pediatr Adolesc Med 1999;153(1):33–7.

93. Ogden CL, Carroll MD, Curtin LR, et al. Prevalence of high body mass index in US children and adolescents, 2007–2008. JAMA 2010;303(3):242–9.

94. Wardle J, Cooke L. The impact of obesity on psychological well-being. Best Pract Res Clin Endocrinol Metab 2005;19(3):421–40.

95. Hart CN, Cairns A, Jelalian E. Sleep and obesity in children and adolescents. Pediatr Clin North Am 2011;58(3):715–33.

96. Guilleminault C, Powell NB, Martinez S, et al. Preliminary observations on the effects of sleep time in a sleep restriction paradigm. Sleep Med 2003;4(3):177–84.

97. Spiegel K, Leproult R, L'hermite-Balériaux M, et al. Leptin levels are dependent on sleep duration: relationships with sympathovagal balance, carbohydrate regulation, cortisol, and thyrotropin. J Clin Endocrinol Metab 2004;89(11):5762–71.

98. Taheri S, Lin L, Austin D, et al. Short sleep duration is associated with reduced leptin, elevated ghrelin, and increased body mass index. PLoS Med 2004;1(3):e62.

99. Wren AM, Seal LJ, Cohen MA, et al. Ghrelin enhances appetite and increases food intake in humans. J Clin Endocrinol Metab 2001;86(12):5992.

100. Levin F, Edholm T, Schmidt PT, et al. Ghrelin stimulates gastric emptying and hunger in normal-weight humans. J Clin Endocrinol Metab 2006;91(9):3296–302.

101. Mars M, de Graaf C, de Groot CP, et al. Fasting leptin and appetite responses induced by a 4-day 65%-energy-restricted diet. Int J Obes (Lond) 2006;30(1):122–8.

102. Buxton OM, Cain SW, O'Connor SP, et al. Adverse metabolic consequences in humans of prolonged sleep restriction combined with circadian disruption. Sci Transl Med 2012;4(129):129–43.

103. Watson NF, Harden KP, Buchwald D, et al. Sleep duration and body mass index in twins: a gene–environment interaction. Sleep 2012;35(5): 597–603.

104. Nedeltcheva AV, Kilkus JM, Imperial J, et al. Sleep curtailment is accompanied by increased intake of calories from snacks. Am J Clin Nutr 2009;89(1):126–33.

105. Brondel L, Romer MA, Nougues PM, et al. Acute partial sleep deprivation increases food intake in healthy men. Am J Clin Nutr 2010;91(6): 1550–9.

106. Snell EK, Adam EK, Duncan GJ. Sleep and the body mass index and overweight status of children and adolescents. Child Dev 2007;78(1): 309–23.

107. Touchette E, Petit D, Tremblay RE, et al. Associations between sleep duration patterns and overweight/obesity at age 6. Sleep 2008;31(11): 1507–14.

108. Rosen CL, Larkin EK, Kirchner HL, et al. Prevalence and risk factors for sleep-disordered breathing in 8- to 11-year-old children: association with race and prematurity. J Pediatr 2003;142(4):383–9.

109. Castronovo V, Zucconi M, Nosetti L, et al. Prevalence of habitual snoring and sleep-disordered breathing in preschool-aged children in an Italian community. J Pediatr 2003;142(4):377–82.

110. Kalra M, Inge T, Garcia V, et al. Obstructive sleep apnea in extremely overweight adolescents undergoing bariatric surgery. Obes Res 2005; 13(7):1175–9.

111. Marcus CL, Curtis S, Koerner CB, et al. Evaluation of pulmonary function and polysomnography in obese children and adolescents. Pediatr Pulmonol 1996;1(3):176–83.

112. Silvestri JM, Weese-Mayer DE, Bass MT, et al. Polysomnography in obese children with a history of sleep-associated breathing disorders. Pediatr Pulmonol 1993;16(2):124–9.

113. Gordon JE, Hughes MS, Shepherd K, et al. Obstructive sleep apnoea syndrome in morbidly obese children with tibia vara. J Bone Joint Surg Br 2006;88(1):100–3.

114. Mortimore IL, Marshall I, Wraith PK, et al. Neck and total body fat deposition in nonobese and obese patients with sleep apnea compared with that in control subjects. Am J Respir Crit Care Med 1998;157(1):280–3.

115. Stauffer JL, Buick MK, Bixler EO, et al. Morphology of the uvula in obstructive sleep apnea. Am Rev Respir Dis 1989;140(3):724–8.

116. Schwab RJ. Imaging for the snoring and sleep apnea patient. Dent Clin North Am 2001;45(4):59–96.

117. Kirkness JP, Schwartz AR, Schneider H, et al. Contribution of male sex, age, and obesity to mechanical instability of the upper airway during sleep. J Appl Physiol 2008;104(6):1618–24.

118. Schwartz AR, Gold AR, Schubert N, et al. Effect of weight loss on upper airway collapsibility in obstructive sleep apnea. Am Rev Respir Dis 1991;144(3 Pt 1):494–8.

119. Arens R, Muzumdar H. Childhood obesity and obstructive sleep apnea syndrome. J Appl Physiol 2010;108(2):436–44.

120. Harsch IA, Konturek PC, Koebnick C, et al. Leptin and ghrelin levels in patients with obstructive sleep apnoea: effect of CPAP treatment. Eur Respir J 2003;22(2):251–7.

121. Ip MS, Lam KS, Ho C, et al. Serum leptin and vascular risk factors in obstructive sleep apnea. Chest 2000;118(3):580–6.

122. Vgontzas A, Papanicolaou DA, Bixler EO, et al. Sleep apnea and daytime sleepiness and fatigue: relation to visceral obesity, insulin resistance, and hypercytokinemia. J Clin Endocrinol Metab 2000;85(3):1151–8.

123. Tauman R, Serpero LD, Capdevila OS, et al. Adipokines in children with sleep disordered breathing. Sleep 2007;30(4):443–9.

124. Costa DJ, Mitchell R. Adenotonsillectomy for obstructive sleep apnea in obese children: a meta-analysis. Otolaryngol Head Neck Surg 2009; 140(4):455–60.

125. Aurora RN, Zak RS, Karippot A, et al. Practice parameters for the respiratory indications for polysomnography in children. Sleep 2011; 34(3):379–88.

126. Downey R 3rd, Perkin RM, MacQuarrie J. Nasal continuous positive airway pressure use in children with obstructive sleep apnea younger than 2 years of age. Chest 2000;117(6):1608–12.

127. Marcus CL, Rosen G, Ward SL, et al. Adherence to and effectiveness of positive airway pressure therapy in children with obstructive sleep apnea. Pediatrics 2006;117(3):e442–51.

128. Massa F, Gonsalez S, Laverty A, et al. The use of nasal continuous positive airway pressure to treat obstructive sleep apnoea. Arch Dis Child 2002;87(5):438–43.

129. Palombini L, Pelayo R, Guilleminault C. Efficacy of automated continuous positive airway pressure in children with sleep-related breathing disorders in an attended setting. Pediatrics 2004;113(5):e412–17.

130. Brouillette RT, Manoukian JJ, Ducharme FM, et al. Efficacy of fluticasone nasal spray for pediatric obstructive sleep apnea. J Pediatr 2001;138(6):838–44.

131. Kheirandish-Gozal L, Gozal D. Intranasal budesonide treatment for children with mild obstructive sleep apnea syndrome. Pediatrics 2008;122(1):e149–55.

132. Goldbart AD, Goldman JL, Veling MC, et al. Leukotriene modifier therapy for mild sleep-disordered breathing in children. Am J Respir Crit Care Med 2005;172(3):364–70.

133. Pirelli P, Saponara M, Guilleminault C. Rapid maxillary expansion in children with obstructive sleep apnea syndrome. Sleep 2004;27(4): 761–6.

134. Villa MP, Malagola C, Pagani J, et al. Rapid maxillary expansion in children with obstructive sleep apnea syndrome: 12-month follow-up. Sleep Med 2007;8(2):128–34.

135. Guilleminault C, Monteyrol PJ, Huynh NT, et al. Adeno-tonsillectomy and rapid maxillary distraction in pre-pubertal children, a pilot study. Sleep Breath 2011;15(2):173–7.

136. Willi SM, Oexmann MJ, Wright NM, et al. The effects of a high-protein, low-fat, ketogenic diet on adolescents with morbid obesity: body composition, blood chemistries, and sleep abnormalities. Pediatrics 1998;101(1 Pt 1):61–7.

137. Allsopp MR, Zaiwalla Z. Narcolepsy. Arch Dis Child 1992;67(3): 302–6.

138. Dahl R, Holttum J, Trubnick L. A clinical picture of child and adolescent narcolepsy. J Am Acad Child Adolesc Psychiatry 1994;3(6): 834–41.

139. Kotagal S, Hartse KM, Walsh JK. Characteristics of narcolepsy in preteenaged children. Pediatrics 1990;85(2):205–9.

139A. Poli F, Pizza F, Mignot E, et al. High prevalence of precocious puberty and obesity in childhood narcolepsy with cataplexy. Sleep 2013; 36(2):175–81.

140. Cave H. Narcolepsy. Arch Neurol Psychiatr 1931;26:50–101.

141. Hara J, Beuckmann CT, Nambu T, et al. Genetic ablation of orexin neurons in mice results in narcolepsy, hypophagia, and obesity. Neuron 2001;30(2):345–54.

142. Chou TC, Lee CE, Lu J, et al. Orexin (hypocretin) neurons contain dynorphin. J Neurosci 2001;21(19):RC168.

143. Broughton R, Krupa S, Boucher B, et al. Impaired circadian waking arousal in narcolepsy-cataplexy. Sleep Res Online 1998;1(4):159–65.

144. Adami GF, Campostano A, Marinari GM, et al. Night eating in obesity: a descriptive study. Nutrition 2002;18(7–8):587–9.

145. Rand CS, Macgregor AM, Stunkard AJ. The night eating syndrome in the general population and among postoperative obesity surgery patients. Int J Eat Disord 1997;22(1):65–9.

146. Winkelman JW, Herzog DB, Fava M. The prevalence of sleep-related eating disorder in psychiatric and non-psychiatric populations. Psychol Med 1999;29(6):1461–6.

147. Schenck CH, Hurwitz TD, Bundlie SR, et al. Sleep-related eating disorders: polysomnographic correlates of a heterogeneous syndrome distinct from daytime eating disorders. Sleep 1991;14(5):419–31.

148. Winkelman JW. Clinical and polysomnographic features of sleep-related eating disorder. J Clin Psychiatry 1998;59(1):14–19.

149. Ford ES, Ajani UA, Mokdad AH, et al. The metabolic syndrome and concentrations of C-reactive protein among U.S. youth. Diabetes Care 2005;28(4):878–81.

150. de Ferranti SD, Gauvreau K, Ludwig DS, et al. Prevalence of the metabolic syndrome in American adolescents: findings from the Third National Health and Nutrition Examination Survey. Circulation 2004;110(16):2494–7.

151. Cruz ML, Weigensberg MJ, Huang TT, et al. The metabolic syndrome in overweight Hispanic youth and the role of insulin sensitivity. J Clin Endocrinol Metab 2004;89(1):108–13.

152. Weiss R, Dziura J, Burgert TS, et al. Obesity and the metabolic syndrome in children and adolescents. N Engl J Med 2004;350(23): 2362–74.

153. Cook S, Weitzman M, Auinger P, et al. Prevalence of a metabolic syndrome phenotype in adolescents: findings from the Third National Health and Nutrition Examination Survey, 1988–1994. Arch Pediatr Adolesc Med 2003;157(8):821–7.

THE HYPERSOMNIAS

Chapter **22**   **Medication-Related Hypersomnia**

Manisha B. Witmans and Rochelle Young

Sleep and wake occur along a complex continuum of biochemical and cellular pathways, the distinction between which is fluid rather than categorical. Both prescription and over-the-counter medications are widely used to treat medical disorders of which the treatment of sleep disorders is no exception. This chapter discusses medications that cause excessive sleepiness or hypersomnia either as an intended or unintended consequence of their use or misuse in children and adolescents for treatment of sleep disorders or other health problems. Use of over-the-counter and prescription medications in and by children and adolescents will be highlighted. Drug classifications associated with hypersomnia will be discussed. Key considerations in assessing adolescents for hypersomnia are reviewed.

Narcolepsy

Suresh Kotagal

INTRODUCTION

In 1880, Gelineau coined the term *narcolepsie* to describe a pathologic condition that was characterized by recurrent, brief attacks of sleepiness.[1] He recognized that the disorder was accompanied by falls or *astasias,* that were subsequently termed cataplexy. Narcolepsy is a lifelong neurologic disorder of rapid eye movement (REM) sleep in which there are attacks of *irresistible daytime sleepiness, cataplexy* (sudden loss of muscle control in the legs, trunk, face or neck in response to emotional stimuli such as laughter, fright, anticipation of reward or rage), *hypnagogic hallucinations* (vivid dreams at sleep onset), *sleep paralysis* (momentary inability to move at the time of sleep onset), and fragmented night sleep.[2] There are two main forms of the disorder: narcolepsy with cataplexy and narcolepsy without cataplexy. This chapter provides an overview of childhood narcolepsy.

EPIDEMIOLOGY

In a community-based survey in Olmsted County, Minnesota, the incidence of narcolepsy was 1.37 per 100 000 persons per year – 1.72 for men and 1.05 for women.[3] It was highest in the second decade of life, followed by a gradual decline. The prevalence was approximately 56 persons per 100 000 persons. In Japan, the prevalence has been estimated at 1 in 600,[4] and in Israel at 1 in 500 000.[5] In Norway, the prevalence of narcolepsy with cataplexy has been estimated at 0.022% based on a survey of 20- to 60-year-olds.[6] The exact prevalence rate of narcolepsy in childhood has been difficult to establish. Some epidemiologic studies have required the presence of cataplexy as a prerequisite for the diagnosis,[7] whereas others[8] have not made this stipulation. This lack of uniformity in clinical diagnostic criteria may explain variability in estimations of the prevalence of narcolepsy.[9] There seems to be a slight male predominance for prevalence – in the Olmsted County study, the male:female ratio was 1.8:1.[3] Narcolepsy has been recognized as early as 1 year of age, though most subjects tend to be adolescents at the time of diagnosis. A seasonal variation in the incidence of narcolepsy has been observed in China, with the lowest incidence in November, and the highest incidence in April.[10] Further, the data from China also indicate an almost threefold increase in the incidence of narcolepsy following the 2009 H1N1 influenza pandemic, which might suggest a role for immune-mediated dysfunction consequent to this infection in the pathogenesis of the disorder.[10] Although the disorder is most often diagnosed in the third and fourth decades, a meta-analysis of 235 subjects derived from three studies by Challamel and coworkers[10] found that 34% of all subjects had onset of symptoms prior to the age of 15 years, 16% prior to age 10 years, and 4.5% prior to age 5 years (Figure 18-1). Increasing awareness of narcolepsy in childhood and the availability of cerebrospinal fluid hypocretin

testing is likely leading to diagnosis at progressively earlier ages, including in preschool-aged children. A lag period of 5 to 10 years between the onset of symptoms and diagnosis has however been observed in adult subjects.[11] Cataplexy, the most specific clinical feature of narcolepsy, is present in only 50% to 70% of all subjects.

CLINICAL FEATURES

Preschool-Aged Children

In their meta-analysis of 235 children, Challamel and colleagues found that 4.6% were below the age of 5 years at the time of diagnosis.[10] Sharp and D'Cruz have described a 12-month-old with hypersomnia who was subsequently confirmed to have narcolepsy.[12] In general, it is difficult to diagnose narcolepsy prior to the age of 4 to 5 years, as even unaffected children of this age tend to take habitual daytime naps and are not able to provide an accurate history of cataplexy, hypnagogic hallucinations, or sleep paralysis. The diagnosis may, however, be facilitated by documentation of cataplexy attacks on video-polysomnography, which shows skeletal muscle atonia and bursts of rapid eye movements coinciding with low-voltage mixed-frequency activity on the electroencephalogram (EEG). The availability of cerebrospinal fluid (CSF) hypocretin analysis also facilitates the diagnosis of narcolepsy–cataplexy in this age group, but this does not apply to narcolepsy without cataplexy, as the latter group is not associated with reduction in CSF hypocretin levels.

School-Aged Children

Daytime sleepiness is an invariant and most disabling feature of narcolepsy. It can manifest itself as early as 5 to 6 years of age. There is a background of a constant, foggy feeling from drowsiness, superimposed on which are periods of more dramatic sleep attacks. Habitual afternoon napping is uncommon in healthy children above age 5 or 6 years, and should raise suspicion of narcolepsy. Lenn reported a 6-year-old who would fall asleep 5 to 10 times a day.[13] Wittig and colleagues have described a 7-year, 5-month-old boy with narcolepsy who tended to fall asleep while watching television for longer than a half hour, at the dinner table, and while seated in his mother's lap at a doctor's office.[14] The naps in children with narcolepsy tend to be longer than those in adult patients (30 to 90 minutes), but they are not consistently followed by a refreshed feeling.[15] These attacks of sleepiness are most likely to occur when the patient is carrying out sedentary activities such as sitting in a classroom or reading a book. Sleepiness occurs regardless of the quantity of night sleep. The daytime sleepiness is frequently associated with automatic behavior of which the subject is unaware, impaired consolidation of memory, decreased concentration, executive dysfunction, and school-related learning problems. The irritability and mood swings that accompany sleepiness may mimic depression.[16,17]

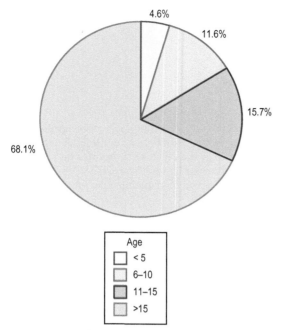

FIGURE 18-1 The age of onset of narcolepsy. *Adapted from Challamel MJ, Mazzola ME, Nevsimalova S, et al: Narcolepsy in children. Sleep 1994;17S:17–20.*

Children with daytime sleepiness may be mistakenly labeled 'lazy' and frequently become the target of negative comments from their peers. Excessive sleepiness might also be overlooked by the parents until it starts adversely impacting mood, behavior, or academic performance. These behavioral changes likely reflect impairment of function of the ventro-lateral prefrontal cortex from sleepiness.[18] Pollack studied the circadian sleep–wake rhythms in subjects with narcolepsy who were isolated from their environmental cues.[19] He found that the major sleep episode was still about 6 hours long, and it occurred about once every 24 hours, thus indicating that the circadian clock was functioning normally. Pollack confirmed that patients with narcolepsy tended to sleep more often, but not longer than people without narcolepsy.

Cataplexy, the second most common but most specific feature of narcolepsy, consists of a sudden loss of muscle tone in the facial muscles, or those of the thighs, back, or neck in response to emotional triggers such as fright, rage, excitement, surprise, or laughter or the anticipation of reward. It is caused by the intrusion of the skeletal muscle atonia of REM sleep into wakefulness.[20,21] Cataplexy is associated with hyperpolarization of spinal alpha motor neurons, with resultant active inhibition of skeletal muscle tone and suppression of the monosynaptic H-reflex and tendon reflexes. A history of cataplexy may be difficult to elicit in young children. The author recalls a 6-year-old girl with proven narcolepsy who denied any episodic muscle weakness but would repeatedly fall down whenever she jumped on a trampoline. Consciousness remains fully intact during the cataplexy episodes, which can last 1 to 30 minutes. Respiration and cardiovascular function remain unaffected. Challamel and coworkers[10] found cataplexy in 80.5% of idiopathic narcolepsy and in 95% of symptomatic narcolepsy subjects.

Hypnagogic halucinations are vivid dreams at sleep onset. Hypnopompic halucinations are vivid and sometimes frightening dreams upon awakening from sleep. Sleep paralysis is the momentary inability to move the body at sleep onset. Halucinations at sleep onset or offset and sleep paralysis are a consequence of intrusion of elements of REM sleep on to wakefulness.

Night-time sleep is also disturbed in narcolepsy with frequent awakenings. Young and colleagues attributed sleep fragmentation in part to periodic limb movements, which were found in five (63%) of eight children with narcolepsy in their series.[22] Periodic limb movements are rhythmic limb muscle contractions of 0.5 to 5 seconds' duration, with an intermovement interval of 5 to 120 seconds, occurring in series of three or more, usually during stage 1 or 2 of non-REM (NREM) sleep. They may or may not be associated with EEG evidence of cortical arousal. They may be a marker for underlying restless legs syndrome. Sleep fragmentation in narcolepsy may also occur unrelated to periodic limb movements or restless leg syndrome. Decreased pressure for NREM sleep homecstasis and altered NREM–REM sleep interaction has also been proposed as underlying the nocturnal sleep disruption of narcolepsy.[89]

Psychosocial problems in children with narcolepsy have been studied.[90] They found that, compared to hypersomnolent controls, children with narcolepsy showed more behavioral difficulties, depressed mood and impaired quality of life.[91]

Obesity may develop at the onset of narcolepsy–cataplexy symptoms, in association with hyperphagia and binge eating. It may be related to loss of the physiological rise in leptin levels at night (leptin acts as an appetite suppressant), or to sedentary behavior and decreased basal metabolism. Obesity does not seem to be related to the use of anticholinergic medications, as it develops even prior to initiation of drug treatment. The obesity may be accompanied by obstructive sleep apnea in 9–19% of subjects.[92] Precocious puberty may also be seen in preteen age boys and girls at onset of narcolepsy–cataplexy.

REM sleep behavior can sometimes be a presenting manifestation of narcolepsy.[93,94] It is characterized by motor dream enactment, typically in the form of flailing of arms and legs and yelling behavior. Simultaneously obtained polysomnogram shows REM sleep without atonia, i.e., persistence of muscle tone during sleep.

PATHOPHYSIOLOGY

The study of narcolepsy in humans has been advanced by the study of the disorder in animals. Narcolepsy has been studied in cats, miniature horses, quarter horses, Brahman bulls, and about 15 breeds of dogs. In animals, it shows a monogenic, autosomal recessive pattern of inheritance.[23–25] Cataplexy can be induced in cats by the injection of carbachol (an acetylcholine-like substance) into the pontine reticular formation.[26] Specifically, muscarinic type-2 receptors of acetylcholine have been implicated.[27,28] The food-elicited cataplexy test, used to study cataplexy in dogs, uses the finding that the time taken for the consumption of food by narcoleptic animals whose eating is interrupted by cataplexy attacks is much longer than in animals without narcolepsy.

In 1999, Lin and coworkers demonstrated that canine narcolepsy is caused by a mutation in the hypocretin receptor-2 (orexin-2) gene.[29] Around the same time, Chemelli and colleagues established that a null mutation for the hypocretin-1 and hypocretin-2 peptides in mice produces aspects reminiscent of human narcolepsy, including cataplexy.[30] The hypocretin-containing neurons are located primarily in the dorsolateral hypothalamus. They have widespread projections to the basal forebrain, amygdala, medial nuclei of the thalamus, periaqueductal gray matter, reticular formation, pedunculopontine nucleus, locus coeruleus, raphe nucleus, pontine tegmentum, and dorsal spinal cord.[29,31] Hypocretins 1 and 2 are peptides that are synthesized from preprohypocretin, and have corresponding receptors. Although the hypocretin type 1 receptor binds only to hypocretin-1, the hypocretin type 2 receptor can bind to both type 1 and type 2 ligands. Hypocretins stimulate food intake, increase the basal metabolic rate, and promote arousal.[31] Decreased activation of the hypocretin system is the underlying theme in canine and murine narcolepsy. This receptor down-regulation may occur as a result of either exon-skipping mutations in the hypocretin receptors (Labrador and Doberman models),[30] or after point mutations in the Hcrt2 receptor gene, with an amino acid change from glutamic acid to lysine in the N-terminus portion of the receptor (Dachshund model).[32] Also of significance is the finding that the intravenous administration of hypocretin-1 (orexin A) in narcoleptic Doberman pinschers reduces cataplexy for up to 3 days, increases activity, promotes waking, and reduces sleep fragmentation in a dose-dependent manner.[33]

Histocompatibility Antigens and Human Narcolepsy

In 1984, an association between narcolepsy and histocompatibility leukocyte antigen (HLA) DR2 was reported in Japan by Juji and coworkers.[34] This association was subsequently observed in other geographic regions of the world as well.[35,36] Consequently, an immunologic mechanism was suspected in the pathogenesis of human narcolepsy, but this has not been established. It was then demonstrated that the association with DR2 is only secondary, and that there is a stronger association of narcolepsy with the HLA DQ antigens, specifically *DQB1*0602* and *DQA1*0102*, which are present in 95% to 100% of patients, as compared to a 12% to 38% prevalence in the general population.[37] In a study of 525 healthy subjects, Mignot and colleagues demonstrated that *DQB1*0602* positivity was linked to shorter REM latency, increased sleep efficiency, and decreased time spent in stage 1 NREM sleep.[38] Pelin and coworkers have demonstrated that homozygosity for these two haplotypes is associated with a twofold to fourfold increase in the likelihood of developing narcolepsy over heterozygotes, but that the presence of these antigens does not influence the *severity* of the disease.[39]

Hypocretins and Human Narcolepsy

Unlike narcolepsy in dogs and mice, human narcolepsy–cataplexy is generally not associated with abnormalities in hypocretin receptors but rather with low to absent levels of cerebrospinal (CSF) hypocretin-1.[40] In a postmortem study of human narcolepsy, Thannickal and colleagues found an 85% to 95% reduction in the number of hypocretin neurons in the hypothalamic region,[41] whereas melanin-concentrating hormone neurons, which are intermingled with the hypocretin neurons, remained unaffected, thus suggesting

a targeted neurodegenerative process. Using a radioimmunoassay, Nishino and coworkers[42] found that the mean CSF level of hypocretin-1 in healthy controls was 230.3 ± 33.0 pg/mL, and in neurologic controls it was 260.5 ± 37.1 pg/mL, whereas in those with narcolepsy, hypocretin-1 was either undetectable or below 100 pg/mL. The diagnostic sensitivity of low levels (less than 100 pg/mL) was 84.2%. Low to absent levels were found in 32 out of 38 patients, who were all HLA *DQB1*0602* positive. HLA-negative narcolepsy patients had normal to high CSF hypocretin-1 levels. In another recent study, 92.3% of patients who were both *DQB1*0602* and cataplexy positive had undetectable CSF hypocretin-1 levels, whereas *DQB1*0602*-negative patients with cataplexy and *DQB1*0602*-negative patients without cataplexy had normal levels.[43] In a study of narcolepsy with cataplexy, narcolepsy without cataplexy and idiopathic hypersomnia, Kanbayashi et al.[44] found that all nine patients who were hypocretin deficient in the cerebrospinal fluid (CSF) were HLA DR2 (i.e. HLA *DQB1*0602*) positive. In contrast, narcolepsy without cataplexy and idiopathic hypersomnia were associated with normal levels of CSF hypocretin (Figure 18-2).

The CSF hypocretin assay is most useful when an HLA *DQB1*0602*-positive patient with suspected narcolepsy–cataplexy is receiving CNS stimulants on initial presentation to the sleep specialist, and when discontinuation of medications for the purpose of obtaining a multiple sleep latency test (MSLT) is inconvenient or impractical.

The Two-Hit Hypothesis

The presence of histocompatibility antigen *DQB1*0602* is, *per se*, insufficient to precipitate narcolepsy. This is substantiated by the fact that *DQB1*0602*-positive monozygotic twins have been incompletely concordant for narcolepsy, with one of the

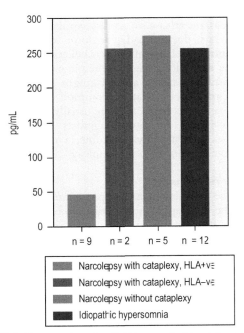

FIGURE 18-2 Mean cerebrospinal fluid hypocretin-1 levels in various categories of hypersomnia. The narcolepsy-cataplexy group included three prepubertal children of ages 6, 7, and 10. *Adapted from Kanbayashi T, Inoue Y, Chiba S, et al: CSF hypocretin-1 (orexin-A) concentrations in narcolepsy with and without cataplexy and idiopathic hypersomnia. J Sleep Res 2002;11:91–93.*

pair developing narcolepsy–cataplexy at age 12 years and the other not until after having suffered emotional stress and sleep deprivation at the age of 45 years.[45] Human narcolepsy is therefore best explained on the basis of a *two-threshold hypothesis*, with an interplay between genetic susceptibility and environmental factors – major life events, such as a systemic illness, an injury, or bereavement, have been reported to be present in 82% of narcolepsy patients, compared with a 44% incidence in controls[46] ($P<0.001$). The combination of genetic susceptibility and an acquired stress seems to trigger most cases of narcolepsy. Recently, there has been documentation of narcolepsy–cataplexy development following H1N1 influenza infection or immunization in children and adults who were positive for the HLA *DQB1*0602* antigen.[95]

Monoamine Disturbances

Hypocretin deficiency in humans leads to down-regulation of arousal-mediating noradrenergic and dopaminergic pathways in the brainstem, and to up-regulation of REM sleep-facilitating cholinergic pathways.[47] Montplaisir and coworkers[48] measured serum and CSF levels of several biogenic amines and their metabolites – dopamine (the metabolite homovanillic acid), norepinephrine (the metabolite 3-methoxy-4-hydroxyphenylethyleneglycol), epinephrine, and serotonin (the metabolite 5-hydroxy indoleacetic acid) – in patients with narcolepsy, in those with idiopathic hypersomnia, and in normal controls. Both narcolepsy and idiopathic hypersomnia patients had significantly decreased concentrations of dopamine and indoleacetic acid, a metabolite of tryptamine. Dopamine and tryptamine are usually present in high concentrations in the basal ganglia. A relative deficiency of these compounds, probably mediated by down-regulation of hypocretin, is involved in the evolution of sleepiness. Stimulants such as dextroamphetamine and methylphenidate, which are used in the treatment of hypersomnolence, are known to enhance dopamine release from presynaptic terminals. Activation of selective dopamine D_2 receptor agonists also suppresses cataplexy.[49] This inhibition is believed to be indirectly mediated via activation of noradrenergic pathways. A reduction in central dopamine activity might also underlie the periodic leg movements that are common in the night sleep of patients with narcolepsy; they are usually relieved by treatment with levodopa or dopamine agonists. A cholinergic disturbance also coexists; physostigmine, a cholinergic agent, leads to a transient increase in cataplexy.

Secondary Narcolepsy

Although the majority of narcolepsy is *idiopathic*, structural lesions of the diencephalon or brainstem may, on rare occasion, precipitate *secondary narcolepsy* in those who are biologically predisposed, perhaps subsequent to disruption of the hypocretin pathways. Cerebellar hemangioblastomas, temporal lobe B-cell lymphomas, pituitary adenoma, third ventricular gliomas, craniopharyngiomas, head trauma, viral encephalitis, ischemic brainstem disturbances, sarcoidosis, and multiple sclerosis have been associated with narcolepsy.[50–57] In such patients, the finding of cataplexy increases the likelihood that the hypersomnolence is narcolepsy-related. Isolated cataplexy has also been observed in Niemann-Pick type C disease,[58] but these patients cannot be labeled as having secondary narcolepsy as they lack other prerequisite clinical and polysomnographic features. Arii and colleagues described a

hypothalamic tumor in a 16-year-old girl who manifested hypersomnolence, obesity, and low CSF hypocretin-1 levels, without cataplexy.[59] Although this patient did not meet the criteria for the diagnosis of narcolepsy, the report highlights the importance of hypocretins in the regulation of alertness.

DIAGNOSIS

The diagnosis of narcolepsy is established on the basis of the history, combined with characteristic findings on the nocturnal polysomnogram and a multiple sleep latency test.[60] In preparation for the sleep studies, the patient should be withdrawn from all central nervous stimulants, hypnotics, antidepressants, and any other psychotropic agents for 2 weeks prior to the sleep studies, as these drugs may impact sleep architecture. In the case of drugs with a long half-life, such as fluoxetine, the drug-free interval may need to be 3 to 4 weeks. In preparation for the sleep studies, the patient should maintain a regular sleep–wake schedule, which can be verified by wrist actigraphy and sleep logs that are maintained by the patient for 1 to 2 weeks prior to the sleep studies.[61] A general physical examination should also be carried out to assess the Tanner stage of sexual development, as normal values for nocturnal total sleep time, daytime sleep latency, and daytime REM sleep latency are closely linked to the Tanner stages.[62]

During the nocturnal polysomnogram, multiple parameters of physiologic activity, such as the EEG (C3-A1, O2-A1 montage), eye movements, chin and leg electromyogram, nasal pressure, thoracic and abdominal respiratory effort, and oxygen saturation, are recorded simultaneously on a computerized sleep monitoring and analysis system.[63] The test helps exclude sleep pathologies such as obstructive sleep apnea, the periodic limb movement disorder,[64,65] and idiopathic hypersomnia[66,67] that can also lead to daytime sleepiness and mimic narcolepsy.

Patients with narcolepsy may exhibit onset of REM sleep within 15 minutes of sleep onset (sleep-onset REM period). Gross sleep efficiency is generally high (greater than 90%), but there may be fragmentation of sleep from an increased number of arousals and periodic limb movements. There is no significant disordered breathing or oxygen desaturation. A useful clue to narcolepsy in adolescents is the presence of decreased nocturnal REM sleep latency (the time between sleep onset and the onset of the first 30-second epoch of REM sleep). For example, in one study,[68] the nocturnal REM sleep latency in narcoleptic subjects was less than 67 minutes (mean, 24.5 minutes; standard deviation, 30; range, 0 to 66.5 minutes; n=8), as compared to a mean nocturnal REM sleep latency of 143.7 minutes in age-matched controls (range, 82.5 to 230.5; SD, 50.9 minutes; $P<0.001$). A similar conclusion was reached by Challamel and coworkers in their meta-analysis of 235 subjects,[10] and in the pioneering work of Carskadon and colleagues.[69]

An MSLT should be started at 2 hours after the final morning awakening. It consists of four to five nap opportunities of 20-minute lengths at 2-hour intervals in a darkened, quiet room (e.g., at 1000, 1200, 1400, and 1600 hours).[60] Eye movements, chin electromyogram and electroencephalogram (generally C3-A2, O2-A1) are recorded. The MSLT provides quantitative information about the degree of sleepiness and qualitative information about the nature of the transition from wakefulness into sleep (i.e., wakefulness to NREM sleep, or wakefulness to REM sleep). The time interval between 'lights out' and sleep onset is termed the *sleep latency*; a *mean sleep latency* is then derived from all the naps. A urine drug screen is obtained between the naps if the patient appears to be falling asleep very quickly. A concerted effort should be made to ensure that the patient does not accidentally fall asleep between the naps. Typically, the mean sleep latency is markedly shortened to less than 5 minutes in patients with narcolepsy, whereas in controls it is generally 15 to 18 minutes (Table 18.1).[63]

In unaffected children, the initial transition is from wakefulness into NREM sleep. Narcolepsy is, however, associated with a transition from wakefulness directly into REM sleep (*sleep-onset REM period* (SOREMP)). This diagnostic feature of two or more SOREMPs may not be consistently present in the early stages of the disorder in children and young adults, and sometimes serial sleep studies are needed to establish a definitive diagnosis (Figure 18-3).[70] Although the normative data derived by Carskadon[62] are widely used, it is conceivable that normal mean sleep latencies in preadolescents may be greater than 20 minutes[71,72]

Serologic testing for the HLA *DQB1*0602* haplotype is sometimes used as an adjunctive test, but it cannot be used to diagnose narcolepsy, as this haplotype is also present in 12% to 38% of the general population.[38] CSF hypocretin analysis is useful in establishing the diagnosis when psychotropic medications cannot be discontinued for safety reasons and for children below the age of 6–7 years because the MSLT is not valid in this age group. Since hypocretin testing is not readily available, nocturnal polysomnography and the MSLT remain the gold standard at this time for making a definitive diagnosis of narcolepsy.

DIFFERENTIAL DIAGNOSIS

By far, the most common disorder leading to excessive daytime sleepiness in an adolescent is *insufficient nocturnal sleep*.[73] To begin with, there is a physiologic shift in the sleep-onset time of most teenagers to between 10:30 and 11:00 p.m.[74] Also, the physiologic delay in the onset of dim-light melatonin secretion to a later time at night and the resultant postponement of sleep onset is associated with a corresponding shift to a later morning awakening time in most adolescents. Linked to this phase shift, Carskadon and coworkers have documented SOREMPs during the MSLT of 12 of 25 healthy students.[75] Superimposed on this may be elements of *abnormal sleep hygiene* (e.g., use of stimulants, late-night television viewing/phone calls/computer chats), or circadian rhythm disturbances such as the *delayed sleep phase syndrome*.[76,77] The use of prescription drugs or over-the-counter sedatives such as antihistamines should also be considered as a possible cause of sleepiness. A high index of suspicion should be maintained for illicit drug use.

It is not uncommon for narcolepsy to present with obesity and nocturnal snoring, thus mimicking *obstructive sleep apnea*. The most common causes of childhood obstructive sleep apnea are adenotonsillar hypertrophy, neuromuscular disorders, and craniofacial anomalies such as Crouzon syndrome and Down syndrome.[78–80] The *upper airway resistance syndrome* is another under-recognized disorder leading to chronic daytime sleepiness. It is characterized by habitual snoring, an increased number of breathing-related microarousals, and increased negative intrathoracic pressures on monitoring of esophageal pressures during polysomnography using balloons.[81]

The *Kleine–Levin syndrome*, or *periodic hypersomnia*, is characterized by recurrent periods of sleepiness.[82] The disorder is common in adolescent males, who manifest 1- to 2-week periods of excessive sleep, in association with hyperphagia and hypersexual behavior. There may be a 2- to 10-pound weight gain during the sleepy periods, which then remits spontaneously, only to reappear a few weeks later. No specific etiology has been found. The disorder subsides gradually over time. The nocturnal polysomnogram shows a high sleep efficiency and a decreased percentage of time spent in stages 3 and 4 of NREM sleep.[83] The MSLT shows moderate daytime sleepiness with a shortened mean sleep latency of 5 to 10 minutes, but fewer than two SOREMPs.

Idiopathic hypersomnia should also be considered in the differential diagnosis of narcolepsy. It is defined as a disorder associated with non-imperative sleepiness, long unrefreshing naps, difficulty reaching full awakening after sleep, and sleep

TABLE 18.1 Normal Values for the Multiple Sleep Latency Test

STAGE OF DEVELOPMENT	MEAN SLEEP LATENCY (MIN)	STANDARD DEVIATION
Tanner stage I	18.8	1.8
Tanner stage II	18.3	2.1
Tanner stage III	16.5	2.8
Tanner stage IV	15.5	3.3
Tanner stage V	16.2	1.5
Older adolescents	15.8	3.5

Adapted from Carskadon MA: The second decade. In Guilleminault C (ed): Sleeping and Waking Disorders: Indications and Techniques. Menlo Park, Calif, Addison-Wesley, 1982, pp 99–125.

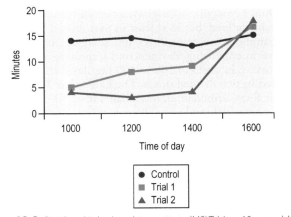

FIGURE 18-3 Serial multiple sleep latency tests (MSLTs) in a 13-year-old child with evolving narcolepsy. MSLT trials 1 and 2 were carried out 9 months apart. They are compared with the MSLT findings of a healthy control. There is progressive decrease over time in the sleep latencies of the patient at 1000, 1200, and 1400 hours, along with an increase in the number of sleep-onset rapid eye movement periods. Sleep latencies in the final nap (1600 hours) may be physiologically prolonged in children as a result of anticipation about going home – the 'last nap' effect. *Reproduced from Kotagal S, Swink TD: Excessive daytime sleepiness in a 13-year old. Semin Pediatr Neurol 1996;3:170–172.*

drunkenness, as well as absence of SOREMPs during the MSLT.[67,84] Night sleep is quantitatively and qualitatively normal. The MSLT shows a short mean sleep latency, generally in the range of 5 to 10 minutes, but two or more SOREMPs, which would be suggestive of narcolepsy, are not seen. The author has studied six children with narcolepsy who underwent serial nocturnal polysomnograms and MSLTs for the assessment of daytime sleepiness.[68] Long, unrefreshing naps were common. Although the initial battery of sleep studies showed shortened mean sleep latencies (less than 10 minutes), suggesting moderate daytime sleepiness, they lacked the necessary (two or more) SOREMPs to diagnose narcolepsy. Initially, therefore, they met the diagnostic criteria for idiopathic hypersomnia. A repeat battery of sleep studies several months later, however, showed the appearance of two or more SOREMPs on the MSLT of each subject, characteristic of narcolepsy. In some children, therefore, idiopathic hypersomnia may be a transitional phase that precedes the development of classic narcolepsy.

CASE PRESENTATION

A 3-year-old girl was evaluated for a 6-week history of sleepiness and unsteadiness while standing and walking, leading to falls, occurring at least 8–10 times per day. The unsteadiness was momentary, and was punctuated with long periods of stable balance and coordination. Her parents noticed that she began to sleep as much as 16 hours per day. She was afebrile. The cranial magnetic resonance imaging scan, electroencephalogram, and serum ammonia, electrolytes, and thyroxine were normal. A lumbar puncture showed normal cerebrospinal fluid cell count and differential, protein and glucose. Video clips of the falls that had been recorded by the father on his cell phone were reviewed – they were suspicious for cataplexy. She was also positive for the histocompatibility antigen *DQB1*0602*. Consequently, 0.7 mL of residual spinal fluid that had been saved and frozen was sent for assessment of cerebrospinal fluid hypocretin, which came back low at 26 pg/mL (reference value is >110 pg/mL). A diagnosis of narcolepsy–cataplexy was established. Upon further questioning, the parents indicated that she had received immunization for influenza A approximately 4 weeks prior to onset of the symptoms. She was provided infusions of intravenous immunoglubulin G every 2 weeks for 3 months, without any benefit. Symptomatic treatment was therefore provided using a combination of methylphenidate 2.5 once a day and sodium oxybate, 2 grams at night in two divided doses, with excellent results. This has now been maintained for about 18 months without any significant side effects.

This case illustrates several aspects of narcolepsy–cataplexy. Children of preschool age can have episodes of abrupt muscle weakness that may or may not be consistently associated with an emotional trigger such as laughter. One needs to keep a high index of suspicion in children who are excessively sleepy. Also, reviewing video clips recorded by the parents can be priceless in pediatric sleep medicine, as exemplified by this case. Further, the diagnosis in children below the age of 5–6 years is problematic because the MSLT can not be applied as it will not be able to distinguish physiological napping from pathologic sleepiness. If cataplexy is present and the patient is positive for HLA *DQB1*0602*, there is a strong likelihood

that spinal fluid hypocretin will be low; thus, assessing its levels becomes important. It is conceivable that in this patient, who was biologically predisposed to develop narcolepsy–cataplexy by virtue of her HLA *DQB1*0602*-positive status, the influenza immunization acted as the 'second hit' that triggered an immune-mediated degenerative process in the hypothalamus that led to reduced central nervous system hypocretin levels and precipitation of narcolepsy–cataplexy. This case also illustrates the challenges pediatric sleep specialists face in treating narcolepsy, as the use of most medications for sleepiness as well as cataplexy remains 'off label.' In the first decade of life, when brain function is most vulnerable and the deleterious effects of hypersomnolence on learning most crucial, ironically, there are no medications approved by the Food and Drug Administration for treating children with narcolepsy!

MANAGEMENT

Because narcolepsy requires lifelong treatment, the nocturnal polysomnogram and MSLT findings should be unequivocally positive before making the diagnosis. Drugs commonly used for treatment are listed in Table 18.2.

General Measures

It is important to maintain regular sleeping and waking schedules. One to two planned naps during the day might help dissipate sleep pressure and daytime sleepiness. Regular exercise during the day might also enhance alertness and prevent excessive weight gain. Attention to comorbid obesity is important as it may predispose to sleep-disordered breathing. Psychiatric consultation should be sought in case of comorbid depression and anxiety.

Daytime sleepiness is countered with stimulants such as methylphenidate (regular or extended-release formulations) or various preparations of amphetamine.[85–88] The half-lives of amphetamine and methylphenidate are 10–12 hours and 3–4 hours, respectively. The side effects of these agents include loss of appetite, nervousness, tics, headache, and insomnia. Modafinil (Provigil), a drug whose mode of action has not been fully defined, but is at least in part related to inhibition of dopamine active transporter, has also been reported to be effective in enhancing alertness and improving psychomotor performance in doses of 100 to 400 mg/day.[92] It works best if provided in two divided doses. The half-life is 3–4 hours. Its racemic form, armodafinil, has a half-life of 10–14 hours and is also now widely utilized. The side effects of modafinil and armodafinil include headache, nervousness, anxiety, and nausea. Stevens–Johnson syndrome is a rare but serious type of delayed hypersensitivity reaction with modafinil that is characterized by a diffuse and progressive vascilitis that involves the skin, mucous membranes and viscera. It requires immediate discontinuation of the drug, assessment for hepatic or renal involvement, and possible treatment with corticosteroids. Modafinil and armodafinil may decrease the potency of concurrently administered oral contraceptives.

Cataplexy seems to be mediated by cholinergic pathways in the brainstem. Drugs with anticholinergic properties such as protryptiline and clomimipramine have been found effective for its control. Unfortunately, these drugs carry significant side effects such as drowsiness, dryness of the mouth and weight gain. Selective serotonin reuptake inhibitors such as fluoxetine

TABLE 18.2   Drugs Commonly Used in the Treatment of Narcolepsy

SYMPTOM	DRUG (TRADE NAME)	DOSAGE	REMARKS
Daytime sleepiness	Modafinil (Provigil)	100–400 mg /day in 2 divided doses	Side effects: headache, nervousness, anxiety, nausea, Stevens Johnson syndrome, lowering efficacy of oral contraceptives
	Armodafinil (Nuvigil)	150–450 mg/day	Side effects: same as with modafinil
	Methylphenidate (Ritalin)	5–60 mg /day in 2–3 divided doses	Side effects: anorexia, weight loss, tremor, worsening of tics, insomnia, agitation, headache – common for all salts of methylphenidate
	Methylphenidate (Ritalin Sr)	20–60 mg /day in 2 divided doses	
	Methylphenidate (Concerta)	18–54 mg/day in 2 divided doses up to age 12; up to 72 mg for those up to age 18 years	
	Methylphenidate (Metadate)	20 mg/day, to a maximum of 60 mg/day	
	Methylphenidate transdermal patch (Daytrana)	10–30 mg; apply 2 hours before need and remove 9 hours after application	Safety and efficacy not established below age 6 years
	Dextroamphetamine (Dexedrine)	5–60 mg/day in 1–2 divided doses	
	Amphetamine/dextroamphetamine mixture (Adderall)	10–40 mg/day in 1–2 divided doses	Side effects: anorexia, weight loss, tremor, worsening of tics, insomnia, agitation, headache – common for all salts of dextroamphetamine
	Lisdexamphetamine (Vyvanse)	30–70 mg/day in 1–2 divided doses	
Cataplexy	Venlafaxine (Effexor) tablets or extended release capsules*	37.5–5 mg/day in 1–2 divided doses	Side effects: nervousness, weight loss, dizziness, headache, constipation, xerostomia
	Fluoxetine (Prozac)	10–30 mg/day every morning	Side effects: insomnia, loss of appetite, somnolence, tremor, anxiety, worsening of depression, suicidal thoughts
	Sertraline (Zoloft)	25–100 mg/day every morning	Same as with fluoxetine
	Clomimipramine (Anafranil)	25–100 mg /day in 1–2 doses	Side effects: weight gain, constipation, nervousness, xerostomia
	Protryptiline (Vivactil)	5–15 mg /day in 1–2 divided doses	Same as with Clomimipramine
	Sodium oxybate (Xyrem)	3–8 g each night in 2 divided doses, with first dose at sleep onset, 2nd dose 2–3 hours later	Use in children is off-label, as it has not been approved by the FDA in this age group. Side effects: worsening of sleep apnea, sleep walking, tremor, constipation, enuresis
Periodic limb movements / restless legs syndrome	Elemental iron	1–2 mg/kg/day with orange juice	Side effects: Constipation and abdominal discomfort
	Gabapentin	100–300 mg at bed time	
	Clonazepam	0.25–0.5 mg at bed time	
	Ropinorole (REQUIP)	0.25–0.5 mg at bed time	Use in children is on an off-label basis
	Pramipexole (MIRAPEX)	0.125–0.25 mg at bed time	Use in children is on an off-label basis

*All antidepressants are associated with a risk of increased suicidal ideation.
Periodic follow-up is needed for all subjects to monitor for improvement and side effects.
Patients may need a combination of drugs for optimum control of symptoms.

may also be utilized to treat cataplexy, especially when there is coexisting depression. Gamma hydroxybutyrate (sodium oxybate) is an endogenous fatty acid with specific affinity for endogenous gamma hydroxybutyrate and gamma amino butyric acid type B receptors.[96] It has a modulating effects on gabaergic, dopaminergic, noradrenergic and serotonergic neurons.[96] The drug is effective against both cataplexy and daytime sleepiness. The half-life is 30–60 minutes. It is typically provided in two divided doses, with the first dose at bed time, and the second dose 2.5–3 hours after initial sleep onset. Sodium oxybate has not been approved by the Food and Drug Administration for use in children; thus, its use in this population is on an off-label basis. Adverse effects include dizziness, nausea, enuresis, exacerbation of sleep apnea, sleep walking and somnolence.[96] Owing to concern about exacerbation of a pre-existing psychiatric condition, its use in narcolepsy–cataplexy subjects with mood or emotional problems should be avoided. It also has a high potential for abuse, and should be avoided in patients who might pose a risk in this regard.

The *Narcolepsy Network* (www.narcolepsynetwork.org) is a private, nonprofit resource for patients, families, and health professionals. Because of the increased risk of accidents from sleepiness, patients should be cautioned against driving long distances and working near sharp, moving machinery. Future treatments might consist of hypocretin analogs.[47]

Clinical Pearls

- Preschool-aged children may not provide accurate information about cataplexy. Reviewing video clips provided by parents may help document cataplexy.
- The manifestations of childhood sleepiness can at times be non-specific, including inattentiveness, mood swings and apathy. These are manifestations of dysfunction of the prefrontal cortex due to sleepiness.
- Spinal fluid hypocretin levels may help make a diagnosis in children below the age of 5–6 years, or when the patient is already receiving medications such as antidepressants that can not be safely stopped.
- Obesity may be present at the onset of childhood narcolepsy–cataplexy.

References

1. Gelineau J. De la narcolepsie. Gaz Hosp (Paris) 1880;53:626–8.
2. American Academy of Sleep Medicine. International classification of sleep disorders. 2nd ed. Diagnostic and coding manual. Westchester, Illinois: American Academy of Sleep Medicine; 2006.
3. Silber M, Krahn L, Olson E, et al. The epidemiology of narcolepsy in Olmsted County, Minnesota: A population-based study. Sleep 2002;25:197–202.
4. Honda Y. Clinical features of narcolepsy: Japanese experience. In: Honda Y, Juji T, editors. Narcolepsy. Springer Verlag; 1988: 1988. p. 2457.
5. Lavie P, Peled R. Narcolepsy is a rare disease in Israel. Sleep 1987;10:608–9.
6. Heier MS, Evsiukova T, Wilson J, et al. Prevalence of narcolepsy with cataplexy in Norway. Acta Neurol Scand 2009;120(4):276–80.
7. Matsuki K, Honda Y, Juji T. Diagnostic criteria for narcolepsy and HLA-DR2 frequencies. Tissue Antigens 1987;30:155–60.
8. Roffwarg HP. Sleep Disorders Classification Committee, Association of Sleep Disorders: Diagnostic classification of sleep and arousal disorders. Sleep 1979;2:1–137.
9. Hublin C, Partinen M, Kaprio J, et al. Epidemiology of narcolepsy. Sleep 1994;17(Suppl. 1):7–12.
10. Challamel MJ, Mazzola ME, Nevsimalova S, et al. Narcolepsy in children. Sleep 1994;17S:17–20.
11. Overeem S, Reading P, Bassetti CL. Narcolepsy. Sleep Med Clin 2012;7(2):263–81.
12. Sharp SJ, D'Cruz OF. Narcolepsy in a 12-month-old boy. J Child Neurol 2001;16:145–6.
13. Lenn NJ. HLA-DR2 in childhood narcolepsy. Pediatr Neurol 1986;2:314–15.
14. Wittig R, Zorick F, Roehrs T, et al. Narcolepsy in a 7-year-old child. J Pediatr 1983;102:725–7.
15. Kotagal S, Hartse KM, Walsh JK. Characteristics of narcolepsy in pre-teen aged children. Pediatrics 1990;85:205–9.
16. Pearl PL, Efron L, Stein MA. Children, sleep, and behavior: A complex association. Minerva Pediatr 2002;54:79–91.
17. Wise MS, Lynch J. Narcolepsy in children. Semin Pediatr Neurol 2001;8(4):198–206.
18. Walker MP. Sleep, memory and emotion. Prog Brain Res 2010;185:49–68.
19. Pollack CP. The rhythms of narcolepsy. Narcolepsy Network 1995;8:1–7.
20. Guilleminault C, Wilson RA, Dement WC. A study of cataplexy. Arch Neurol 1974;31:255–61.
21. Guilleminault C, Pelayo R. Narcolepsy in prepubertal children. Ann Neurol 1998;43:135–42.
22. Young D, Zorick F, Wittig R, et al. Narcolepsy in a pediatric population. Am J Dis Child 1988;142:210–14.
23. Foutz AS, Mitler MM, Cavalli-Sforza LL, et al. Genetic factors in canine narcolepsy. Sleep 1979;1:413–21.
24. Knecht CD, Oliver JE, Redding R, et al. Narcolepsy in a dog and a cat. J Am Vet Med Assoc 1984;162:1052–3.
25. Strain GM, Olcott BM, Archer RM, et al. Narcolepsy in a Brahmin bull. J Am Vet Med Assoc 1984;185:538–41.
26. Mitler MM, Dement WC. Cataplectic-like behavior in cats after micro-injection of carbachol in the pontine reticular formation. Brain Res 1974;68:335–43.
27. Nishino S, Reid MS, Dement WC, et al. Neuropharmacology and neurochemistry of narcolepsy. Sleep 1994;17(Suppl. 1):S84–92.
28. Reid MS, Tafti M, Geary JN, et al. Cholinergic mechanisms in cataplexy: I. Modulation of cataplexy via local drug administration into the paramedian pontine reticular formation. Neuroscience 1994;59:511–22.
29. Lin L, Faraco J, Li R, et al. The sleep disorder, canine narcolepsy, is caused by a mutation in the hypocretin (orexin) receptor 2 gene. Cell 1999;98:365–76.
30. Chemelli RM, Willie JT, Sinton CM, et al. Narcolepsy in orexin knock-out mice: Molecular genetics of sleep regulation. Cell 1999;98:437–51.
31. Silber MH, Rye DB. Solving the mysteries of narcolepsy: The hypocretin story. Neurology 2001;56:1616–18.
32. Hungs Fan J, Lin X, Maki RA, et al. Identification and functional analysis of mutations in the hypocretin (orexin) genes of narcoleptic canines. Genome Res 2001;11:531–9.
33. John J, Wu M-F, Siegel JM. Systemic administration of hypocretin-1 reduces cataplexy and normalizes sleep and waking durations in narcoleptic dogs. Sleep Res Online 2000;3:23–8.
34. Juji T, Satake M, Honda Y, et al. HLA antigens in Japanese patients with narcolepsy. Tissue Antigens 1984;24:316–19.
35. Billiard M, Seignalet J, Besset A, et al. HLA DR2 and narcolepsy. Sleep 1986;9:149–52.
36. Langdon N, Lock C, Welsh K, et al. Immune factors in narcolepsy. Sleep 1986;9:143–8.
37. Mignot E, Lin L, Rogers W, et al. Complex HLA-DR and -DQ interactions confer risk of narcolepsy-cataplexy in three ethnic groups. Am J Hum Genet 2001;68:686–99.
38. Mignot E, Young T, Lin L, Fin L. Nocturnal sleep and daytime sleepiness in normal subjects with HLA-DQB1*0602. Sleep 1999;22:347–52.
39. Pelin Z, Guilleminault C, Risch N, et al. HLA DQB1*0602 homozygosity increases relative risk for narcolepsy but not disease severity in two ethnic groups. Tissue Antigens 1998;51:96–100.
40. Nishino S, Ripley B, Overeem S, et al. Hypocretin (orexin) deficiency in human narcolepsy. Lancet 2000;355:39–40.
41. Thannickal TC, Moore RY, Nienhuis R, et al. Reduced number of hypocretin neurons in human narcolepsy. Neuron 2000;27:469–74.
42. Nishino S, Ripley B, Overeem S, et al. Low cerebrospinal fluid hypocretin (orexin) and altered energy homeostasis in human narcolepsy. Ann Neurol 2001;50:381–8.
43. Krahn LE, Pankrantz VS, Oliver L, et al. Hypocretin (orexin) levels in cerebrospinal fluid of patients with narcolepsy: Relationship to cataplexy and DQB1*0602. Sleep 2002;25:733–8.
44. Kanbayashi T, Inoue Y, Chiba S, et al. CSF hypocretin-1 (orexin-A) concentrations in narcolepsy with and without cataplexy and idiopathic hypersomnia. J Sleep Res 2002;11:91–3.
45. Honda M, Honda Y, Uchida S, et al. Monozygotic twins incompletely concordant for narcolepsy. Biol Psychiatr 2001;49:943–7.
46. Orellana C, Villemin E, Tafti M, et al. Life events in the year preceding the onset of narcolepsy. Sleep 1994;17(Suppl. 1):50–3.
47. Mignot E, Taheri S, Nishino S. Sleeping with the hypothalamus: Emerging therapeutic targets for sleep disorders. Nat Neurosci 2002;5(Suppl.):1071–5.
48. Montplaisir J, de Champlain J, Young SN, et al. Narcolepsy and idiopathic hypersomnia: Biogenic and related compounds in CSF. Neurology 1982;32:1299–302.
49. Nishino S, Arrigoni J, Valtier D, et al. Dopamine D2 mechanisms in canine narcolepsy. J Neurosci 1991;11:2666–71.
50. Autret A, Lucas F, Henry-Lebras F, et al. Symptomatic narcolepsies. Sleep 1994;17S(Suppl. 1):21–4.
51. Tridon P, Montaut J, Picard L, et al. Syndrome de Gelineau et hemangioblastome kystique u cervelet. Rev Neurol 1969;121:186–9.
52. Onofrj M, Curatola L, Ferracci F, et al. Narcolepsy associated with primary temporal lobe B-cell lymphoma in a HLA DR2 negative subject. J Neurol Neurosurg Psychiatry 1992;55:852–3.
53. Schwartz WJ, Stakes JW, Hobson JA. Transient cataplexy after removal of craniopharyngoma. Neurology 1984;34:1372–5.
54. Lankford DA, Wellman JJ, Ohara C. Post-traumatic narcolepsy in mild to moderate closed head injury. Sleep 1994;17S(Suppl. 1):25–8.
55. Bonduelle C, Degos C. Symptomatic narcolepsies: A critical study. In Guilleminault C, Dement WC, Passouant P, editors. Narcolepsy. New York: Spectrum; 1976. p. 312–32.
56. Rivera VM, Meyer JS, Hata T, et al. Narcolepsy following cerebral ischemia. Ann Neurol 1986;19:505–8.
57. Schrader H, Gotlibsen OB. Multiple sclerosis and narcolepsy-cataplexy in a monozygotic twin. Neurology 1980;30:105–8.
58. Kandt RS, Emerson RG, Singer HS, et al. Cataplexy in variant forms of Niemann–Pick disease. Ann Neurol 1982;12:284–8.
59. Arii J, Kanbayashi T, Tanabe Y, et al. A hypersomnolent girl with decreased CSF hypocretin level after removal of a hypothalamic tumor. Neurology 2001;56:1775–6.
60. Carskadon MA, Dement WC, Mitler MM, et al. Guidelines for the multiple sleep latency test (MSLT): A standard measure of sleepiness. Sleep 1986;9:519–24.
61. Sadeh A, Hauri PJ, Kripke DF, et al. The role of actigraphy in the evaluation of sleep disorders. Sleep 1995;18:288–302.
62. Carskadon MA. The second decade. In: Guilleminault C, editor. Sleeping and waking disorders: indications and techniques. Menlo Park, Cal. Addison-Wesley; 1982. p. 99–125.
63. Kotagal S, Goulding PM. The laboratory assessment of daytime sleepiness in childhood. J Clin Neurophysiol 1996;13:208–18.
64. American Sleep Disorders Association. Periodic limb movement disorder. In: The international classification of sleep disorders: diagnostic and coding manual. Rochester, Minn: American Sleep Disorders Association. 1997. p. 5–8.

65. Chervin RD, Archbold KH, Dillon JE, et al. Association between symptoms of inattention, hyperactivity, restless legs syndrome, and periodic leg movements. Sleep 2002;25:213–18.
66. Roth B. Narcolepsy and hypersomnia: Review and classification of 642 personally observed cases. Scweiz Arch Neurol Neurochir Psychiatr 1976;119:31–41.
67. Basetti C, Aldrich MS. Idiopathic hypersomnia: A series of 42 patients. Brain 1997;120:1423–35.
68. Kotagal S. A developmental perspective on narcolepsy. In: Loughlin GM, Carroll JL, Marcus CL, editors. Sleep and breathing in children. New York: Marcel Dekker; 2000. p. 347–62.
69. Carskadon MA, Harvey K, Dement WC. Multiple sleep latency tests during the development of narcolepsy. West J Med 1981;135:414–18.
70. Kotagal S, Swink TD. Excessive daytime sleepiness in a 13-year-old. Semin Pediatr Neurol 1996;3:170–2.
71. Gozal D, Wang M, Pope DW. Objective sleepiness measures in pediatric obstructive sleep apnea. Pediatrics 2001;108:693–7.
72. Palm L, Persson E, Elmquist D, et al. Sleep and wakefulness in normal pre-adolescents. Sleep 1989;12:299–308.
73. Brown LW, Billiard M. Narcolepsy, Kleine–Levin syndrome, and other causes of sleepiness in children. In: Ferber R, Kryger M, editors. Principles and practice of sleep medicine in the child. Philadelphia: WB Saunders; 1995. p. 125–34.
74. Carskadon MA. Factors influencing sleep patterns of adolescents. In: Carskadon MA, editor. Adolescent sleep patterns: biological, social, and psychological perspectives. Cambridge, Mass: Cambridge University Press; 2002. p. 18–9.
75. Carskadon MA, Wolfson AR, Acebo C, et al. Adolescent sleep patterns, circadian timing, and sleepiness at a transition to early school days. Sleep 1998;21:871–81.
76. Garcia J, Rosen G, Mahowald M. Circadian rhythms and circadian rhythm disorders in children and adolescents. Semin Pediatr Neurol 2001;8:229–40.
77. Dijk DJ, Bolos Z, Eastman CI, et al. Light treatment of sleep disorders: Consensus report: II. Basic properties of circadian physiology. J Biol Rhythms 1995;10:113–25.
78. Marcus CL. Sleep architecture and respiratory disturbance in children with obstructive sleep apnea. Am J Respir Crit Care Med 2000;162(Part 1):682–6.
79. Marcus CL. Obstructive sleep apnea symptoms: Difference between children and adults. Sleep 2000;23(Suppl. 4):S140–1.
80. Brooks LJ. Genetic syndromes affecting breathing during sleep. In: Loughlin GM, Carroll JL, Marcus CL, editors. Sleep and breathing in children. New York: Marcel Dekker; 2000. p. 737–54.
81. Guilleminault C, Pelayo R, Leger D, et al. Recognition of sleep-disordered breathing in children. Pediatrics 1996;98:871–82.
82. Papacostas SS, Hadjivasilis V. Klein–Levin syndrome: Report of a case and review of literature. Eur Psychiatr 2000;15:231–5.
83. Gadoth N, Kesler A, Vainstein G, et al. Clinical and polysomnographic characteristics of 34 patients with Klein Levin syndrome. J Sleep Res 2001;10:337–41.
84. Billiard M, Rondouin G, Espa F, et al. Pathophysiology of idiopathic hypersomnia: Current studies and new orientation. Rev Neurol (Paris) 2001;157(Part 2):S101–6.
85. Stahl SM. Awakening to the psychopharmacology of sleep and arousal: Novel neurotransmitters and wake-promoting drugs. J Clin Psychiatr 2002;63:467–8.
86. Mitler MM. Evaluation of treatment with stimulants in narcolepsy. Sleep 1994;17(Suppl. 1):103–6.
87. Billiard M, Besset A, Montplaisir F, et al. Modafinil: A double blind multicentric study. Sleep 1994;17S:107–12.
88. Littner M, Johnson SF, McCall WV, et al. Practice parameters for treatment of narcolepsy: An update for 2000. Sleep 2001;24:451–66.
89. Khatami R, Landolt HP, Acherman P, et al. Challenging sleep homeostasis in narcolepsy-cataplexy: implications for non-REM and REM sleep regulation. Sleep 2008;31:859–67.
90. Stores G, Montgomery P, Wiggs L. The psychosocial problems of children with narcolepsy and those with excessive daytime sleepiness of uncertain origin. Pediatrics 2006;118:e1116–23.
91. Kotagal S, Krahn LE, Slocumb N. A putative link between childhood narcolepsy and obesity. Sleep Med 2004;5:147–50.
92. Poli F, Pizza F, Mignot E, et al. High prevalence of precocious puberty and obesity in childhood narcolepsy with cataplexy. Sleep 2013;36:175–81.
93. Nevsimalova S, Prihodova I, Kemlink D, et al. REM sleep behavior disorder (RBD) can be one of the first symptoms of childhood narcolepsy. Sleep Med 2007;7–8:784–6.
94. Lloyd R, Tippman-Peikert M, Slocumb N, et al. Characteristics of REM sleep behavior disorder in childhood. J Clin Sleep Med 2012;8:127–31.
95. Dauvilliers Y, Montplaisir J, Cochen V, et al. Post-H1N1 narcolepsy-cataplexy. Sleep 2010;33:1428–30.
96. Alshaikh MK, Tricco AC, Tashkandi M, et al. Sodium oxybate for narcolepsy with cataplexy: systematic review and meta-analysis. J Clin Sleep Med 2012;8:451–8.

Idiopathic Hypersomnia

Michael Kohrman

INTRODUCTION

Excessive daytime sleepiness in the adolescent is epidemic in our society. In the adolescent population, hypersomnolence manifests primarily as excessive daytime sleepiness. In part, symptoms are the result of school and lifestyle pressures. This is in combination with changes in circadian phase and total sleep time. In contrast, excessive daytime sleepiness manifesting as hypersomnolence is uncommon in young children. The primary manifestation of sleepiness in young children is hyperactivity. Young children respond to the symptom of sleepiness by increasing their motor activity to maintain alertness. However, even in this group, careful questioning does reveal symptoms of daytime sleepiness. The clinical definition of idiopathic hypersomnolence in childhood must take into account this difference in the clinical response of children to the same 'sleep pressure' manifested as excessive daytime sleepiness in adults.

Idiopathic hypersomnia (IH) is characterized by excessive daytime sleepiness and normal or long nocturnal sleep times, along with frequent and often prolonged naps. Both major sleep period and naps are typically unrefreshing.[1] PSG and MSLT demonstrate the absence of frequent periods of sleep onset with REM (SOREMP). The second edition of *The International Classification of Sleep Disorders: Diagnostic and Coding Manual* divides IH based on nocturnal sleep time: idiopathic hypersomnia with long sleep time (ICD-10-CM G47.11) and idiopathic hypersomnia without long sleep time (ICD-10-CM G47.11). Table 19.1 contrasts the clinical criteria between these two diagnoses and narcolepsy without cataplexy (ICD-10-CM G47.419).[1] The key objective difference between narcolepsy and IH is SOREMP in two or more MSLT naps associated with narcolepsy.

Both disorders of IH are associated with difficult awakenings, sleep drunkenness, and unrefreshing primary sleep periods/naps.[1,2] Guilleminault and Pelayo have divided idiopathic hypersomnia into three types based on etiology: those patients with a positive family history and positive HLA Cw2 antigen, a second type with history of viral infection, and a third group of those patients not included in the first two groups.[3] Bassetti and Aldrich divided their patients into three groups based on clinical symptoms.[2] The 'classic idiopathic hypersomnia' group tended to have sleepiness that was not overwhelming, take unrefreshing naps of up to 4 hours, have prolonged nighttime sleep, and difficulty awakening. The second group they termed a 'narcoleptic type' presented with overwhelming excessive daytime sleepiness, took short refreshing naps, and awakens without sleepiness. Their third group was a 'mixed group' with features of both syndromes.

Idiopathic hypersomnolence is a diagnosis of exclusion. A complete evaluation of other causes of hypersomnolence must be undertaken. The differential diagnosis of hypersomnolence is quite broad, ranging from mood disorders, to narcolepsy, to circadian rhythm disturbances or primary sleep disorders that cause excessive daytime sleepiness. Table 19.1 provides a framework based on etiology for further discussion of the differential diagnosis below.

EPIDEMIOLOGY

The incidence of diagnosis at major sleep centers varies from approximately 10% to 60% that of narcolepsy.[4,5] Anderson et al., in their series of 77 patients, noted that hypersomnia began at an age of 16.6 ± 9.4 years. Approximately two thirds of patients developed symptoms before the age of 18. The mean age of diagnosis was 30 years.[4] In addition, Anderson et al. found 34% had a family history of similar symptoms, and, in eight cases, more than one family member was affected. Ali et al. in their series of 85 patients, found a familial incidence of 58%.[6]

Anderson found that 18% of IH patients were positive for the HLA *DQB1*0602* antigen compared to 98% of patients with narcolepsy.[4] The Cw2 antigen was observed in 10% of IH patients. A case report of three adolescent-onset cases of IH in a two-generation family raises the question of autosomal dominant inheritance.[7]

PATHOPHYSIOLOGY

The underlying cause of the sleepiness in IH continues to be an active area of inquiry. Kanbayashi et al.[8] examined CSF levels of histamine in patients with IH, narcolepsy, OSA and normal neurologic controls. They found that low CSF histamine levels were mostly observed in non-medicated patients, and significant reductions compared to controls in histamine levels were observed only in non-medicated patients with hypocretin deficiency and with IH. In contrast, the levels in the medicated subjects with hypocretin deficiency and with IH did not differ significantly from those in control subjects. The authors also note that hypocretin-1 levels did not differ between medicated and non-medicated subjects in any of the hypersomnia categories.

Scammell and Mochizuki[9] note in an editorial in *Sleep* that reduced histamine signaling is an attractive explanation for the sleepiness of idiopathic hypersomnia. Parallel behavior between individuals with IH and mice with central histamine knockout (humans have great difficulty rousing from sleep in the morning, and mice lacking histamine exhibit a reduction in wake at the beginning of the usual active period).[10] Histamine H_3 receptors are inhibitory, exclusively located in the CNS.[8] H_3 receptor antagonists enhance central histaminergic neurotransmission specifically and are reported to enhance alertness in mouse models of narcolepsy. Kanbayashi's finding that low CSF histamine levels are observed in hypersomnia of central origin, regardless of hypocretin-1 status suggests a wider role for this mechanism in the treatment of hypersomnia.[8]

TABLE 19.1 Diagnostic Criteria

NARCOLEPSY WITHOUT CATAPLEXY	IDIOPATHIC HYPERSOMNIA WITH LONG SLEEP TIME	IDIOPATHIC HYPESOMNIA WITHOUT LONG SLEEPTIME
Complaint of EDS almost daily for more than 3 months	Complaint of EDS almost daily for more than 3 months	Complaint of EDS almost daily for more than 3 months
Typical cataplexy not reported	Prolonged nocturnal sleep greater than 10 h	Nocturnal sleep Duration normal (6–10 h)
PSG demonstrates at least 6 h sleep and no other cause for EDS	PSG demonstrates at least 6 h sleep and no other cause for EDS	PSG demonstrates at least 6 h sleep and no other cause for EDS
Mean sleep latency less than 8 min and 2 or more SOREMPs	Mean sleep latency less than 8 min and less than 2 SOREMPs	Mean sleep latency less than 8 min and less than 2 SOREMPs
Hypersomnia not better explained by another sleep disorder, medical condition, behavioral problem or substance abuse	Hypersomnia not better explained by another sleep disorder, medical condition, behavioral problem or substance abuse	Hypersomnia not better explained by another sleep disorder, medical condition, behavioral problem or substance abuse

Based on American Academy of Sleep Medicine. International classification of sleep disorders 2nd ed. Diagnostic and Coding manual. Westchester Illinois: American Academy of Sleep Medicine 2005.

Box 19-1   Diagnostic Studies to Define Idiopathic Hypersomnia

- Sleep log
- PSG
- Multipe Sleep Latency Test/Maintenance of Wakefulness Test
- Actigraphy
- MRI
- EEG
- Psychological testing
- Pediatric sleepiness scale

EVALUATION OF SLEEPINESS IN CHILDREN

Objective evaluation of sleepiness begins with a complete sleep history and physical examination to eliminate other causes of excessive daytime sleepiness (see Box 19-1). Sleep logs should be obtained to document sleep times, and actigraphy may be utilized to confirm the sleep log data. On the night prior to laboratory testing for daytime sleepiness, a polysomnogram should be obtained to confirm the absence of a primary sleep disorder. Hypersomnolence can be characterized quantitatively via the multiple sleep latency test (MSLT)[11] or maintenance of wakefulness test (MWT).[12] Both tests measure the time to fall asleep during the daytime. The MSLT requires the patient to fall asleep while the MWT requires the patient to stay awake. The mean adult sleep latency is 18.7 minutes. It is generally accepted that in the adult population the pathologic average sleep latency is 8 minutes or less as the result of the MSLT with an average sleep latency of 13.4 minutes.[13] Results from the MSLT and MWT often differ. Bonnet and Arand suggest that the MWT measures the sleep propensity and also the arousal system secondary to motivation and posture, while the MSLT is done supine and only measures sleep propensity.[14] Carskadon and Dement have demonstrated that sleep latency in children is age-dependent.[15] Using Tanner stages to group children during

adolescence, they observed a drop in average sleep latency on the MSLT of 20% between Tanner stages 1 and 3. This decreased sleep latency persisted in later adolescence (Tanner 4 and 5). In the same subjects, total sleep time and total REM time remained constant but total slow wave sleep time deceased by 70%. Mean sleep latency of Tanner 1 and 2 children (mean age 12 years sleeping their habitual average of 9.1 h) is 18 min. Compared to the college student (mean age 19 y, habitual sleep 7.1 h) of less than 5.5 minutes. The definition of pathological sleepiness in children must account for this age difference.

A number of pediatric sleepiness scales have been developed over the past 10 years. Lewandowski et al. reviewed 21 measures and found that only six met 'well-established' evidence-based assessment criteria.[16] Of these, only two: the Pediatric Daytime Sleepiness Scale (PDSS)[17] and the Sleep Disturbance Scale for Children (SDSC),[18] assessed EDS.

CLINICAL PRESENTATION

Bassetti and Aldrich reviewed 42 cases of idiopathic hypersomnia.[2] Onset of hypersomnolence was a mean age of 19 ± 8 years (range 6–43). Onset was associated with insomnia in five, weight gain in two, viral illness in four, and minor head trauma in three. Forty-five percent of patients snored. Sixty percent took one or more involuntary naps during the day. Over half the subjects took naps of 30 minutes or longer, and ¾ reported the naps were unrefreshing. Over half of the patients had psychiatric problems. Polysomnographic recordings demonstrated short sleep latency of 6.6 ± 5.7 min. Mean latency on the MSLT was 4.3 ± 2.1 minutes. In 5 of 12 patients who underwent esophageal pressure monitoring were found to have upper airway resistance syndrome. None of these patients reported improved sleep with CPAP.

In their series of 77 patients with IH, Ali et al.[6] found that hypersomnia began at a mean$\pm$SD age of 16.6 ± 9.4 years (range 0–46 years). Symptoms began before 18 years of age in 49 of 77 patients. Some patients and their families believed that the symptoms had been present from the first year of life, and, in 7 cases, worsening occurred over a period of several years. The mean age of diagnosis in this group was 30 years.[6] Precipitants were described by three subjects who reported a transient viral illness at the time of symptom onset, and one subject reported onset of symptoms over a day. The mean ESS score at initial presentation prior to treatment was 16.3±3.3 (range 11–24). In their study, Ali et al. noted that daytime somnolence interfered with work and social activities. The mean length of nighttime sleep reported was 9.2±1.8 hours, and this did not correlate with EES score.[6] There was no significant difference in MSLT between those with a long sleep time and those with a sleep time shorter than 10 hours. Seventy-six patients took nighttime sleep and sleep drunkenness was not observed.[6]

Typically, symptoms begin during childhood including prolonged nighttime sleep, and awakening difficulties often precede the onset of daytime sleepiness. Roth reported continuous non-imperative sleepiness prolonged unrefreshing naps without dreaming and difficult arousal.[19] The risk of automobile accident or near-miss event was reported in 50% of 50 adult patients with IH over a 5-year period in Japan.[10]

Polysomnographic studies from Baseetti and Aldrich's 42 patients demonstrated a sleep efficiency of 93%, mean of 20 total awakenings greater than 1 minute, 8% slow wave sleep, 18% REM sleep, automatic behaviors in 61%, and sleep paralysis in 40%.[2] Hours of sleep per day were 8.4±1.9 and time to activity in the morning 42 min. Forza et al. studied 10 patients with IH.[20] All had onset before age 21. There was no statistical difference between IH patients and controls for TST or sleep latency. Mean sleep latency was 9.1 minutes. IH patients demonstrated decreased SWS and increased REM sleep percent with a sleep latency of 5. ±0.7 min.

Anderson et al.,[4] in their study of 77 IH patients, found a mean sleep latency of 11.5 minutes ±8.2, increased mean slow wave sleep of 22.9%±8.7, and mean sleep efficiency of 94.3%. Ten patients had a sleep efficiency of less than 89%, and none. REM sleep latency and percentages of light sleep and REM sleep were normal. Results from MSLT in this group of IH patients demonstrated that a mean sleep latency in patients with idiopathic hypersomnia was 8.3±3.1 minutes, versus the narcolepsy group (4.1±2.6; P<0.001). Comparison of the IH grouped by MSLT with sleep latency ≥8 min or <8 min demonstrated no differences between these two groups in the duration of light sleep, slow-wave sleep, REM sleep, sleep latency, sleep efficiency, REM sleep latency, body mass index, or untreated ESS.

Ali et al.[6] found the median nocturnal sleep latency was similar for males and females, but on MSLT, the mean sleep latency for males was lower than that for females. Thirteen patients had one sleep-onset REM period (SOREMP) on either overnight polysomnography or MSLT, but none had two or more SOREMPs.

In a study of 75 patients with idiopathic hypersomnia with and without long sleep time, Vernet and Arnulf[21] found that hypersomniacs had more fatigue, higher anxiety and depression scores, and more frequent hypnagogic hallucinations (24%), sleep paralysis (28%), sleep drunkenness (36%), and unrefreshing naps (46%) than controls. *DQB1*0602* genotype was similar observed in 19% of controls and 24% of IH patients. Comparing the IH patients with long versus normal sleep time, those with long sleep time were younger, slimmer and more evening type characteristics and higher

sleep efficiencies than those without long sleep time. MSLT latencies were normal (>8 min) in 71% of IH patients with long sleep time.[21]

Box 19-2   Differential Diagnosis of Hypersomnolence

- Neurologic disorders
  - Epilepsy and anticonvulsant therapy
  - Stroke
  - Tumor/increased intracranial pressure
  - Narcolepsy
- Primary sleep disorders
  - Insufficient sleep syndrome
  - Insomnia
  - Upper airway resistance syndrome
  - OSAS
  - RLS
- Circadian disorders
  - Delayed phase syndrome
- Medical disorders
  - Infection: acute and chronic
  - Muscle diseases
  - Metabolic disorders
  - Prader–Willi syndrome
- Other disorders
  - ADHD
  - Chronic fatigue syndrome/fibromyalgia
  - Kleine-Levin syndrome
  - Mood disorders
  - Drug dependance/abuse

DIFFERENTIAL DIAGNOSIS OF IDIOPATHIC HYPERSOMNOLENCE

The differential diagnosis of idiopathic hypersomnolesence includes those disorders that can produce excessive daytime sleepiness. A list based on etiology is seen in Box 19-2. History, physical examination, polysomnography, and assessment of daytime sleep latency can usually exclude most of these diagnoses. Other chapters in this text cover most of these diagnoses and this chapter will only touch on those that are outside of the primary sleep disorders.

Primary Sleep Disorders

While diagnostic criteria are well established for the primary sleep disorders in adults, normative data on which to base clinical decisions are only recently available for children. Thus, the reader must apply pediatric normative values when diagnosing sleep-disordered breathing[22] or restless leg syndrome/periodic leg movement disorder.[23] Insufficient sleep syndrome is still the primary cause of daytime somnolence in most children. A number of studies have led to conflicting results with regards to school start times and daytime somnolence. Epstein et al. in Israel found decreased total sleep time and increased somnolence in fifth-grade pupils who started school at 7:10 a.m. versus 8 a.m.[24] A study in Maryland demonstrated no correlation of total sleep time with academic performance.[25]

Upper airway resistance syndrome remains a diagnosis that must be excluded in this patient population. The use of esophageal pressure manometry is controversial and consensus as to the usefulness of non-invasive measures nasal pressure, and arterial tonometry has not been established in evaluation of upper airway resistance.

Neurologic Disorders

Narcolepsy remains the most difficult clinical syndrome to exclude in this group of disorders. It can present as young as 4 years of age and often cataplexy may not appear until later in life. However, the recent understanding that the absence of orexin/hypocretin as the pathophysiologic cause will facilitate accurate diagnosis of this patient group. CSF assay for the absence of orexin is becoming a routine clinical test.[26]

Heier et al. looked at CSF hypocretin-1 levels in patients with IH and those with narcolepsy with or without cataplexy. None of the patients with IH, narcolepsy without cataplexy and those patients with HLA-negative narcolepsy with cataplexy had hypocretin levels less than 200 000 pg/mL. In contrast, 31/43 patients in the HLA-positive group had hypocretin levels less than 200 000 pg/mL.[27]

CNS lesions that produce increased intracranial pressure can be associated with hypersomnia. Poca et al. determined hypocretin levels in 26 patients with idiopathic intracranial hypertension and found no difference in these patients and their control group.[28] Subdural hematomas can produce an indolent syndrome of decreasing mental status and lethargy. Headache and vomiting are often associated with increased intracranial pressure. Epilepsy can produce a state in which the patient becomes lethargic and less responsive, the so-called petit-mal status or spike and wave stupor. During these periods, a pattern of the atypical continuous spike and wave discharges is observed on EEG. Petit-mal status is often responsive to valproic acid with rapid return to normal state. Anticonvulsants also can produce sedation and excessive daytime sleepiness or paradoxical hyperactivity in children. Sedation appears to be common with carbamazepine, while hyperactivity is more common with phenobarbital.

Other Disorders

Attention deficit hyperactivity disorder is an active area of investigation as to its relationship to sleep disruption. While both OSAS and RLS/PLMD are associated with hyperactivity in children, attention deficit hyperactivity disorder is multi-factorial in origin and sleep disorders and account for the etiology in a significant fraction of children with ADHD.

Chronic fatigue/fibromyalgia syndrome is also a diagnosis of exclusion. Children often complain of diffuse muscle aches, trigger points may be observed. The symptom is described as tiredness rather than true hypersomnia. Polysomnography may demonstrate an alpha–delta pattern on EEG.[29] Depression and upper airway resistance syndrome must be excluded in chronic fatigue patients as well.

Childhood mood disorders are commonly associated with sleep difficulties. Symptoms often manifest as insomnia, early morning awakenings, daytime sleepiness or hypersomnia. Vgontzas et al. found increased sleep latency (54 vs 15 min), increased wake time after sleep onset (79 vs 56.8 min), and increase total wake time (134 vs 72 min) in patients with psychiatric etiologies for their hypersomnia compared to patients with idiopathic hypersomnia. In patients with psychiatric disorders, REM sleep was decreased, compared to patients with idiopathic hypersomnia.[30] Bipolar disorder may also present with hypersomnia during the depression phase of

the illness. At times, there may be overlap with Kleine–Levin syndrome (see Chapter 20).

Circadian Disorders

Delayed-phase syndrome may also produce hypersomnolence. Affected children, however, report normal total sleep times in the presence of delayed sleep onset and morning hypersomnia (see Chapter 5). Non–24-hour sleep–wake cycles as well as advanced sleep-phase syndrome may also produce hypersomnolence. Sleep logs and/or actigraphy are often helpful in differentiating these problems.

Medical Disorders

Recovery from acute viral or bacterial illness often results in hypersomnolence. Hypersomnolence associated with fever and stiff neck should alert the examiner to possible meningitis. Stiff neck and other meningeal signs may be absent in children under 1 year of age. Lumbar puncture should always be performed if any question of meningitis exists. Kuboto et al. report a case of acute disseminated encephalomyelitis associated with hypersomnolence as the major presenting feature and low hypocretin levels in the CSF.[31] Arii et al. describe hypersomnolence and low hypocretin levels in a child after removal of a hypothalamic tumor.[32]

Metabolic disorders may produce episodic mental status changes that produce sleepiness and altered mental status. Disorders of ammonia metabolism, lactate and pyruvate metabolism, and mitochondrial metabolism can be associated with episodic hypersomnia. Acute infection or other metabolic stress often precipitates these episodes. Muscle weakness can also be a source of hypersomnolence. In primary muscle disease, the dystrophies are often associated with decreased respiratory effort secondary to fatigue. Polysomnography demonstrates increasing REM-related central apnea as the first sign of weakness and need for nocturnal respiratory support.[33]

Prader–Willi syndrome is associated with obesity, cranial-facial dysmorphyism, hypotonia, hyperphasia, hypersomnia, and hypothalamic dysfunction. Manni et al. found sleep-onset REM periods in 5 of 10 children with Prader–Willi syndrome on MSLT.[34] None of the patients was Dr 15 or Dq 6 positive. Hypersomnia and SOREMPs could not be accounted for by sleep-disordered breathing alone; however, UARS was not excluded in these patients.

TREATMENT

The goal in IH is improvement in quality of life and improvement in symptoms of excessive daytime sleepiness. In untreated IH patients greater than 20 years of age, Özaki et al.[35] found decreased subscale scores in 7/9 domains of the SF-36, compared to normal. The changes did correlate with ESS scores in domains of autonomy, in controlling one's own job schedule, experience of divorce or break-up with a partner due to symptoms, experience of being forced to relocate or being dismissed due to symptoms and perception of support of others. Treatment improved ESS scores. They concluded that the decrease of HRQOL could be attributed to psychological, social, and environmental factors, such as lifestyle or social support rather than subjective sleepiness.[35] Comparing patients with IH and narcolepsy without cataplexy Dauvilliers

TABLE 19.2 Stimulants Used for Treatment of Idiopathic Hypersomnolence

NAME	DURATION OF ACTION	CONTRAINDICATIONS	SPECIAL CONSIDERATIONS
Methylphenidate	4–6 h	Increased risk of cardiac arrhythmias	
Time release preps	8–12 h		Longer action
Dexmethylphenidate	4–6 h		Isomer of parent compound
Dextroamphetamines	4–6 h		
Time spans	6–12 h		
Mixed salts	4–6 h		
Extended release preps	8–12 h		Longer duration of action
Modafinil	6–8 h		Non amphetamine drugs
Armodafinil	6–8 h		
Pemoline	12 h	High risk of liver disease	Rarely used

et al. found similar results of the Beck Depression Scale and SF36 in both groups. These results contrasted with the narcolepsy with cataplexy group who demonstrated higher mean scores and increased percentage with a score greater than 7 (31.8% vs 18.1% in the IH group) on the Beck inventory.[36]

Treatment of idiopathic hypersomnia is focused on symptom control, as the primary etiology remains unknown. The goal of therapy is to allow the patient to enjoy normal alert functioning and restful nocturnal sleep.

The approach to therapy is sleep hygiene, appropriate use of stimulant medication and safety for the patient. Sleep hygiene measures should include scheduled naps and regular sleep periods of 8–10 hours nightly. Medications, drugs or alcohol that promote sleepiness should be avoided. Stimulant medication should be used at the lowest effective doses tolerated. Growth problems secondary to anorexia can be a limiting factor for stimulant use is some children. In addition, a balanced plan of stimulant use must be maintained so as not to interfere with nighttime sleep. The newer longer-acting stimulants (Table 19.2) have been beneficial in management, keeping medicine out of the school setting and decreasing the need for late afternoon dosing. The American Academy of Child and Adolescent Psychiatry has produced a practice parameter for stimulant use in children, adolescents, and adults.[37] In 2007, the American Academy of Sleep Medicine produced a practice parameter for the treatment of narcolepsy and other hypersomnias of central origin.[38] They concluded, 'Treatment of hypersomnia of central origin with methylphenidate or modafinil in children between the ages of 6 and 15 appears to be relatively safe.' They recommend regular follow-up of patients to monitor response to treatment and side effects and to enhance the patient's adaptation to the disorder.[38]

A number of retrospective studies examined modafinil versus methylphenidate. Ali et al.[6] followed 85 patients for a median duration of 2.4 years. In their group, 65% of patients demonstrated a 'complete response' to pharmacotherapy. Methylphenidate was the most commonly used as a first-line agent prior to December 1998, but after its approval modafinil became the most commonly used first drug. At the last visit, 92% of patients were on monotherapy, 51% on methylphenidate versus 32% on modafinil. No difference in the response rate between the two drugs was demonstrated.[6] Adult dosing in this study was 367.4±140.9 mg for modafinil and 50.9±27.3 mg for methylphenidate.[6] Lavault et al.[39] reviewed response to therapy with modifinil in 104 patients with IH (59 with long sleep time compared to patients with narcolepsy with cataplexy). They found similar response to modifinil in both patient populations. Improvement in ESS scores was greater in the IH group without long sleep time compared to those with long sleep time. Loss of efficacy and habituation were rare. Adult doses of modifinil in this study ranged from 50 to 600 mg.[39] In 66 patients with IH, Anderson et al. found that 11 had spontaneous remission. No clinical characteristics could be identified to differentiate the spontaneous remitters.[4] In this study, 24/39 patients treated with modinifinil had a 4-point or greater reduction in ESS.[4]

SUMMARY

Idiopathic hypersomnia remains a diagnosis of exclusion, and at times it can be difficult to differentiate from the other disorders producing hypersomnolence in (see Table 19.1). Continued research is necessary to better characterize this disorder in children. Treatment should be symptomatic; naps, improved sleep hygiene and stimulants should be used in concert to improve quality of life in affected children. While no dosing studies are available for children, both modifinil and methylphenidate appear to be safe and effective treatments. The role of histamine in the etiology of idiopathic hypersomnia in children requires further exploration and may lead to future treatment in hypersomnias of central origin.

Clinical Pearls

- Idiopathic hypersomnia is a diagnosis of exclusion.
- Narcolepsy without cataplexy can be distinguished by sleep-onset REM periods.
- Inadequate sleep hygiene is the most common cause of daytime sleepiness in adolescents and adults.
- Use of actigraphy may be helpful to distinguish the disorder from the consequences of inadequate sleep.

References

1. American Academy of Sleep Medicine. International classification of sleep disorders 2nd ed. Diagnostic and coding manual. Westchester Illinois: American Academy of Sleep Medicine; 2005.
2. Bassetti C, Aldrich MS. Idiopathic hypersomnia aseries of 42 patients. Brain 1997;120:1423–35.
3. Guilleminault C, Pelayo R. Idiopathic central nervous system hypersomnia. In: Kryger MH, Roth T, Dement WC, editors. Practice and principles of sleep medicine. 3rd ed. W.B. Saunders; 2000. p. 687–92.
4. Anderson KN, Pilsworth S, Sharples LD, et al. Idiopathic hypersomnia: a study of 77 cases. Sleep 2007;30(10):1274–81.
5. Han F, Lin L, Li J, et al. Presentations of primary hypersomnia in Chinese children. Sleep 2011;34(5):627–32.
6. Ali M, Auger RR, Slocumb NL, et al. Idiopathic hypersomnia: clinical features and response to treatment. J Clin Sleep Med 2009;5(6):562–8.
7. Janackova S, Motte J, Bakchine S, et al. Idiopathic hypersomnia: a repot of three adolescent-onset cases in a two-generation family. J Child Neurol 2011 Apr;26(4):522–5.
8. Kanbayashi T, Kodama T, Kondo H, et al. CSF histamine contents in narcolepsy, idiopathic hypersomnia and obstructive sleep apnea syndrome. Sleep 2009;32(2):181–7.
9. Scammell TE, Mochizuki T. Is low histamine a fundamental cause of sleepiness in narcolepsy and idiopathic hypersomnia? Sleep 2009;32(2):133–4.
10. Parmentier R, Ohtsu H, Djebbara-Hannas Z, et al. Anatomical, physiological, and pharmacological characteristics of histidine decarboxylase knock-out mice: evidence for the role of brain histamine in behavioral and sleep-wake control. J Neurosci 2002;22:7695–711.
11. Carskadon MA, Dement WC, Mitler MM, et al. Guidelines for the multiple sleep latency test (MSLT): a standard measure of slepiness Sleep 1986;9:519–24.
12. Mitler MM, Gujavarti KS, Browman CP. Maintenance of wakefulness test: a polysomnographic technique for evaluation of treatment efficacy in patients with excessive somnolence. Electroencephalogr Clin Neurophysiol 1982;53:658–61.
13. Mitler MM, Carskadon MA, Hirshkowitz M. Evaluating sleepiness. In: Kryger MH, Roth T, Dement WC, editors. Practice and principles of sleep medicine. 3rd ed. Philadelphia: W.B. Saunders; 2000.
14. Bonnet MH, Arand DL. Arousal components which differentiate the MWT from the MSLT. Sleep 2001;24:441–7.
15. Carskadon MA, Dement WC. Sleepiness in the normal adolescent. In: Guilleminault C, editor. Sleep and its disorders in children. New York: Raven Press; 1987. p .53–66.
16. Lewandowski AS, Toliver-Sokol M, Palermo TM. Evidence-based review of subjective pediatric sleep measures. J Pediatr Psychol 2011;36(7):780–93.
17. Drake C, Nickel C, Burduvali E, et al. The Pediatric Daytime Sleepiness Scale (PDSS): Sleep habits and school outcomes in middle-school children. Sleep 2003;26(4):455–8.
18. Bruni O, Ottaviano S, Guidetti V, et al. The Sleep Disturbance Scale for Children (SDSC). Construction and validation of an instrument to evaluate sleep disturbances in childhood andadolescence. J Sleep Res1996;5(4):251–61.
19. Roth B. Narcolepsy and hypersomnia. Basel: Karger; 1980.
20. Forza E, Gaudreau H, Petit D, et al. Homeostatic sleep regulation in patients with idiopthic hypersomnia. Clin Neurphysiol 2000;111:277–82.
21. Vernet C, Arnulf I. Idiopathic hypersomnia with and without long sleep time: a controlled series of 75 patients. Sleep 2009;32(6):753–9.
22. Goodwin JL, Enright PL, Morgan WJ, et al. Correlates of obstructive sleep apnea in 6–12 year old children. The Tucson Children Assessment of Sleep Apnea Study (TUCASA). Sleep 2002;25 abstract supplement:A80.
23. Kohrman MH, Kerr SL, Schumacher S. Effect of sleep disordered breathing on periodic leg movements of sleep in children. Sleep 1997;20:abstract supplement.
24. Epstein R, Chillag N, Lavie P. Starting times of school: effects on daytime functioning of fifth grade children in Israel. Sleep 1998;21:250–6.
25. King J, Gould B, Eliasson A. Association of sleep and academic performance. Sleep Breath 2002;45–8.
26. Nishino S, Ripley B, Overeem S, et al. Hypocretin (orexin) deficency in human narcolepsy. Lancet 2000;355:39–40.
27. Heier MS, Evsiukova T, Vilming S, et al. CSF hypocretin-1 levels and clinical profiles in narcolepsy and idiopathic CNS hypersomnia in Norway. Sleep 2007;30(8):969–73.
28. Poca MA, Galard R, Serrano E, et al. Normal hypocretin-1 (orexin A) levels in cerebrospinal fluid in patients with idiopathic intracranial hypertension. Acta Neurochir Suppl 2012;114:221–5.
29. Whelton CL, Salit I, Moldofsky H. Sleep, Epstein–Barr virus infection, musculotal pain and depressive symptons in chronic fatigue syndrome J Rheumatol 1992;19:939–43.
30. Vgontzas AN, Bixler EO, Kales A, et al A. Differences in nocturnal and daytime sleep between primary and psychiatric hypersomnia: diagnostic and treatment implications. Psychosomatic Med 2000;62:220–6.
31. Kubota H, Kanbayashi T, Tanabe Y, et al. A case if acute disseminrated encephalomyletis presenting hypersomnia with decreased hypocretin level in cerebrospinal fluid. J Child Neuro 2002;17:537–9.
32. Arii J, Kanbayashi T, Tababe Y, et al. A hypersomnolent girl with decreased CSF hypocretin level after removal of a hypothalamic tumor. Neurology 2001;56:1775–6.
33. Kerr SL, Kohrman MH. Polysomnogram in Duchenne muscular dystrophy. J Child Neurol 1994;9:332–4.
34. Manni R, Politini L, Nobili L, et al. Hypersomnia in the Prader-Willi syndrome:clinical – electrophysiological features and underlying factors. Clin Neurophysiol 2001;112:800–5.
35. Ozaki A, Inoue Y, Nakajima T, et al. Health-related quality of life among drug-naïve patients with narcolepsy with cataplexy, narcolepsy without cataplexy, and idiopathic hypersomnia without long sleep time. J Clin Sleep Med 2008;4(6):572–8.
36. Dauvilliers Y, Paquereau J, Bastuji H, et al. Psychological health in central hypersomnias: the French Harmony study. J Neurol Neurosurg Psychiatry 2009;80:636–41.
37. Greenhill LL, Plixzka S, Dulcan MK, Work Group on Quality Issues. Practice parameter for the use of stimulant medications in the treatment of children, adolescents, and adults. J Am Acad Child Adolesc Psychiatry 2002;41:26S–49S.
38. Kapur VK, Brown T, Swick TJ, et al. Standards of Practice Committee of the AASM. Practice parameters for the treatment of narcolepsy and other hypersomnias of central origin. Sleep 2007;30(12):1705–11.
39. Lavault S, Dauvilliers Y, Drouot X, et al. Benefit and risk of modafinil in idiopathic hypersomnia vs. narcolepsy with cataplexy. Sleep Med 2011;12:550–6.

Kleine-Levin Syndrome and Recurrent Hypersomnias

Stephen H. Sheldon

INTRODUCTION

Kleine-Levin syndrome is an unusual disorder of recurrent episodes of excessive sleepiness and prolonged total sleep time. It is a rare syndrome with an onset typically in late adolescence, but younger and older cases have been reported. It has been suggested that a predisposing event occurs prior to onset of symptoms.[1] This may occur in nearly half of the reported cases. Most commonly, a flu-like syndrome precedes the onset of symptoms.

CLINICAL CHARACTERISTICS

Hypersomnia is the characteristic symptom of the Kleine–Levin syndrome. Sleepiness is profound and, during spells, patients may sleep continuously for more than 20 hours. This excessive sleepiness and true hypersomnia can develop suddenly. However, symptoms typically have a more gradual onset of 1–7 days. During spells of hypersomnia, patients rarely leave their beds and sleep continuously. Sleep may be calm, but at times agitated, restless sleep occurs and vivid dreams are occasionally reported.

In addition to excessively long sleep episodes, abnormal behaviors, including but not limited to compulsive and excessive overeating and sexually acting-out behaviors occur. Other mental disturbances may be present. Compulsive overeating and hypersexuality may not be present with each episode. Excessive caloric intake during spells frequently results in weight gain by the end of the spell.

Overt expression of hypersexuality may include indiscriminate sexual advances, masturbation, and/or public display of sexual fantasy. Sexually acting-out is reported in approximately one-third of males with Kleine–Levin syndrome. Hypersexuality is less often reported in females. The presence of excessive eating and/or hypersexuality is not required for the diagnosis of Kleine–Levin syndrome. In many cases, hypersomnia and its recurrence may be the only symptom.[2] Psychological symptoms vary considerably. Irritability is common. Confusion, visual hallucinations, or auditory hallucinations frequently occur.

Recurrent episodes of hypersomnia may be brief and last less than 1 week or may be prolonged and last up to 30 days. Characteristic of the Kleine–Levin syndrome is recurrence of episodes of hypersomnia and behavioral abnormalities. Patients are normal between episodes. Nevertheless, neuropsychological sequelae, changes in personality, and decrease in school performance have been reported after a second hypersomnolent episode. Physical examination is generally normal.

Although Kleine–Levin syndrome is characterized by the triad of recurrent spells of hypersomnolence, hyperphagia, and hypersexuality, it is likely that incomplete manifestation is more common than the complete triad. Isolated abnormal sleepiness and recurrent periods of hypersomnia without associated symptoms may be a more common manifestation.

Periods of hypersomnia gradually decrease in frequency as the youngster ages. Spells gradually become less severe and eventually resolve.[3] Nonetheless, patients have been reported with recurrent episodes of hypersomnia occurring 20 years after the initial onset of symptoms.[4,5]

Menstruation-associated hypersomnia has been reported in female patients. Recurrent periods of hypersomnolence occur and are coupled to menses. Occasionally, mental disturbances also occur, and also occur with the menstrual cycle.[6] (Several female patients with recurrent hypersomnia had notable absence of symptoms.[1]) Prognosis of menstrual-related hypersomnia is similar to that of the Kleine–Levin syndrome.

ETIOLOGY

The cause of recurrent hypersomnia is unknown. A possible viral etiology may be present in some cases. In other cases, there may be a suggestion of a local encephalitis in the region of the diencephalon.[7-9] Recurrent transient episodes of unresponsiveness and clearly identified stage 2 sleep pattern with the presence of sleep spindles has also been reported due to bilateral paramedian thalamic infarctions.[10] Although the exact cause of recurrent hypersomnia and other manifestations is still unclear, the symptoms of hypersomnolence, excessive and compulsive eating, hypersexuality, recurrence, and absence of any identifiable abnormalities between spells is suggestive of a functional abnormality at the level of the diencephalon. The hypothalamus may also be involved. Indeed, identical symptoms have been reported in patients with tumors of the hypothalamus or third ventricle and in patients with epidemic encephalitis. Most literature and case reports suggest that this recurrent hypersomnia is caused by dysfunction of the hypothalamus and midbrain limbic system. There is also evidence that brainstem dysfunction may also be involved. Recurrent hypersomnia associated with decreased blood flow in the thalamus on single photon emission computed tomography has also been reported.[11] During the remission period, there were no abnormal data in these tests.

Social and professional consequences are not negligible. Students miss classes and young workers may be fired because of repeated absences.

Neuroendocrine function in patients with Kleine–Levin syndrome has been assessed; however, only a limited number of subjects have been investigated and most literature consists of case reports. Investigation is complicated by the inability to predict timing of episodes, lack of a prodromal period and relatively rapid recovery once symptoms begin.

Nonetheless, some abnormal laboratory data reported to date include a paradoxical growth hormone response to thyroid-releasing hormone stimulation,[12] a blunted cortisol response to insulin-induced hypoglycemia,[13,14] and an absent thyroid-stimulating hormone response to thyroid-releasing hormone.[13] These findings suggest a possible dysfunction within the hypothalamic–pituitary axis. However, other basal and post-stimulation values of hormones are usually normal and laboratory values are normal during the asymptomatic periods between spells.

Studies of nocturnal or 24-hour secretory patterns of pituitary hormones have been conducted in a limited number of patients. Normal secretory pattern of growth hormone was reported in one patient, but the sampling at 4-hour intervals was sparse.[15] On the other hand, an elevated growth hormone secretory pattern was reported in two patients.[16] A normal secretory pattern of cortisol and somewhat abnormal patterns of growth hormone have been identified in four other patients.[17] Normal 24-hour patterns of melatonin, prolactin, and cortisol secretion have been reported.[18] Gadoth and colleagues found an increased nocturnal prolactin secretory pattern and an abnormally flat nocturnal luteinizing hormone secretory pattern, whereas follicle-stimulating hormone and thyroid-stimulating hormone secretory patterns were normal.[12] Chesson and Levine compared 24-hour secretions in the symptomatic and the asymptomatic period and found that values obtained during nocturnal sleep showed a significantly decreased growth hormone, but increased prolactin and thyroid-stimulating hormone, in a direction that supports the hypothesis that dopamine tone is reduced during the symptomatic period in Kleine–Levin syndrome.[19] However, Mayer and colleagues found only minor hormonal changes in five patients.[20] Altogether, these data suggest some functional disturbance in the hypothalamic–pituitary axis in Kleine–Levin syndrome, but the disturbance may be in response to the sleep-related and behavioral changes rather than a cause. An observation supporting a diencephalic dysfunction is the occurrence of dysautonomic features in some patients.[21] Differentiating Kleine–Levin syndrome from organic etiologies is often difficult. Diagnosis is often based on clinical presentation of recurrence of symptoms with asymptomatic intervals and progressive improvement to resolution. In addition, it is often a diagnosis of exclusion. Recurrent hypersomnia may occur with space-occupying lesions of the central nervous system, idiopathic recurring stupor, and certain psychological/psychiatric conditions.

Tumors in the region of the third ventricle, such as cysts, astrocytomas, and/or craniopharyngiomas, may be responsible for intermittent obstruction of the third ventricle leading to headache, vomiting, sensory disturbances, and intermittent impairment of alertness. Less frequently, tumors in other CNS locations may result in hypersomnia. Tumors in the middle fossa may disrupt the suprachiasmatic nucleus and an irregular sleep–wake pattern or a free-running state might occur. If a free running state occurs, hypersomnia may alternate with sleeplessness at a regular interval as the pacemaker cycles at its inherent rhythm. Recurrent hypersomnia may also develop after encephalitis or head trauma. Periodic hypersomnia has also been reported in a patient with a Rathke's cleft cyst.[22]

Major recurrent depression and bipolar affective disorder can be associated with excessive sleepiness.[23] Patients with psychogenic recurrent hypersomnia complain of extreme sleepiness and fatigue, and may spend many hours in bed. Continuous night-and-day polygraphic recording often fails to demonstrate increased total sleep time despite the complaint of sleepiness.[24]

EVALUATION

The diagnosis of Kleine–Levin syndrome is typically based on clinical features. Laboratory evaluations are occasionally useful, since the diagnosis may be one of exclusion of other similar pathology. CBC, platelet count, electrolytes, renal and liver function tests, calcium, phosphorus, serum protein electrophoresis, immunoglobulins, antinuclear antibodies, rheumatoid factor, and serum titers for herpes simplex, Epstein–Barr virus, cytomegalovirus, varicella-zoster, mumps, and measles have all been found to be normal in patients with Kleine–Levin syndrome both during episodes and between episodes. Cerebrospinal fluid evaluation with cultures for bacteria, mycobacterium, virus, and fungi have also been shown to be negative.

Routine EEG obtained during attacks may show generalized slowing of background activity or may be unremarkable. MRI is normal during and between spells of hypersomnia.[19] Prolonged polysomnographic monitoring may reveal the increased total sleep time. During symptomatic periods, the multiple sleep latency test (MSLT) can reveal abnormal sleep latencies and sleep-onset REM periods (SOREMPS). Therefore, it has been suggested the multiple sleep latency test may be useful in diagnosis, especially when the PSG and multiple sleep latency test are performed no earlier than the second night after the onset of hypersomnolent.[25] During asymptomatic periods polysomnography and MSLT are both normal.[26]

TREATMENT

Kleine–Levin syndrome is typically treated symptomatically.[27,28] Interventions are focused on terminating the hypersomnia episode. Amphetamines and methylphenidate, and modafinil have been utilized in both treatment and prevention.[29] No treatment has been consistently successful. Gabapentin has been effective in preventing symptoms in some patients.[30] Generally, the effectiveness of maintaining wakefulness, treating symptoms, and prevention of recurrences using a variety of therapeutic approaches does not seem effective.

Clinical Pearls

- Kleine–Levin syndrome is an uncommon disorder occurring most often in males (but can occur in females) during middle adolescence.
- It is characterized by recurrent hypersomnia, hyperphagia, and hypersexual behavior.
- Underlying etiology is unclear and the exact pathophysiological mechanism is still to be determined.
- Treatment and prevention are based on symptomatology, and therapeutic response varies.
- Most often, there is spontaneous resolution of symptoms without noted sequelae.

References

1. Huang YS, Guilleminault C, Lin KL, et al. Relationship between Kleine–Levin syndrome and upper respiratory tract infection in Taiwan. Sleep 2012;35(1):123–9.
2. Kesler A, Gadoth N, Vainstein G, et al. Kleine–Levin syndrome (KLS) in young females. Sleep 2000;23(4):563–7.
3. Critchley M. Periodic hypersomnia and megaphagia in adolescent males. Brain 1962;85:627–56.
4. Gran D, Begemann H. Neue Beobachtungen bei einem fall von Kleine–Levin Syndrom Munch Med Wochenschr 1973;115:1098–102.
5. Bucking PH, Palmer WR. New contribution to the clinical aspects and pathophysiology of the Kleine–Levin syndrome. MMW Munch Med Wochenschr 1978;120(47):1571–2.
6. Billiard M, Guilleminault C, Dement WC. A menstruation-linked periodic hypersomnia. Neurology 1975;25:436–43.
7. Kesler A, Gadoth N, Vainstein G, et al. Kleine-Levine syndrome (KLS) in young female. Sleep 2000;23(4):563–7.
8. Carpenter S, Yassa R, Ochs R. A pathological basis for Kleine–Levin syndrome. Arch Neurol 1982;39:25–8.
9. Fenzi F, Simonati A, Crosato F, et al. Clinical features of Kleine–Levin syndrome with localized encephalitis. Neuropediatrics 1993;24:292–5.
10. Bjornstad B, Goodman SH, Sirven JI, et al. Paroxysmal sleep as presenting symptom of bilateral paramedian thalamic infarction. Mayo Clin Proc 2003;78:347–9.
11. Nose I, Ookawa T, Tanaka J, et al. Decreased blood flow of the left thalamus during somnolent episodes in a case of recurrent hypersomnia. Psychiatr Clin Neurosci 2002;56:277–8.
12. Gadoth N, Dickerman Z, Bechar M, et al. Episodic hormone secretion during sleep in Kleine–Levin syndrome: evidence for hypothalamic dysfunction. Brain Dev 1987;9:309–15.
13. Koerber RK, Torkelson R, Haven G, et al. Increased cerebrospinal fluid 5-hydroxytryptamine and 5-hydroxyindoleacetic acid in Kleine–Levin syndrome. Neurology 1984;34:1597–600.
14. Fernandez JM, Lara I, Gila L, et al. Disturbed hypothalamic-pituitary axis in idiopathic recurring hypersomnia syndrome. Acta Neurol Scand 1990;82(6):361–3.
15. Gilligan BS. Periodic megaphagia and hypersomnia – an example of the Kleine–Levine syndrome in an adolescent girl. Proc Aust Assoc Neurol 1973;9:67–72.
16. Kaneda H, Sugita Y, Masoaka S, et al. Red blood cell concentration and growth hormone release in periodic hypersomnia. Waking Sleeping 1977;1:369–74.
17. Hishikawa Y, Iijima S, Tashiro T, et al. Polysomnographic findings and growth hormone secretion in patents with periodic hypersomnia. In: Koella WP, editor. Sleep. Basel: Karger; 1981. p. 128–33.
18. Thompson C, Obrecht R, Franey C, et al. Neuroendocrine rhythms in a patient with the Kleine–Levin syndrome. Br J Psychiatry 1985;147:440–3.
19. Chesson AL, Levine SN. Neuroendocrine evaluation in Kleine–Levin syndrome: evidence of reduced dopaminergic tone during periods of hypersomnolence. Sleep 1991;14:226–32.
20. Mayer G, Leonhard E, Krieg J, et al. Endocrinological and polysomnographic findings in Kleine–Levin syndrome: no evidence for hypothalamic and circadian dysfunction. Sleep 1998;21:278–84.
21. Hegarty A, Merriam AE. Autonomic events in Kleine–Levin syndrome. Am J Psychiatry 1990;147:951–2.
22. Autret A, Lucas B, Mondon K, et al. Sleep and brain lesions: a critical review of the literature and additional new cases. Neurophysiol Clin 2001;31(6):356–75.
23. Jeffries JJ, Lefebvre A. Depression and mania associated with Kleine–Levin–Critchley syndrome. Can Psychiatr Assoc J 1973;18:439–44.
24. Billiard M, Cadilhac J. Les hypersomnies recurrentes. Rev Neurol (Paris) 1988;144:249–58.
25. Rosenow F, Kotagal P, Cohen BH, et al. Multiple sleep latency test and polysomnography in diagnosing Kleine–Levin syndrome and periodic hypersomnia. J Clin Neurophysiol 2000;17(5):519–22.
26. Huang YS, Lin YH, Guilleminault C. Polysomnography in Kleine–Levin syndrome. Neurology 2008;70(10):795–801.
27. Oliveria MM, Conti C, Saconato H, et al. Pharmacological treatment for Kleine-Levin syndrome. Cochrane Database of Systematic Reviews 2009;(2):CD006685.
28. Arnulf I, Lecendreux M, Franco P, et al. Kleine–Levin syndrome: state of the art. Revue Neurologique 2008;164(8–9):658–68.
29. Huang YS, Lakkis C, Guilleminault C. Kleine–Levin syndrome: current status. Med Clin N Am 2010;94(3):557–62.
30. Itokawa K, Fukui M, Ninomiya M, et al. Gabapentin for Kleine–Levin syndrome. Intern Med 2009;48(13):1183–5.

Post-Traumatic and Post-Neurosurgical Hypersomnia

Rafael Pelayo

For children with post-traumatic and post-neurosurgical hypersomnia the best-fitting diagnosis within the International Classification of Sleep Disorders (ICSD) 2e is hypersomnia due to a medical condition.[1] By definition, excessive sleepiness is described as having a duration of more than 3 months, although it may be more pragmatic to make this clinical diagnosis earlier. References cited in the ICSD are more applicable for adults. There is no clear distinction made for post-traumatic hypersomnia in children. Children who suffer significant head injury frequently experience significant sleep disturbances, particularly when the injury is severe enough to result in major loss of consciousness. Nonetheless, sleep disturbances may follow minor trauma in which a brief loss of consciousness occurs. In all instances, sleep patterns after the injury vary notably from the pre-trauma sleep habits.

Closed-head trauma is the most common event resulting in post-traumatic hypersomnia. Similar symptoms may occur after neurosurgical procedures and other brain traumas. It appears that the cause is less important than the location. Symptomatically, there is a variable period of initial coma that evolves into a post-traumatic hypersomnolence and excessive daytime sleepiness with or without sleep attacks or unintentional sleep episodes. Nocturnal sleep may or may not be prolonged compared with the pre-injury period. When total sleep time within each 24-hour day is increased, the term 'post-traumatic hypersomnia' is fitting. Associated symptoms are typically due to daytime sleepiness (e.g., concentration difficulties, amnesia of recent events, fatigue, and occasional visual problems). Chronic headache and minor neurologic signs of traumatic brain injury may also be present.

Every year in the United States, 50 000 people die and more than 1.4 million seek medical care for traumatic brain injuries (TBI). Approximately 5.3 million Americans live with brain-injury-associated long-term disabilities, such as seizure disorders and cognitive and psychosocial impairments.[2] TBI is a leading cause of morbidity and mortality in children. Each year, almost half a million children seek emergency care because of head trauma. Fortunately, the majority of children (90%) suffer only from minor injuries. Nevertheless, 37 000 children require hospitalization, and up to 2685 children per year do not survive their sustained injuries.[3] The CDC (Centers for Disease Control and Prevention in the United States) reports TBI-related death rates for the different age groups as follows: 5.7/100 000 (0–4 years), 3.1/100 000 (5–9 years), and 4.8/100 000 (10–14 years). This rate increases approximately fivefold (24.3/100 000) for patients between 15 and 19 years. Pediatric TBI is most commonly caused by falls and non-accidental injury in younger children, and road traffic accidents (as pedestrians or passengers) in older children and adolescents.[4]

Head trauma has been reported to increase the likelihood of sleep-disordered breathing.[5] A polysomnogram may be necessary to exclude this etiology for the hypersomnia. The mechanism by which head trauma may result in sleep-disordered breathing is not clear. It is hypothesized that a whiplash type of injury may damage the pharyngeal nerves, which would alter some of the airway reflexes. Performing a polysomnogram may not be clinically possible in a child after a head injury. Empiric use of positive airway pressure (PAP) therapy should be used very cautiously since basilar skull fractures are a contraindication to PAP due to potential pneumocephaly.

Ideally, quantification of hypersomnia with a multiple sleep latency test, MSLT, may be helpful, especially to distinguish true sleepiness from fatigue or depression. However, in the presence of severe trauma, conducting and interpreting an MSLT may not be possible. The ICSD specifically states that a clinical complaint of excessive sleepiness is 'far more important' than a short sleep latency on an MSLT.[1]

A key question asked by patients and family members when addressing post-traumatic or post-neurosurgical hypersomnia is how long will the condition last and will it spontaneously resolve with time. To evaluate the prevalence and natural history of sleepiness following traumatic brain injury, Watson and colleagues undertook a prospective cohort study of 514 young men and adolescents with traumatic brain injury (TBI). The TBI group was compared to 132 non-cranial trauma controls, and 102 trauma-free controls. Subjects were evaluated at 1 month and 1 year after injury. Sleepiness was measured subjectively with a self-administered questionnaire from which the following four questions were asked: (1) I am sleeping or dozing most of the time – day or night, (2) I sit around half-asleep, (3) I sleep or nap more during the day, and (4) I sleep longer during the night. At the 1-month time point more than half of the TBI subjects reported sleepiness (55%). Of interest, 41% of non-cranial trauma controls also reported sleepiness, as did only 3% of trauma-free controls. The TBI group was not only more likely to report being sleepy but the severity of the sleepiness was also greater since a greater percentage of subjects with TBI endorsed each of the four sleepiness items than did both the trauma controls and trauma-free controls at 1 month. One year following injury, 27% of TBI subjects, 23% of non-cranial trauma controls, and 1% of trauma-free controls reported sleepiness.[2]

In this study, patients with TBI were sleepier than non-cranial trauma controls at 1 month but not 1 year after injury. The cause of the residual sleepiness is unclear. One important factor in predicting persistent sleepiness is the severity of trauma. The brain injury of the majority of patients in this study was considered mild. To better understand the role of severity, the brain-injured subjects were divided into injury-severity groups based on time to follow commands (TFC) after the injury. The subgroup that was able to follow commands less than 24 hours after injury was less sleepy at the 1-month measurement than the 7- to 13-day and 14-day or longer TFC groups. At 1 year, the non-cranial trauma control group and the ≤24-hour TFC group were less sleepy than the 14-day or longer TFC group. Overall sleepiness improved in many patients in this study, with the TBI group more likely to improve than the non-cranial trauma group. Sleepiness improved in 84% to 100% of TBI patients as compared with 78% of the non-cranial trauma control group. However, about a quarter of TBI subjects remained sleepy 1 year after injury. In addition, patients with more severe brain injuries were unable to participate in the study and the authors felt this could have resulted in an underestimation of the true extent of sleepiness in the TBI group.[2]

It is of interest that significant and persistent hypersomnia was present in the non-brain trauma group even though the sleepiness was not as severe as the TBI group. No details about the type of trauma in the former group are provided.[2] This raises the question of what is the cause of the hypersomnia. We can speculate that perhaps adolescents' and young adults' whiplash-type injuries were included in the non-brain trauma group which, as mentioned above, can develop sleep-disordered breathing. Non-brain trauma victims may have poor sleep for other reasons that can lead to daytime hypersomnia. For example, chronic pain and insomnia may develop in this population.

Symptoms resulting from closed-head injury depend on the location of injury within sleep-regulating brain areas. Areas of the brain expected to be involved are those most commonly related to maintaining wakefulness, including but not limited to the brainstem reticular formation, posterior hypothalamus, and the region of the third ventricle. Shearing forces along the direction of main fiber pathways can lead to microhemorrhages in these areas. High cervical cord trauma has also been known to cause sleepiness and unintentional sleep episodes.[6,7] Whiplash injury may result in hypersomnia, with consequent sleep-disordered breathing. In these cases, the hypersomnolence appears to be secondary to the respiratory abnormality.[5] Countercoup injuries commonly occur at the base of the skull and may result in organic post-traumatic sleeplessness. These types of injury occur in areas of bony irregularities (especially the sphenoid ridges), with consequent damage to the inferior frontal and anterior temporal regions, including the basal forebrain.[8] Injury to the posterolateral hypothalamus provides a potential physiologic explanation for post-injury sleepiness. Levels of hypocretin, an alerting neuropeptide, have been shown to be lower in patients with acute moderate to severe TBI.[9,10] Thus, trauma-induced transient reductions in hypocretin may be an unappreciated cause for hypersomnia. This would be consistent with case reports of post-traumatic narcolepsy and cataplexy.[11] Hypersomnia and insomnia are not the only sleep symptoms that can develop after a traumatic brain injury. Rodrigues and Silva have reported a patient with aggressive body movements during rapid eye movement (REM) sleep and periodic limb movements after a traumatic brain injury consistent with REM sleep-behavior disorder.[12]

A more recent multi-center prospective study was performed on sleep disturbances in children with TBI by Tham and colleagues.[13] This study followed 729 children for 24 months following a TBI) and compared them to 197 children with orthopedic injury (OI), who served as controls. Sleep disturbance was assessed using only one question from a standardized questionnaire completed by the parents. Specifically, 'How often did he/she have a problem with trouble sleeping in the last 4 weeks?' Response options include 'never'

=0, 'almost never' =1, 'sometimes' =2, 'often' =3, and 'almost always' =4. Additional data were collected to determine functional outcomes in the areas of adaptive behavior skills and activity participation. Parental reports of pre-injury sleep disturbances were compared to reports of post-injury changes at 3, 12, and 24 months. The average age of the patients was 9 years. Both cohorts (children with TBI and OI) displayed increased sleep disturbances after injury. However, children with TBI experienced higher severity and more prolonged duration of sleep disturbances compared to children with OI. Risk factors for disturbed sleep included mild TBI, psychosocial problems, and frequent pain. Sleep disturbances emerged as significant predictors of poorer functional outcomes in children with moderate or severe TBI. The authors found that using a multivariate model with demographic and psychosocial factors, mild TBI was a significant predictive factor for sleep disturbances in their cohort. The authors proposed as an explanation that persons with mild TBI may have increased recognition of post-injury impairments, and therefore may be more likely to report sleep disturbances as an injury complication. In children with mild TBI, sleep disturbances may also be a symptom of increased awareness of post-injury changes subsequently reported by parents and caregivers. The other important predictors of sleep disturbances in the TBI cohort were frequent pain and the presence of psychosocial problems.

An important distinction between children and adults with TBI is that the neurosystem is maturing but not yet completely developed. The timing of the injury relative to the child's age and maturation needs to be considered. Crowe and colleagues studied participants injured across various stages of childhood to examine the influence of age on recovery and see if it fits an early vulnerability or critical developmental periods model. A total of 181 children with TBI were categorized into 4 age-at-injury groups – infant, preschool, middle childhood, and late childhood – and were evaluated at least 2 years post-TBI with neurocognitive testing (IQ). The study found that overall, the middle childhood group had lower IQ scores across all domains. The authors concluded that contrary to expectations, children injured in middle childhood demonstrated the poorest outcomes which may coincide with a critical period of brain and cognitive development.[14]

A consistent finding in the literature is that children with more severe traumatic brain injury have a greater likelihood of neurocognitive deficits than children with mild TBI. Longitudinal data with 10-year post-injury follow-up confirm this.[15–18] Children with mild TBI tend not to exhibit long-lasting impairment. However, some children even with relatively mild trauma can have persistent cognitive problems. Babikian and colleagues studied predictors of these persistent problems. They found that pre-injury variables such as parental education, premorbid behavior and/or learning problems, and school achievement predicted cognitive impairments in children with otherwise mild TBI.[19] Given this information, it might be expected that children with prior subacute sleep disturbances are more likely to report sleep problems with mild TBI than children who otherwise slept well pre-injury.

In evaluating a child with sleep disturbances after a traumatic brain injury, the possibility of confounding depression should be considered. Max and colleagues prospectively studied 177 children with TBI and measured emergence of new-onset depression symptoms 6 months after TBI The population studied was predominately male with a mean age of 10 years. The authors found an incidence of 11% of 'novel definite/subclinical depressive disorders.' Among these children, they further identified subsets of children with non-anxious depression and anxious depression. Emergence of depressive disorder was significantly associated with older age at the time of injury, family history of anxiety disorder, left inferior frontal gyrus (IFG) lesions, and right frontal white matter lesions.[20]

Children with TBI have been described as having symptoms consistent with attention deficit hyperactivity disorder (ADHD).[21] A prospective study of 82 children with TBI with a mean age of 5 found that, compared to a control group of children with orthopedic injuries, severe TBI was associated with significantly greater anxiety problems. In addition, over time, children who sustained a severe TBI at an earlier age had significantly higher levels of parent-reported symptoms of ADHD and anxiety.[22] Unfortunately, sleep disorders were not specifically evaluated in the methods described.

In the hypersomnolent patient, polysomnography and multiple sleep latency testing should be considered in order to determine the nature of the post-traumatic nocturnal sleep disturbances as well as rule out coexisting pathologies such as obstructive sleep apnea syndrome and periodic limb movement disorder. Comprehensive treatment of hypersomnia in this population will require evaluating the underlying cause of hypersomnia. In children with TBI who have lost consciousness or are recovering from coma it may seem obvious that the hypersomnia is due to the brain injury. However, a careful history must always be taken, and the presence or absence of prior sleep disturbances should be determined. Other causes of hypersomnolence should also be considered in the evaluation of the patient with suspected post-traumatic hypersomnia. Hydrocephalus, subdural hematoma, meningitis, encephalitis, and seizure disorders should be considered as contributing to sleep disturbances.[23] Physical examination can reveal the possibility of minor focal neurologic signs, especially those of brainstem origin. Daytime fatigue may be due to insomnia. The possibility of a medication effect should also be considered. When comprehensive nocturnal polysomnography reveals the presence of sleep-disordered breathing after head trauma, the sleep-related breathing disorders must first be managed before determining the extent to which each comorbid condition contributes to the hypersomnolence. The recognition that head trauma can be a precipitating factor to syndromes leading to excessive daytime sleepiness is important, and a comprehensive evaluation of all patients who exhibit excessive sleepiness after head trauma is needed.

Galland and colleagues conducted a systematic literature review on interventions for sleep problems in children with TBI and found very little evidence-based data in this population.[24] They did describe a case report of a 6-year-old boy with a traumatic right-sided hemorrhage in the basal ganglia with pathological crying and poor sleep. The crying decreased and the sleep improved with the use of citalopram.[25]

Given the description of ADHD complaints in children with TBI, it is not surprising that the use of stimulants in children with TBI has been described and reviewed.[26–29] No specific trials of stimulants for hypersomnia in children with TBI were located. In adults, modafinil for hypersomnia associated with TBI has been reported with mixed results.[29] The use of modafinil in children has been discouraged due to

cutaneous adverse reactions.[30] Methylphenidate has been studied in children with TBI predominantly to treat cognitive and behavioral difficulties.[26,27,31–33] A small randomized trial by Williams and colleagues failed to find a significant improvement of cognitive function in children with TBI using methylphenidate. These children only received 4 days of treatment.[32] In a treatment trial by Mahalick and colleagues using methylphenidate in children with TBI a significant improvement in attention and concentration on neuropsychological tests was found. In this placebo-controlled trial, methylphenidate was given for 14 days.[33] Clearly, further research is needed before the use of stimulants in this pediatric population can unequivocally be recommended. A behavioral approach to sleep disorders, especially if insomnia is present, may be a better alternative.

In the absence of sufficient evidence-based research to standardize the treatment of children with post-traumatic and post neurosurgical hypersomnia, patients are forced to rely on available resources and variable regional sleep medicine expertise. Fortunately, newer techniques such as brain tissue oxygenation monitoring are being applied to children after TBI to maximize neurological outcome.[34] More recent information allows us to anticipate, for patients and families, possible likelihood of recovery and of persistent symptoms. Given the ongoing neurocognitive development of children, we cannot continue to merely extrapolate medical decisions based on studies in adults! Traumatic brain injuries are among the most common and tragic events that can befall an otherwise healthy child. We need further research, specifically treatment intervention trials for a wide age range of children to develop appropriate management protocols.

Clinical Pearls

- Children who suffer significant head trauma frequently experience significant sleep disturbances after the injury, particularly when the trauma is severe enough to result in major loss of consciousness, although sleep disturbances may also follow minor trauma with only a brief loss of consciousness.
- Head trauma has been reported to increase the likelihood of sleep-disordered breathing.
- In the presence of severe trauma, conducting and interpreting an MSLT may not be possible.
- Confounding depression and anxiety should be considered in a child with sleep disturbances after a traumatic brain injury.
- No specific medication trials for post-traumatic hypersomnia are available; however, stimulants for cognitive deficits in this population have been reported to have mixed results.

References

1. International classification of sleep disorders. 2nd ed. Westchester, Illinois: American Academy of Sleep Medicine; 2005.
2. Watson NF, Dikmen S, Machamer J, et al. Hypersomnia following traumatic brain injury. J Clin Sleep Med 2007;3:363–8.
3. Pinto PS, Poretti A, Meoded A, et al. The unique features of traumatic brain injury in children. Review of the characteristics of the pediatric skull and brain, mechanisms of trauma, patterns of injury, complications and their imaging findings – part 1. J Neuroimaging 2012;22:e1–e17.
4. Pinto PS, Meoded A, Poretti A, et al. The unique features of traumatic brain injury in children. review of the characteristics of the pediatric skull

and brain, mechanisms of trauma, patterns of injury, complications, and their imaging findings – part 2. J Neuroimaging 2012;22:e18–41.

5. Guilleminault C, Yuen KM, Gulevich MG, et al. Hypersomnia after head-neck trauma: a medicolegal dilemma. Neurology 2000;54:653–9.

6. Adey W, Porter RW. EEG patterns after high cervical lesions in man. Arch Neurol 1968;19:377–83.

7. Hall CS. Sleep attacks: Apparent relationship to atlantoaxial dislocation. Arch Neurol 1975;32:58–9.

8. Ommaya AK, Grubb RL Jr, Naumann RA. Coup and contre-coup injury: observations on the mechanics of visible brain injuries in the rhesus monkey. J Neurosurg 1971;35:503–16.

9. Baumann CR, Bassetti CL, Valko PO, et al. Loss of hypocretin (orexin) neurons with traumatic brain injury. Ann Neurol 2009;66:555–9.

10. Baumann CR, Stocker R, Imhof HG, et al. Hypocretin-1 (orexin A) deficiency in acute traumatic brain injury. Neurology 2005;65:147–9.

11. Lankford DA, Wellman JJ, O'Hara C. Posttraumatic narcolepsy in mild to moderate closed head injury. Sleep 1994;17:S25–8.

12. Rodrigues RN, Silva AA. [Excessive daytime sleepiness after traumatic brain injury: association with periodic limb movements and REM behavior disorder: case report]. Arquivos de Neuro-psiquiatria. 2002;60:656–60.

13. Tham SW, Palermo TM, Vavilala MS, et al. The longitudinal course, risk factors, and impact of sleep disturbances in children with traumatic brain injury. J Neurotrauma 2012;29:154–61.

14. Crowe LM, Catroppa C, Babl FE, et al. Timing of traumatic brain injury in childhood and intellectual outcome. J Pediatr Psychol 2012;37:745–54.

15. Catroppa C, Godfrey C, Rosenfeld JV, et al. Functional recovery ten years after pediatric traumatic brain injury: outcomes and predictors. J Neurotrauma 2012;29:2539–47.

16. Anderson V, Godfrey C, Rosenfeld JV, et al. 10 years outcome from childhood traumatic brain injury. Int J Dev Neurosci 2012;30:217–24.

17. Anderson V, Godfrey C, Rosenfeld JV, et al. Predictors of cognitive function and recovery 10 years after traumatic brain injury in young children. Pediatrics 2012;129:e254–61.

18. Anderson V, Catroppa C, Godfrey C, et al. Intellectual ability 10 years after traumatic brain injury in infancy and childhood: what predicts outcome? J Neurotrauma 2012;29:143–53.

19. Babikian T, McArthur D, Asarnow RF. Predictors of 1-month and 1-year neurocognitive functioning from the UCLA longitudinal mild, uncomplicated, pediatric traumatic brain injury study. J Int Neuropsychol Soc: JINS 2012;1–10.

20. Max JE, Keatley E, Wilde EA, et al. Depression in children and adolescents in the first 6 months after traumatic brain injury. Int J Dev Neurosci 2012;30:239–45.

21. Levin H, Hanten G, Max J, et al. Symptoms of attention-deficit/hyperactivity disorder following traumatic brain injury in children. J Dev Behavioral Pediatr: JDBP 2007;28:108–18.

22. Karver CL, Wade SL, Cassedy A, et al. Age at injury and long-term behavior problems after traumatic brain injury in young children. Rehabil Psychol 2012;57:256–65.

23. Grigg-Damberger M. Neurologic disorders masquerading as pediatric sleep problems. Pediatr Clin North Am 2004;51:89–115.

24. Galland BC, Elder DE, Taylor BJ. Interventions with a sleep outcome for children with cerebral palsy or a post-traumatic brain injury: a systematic review. Sleep Med Rev 2012;16:561–73.

25. Andersen G, Stylsvig M, Sunde N. Citalopram treatment of traumatic brain damage in a 6-year-old boy. J Neurotrauma 1999;16:341–4.

26. Jin C, Schachar R. Methylphenidate treatment of attention-deficit/ hyperactivity disorder secondary to traumatic brain injury: a critical appraisal of treatment studies. CNS Spectrums 2004;9:217–26.

27. Nicholls E, Hildenbrand AK, Aggarwal R, et al. The use of stimulant medication to treat neurocognitive deficits in patients with pediatric cancer, traumatic brain injury, and sickle cell disease: a review. Postgrad Med 2012;124:78–90.

28. Castriotta RJ, Murthy JN. Sleep disorders in patients with traumatic brain injury: a review. CNS Drugs 2011;25:175–85.

29. Castriotta RJ, Atanasov S, Wilde MC, et al. Treatment of sleep disorders after traumatic brain injury. J Clin Sleep Med 2009;5:137–44.

30. Kumar R. Approved and investigational uses of modafinil: an evidence-based review. Drugs 2008;68:1803–39.

31. Hornyak JE, Nelson VS, Hurvitz EA. The use of methylphenidate in paediatric traumatic brain injury. Pediatr Rehabil 1997;1:15–17.

32. Williams SE, Ris MD, Ayyangar R, et al. Recovery in pediatric brain injury: is psychostimulant medication beneficial? J Head Trauma Rehabil 1998;13:73–81.

33. Mahalick DM, Carmel PW, Greenberg JP, et al. Psychopharmacologic treatment of acquired attention disorders in children with brain injury. Pediatr Neurosurg 1998;29:121–6.

34. Stippler M, Ortiz V, Adelson PD, et al. Brain tissue oxygen monitoring after severe traumatic brain injury in children: relationship to outcome and association with other clinical parameters. J Neurosurg Pediatr 2012;10:383–91.

Medication-Related Hypersomnia

Manisha B. Witmans and Rochelle Young

INTRODUCTION

Sleep and wake states occur along a continuum which is a complex biological process involving the integration and orchestration of neurochemical substances across various regions of the human brain. Regulators and modulators within the brain may act to either promote sleep or wake states depending upon the interactions of multiple biochemical and cellular pathways. Hence, the distinction between the neurological states of wake and sleep is rather more fluid than categorical. Despite the essential need for sleep, its true function remains elusive. What evidence exists suggests that sleep plays a role in biological function, cellular repair, memory and learning. Investigations into sleep deprivation have yielded data that suggest physiological consequences across behavioral, physical and emotional domains in correlational and experimental studies. Disorders of hypersomnia, such as narcolepsy and the mechanisms involved, have improved our current understanding of several neuroanatomic pathways in the brain as well as the molecular mechanisms involved in sleep–wake regulation. Many commonly used medications can similarly affect sleep–wake regulation as sleep disorders have been shown to do, either as a treatment of sleep disorders, or those used socially or recreationally. Furthermore, the utilization of genetic information and pharmaceutical agents has narrowed the target as such that our ability to regulate sleep–wake states has become more precise, while minimizing unpleasant side effects. The aim of this chapter is to provide an overview of medications that cause excessive sleepiness or hypersomnia as an intended or unintended consequence of their use and/or misuse in children and adolescents for treatment of sleep disorders or other health problems that affect sleep–wake regulation. Despite the widespread and common use of complementary alternative medications, hypersomnia is not a specifically reported side effect despite their use as a hypnotic to promote sleep, and therefore will not be reviewed.

HYPERSOMNIA

Hypersomnia is defined as excessive sleepiness out of proportion for age, gender and development in any given individual. Features that may be used to describe hypersomnia include persistent sleepiness, sleep episodes that may be resistible, non-refreshing and long-lasting periods of sleep without associated sleep-onset REM periods which characterize narcolepsy. The excessive sleepiness may be associated with increased sleep time, even sleep drunkenness, or difficulty waking. That hypersomnia is a significant finding is underscored by the International Classification of Sleep Wake Disorders manual (ICSD-2), which includes a section specifically related to hypersomnia disorders which are not in context with sleep-related breathing disorders. Among the well-described categories are narcolepsy with and without

cataplexy, recurrent hypersomnia and idiopathic hypersomnia.[1] Sleepiness is children and adolescents is more commonly related to a multitude of factors (imposed academic, social or work-related schedules), actual sleep disorders, such as behaviorally induced insufficient sleep syndrome, poor sleep hygiene, sleep-related breathing disorder, restless legs syndrome, or even circadian rhythm disorder, rather than a disorder of sleepiness itself.[2] As such, disorders of sleepiness have been increasingly recognized by clinicians around the world, particularly over the past decade. What makes hypersomnia challenging to recognize is that children may not present clinically as adults do, and often the hypersomnia becomes a concern only when it interferes with academic performance or societal expectations of the child, adolescent or their caregivers. In addition to defined disorders of hypersomnia, hypersomnia itself can occur due to the ingestion of a drug or substance. Related to the use of medications, hypersomnia may be observed with the abrupt cessation of excessive stimulant use (abuse) or, alternatively, the sleepiness complaint may result from previous long-term use of stimulants with termination of use (chronic use). Hypersomnia may also result from use of sedatives such as benzodiazepines, barbiturates, gamma hydroxybutyrate or alcohol. Other medications that may result in sleepiness include high doses of anticonvulsant medications or even opioid analgesics. Another overlooked category are over-the-counter medications such as sedating antihistamines, or anti-emetics which are often used as sleep aids but also as agents of abuse. In addition, medications used in combination may compound the hypersomnia effects such as the combinations of alcohol mixed with sedatives. Medications used for other medical problems that may cause hypersomnia such as varenicline (Chantix), a smoking cessation medication, or some chemotherapeutic agents will not be discussed. The chapter will discuss some of the available evidence related to these medications and highlight important clinical considerations. The increasing use of medication in general has resulted, predictably, in the unintended uses of said medications, possibly increasing the incidence of sleepiness in children and especially adolescents. Many different medications have associated reports of hypersomnia as an adverse drug event related to their use. The lengthy list of potential culprits will not be reviewed here but the interested reader can search other sources such as drug monographs or drugcite.com.

SLEEP–WAKE CONTINUUM: ANATOMY AND ITS SUBSTRATES

From historical experiments involving the introduction of brain lesions in animals to facilitate the study of sleep and wake behaviors, the field of inquiry has evolved. Findings now suggest that sleep and wake states are generated by specific neurotransmitters in specific neuronal systems which together have widespread projections in the brain. Sleep and waking behavior can occur in the absence of the cortex, but the cortex is involved in coordination with the ascending reticular activating system to maintain arousal and alertness. Sleep regulatory substances (SRS) are considered to occur apart from these mechanisms and felt to be contributing factors to the sleep–wake continuum. It has been found that wakefulness increases SRS production while SRS themselves promote and alter sleep. For a substance or neurotransmitter to be considered a sleep regulatory factor it must meet the following criteria: (1) the substance and/or its receptor oscillates with sleep propensity, (2) sleep is increased or decreased with administration of the substance, (3) blocking the action or inhibiting the production of the substance changes sleep, (4) disease states, e.g., infection, associated with altered sleep also change levels of the putative SRS, and finally (5) the substance acts on known sleep regulatory circuits.[3] Medications may exert their effects along various aspects of the same pathway as SRS function to inhibit or enhance sleep. The molecular basis of medications from microinjection studies are well established from various drug classes. What are less well known are the anatomic sites where different medications work to induce sleep. Just as a single EEG measure is insufficient to differentiate sleepiness, various medications uniquely affect the degrees of sleepiness in different populations. As a result of hypersomnia, manifestations of sleepiness may include hyperactivity, motor restlessness, behavioral problems and poor academic performance, particularly in children.

No specific structure of the brain is independently involved in the maintenance of sleep or wake states. Rather, it is unique types of neurons within the same structure which may be playing a role in maintaining the state of sleep or wakefulness. Wakefulness and alertness are maintained by neurons within the brainstem ascending reticular formation that send projections to the thalamocortical pathways via two routes, the dorsal pathway and in the posterior thalamus, and the basal forebrain in the ventral pathway.[3,4] Neurons that are involved in activation and wake promotion are concentrated in certain regions of the brain including the oral pontine, midbrain tegmentum and posterior hypothalamus. In contrast, the sleep-promoting regions are in the brainstem, dorsolateral medullary reticular formation, basal forebrain, and anterior hypothalamus ventrolateral preoptic area. Sleep is promoted through the inhibitory neurotransmitters, gamma-hydroxybutyric acid (GABA) and galanin. Experiments in the 1950s and 1960s showed that acetylcholine is important for vigilance and cortical activation. Locus coeruleus neurons using norepinephrine project diffusely to the forebrain and brainstem to maintain cortical activation. Further studies suggest that norepinephrine and adrenergic receptors are important for stimulating and maintaining activating processes, whereas dopaminergic nuclei in the midbrain ventral tegmental areas are important in stimulating behavioral arousal. The posterior thalamic neurons have histamine, which has been long assumed to play a role in vigilance, and have widespread projections to areas of the hypothalamus and cortex. Orexin (hypocretin) also has widespread projections across the forebrain and cortex is involved in maintaining wakefulness. Serotonergic neurons from the raphe nuclei are also important in maintaining wakefulness. Adenosine is another neurotransmitter involved in sleep–wake regulation in the homeostatic process, and may promote sleep through

anticholinergic activity in the basal forebrain and brainstem There may be many other neuroactive substances such as cytokines that alone or in combination with some of these established neurotransmitters further mediate sleep and wake states. Medications may cause hypersomnia by different mechanisms, by either promoting sleep-activating neurons (GABA), or inhibiting the wake-promoting regions (antihistamines).[4] Medications may cause hypersomnia if they impair wakefulness either by the sedating effect lasting longer or prolonged action lasting into waking hours. Medications that promote alertness may impair sleep continuity. Much of the available data on use of these psychoactive medications are from adults, and effects on children may not be the same.[5] Table 22.1 provides a simplistic categorization of the neurotransmitter role in sleep and wake determination and primary anatomic location that is involved. Different classes of medications and the associated evidence in children and adolescents are discussed below.

ABUSE OR MISUSE OF PRESCRIPTION AND OVER-THE-COUNTER MEDICATIONS

The use of medications has climbed steadily over the years in all fields of medicine, particularly in sleep medicine, either to promote wakefulness or sleepiness, depending on the presenting problem. As a result of this, our collective desire to manipulate and regulate sleep–wake cycles as much as we dictate personal schedules is rampant across society, and children are no exception, either because of parental or societal expectations or their own in meeting all their social and personal demands. Strategic and direct marketing to consumers and prescribers has contributed to the widespread use of pharmacological agents to manipulate and treat sleep. Compounding this problem is that medications are no longer available just to those with prescribing authority. Internet access has enhanced the spread of drug information as well as the distribution of medications themselves, fuelling the phenomenon. One could also surmise that the current cultural ideation of a 'magic pill' or cure-all for any ailment has resulted in the development of a focused pharmaceutical industry promoting medications for actual or perceived medical conditions According to the FDA, from 1960 to 2004, the amount spent on prescription drugs increased from $2.7 billion to over $200 billion with no expected reduction, as more sophisticated medications are developed for targeted use.[6] Most importantly, the misperception, particularly in adolescents, that medications prescribed by physicians and dispensed by pharmacists are safer than illicit drugs has resulted in a widespread epidemic of misuse of prescription and over-the-counter medications.[7]

Society's ever-increasing use of medications has resulted in the intentional abuse of prescribed and over-the-counter (OTC) medications to affect mood, performance, and sleep–wake state. A wide variety of classes of medications contain the potential for abuse including: sedatives, opioids and derivatives, stimulants, tranquilizers and muscle relaxants, as well as centrally acting agents. Data from the National Survey on Drug Use and Health in 2010 showed that almost one-third of individuals over age 12 who used drugs for the first time in 2009 had begun by using a prescription drug non-medically.[5] Data also showed that prescription drugs account for the second

TABLE 22.1   Neurotransmitters and Neuroanatomic Associations and their Rates of Discharge

NEUROTRANSMITTER	LOCATION	PROJECTION	AWAKE	REM	NREM	DRUG CLASS
Gamma aminobutyric acid (GABA)		Widespread	−	−	++	Benzodiazepine receptor agonists and antagonists promote sleepiness
Serotonin (5-HT)	Dorsal raphe and median raphe nuclei in the midbrain	Diencephalon, limbic system and neocortex	+++	−	++	Selective serotonin reuptake inhibitors, many can cause daytime sedation
5-HT$_{1A}$				−		
5-HT$_{2A}$				−	++	Serotonin antagonist/reuptake inhibitor (trazadone and nefazadone)
Norepinepherine	throughout the brainstem, primarily Locus ceoruleus (LC)	Diencephalon, forebrain, cerebellum	+++	−	++	Tricyclic antidepressant medications
Various receptor types: norepinephine alpha-1, alpha-2, and beta NE	Preoptic area and basal forebrain		+++	++	−	Tricyclic antidepressant medications
Histamine	Tuberomamillary nucleus (TMN) and posterior hypothalamus (PH)	Hypothalamus and forebrain and neocortex	+++	−	++	Antihistamines
Orexin	Midlateral hypothalamus	All brain regions including brainstem	+++	++	−	

(Data from Priniciples and Practice of Sleep Medicine.)

most commonly abused category of drugs after marijuana but ahead of cocaine, heroin and methamphetamines.[9] The National Survey on Drug Use and Health revealed in 2010, about 22.6 million Americans aged 12 and older had used illicit drugs during the past month, including prescription-type psychotherapeutics non-medically.[8] When lifetime prevalence of misuse of medications is considered, the number is a staggering 52 million individuals aged 12 and older, representing 20.6% of the US population.[10] The majority of these medications are obtained from friends or relatives (55%), and 17.3% from physicians, 4.4% from strangers; 0.4% reported buying the drug on the internet. Non-medicinal use of psychotherapeutics occurred in 7.0 million (2.7%) children 12 and older compared to 6.3 million in 2002.[9] The types of medications used non-medicinally were: pain relievers (5.1 million), tranquilizers (2.2 million), stimulants (1.1 million), and sedatives/hypnotics (374,000). The rates of use of these medications do vary by age, with increasing prevalence of use with age (4.0% in children age 12–13 years, to 9.3% in those age 14–15 years, to 16.6% in 16–17-year-olds).[9] These data suggest that use of psychoactive medications for non-medicinal purposes is common among youth. For the clinician, the challenge lies in trying to differentiate not only what the complaint of hypersomnia is as a result of the complex interplay of development, socio-cultural influence on sleep–wake regulation and a possible sleep disorder, but also being able to differentiate iatrogenic causes of sleepiness that may further compound the presenting complaint. For example, the multiple sleep latency test may be positive, not because of the true hypersomnia or associated disorder, but rather the use of the medications that are used in combination with the given youth's circadian rhythm that may be influencing the findings. Conversely, use of stimulant medication or caffeine, either in the form of energy drinks or excessive use of other forms of caffeine, as a countermeasure may mask the true sleepiness that is present for the given adolescent. For patients on anticonvulsant medications, either as a mood stabilizer or for their epilepsy, teasing apart the true sleepiness versus the sleepiness resulting from medications or even psychiatric disorder can be quite challenging.

The inappropriate use of medications has significant consequences ranging from increased healthcare utilization to policy-level regulations for drug dispensation. The overall dependence on a specific medication may very well be therapeutic regardless of the class of said medication. The challenge often lies in the distinction and what it means for the functioning for the given individual. For example, a person may be pseudo-addicted when a patient requiring a stimulant for narcolepsy engages in drug-seeking behavior to obtain a therapeutic and effective dose of medications. Conversely, a drug-addicted person may have underlying medical issues that have been untreated, as the person was engaged in abuse to self treat the problem without seeking appropriate advice. A person on long-term anxiolytics for symptoms related to insomnia may turn to other agents such as alcohol to cope with the symptoms of withdrawal or for the desired effect of sedation.

With increasingly rapid advances in technology, access to medical services and information has also advanced. Previously, prescriptions or medications were either prescribed or bought directly from a pharmacy. Presently, any individual with access to the internet may order a variety of prescription and over-the-counter medications, delivered straight to their home. Many sites that sell medications on the internet may or may not require a prescription, or have opportunities for individuals to gain inappropriate access to these medications. The lack of regulation also does not guarantee that the consumer is getting appropriate or the actual medication that is prescribed. There were over 340 online 'approved pharmacies' in 2010 and many rogue pharmacies (FDA website).[11] Increased travel to countries where access to prescription medications is less diligently controlled also increases the individual's chances of obtaining potentially harmful medications. The widespread availability of these agents not only improves access to, but provides more opportunities for those who are prone to abuse the medications, to obtain them or seek out these agents as substitutes when the drug of choice is not available.

A particular abuse of medications in adolescents, referred to as 'pharming,' warrants special consideration, particularly as the prescription and over-the-counter medication abuse of cough and cold preparations is becoming more common. Factors that promote the likelihood of abuse include the ease of accessibility, since most of these medications are widely available in homes, are relatively inexpensive, and decreased perception of potential harm because they are legal.[12] The abuse of these drugs is strongly associated with abuse of alcohol and other illicit substances.[13] Data from a self-administered study of 7300 adolescents from grade 7–12 revealed that one in five (19%) of 4.5 million reported abusing prescription medications to 'get high' while one in ten (10% or 2.4 million) reported abusing cough medications to 'get high.' These findings exceed rates of abuse from illicit substances such as methamphetamines (8%).[13] In addition, a nationwide survey among 50 000 students from grade 8 revealed a higher use of narcotic pain relievers than previous years in grades 8 and 10.[14] Data from the California Poison Control Center showed dexomethorphan abuse increased 10-fold from 1999 to 2004, with a 15-fold increase in adolescents aged 9–17 years.[15] Many adolescents obtain these medications from their peers[16] or from their social network of friends, relatives, physicians.[17] These medications may be used as sleep aids or study aids. There is also less social stigma for use of these medications rather than street drugs.[13] Prescription medications abused by adolescents including opioid analgesic agents, sedative hypnotics and stimulants are discussed below.

COMPLEMENTARY ALTERNATIVE MEDICATIONS

Complementary alternative medication (CAM) use has increased substantially over the past decade. In sleep medicine, many of these agents are used as sleep aids and are discussed in the associated relevant chapters. The 2001 National Health Interview Survey gathered information on CAM use among more than 9000 children younger than 18 years of age. It was found that nearly 12% of the children had used some form of CAM during the past 12 months. CAM use was much more likely to occur among children whose parents also used CAM. Adolescents aged 12–17 years, children with multiple health conditions, and those whose families delayed or did not use conventional medical care because of cost were also more likely to use CAM,[18] suggesting that CAM use may be more common than reported in the literature. Review of multiple data sources did not reveal any CAM therapies that list hypersomnia as a concerning symptom, either as a cause or side effect of the medication.

CATEGORIES OF MEDICATION THAT RESULT IN SLEEPINESS AS EITHER AN INTENDED OR UNINTENDED CONSEQUENCE

Sedative-Hypnotics

Sedatives and hypnotics have really transformed from the initial agents that used to include barbiturates. Virtually all of the sedative, hypnotic and anxiolytic agents bind to GABA moieties at the benzodiazepine receptor.[19] Barbiturates, for example, increase stage 1 sleep, and decrease REM sleep; thus, these could affect the findings of the multiple sleep latency test, and even either mask or underestimate the severity of sleep-disordered breathing. The use of some of these agents has, in general, decreased because of the availability of better agents with fewer side effects, higher therapeutic window, and less toxicity. Chloral hydrate has been widely used in medicine for sedating children for procedures and has been used as a hypnotic. (However, Chloral hydrate has been discontinued in the US.) Excessive doses result in hypersomnia. Respiratory depression can occur when combined with other sedatives and hypnotics. Case reports of death exist at doses of 100 mg/kg.[20,21] The medication is no+ longer available because of a production shortage, and clinicians are faced with a challenge of finding suitable alternatives, especially because it is widely used for sedated procedures in pediatrics.[22] Long-term use has been reported in children with neurodevelopmental disabilities. Tolerance may develop to the medication. Notable effects of this class of medication include: reduced anxiety, anterograde amnesia, and sedation as well as memory impairment.

GABA$_A$ Agonists: Benzodiazepines and the Non-Benzodiazepines

The 35 benzodiazepine compounds currently available are the most widely prescribed and used hypnotic agents in clinical practice. This class of medication is typically utilized by practitioners as hypnotics, sedatives and anxiolytics. The receptor complex of GABA agonists includes a group of ligand-gated ion channels, the mechanism of which is at the benzodiazepine binding site on GABA$_A$ receptor and its associated chloride channel. Each of these compounds displays unique aspects pertaining to their individual receptor subtype involved in binding and the resultant half-life. As such, GABA agonists with a shorter half-life tend to be used in practice as amnestics for invasive procedures, such as midazolam, while the longer-acting medications result in more daytime sleepiness. Given these traits, it is not surprising to find that those benzodiazepines with longer half-lives are typically prescribed as sleep aids. Caution in prescribing should be exercised, as overdose of this class of medications can result in respiratory depression, especially when combined with other sedative medications or alcohol.[23] Benzodiazepines may be used in isolation for the euphoric effects or combined in different forms to augment the effects of other medications.

In particular, two medications in this category deserve special mention as they are widely used in the adult sleep medicine for the treatment of insomnia.[2] Zaleplon (Sonata) is a non-benzodiazepine which binds to the benzodiazepine receptor with a resulting ultra-short half-life, making it the agent of choice for sleep-onset insomnia and may actually induce slow wave sleep, unlike the other benzodiazepine agents. Zaleplon has been found to have greater efficacy in children compared to zolpidem. Zolpidem (Ambien) also has a relatively short half-life and is another non-benzodiazepine agent different from similar drugs in that it binds to the benzodiazepine receptor site, and as a result has excellent hypnotic properties. In general, agents with a longer half-life are more likely to cause daytime sleepiness, and the inappropriate timing of administration can lead to drug-induced hypersomnia. In comparison to the other sedative-hypnotics, these cause the least amount of sleepiness.

Opioids and Morphine Derivatives

As the management of chronic pain has garnered more attention and awareness, there has been a steady increase in use of prescription pain medications, including over-the-counter remedies. The neurobiology of pain is complex and involves both central and peripheral mechanisms. Simply, pain disrupts sleep while sleep deprivation may increase pain sensitivity.[24] Opioid peptides may be involved in modulation of various biological processes including sleep, which is how they mediate their effect, and somnolence is a common side effect.[25] Sleep medicine has also embraced the use of opioids and derivatives as second-line agents for treating restless legs syndrome or Willis–Ekbom disease. Opioids and their derivatives are the most commonly abused prescription medications, resulting in social programs and dispensary interventions to stave off the epidemic. In 2009, about 9.7% of 12th-graders reported misuse of Vicodin (an opiate narcotic) in the past year in a national survey[26] while up to 18% of 11th-graders used opiates without a prescription.[27] Opioids bind to receptors across various regions in the brain, and, in high enough doses, cause sleepiness and respiratory depression. Long-term use can lead to physical dependence, tolerance and addiction. Combination of opioids in addition to other agents such as alcohol, antihistamines, or sedatives can result in life-threatening respiratory depression, coma and death.

Antidepressants

Dependent upon the specific antidepressant agent chosen, medications in this category can be either activating or sedating. Sleep-enhancing antidepressants may result in hypersomnia even at clinically therapeutic doses, such as mirtazepine (remeron) which is a serotonin $5\text{-}HT_{2A}$ antagonist/reuptake inhibitor. This medication has widespread effects on norepinephrine, histamine and alpha adrenergic systems. In contrast, nefazadone inhibits norepinephrine reuptake and is antagonistic at the $5\text{-}HT_{2A}$ receptor and is a bit more alerting in comparison. Trazadone enhances sleep by acting at $5\text{-}HT_{2A}$ as an antagonist and blocks histamine receptors and, as a result, it is the most sedating antidepressant, often used for insomnia. A relatively newer antidepressant, escitalopram (Cipralex), is an antidepressant belonging to the selective serotonin reuptake inhibitors. Somnolence has been reported as a side effect, but less so than with others.[4] If combined with dextromethorphan, it can cause serotonin syndrome, which is an idiosyncratic, potentially life-threatening adverse drug reaction, from excess serotonergic activity at the central nervous system.

Antihistamines

Antihistamines are available as both prescription and over-the-counter preparations and are used for treatment of allergies, cold symptoms, and as sleep aids, commonly off-label in children because of their sedating properties. A novel

technique in neuroimaging, including PET scanning, has enabled specific identification of H1 receptor occupancy in the brain. This can be linked to cognitive processing to be able to determine where and how H1 receptors are activated or inhibited and how that might affect the cognitive tasks that an individual performs.[28] Most first-generation antihistamines cause drowsiness, sleepiness or sedation as a side effect because they are lipophilic and cross the blood–brain barrier. The effects may be augmented when used in conjunction with alcohol, sedative hypnotics or narcotic agents. These agents are generally regarded as less harmful because they are readily available and widely used, but their effects can be profound and they do have addictive potential. Diphenhydramine is a commonly available antihistaminic drug that is often used off-label for sedation and hypnotic for children. Diphenhydramine is typically used for allergy and atopic disorders with such regularity by practitioners and the public, and is largely regarded as being harmless. Interestingly, in those with a genetic predisposition to addiction, this medication is often used to 'get high,' similar to use of a stimulant, and can be associated with significant sequelae.[29] In most of the rest of the population, it is used as a hypnotic, even in very young children for insomnia of childhood. The reported effect can be quite inconsistent, ranging from paradoxical excitation to somnolence and sedation.

Dimenhydrinate is another over-the-counter antihistamine for nausea and is highly valued for its sedative properties. The effects are similar to those of diphenhydramine. Dimenhydrinate is an H1 histamine receptor antagonist and interacts with other neurotransmitters, either directly or indirectly. Some of the neurotransmitters it can interact with include: acetylcholine, serotonin, norepinepherine, dopamine, opioids, or adenosine.[31] Although it is available over the counter, and appears to be benign, this drug also has abuse potential and does result in hypersomnia.

Hydroxyzine is also a centrally acting H1 histamine receptor antagonist that is used for sedation, as an anxiolytic and for atopic disorders for pruritus. Off label, this agent can be used for sedation. This medication, like other sedating antihistamines, can result in hypersomnia if used inappropriately during the day. The newer-generation antihistamines (certirizine, desloratidine, loratidine) are hydrophilic and do not cross the blood–brain barrier and are much more selective, enabling treatment of atopy without associated sedation.

Dextromethorphan

Dextromethorphan hydrobromide is common in more than 150 over-the-counter cough and cold remedies in the United States.[23] Dexamethorphan is a synthetic opioid and is the dextroisomer of the codeine analog, levorphenol. This is commonly used to treat cough as a cough suppressant at doses of 15–30 mg. Use of this medication at higher doses, referred to as 'sheeting,' where upwards of 8–16 tablets are consumed at once, has been reported.[12,30] At very high doses of 600–1500 mg, it can result in symptoms similar to phencyclidine or ketamine as the dextromethorphan is converted to dextrophan, causing dissociative effects by antagonizing N-methyl-D-aspartate (NMDA).[12] A small portion of Caucasian individuals have difficulty metabolizing this medication, resulting from a genetic polymorphism and may not experience the dissociative effects.[30] This medication can induce addiction and can cause cravings with sustained use.

In addition, many cough syrup preparations contain additionally significant active ingredients. For example, Coricidin, a common and popular over-the-counter antihistamine and decongestant, contains dextromethorphan, chlorpheniramine, phenylpropranolamine and acetaminophen. Intoxication with this medication presenting to the emergency room can be associated with sleepiness in up to 24%.[23]At high doses, the effects can be profound and life-threatening.

Amphetamines and Other Stimulants

Amphetamines and stimulants are used primarily for the treatment of attention deficit hyperactivity disorder and for narcolepsy in conjunction with anti-cataplectic agents. Various agents are available including: amphetamine, dextroamphetamine, methamphetamine, methylphenidate, or their derivatives. Abrupt withdrawal of amphetamines may unmask unwanted symptoms such as depression, irritability, psychomotor agitation or even hypersomnia and disturbed sleep. Conversely, large doses of amphetamines may also cause mental depression, disorientation, hallucinations and even coma. In addition to prescription use, these drugs are also often used inappropriately for non-medicinal purposes. Ritalin has the highest rates of non-medicinal use. The National Survey on Drug Use and Health revealed from 2005 that 6.4 million (2.6%) people aged 12 and older had used prescription medications within a month, stimulants were used by 1.1 million people (512000 used methamphetamines), and suggested ongoing gradual increase in use of stimulant medications.[9,23] The use of such medications recreationally or socially, without a medical indication, makes the issue of evaluating a sleep disorder quite challenging because the fragmentation of nighttime sleep can result in daytime somnolence, and a disorder of hypersomnia may be masked by the use of such agents. These medications, when prescribed with others which are sedating, also have to be timed appropriately for optimal benefit and sleep–wake regulation.

Anticonvulsant Medications and Hypersomnia

Medications used in the treatment of epilepsy have been found to be sedating, thus challenging the clinician to distinguish sleepiness related to epilepsy control from sleepiness due to drug therapy. Several medications in this category include: valproic acid (Depakene), carbamazepine (Tegretol) and Gabapentin (Neurontin).[3] These medications may be used to optimize sleep or to induce hypersomnia due to their sedating properties.

Sodium Oxybate

Sodium oxybate (gamma hydroxybutyrate: Xyrem) is a central nervous system depressant that exhibits potent hypnotic activity.[32,33] Although the exact mechanism of action has not been fully elucidated, sodium oxybate is thought to act on $GABA_B$ receptors.[34] Used to treat narcolepsy with cataplexy, sodium oxybate has been shown to be an effective treatment,[35] and has been used off-label for narcolepsy with cataplexy in children. No tolerance was reported in a small level-IV evidence study of 15 adolescents (mean age 11 years) on sodium oxybate with a mean follow-up of 33 months.[36] Only one patient discontinued the medication because of a dissociative state.[36] The subjects did, however, show a need for less other medications after the initiation of sodium oxybate for cataplexy. Recreational use of this medication has been associated with

significant sequelae including respiratory depression, loss of consciousness, coma and death.[37-39] The concern for potential abuse has resulted in restricted access to the medication by way of a central dispensing pharmacy following the intensive education of the patient. Even at therapeutic doses, the sodium oxybate is associated with confusion, increased parasomnias, depression and other neuropsychiatric symptoms.[43] Concerns surrounding potential abuse of sodium oxybate should be taken into consideration when prescribing this particular drug.

Dopaminergic Medications

As the precursor of dopamine, dopaminergic agents such as levodopa act by repleting dopamine to treat dystonic disorders. They are considered first-line agents for the treatment of restless legs syndrome and periodic limb movements (see Chapter 43). There is a dopa-decarboxylase inhibitor which reduces the peripheral conversion of levodopa to dopamine helping to prevent untoward side effects that can occur. In addition, the enzymatic breakdown enables the medication to be used at lower doses centrally to produce effective outcomes. The extracerebral dopa-decarboxylase inhibitor most commonly used in children is carbidopa. This has been used in dystonias associated with cerebral palsy and certain metabolic disorders. Excessive daytime sleepiness and sudden onset of sleep can occur with this agent and therefore it should be used with caution.[4]

Atypical Antipsychotic Agents

Some of the more commonly used atypical antipsychotic agents including ziprasidone, quetiapine, and olanzepine can be significantly sedating. Respiridone, another atypical antipsychotic, which is increasingly used in children for agitation associated with insomnia, has also been utilized by clinicians for the side benefit of sedation. While weight gain is a common side effect, atypical antipsychotic agents have much fewer side effects than typical neuroleptics used for schizophrenia. Quetiapine has been widely used off-label for its sedation properties in children and adolescents because it is a dopamine, serotonin, and adrenergic antagonist with potent antihistamine properties.[41] Lurasidone is an atypical second-generation antipsychotic agent approved for use in adults for long-term symptom control of schizophrenia, but safety and efficacy of its use in children has not been established. Like other antipsychotic agents, it may impair judgment and can result in hypersomnia, hypersomnolence and sedation.[42,43]

EVALUATING HYPERSOMNIA RESULTING FROM MEDICATIONS: CONSIDERATIONS FOR THE CLINICIAN

Pharmacological treatments required in the management of medical conditions in children and adolescents may result in a clinical presentation of hypersomnia. In addition, medications used for the treatment of disorders of sleepiness and/or sleeplessness may confound the clinical picture, leaving the sleep specialist with the challenge of evaluating the role of medication in relation to sleep–wake regulation. A thorough review of prescribed medications, over-the-counter medication, dosage, frequency and timing and associated countermeasures used to manage sleepiness, such as caffeine in its various forms, should be undertaken. It is important to consider the medications in view of the circadian factors that may enhance or inhibit the effect of medication, such as the use of stimulants in the late afternoon versus a morning dosage. Teenagers should specifically be asked about use of prescription, non-prescription or over-the-counter medications, complementary alterative substances, as well as illicit drug use, in a non-threatening or judgmental manner. Given the high prevalence of abuse of some of these agents amongst adolescents, additional history about associated mood problems, learning disabilities and sleep disorders should be sought. Management of the abuse of these medications, either acutely, which is often symptomatic, or as a result of chronic use, is beyond the scope of this chapter, but other excellent resources are available. Teenagers and their parents should be cautioned about the safety profile of medications, encouraged to avoid sharing medications, and warned about signs suggesting abuse, such as frequent prescription refills or altered academic performance at school. Pharmacists should equally be vigilant in questioning refills, and store the medications appropriately behind the counter. Internet shopping for medications should be banned for children less than 18 years of age, with strict legislation.

SUMMARY

Sleep–wake regulation is a complex process with the potential to be further confounded by the use of prescription or non-prescription drugs. Resulting hypersomnia must be evaluated by the clinician in the context of the social, medical and physical parameters of the presenting patient, with particular diligence applied to the adolescent. With the large number of medications available that may result in a presentation of hypersomnia, it is the role of medical personnel to remain diligent in their assessment of the sleepy patient. Ultimately, it is imperative for the clinician to be aware of the different classes of medications, their associated effects, and the trends of use of these medications by children and adolescents.

Clinical Pearls

- The possibility of hypersomnia associated with medications should be explored in children and adolescents presenting with excessive sleepiness.
- Medications used to treat various different medical or sleep disorders may result in sleepiness being an intended/ unintended consequence.
- Use of medications by adolescents should prompt the clinician to inquire about what pharmacological or non-pharmacological agents are being used to affect the sleep–wake continuum.
- A detailed inquiry will help the physician determine appropriate targets for intervention.

References

1. American Academy of Sleep Medicine. The international classification of sleep disorders, 2nd edn. Diagnostic and coding manual. Westchester, IL; 2005. p. 79–115.
2. Sheldon SH. Introduction to pediatric sleep medicine. In: Sheldon SH, Ferber R, Kryger MH, editors. Principles and practice of pediatric sleep medicine. Philadelphia: Elsevier Saunders; 2005. p. 1–23.
3. Saper CB, Scammell T, Lu J. Hypothalamic regulation of sleep and circadian rhythms. Nature 2005;437:1257–63.
4. Herman JH, Sheldon SH. Pharmacology of sleep disorders in children. In: Sheldon SH, Ferber R, Kryger MH, editors. Principles and practice of pediatric sleep medicine. Philadelphia: Elsevier Saunders; 2005. p. 327–38.
5. Doloresco F, Fominaya C, Schumock GT, et al. Projecting future drug expenditures – 2011. Am J Health-Syst Pharm 2011;58:e1–12.
6. Johnston LD, O'Malley PM, Bachman JG, et al. Monitoring the future national results on adolescent drug use: overview of key findings 2009. NIH Publication Number 10-7583). Bethesda, MD: National Institute on Drug Abuse; 2010.
7. Substance Abuse and Mental Health Services Administration. Results from the 2009 National Survey on Drug Abuse and Health II: technical appendices and selected tables (NSDUH series H-38A, HHS publ. no, SMA 10-4b56A Appendices
8. Office of the National Drug Control Policy (ONDCP). Teens and prescription drugs: An analysis of recent trends on the emerging drug threat. Washington D.C.: Executive Office of the President; 2007.
9. Substance Abuse and Mental Health Services Administration. Results from the 2010 National Survey on Drug Use and Health: Summary of National Findings, NSDUH Series H-41, HHS Publication No. (SMA) 11-4658. Rockville, MD: Substance Abuse and Mental Health Services Administration; 2011.
10. Gonzales R, Brecht ML, Mooney L, et al. Prescription and over the counter drug treatment admissions to the California public treatment system. J Subst Abuse Treat 2011;40:224–9.
11. FDA approved sites for internet medication access. http://www.fda.gov/Drugs/ResourcesForYou/Consumers/BuyingUsingMedicineSafely/EnsuringSafeUseofMedicine/.
12. Levine D. 'Pharming': the abuse of prescription and over-the counter drugs in teens. Curr Opin Pediatr 2007;19:270–4.
13. Partnership in Drug Free America. The Partnership Attitude Tracking Study. New York: Partnership for Drug Free America; 2005. http://www.drug-free.org/files/full_Teen_report.
14. Johnson LD, O'Malley PM, Bachman JG, et al. Monitoring the future national results on adolescent drug use: overview of key findings 2005 (NIH pub no 06-5882). Bethesda: National Institute on Drug Abuse; 67 pp. http://www.monitoringthefuture.org/pubs/monographs.
15. Bryner JK, Wang UK, Hiu JW, et al. Dextromethorphan abuse in adolescence: an increasing trend 1999–2004. Arch Pediatr Adolsec Med 2006;160:1217–22.
16. McCabe SE, Boyd CJ. Sources of prescription drugs for illicit use. Addict Behav 2005;30:1342–50.
17. Arria AM, Calderia KM, Vincent KB, et al. Perceived harmfulness predicts non-medicinal use of prescription drugs among college students: Interactions with sensation seeking. Prevent Sci 2008;9:191–201.
18. Davis MP, Darden PM. Use of complementary and alternative medicine by children in the United States. Arch Pediatr Adolesc Med 2003;157(4):393–6.
19. Lu J, Greco MA. Sleep circuitry and the hypnotic mechanism of GABAA drugs. J Clin Sleep Med 2006;2(2):S19–26.
20. Seger D, Schwartz G. Chloral hydrate: A dangerous sedative for overdose patients? Pediatr Emerg Care 1994;10(6):349–50.
21. Kupiec TC, Kemp P, Raj V, et al. A fatality due to an accidental methadone substitution in a dental cocktail. J Anal Toxicol 2011;35(7):515–25.
22. Cote CJ, Karl HW, Notterman DA, et al. Adverse sedation events in pediatrics: analysis of medications used for sedation. Pediatrics 2000;106:633–44.
23. Lessenger JE, Feinberg SD. Abuse of prescription and over the counter medications. J Am Board Fam Med 2008;21:45–54.
24. Schug S, Garrett W, Gillespie G. Opioid and non-opioid anagesics. Best Pract Resd Clin Anaesthesiol 2003;17:91–110.
25. Inturrisi C. Clinical pharmacology of opioids for pain. Clin J Pain 2002;18:S3–13.
26. Johnson LD, O'Malley PM, Bachman JG, et al. Monitoring the future national results on adolescent drug use: overview of key findings 2009 (NIH pub no 10-7583). Besthesda: National Institute on Drug Abuse; 77 pp.
27. Austin G, Skager R. Highlight: 12th Biennial California Student Survey Drug, Alcohol and Tobacco Use 2007–2008. Sacremento, CA: California Attorney General's Office.
28. Yanaki K, Zhang D, Tashiro M, et al. Positron emission tomography evaluation of sedative properties of antihistamines. Exp Opinn Drug Saf 2011;10(4):613–22.

29. Griffiths RR, Johnson MW. Relative abuse liability of hypnotic drugs: a conceptual framework and algorithm for differentiating among compounds. J Clin Psychiatry 2005;66:31–41.

30. Schwartz RH. Adolescent abuse of dextromethorphan. Clin Pediatr (Phil) 2005;44:565–8.

31. Halpert AG, Olmstead MC, Beninger RJ. Mechanisms and abuse liability of the anti-histmaine dimenhydrinate. Neurosci Behav Rev 2002; 26:61–7.

32. Jazz Pharmaceuticals. Xyrem® (sodium oxybate) oral solution prescribing information. Palo Alto, CA: Jazz Pharmaceuticals; 2005.

33. Sweetman SC, editor. Martindale: the complete drug reference. 33rd ed. London: The Pharmaceutical Press; 2002. p. 1268.

34. Koek W, Mercer SL, Coop A, et al. Behavioral effects of gamma hydroxybutyrate, its precursor gamma-butyrolactone, and GABA-B receptor agonists; time course and differential antagonism by the GABA (B) receptor antagonist 3-aminopropyl (diethoxymethyl) phsophinic acid (CGP35348). J Pharmacol Exp Therap 2009;330(3):876–83.

35. Aren A, Einen M, Lin L, et al. Clinical and therapeutic aspects of childhood narcolepsy-cataplexy: A retrospective study of 51 children. Sleep 2010;33(11):1457–64.

36. Mansukhani MP, Kotagal S. Sodium oxybate in the treatment of childhood narcolepsy-cataplexy: A retrospective study. Sleep Med 2012. 13:606–10.

37. Nightingale SL. Warning about GHB. JAMA 1991;265:1802.

38. Anon. Multistate outbreak of poisonings associated with illicit use of gammy hydroxy butyrate. JAMA 1991;265:447–8.

39. Galloway GP, Frederick SL, Staggers F Jr. Physical dependence or sodium oxybate. Lancet 1994;343:57.

40. Zeman A, Britton T, Douglas N, et al. Narcolepsy and excessive daytime sleepiness. BMJ 2004;329:724–8.

41. Richelson E, Souder T. Binding of antipsychotic drugs to human brain receptors focus on newer generation compounds. Life Sci 2000;68(1): 29–39.

42. Sunovion Pharmaceuticals Inc. Latuda® (lurasidone hydrochloride tablets prescribing information. Marlborough, MA: Sunovion Pharmaceuticals; 2010.

43. Ishibashi T, Horisawa T, Tokuda K, et al. Pharmacological profile of lurasidone, a novel antipsychotic agent with potent 5-hydroxytryptamine 7 (5-HT7) and 5-HT1A receptor activity. J Pharmacol Exp Ther 2010;334:171–81.

SLEEP AND BREATHING DISORDERS

Rapid-Onset Obesity with Hypothalamic Dysfunction, Hypoventilation, and Autonomic Dysregulation (ROHHAD)

Pallavi P. Patwari and Casey M. Rand

Rapid-onset obesity with hypothalamic dysfunction, hypoventilation, and autonomic dysregulation (ROHHAD) is a rare and devastating disorder involving variable dysfunction of control of breathing, the endocrine system, and autonomic nervous system (ANS) regulation. Despite distinct clinical criteria, the spectrum and complexity of ROHHAD in regards to the multi-system involvement, severity, and timing can be quite perplexing. In mild cases and conservative management, children can have excellent neurocognitive outcome and be supported with night-only, non-invasive positive-pressure ventilation. However, in severe cases, clinical features can reach extremes in regards to hypoventilation requiring tracheostomy and 24-hour supported ventilation, marked swings in serum sodium levels (hyper- or hyponatremia), body temperature, bradycardia, and behavioral problems. Overall, it is expected that in order to reduce morbidity and mortality, these children require early diagnosis and periodic comprehensive evaluation with attention to all affected systems.

Chapter 23

Respiratory Physiology and Pathophysiology During Sleep

John L. Carroll and David F. Donnelly

INTRODUCTION

In mammals, the respiratory pump and upper airway muscles are under continuous, dynamic central nervous system (CNS) control by neurons that are, in turn, heavily modulated by states of wakefulness, NREM and REM sleep. Neural control of breathing consists not only of phasic activity driving rhythmic breathing movements, but also tonic modulation of muscle activity to maintain optimum thoracic cage configuration, lung volumes and upper airway patency. Central drive to respiratory pump and upper airway muscles is modulated dynamically by sensory information provided to the central (breathing) pattern generator from a complex system of mechano- and chemosensors, the input of which may be gated by sleep state. The central respiratory pattern generator (CPG) itself comprises a highly complex network of interacting neuronal groups that exhibit oscillatory firing behavior resulting from their reciprocal, cyclical interactions. The CPG is subject to modulation by wakefulness and sleep states not only via mechano- and chemoreceptor inputs, but also via inputs from other neurons in the brainstem, hypothalamus and cortex. Given the extent to which normal breathing is dependent on real-time neural modulation, the profound effects of sleep on breathing pattern and ventilation are a key component of normal respiratory physiology and play an important role in sleep-disordered breathing.

All aspects of the human respiratory system, including structural, mechanical and neural control, undergo profound maturational changes during growth and development. Breathing begins before birth, with fetal breathing movements *in utero*, and respiratory system maturation continues throughout childhood, with different developmental time frames for individual components, as body size increases ≈20-fold from infancy to late adolescence. Concurrent maturation of the nervous system, including the effect of wakefulness and sleep state on respiratory control, imposes another layer of important functional changes during growth and development. Thus, respiratory system physiology and the effects of sleep on breathing vary throughout life, from infancy through elderly adulthood and these changes are highly relevant to sleep medicine.

As pointed out by previous authors, several factors frustrate attempts to summarize the normal effects of sleep on breathing during postnatal development.[1] Although numerous articles explore respiratory system mechanics and respiratory control maturation in sleeping children, there are significantly fewer that explore the effects of sleep, *per se*, on breathing. Another frustrating reality is the heavily skewed focus on infants, especially preterm infants, while large gaps exist in the literature on sleep and breathing in older infants, children and adolescents. Studies that span the entire developmental age range, from infancy through late adolescence, are rare. The methods used to assess state in these studies vary from full polysomnography to simple observation, often relying on indirect indicators of sleep state. Finally, there is enormous variation in the methods and techniques used to assess respiratory system function, which have evolved over time and vary between studies. In this chapter we will selectively highlight important effects of sleep on normal respiratory physiology during childhood.

THORACIC CAGE AND PULMONARY MECHANICS

The mammalian respiratory system consists of a gas exchanger (the lungs), which are cyclically inflated and deflated by a pump (the diaphragm, rib cage and intercostal, accessory and abdominal muscles), via a single partially collapsible intake manifold (the nose, mouth and upper airway). The ability of the respiratory pump to achieve adequate gas exchange depends, in part, on resistive and elastic loads imposed and the real-time response of the system. Although the rib cage is commonly thought of as a 'structural' element of the respiratory system, the muscular components are all under continuous neural modulation and subject to further modulation by state.

Chest Wall Mechanics

Rib cage geometry in infants and children differs markedly from that of adults. Openshaw and colleagues, using chest radiographs and CT scans from individuals 1 month to 31 years of age, found that the dome of the diaphragm and head of the sternum were higher in children, relative to thoracic vertebrae.[2] The ribs of infants and young children were more horizontal (less downward slope) compared to older children and adults, and downward slope of the ribs increased with age. These changes occurred primarily between infancy and 2–3 years. The cross-sectional shape of the thorax also changed, being more rounded in infancy and becoming more ovoid (adult pattern) by about 3 years of age.[2]

In infancy, chest wall compliance is several-fold higher than lung compliance and is even higher, relative to lung compliance, in preterm infants.[3–6] With age, chest wall compliance decreases relative to lung compliance; thus, the chest wall becomes stiffer with age while lung compliance changes little. Chest wall compliance becomes approximately equal to lung compliance, as in adults, by the second year of life due to bone ossification and increased muscle mass.[4,7]

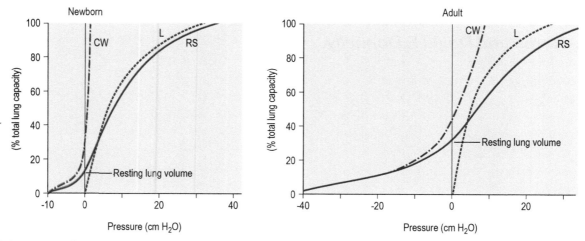

FIGURE 23-1 **Pressure volume curves of the respiratory system.** The solid line represents the compliance of the respiratory system (RS). The chest wall (CW, dash-dot line) is highly compliant in the newborn compared to the adult, while lung compliance (dashed line) changes little with age. *Adapted from Agostoni E, Mead J. Statics of the respiratory system. In: Fenn WO, Rahn H, eds. Handbook of Physiology. Washington, D.C.: American Physiological Society 1964:401.*

The high chest wall compliance of the neonate has clinical relevance. Passive (relaxed) resting lung volume (V_r) is determined by the balance between the outward recoil of the chest wall and the inward recoil of the lungs. Figure 23-1 shows the static volume pressure curves of the lung (L) and chest wall (CW) typical of a newborn and an adult.[8] Note that lung compliance is quite similar at both ages, while the chest wall is much less stiff (more compliant) in the newborn (Fig. 23-1, left panel). When the chest wall is highly compliant, the inward recoil of the lungs (L) is less opposed, resulting in a lower resting lung volume (Fig. 23-1, left panel). As the lungs are the major reservoir for oxygen, low resting lung volume predisposes infants to rapidly developing hypoxemia and atelectasis.[9,10]

Paradoxical Inward Rib Cage Motion (PIRCM)

In normal infants, without lung disease or upper airway obstruction, the highly compliant infant chest wall leads to the well-known phenomenon of 'paradoxical inward rib cage motion' (PIRCM; also called thoraco-abdominal asynchrony) during the inspiratory phase of breathing. Multiple studies during the 1970s showed that the rib cage of otherwise normal infants collapses during the inspiratory descent of the diaphragm and is associated with deflation of the rib cage, independent of upper airway obstruction.[11-13] The degree of thoraco-abdominal asynchrony is significantly greater in preterm versus full-term infants.

As expected, given the normal atonia that occurs during REM[a] sleep, PIRCM is more likely to occur during REM sleep. Even in full-term normal infants, PIRCM occurs during REM sleep and is associated with a lower and more variable PaO_2.[14] In mature, healthy, full-term infants with PIRCM during REM sleep, thoracic gas volume (TGV) was 31% reduced compared to TGV during NREM sleep.[13] As noted above, such a large decrease in TGV during REM sleep

markedly increases the probability of hypoxia with brief respiratory events, especially given that REM is the predominant sleep stage in infants, and O_2 stores (primarily the lungs) are low relative to metabolic rate.[9,10]

At what age do normal infants stop exhibiting PIRCM during childhood? This is a key question for sleep medicine specialists, as PIRCM is considered a sign of increased upper airway resistance or obstruction in older children and adults. Gaultier and colleagues studied healthy infants between 7 and 31 months of age using polysomnography and diaphragmatic EMG during a daytime nap. The duration of PIRCM during sleep decreased as postnatal age increased.[15] By 3 years of age, PIRCM is 'rare or absent' in normal children[16] and does not occur during REM sleep in normal adolescents.[17] Therefore, finding PIRCM in a child older than 3 years of age (with normal neuromuscular function) should raise suspicion for increased upper airway resistance or obstruction. However, it is important to note that the amount of measured 'paradoxical breathing' (PIRCM) might depend heavily on the technology used to detect it. In a study of 55 normal children 2–9 years of age without sleep-disordered breathing, PIRCM was detected in 40% of 30 s sleep epochs when piezo technology was used versus only 1.5% of epochs when respiratory inductance plethysmography (RIP) was used to detect thoraco-abdominal motion.[18]

Dynamic Maintenance of End Expiratory Lung Volume

Inhibition of respiratory muscle tone at any age results in a decrease in lung volume.[19-22] In other words, lung volume is maintained, in part, by respiratory muscle activity. In full-term infants, during tidal breathing in NREM sleep, end-expiratory lung volume (EEV) is maintained above the passive relaxed lung volume (V_r).[23] This is accomplished by multiple mechanisms including expiratory 'braking' using muscles of the upper airway, and post-inspiratory inspiratory activity (PIIA) of the diaphragm, which alter expiratory time constant-Te relationship such that expiration is terminated (interrupted) before reaching V_r.[23-25]

---

[a]*Sleep is typically staged as 'active' and 'quiet' in infants and 'REM' and 'NREM' in older children and adults. However, for clarity, in this chapter we use the terms REM and NREM for all ages.*

The strategy of maintaining EEV above V_r is sleep-state-dependent. Several studies of EEV in full-term infants were performed during behavioral NREM sleep but did not study the effects of sleep *per se*. When sleep state was studied, TGV was found to be greater in NREM sleep compared to REM sleep in full-term infants, suggesting that EEV was better maintained in NREM sleep.[13] Preterm infants also maintain EEV above passive V_r, also with clear sleep-state dependency. Preterm infants ≈32 weeks' gestational age were studied during the first week of life during REM and NREM sleep. In NREM sleep, a shortened expiratory time (T_E) and diaphragmatic braking resulted in maintenance of EEV above V_r. In contrast, during REM sleep, T_E was longer and expiratory braking was reduced such that EEV approached V_r.[25]

The dynamically maintained EEV, which helps maintain SpO_2 in infants, may be lost during apnea. Preterm infants ≈29 weeks' gestational age were studied during central apnea using intercostal muscle and diaphragm surface EMG activity as well as anterior–posterior (AP) diameter of the rib cage and abdomen (as a measure of EEV).[21] During apnea, decreased activity of the respiratory muscles correlated with loss of EEV. The apnea-related drop in EEV was greater during NREM sleep, suggesting that EEV was better maintained during NREM compared to REM sleep.[21] Thus, infants are able to compensate for their 'mechanical disadvantage' by maintaining EEV above passive V_r during sleep, although they do this less effectively during REM sleep. This has important clinical implications, given the importance of lung O_2 stores in infants for maintaining normal SpO_2. The loss of EEV in infants during apnea increases the probability of, and potentially the rapidity of, O_2 desaturation.

How long does the active maintenance of EEV above V_r persist during infancy? In healthy infants and children aged 1 month to 8 years, studied using RIP-derived tidal breathing flow-volume loops to assess breathing strategy, the flow-volume pattern during expiration was 'interrupted' up to 6 months of age, consistent with dynamic maintenance of an elevated EEV during this period.[26] Between 6 and 12 months, expiratory flow-volume patterns were a mixture of 'interrupted' and 'uninterrupted,' indicating a transitional period. After 1 year of age, expiratory flow-volume patterns were 'uninterrupted,' consistent with relaxed or passive end expiratory lung volume.[26] Thus, the transition from dynamic maintenance of EEV to the mature, adult-like, passive or relaxed EEV occurs during the second half of the first year of life.

Relative Contribution of Rib Cage and Abdomen to Tidal Volume

Postnatal developmental changes in chest wall compliance and active maintenance of EEV predict that the relative contributions of the rib cage (RC) and abdomen (ABD) to tidal volume, and the effects of sleep, are likely to change with maturation. In studies of normal supine adults, the average rib cage contribution to V_T fell by 25–32% during REM sleep compared to waking, consistent with the normal skeletal muscle atonia that occurs during REM sleep.[22,27] Similarly, in healthy term infants, the RC contribution to V_T was found to be lower in REM versus NREM sleep.[28] As anticipated, based on normal maturation of chest wall compliance, the contribution of the rib cage to V_T during NREM sleep (measured using RIP) increases during infancy between 1 and 26 months of age.[29]

RESPONSE TO MECHANICAL LOADING OF THE RESPIRATORY SYSTEM DURING SLEEP

Elastic and resistive loads on the respiratory system are intrinsic to the normal lungs, chest wall and upper airway. In adults, nasal and upper airway resistance increases during normal sleep, although with considerable individual variation.[30–32] Numerous disorders impose additional loading on the respiratory system, including lung disease and sleep-related upper airway obstruction, and the normal respiratory system responds with load compensation strategies that vary with type of load, age, position and state.

An added load is typically defined as anything that requires increased respiratory muscle effort in order to maintain minute ventilation. The ability of the system to compensate for increased loading can be studied using externally imposed elastic or resistive loads. Unfortunately, although most of the available studies in children have been performed *during* sleep, few have examined the effects of sleep *per se* on the respiratory system response to loading. In addition, it is difficult to compare studies due to the variety of methodologies used. Nevertheless, these studies have relevance in the context of sleep-disordered breathing, which imposes abnormal mechanical loads on the respiratory system. The key points highlighted here are (1) developmental changes in compensation for resistive loading and (2) how load compensation is affected by sleep.

Resistive Loading

Awake, normal adults are able to compensate for added resistive loads and maintain minute ventilation (V_E) and tidal volume (V_T).[33,34] This compensatory ability depends on the adequacy of the respiratory control system response as well as chest wall stability and respiratory muscle strength.[33,35] During REM and NREM sleep in normal adults, progressive addition of inspiratory resistive loads decreases V_E, largely due to inadequate prolongation of inspiratory time (T_I) in the presence of increased inspiratory resistance.[34]

The much greater compliance of the chest wall during infancy, especially in preterm infants, predicts that infants may not cope well with inspiratory resistive loading. Preterm and full-term infants during NREM sleep exhibited similar lung resistance and compliance, although the preterm infants exhibited greater thoraco-abdominal asynchrony prior to loading compared to full-term.[35] When presented with an inspiratory resistive load, full-term infants were able to maintain V_E and V_T with little effect on thoraco-abdominal synchrony. In contrast, identical inspiratory loading in preterm infants resulted in decreased V_T and V_E as well as increased chest wall asynchrony, suggesting that the preterm infant is less able to compensate due to chest wall instability.[35]

Resistive loading alters vagally mediated reflexes that modify mechanical and neural inspiratory duration. For example, in a study of full-term, 2–3-day-old infants during NREM sleep, application of increasing inspiratory resistive loads (to a single breath) resulted in progressive prolongation of T_I, shortening of expiratory time (T_E) and decreasing V_T.[36] These changes were also reflected in 'neural' V_T, T_I and T_E as measured by EMG.[36] In the same group of infants (during NREM sleep), increasing expiratory resistive loading was associated with progressive decrements in V_E and prolongation of (neural and mechanical) T_E, with little effect on T_I.[37]

In summary, both inspiratory and expiratory resistive loading decrease minute ventilation in infants, but effects on breathing pattern differ. In addition, the effects of mechanical loading on respiratory timing in infants tend to be more pronounced with resistive loads versus elastic loads.[36–38] Unfortunately, although studies were often performed during sleep, the effects of sleep *per se* were typically not examined.

Very few studies have reported the effects of respiratory mechanical loading in older normal children. Marcus and co-workers studied the effects of inspiratory resistive loading in normal children ≈9 years of age.[39] When presented with a flow-resistive load for 3 minutes during sleep, in both REM and NREM sleep there was an immediate fall in V_T and V_E, which was proportional to the magnitude of the resistance and associated with a small increase in the ratio of T_I to total breath time (T_{TOT}) due to shortening of T_E.[39] A similar study of inspiratory resistive loading during NREM sleep in normal young adults (mean age 20.5 years) also reported a marked drop in V_T (and V_E), proportional to the magnitude of the resistive load.[40] This was associated with significant prolongation of T_I and increase of T_I/T_{TOT}, with no change in respiratory rate.[40]

Elastic Loading

Although there are multiple ways to impose an elastic load on the respiratory system, a common approach is to have the subject breathe from a closed volume reservoir (elastic load varies with the size of the reservoir). In normal adults, during wakefulness, application of an inspiratory elastic load is compensated immediately such that V_T and V_E are preserved.[41] However, during NREM sleep, sustained inspiratory elastic loading caused a sustained drop in V_T and V_E until they were restored by increasing PCO_2.[41] Thus, during NREM sleep in adults, compensatory responses to elastic loading only occur when respiratory effort is increased by chemical stimuli.

In full-term, quietly sleeping infants, application of an elastic load during inspiration caused a marked fall in V_T and prolongation of T_I, with little effect on T_E.[36] Application of an elastic load during expiration in infants of the same age also caused a marked drop in V_T and prolongation of T_E, with little effect on T_I.[37] Similarly, in preterm infants ≈31 weeks' gestational age and ≈8 days' postnatal age, addition of external elastic loads caused a marked drop in V_T and prolongation of T_I and T_E, the magnitude of which increased progressively with the magnitude of the elastic load.[38]

When application of respiratory elastic loading during sleep is prolonged in term and preterm infants, V_T initially drops but progressively increases during subsequent breaths, indicating a compensatory response.[12] In both term and preterm infants, load compensation was more effective during NREM sleep. During REM sleep, elastic loading increased rib cage distortion, which limited compensation.[12] Increased respiratory elastic load occurs in numerous clinical conditions, including hyperinflation, obesity and neuromuscular disorders, and compensatory responses may be blunted by sleep, especially REM sleep.

Complete Airway Occlusion – Effects on Breathing during Sleep

Although review of the extensive literature on the Hering–Breuer (HB) and other lung-inflation reflexes is beyond the scope of this chapter, several points about the respiratory timing effects of total airway occlusion in children will be highlighted here. In 1868, Breuer and Hering described the role of the pulmonary slowly adapting stretch receptors (fibers carried in the vagus nerves) in determining the rate, depth and timing of tidal breathing.[42] The HB reflexes are classically elicited in several ways; occlusion of the airway at the beginning of inspiration prolongs T_I, while airway occlusion at end inspiration prolongs T_E. The HB reflexes can be elicited in normal, unsedated adults, but volumes larger than the normal tidal volume range are required and evidence for the persistence of HB reflexes beyond infancy is controversial.[43] In spite of multiple early studies suggesting that the HB reflexes participate in controlling tidal breathing during infancy, their role during postnatal development remains controversial.[36,37,44,45]

In full-term infants 2–3 days of age, during NREM sleep, total occlusion of the airway during inspiration (for a single breath) resulted in marked prolongation of mechanical and neural (EMG) T_I, as expected due to removal of vagally mediated feedback from pulmonary slowly adapting stretch receptors, without effect on T_E.[36] In the same group of infants, total airway occlusion during expiration (for a single breath) led to marked prolongation of T_E, without effect on T_I.[37] Beyond the newborn period, prolongation of T_E by end-inspiratory occlusion persisted throughout the first year although the magnitude of the T_E prolongation decreased with age.[46,47]

Studies in preterm infants indicate that reflex effects of inspiratory airway occlusion on timing depend on gestational age at birth and chronological age. In one study of preterm infants, ≈30 weeks' gestational age and ≈8 days old, the prolongation of T_I was similar to that seen in term infants.[48] Closer examination of the effects of maturity and age yielded different results. Preterm infants born at 27–32 weeks' gestational age and studied within the first 3–4 days exhibited wide variation in the response to inspiratory occlusion.[49] T_I was prolonged in some and shortened in others, while the overall magnitude of prolongation was much less than the ≈30% prolongation of T_I observed in full-term infants.[49] In the same group of infants, the response to inspiratory occlusion was still immature at 7–10 days, but was similar to the full-term response by 14 days. In preterm infants born at 33–36 weeks' gestational age, the T_I prolongation with inspiratory occlusion was mature by 7–10 days, suggesting that the rapidity of maturation depends on the degree of maturity at birth.[49]

Sleep may profoundly affect Hering–Breuer reflexes in infants. In a study of preterm infants 30–36 weeks' postconceptual age' (sic), using observational sleep staging, occlusion of a normal tidal breath at end inspiration resulted in an average T_E prolongation of 87% in NREM sleep compared to 419% in REM sleep.[45] However, another study, using single-breath inspiratory occlusions in term newborns, found increased Hering–Breuer activity in NREM compared to REM sleep.[50]

Caution should be exercised in the interpretation of studies using mechanical loading or total airway occlusion. As noted above, most studies only studied infants during NREM sleep. Many studies only examined the effects of occlusion for brief durations, even a single breath or parts of a breath. Reflex effects during longer occlusions may lead to increasing compensatory adaptations over time. In addition, these methods may evoke other reflex effects from face masks used and some authors have suggested that the upper airway

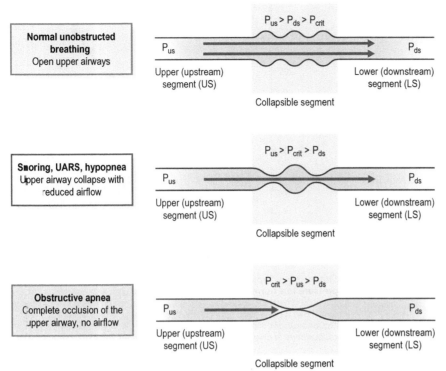

FIGURE 23-2 The upper airway modeled as a Starling resistor; airflow through a tube with rigid upstream (nasal airway) and downstream (hypopharyngeal airway) segments, and a collapsible segment in a sealed box in between (pharyngeal airway). The upstream and downstream segments have defined resistances and fixed diameters. Pus = pressure upstream. Pds = pressure downstream. The patency of the collapsible segment depends on the pressure exerted by the surrounding tissues (Pcrit). See text for explanation. *From Kirkness JP, Krishnan V, Patil SP, Schneider H. Upper Airway Obstruction in Snoring and Upper Airway Resistance Syndrome. In: Randerath WJ, Sanner BM, Somers VK, eds. Sleep Apnea. Basel: Karger; 2006:79–89.*

negative pressure and other reflexes may contribute, potentially confounding interpretation.[51]

MAINTENANCE OF UPPER AIRWAY PATENCY DURING SLEEP IN NORMAL CHILDREN

The pharyngeal airway, extending from the nasal choanae to the epiglottis, is a collapsible tube composed of muscle and soft tissues, without support from bony structures except for the posterior pharyngeal wall.[52] Pharyngeal patency depends on mechanical factors (muscle mass, connective tissue, submucosal fat, mucosal edema, perfusion, position, etc.) as well as activity of the muscles that compose and surround the airway.[52,53] The pharyngeal muscles may act to stiffen the airway soft tissues, making them less deformable by intraluminal negative pressure, or actively dilate the airway and change its caliber.[52]

The pharyngeal airway is bounded by the posterior pharyngeal wall, anchored at the top by the palatal muscles (musculus uvulae, palatoglossus, palatopharyngeus, tensor veli palatine and levator veli palatine), at the bottom by the hyoid muscles (thyrohyoid, mylohyoid, stylohyoid, geniohyoid and sternohyoid) and anteriorly by the genioglossus muscle.[52,54] The activity of these muscle groups is largely responsible for the maintenance of airway patency during sleep. It is important to note that, although most studies to date have focused on the genioglossus muscle, innervated by the hypoglossal nerve (XII), upper airway tone is influenced by input from other motoneuron groups including the motor vagus (X), glossopharyngeal (IX), facial (VII) and motor trigeminal (V).[53] In addition, motoneurons of the cervical ventral horn may contribute to airway patency via their influence on neck

and jaw position as well as lung volume.[53] As these muscles are modulated by state, sleep may profoundly affect pharyngeal patency and reflex responses (e.g., to negative pressure).

A full review of normal upper airway structure, physiology and its development is beyond the scope of this chapter. The reader is referred to several excellent reviews of upper airway structural development during childhood.[55–57] Here, we review what is known about the physiology of upper airway collapsibility in infants and children, how it can be measured, how airway patency is affected by sleep and the effects of puberty and age.

Critical Closing Pressure, P_{crit}

The human upper airway behaves as a Starling resistor, modeled as a tube with rigid segments on either end and a collapsible segment in a sealed box in between (representing the collapsible pharynx and surrounding tissue mass).[58] The patency of the collapsible segment is determined by the mechanical factors noted above and by the activity of upper airway muscles. P_{crit}, the *critical closing pressure* of the collapsible segment, is the pharyngeal lumenal pressure when collapse occurs (Figure 23-2). In this model, the upstream (nasal) and downstream (hypopharyngeal/tracheal) segments have defined resistances and fixed diameters.

During inspiration, diaphragm contraction and thoracic cage expansion lower pressure in the downstream segment, creating a pressure gradient for inspiratory airflow. The degree of inspiratory airflow limitation (if any) depends on the pressure gradient between the upstream segment (P_{us}) and P_{crit}, and is independent of downstream pressure (P_{ds}). P_{us} at the nares is atmospheric pressure (zero cmH_2O, reference) and P_{crit}, in normals, is typically less than -10 cmH_2O. Therefore, although there is a small pressure drop across the upstream segment, in normal subjects upstream pressure remains sufficiently greater than the pressure in the collapsible segment such that inspiratory airflow is unimpeded (Figure 23-2, upper panel).[58,59]

Any condition that increases P_{crit} (upper airway dilator muscle hypotonia, sedation, anesthesia, obesity, edema) may reduce the difference between P_{us} and P_{crit}, with resulting inspiratory airflow limitation (Figure 23-2, middle panel). When P_{crit} exceeds P_{us}, complete obstruction occurs (Figure 23-2, lower panel).[52,53,58,59] In simple terms, when pharyngeal critical closing pressure is positive to atmospheric pressure, complete airway collapse occurs during inspiration and upstream (nasal) positive pressure (greater than P_{crit}) is required to restore pharyngeal patency (e.g., nasal continuous positive airway pressure (CPAP)). In normal infants, children and adults, Pcrit is negative during wakefulness and sleep, usually ≤ 10 cmH$_2$O, and the pharyngeal airway is always patent, with no inspiratory airflow limitation.

Variations in P_{crit} during wakefulness and sleep are due largely to its dependence on upper airway dilator muscle activity. During normal breathing, airway patency is heavily influenced by state-dependent activity of the upper airway dilator muscles. In addition, upper airway dilator muscles are activated by negative pressure in the airway, sensed by negative pressure receptors primarily in the larynx.[52,60] Finally, the negative pressure reflex and respiratory drive to the upper airway dilator muscles are strongly influenced by the levels of chemical respiratory drive (PaO$_2$ and PaCO$_2$) from the peripheral and central chemoreceptors.[61–65] All of these factors combine to make P_{crit} dynamic, varying with position, sleep state, levels of chemical stimuli and other factors that affect pharyngeal deformability.

Measurement of Upper Airway Collapsibility

Upper airway collapsibility can be well-characterized by two values: (1) the slope of the linear relationship between maximal inspiratory flow (y-axis) and upstream (nasal) pressure (x-axis), and (2) P_{crit}, the x-axis intercept (zero flow). The relationship between upper airway maximal inspiratory flow (V_{Imax}) and nasal pressure (P_N) may be termed V_{Imax}/P_N and is also termed 'S_{PF}' (slope of the pressure–flow relationship) in the pediatric literature.[66] P_{crit} and V_{Imax}/P_N can be determined experimentally in individual subjects to obtain numerical measures of upper airway collapsibility. Their classic laboratory measurement yields values that 'characterize' upper airway collapsibility during sleep for a particular sleep stage and specific method of measurement, in an individual subject. P_{crit} and V_{Imax}/P_N are typically measured during slow wave sleep and are difficult to measure during wakefulness or REM sleep.

In humans, P_{crit} of the upper airway is typically measured during tidal breathing, using a nasal mask attached to source of negative or positive pressure. A pneumotachograph is used to measure inspiratory airflow and P_N is measured at the mask.[67,68] In normal subjects there is no inspiratory flow limitation when nasal pressure is zero (atmospheric pressure), so negative pressure is applied via the nasal mask and made more negative in steps to produce a V_{Imax} vs. P_N relationship as shown in Figure 23-3. When maximal inspiratory airflow (for tidal breaths at a given pressure) is plotted versus nasal mask pressure, a linear relationship is obtained and extrapolated to zero flow. The slope of the V_{Imax}/P_N relationship (aka 'slope of

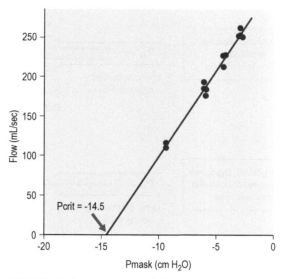

FIGURE 23-3 Typical measurement of pharyngeal critical closing pressure in a normal subject. The slope of the pressure–flow relationship (in mL/sec/cmH$_2$O) represents airway conductance and the x-axis intercept (zero flow) represents critical closing pressure (P_{crit}). *From Litman RS, McDonough JM, Marcus CL, Schwartz AR, Ward DS. Upper airway collapsibility in anesthetized children. Anesth Analg 2006;102:750–4.*

the pressure–flow relationship' (S_{PF}) in the literature) represents the collapsibility of the upper airway and the x-axis (zero flow) intercept represents P_{crit} (Figure 23-3). This approach has been used to characterize upper airway collapsibility in numerous studies of normal children[69] and adults.[67,68] In children with sleep-disordered breathing (SDB), when airflow limitation or obstructive apnea are already present at baseline (nasal mask pressure $=0$), a linear pressure–flow relationship can be obtained in a similar manner by applying positive pressure via nasal mask, increasing in steps until airflow limitation is abolished.

Dynamic Upper Airway Negative Pressure Reflexes: Active Versus Passive P_{crit}

In normal children during neuromuscular paralysis P_{crit} is about -7.5 cmH$_2$O,[70] much higher than the P_{crit} of normal children during sleep, which is about -25 cmH$_2$O using the 'gradual' method of measurement (see below).[66,71,72] Loads imposed on the upper airway that generate negative pressure in the pharynx and larynx may cause reflex activation of upper airway dilator muscles to stiffen and/or alter the caliber of the airway.[52] This has very important implications for the measurement of the V_{Imax}/P_N relationship and P_{crit}. When upper airway collapsibility is measured in the classic way, by progressively stepping down nasal (mask) pressure, the upper airway dilator muscles are reflexly activated as nasal pressure is decreased (made more negative). Figure 23-4 shows a normal subject, in stage 2 NREM sleep, starting from a nasal mask holding pressure of 5 cmH$_2$O.[73] The left panel shows the 'gradual' approach, in which P_N is decreased 1–2 cmH$_2$O every 10 minutes, without returning to baseline holding pressure. This results in recruitment of compensatory upper airway dilator muscle activity, as evidenced by the marked genioglossus muscle EMG activity (Figure 23-4). The P_{crit} and V_{Imax}/P_N relationships measured using the 'gradual' approach include

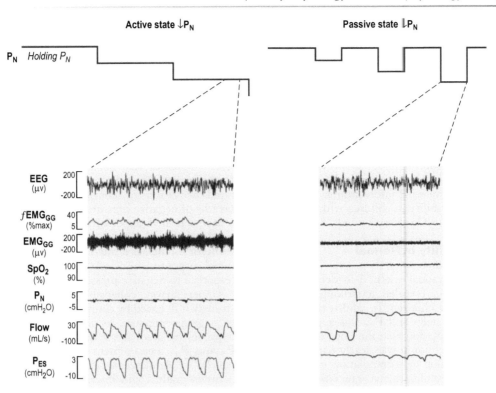

FIGURE 23-4 Comparison of the two methods of measuring upper airway collapsibility in a control subject. *Left panel:* 'Gradual' method. *Left upper:* From holding pressure of 5 cmH₂O during stage 2 NREM sleep, nasal mask (P_N) pressure is lowered in steps about every 10 minutes. *Left lower:* At –3 cmH₂O nasal pressure, inspiratory flow limitation occurs and compensatory dilator muscle activity (EMG_{GG}) is markedly increased. *Right panel:* 'Intermittent' method. *Right upper:* Starting from the same holding pressure (5 cm H₂O) in stage 2 NREM sleep, nasal mask pressure is lowered intermittently for five breaths only and then returned to the baseline holding pressure. *Right lower:* At –3 cmH₂O, in sharp contrast to the 'gradual' method (*left*), there is no compensatory upper airway dilator muscle activation. **Modified from McGinley BM, Schwartz AR, Schneider H, Kirkness JP, Smith PL, Patil SP. Upper airway neuromuscular compensation during sleep is defective in obstructive sleep apnea. J Appl Physiol 2008;105:197–205.**

the effects of compensatory dilator muscle activity and are therefore also known as 'active' or 'activated' pressure–flow measurements.[66]

The 'intermittent' method of measuring the V_{Imax}/P_N relationship and P_{crit} was developed to avoid the effects of upper airway dilator muscle recruitment during the measurement. This method, shown in the right panel of Figure 23-4, also starts from a holding pressure but decreases P_N for only 5 breaths and then returns to baseline holding pressure. In the example shown in Figure 23-4, right panel, nasal mask pressure was lowered without activation of compensatory upper airway dilator muscle activity, as indicated by the absence of genioglossus muscle activation (EMG_{GG}).[73] The 'intermittent' approach is also known as the 'passive' or 'hypotonic' method, as it characterizes upper airway collapsibility without the effects of compensatory dilator muscle activity.[66]

When both the 'gradual' and 'intermittent' methods of upper airway pressure–flow measurement are used in the same individual, important additional information is gained. Differences in P_{crit} and the slope of V_{Imax}/P_N, measured using the 'gradual' and 'intermittent' method, reflect the magnitude of compensatory upper airway dilator muscle responses. As illustrated in Figure 23-5, use of the intermittent method results in a higher (less negative) P_{crit} and steeper slope of the V_{Imax}/P_N relationship, compared to the gradual method. In sharp contrast, the gradual method applied to the same child results

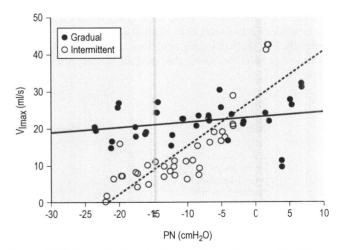

FIGURE 23-5 Example of 'gradual' versus 'intermittent' method of measuring upper airway pressure–flow relationships in a child. With the 'gradual' method compensatory muscle responses decreased airway collapsibility. With the intermittent technique, compensatory dilator muscle responses are not activated; resulting in a higher P_{crit} and steeper slope (SPF). *From Marcus CL, Fernandes Do Prado LB, Lutz J, et al. Developmental changes in upper airway dynamics. J Appl Physiol 2004;97:98–108.*

in a much flatter slope of the V_{Imax}/P_N relationship and P_{crit} is shifted far to the left (more negative) (Figure 23-5).[66] Thus, when the gradual method was used, upper airway dilator muscle recruitment preserved V_{Imax} in spite of increasingly negative P_N, indicating strong dynamic regulation of airway patency.

P_{crit} and the slope of the V_{Imax}/P_N relationship have been studied extensively in normal adults and children and in subjects with SDB, before and after airway surgery, pre- and post-weight loss, before and after puberty and a variety of other conditions. Both measures of upper airway collapsibility correlate strongly with apnea–hypopnea index (AHI) in subjects with SDB and improve with interventions that reduce AHI. Upper airway collapsibility in children with pathological conditions is discussed in Chapters 27 and 28.

Upper Airway Collapsibility in Normal Children – Effects Of Age

Early studies, using the 'gradual' method to determine P_{crit} and the slope of V_{Imax}/P_N, revealed a striking difference between normal adults and children. In adults, the V_{Imax}/P_N relationship was relatively steep and P_{crit} was approximately -5 to -30 cmH$_2$O.[74] In sharp contrast, the slope of the V_{Imax}/P_N relationship in normal children was nearly flat, making it difficult to obtain a P_{crit} value by extrapolation to zero flow. This indicated that normal children have a remarkable ability to maintain upper airway patency in spite of increasingly negative pressure in the airway lumen. The slope of the V_{Imax}/P_N relationship averaged ≈ 8.5 mL/s/cmH$_2$O in children compared to ≈ 30 mL/s/cmH$_2$O in adults.[74]

Later studies covered a larger age range and used both the 'gradual' and the 'intermittent' methods for determining upper airway collapsibility. In adults, the V_{Imax}/P_N relationship is steeper than in children, indicating that the adult airway is more collapsible compared to infants and children (Figure 23-6).[66] Figure 23-6, right panel, shows that the method used ('gradual' vs. 'intermittent') had little effect on the slope or on P_{crit} in adults. Other studies in normal adults suggest that P_{crit} is slightly left-shifted (more negative) by 5–10 cmH$_2$O, with little change in slope, using the 'gradual' versus 'intermittent' approach.[73,75]

The V_{Imax}/P_N relationship in infants is relatively flat, P_{crit} is much more negative compared to adult values, and neither is affected by the 'gradual' versus 'intermittent' method (Figure 23-6, left panel). This indicates that the infant upper airway is far less collapsible compared to the adult airway, in spite of being narrower.[66] The lack of difference between the 'gradual' and 'intermittent' approaches in infants (Figure 23-6, left panel) should not be interpreted as a lack of compensatory upper airway muscle activity during infancy. Indeed, the infant airway is heavily dependent upon dilator muscle activity.[76] The reason that the 'gradual' versus 'intermittent' V_{Imax}/P_N curves are about the same in infants is likely due to very rapid activation of compensatory responses, within 1–2 breaths of negative pressure application, such that *both curves* reflect activated upper airway dilator muscles.[77,78] In other words, the 'gradual' versus 'intermittent' approach does not work for infants, as a way to separate 'activated' versus 'hypotonic' responses, because the timing of their compensatory responses to negative pressure is so rapid.[66]

Upper airway collapsibility in school-aged children is strongly influenced by compensatory dilator muscle responses to negative pressure, as indicated by the large difference between the 'gradual' versus 'intermittent' approach to V_{Imax}/P_N and P_{crit} measurement (Figures 23-5 and 23-6, middle panel).[66,72] Adolescents also exhibit a marked difference between 'gradual' and 'intermittent' measurement approaches in the slope of the upper airway V_{Imax}/P_N relationship and P_{crit} which increases with age.[79] The increase in adolescent upper airway collapsibility with age, approaching adult values by late adolescence, is independent of Tanner stage.[80] Normal, nonsnoring obese adolescents exhibit normal, vigorous upper airway neuromotor responses to negative pressure loading (using the 'gradual' and 'intermittent' methods) that are nearly identical to those of lean controls.[79]

In summary, with increasing age, from infancy through adolescence, P_{crit} becomes less negative and the slope of the VI_{max}/P_N relationship becomes steeper. Thus, compared to adults, the upper airway of infants and children is relatively resistant to collapse, largely due to highly effective compensatory neuromotor responses to negative pressure during sleep. This may explain, in part, why children have less obstructive

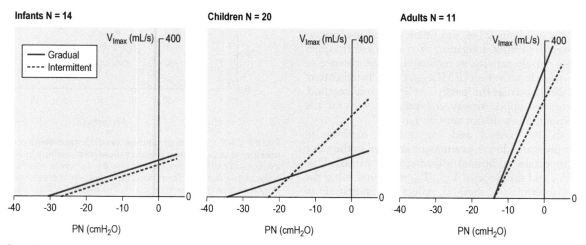

FIGURE 23-6 Median V_{Imax}/P_N relationships for normal infants, children and adults using the 'gradual' and 'intermittent' methods. See text for explanation. *From Marcus CL, Fernandes Do Prado LB, Lutz J, et al. Developmental changes in upper airway dynamics. J Appl Physiol 2004;97:98–108.*

SDB and snore less than adults, in spite of having a smaller, narrower upper airway. Indeed, defective upper airway neuromotor responses to loading are believed to be a major factor in the pathophysiology of obstructive SDB in children.[81,82]

Effects of Sleep Stage on Maintenance of Upper Airway Patency

It is well known that obstructive sleep-disordered breathing usually occurs during REM sleep in children,[83] possibly related to decreased upper airway dilator muscle activity,[84-86] decreased sensitivity of upper airway reflexes to chemical stimuli,[63] or other factors. Unfortunately, little is known about the physiology of upper airway collapsibility during REM sleep. The earliest studies in this area found that arousal tends to occur with negative pressure or occlusion challenges during REM sleep and therefore studies are typically performed only during stage 2 NREM sleep.[69] Therefore, most data on effects of wakefulness, REM and NREM sleep on upper airway physiology have been performed using non-challenge protocols, typically by measuring genioglossus muscle EMG during sleep. In normal, non-snoring, asymptomatic children studied using EMG_{GG} during polysomnography, tonic EMG_{GG} activity was highest during wakefulness, decreased to 65% of wakefulness level during NREM sleep and further decreased to about half of wakefulness level during REM sleep.[84] In normal children, no phasic EMG_{GG} activity was observed during sleep.[84]

Dynamic Neuromotor Responses to Upper Airway Negative Pressure Loading

Dynamic upper airway responses have been studied in normal children ($\approx$9–16 years of age) using negative pressure challenges (via nasal mask) during polysomnography, while recording EMG_{GG}.[87] As illustrated in Figure 23-7, the upper airway neuromotor responses to negative pressure may develop quite rapidly. In this example, phasic EMG_{GG} activity can be observed even on breath 1 of the negative pressure challenge (Figure 23-7). As EMG_{GG} activity increases progressively breath by breath, inspiratory flow limitation decreases until flow limitation is abolished by breath 5 (Figure 23-7). These rapid-onset EMG_{GG} responses to negative pressure were

highly variable between individuals.[87] In another study, adolescents exposed during NREM sleep to 'gradual' stepping down of nasal pressure or the 'intermittent' method showed greater activation of EMG_{GG} using the 'gradual' method compared to the 'intermittent' approach. Normal, non-snoring obese adolescents showed much greater activation of EMG_{GG} during sleep compared to lean controls, suggesting that they maintain upper airway patency during sleep via increased compensatory upper airway neuromotor activity compared to lean controls.[79]

Effects of Chemical Stimuli on Upper Airway Collapsibility

The effect of chemical stimuli on the upper airway muscles is a complex topic, beyond the scope of this chapter. Suffice it to say that both hypoxia and hypercapnia increase the activity of some (but not all) of the upper airway dilator muscles.[52,88,89] In humans, although stimulation of the upper airway muscles by CO_2 in adults is greatly reduced during sleep (compared to wakefulness), this response appears to be preserved during sleep in children.[66] The main effect of increased PCO_2, studied in normal school-aged children during NREM sleep, using the 'gradual' approach for measuring upper airway collapsibility, was an increase in inspiratory flow at a given nasal pressure. This effect was greatest for mild negative nasal pressures and diminished with increasingly negative P_N.[56]

VENTILATION DURING SLEEP IN NORMAL CHILDREN

Respiratory Frequency

Breathing pattern becomes more regular with age. Parmelee et al. studied a group of premature infants from 30 weeks' gestation and a group of term infants. In preterm infants, regular breathing occurs only 10% of the time at 36 weeks' gestation and 30% of the time in infants at 40 weeks' gestation.[90] For both premature and term infants, respiration became more regular over the 8-month period studied. In general, respiratory rate is lower during sleep than during wakefulness.[91] There is a general consensus that the respiratory rate,[50,92-96] and particularly the variability of respiratory

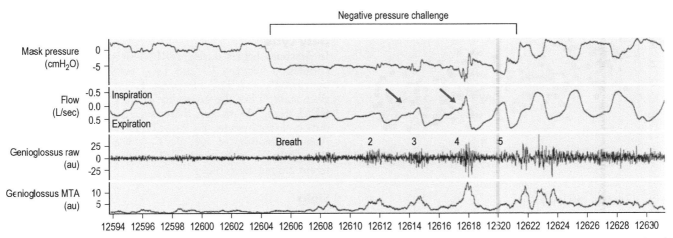

FIGURE 23-7 Dynamic, breath-by-breath response to negative pressure challenge in a normal child. See text for explanation. *From Katz ES, Marcus CL, White DP. Influence of airway pressure on genioglossus activity during sleep in normal children. Am J Respir Crit Care Med 2006;173:902–9.*

frequency,[92] is higher in REM sleep compared to NREM sleep. This is likely due to direct stimulation of brainstem respiratory neurons during REM sleep.[97] Breathing frequency is not different between sexes,[98-100] at least in the first weeks of life. However, the range of respiratory frequencies is quite large, ranging from 40–60 breaths/min for infants less than 10 days old.[96,98-100] In addition to variability in recording methodologies and time of day of recordings, ambient temperature and even the type of feeding[101] may have influenced the measurement and contributed to the large range of observations.

Over the first year of life, there is a general trend towards lower respiratory rates,[102] an increase in regular breathing,[90] and a smaller difference in respiratory frequency between NREM and REM sleep.[90] For instance, in one longitudinal study respiratory frequency declined from 41 breaths/min at 1 month of age to 31 breaths/min at 5–6 months for both sleep states[101] but others have found the decrease in respiratory rate is primarily in REM sleep.[103] In another study, which examined 57 normal infants, respiratory frequency was higher at 2–5 weeks, and 6–10 weeks compared to newborns or 11–18-week-old infants.[95] Beyond 1 month of age, males breathe more rapidly than females, suggesting a slower maturation of the respiratory control system in males.[104]

A recent, large, multicenter study of over 200 Caucasian children 1–18 years of age, found that respiratory rate during NREM sleep declined steadily over the entire age range, from 1 to 18 years (Figure 23-8).[105] Average respiratory frequency declined from ≈22 breaths/min at 1–1.5 years to ≈15 breaths/min at 16–18 years of age. The scatter in normal respiratory rate values was large over the entire age range, such that there is substantial overlap in the normal range for a normal 1-year-old and 17-year-old (Figure 23-8).[105]

In older children between 9 and 13 years, respiratory rate is highest in wakefulness and stage 1 sleep and lowest in stage 2 sleep.[106] While the average respiratory rate is the same in males and females, the variance of rate is higher in males.[102,106] In a study of adolescents, respiratory rate decreased in going from wakefulness to NREM sleep and increased during REM sleep;[17] in another, respiratory frequency was not different between NREM and REM sleep.[107]

Tidal Volume

In preterm infants ≈31 weeks' gestational age, studied at ≈3 weeks of age, average tidal volume during sleep was 6.7–7.0 mL/kg during sleep and did not differ between REM and NREM sleep.[108] Average tidal volume for term infants during the first week of life is about 4.6–4.9 mL/kg.[93,109] In contrast to respiratory frequency, generally no significant difference was observed in tidal volume between REM and NREM sleep in babies[50,92,93] or only a slight decrease in V_T was observed.[93] This is perhaps surprising since the chest wall and abdominal wall are more synchronous in NREM sleep, but during REM sleep abdominal wall and chest wall are asynchronous, and tidal volume is negatively correlated with the phase shift between the two.

In older babies at 2 months of age, using barometric plethysmography, V_T was greater in NREM sleep than REM sleep.[102] In adolescents, tidal volume was not significantly changed between wakefulness, NREM sleep and REM sleep.[17]

Minute Ventilation

As expected for an increase in breathing frequency and little or no change in V_T, minute ventilation is generally increased in REM sleep compared to NREM sleep,[50,92,93,108] but this was not found uniformly in all studies.[94,102] This is perhaps surprising because of the thoraco-abdominal asynchrony in REM sleep, but an increase in minute ventilation is even observed in preterm infants in which the chest wall is most compliant.[109] As expected from the greater variability of respiratory frequency in REM sleep, minute ventilation also showed higher variability in REM sleep.[92]

In adolescents, minute ventilation decreased by 8% in going from wakefulness to NREM sleep and increased by 4% in going from NREM to REM sleep.[17] In another study of older children, minute ventilation was not different between NREM and REM sleep.[107] In adults, data from numerous studies indicate that V_E falls about 15–18% in NREM and REM sleep, due largely to a decrease in V_T without a change in respiratory rate, although variability is higher between studies.[110] Some of the variation between studies may be due to measurement of respiratory rate during tonic versus phasic REM sleep.

Duty Cycle

In newborn babies during NREM sleep, there is a positive correlation between V_T and T_{TOT}, between T_I and T_E and between V_T and T_I.[93] However, T_I/T_{TOT} does not vary with sleep state,[102] but the variability of T_I/T_{TOT} was increased in REM sleep.[94] With age, there is a general increase in most duty cycle parameters: V_T, V_{TOT}, T_I, T_E, V_T/T_I and V_T/T_{TOT}.[102] Above 2 months of age, V_T/T_{TOT} was smaller in NREM sleep.[102] In adolescents, the T_I/T_{TOT} was not significantly different among sleep states.[17]

Sighs

Sighs or augmented breaths are spontaneous deep breaths several times larger than regular tidal breaths. Some sighs appear to be a 'breath on top of a breath,' which is characterized by a biphasic respiratory pattern; a long inspiratory

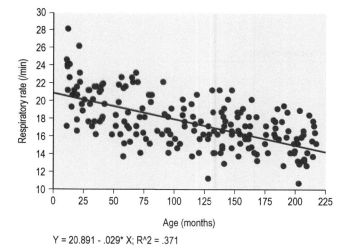

$$Y = 20.891 - .029 * X; R^2 = .371$$

FIGURE 23-8 Respiratory rate in normal children 1–18 years of age and results of linear regression. *From Scholle S, Wiater A, Scholle HC. Normative values of polysomnographic parameters in childhood and adolescence: cardiorespiratory parameters. Sleep Med 2011;12:988–96.*

duration with an abrupt change in inspiratory flow rate halfway through the inspiratory phase.[111] These intermittent deep breaths are believed to serve an important function in re-expanding collapsed lung segments. Sighs are common in the newborn period, particularly during REM sleep, and are associated with periodic breathing which occurs in about half the subjects and is unrelated to sleep stage.[112] The frequency of sighs decreases with postnatal age.[111,113] It is unclear whether they are more numerous in NREM sleep – one study concluded that they are[114] while another concluded that they are not.[113] Retarded expiratory flow, possibly due to post-inspiratory inspiratory diaphragmatic activity, is also mostly encountered in NREM sleep.[114] Spontaneous sighs appear to increase the probability of a subsequent apnea along with oscillatory respiratory efforts.[115]

Normal Apnea

Apneas are common in the newborn period,[91,116,117] decrease in frequency with age,[96,118] and are often associated with body movements.[112] They are especially prevalent in preterm newborns,[116,119] they occur more often in REM than NREM sleep,[95,100,101,120–124] and last longer in REM sleep.[101] Apnea also appeared to occur more commonly in breast-fed infants[101] and may occur more in females than males beyond 1 month of age.[101,104,122]

Apnea durations of 6–10 s are especially common during infancy, generally considered to be normal,[91,112,125] and are more likely to occur during REM sleep (Figure 23-9).[96] Most apneas are central apneas and obstructive or mixed apneas are infrequent in the newborn period,[121] but increase between 3 and 6 weeks and then diminish by 3 months.[118] Their incidence is affected by sleep position, being more common in the prone position.[126] Others have found that in young infants obstructive apneas are more common than central apneas.[124] In a study of 88 full-term healthy infants between 12 and 18 months/age, apnea density (minutes of apnea/100 min of quiet time) remained constant at 0.5 and did not differ across ages or between sexes.[127]

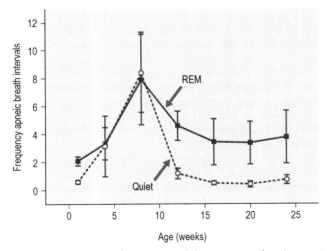

FIGURE 23-9 Frequency of apneic intervals lasting greater than 4 sec as a function of age and sleep state. *Adapted from Adamson TM, Cranage S, Maloney JE, Wilkinson MH, Wilson FE, Yu VY. The maturation of respiratory patterns in normal full term infants during the first six postnatal months. II: Sleep states and apnoea. Australian Paediatric Journal 1981;17:257–61.*

Apneas become less common at older ages[121] and cannot be reliably predicted from recordings from the first week of life.[91] By 1 year of age, no apneas greater than 20 seconds were observed in a population of infants.[120] Here, the time and duration of recording may play a role since greater recording times are associated with an increase in apnea index, perhaps due to the influence of circadian rhythms.[123] Again, there appears to be a prevalence of central apneas over obstructive apneas in children 2–9 years old with an apnea index of 0.08/hour for central apneas and 0.01/hour for obstructive apneas.[18]

In normal children 9–13 years of age, apnea lasting five seconds or longer was observed in all subjects ranging from 3 to 40/night, with an average of about 18/night.[106] Some of these central pauses lasted up to 25 seconds and were most prevalent in stage 1 and REM sleep compared to stages 2–4.[106] In children 1–18 years old, the prevalence of central apneas lasting longer than 10 seconds was 30%.[129] No mixed apneas were observed in any normal children or adolescents.[129]

In contrast to obstructive apnea, central apneas lasting >10 s occurs frequently in children and occur slightly more commonly in NREM sleep compared to REM sleep.[129] Often, central apnea was not associated with significant O_2 desaturation, which was observed with only 19% of central apneas.[130] The lowest O_2 desaturation observed was 88%. There was no apparent difference between children demonstrating apneas and those that did not. Both groups spent the same amount of time in REM sleep (18% of total sleep time).

In a study of normal children aged 1–18 years, 18% had obstructive apneas, but they were rare; averaging only 0.1 obstructive apneas per sleep hour, never longer than 10 seconds duration and not correlated with age.[129] In normal children 1–15 years of age, central apneas were much more common compared to obstructive apneas (89% incidence).[130] Obstructive apneas were observed in only 4% of normal children and were not associated with a specific sleep stage.[130] Of those normal children exhibiting obstructive apneas, the apnea index was about 0.37[130] to 0.56.[129] Compared to normal children, obstructive apneas in adults are more common and increase with advancing age.[131]

The physiologic and clinical importance of normal apnea pauses is uncertain. Analysis of event recording in infants (about 6–7 months of age) demonstrates that out of 1306 apneic events lasting longer than 15 seconds, only 14.9% were associated with bradycardia.[132] Follow-up on patients who demonstrated prolonged apneas, some exceeding 25 seconds, indicated that none had subsequent life-threatening events.[132] In older children (9–13 years), apneas lasting greater than 5 seconds also occurred frequently.[106] These pauses were most frequent in stage 1 and REM sleep compared to stages 2, 3 and 4,[106] and most occurred in association with sigh or movement.[17] Another study in adolescents recorded 5.5 central apneas lasting longer than 10 s per night,[17] but these were not associated with an O_2 desaturation below 90%.[129]

Over multiple studies, the overall apnea index is near 1,[130,133] which is considerably less than that observed in adults.[131] This underscores the conclusion that normative data developed in adults do not well apply to the pediatric population,[134] although it may apply to adolescents in some cases.[135]

Periodic Breathing

Periodic breathing, characterized by periodic respiratory pauses, is common in the newborn period, especially in preterm infants.[90] As with apnea, periodic breathing is more common in REM sleep compared to NREM sleep.[136] The incidence of periodic breathing appears to decrease over the first 3 months of life.[100,121]

CONTROL OF VENTILATION DURING SLEEP

Ventilatory Response To Hypoxia

The hypoxic ventilatory response normalized to weight decreases with age, from -0.035 $L\cdot kg^{-1}\cdot min^{-1}\cdot SaO_2^{-1}$ in children to -0.024 $L\cdot kg^{-1}\cdot min^{-1}\cdot SaO_2^{-1}$ in adults, similar to the age-dependent decrease in hypercapnic ventilatory response.[137] This may serve an important purpose in promoting respiratory stability since high levels of peripheral chemoreceptor responsiveness are correlated with respiratory instabilities, particularly apnea and oscillatory breathing patterns.[138,139] This is consistent with an age-dependent decrease in peripheral chemoreceptor drive to breath which continues at least through 28 years.[140]

In adult men, the hypoxic ventilatory response decreased to two-thirds of waking value in NREM sleep and to one-third of waking value in REM sleep,[141] although another study found similar values in NREM sleep and wakefulness.[142] The response appears to be state-dependent. Stimulation of breathing with 15% O_2 caused a biphasic response in wakefulness and REM but a sustained increase in NREM sleep.[143]

Ventilatory Response to Hyperoxia

In premature infants, the response to reducing peripheral chemoreceptor input by breathing 100% O_2 caused ventilation to drop by 28% in wakefulness, 39% in REM sleep and 37% in NREM sleep and often caused an apnea lasting 8–11 seconds.[143] In older infants, the drop in minute ventilation in response to a step increase in inspired O_2 is similar in REM and NREM sleep, primarily due to a decrease in V_T compared to F.[92]

Ventilatory Response to Hypercapnia

The absolute ventilatory response to hypercapnia during wakefulness increases with the weight of the subject over the period of 4–49 years, but when normalized to body weight, the ventilatory response decreases with age.[137,144] The normalized ventilatory response in children was $0.056\,L\cdot kg^{-1}\cdot min^{-1}\cdot torr$ $P_{ET}CO_2^{-1}$ and in adults was $0.032\,L\cdot kg^{-1}\cdot min^{-1}\cdot torr\,P_{ET}CO_2^{-1}$. The ventilatory response to CO_2 is generally linear and, thus, may be extrapolated to the point where ventilation is zero, the CO_2 threshold. The CO_2 threshold was also lower in children compared to adults, 36 versus 40 torr. When normalized to weight, there are no significant ventilatory differences between males and females, except for a slightly lower CO_2 threshold in females.[137] The decrease in hypercapnic ventilatory response is paralleled by a decrease in airway occlusion pressure ($P_{0.1}$) during hypercapnic stimulation, a measure of ventilatory drive, which also decreases with age.[145]

Control of $PaCO_2$ appears to be sleep-stage-dependent. End-tidal CO_2 for older children (1–15 years) exceeds 45 mmHg about 1.6–2% of total sleep time.[130] $P_{ET}CO_2$ was >50 mmHg for 0.3% total sleep time[130] similar to the conclusion of Brouillette et al., who consider 45 mmHg to be the upper limit of normal.[146] This is less than earlier values, where Marcus et al.[129] found >45 mmHg some 7% of the time and

>50 mmHg 0.5% of the time. Despite the hypoventilation, as indicated by CO_2 values, desaturation events (lower than 92%) are very rare in the normal population and may represent the most accurate parameter to determine whether respiratory pathology exists.[129,147] While being different in sleep, the ventilatory response to CO_2 was the same in both NREM and REM sleep.[108]

NORMAL AROUSAL FROM SLEEP

Arousal from sleep represents an important defense response against an ongoing respiratory challenge. Spontaneous arousals are a normal part of REM and NREM sleep.[148] For instance, in preterm and term infants, arousals (as defined by behavior) not associated with apnea occurred at a rate of 0.23/minute.[149] The frequency increased to 0.59/minute in sleep periods with apnea and was significantly higher during long apneic periods, during mixed versus central apnea and during severe versus mild apnea.[149] The arousal frequency may be influenced by sleep position. In healthy term infants, during REM sleep the prone position is associated with significantly fewer arousals compared to supine; however, the rate of arousal is the same (prone versus supine) in NREM sleep.[150] Overall, the rate of arousals is lower in the prone compared to supine positions at 3 months of age.[151]

Despite their association with apnea termination, arousal may not be essential since most apneic events appear to terminate without arousals, at least in younger infants.[149] In older (pre-pubertal) children during NREM sleep, termination of obstructive apnea events was associated with EEG arousal in only 12%, with movement in the rest.[152] Here, movement occurred in the absence of EEG changes. In comparison, all REM sleep apneas were terminated with a movement.[152] Thus, arousal as defined by EEG changes does not appear to be a prerequisite for apnea termination.

Hypercarbia is a strong stimulus for arousal and probably plays a critical role in apnea termination. In a group of normal infants aged 7.3 weeks, the arousal threshold to increased CO_2 was 48.4 torr.[153] An even lower arousal threshold, 40.1 torr, was reported for 1–25 months of age.[154] This CO_2 threshold is only slightly above the normal resting level of CO_2. Similarly, in children 9 weeks of age, raising CO_2 to 60 torr by adding CO_2 to the inspired air caused arousal in all children.[155] In older children at 4.4 years of age, every child aroused when CO_2 was increased to 60 torr.[156] Although most of the ventilatory drive due to CO_2 is due to central chemoreceptors, arousal from sleep due to increased CO_2 appears to be dependent on peripheral chemoreceptors, at least in experimental models where it may be reduced by carotid sinus nerve section or hyperoxia.[157,158]

In comparison to hypercarbia, hypoxia appears to be a weaker stimulus for arousal. In normal infants, arousal was observed 70% of the time when FiO_2 was decreased to 0.15.[153] In another study, an FiO_2 of 0.15 caused arousal in only 32% of the trials.[159] In infants of 9 weeks of age, hypoxia (80 torr) failed to cause arousal in most cases, and in a group of infants averaging 12 weeks of age, hypoxia (80 torr) caused arousal in only 8 of 18 infants.[155] Arousal to hypoxia appears to occur more frequently in the older infant. In infants 1–25 months (average age 8 months) arousal to hypoxia (78 torr) occurred in all instances.[154] Position also has a significant influence.

Hypoxia-induced arousal threshold is higher in the prone position compared to the supine position.[160]

There is limited information on the state dependence of hypoxia-induced arousal from sleep in humans. In normal term infants, the level of PaO_2 is significantly lower and more variable in REM sleep compared to NREM sleep.[14] However, the frequency of arousal during hypoxia is higher in REM compared to NREM sleep for infants studied at 2–5 weeks, 2–3 months and 5–6 months.[161–163] This difference may be related to the rate of O_2 desaturation in the two states since no difference in level of O_2 saturation at the time of arousal was observed between the sleep states.[164]

The rate of desaturation may also be important. In lambs, where the rate of desaturation could be experimentally controlled, arousal from NREM sleep occurred at an SaO_2 of 80–83%;[165] however, during REM sleep arousal occurred between 44–76% SaO_2, with the lower value associated with the most rapid development of hypoxia.[165] Similar results were found in other laboratories where the SaO_2 at arousal was lower in REM than NREM sleep[166] and significantly reduced by carotid nerve denervation.[167]

State-related differences in arousal threshold have been observed for other stimuli. Arousal threshold in response to a nasal air-jet is significantly higher (i.e., stronger jet pressure required) in NREM sleep compared to REM sleep at 2–3 weeks and at 2–3 months,[168] but the difference is absent in the premature infant.[169] This is similar to the higher threshold for arousal from air-jet stimulation in the prone position during both NREM and REM sleep,[170,171] but this may be dependent on age since it was not observed at 2–3 weeks or 5–6 months post term.[172]

In conclusion, arousal serves an important function in the termination of some apneic events but does not appear to be involved in the majority of cases. Increases in CO_2 in particular can initiate arousal but decreases in SaO_2 may also evoke arousal. In general, the threshold for arousal is higher in NREM sleep compared to REM sleep.

SUMMARY

With respect to normal respiratory physiology during sleep, infancy is a time of rapid central nervous system, neural respiratory control, respiratory system structural and mechanical maturation, as well as developmental plasticity and vulnerability. Rib cage geometry, which differs markedly in infants compared to that of adults, becomes more adult-like by about 3 years of age. The high chest wall compliance of the newborn decreases with age and becomes approximately equal to lung compliance, as in adults, by the second year of life, resulting in higher resting lung volume. Concurrently, the contribution of the rib cage to tidal volume during sleep increases over the first 26 months of life. Paradoxical inward rib cage motion (thoracoabdominal asynchrony), so commonly observed in term newborns, and even more so in preterm newborns, decreases with age over the first 2–3 years of life. PIRCM after age 3 is abnormal and can be reliably used as a sign of abnormal physiology (e.g., increased upper airway resistance). The dynamic maintenance of end-expiratory lung volume above passive V_r, characteristic of the newborn and infants up to ≈6 months of life, transitions to passive or relaxed end-expiratory lung volume by about 1 year of age. Mechanical

loading of the respiratory system reveals infant vulnerability, especially in preterm newborns due, in part, to their high chest wall compliance. Infancy is also a time of respiratory control immaturity and instability, frequent central apnea and periodic breathing, all of which resolve or decline with maturation.

Childhood, between infancy and adolescence, continues to be a time of rapid growth, and maturation of neural respiratory control continues across childhood. Ventilatory drive decreases with age. Ventilatory responses to both hypoxia and hypercapnia (adjusted for body weight) decrease with age. Although the upper airway is smaller in young children and increases in size throughout childhood, the upper airway is much less collapsible in infants and children compared to adults. This is due to robust, dynamic, reflex regulation of upper airway collapsibility, likely mediated by negative pressure reflexes that persist throughout childhood and into adolescence, but are greatly reduced in adults. Central apnea continues to occur normally in children, but is less frequent than in the newborn. Obstructive apnea is uncommon in infants and children but becomes more common in adults and continues to increase with age throughout the entire lifespan, into elderly adulthood.

Adolescence is a time of physiological transition as children literally become adults over a 6–7-year time period. Thus, there may be very large differences in normal respiratory physiology between a 13- and an 18-year-old. The upper airway, for example, is 'child-like' in early adolescence and collapsibility (e.g., as characterized by V_{Imax}/P_N and P_{crit}) progressively increases during adolescence to 'adult-like' values by late adolescence.

Understanding normal respiratory physiology during sleep is absolutely essential to advance understanding of sleep-related breathing disorders, as well as to understand the effects of sleep on pulmonary and respiratory system disorders. A deep understanding of normal respiratory physiology during sleep is also clinically useful and greatly strengthens mechanistic insights into sleep-related breathing disorders. Taken together, the studies reviewed in this chapter constitute an impressive wealth of important knowledge and paint a relatively clear picture of normal respiratory physiology maturation. However, as noted in the introduction, there are still major gaps and inconsistencies, in part due to the enormous variation in and lack of standardization of definitions, experimental approaches, methodologies, etc. The increasing number of mechanistic studies and life-spanning studies from infancy to late adolescence are, perhaps, promising signs.

References

1. Gaultier C. Repiratory adaptation during sleep from the neonatal period to adolescence. In: Guilleminault C, editor. Sleep and it disorders in children. New York: Raven, Press; 1987. p. 97.
2. Openshaw P, Edwards S, Helms P. Changes in rib cage geometry during childhood. Thorax 1984;39:524–7.
3. Gerhardt T, Bancalari E. Chestwall compliance in full-term and premature infants. Acta Paediatr Scand 1980;69:359–64.
4. Papastamelos C, Panitch HB, England SE, et al. Developmental changes in chest wall compliance in infancy and early childhood. J Appl Physiol 1995;78:179–84.
5. Richards CC, Bachman L. Lung and chest wall compliance of apneic paralyzed infants. J Clin Invest 1961;40:273–8.
6. Davis GM, Coates AL, Papageorgiou A, et al. Direct measurement of static chest wall compliance in animal and human neonates. J Appl Physiol 1988;65:1093–8.
7. Allen J, Gripp KW. Development of the thoracic cage. In: Haddad GG, Abman SH, Chernick V, editors. Chernick-Mellins basic mechanisms

of pediatric respiratory disease. 2nd ed. Hamilton-London: BC Decker; 2002. p. 124–38.

8. Agostoni E, Mead J. Statics of the respiratory system. In: Fenn WO, Rahn H, editors. Handbook of physiology. Washington, D.C.: American Physiological Society; 1964. p. 401.

9. Cherniack NS, Longobardo GS. Oxygen and carbon dioxide gas stores of the body. Physiol Rev 1970;50:196–243.

10. Cook CD, Cherry RB, O'Brien D, et al. Studies of respiratory physiology in the newborn infant. I. Observations on normal premature and full-term infants. J Clin Invest 1955;34:975–82.

11. Henderson-Smart DJ, Read DJ. Depression of respiratory muscles and defective responses to nasal obstruction during active sleep in the newborn. Australian Paediatr J 1976;12:261–6.

12. Knill R, Andrews W, Bryan AC, et al. Respiratory load compensation in infants. J Appl Physiol 1976;40:357–61.

13. Henderson-Smart DJ, Read DJ. Reduced lung volume during behavioral active sleep in the newborn. J Appl Physiol 1979;46:1081–5.

14. Martin RJ, Okken A, Rubin D. Arterial oxygen tension during active and quiet sleep in the normal neonate. J Pediatr 1979;94:271–4.

15. Gaultier C, Praud JP, Canet E, et al. Paradoxical inward rib cage motion during rapid eye movement sleep in infants and young children. J Dev Physiol 1987;9:391–7.

16. Gaultier C. Cardiorespiratory adaptation during sleep in infants and children. Pediatr Pulmonol 1995;19:105–17.

17. Tabachnik E, Muller NL, Bryan AC, et al. Changes in ventilation and chest wall mechanics during sleep in normal adolescents. J Appl Physiol 1981;51:557–64.

18. Traeger N, Schultz B, Pollock AN, et al. Polysomnographic values in children 2–9 years old: additional data and review of the literature. Pediatr Pulmonol 2005;40:22–30.

19. Muller N, Volgyesi G, Becker L, et al. Diaphragmatic muscle tone. J Appl Physiol 1979;47:279–84.

20. Muller NL, Bryan AC. Chest wall mechanics and respiratory muscles in infants. Pediatr Clin North Am 1979;26:503–16.

21. Lopes J, Muller NL, Bryan MH, et al. Importance of inspiratory muscle tone in maintenance of FRC in the newborn. J Appl Physiol 1981;51:830–4.

22. Tusiewicz K, Moldofsky H, Bryan AC, et al. Mechanics of the rib cage and diaphragm during sleep. J Appl Physiol 1977;43:600–2.

23. Kosch PC, Stark AR. Dynamic maintenance of end-expiratory lung volume in full-term infants. J Appl Physiol 1984;57:1126–33.

24. Kosch PC, Hutchinson AA, Wozniak JA, et al. Posterior cricoarytenoid and diaphragm activities during tidal breathing in neonates. J Appl Physiol 1988;64:1968–78.

25. Stark AR, Cohlan BA, Waggener TB, et al. Regulation of end-expiratory lung volume during sleep in premature infants. J Appl Physiol 1987;62:1117–23.

26. Colin AA, Wohl ME, Mead J, et al. Transition from dynamically maintained to relaxed end-expiratory volume in human infants. J Appl Physiol 1989;67:2107–11.

27. Stradling JR, Chadwick GA, Frew AJ. Changes in ventilation and its components in normal subjects during sleep. Thorax 1985;40:364–70.

28. Hershenson MB, Stark AR, Mead J. Action of the inspiratory muscles of the rib cage during breathing in newborns. Am Rev Respir Dis 1989;139:1207–12.

29. Hershenson MB, Colin AA, Wohl ME, et al. Changes in the contribution of the rib cage to tidal breathing during infancy. Am Rev Respir Dis 1990;141:922–5.

30. Wiegand L, Zwillich CW, White DP. Collapsibility of the human upper airway during normal sleep. J Appl Physiol 1989;66:1800–8.

31. Hudgel DW, Martin RJ, Johnson B, et al. Mechanics of the respiratory system and breathing pattern during sleep in normal humans. J Appl Physiol 1984;56:133–7.

32. Hudgel DW, Robertson DW. Nasal resistance during wakefulness and sleep in normal man. Acta Otolaryngol 1984;98:130–5.

33. Freedman S, Campbell EJ. The ability of normal subjects to tolerate added inspiratory loads. Respir Physiol 1970;10:213–35.

34. Wiegand L, Zwillich CW, White DP. Sleep and the ventilatory response to resistive loading in normal men. J Appl Physiol 1988;64:1186–95.

35. Deoras KS, Greenspan JS, Wolfson MR, et al. Effects of inspiratory resistive loading on chest wall motion and ventilation: differences between preterm and full-term infants. Pediatr Res 1992;32:589–94.

36. Kosch PC, Davenport PW, Wozniak JA, et al. Reflex control of inspiratory duration in newborn infants. J Appl Physiol 1986;60:2007–14.

37. Kosch PC, Davenport PW, Wozniak JA, et al. Reflex control of expiratory duration in newborn infants. J Appl Physiol 1985;58:575–81.

38. Boychuk RB, Seshia MM, Rigatto H. The immediate ventilatory response to added inspiratory elastic and resistive loads in preterm infants. Pediatr Res 1977;11:276–9.

39. Marcus CL, Moreira GA, Bamford O, et al. Response to inspiratory resistive loading during sleep in normal children and children with obstructive apnea. J Appl Physiol 1999;87:1448–54.

40. Pillar G, Schnall RP, Peled N, et al. Impaired respiratory response to resistive loading during sleep in healthy offspring of patients with obstructive sleep apnea. Am J Respir Crit Care Med 1997;155:1602–8.

41. Wilson PA, Skatrud JB, Dempsey JA. Effects of slow wave sleep on ventilatory compensation to inspiratory elastic loading. Respir Physiol 1984;55:103–20.

42. Schelegle ES. Functional morphology and physiology of slowly adapting pulmonary stretch receptors. Anat Rec A Discov Mol Cell Evol Biol 2003;270:11–16.

43. Hamilton RD, Winning AJ, Horner RL, et al. The effect of lung inflation on breathing in man during wakefulness and sleep. Respir Physiol 1988;73:145–54.

44. Trippenbach T. Pulmonary reflexes and control of breathing during development. Biol Neonate 1994;65:205–10.

45. Hand IL, Noble L, Wilks M, et al. Hering–Breuer reflex and sleep state in the preterm infant. Pediatr Pulmonol 2004;37:61–4.

46. Rabbette PS, Fletcher ME, Dezateux CA, et al. Hering–Breuer reflex and respiratory system compliance in the first year of life: a longitudinal study. J Appl Physiol 1994;76:650–6.

47. Rabbette PS, Costeloe KL, Stocks J. Persistence of the Hering–Breuer reflex beyond the neonatal period. J Appl Physiol 1991;71:474–80.

48. Gerhardt T, Bancalari E. Apnea of prematurity: II. Respiratory reflexes. Pediatrics 1984;74:63–6.

49. Thach BT, Frantz ID 3rd, Adler SM, et al. Maturation of reflexes influencing inspiratory duration in human infants. J Appl Physiol 1978;45:203–11.

50. Finer NN, Abroms IF, Taeusch HW Jr. Ventilation and sleep states in newborn infants. J Pediatr 1976;89:100–8.

51. Mathew OP. Apnea of prematurity: pathogenesis and management strategies. J Perinatol 2011;31:302–10.

52. Jordan AS, White DP. Pharyngeal motor control and the pathogenesis of obstructive sleep apnea. Respir Physiol Neurobiol 2008;160:1–7.

53. Dempsey JA, Veasey SC, Morgan BJ, et al. Pathophysiology of sleep apnea. Physiol Rev 2010;90:47–112.

54. Horner RL. Motor control of the pharyngeal musculature and implications for the pathogenesis of obstructive sleep apnea. Sleep 1996;19:827–53.

55. Arens R, Marcus CL. Pathophysiology of upper airway obstruction: a developmental perspective. Sleep 2004;27:997–1019.

56. Pohunek P. Development, structure and function of the upper airways. Paediatr Resp Rev 2004;5:2–8.

57. Praud JP, Reix P. Upper airways and neonatal respiration. Respir Physiol Neurobiol 2005;149:131–41.

58. Gold AR, Schwartz AR. The pharyngeal critical pressure. The whys and hows of using nasal continuous positive airway pressure diagnostically. Chest 1996;110:1077–88.

59. Kirkness JP, Krishnan V, Patil SP, et al. Upper airway obstruction in snoring and upper airway resistance syndrome. In: Randerath WJ, Sanner BM, Somers VK, editors. Sleep apnea. Basel: Karger; 2006. p. 79–89.

60. Chamberlin NL, Eikermann M, Fassbender P, et al. Genioglossus premotoneurons and the negative pressure reflex in rats. J Physiol 2007;579:515–26.

61. Gauda EB, Carroll JL, McColley S, et al. Effect of oxygenation on breath-by-breath response of the genioglossus muscle during occlusion. J Appl Physiol 1991;71:1231–6.

62. Pillar G, Malhotra A, Fogel RB, et al. Upper airway muscle responsiveness to rising PCO_2 during NREM sleep. J Appl Physiol 2000;89:1275–82.

63. Horner RL, Liu X, Gill H, et al. Effects of sleep-wake state on the genioglossus vs.diaphragm muscle response to CO_2 in rats. J Appl Physiol 2002;92:878–87.

64. Lo YL, Jordan AS, Malhotra A, et al. Genioglossal muscle response to CO_2 stimulation during NREM sleep. Sleep 2006;29:470–7.

65. Weiner D, Mitra J, Salamone J, et al. Effect of chemical stimuli on nerves supplying upper airway muscles. J Appl Physiol 1982;52:530–6.

66. Marcus CL, Fernandes Do Prado LB, Lutz J, et al. Developmental changes in upper airway dynamics. J Appl Physiol 2004;97:98–108.

67. Smith PL, Wise RA, Gold AR, et al. Upper airway pressure-flow relationships in obstructive sleep apnea. J Appl Physiol 1988;64:789–95.

68. Schwartz AR, Smith PL, Wise RA, et al. Induction of upper airway occlusion in sleeping individuals with subatmospheric nasal pressure. J Appl Physiol 1988;64:535–42.

69. Marcus CL, McColley SA, Carroll JL, et al. Upper airway collapsibility in children with obstructive sleep apnea syndrome. J Appl Physiol 1994;77:918–24.

70. Isono S, Shimada A, Utsugi M, et al. Comparison of static mechanical properties of the passive pharynx between normal children and children with sleep-disordered breathing. Am J Respir Crit Care Med 1998;157:1204–12.

71. Schultz HD, Del Rio R, Ding Y, et al. Role of neurotransmitter gases in the control of the carotid body in heart failure. Respir Physiol Neurobiol 2012;184(2):197–203.

72. Marcus CL, Katz ES, Lutz J, et al. Upper airway dynamic responses in children with the obstructive sleep apnea syndrome. Pediatr Res 2005;57:99–107.

73. McGinley BM, Schwartz AR, Schneider H, et al. Upper airway neuromuscular compensation during sleep is defective in obstructive sleep apnea. J Appl Physiol 2008;105:197–205.

74. Marcus CL, Lutz J, Hamer A, et al. Developmental changes in response to subatmospheric pressure loading of the upper airway. J Appl Physiol 1999;87:626–33.

75. Patil SP, Schneider H, Marx JJ, et al. Neuromechanical control of upper airway patency during sleep. J Appl Physiol 2007;102:547–56.

76. Wilson SL, Thach BT, Brouillette RT, et al. Upper airway patency in the human infant: influence of airway pressure and posture. J Appl Physiol 1980;48:500–4.

77. Carlo WA, Miller MJ, Martin RJ. Differential response of respiratory muscles to airway occlusion in infants. J Appl Physiol 1985;59:847–52.

78. Gauda EB, Miller MJ, Carlo WA, et al. Genioglossus response to airway occlusion in apneic versus nonapneic infants. Pediatr Res 1987;22:683–7.

79. Huang J, Pinto SJ, Yuan H, et al. Upper airway collapsibility and genioglossus activity in adolescents during sleep. Sleep 2012;35:1345–52.

80. Bandla P, Huang J, Karamessinis L, et al. Puberty and upper airway dynamics during sleep. Sleep 2008;31:534–41.

81. Carrera HL, McDonough JM, Gallagher PR, et al. Upper airway collapsibility during wakefulness in children with sleep disordered breathing, as determined by the negative expiratory pressure technique. Sleep 2011;34:717–24.

82. Gozal D, Burnside MM. Increased upper airway collapsibility in children with obstructive sleep apnea during wakefulness. Am J Respir Crit Care Med 2004;169:163–7.

83. Goh DY, Galster P, Marcus CL. Sleep architecture and respiratory disturbances in children with obstructive sleep apnea. Am J Respir Crit Care Med 2000;162:682–6.

84. Katz ES, White DP. Genioglossus activity during sleep in normal control subjects and children with obstructive sleep apnea. Am J Respir Crit Care Med 2004;170:553–60.

85. Schwartz AR, O'Donnell CP, Baron J, et al. The hypotonic upper airway in obstructive sleep apnea: role of structures and neuromuscular activity. Am J Respir Crit Care Med 1998;157:1051–7.

86. Horner RL. Emerging principles and neural substrates underlying tonic sleep-state-dependent influences on respiratory motor activity. Philos Trans R Soc Lond B Biol Sci 2009;364:2553–64.

87. Katz ES, Marcus CL, White DP. Influence of airway pressure on genioglossus activity during sleep in normal children. Am J Respir Crit Care Med 2006;173:902–9.

88. Onal E, Lopata M, O'Connor TD. Diaphragmatic and genioglossal electromyogram responses to isocapnic hypoxia in humans. Am Rev Respir Dis 1981;124:215–17.

89. Onal E, Lopata M, O'Connor TD. Diaphragmatic and genioglossal electromyogram responses to CO_2 rebreathing in humans. J Appl Physiol 1981;50:1052–5.

90. Parmelee AH, Stern E, Harris MA. Maturation of respiration in prematures and young infants. Neuropadiatrie 1972;3:294–304.

91. Hoppenbrouwers T, Hodgman JE, Arakawa K, et al. Respiration during the first six months of life in normal infants. III. Computer identification of breathing pauses. Pediatr Res 1980;14:1230–3.

92. Bolton DP, Herman S. Ventilation and sleep state in the new-born. J Physiol 1974;240:67–77.

93. Hathorn MK. The rate and depth of breathing in new-born infants in different sleep states. J Physiol 1974;243:101–13.

94. Andersson D, Gennser G, Johnson P. Phase characteristics of breathing movements in healthy newborns. J Dev Physiol 1983;5:289–98.

95. Curzi-Dascalova L, Gaudebout C, Dreyfus-Brisac C. Respiratory frequencies of sleeping infants during the first months of life: correlations between values in different sleep states. Early Hum Dev 1981;5:39–54.

96. Adamson TM, Cranage S, Maloney JE, et al. The maturation of respiratory patterns in normal full term infants during the first six postnatal months. II: Sleep states and apnoea. Austr Paediatr J 1981;17:257–61.

97. Orem JM, Lovering AT, Vidruk EH. Excitation of medullary respiratory neurons in REM sleep. Sleep 2005;28:801–7.

98. Curzi-Dascalova L, Lebrun F, Korn G. Respiratory frequency according to sleep states and age in normal premature infants: a comparison with full term infants. Pediatr Res 1983;17:152–6.

99. Haddad GG, Lai TL, Mellins RB. Determination of ventilatory pattern in REM sleep in normal infants. J Appl Physiol 1982;53:52–6.

100. Hoppenbrouwers T, Harper RM, Hodgman JE, et al. Polygraphic studies on normal infants during the first six months of life. II. Respiratory rate and variability as a function of state. Pediatr Res 1978;12:120–5.

101. Steinschneider A, Weinstein S. Sleep respiratory instability in term neonates under hyperthermic conditions: age, type of feeding, and rapid eye movements. Pediatr Res 1983;17:35–41.

102. Haddad GG, Epstein RA, Epstein MA, et al. Maturation of ventilation and ventilatory pattern in normal sleeping infants. J Appl Physiol 1979;46:998–1002.

103. Carse EA, Wilkinson AR, Whyte PL, et al. Oxygen and carbon dioxide tensions, breathing and heart rate in normal infants during the first six months of life. J Dev Physiol 1981;3:85–100.

104. Hoppenbrouwers T, Hodgman JE, Harper RM, et al. Respiration during the first six months of life in normal infants: IV. Gender differences. Early Hum Dev 1980;4:167–77.

105. Scholle S, Wiater A, Scholle HC. Normative values of polysomnographic parameters in childhood and adolescence: cardiorespiratory parameters. Sleep Med 2011;12:988–96.

106. Carskadon MA, Harvey K, Dement WC, et al. Respiration during sleep in children. West J Med 1978;128:477–81.

107. Huang J, Colrain IM, Panitch HB, et al. Effect of sleep stage on breathing in children with central hypoventilation. J Appl Physiol 2008;105:44–53.

108. Davi M, Sankaran K, Maccallum M, et al. Effect of sleep state on chest distortion and on the ventilatory response to CO_2 in neonates. Pediatr Res 1979;13:982–6.

109. Cross KW. The respiratory rate and ventilation in the newborn baby. J Physiol 1949;109:459–74.

110. Krieger J, Maglasiu N, Sforza E, et al. Breathing during sleep in normal middle-aged subjects. Sleep 1990;13:143–54.

111. Thach BT, Taeusch HW Jr. Sighing in newborn human infants: role of inflation-augmenting reflex. J Appl Physiol 1976;41:502–7.

112. Ellingson RJ, Peters JF, Nelson B. Respiratory pauses and apnea during daytime sleep in normal infants during the first year of life: longitudinal observations. Electroencephalography Clinl neurophysiol 1982;53:48–59.

113. Curzi-Dascalova L, Plassart E. Respiratory and motor events in sleeping infants: their correlation with thoracico-abdominal respiratory relationships. Early Hum Dev 1978;2:39–50.

114. Radvanyi-Bouvet MF, Monset-Couchard M, Morel-Kahn F, et al. Expiratory patterns during sleep in normal full-term and premature neonates. Biol Neonate 1982;41:74–84.

115. Fleming PJ, Goncalves AL, Levine MR, et al. The development of stability of respiration in human infants: changes in ventilatory responses to spontaneous sighs. J Physiol 1984;347:1–16.

116. Southall DP, Richards J, Brown DJ, et al. 24-hour tape recordings of ECG and respiration in the newborn infant with findings related to sudden death and unexplained brain damage in infancy. Arch Dis Child 1980;55:7–16.

117. Hoppenbrouwers T, Hodgman JE, Harper RM, et al. Polygraphic studies of normal infants during the first six months of life: III. Incidence of apnea and periodic breathing. Pediatrics 1977;60:418–25.

118. Guilleminault C, Ariagno R, Korobkin R, et al. Mixed and obstructive sleep apnea and near miss for sudden infant death syndrome: 2. Comparison of near miss and normal control infants by age. Pediatrics 1979;64:882–91.

119. Gabriel M, Albani M, Schulte FJ. Apneic spells and sleep states in preterm infants. Pediatrics 1976;57:142–7.

120. Gould JB, Lee AF, James O, et al. The sleep state characteristics of apnea during infancy. Pediatrics 1977;59:182–94.

121. Flores-Guevara R, Plouin P, Curzi-Dascalova L, et al. Sleep apneas in normal neonates and infants during the first 3 months of life. Neuropediatrics 1982;13(Suppl):21–8.

122. Waite SP, Thoman EB. Periodic apnea in the full-term infant: individual consistency, sex differences, and state specificity. Pediatrics 1982;70:79–86.

123. Rigatto H. Breathing and sleep in preterm infants. In: Loughlin GM, Marcus, CL, editors. Sleep and breathing in children: a developmental approach. New York: Dekker; 2000. p. 495–523.

124. Vecchierini MF, Curzi-Dascalova L, Trang-Pham H, et al. Patterns of EEG frequency, movement, heart rate, and oxygenation after isolated short apneas in infants. Pediatr Res 2001;49:220–6.

125. Stein IM, White A, Kennedy JL Jr, et al. Apnea recordings of healthy infants at 40, 44, and 52 weeks postconception. Pediatrics 1979;63:724–30.

126. Fernandes do Prado LB, Li X, Thompson R, et al. Body position and obstructive sleep apnea in children. Sleep 2002;25:66–71.

127. Kelly DH, Riordan L, Smith MJ. Apnea and periodic breathing in healthy full-term infants, 12–18 months of age. Pediatr Pulmonol 1992;13:169–71.

128. Hoppenbrouwers T, Jensen D, Hodgman J, et al. Respiration during the first six months of life in normal infants: II. The emergence of a circadian pattern. Neuropadiatrie 1979;10:264–80.

129. Marcus CL, Omlin KJ, Basinki DJ, et al. Normal polysomnographic values for children and adolescents. Am Rev Respir Dis 1992;146:1235–9.

130. Uliel S, Tauman R, Greenfeld M, et al. Normal polysomnographic respiratory values in children and adolescents. Chest 2004;125:872–8.

131. Berry RB, Block AJ. Positive nasal airway pressure eliminates snoring as well as obstructive sleep apnea. Chest 1984;85:15–20.

132. Weese-Mayer DE, Morrow AS, Conway LP, et al. Assessing clinical significance of apnea exceeding fifteen seconds with event recording. J Pediatr 1990;117:568–74.

133. Acebo C, Millman RP, Rosenberg C, et al. Sleep, breathing, and cephalometrics in older children and young adults. Part I – Normative values. Chest 1996;109:664–72.

134. Rosen CL, D'Andrea L, Haddad GG. Adult criteria for obstructive sleep apnea do not identify children with serious obstruction. Am Rev Respir Dis 1992;146:1231–4.

135. Accardo JA, Shults J, Leonard MB, et al. Differences in overnight polysomnography scores using the adult and pediatric criteria for respiratory events in adolescents. Sleep 2010;33:1333–9.

136. Fenner A, Schalk U, Hoenicke H, et al. Periodic breathing in premature and neonatal babies: incidence, breathing pattern, respiratory gas tensions, response to changes in the composition of ambient air. Pediatr Res 1973;7:174–83.

137. Marcus CL, Glomb WB, Basinski DJ, et al. Developmental pattern of hypercapnic and hypoxic ventilatory responses from childhood to adulthood. J Appl Physiol 1994;76:314–20.

138. Nock ML, Difiore JM, Arko MK, et al. Relationship of the ventilatory response to hypoxia with neonatal apnea in preterm infants. J Pediatr 2004;144:291–5.

139. Al-Matary A, Kutbi I, Qurashi M, et al. Increased peripheral chemoreceptor activity may be critical in destabilizing breathing in neonates. Semin Perinatol 2004;28:264–72.

140. Springer C, Cooper DM, Wasserman K. Evidence that maturation of the peripheral chemoreceptors is not complete in childhood. Respir Physiol 1988;74:55–64.

141. Douglas NJ, White DP, Weil JV, et al. Hypoxic ventilatory response decreases during sleep in normal men. Am Rev Respir Dis 1982;125:286–9.

142. Hedemark LL, Kronenberg RS. Ventilatory and heart rate responses to hypoxia and hypercapnia during sleep in adults. J Appl Physiol 1982;53:307–12.

143. Rigatto H, Kalapesi Z, Leahy FN, et al. Ventilatory response to 100% and 15% O_2 during wakefulness and sleep in preterm infants. Early Hum Dev 1982;7:1–10.

144. Avery ME, Chernick V, Dutton RE, et al. Ventilatory response to inspired carbon dioxide in infants and adults. J Appl Physiol 1963;18:895–903.

145. Gaultier C, Perret L, Boule M, et al. Occlusion pressure and breathing pattern in healthy children. Respir Physiol 1981;46:71–80.

146. Brouillette RT, Weese-Mayer DE, Hunt CE. Breathing control disorders in infants and children. Hosp Pract (Off Ed) 1990;25:82–5, 88, 93–6 passim.

147. Chipps BE, Mak H, Schuberth KC, et al. Nocturnal oxygen saturation in normal and asthmatic children. Pediatrics 1980;65:1157–60.

148. Thach BT, Lijowska A. Arousals in infants. Sleep 1996;19:S271–3.

149. Thoppil CK, Belan MA, Cowen CP, et al. Behavioral arousal in newborn infants and its association with termination of apnea. J Appl Physiol 1991;70:2479–84.

150. Kato I, Scaillet S, Groswasser J, et al. Spontaneous arousability in prone and supine position in healthy infants. Sleep 2006;29:785–90.

151. Kahn A, Groswasser J, Sottiaux M, et al. Prone or supine body position and sleep characteristics in infants. Pediatrics 1993;91:1112–15.

152. Praud JP, D'Allest AM, Nedelcoux H, et al. Sleep-related abdominal muscle behavior during partial or complete obstructed breathing in prepubertal children. Pediatr Res 1989;26:347–50.

153. McCulloch K, Brouillette RT, Guzzetta AJ, et al. Arousal responses in near-miss sudden infant death syndrome and in normal infants. J Pediatr 1982;101:911–17.

154. van der Hal AL, Rodriguez AM, Sargent CW, et al. Hypoxic and hypercapneic arousal responses and prediction of subsequent apnea in apnea of infancy. Pediatrics 1985;75:848–54.

155. Ward SL, Bautista DB, Woo MS, et al. Responses to hypoxia and hypercapnia in infants of substance-abusing mothers. J Pediatr 1992;121:704–9.

156. Marcus CL, Bautista DB, Amihyia A, et al. Hypercapneic arousal responses in children with congenital central hypoventilation syndrome. Pediatrics 1991;88:993–8.

157. Fewell JE, Kondo CS, Dascalu V, et al. Influence of carotid-denervation on the arousal and cardiopulmonary responses to alveolar hypercapnia in lambs. J Dev Physiol 1989;12:193–9.

158. Baker SB, Fewell JE. Effects of hyperoxia on the arousal response to upper airway obstruction in lambs. Pediatr Res 1987;21:116–20.

159. Milerad J, Hertzberg T, Wennergren G, et al. Respiratory and arousal responses to hypoxia in apneic infants reinvestigated. Eur J Pediatr 1989;148:565–70.

160. Martin RJ, Herrell N, Rubin D, et al. Effect of supine and prone positions on arterial oxygen tension in the preterm infant. Pediatrics 1979;63:528–31.

161. Parslow PM, Cranage SM, Adamson TM, et al. Arousal and ventilatory responses to hypoxia in sleeping infants: effects of maternal smoking. Respir Physiol Neurobiol 2004;140:77–87.

162. Verbeek MM, Richardson HL, Parslow PM, et al. Arousal and ventilatory responses to mild hypoxia in sleeping preterm infants. J Sleep Res 2008;17:344–53.

163. Parslow PM, Harding R, Cranage SM, et al. Arousal responses to somatosensory and mild hypoxic stimuli are depressed during quiet sleep in healthy term infants. Sleep 2003;26:739–44.

164. Horne RS, Parslow PM, Harding R. Postnatal development of ventilatory and arousal responses to hypoxia in human infants. Respir Physiol Neurobiol 2005;149:257–71.

165. Fewell JE, Baker SB. Arousal from sleep during rapidly developing hypoxemia in lambs. Pediatr Res 1987;22:471–7.

166. Davidson TL, Fewell JE. Arousal response from sleep to tracheal obstruction in lambs during postnatal maturation. Pediatr Res 1994;36:501–5.

167. Fewell JE, Taylor BJ, Kondo CS, et al. Influence of carotid denervation on the arousal and cardiopulmonary responses to upper airway obstruction in lambs. Pediatr Res 1990;28:374–8.

168. Read PA, Horne RS, Cranage SM, et al. Dynamic changes in arousal threshold during sleep in the human infant. Pediatr Res 1998;43:697–703.

169. Horne RS, Sly DJ, Cranage SM, et al. Effects of prematurity on arousal from sleep in the newborn infant. Pediatr Res 2000;47:468–74.

170. Horne RS, Ferens D, Watts AM, et al. The prone sleeping position impairs arousability in term infants. J Pediatr 2001;138:811–16.

171. Horne RS, Bandopadhayay P, Vitkovic J, et al. Effects of age and sleeping position on arousal from sleep in preterm infants. Sleep 2002;25:746–50.

172. Litman RS, McDonough JM, Marcus CL, et al. Upper airway collapsibility in anesthetized children. Anesth Analg 2006;102:750–4.

Apnea of Prematurity

Christian F. Poets

INTRODUCTION

Apnea of prematurity (AOP) affects almost every extremely low gestational age neonate (ELGAN) and also many less immature infants. Its pathophysiology, however, is incompletely understood. This chapter reviews observational studies better to understand the pathophysiology of AOP, focusing on bradycardia and hypoxemia because they, and not apnea duration, are relevant to the well-being of an infant. Based on these data, current strategies to treat or prevent AOP will be reviewed.

PATHOPHYSIOLOGY

The Role of Upper Airway Obstruction

Traditionally, apnea is divided into central, obstructive and mixed. Many apparently 'central' apneas, however, involve a loss of airway tone that results in intermittent airway obstruction,[1] while active glottic closure, similar to that preventing outflow of lung water during *in utero* apnea,[2] has also been observed in AOP, potentially preserving lung volume during apnea also *ex utero*. Airway obstruction may also prolong initially short respiratory pauses.[3] Thus, the narrow upper airways of preterm infants might be actively maintained open via a respiratory center input, and it simply depends on which component of this input is activated first (diaphragm or upper airway) whether an apnea will appear as central or obstructive.[4]

Relationship between Apnea, Bradycardia and Desaturation

Apnea, bradycardia and desaturation during AOP are closely temporally related.[5] According to the author's data on 80 preterm infants, 83% of bradycardias (heart rate less than two-thirds of baseline) were accompanied by an apnea (≥4 s), 86% by a fall in pulse oximeter saturation (SpO$_2$) to ≤80%, and 79% by both apnea and desaturation.[6] The interval between apnea and bradycardia was extremely short (median, 4.8 s), as was that between bradycardia and desaturation (median, 4.2 s). This was predominantly because the interval between the onset of apnea and that of desaturation, corrected for the time it takes for the blood to travel from the lung to the pulse oximeter sensor site, was only 0.8 s (Figure 24-1).[6]

These observations support the concept that hypoxemia causes bradycardia, e.g., via stimulation of peripheral chemoreceptors,[7] the occurrence of which is facilitated by the absence of the pulmonary inflation reflex during apnea. The latter would also explain why, despite a similar severity of the accompanying hypoxemia, bradycardia is more common with central than with mixed or obstructive apnea.[8]

Changes in Lung Volume, Apnea and Desaturation

Why is the interval between apnea and desaturation onset so short? This may be related to a reduced functional residual capacity (FRC). In preterm infants, relaxation volume is only 10–15% of total lung capacity and thus very close to residual volume, predisposing them to the development of peripheral airway closure.[9] To compensate for this disadvantage, these infants actively maintain their end-expiratory lung volume above relaxation volume, which is one reason for their high respiratory rate.[10] In fact, lung volume is 20% lower after an apnea than after a sigh, i.e., apnea results in a loss of FRC, which is restored by a sigh. This suggests that one of the main functions of sighs in preterm infants is to reverse falls in lung volume caused by apneas.[11,12]

During periodic apnea, SpO$_2$ falls twice as fast as during isolated apneas.[5] Although a reduced mixed venous SO$_2$ following a prior fall in SpO$_2$ may also contribute to this, another reason for this is a progressive fall in lung volume during the repeated apneas, resulting in peripheral airway closure. The complex interrelations of the factors influencing the speed of the fall in SpO$_2$ during AOP have recently been modeled mathematically.[13]

A loss in lung volume may also be decisive for the development of hypoxemia following abdominal muscle contractions in ELGANs, being involved in 80% of their desaturations to <75% SpO$_2$ in one study, and being associated with an average decrease in resting lung volume by 69% of tidal volume.[14]

A potential consequence of a reduction in lung volume is a (further) inhibition of respiration via activation of the Hering–Breuer deflation reflex. In term infants, this vagally mediated reflex terminates expiration while initiating inspiration. In preterm infants, however, induction of this reflex via chest compression resulted in a shortening of inspiratory time and a tendency to have short apneas (2–5 s).[15] The same may occur if lung volume falls spontaneously, e.g., during apnea.

Conversely, an increase in lung volume was recently found to stabilize breathing by reducing loop gain, i.e., the sensitivity of the negative feedback loop of the chemoreflex control of the respiratory system, while a reduced lung volume will increase the instability of the respiratory control system, as evident during periodic breathing.[16]

These considerations provide a theoretical basis for the effectiveness of strategies that increase lung volume in reducing the frequency and/or severity of AOP in preterm infants.[17]

The Role of Feeding and Gastro-Esophageal Reflux

Symptoms of AOP often increase in relation to feeding. We studied the effect of bottle feeding, as compared to slow (1 h) and bolus (10 min) gavage feeding, on AOP and found three times more desaturations to ≤80% with bottle than with bolus gavage feeding, but no further reduction with slow gavage

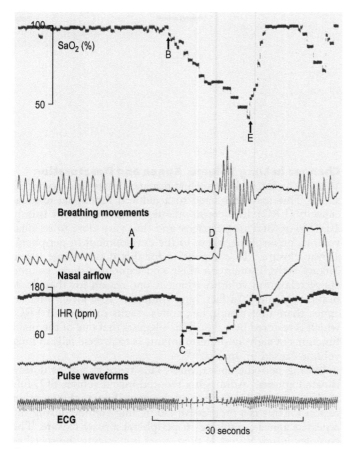

FIGURE 24-1 Example for the close temporal relationship between apnea, bradycardia and desaturation. The delay caused by the time it takes for the blood to travel from the lung to the pulse oximeter sensor attached to the foot can be estimated from the delay between the first breath following an apnea and the onset of the recovery in SpO₂ (D to E). This must be subtracted from the interval between the onset of apnea and that of desaturation (A to B) and from the interval between the onset of bradycardia and that of desaturation (B to C). *Reproduced from Poets CF. Pathophysiology of Apnea of Prematurity: Implications from Observational Studies. In: Mathew OP. Respiratory control and its disorders in the newborn. Marcel Dekker, Inc, New York 2003,295–316, with permission.*

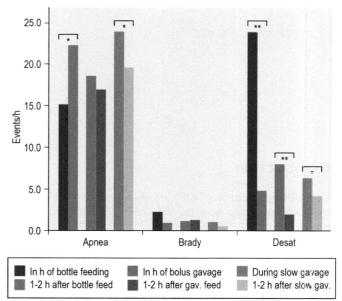

FIGURE 24-2 Apnea, bradycardia (Brady) and desaturation (Desat) rates during the hour feedings were given compared to the following 2 hours in 30 preterm infants studied at 34 wk (SD 1.4) gestational age. * $p < 0.05$. ** $p < 0.01$. *Reproduced from Poets C. Apnea of Prematurity. In: Kheirandish-Gozal L, Gozal, D., editor. Sleep-Disordered Breathing in Children: A Comprehensive Clinical Guide to Evaluation and Treatment. New York: Humana press, Springer; 2012. p. 263–78, with permission.*

feeding. There were always significantly more desaturations in the hour feeds were given than during the following 2 hours, but the effect of feeding method persisted throughout these 3-h feeding intervals. Interestingly, there was no significant effect of feeding technique on the frequency of apnea or bradycardia (Figure 24-2).[18]

Thus, bottle feeding may confer a significantly increased risk of episodic desaturation, which may be quite long-lasting. It is puzzling that slow gavage feeding offered no advantage over bolus gavage feeding. Might gastro-esophageal reflux (GER), occurring with either feeding method, be an explanation for this?

With the new multiple intraluminal impedance (MII) technique, GER can now be detected, independent of acidity, via changes in impedance caused by a liquid bolus inside the esophagus. We recorded MII, together with cardiorespiratory (CR) signals, in 19 infants with AOP.[19] MII signals were analyzed, independently of CR signals, for reflux episodes.

CR signals were analyzed for apneas (≥4 s), desaturations to ≤80%, and bradycardias to ≤100 bpm. A temporal relationship between GER and a CR event was considered present if both commenced within 20 s of each other. We found a high rate of both apnea and GER, but the apnea frequency within 20 s of a reflux episode was not significantly different from that during reflux-free epochs (mean, 0.19/min. vs. 0.25/min); the same was true for desaturations and bradycardias. Also, GER occurred similarly often before as after an apnea. Only in the few apneas (3.5%) that were associated with GER reaching the pharyngeal level, significantly more (45 vs. 26) occurred after rather than before GER. Thus, while both CR events and GER were common, they did not, with few exceptions, appear to be temporally related.[19] Similar results have since been reported by others.[20,21] Thus, the widespread practice[22] of giving antireflux medications to infants with AOP is futile.

Chest Wall Distortion, Anatomic Dead Space and Diaphragmatic Fatigue

Chest wall distortion, clinically apparent as paradoxical breathing, is common in infants and is especially visible in preterm infants. It has been suggested that this distortion increases the volume displacement of the diaphragm during inspiration.[23,24] In longitudinal studies, Heldt showed that the minute volume displacement of the diaphragm was almost twice as large as pulmonary ventilation at 29–30 weeks' gestational age (GA) and fell to approximately 90% of pulmonary ventilation at 36 weeks' GA. Concomitantly, diaphragmatic work was almost halved.[24] The author speculated that this additional workload may represent not only a significant calorie expenditure in these infants, but contributes to the development of diaphragmatic fatigue and apnea.[24] Further contributing is that, because of their relatively large head size, anatomic dead space is approximately 45% of tidal volume in neonates, but only 25% in adults.[25,26]

Circumstantial evidence that muscle fatigue may indeed be involved in neonatal apnea stems from the time course of apnea in term and preterm infants. AOP becomes more problematic towards the end of the first or during the second week of life,[27] while chemoreceptor resetting, which otherwise might also explain this phenomenon, is essentially complete within approximately 24–48 h after birth.[27] We confirmed this observation for desaturation rates in both term and preterm infants.[28,29] A mechanism through which labored breathing may produce apnea in preterm infants is the intercostal–phrenic inhibitory reflex. This may be elicited both by rib cage distortion[30] and respiratory loading,[31] and is known to inhibit respiratory effort in infants.

Thus, it is conceivable that similar to the obstructive sleep apnea syndrome in adults, where an increased work of breathing resulting from upper airway obstruction may lead to an increased rate of central apneas, the same mechanism may also play a role in AOP.

Hypoxic Ventilatory Depression

Fetal breathing is diminished if oxygen supply via the placenta is reduced.[32] For the fetus, respiratory movements are a waste of energy that cannot be afforded if oxygen supply via the placenta is reduced. This behavior, however, although counterproductive *ex utero*, continues after preterm birth,[33,34] switching to a mature hypoxic ventilatory response only at approximately 35 weeks' PCA. This correlates well with the natural course of AOP.[35] While the classic hypoxic response is biphasic, consisting of an initial increase followed by a decrease in ventilation,[33,35] ELGANs show an immediate reduction in minute ventilation during hypoxia, which is mainly due to a fall in respiratory rate.[36]

The clinical relevance of this maturational phenomenon was recently demonstrated in a substudy of SUPPORT, a large multicenter study comparing the effects of a high (91–95% SpO_2) versus a low (85–89%) target range for SpO_2 in ELGANs.[37] By recording desaturation rates until 36 wk PCA in infants randomized in their center, the authors found significantly (2–3 times) more desaturations to ≤80% for ≥10 s in the first 11 days of life and again between 8 weeks of age and reaching 36 wk PCA in those infants who had been randomized to the lower SpO_2 target group.[38] This observation is best explained by the effects seemingly small decreases in baseline SpO_2 have on hypoxic ventilatory depression.[39]

As mentioned above, an important question is which molecular mechanisms are responsible for the hypoxic ventilatory depression. One candidate is the creatine–phosphocreatine (PCr) system. In the absence of oxidative phosphorylization, provision of phosphate for generation of adenosine-triphosphate (ATP) relies predominantly on the PCr pool, before anaerobic glycolysis, with increased production of lactate and H^+, is activated.[40] This is particularly relevant to tissues with a high energy metabolism such as the central nervous system. A fall in intracellular ATP is an important trigger for hypoxia-induced neuronal damage, and maintenance of ATP levels is therefore of fundamental importance for neuronal protection from hypoxic insult.[41] The neonatal brain is relatively deficient in creatine, and it is tempting to speculate that the much earlier onset of the hypoxic ventilatory depression in this age group is related to a decreased availability of PCr in the neonatal brainstem.

Brainstem slices from pups of creatine-fed mice (2 g/kg/d) did indeed show higher phosphocreatine contents and significantly less hypoxic ventilatory depression (−14% vs. −41%), than those from non-supplemented control animals. This corresponded to nearly constant cerebral ATP levels in the former versus a 54% decrease in the latter animals after 30 min of anoxia.[42] Also, measurements of the maximal respiratory amplitudes in such pups during hypoxia showed an increase by 51%, compared to 22% in control animals.[43] A randomized, controlled trial of creatine supplementation (200 mg/kg/d) to preterm infants with AOP, however, starting at around 2 wk of age and being administered for 14 d, showed no effect at all on AOP,[44] although this could have also been due to an insufficient dose and/or duration of treatment. This issue deserves further study.

Relevance of the pCO₂ Apneic Threshold

Respiratory drive also depends on CO_2. A baseline concentration of pCO_2 is essential for breathing to occur; conversely, if pCO_2 falls considerably below its eupneic baseline, apnea sets in. The pCO_2 value at which this occurs is called the apnea–hypopnea threshold; it is approximately 3.5 Torr below eupneic pCO_2 in healthy adults.[45] The closer this eupneic pCO_2 is to apneic threshold pCO_2, the more unstable breathing likely gets, as minor behavioral changes in ventilation would be sufficient to propel the pCO_2 to below threshold, inducing apnea.[45] The spontaneous pre-apneic threshold in term and preterm neonates is only 1–1.3 mmHg below eupneic values, potentially destabilizing respiration in neonates compared to older subjects.[45] The logical clinical consequence of these findings, namely CO_2 inhalation as a treatment for AOP, was recently tested and shown to be effective, but less than treatment with theophylline.[46]

Influence of the Thermal Environment

There are several case studies suggesting that overheating causes apnea in infants,[47,48] but there have been surprisingly few studies to prove the opposite, i.e., that cold stress stimulates breathing. One study, performed in three preterm infants, showed that apnea was more likely to occur during a decrease rather than an increase in incubator temperature.[49] Recently, Tourneux et al. measured energy expenditure and apnea rate in 22 preterm infants at thermoneutrality (32.5°C) and at ambient temperatures 2°C below and above this level. Apneas were less frequent and shorter in duration with cold exposure (during which oxygen consumption increased), but there was no association between body temperature and apnea rate.[50] Thus, the likelihood of apnea to occur seems to be inversely related to metabolic drive, although not necessarily to ambient temperature.

Termination of Apnea

As important as the question of what *causes* an apnea is that of what *terminates* it. In adults, recovery from apnea is usually associated with arousal from sleep, probably via activation of peripheral chemoreceptors. In preterm infants, the situation is more complex as here, motor activity may *precede* the onset of apnea and continues during apnea, i.e., apnea occurs *after* arousal rather than resulting in it.[51] In contrast, when looking for signs of behavioral arousal in sleep-related apneas, this may be more likely to occur with longer (>15 s) compared to shorter (5–15 s) apneas, with those that are associated with hypoxemia (SpO$_2$<80%) or bradycardia (HR<100/min), and with mixed compared to central apneas.[52] Thus, several factors may affect the occurrence of arousal during apneas in preterm infants: sleep state, severity of hypoxia/hypercapnia, airway afferent input and sleep fragmentation/habituation resulting from previous apneic episodes.[52] Whatever the precise mechanism, it seems that chemoreceptor activation, but not cortical arousal, is required for apnea termination.

TREATMENT

For space constraints, this review will focus on interventions for AOP that have already been proven beneficial, except for Doxapram (see below).

Prone Head-Elevated Positioning
In the prone position, the chest wall is stabilized and thoraco-abdominal asynchrony reduced. Several studies have demonstrated that the prone position reduces the apnea rate in preterm infants.[53,54] A 15° head-elevated tilt prone position was even associated with a 49% reduction in desaturations to <85%.[55] Recently, however, two studies re-investigated the issue, and found only a slight (−13%) reduction in the frequency of desaturation/bradycardia compared to the horizontal position; one found no advantage even for the head-up tilt position.[56,57] This much less clear advantage of the head-up tilt position may be due to the fact that infants in the earlier study[55] had received no other treatment for AOP, whereas in the more recent ones all had received caffeine, and most CPAP. Thus, positional effects on AOP may be less pronounced in infants already receiving caffeine. The prone, head-up tilt position may therefore be considered as a first-line intervention for AOP, but offers little additional effect in infants already treated with caffeine or CPAP.

Continuous Positive Airway Pressure and Synchronized Nasal Ventilation
Continuous positive airway pressure (CPAP) has been shown to reduce extubation failure in preterm infants, despite the fact that most systems currently available do *not* reduce the work of breathing.[58] CPAP can be applied via a nasopharyngeal tube or (bi-)nasal prongs. Reintubation rates are 40% lower with the latter devices (relative risk (RR) 0.59 (0.41;0.85), number needed to treat (NNT) 5).[59] They are thus the preferred mode when applying CPAP. An extension to CPAP is nasal intermittent positive pressure ventilation (N-IPPV), which has a high effectiveness over CPAP in preventing extubation failure (RR 0.21 (0.10–0.45), NNT 3).[60] Typically, an inspiratory pressure of 15–20 cmH$_2$O, applied at a rate of 10–20/min, is combined with a CPAP level of 5–6 cmH$_2$O. There is theoretical concern that this might result in gastric distension, but this has not been confirmed in meta-analysis.[60] Importantly, studies showing superiority of N-IPPV in meta-analysis used *synchronized* N-IPPV. When we compared non-synchronized N-IPPV, the only mode currently available with most ventilators, with nasal CPAP delivered via a variable flow device that reduces the work of breathing (InfantFlow, EME, Brighton, UK), the rate of bradycardia

and desaturation was 50% lower with the latter device than with N-IPPV.[58] Thus, use of a technique that reduces the work of breathing, or synchronized N-IPPV, may be key to success for nasal ventilatory support to improve AOP.[61]

Caffeine
Methylxanthines increase chemoreceptor sensitivity as well as respiratory drive and can also improve diaphragmatic function. Of the substances available, caffeine has a wider therapeutic range and fewer side effects than theophylline. In the large randomized Caffeine for Apnea of Prematurity (CAP) study, caffeine (or placebo) was started during the first 10 days of life in infants of 500–1250 g birth weight until no longer considered necessary for AOP treatment. Mechanical ventilation, CPAP, and oxygen administration could be discontinued 7–10 days earlier in infants treated with caffeine. Most important, however, are the data on the primary outcome, i.e., death or disability at 18 months corrected age. These showed that caffeine was associated with a 23% reduction in this outcome (OR 0.77; 95% CI 0.64–0.93). This benefit was particularly strong for cerebral palsy: 4.4% versus 7.3% of infants had this outcome (RR 0.58; 0.39–0.87).[62] Somewhat unexpectedly, and not primary end points, were the findings of a 40% lower risk of bronchopulmonary dysplasia (BPD; 36% vs. 47%: OR 0.6; 95% CI 0.5–0.8), a 30% lower risk of developing a symptomatic patent ductus arteriosus (OR 0.7; 0.5–0.8), and a 40% reduction in the risk of developing stage 4 or 5 retinopathy of prematurity (ROP) or requiring treatment for ROP (5 vs. 8%; OR 0.6; 0.4–0.9) in the caffeine group.[63] Recently, data from the 5-year follow-up to this study showed that the preventive effect of caffeine on motor impairment persists even into middle childhood.[64]

In subgroup analyses, the effect of caffeine on the primary outcome was found to be restricted to infants requiring respiratory support at randomization; i.e., caffeine had no effect on death or disability in infants *not* requiring CPAP or IPPV.[55] Interestingly, the reduced duration of the need for ventilatory support was only evident in those who were randomized within their first 3 days of life.

Because of the above data, and because ≥90% of infants <1250 g birth weight are considered candidates for caffeine administration, the latter may be considered within the first 3 days of age in any infant <1250 g who requires respiratory support and suffers from, or is likely to develop, AOP (i.e., is very immature and still being ventilated). It is important, however, also to consider when to discontinue caffeine treatment. Here, CAP study infants received caffeine up to a median GA of 34 wk. It is possible, however, that a longer duration of treatment will be even more beneficial, particularly given that the more mature brain is less tolerant to the detrimental effects of intermittent hypoxia, but longer duration of treatment may equally well be detrimental. This must therefore be tested in further RCTs.

In the CAP study, a loading dose of 10 mg/kg caffeine base (IV or orally) and a maintenance dose of 2.5–5 mg/kg once daily were used. Subgroup analysis, however, revealed that the reduction in death or disability was more pronounced in infants receiving an average dose of >3.5 mg/kg/d than it was in infants receiving caffeine at a lower dose.[66] Another RCT compared a loading dose of 40 mg/kg caffeine base (maintenance dose 10 mg/kg/d) with a 'conventional' 10/2.5 mg/kg regimen in 234 infants born at a mean GA of 27 wk. Infants in the high-dose group had only half the risk of failing extubation within 48 h of caffeine loading or to require reintubation and mechanical ventilation or doxapram within 7 d of caffeine loading (15.0 vs. 29.8%, RR 0.51 (0.31–0.85)).[67] This better efficacy was not at the expense of an increased risk of side effects. Given the extremely sparse data on doxapram (see below), clinicians may consider to give an extra dose of caffeine if AOP persists at the standard dose in an occasional infant. It has to be kept in mind, however, that caffeine may also be neurotoxic.[68] Higher doses and a 12-h dosing interval may be necessary in infants approaching term-equivalent age because of a more rapid caffeine metabolism in this age group.[69]

Doxapram

Doxapram stimulates peripheral chemoreceptors at low and central ones at high doses. It shows a clear dose–response curve, with a 50% reduction in apnea rate occurring in 47%, 65%, 82% and 89% of infants at doses of 0.5, 1.5, 2.0 and 2.5 mg/kg/h, respectively.[70] Most studies used a continuous intravenous infusion, although some suggest that the IV solution might also be given orally at twice the dose with good effect (enteral absorption is approximately 50%).[71] Short-term side effects become quite common at doses above 1.5 mg/kg/h and include irritability, myoclonus, elevated blood pressure and gastric residuals. Of concern is the fact that the long-term effects of doxapram are unknown. This is particularly worrying given that in a study on factors associated with poor development in extremely low birth weight infants, the only difference found was that infants with a mental development index (MDI) <70 had received a mean cumulative doxapram dose of 2233 mg, compared to 615 mg in matched controls without developmental delay ($p < 0.01$).[72] Although such a retrospective analysis cannot distinguish whether this reflects sequelae of severe AOP (for which doxapram had been given) or a direct drug effect, it clearly raises concern. In the CAP trial,[63] infants in the placebo group had not only been more likely to develop cerebral palsy, but were also three times more likely to receive doxapram. Given these data (or lack thereof), doxapram cannot be recommended as a standard treatment for AOP.

In summary, treatment for AOP may follow an incremental approach, starting with infant care procedures such as prone positioning, followed by caffeine and CPAP/N-IPPV (Box 24-1). We urgently need data on how much intermittent hypoxia/bradycardia can be tolerated in an individual infant without putting her/him at risk of developmental impairment, and on the efficacy and side effects of pharmacological treatments such as high-dose caffeine or doxapram, or new treatment modalities that may be based on the pathophysiology of this condition, as summarized above.

Box 24-1   Suggested Incremental Treatment Plan for AOP

- 1st step: Prone, 15° head-up tilt position
- 2nd step: Caffeine*
- 3rd step: Variable flow CPAP or synchronized N-IPPV
- 4th step: Intubation and mechanical ventilation**

*Consider caffeine as first-line treatment in infants <29 weeks GA/<1250 g.
**Caffeine at a higher dose or doxapram may be considered by some neonatologists prior to intubation, but data are insufficient to give a clear recommendation.

Clinical Pearls

- Understanding that the respiratory pattern of the preterm neonate largely resembles the fetal breathing pattern will help better to understand many of the phenomena seen with apnea of prematurity (AOP).
- Our treatment approach should keep this in mind, i.e., it should be directed at reducing chest wall distortion, avoiding hypoxia (and thereby hypoxic ventilatory depression) and preserving lung volume.
- Pharmacologically, caffeine citrate is the only substance used for AOP that has been thoroughly studied and shown to be neuroprotective, at least in infants of <1250 g birth weight; it may thus be considered in any such infant at risk of AOP.
- Otherwise, treatment should be incremental, starting with prone, head-up tilt positioning, moving on to caffeine and nasal continuous or intermittent airway pressure.

References

1. Lemke RP, Idiong N, Al-Saedi S, et al. Evidence of a critical period of airway instability during central apneas in preterm infants. Am J Respir Crit Care Med 1998;157:470–4.
2. Kianicka I, Diaz V, Dorion D, et al. Coordination between glottic adductor muscle and diaphragm EMG activity in fetal lambs in utero. J Appl Physiol 1998;84(5):1560–5.
3. Abu-Osba YK, Mathew OP, Thach BT. An animal model for airway sensory deprivation producing obstructive apnea with postmortem findings of sudden infant death syndrome. Pediatrics 1981;68:796–801.
4. Poets C. Apnea of prematurity. In: Kheirandish-Gozal L, Gozal D, editors. Sleep-disordered breathing in children: a comprehensive clinical guide to evaluation and treatment. New York: Humana Press, Springer; 2012. p. 263–78.
5. Poets CF, Southall DP. Patterns of oxygenation during periodic breathing in preterm infants. Early Hum Dev 1991;26:1–12.
6. Poets CF, Stebbens VA, Samuels MP, et al. The relationship between bradycardia, apnea, and hypoxemia in preterm infants. Pediatr Res [Research Support, Non-U.S. Gov't] 1993;34(2):144–7.
7. Daly M. Interactions between respiration and circulation. Bethesda, MD: American Physiological Society; 1986. p. 529–94.
8. Finer NN, Barrington KJ, Hayes BJ, et al. Obstructive, mixed, and central apnea in the neonate: physiologic correlates. J Pediatr 1992;121:943–50.
9. Olinsky A, Bryan MH, Bryan AC. Influence of lung inflation on respiratory control in neonates. J Appl Physiol 1974;36:426–9.
10. Kosch PC, Stark AR. Dynamic maintenance of end-expiratory lung volume in full-term infants. J Appl Physiol: Respirat Environ Exercise Physiol 1984;57:1126–33.
11. Poets CF, Rau GA, Neuber K, et al. Determinants of lung volume in spontaneously breathing preterm infants. Am J Respir Crit Care Med 1997;155(2):649–53.
12. Tourneux P, Leke A, Kongolo G, et al. Relationship between functional residual capacity and oxygen desaturation during short central apneic events during sleep in 'late preterm' infants. Pediatr Res 2008;64(2):171–6.
13. Sands SA, Edwards BA, Kelly VJ, et al. A model analysis of arterial oxygen saturation during apnea in preterm infants. PLoS Comput Biol 2010;54:429–48.
14. Esquer C, Claure N, D'Ugard C, et al. Mechanisms of hypoxemia episodes in spontaneously breathing preterm infants after mechanical ventilation. Neonatology 2008;94(2):100–4.
15. Hannam S, Ingram DM, Milner AD. A possible role for the Hering-Breuer deflation reflex in apnea of prematurity. J Pediatr 1998;132:35–9.
16. Edwards BA, Sands SA, Feeney C, et al. Continuous positive airway pressure reduces loop gain and resolves periodic central apneas in the lamb. Respir Physiol Neurobiol 2009;168(3):239–49.
17. Speidel BD, Dunn PM. Use of nasal continuous positive airway pressure to treat severe recurrent apnea in very preterm infants. Lancet 1976: 658–60.
18. Poets CF, Langner M, Bohnhorst B. Effects of nipple feeding and 2 different methods of gavage feeding on oxygenation in preterm infants. Acta Paediatr 1997;86:419–23
19. Peter CS, Bohnhorst B, Silny J, et al. Gastroesophageal reflux and apnea of prematurity: no temporal relationship. Pediatrics 2002;109:8–11.

20. Dorostkar PC, Baird TM, Rodriguez S, et al. Asystole and severe bradycardia in preterm infants. Biol Neonate 2005;88:299–305.
21. Di Fiore JM, Arko M, Whitehouse M, et al. Apnea is not prolonged by acid gastroesophageal reflux in preterm infants. Pediatrics 2005;116(5):1059–63.
22. Ward RM, Lemons JA, Molteni RA. Cisapride: a survey of the frequency of use and adverse events in premature newborns. Pediatrics 1999;103:469–72.
23. Lopes JM, Muller NL, Bryan MH, et al. Synergistic behavior of inspiratory muscles after diaphragmatic fatigue in the newborn. J Appl Physiol Respirat Environ Exercise Physiol 1981;51:547–51.
24. Heldt GP. Development of stability of the respiratory system in preterm infants. J Appl Physiol 1988;65:441–4.
25. Adams JA, Zabaleta IA, Sackner MA. Hypoxemic events in spontaneously breathing premature infants: etiologic basis. Pediatr Res 1997;42:463–71.
26. Numa AH, Newth CJL. Anatomic dead space in infants and children. J Appl Physiol 1996;80:1485–9.
27. Fenner A, Schalk U, Hoenicke H, et al. Periodic breathing in premature and neonatal babies: incidence, breathing pattern, respiratory gas tensions, response to changes in the composition of ambient air. Pediatr Res 1973;7:174–83.
28. Poets CF, Stebbens VA, Alexander JR, et al. Arterial oxygen saturation in preterm infants at discharge from the hospital and six weeks later. J Pediatr 1992;120:447–54.
29. Richard D, Poets CF, Neale S, et al. Arterial oxygen saturation in preterm neonates without respiratory failure. J Pediatr 1993;123:963–8.
30. Knill R, Bryan AC. An intercostal–phrenic inhibitory reflex in human newborn infants. J Appl Physiol 1976;40:352–61.
31. Knill R, Andrews W, Bryan AC. Respiratory load compensation in infants. J Appl Physiol 1976;40(3):357–61.
32. Eastman NJ. Fetal blood studies. Am J Obstetr Gynecol 1936:563–72.
33. Rigatto H, Brady JP, de la Torre Verduzco R. Chemoreceptor reflexes in preterm infants: I. The effect of gestational and postnatal age on the ventilatory response to inhalation of 100% and 15% oxygen. Pediatrics 1975;55:604–13.
34. Verbeek MM, Richardson HL, Parslow PM, et al. Arousal and ventilatory responses to mild hypoxia in sleeping preterm infants. J Sleep Res 2008;17(3):344–53.
35. Martin RJ, Di Fiore JM, Davis RL, et al. Persistence of the biphasic ventilatory response to hypoxia in preterm infants. J Pediatr 1998;132:960–4.
36. Alvaro R, Alvarez J, Kwiatkowski K, et al. Small preterm infants (<1500 g) have only a sustained decrease in ventilation in response to hypoxia. Pediatr Res 1992;32:403–6.
37. Carlo WA, Finer NN, Walsh MC, et al. Target ranges of oxygen saturation in extremely preterm infants. N Engl J Med 2010;362(21):1959–69.
38. Di Fiore JM, Walsh M, Wrage L, et al. Low oxygen saturation target range is associated with increased incidence of intermittent hypoxemia. J Paediatr 2012;Jun 26, epub ahead of print.
39. Lagercrantz H, Ahlstrøm H, Jonson B, et al. A critical oxygen level below which irregular breathing occurs in preterm infants. Oxford: Pergamon Press; 1978. p. 161–4.
40. Bessman SP, Carpenter CL. The creatine-creatine phosphate energy shuttle. Annu Rev Biochem 1985;54:831–62.
41. Wilken B, Ramirez JM, Probst I, et al. Creatine protects the central respiratory network of mammals under anoxic conditions. Pediatr Res 1998;43:8–14.
42. Wilken B, Ramirez JM, Probst IR, et al. Anoxic ATP depletion in neonatal mice brainstem is prevented by creatine supplementation. Arch Dis Child Fetal Neonatal Ed 2000;82:F224–7.
43. Wilken B, Ramirez JM, Richter DW, et al. Supplemental creatine enhances hypoxic augmentation in vivo by preventing ATP depletion (abstract). Eur J Pediatr 1998;157:178.
44. Bohnhorst B, Geuting T, Peter CS, et al. Randomized, controlled trial of oral creatine supplementation (not effective) for apnea of prematurity. Pediatrics 2004;113:e303–7.
45. Khan A, Qurashi M, Kwiatkowski K, et al. Measurement of the CO_2 apneic threshold in newborn infants: possible relevance for periodic breathing and apnea. J Appl Physiol 2005;98(4):1171–6.
46. Alvaro RE, Khalil M, Qurashi M, et al. CO(2) inhalation as a treatment for apnea of prematurity: a randomized double-blind controlled trial. J Pediatr 2012;160(2):252–7.
47. Tappin DM, Ford RPK, Nelson KP, et al. Breathing, sleep state, and rectal temperature oscillations. Arch Dis Child 1996;74:427–31.
48. Gozal D, Colin A, Daskalovic YI, et al. Environmental overheating as a cause of transient respiratory chemoreceptor dysfunction in an infant. Pediatrics 1988;82:738–40.
49. Perlstein PH, Edwards NK, Sutherland JM. Apnea in premature infants and incubator-air-temperature changes. N Engl J Med 1970;282:461–6.
50. Tourneux P, Cardot V, Museux N, et al. Influence of thermal drive on central sleep apnea in the preterm neonate. Sleep 2008;31(4):549–56.
51. Mathew OP, Thoppil CK, Belan M. Motor activity and apnea in preterm infants. Am Rev Respir Dis 1991;144:842–4.
52. Thoppil CK, Belan MA, Cowen CP, et al. Behavioral arousal in newborn infants and its association with termination of apnea. J Appl Physiol 1991;70:1479–84.
53. Heimler R, Langlois J, Hodel DJ, et al. Effect of positioning on the breathing pattern of preterm infants. Arch Dis Child 1992;67:312–14.
54. Martin RJ, Herrell N, Rubin D, et al. Effect of supine and prone positions on arterial oxygen tension in the preterm infant. Pediatrics 1979;63:528–31.
55. Jenni OG, von Siebenthal K, Wolf M, et al. Effect of nursing in the head elevated tilt position (15) on the incidence of bradycardic and hypoxemic episodes in preterm infants. Pediatrics 1997;100:622–5.
56. Reher C, Kuny KD, Pantalitschka T, et al. Randomised crossover trial of different postural interventions on bradycardia and intermittent hypoxia in preterm infants. Arch Dis Child Fetal Neonatal Ed 2008;93(4):F289–91.
57. Bauschatz AS, Kaufmann CM, Haensse D, et al. A preliminary report of nursing in the three-stair-position to prevent apnoea of prematurity. Acta Paediatr 2008;97(12):1743–5.
58. Pantalitschka T, Sievers J, Urschitz MS, et al. Randomised crossover trial of four nasal respiratory support systems for apnoea of prematurity in very low birthweight infants. Arch Dis Child Fetal Neonatal Ed 2009;94(4):F245–8.
59. De Paoli AG, Davis PG, Faber B, et al. Devices and pressure sources for administration of nasal continuous positive airway pressure (NCPAP) in preterm neonates. Cochrane Database Syst Rev 2008;(1):CD002977.
60. Lemyre B, Davis PG, De Paoli AG. Nasal intermittent positive pressure ventilation versus nasal continuous positive airway presssure for apnea of prematurity. Available at: http://wwwnichdnihgov/cochranenematal/lemyre/review01htm. 2000.
61. Moretti C, Giannini L, Fassi C, et al. Nasal flow-synchronized intermittent positive pressure ventilation to facilitate weaning in very low-birthweight infants: unmasked randomized controlled trial. Pediatr Int 2008;50(1):85–91.
62. Schmidt B, Roberts RS, Davis P, et al. Long-term effects of caffeine therapy for apnea of prematurity. N Engl J Med 2007;357(19):1893–902.
63. Schmidt B, Roberts RS, Davis P, et al. Caffeine therapy for apnea of prematurity. N Engl J Med 2006;354(20):2112–21.
64. Schmidt B, Anderson PJ, Doyle LW, et al. Survival without disability to age 5 years after neonatal caffeine therapy for apnea of prematurity. JAMA 2012;307(3):275–82.
65. Davis PG, Schmidt B, Roberts RS, et al. Caffeine for Apnea of Prematurity trial: benefits may vary in subgroups. J Pediatr 2010;156(3):382–7.
66. Barrington KJ, Roberts R, Schmidt B, et al. The Caffeine for Apnea of Prematurity (CAP) Trial, analyses of dose effect. PAS 2010, Abstract-CD 2010;Abstr 4350.4.
67. Steer PA, Shearman A, Lee TC, et al. Periextubation caffeine in preterm neonates: a randomized dose response trial. J Paediatr Child Health 2003;39:511–15.
68. Schmidt B. Methylxanthine therapy in premature infants: Sound practice, disaster, or fruitless byway? J Pediatr 1999;135:526–8.
69. Charles BG, Townsend SR, Steer PA, et al. Caffeine citrate treatment for extremely premature infants with apnea: population pharmacokinetics, absolute bioavailability, and implications for therapeutic drug monitoring. Ther Drug Monit 2008;30(6):709–16.
70. Barrington KJ, Finer NN, Torok-Both G, et al. Dose-response relationship of doxapram in the therapy for refractory apnea of prematurity. Pediatrics 1987;80:22–7.
71. Poets CF, Darraj S, Bohnhorst B. Effect of doxapram on episodes of apnoea, bradycardia and hypoxaemia in preterm infants. Biology of the Neonate [Clinical Trial Randomized Controlled Trial] 1999;76(4):207–13.
72. Sreenan C, Etches PC, Demianczuk N, et al. Isolated mental developmental delay in very low birth weight infants: Association with prolonged doxapram therapy for apnea. J Pediatr 2001;139:832–7.

Apparent Life Threatening Events (ALTE)

Rosemary S.C. Horne

DEFINITION OF APPARENT LIFE-THREATENING EVENTS (ALTE)

In the 1970s, it was thought that apparent life-threatening events (ALTE) were precursors to the sudden infant death syndrome (SIDS). These events, which were characterized by an acute and unexpected change in behavior with or without witnessed apnea, were referred to as near-miss for SIDS events.[1] In 1987, an expert panel sponsored by the National Institutes of Health developed the now widely accepted definition of ALTE as 'an episode that is frightening to the observer and that is characterized by some combination of apnea (central or occasionally obstructive), color change (usually cyanotic, but occasionally erythematous or plethoric), marked change in muscle tone (usually marked limpness), choking, or gagging.'[2] The term ALTE has been adopted to replace the term near-miss for SIDS as no substantial evidence has been found to link the two conditions.[2] During the 1980s and 1990s, numerous studies were carried out investigating infants who presented with ALTE to try to identify causes and risk factors for SIDS; however, a link between the two has never been proven and there is substantial evidence that the two conditions are, in fact, not related.

RELATIONSHIP BETWEEN ALTE AND SIDS

There is no evidence that ALTE is a precursor to SIDS.[2,3] This lack of association is evidenced by a number of findings including the temporal occurrence of the two events. SIDS invariably occurs during sleep and this finding has been included in the recent definition of the event.[4] An ALTE can occur during sleep, when awake or during feeding,[5] and in contrast to SIDS, most ALTE have been reported to occur during the daytime[6–8] and whilst awake.[9] In most cases, observers of an infant experiencing an ALTE report that the event appeared life-threatening or that they thought that the infant had died, but that prompt intervention resulted in normalization of the child's appearance.[5]

This lack of association is further supported by the evidence that SIDS incidence has significantly decreased since the early 1990s in Western countries where campaigns to reduce the risks were introduced, while the incidence of ALTE has remained unchanged.[10] In a study of 153 cases of ALTE that were enrolled in the Collaborative Home Infant Monitoring Evaluation (CHIME) between 1994 and 1998 it was reported that ALTE infants differed significantly from SIDS infants in four respects.[8] Fewer ALTE infants (9%) were small for gestational age at birth compared with 19% of SIDS infants,[11] fewer ALTE infants (19 %) were born to teenage mothers and this distribution was similar to the general population compared to 25% of SIDS mothers,[11] and ALTE infants were of

a younger age, 74% under 2 months of age compared to 27%[12] and 24%.[13] SIDS and ALTE infants had similar rates of prematurity (≈20%) and exposure to maternal smoking (ALTE infants 36%[8] and SIDS infants 30–56%).[11–15] One estimate has suggested that 7% of SIDS cases are preceded by ALTE;[2] however, in the CHIME study only 1 of 153 ALTE infants subsequently died[8] and in a review of 8 studies and 643 infants 5 deaths (0.8%) were reported, with all infants having an underlying medical problem.[16]

Although ALTE is not a precursor to SIDS, one study found that the SIDS rate for infants with ALTE was 10% and in those infants who had experienced multiple ALTE it rose to 28%.[17] The two entities do, however, share some common risk factors. In a study of 244 SIDS cases and 868 SIDS controls, the incidence of ALTE was 1.9% in SIDS controls compared to 7.4% in the infants who subsequently died of SIDS.[18] Furthermore, 33.3% of infants with ALTE who subsequently died from SIDS where exposed to both prenatal smoking and the prone sleeping position compared to 13% of ALTE survivors.[18] The study suggested that there may be a subpopulation of ALTE infants who do not go on to die from SIDS because they were sleeping supine and not exposed to maternal smoking. In a recent study of 35 ALTE infants and 19 healthy control infants who underwent overnight polysomnography at 2–3 months, 5–6 months and 8–9 months of age, arousal characteristics were examined.[19] All infants were born at term and were usual supine sleepers, and 18 of the ALTE infants had mothers who smoked. During non-rapid eye movement (NREM) sleep the ALTE infants had fewer total spontaneous arousals, cortical arousals and subcortical activations at both 2–3 and 5–6 months of age than control infants. ALTE infants with mothers who smoked had more obstructive apneas and more subcortical activations during rapid eye movement (REM) sleep. The same authors had previously reported that infants who subsequently died from SIDS had fewer cortical arousals and more subcortical activations, especially during REM sleep;[20] thus, they concluded that ALTE and SIDS victims had distinctly different arousal characteristics. In contrast, another polysomnographic study of 26 ALTE infants and 36 age-matched control infants studied at 3 months of age found that ALTE infants exhibited enhanced arousal mechanisms and increased NREM sleep discontinuity compared to controls.[21] Furthermore, normal infants showed a significant increase in cyclic alternating pattern (CAP) rate and a decrease in arousal index with age, while the ALTE infants showed no such correlation. The differences between the studies may have been due to the much lower incidence of maternal smoking (1/26) and the higher frequency of respiratory events (obstructive sleep apnea and periodic breathing) in the Miano et al. study.[21] Despite these differences, both studies identified that ALTE infants demonstrated an immaturity of sleep EEG patterns that was most marked in NREM sleep, and both showed significant differences in arousal patterns from previous studies of SIDS infants.

THE INCIDENCE OF ALTE

The incidence of ALTE has been estimated to be between 0.6 and 2.46 per 1000 live births.[10,22,23] ALTE account for 0.6% to 1.7% of all emergency department visits of patients less than 1 year of age[22-24] and 2.3% of pediatric hospitalizations in the USA.[25] The majority of ALTEs occur in infants younger than 1 year of age, with a median age of 1-3 months[16,26,27] and prematurely born infants are at increased risk.[28]

CAUSES OF ALTE

Over 80% of infants with ALTE appear to have no acute distress when they are seen at the emergency department[29] and no specific diagnosis can be found in up to 30% of those infants seen.[26] The common causes of ALTE are listed in Table 25.1.

In a systematic review of 23 publications with 20 different cohorts from 9 different countries and a total of 6849 infants presenting with ALTE, 3.2% of infants were diagnosed with a serious bacterial infection, 5.0% with seizures, 0.4% as child abuse and 0.3% with a metabolic disorder.[30] In another systematic review of eight non-randomized descriptive studies[22,23,31-35] the most common diagnoses were gastro-esophageal reflux disease (GERD), which was reported in all studies and comprised 31% of total diagnoses, lower respiratory tract infection (LRTI) including 'pertussis' and 'respiratory syncytial virus infection' were reported in 5 studies and 8% of all diagnoses, and seizure was reported in 7 studies and 11% of diagnoses.[16] Other diagnoses were problems with ear, nose and throat (3.6% of all diagnoses), cardiac problems (0.8%), urinary tract infection (1.1%), metabolic disease (1.5%), ingestion of drugs or toxins (1.5%), breath holding (2.3%), and factitious illness (0.3%). Only five ALTE episodes (0.7%) were completely benign. Unknown diagnoses were reported in 7/8 studies and made up 23% of all diagnoses, and this varied widely from 9% to 83% between studies.[16]

When investigating the underlying causes of ALTE, child abuse should also be considered, as studies have reported figures of up to 11%,[36] although other studies have reported the incidence to be around 2%.[37,38] In a study of infants diagnosed with abusive head trauma, over 30% of infants had been seen in the previous 3 weeks for other complaints including ALTE.[39]

RISK FACTORS FOR ALTE

Studies have consistently identified a number of risk factors for ALTE. ALTE typically affects infants under the age of 1 year and usually under 10 weeks of age, and there is a predisposition for more male infants to be affected.[40] Premature infants are at twice the risk, with a national survey in the Netherlands reporting that 29.5% of ALTE infants were born preterm compared with 13% being born preterm in the general population.[41] In a study of 625 infants admitted to Montreal

TABLE 25.1 Common Causes of ALTE

Most Common Causes

Gastro-esophogeal reflux
Infection (septicaemia, urinary tract infection, gastroenteritis)
Volvulus
Intussusception
Dumping syndrome
Chemolaryngeal reflex
Aspiration and choking

Neurological Problems

Convulsive disorders
Intracranial infection
Intracranial hypertension
Vasovagal reflexes
Congenital malformations of the brainstem
Muscular problems
Congenital central alveolar hypoventilation

Respiratory Problems

Apnea of infancy/breath-holding spells
Airway and pulmonary infection (respiratory syncytial virus, pertussis, pneumonia)
Congenital airway abnormalities
Airway obstruction
Obstructive sleep apnea

Cardiovascular Problems

Heart rhythm problems
Urea cycle defects
Galactosemia
Leigh or Reye syndrome
Neisidioblastosis
Menkes syndrome

Other Conditions

Excessive feeding volumes
Medications
Accidental smothering or asphyxia
Accidental carbon monoxide intoxication
Drug toxicity
Child abuse
Munchausen by proxy syndrome
Idiopathic ALTE

Adapted from Kahn A. Recommended clinical evaluation of infants with an apparent life-threatening event. Consensus document of the European Society for the Study and Prevention of Infant Death, 2003. Eur J Pediatr. 2004;163(2):108–115; Fu LY, Moon RY. Apparent life-threatening events: an update. Pediatr Rev. 2012;33(8):361–368; quiz 368–369 and Samuels MP. Apparent Life-Threatening Events: Pathogenesis and Management. In: C.L Marcus JLC, D.F. Donnelly, G.M. Loughlin, editor. Sleep and Breathing in Children. Second ed. New York: Informa Healthcare; 2008. p. 229–254.

Children's Hospital between 1996 and 2006 for ALTE a similar proportion of 21% were born preterm.[24] Furthermore, the relative risk of having an extreme event (either a central apnea lasting >30 s or an extreme bradycardia HR <60 bpm for 10 s) in infants <44 weeks post conceptional age (PCA) and HR <50 bpm for 10s in infants ≥44 weeks PCA whilst on a cardio-respiratory monitor was 6.3 (95% CI 3.6–11.0) for preterm born infants. Other risk factors include exposure to second-hand cigarette smoke, exposure to pertussis, respiratory syncytial virus or recent general anesthesia.[16,22,42]

ALTE IN THE FIRST 24 HOURS AFTER BIRTH

Recently, there have been reports of infants with ALTE within the first day of life. A nationwide retrospective German study reported a rate of 2.6 per 100 000 live births of severe ALTE requiring resuscitation and SIDS in the first 24 hours after birth.[43] Of the 17 infants who met the inclusion criteria 7 infants died; 3 after unsuccessful resuscitation and 4 had initially been resuscitated but had treatment discontinued because of severe hypoxic brain damage. Of the 10 survivors, 6 were neurologically abnormal on discharge. Twelve infants were found lifeless, lying on their mother's breast/abdomen or very close to and facing her, two were supine in their cots, two were being held by their fathers and one was lying supine next to their mother. Among the 26 cases excluded from the analysis, 4 were preterm but otherwise met the inclusion criteria. A further 3 infants were resuscitated with vigorous stimulation only. Another study published in the same year reports 6 cases of healthy term newborns (all with Apgar scores of 10 at both 5 and 10 minutes) who suffered an ALTE within 2 hours of delivery whilst in skin-to-skin contact with their mother; 3 of 6 infants died.[44] A prospective French regional study reported a rate of ALTE and SIDS of 0.032 deaths per 1000 live births within the first 2 hours after birth.[45] These studies highlight that there are risks associated with early skin-to-skin contact or breast feeding, especially when infants are not being closely observed by healthcare professionals.

INITIAL ASSESSMENT FOR ALTE

In a consensus statement from the European Society for the Study and Prevention of Infant Death in 2004 it was concluded that, 'There was no standard minimal workup in the evaluation of ALTE.'[5] The assessment of an infant who presents with an ALTE has been well reviewed in the literature recently.[5,9,30,46–49] A number of protocols for the initial examination have been published.[5,9,30,46,49–51] Details of the recommendations for the initial assessment are provided in Table 25.2.

In summary, any evaluation should always start with a careful history of the event as reported by the observer, a review of the infant's past medical history and a physical examination focusing on any evidence that might have caused or contributed to the event. Details of questions to be asked about the history of the ALTE infant and the event are listed in Table 25.3. If the event fits the definition of an ALTE, a full blood examination, blood glucose, serum electrolytes including calcium and blood gases with serum bicarbonate and lactate should be done as soon as possible. A urinary analysis and culture should also be performed. In most reviews a chest X-ray and tests to identify common respiratory viruses are also recommended. These tests are aimed at identifying a potential cause such as infection, hypocalcemia, hypomagnesemia, hypo- or hypernatremia leading to seizures or hypo- or hyperkalemia leading to cardiac arrhythmias. Metabolic disorders account for 2–5% of all cases of ALTE and, if not identified and treated, can lead to long-term sequelae. As these serum biochemistry tests are routinely available and relatively inexpensive, they are recommended.[49] Urine toxicology screening is also important to identify both intentional and unintentional poisoning.[49] In a retrospective study of children under 2 years of age presenting with ALTE, 8.4% had been given a medication that could have caused apnea, with 4.7% of children receiving over-the-counter cough and cold medication.[52] Importantly, none of the parents admitted to

TABLE 25.2	Recommendations for Initial Assessment

If the Event was:

- the first the infant had experienced
- was short
- the infant recovered spontaneously
- associated with feeding
- infant was awake
- physical examination was normal

Recommend that the infant be discharged home after parent's fears have been addressed, notify the family primary care physician and advise follow-up, advise to re-consult if recurrence.

If Event was as above but Physical Examination was Not Normal

- carry out investigation and manage as clinically indicated, usually with admission for at least 24 hours:
  - cardio-respiratory monitoring and saturation recording
  - complete blood count and differential
  - C-reactive protein levels
  - sodium and potassium
  - glucose and electrolytes
  - magnesium and calcium
  - blood glucose levels
  - serum lactate
  - urinalysis
  - toxicology screen
  - blood culture
  - chest X-ray
  - ECG, CT or MRI
  - consider dilated fundoscopy or swallowing test or esophageal pH monitoring

If Event was Prolonged, Infant had had Repetitive Events and Perceived need for Strong Stimulation to Terminate Event:

- as above
- if infant has fever or lethargy and does not appear normal on examination
- also consider brain imaging
- blood ammonia level
- full metabolic work-up

Adapted from McGovern MC, Smith MB. Causes of apparent life threatening events in infants: a systematic review. *Arch Dis Child*. 2004;89(11):1043–1048 and Al Khushi N, Cote A. Apparent life-threatening events: assessment, risks, reality. *Paediatr Respir Rev.* 2011;12(2):124–132

giving their children the medications, which were not recommended in children under 2 years of age.

Around 30% of ALTE cases are attributed to GERD[6] and about 25% of children admitted for ALTE undergo an upper gastrointestinal fluoroscopy or swallowing test.[49] These tests are useful for diagnosing anatomical abnormalities which could contribute to ALTE but, as many normal infants suffer from reflux, they are not specific to ALTE. Esophageal pH monitoring with concurrent cardio-respiratory monitoring can identify periods of reflux associated with apnea and/or hypoxemia. As these tests are uncomfortable for the patient and not inexpensive, it has been suggested that these tests only be recommended if the ALTE infant history indicated frequent bouts of reflux, if the event was immediately following a feed, or if gastric contents were noted in the infant's mouth or nose by the caregiver during the event.[49]

In a review of 36 children's hospitals across the USA, there was large inter-hospital variability in all aspects of ALTE infant care; however, the most common tests requested after an ALTE were a full blood examination (70%) and

Table 25.3 Details to Record of the History of the ALTE

Personal and Family History:

- details of pregnancy, gestation at birth, delivery and neonatal health, usual sleeping and feeding habits, method of feeding
- any medical or surgical problems and previous evaluations
- characteristics of other siblings with an ALTE, early death, SIDS, family history of genetic, metabolic, cardiac or neurological problems
- parents' age, smoking and drinking habits. Usual medical treatments in the past 7 days. Details also of any other care giver

Daily Routine:

- usual sleep conditions, including position put down and when found if event occurred during sleep. Bed/cot and bedding, sleep attire room temperature, use of dummy/pacifier or any sedative medications
- in breast feeding mothers, did they take any prescription, over-the-counter or herbal remedies within 24 hours of the event?

Events Immediately Preceding ALTE:

- the events and minor symptoms that preceded the ALTE
- including any episodes of fever, illness, medications, immunization, sleep restriction, or change in daily routine

Detailed Description of the ALTE Event:

- precise timing of ALTE
- relationship to feeding
- exact place of ALTE (child's cot, parent's bed, car seat, parent's arms)
- the state of the infants when the event began – awake or asleep
- if asleep, infant's body position, type of bedding, whether face was covered or not. Specific details of the sleeping arrangements, own cot, parental bed, sofa, pram, etc. Was the infant in a co-sleeping situation?
- if awake, whether the infant was being fed, handled, crying, being bathed
- the reason the event was noticed – infant cry or other noise
- did the infant fall or experience any other trauma?
- who discovered the infant or witnessed the event?
- the infant's appearance when found: were they conscious or not, muscle tone (rigid or floppy), vomiting, foreign body or milk in mouth or nose, sweating, skin temperature, lethargy, pupil size?
- color (pallor, red, purple, blue), location of color changes – peripheral, whole body, around the mouth, tongue and palate, symmetric or asymmetric
- respiratory effort – none, shallow, chocking, gasping, increased effort, nasal flaring, stridor, wheeze
- movement and muscle tone – rigid, floppy, limp, jerking, convulsions
- interventions – the event resolved spontaneously, required gentle stimulation, blowing air on face, vigorous stimulation, CPR
- child's response to intervention
- estimated time to recovery and duration of event
- was there anything unusual about the child before the event?

Adapted from Kahn A. Recommended clinical evaluation of infants with an apparent life-threatening event. Consensus document of the European Society for the Study and Prevention of Infant Death, 2003. Eur J Pediatr. 2004;163(2):108–115; Scollan-Koliopoulos M, Koliopoulos JS. Evaluation and management of apparent life-threatening events in infants. Pediatr Nurs. 2010;36(2):77–83; quiz 84; and Fu LY, Moon RY. Apparent life-threatening events: an update. Pediatr Rev. 2012;33(8):361–368; quiz 368–369.

electrolytes (65%), chest X-ray (69%), electrocardiogram (36%) and upper gastrointestinal fluoroscopy or swallow testing (26%).[25]

Previously, McGovern and Smith[16] recommended inclusion of an EEG assessment in the initial investigation of ALTE based on the findings of their study that 11% of infants were diagnosed with seizures. However, in their review only two of seven revealed that the diagnosis of epilepsy was made from EEG. In a more recent study, only 3.6% of ALTE infants were diagnosed with epilepsy[36] and EEG only had a sensitivity for diagnosis of 15%. The majority of infants diagnosed had recurrent ALTE events within 1 month (71%) and 41% were diagnosed as having seizures within 1 week of the initial event. Recent recommendations suggest that, given the difficulty of obtaining an EEG in the emergency department setting and the low sensitivity for diagnosing epilepsy, EEG monitoring be reserved for infants presenting with recurrent ALTE events.[49] In addition to EEG, neuroimaging can be used to help diagnose chronic epilepsy by identifying underlying brain anatomical abnormalities. Neuroimaging is also useful for identifying abusive head trauma. However, in a study by the Bonkowsky et al., when combined all neuroimaging techniques (cranial computed tomography (CT), magnetic resonance imaging (MRI) and ultrasound) they only had a sensitivity of 6.7% for detecting chronic epilepsy.[36] Head CT is the most commonly ordered imaging study to investigate ALTE,[49] and one study found that ordering a head CT for all asymptomatic ALTE infants actually saved money from a medical payer perspective for identifying abusive head trauma.[53] However, as only 1–3% of all ALTE cases are due to abusive head trauma, many infants would be subjected to unnecessary irradiation if this practice was to be adopted, and it has been recommended that this assessment only be performed where abuse is suspected.[49] Two separate studies have identified that discrepancies in the reported history of the ALTE by different caregivers, or that the history changes over time or is confusing, was highly predictive of physical abuse.[54,55] In addition, delays in seeking medical attention, vomiting and irritability were also predictive. It has been suggested that having multiple emergency department staff taking the history, looking for inconsistencies and for other symptoms of abuse such as retinal examinations and recent fractures, may help identify those infants who should be referred for CT scans.[49]

SHOULD ALL ALTE INFANTS BE ADMITTED?

The question of whether an infant presenting at the emergency department with ALTE routinely requires hospital admission is controversial. In the past, as it was thought that infants who had experienced an ALTE might subsequently go on to die from SIDS, infants were routinely admitted to hospital for diagnostic monitoring and frequently discharged home on an apnea/bradycardia monitor.[56] Some recent reviews of treatment for ALTE still strongly recommend admission.[22,50] It has been reported that in the USA the average length of hospital stay of an ALTE infant is 4.4±5.6 (SD) days with total charges of $15 567±$28 510 (SD).[25] In a retrospective study of 625 infants admitted following an ALTE, 13.6% had a subsequent extreme cardio-respiratory event and 85% of these occurred within the first 24 hours after admission and were attributed to respiratory tract infection.[24] In a prospective study of 66 infants, 14 of whom had perinatal risk factors and 16 had had a previous ALTE, 12% had recurrent events within 24 hours of admission, 9% had events requiring moderate stimulation and 3% required resuscitation.[57]

In the majority of cases presenting in the emergency department, the infants appear normal after a suspected ALTE at home, and there have been few studies to evaluate the benefit of hospital admission. In a recent multicenter observational cohort study of 832 infants, 84.4% of infants appeared well in the emergency department and 16.5% obviously required patient admission.[9] Criteria for 'obviously needed admission' were: required supplemental oxygen for non-self-resolving hypoxia, intubation, ventilation, intravenous antibiotics for confirmed serious bacterial infection, antiepileptic drugs or a positive test for respiratory syncytial virus or pertussis. Nearly 80% of infants were admitted, with more than 40% admitted to a monitored bed. Together with this criterion, two other factors, significant medical history and >1 ALTE in 24 hours, identified 89% of infants who ultimately had justifications for hospitalization. The use of the authors' published decision tree would have potentially reduced the number of admissions by 27% while missing 2% of patients who required hospital admission. In another large study of 300 infants, 76% were admitted but only 12% required significant intervention.[26] None of the infants died during their hospital stay or with 72 hours of discharge. Logistic regression identified prematurity, abnormal result on physical examination, color change to cyanosis, absence of symptoms of upper respiratory tract infection, and the absence of choking as predictors of significant intervention. When these predictors were used to form a clinical decision rule, 64% of infants could have been discharged home safely from the emergency department, reducing the hospitalization rate to 36%.[26] In an earlier smaller study of 59 patients, two 'high-risk' factors that predicted the need for hospital admission were age less than 1 month and multiple ALTE in the past 24 hours.[58] They concluded that infants older than 1 month who had experienced a single ALTE could safely be discharged from the emergency department.

From the above literature, it can be seen that there is still debate regarding whether or not all ALTE infants should be admitted. A recent review suggested that, in the light of findings that repeat events usually occurred within 24 hours, the majority of ALTE infants should be admitted for at least 23 hours with continuous cardio-respiratory monitoring, ideally with pulse oximetry and event recording.[49] However, if the event was the first ALTE experienced, when infants were not premature, had suffered a single event which was brief, not severe and self-resolving and if there was a probable cause such as GERD, it was reasonable for the infant not to be admitted.[49]

LONG-TERM FOLLOW-UP – HOME MONITORING

If it is decided that cardio-respiratory monitoring is required after discharge home, it should be aimed at assisting with diagnosis and management of ALTE.[59] It is therefore important to use monitors that record respiration and heart rate in conjunction with oxygen saturation so that central and obstructive respiratory events can we distinguished. In the CHIME study, the majority of significant events had a central component.[60]

There is still debate as to whether or not polysomnography should be routinely requested when investigating ALTE.[5,59] Disadvantages of polysomnography are that it is not readily available in all centers where ALTE infants might present, it frequently cannot be arranged immediately after admission, it is only for one night in duration and it is costly to perform. It is, however, the gold standard for distinguishing central and obstructive events.

There is also still debate as to whether or not ALTE infants should be sent home on cardio-respiratory monitors. In the 1980s, home cardio-respiratory monitoring became widely used in order to try to prevent SIDS; however, it is now no longer recommended.[3] Furthermore, the frequency of false alarms has the undesired effect of causing more anxiety for parents. For those infants who have suffered severe ALTE at home and who have underlying cardio-respiratory abnormalities which are not immediately treatable, home monitoring may be beneficial. Short periods of home monitoring with devices in which events can subsequently be downloaded can also assist with diagnosis. It has been documented that seizures, metabolic disorders and Munchausen by proxy syndrome can be distinguished in infants who have had recurrent ALTE.[61,62]

SUMMARY

ALTE is common in infancy and it is often difficult to diagnose the cause, as most infants appear well by the time they present at the emergency department. The definition of ALTE is also very subjective and depends on the first-hand report of the event by parents/caregivers and this adds to the difficulty of diagnosis. A thorough history and details of the event together with a careful physical examination of the infant may provide clues to the underlying cause. Most frequently, no cause can be determined and it is therefore difficult for clinicians to decide how intensively the infant should be investigated and for how long they should be monitored. The most common causes of ALTE are gastro-esophageal reflux, lower respiratory tract infection and seizure. Premature infants and those exposed to second-hand smoke are at increased risk. Most ALTE do not result in a serious diagnosis, and a single episode in a young infant usually does not require prolonged investigation. If the infant has had recurrent events and/or required vigorous stimulation, then admission and a battery of appropriate tests are required. It is no longer recommended that infants be monitored at home long-term.

Clinical Pearls

- Apparent life-threatening events (ALTE) are relatively common in infancy, particularly in infants under 10 weeks of age and those born preterm.
- Diagnosis of the underlying cause is difficult.
- A thorough case history and detailed description of the event are essential.
- Most ALTE do not result in a serious diagnosis and a single episode in a young infant usually does not require prolonged investigation.

References

1. American Academy of Pediatrics. Task Force on Prolonged Infantile Apnea. Prolonged infantile apnea: 1985. Pediatrics 1985;76(1):129–31.
2. National Institutes of Health Consensus Development Conference on Infantile Apnea and Home Monitoring, Sept 29 to Oct 1, 1986. Pediatrics 1987;79(2):292–9.
3. American Academy of Pediatrics Apnea, sudden infant death syndrome, and home monitoring. Pediatrics 2003;111(4 Pt 1):914–17.
4. Krous HF, Beckwith JB, Byard RW, et al. Sudden infant death syndrome and unclassified sudden infant deaths: a definitional and diagnostic approach. Pediatrics 2004;114(1):234–8.
5. Kahn A. Recommended clinical evaluation of infants with an apparent life-threatening event. Consensus document of the European Society for the Study and Prevention of Infant Death, 2003. Eur J Pediatr 2004;163(2):108–15.
6. Wennergren G, Milerad J, Lagercrantz H, et al. The epidemiology of sudden infant death syndrome and attacks of lifelessness in Sweden. Acta Paediatr Scand 1987;76(6):898–906.
7. Kahn A, Blum D, Hennart P, et al. A critical comparison of the history of sudden-death infants and infants hospitalised for near-miss for SIDS. Eur J Pediatr 1984;143(2):103–7.
8. Esani N, Hodgman JE, Ehsani N, et al. Apparent life-threatening events and sudden infant death syndrome: comparison of risk factors. J Pediatr 2008;152(3):365–70.
9. Kaji AH, Claudius I, Santillanes G, et al. Apparent life-threatening event: multicenter prospective cohort study to develop a clinical decision rule for admission to the hospital. Ann Emerg Med 2013;61(4):379–87.
10. Kiechl-Kohlendorfer U, Hof D, Peglow UP, et al. Epidemiology of apparent life threatening events. Arch Dis Child 2004;90(3):297–300.
11. Getahun D, Demissie K, Lu SE, et al. Sudden infant death syndrome among twin births: United States, 1995–1998. J Perinatol 2004;24(9):544–51.
12. Leach CE, Blair PS, Fleming PJ, et al. Epidemiology of SIDS and explained sudden infant deaths. CESDI SUDI Research Group. Pediatrics 1999;104(4):e43.
13. Li DK, Petitti DB, Willinger M, et al. Infant sleeping position and the risk of sudden infant death syndrome in California, 1997–2000. Am J Epidemiol 2003;157(5):446–55.
14. Malloy MH. Size for gestational age at birth: impact on risk for sudden infant death and other causes of death, USA 2002. Arch Dis Child Fetal Neonatal Ed 2007;92(6):F473–8.
15. Hauck FR, Herman SM, Donovan M, et al. Sleep environment and the risk of sudden infant death syndrome in an urban population: the Chicago Infant Mortality Study. Pediatrics 2003;111(5 Pt 2):1207–14.
16. McGovern MC, Smith MB. Causes of apparent life threatening events in infants: a systematic review. Arch Dis Child 2004;89(11):1043–8.
17. Samuels MP, Poets CF, Noyes JP, et al. Diagnosis and management after life threatening events in infants and young children who received cardiopulmonary resuscitation. BMJ 1993;306(6876):489–92.
18. Edner A, Wennborg M, Alm B, et al. Why do ALTE infants not die in SIDS? Acta Paediatr 2007;96(2):191–4.
19. Franco P, Montemitro E, Scaillet S, et al. Fewer spontaneous arousals in infants with apparent life-threatening event. Sleep 2011;34(6):733–43.
20. Kato I, Franco P, Groswasser J, et al. Incomplete arousal processes in infants who were victims of sudden death. Am J Respir Crit Care Med 2003;168(11):1298–303.
21. Miano S, Castaldo R, Ferri R, et al. Sleep cyclic alternating pattern analysis in infants with apparent life-threatening events: a daytime polysomnographic study. Clin Neurophysiol 2012;123(7):1346–352.
22. Davies F, Gupta R. Apparent life threatening events in infants presenting to an emergency department. Emerg Med J 2002;19(1):11–16.
23. Gray C, Davies F, Molyneux E. Apparent life-threatening events presenting to a pediatric emergency department. Pediatr Emerg Care 1999;15(3):195–9.
24. Al-Kindy HA, Gelinas JF, Hatzakis G, et al. Risk factors for extreme events in infants hospitalized for apparent life-threatening events. J Pediatr 2009;154(3):332–7, 337 e331–2.
25. Tieder JS, Cowan CA, Garrison MM, et al. Variation in inpatient resource utilization and management of apparent life-threatening events. J Pediatr 2008;152(5):629–35, 635 e621–2.
26. Mittal MK, Sun G, Baren JM. A clinical decision rule to identify infants with apparent life-threatening event who can be safely discharged from the emergency department. Pediatr Emerg Care 2012;28(7):599–605.
27. DiMario FJ Jr. Apparent life-threatening events: so what happens next? Pediatrics 2008;122(1):190–1.
28. Myerberg DZ, Carpenter RG, Myerberg CF, et al. Reducing postneonatal mortality in West Virginia: a statewide intervention program targeting risk identified at and after birth. Am J Public Health 1995;85(5):631–7.
29. Southall DP, Plunkett MC, Banks MW, et al. Covert video recordings of life-threatening child abuse: lessons for child protection. Pediatrics 1997;100(5):735–60.
30. Al Khushi N, Cote A. Apparent life-threatening events: assessment, risks, reality. Paediatr Respir Rev 2011;12(2):124–32.
31. Laisne C, Rimet Y, Poujol A, et al. [Apropos of 100 cases of malaise in infants]. Ann Pediatr (Paris) 1989;36(7):451–4.
32. Tal Y, Tirosh E, Even L, et al. A comparison of the yield of a 24 h versus 72 h hospital evaluation in infants with apparent life-threatening events. Eur J Pediatr 1999;158(11):954.
33. Veereman-Wauters G, Bochner A, Van Caillie-Bertrand M. Gastroesophageal reflux in infants with a history of near-miss sudden infant death. J Pediatr Gastroenterol Nutr 1991;12(3):319–23.
34. Tsukada K, Kosuge N, Hosokawa M, et al. Etiology of 19 infants with apparent life-threatening events: relationship between apnea and esophageal dysfunction. Acta Paediatr Jpn 1993;35(4):306–10.
35. Sheikh S, Stephen T, Frazer A, et al. Apparent life-threatening episodes in infants. Clin Pulm Med 2000;7(2):81–4.
36. Bonkowsky JL, Guenther E, Filloux FM, et al. Death, child abuse, and adverse neurological outcome of infants after an apparent life-threatening event. Pediatrics 2008;122(1):125–31.
37. Altman RL, Brand DA, Forman S, et al. Abusive head injury as a cause of apparent life-threatening events in infancy. Arch Pediatr Adolesc Med 2003;157(10):1011–15.
38. Pitetti RD, Maffei F, Chang K, et al. Prevalence of retinal hemorrhages and child abuse in children who present with an apparent life-threatening event. Pediatrics 2002;110(3):557–62.
39. Jenny C, Hymel KP, Ritzen A, et al. Analysis of missed cases of abusive head trauma. JAMA 1999;281(7):621–6.
40. Scollan-Koliopoulos M, Koliopoulos JS. Evaluation and management of apparent life-threatening events in infants. Pediatr Nurs 2010;36(2):77–83; quiz 84.
41. Semmekrot BA, van Sleuwen BE, Engelberts AC, et al. Surveillance study of apparent life-threatening events (ALTE) in the Netherlands. Eur J Pediatr 2010;169(2):229–36.
42. Carroll JL. Apparent life threatening event (ALTE) assessment. Pediatr Pulmonol Suppl 2004;26:108–9.
43. Poets A, Steinfeldt R, Poets CF. Sudden deaths and severe apparent life-threatening events in term infants within 24 hours of birth. Pediatrics 2011;127(4):e869–73.
44. Andres V, Garcia P, Rimet Y, et al. Apparent life-threatening events in presumably healthy newborns during early skin-to-skin contact. Pediatrics 2011;127(4):e1073–6.
45. Dageville C, Pignol J, De Smet S. Very early neonatal apparent life-threatening events and sudden unexpected deaths: incidence and risk factors. Acta Paediatr 2008;97(7):866–9.
46. Hall KL, Zalman B. Evaluation and management of apparent life-threatening events in children. Am Fam Physician 2005;71(12):2301–8.
47. Brand DA, Altman RL, Purtill K, et al. Yield of diagnostic testing in infants who have had an apparent life-threatening event. Pediatrics 2005;115(4):885–93.
48. Dewolfe CC. Apparent life-threatening event: a review. Pediatr Clin North Am 2005;52(4):1127–146, ix.
49. Fu LY, Moon RY. Apparent life-threatening events: an update. Pediatr Rev 2012;33(8):361–8; quiz 368–9.

50. De Piero AD, Teach SJ, Chamberlain JM. ED evaluation of infants after an apparent life-threatening event. Am J Emerg Med 2004;22(2):83–6.
51. Reix P, St-Hilaire M, Praud JP. Laryngeal sensitivity in the neonatal period: from bench to bedside. Pediatr Pulmonol 2007;42(8):674–82.
52. Pitetti RD, Whitman E, Zaylor A. Accidental and nonaccidental poisonings as a cause of apparent life-threatening events in infants. Pediatrics 2008;122(2):e359–62.
53. Campbell KA, Berger RP, Ettaro L, et al. Cost-effectiveness of head computed tomography in infants with possible inflicted traumatic brain injury. Pediatrics 2007;120(2):295–304.
54. Vellody K, Freeto JP, Gage SL, et al. Clues that aid in the diagnosis of nonaccidental trauma presenting as an apparent life-threatening event. Clin Pediatr (Phila) 2008;47(9):912–18.
55. Guenther E, Powers A, Srivastava R, et al. Abusive head trauma in children presenting with an apparent life-threatening event. J Pediatr 2010;157(5):821–5.
56. Oren J, Kelly D, Shannon DC. Identification of a high-risk group for sudden infant death syndrome among infants who were resuscitated for sleep apnea. Pediatrics 1986;77(4):495–9.
57. Santiago-Burruchaga M, Sanchez-Etxaniz J, Benito-Fernandez J, et al. Assessment and management of infants with apparent life-threatening events in the paediatric emergency department. Eur J Emerg Med 2008;15(4):203–8.
58. Claudius I, Keens T. Do all infants with apparent life-threatening events need to be admitted? Pediatrics 2007;119(4):679–83.
59. Cote A. Home and hospital monitoring for ALTE. Paediatr Respir Rev 2006;7(Suppl 1):S199–201.
60. Ramanathan R, Corwin MJ, Hunt CE, et al. Cardiorespiratory events recorded on home monitors: Comparison of healthy infants with those at increased risk for SIDS. JAMA 2001;285(17):2199–207.
61. Cote A, Hum C, Brouillette RT, et al. Frequency and timing of recurrent events in infants using home cardiorespiratory monitors. J Pediatr 1998;132(5):783–9.
62. Poets CF, Samuels MP, Noyes JP, et al. Home event recordings of oxygenation, breathing movements, and heart rate and rhythm in infants with recurrent life-threatening events. J Pediatr 1993;123(5):693–701.

Primary Snoring

Susanna McColley and Mark Haupt

PRIMARY SNORING

Snoring is an inspiratory noise produced by vibration of the soft tissues of the oropharyngeal walls that occurs because of changes in the configuration and properties of the upper airway during sleep (Figures 26-1 and 26-2). Snoring is the most common, and sometimes, the only presenting symptom of sleep-disordered breathing (SDB). A spectrum of SDB exists and is viewed on a continuum of severity based on the degree of upper airway narrowing, arousals, and gas exchange abnormalities. The spectrum ranges from primary snoring to the upper airway resistance syndrome (UARS) to obstructive sleep apnea syndrome (OSAS).

Primary snoring (PS) is traditionally defined as nightly or frequent snoring that is not associated with hypoxemia, hypercapnia, sleep disruption or daytime symptoms.[1] For the child with habitual snoring, it is essential to discriminate PS from OSAS so that appropriate treatment can be provided. By definition, the diagnosis of PS is made by polysomnographic criteria with objective measurement of sleep and respiratory function, as clinical history alone cannot differentiate PS from OSAS.[2]

In a study of 83 snoring children referred to a tertiary pediatric sleep clinic, parents completed a standardized, nurse-administered questionnaire that asked questions regarding snoring frequency, observed apnea, struggling to breathe, and other daytime and nighttime symptoms. Children then underwent nocturnal polysomnography to assess for sleep-disordered breathing. Although there were several differences in symptom frequencies between the children with PS and those with OSAS, both single and multiple questions showed poor sensitivity and specificity in differentiating PS and OSAS. Other studies demonstrate a similar inability of clinical history to differentiate PS from OSAS.[3–8]

Upper Airway Resistance Syndrome

Although PS is a polysomnographic diagnosis, the diagnosis of PS suggests that it is a benign condition, without adverse sleep-related or daytime sequelae since there are no aberrations in gas exchange abnormalities or sleep architecture. In other words, children with primary snoring have no disruption of normal sleep patterns, no cardiorespiratory compromise, and no neuropsychological morbidity. Since snoring affects approximately 10% of children, the presence of snoring without consequence is likely to occur. However, the original descriptions of PS occurred prior to description of the upper airway resistance syndrome (UARS) as a distinct clinical entity. Although the consensus on the definition of UARS is still lacking, interpretation of the literature can be difficult, since some children previously characterized as having PS may have actually had UARS.

UARS is defined as partial upper airway obstruction that is not associated with gas exchange abnormalities but is accompanied by increased respiratory effort (initially measured by changes in intrathoracic pressure via esophageal manometry) terminated by electroencephalographic arousal and responds positively to treatment in the same manner as OSAS.[9] Snoring occurs in most affected individuals, but physiologic findings of UARS have been noted in patients without snoring, particularly in those who have had palatal surgery for upper airway obstruction. UARS is associated with increased upper airway collapsibility during sleep.[10] Guilleminault and colleagues reported the clinical and polysomnographic characteristics of UARS in 25 children who were referred for snoring, excessive daytime somnolence, and behavioral problems.[11] They demonstrated marked difference in the referred group compared to 25 healthy control children. Subsequently, numerous studies have demonstrated these polysomnographic findings of UARS in adults with daytime somnolence. Daytime somnolence in adults with UARS is significantly improved with nasal continuous positive airway pressure therapy, as objectively measured by the multiple sleep latency test.[12]

In adults, excessive daytime somnolence has a number of significant sequelae, including an increased risk of motor vehicle and work-related accidents and impaired mood. Hypertension is also frequently seen in adults with UARS. Children identified as having UARS have a variety of daytime symptoms, including symptoms of attention deficit hyperactivity disorder and academic problems. Most studies of snoring have not defined or described UARS as a distinct clinical entity and the true prevalence of UARS is unknown.[9] However, studies now suggest significant neurocognitive abnormalities in children with habitual snoring occur, including attention deficit hyperactivity disorder, academic problems and behavior problems.[13–15] Children with polysomnographically confirmed PS may demonstrate reduced neurocognitive capabilities, particularly in the domains of attention, memory and intelligence,[16] and decreased performance in several measures of language and visuospatial ability.[17] Available data, however, do not allow clear separation between patients with UARS and those with OSAS.

Although sleep physiologists often view sleep-disordered breathing as a spectrum with primary snoring being the mildest and OSAS the most severe form, no studies demonstrate a clear relationship between the degree of sleep-disordered breathing and symptoms or physiologic sequelae. Furthermore, although the diagnosis of primary snoring has traditionally been made on the basis of polysomnographic findings alone, available evidence suggests the absence of daytime somnolence should be an additional diagnostic criterion. In addition, children with primary snoring may demonstrate daytime symptoms in the form of habitual mouth breathing or a dry mouth, symptoms that might reduce quality of life.[18,19]

Epidemiology

A number of epidemiological studies from diverse geographic locations have been published describing the prevalence of snoring in children. Most of these have used parental

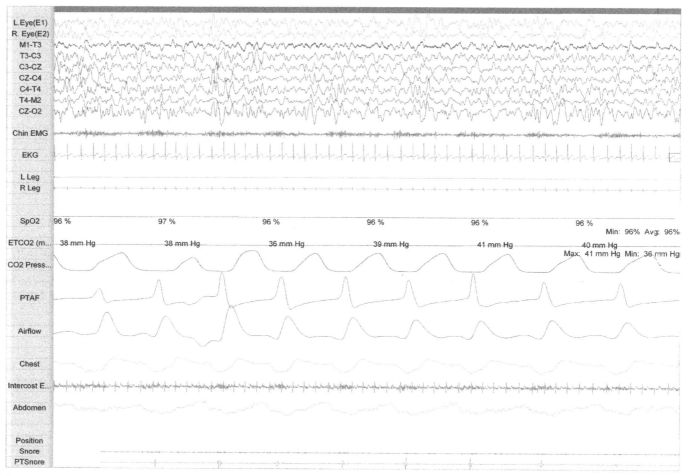

FIGURE 26-1 Thirty-second epoch in N3 sleep from a 4-year-old girl referred for evaluation of snoring. Note the presence of snore artifact present in the Chin EMG. This epoch demonstrates primary snoring without classic changes on EEG suggestive of an arousal.

report by way of either questionnaire or interview format. Most have not included objective measurements of respiration during sleep, or they have included such measures on only a subset of children felt to be at high risk for OSAS. Additionally, there is no universally accepted, clear definition of snoring. Thus, the prevalence of the condition may differ based on varying interpretations of the term 'snoring' across cultures.[9]

A summary of representative epidemiological studies of snoring in children is presented in Table 26.1. A recent meta-analysis by Lumeng and Chervin suggests the overall prevalence, as reported by parents, is 7.45%,[9] contrasting the 40% frequency of regular snoring in adults. The same authors reported that prevalence of habitual snoring ranges from a minimum of 2.4% in Turkey to a maximum of 34.5% in Italy. Within the same meta-analysis, the prevalence of OSAS is 0.1% to 13%. The study presenting the prevalence of OSAS as 13% is a significant outlier, with the diagnosis of OSAS based on oxygen desaturation index rather than standard measures. Excluding the 13%, the prevalence of OSAS ranges from 0.1% to 5.7%. None of these epidemiological studies has attempted to distinguish UARS from PS. Rosen[20] studied 326 otherwise healthy children with snoring. Fifty-nine percent of children had OSAS, 25% had PS, 6% had UARS and 10%

had no snoring. It is notable that 28% of the children in the study were obese. Racial and ethnic differences also contribute to varying prevalence of snoring in a given population.[7]

Natural History

Limited data are available regarding the natural history of primary snoring in children. Marcus and co-workers repeated polysomnography in 20 children 1 to 3 years after the initial diagnosis of PS; none had undergone airway surgery.[21] All of these children had persistent snoring; in 20% snoring had increased, and in 70% there had been no change. Overall, there was no change in apnea index, oxyhemoglobin saturation, or peak end-tidal Pco_2. However, two children had mild OSAS on repeat testing. The authors concluded that most children with PS do not progress to having OSAS, and those who do progress have only mild OSAS. Daytime symptoms in persistently snoring children were not reported.

Topol and Brooks studied nine children with primary snoring 3 years after initial polysomnographic diagnosis of PS; a control group of nine age-matched, non-snoring subjects was studied for comparison.[22] As in the study by Marcus and colleagues, there was no overall change in respiratory parameters between the first and second polysomnogram; one snoring subject had significant worsening of the respiratory

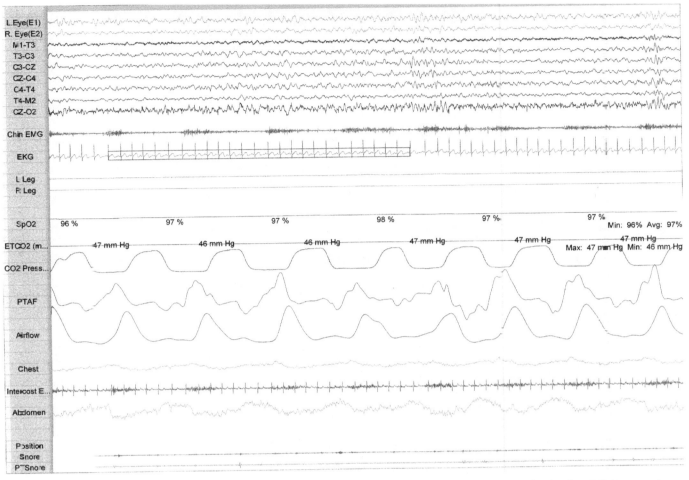

FIGURE 26-2 Thirty-second epoch in N2 sleep from the same 4-year-old girl as in Figure 26-1. Snore artifact is again noted in the Chin EMG. However, theta bursts are associated with the snoring, suggestive of arousal and upper airway resistance.

disturbance index. Interestingly, the control group had significantly better sleep efficiency and fewer brief arousals than the snoring group, which suggests that some of the children with PS may actually have been affected by UARS. Supporting the notion that PS may affect sleep architecture, O'Brien and colleagues recently demonstrated that children with PS exhibited a lower percentage of rapid eye movement (REM) sleep.[17]

Urschitz and colleagues presented similar findings from a large-scale questionnaire-based study of 1144 preschool children in Germany who were followed over a 1-year period.[19] Ten percent of the children in this particular study demonstrated habitual snoring. Forty-nine percent of respondents continued to snore after 1 year. Predictors of long-term habitual snoring included decreased maternal education, the presence of a smoker in the household, loud snoring and surgical intervention for snoring since the initial survey.

While most children with primary snoring demonstrate resolution of their symptoms, Gozal and Pope demonstrated that a 'learning debt' may develop in children who snore during early childhood.[15] In this large survey-based study, children in the bottom quartile of their seventh- or eighth-grade class were more likely to have snored during early childhood (OR 2.79, confidence interval: 1.88–4.15) and required

a tonsillectomy for snoring as compared to the top-performing quartile members of their class. The authors suggested that children who experienced sleep-disordered breathing during a period traditionally associated with major brain growth and substantial acquisition of cognitive and intellectual capabilities may in part undermine their capacity for future academic achievement. These findings are consistent with the principle, suggested by Topol and Brooks, that some children may be experiencing UARS or that PS may have more significant consequences than originally appreciated.

Along with the potential long-term neurologic effects of PS, cardiovascular disturbances may be associated with PS. Initial conflicting studies regarding blood pressure changes in primary snoring exist. Kwok et al. demonstrated significantly increased systolic, diastolic and mean blood pressure in 30 children with PS as compared to age-, sex- and body-size-matched healthy controls.[23] The TuCASA Study, a community-based sample of 239 white and Hispanic preadolescent children, demonstrated an association between sleep-disordered breathing, as diagnosed by unattended home polysomnography, and elevated blood pressure.[24] Kaditis et al.[25] and Amin et al.[26] demonstrated no association between sleep-disordered breathing and blood pressure. However, each of these studies had design limitations.

TABLE 26.1   Epidemiology of Snoring in Children

FIRST AUTHOR (YEAR)	NUMBER (AGE RANGE)	COUNTRY	METHODS*	HABITUAL SNORING[‡] PREVALENCE	OSAS PREVALENCE
Corbo (1989)[31]	1615 (6–13 yr)	Italy	Self-administered questionnaire	7.3%	Not examined
Teculescu (1992)[39]	190 (5–6.4 yr)	France	Interview Questionnaire	10%	Not examined
Ali (1993)[40]	782 (4–5 yr)	England	Postal questionnaire; home overnight video and oximetry in a subset of 'high risk' and control	12.1%	0.7%
Ali (1994)[41]	504 (7–10 yr)	England	Follow up study of children in preceding study; repeat postal questionnaire only	11.4%	Not examined
Gislason (1995)[42]	454 (6mo–6 yr)	Iceland	Postal questionnaire; overnight respiratory monitoring in children suspected of having sleep apnea	3.2%	2.9%
Hultcrantz (1995)[43]	500 (4 yr)	Sweden	Interview; PSG in children with habitual snoring	6.2%	Data incomplete
Smedje (1999)[44]	1844 (5–7 yr)	Sweden	Self-administered questionnaire	7.7%	Not examined
Ferreira (2000)[45]	976 (6–11 yr)	Portugal	Self-administered questionnaire	8.6%	Not examined
Corbo (2001)[46]	2209 (10–15 yr)	Italy	Self-administered questionnaire	5.6%	Not examined
Anuntaseree (2001)[47]	1008 (6–13 yr)	Thailand	Self-administered questionnaire; PSG in patients snoring 'most nights'	8.5%	0.7%
Zhang (2004)[38]	996 (4–12 yr)	Australia	Self-administered questionnaire	15.2%	Not examined
Tafur (2009)[48]	1193 (6–12 yr)	Ecuador	Self-administered questionnaire	15.1%	Not examined
Li (2010)[49]	6349 (5–14 yr)	China	Self-administered questionnaire	7.2%	Not examined
Goldstein (2011)[7]	346 (2–6 yr)	United States	Self-administered questionnaire	13.9%	Not examined

*All questionnaire and interview data were obtained from parents.
[‡]Habitual snoring is defined as frequent or nightly snoring, or snoring at least 3 nights per week, in the absence of upper respiratory infection.
OSAS, obstructive sleep apnea syndrome; PSG, polysomnography.

Li and colleagues[27] evaluated 190 children aged 6 to 13 years via overnight attended polysomnography and ambulatory blood pressure monitoring. Systolic blood pressure, diastolic blood pressure and mean arterial pressure were significantly increased in snoring subjects with PS as compared to healthy controls. As the severity of SDB increased, blood pressure abnormalities worsened. Particularly notable was the increase in nocturnal diastolic blood pressure in children with PS, which the authors attributed to an increase in sympathetic tone, similar to what is seen in OSAS. The authors conclude by stating that PS should no longer be considered entirely benign. Furthermore, there are now data to suggest that growth hormone secretion is impaired in children with PS,[28] illustrating a point made by Guilleminault and Lee: 'chronic regular snoring always has had a health impact when we have investigated a child appropriately.'[29]

Diagnosis

History and Physical Examination

A sleep history that includes questions regarding nocturnal snoring should be included in health maintenance and well-child care visits.[30] The hallmark of PS is nightly or near-nightly snoring without physiologic or neurologic consequences. Verifying the latter, however, may be difficult without objective neuropsychological testing. Once a history of habitual snoring is elicited, additional history taking and physical examination serve to assess sleep-related or daytime symptoms that may be associated with significant upper airway

obstruction during sleep. The sleep history should include questions about labored breathing during sleep, observed apnea, restless sleep, diaphoresis, enuresis, cyanosis, and behavior or learning problems. A history of recurrent otitis media or typanostomy tube placement may suggest habitual snoring.[31] A history of allergic rhinitis, wheezing, tonsillitis within the last 12 months, maternal education, atopy and a parent with habitual snoring are risk factors for habitual snoring and should be identified.[19,32,33] An environmental history should be solicited for environmental tobacco smoke exposure and other particulate matter as air pollutants are associated with snoring.[31,33] Children who have numerous episodes of observed obstructive apnea, daytime somnolence, and problems with behavior, attention, or school performance require prompt referral for diagnostic testing and treatment for OSAS or UARS.

The physical examination may be normal, or it may reveal signs of upper airway obstruction such as mouth breathing and tonsilar hypertrophy. Dolichocephaly and midface hypoplasia are associated with snoring and OSAS. Obesity is a predisposing factor to both snoring and OSAS, whereas growth failure may signify severe sleep-disordered breathing.

Nocturnal Polysomnography

Primary snoring is defined by polysomnographic criteria. To differentiate PS from OSAS or UARS, it is important to carefully evaluate sleep staging and the frequency of electroencephalographic arousals. It is also essential to use pediatric scoring criteria as pediatric normative values are different from those of adults. Normal polysomnographic findings, including the absence of increased arousal frequency or abnormal tachypnea during sleep, suggest PS. Although the gold standard for diagnosis of UARS is measurement of esophageal pressure, this technique is invasive. Other techniques have been evaluated but are not in widespread clinical use. There is evidence, however, suggesting the flattening of nasal pressure signal may be a useful tool in identifying upper airway resistance.[34] The diagnosis of UARS is suggested by the presence of frequent arousals during the night. A diagnosis of UARS should not be dependent only on the presence of visual EEG changes. Sophisticated assessments demonstrate sympathetic surges, EEG spectral power or CAP score may change in the absence of typical EEG changes suggestive of an arousal.[35–37] Careful interpretation of the polysomnogram is necessary to appreciate these changes and distinguish between primary snoring and UARS. An otherwise asymptomatic snorer who has a normal polysomnogram is diagnosed with PS. Normal cardiorespiratory function with frequent arousals is consistent with UARS. We propose that a child with normal polysomnographic findings and abnormal daytime symptoms be given a working diagnosis of UARS, and treatment should be considered.

Treatment

By definition, primary snoring requires no specific treatment. Because of the rare progression from primary snoring to OSAS, children should be monitored clinically and reevaluated if symptoms increase over time. Because pediatric sleep-disordered breathing is a spectrum, individual treatment decisions must be based on individual symptoms and physical findings, not on polysomnographic findings alone.

FUTURE DIRECTIONS

Further studies of snoring in children are needed. The wide variability in published prevalence may be secondary to the influence of ethnicity and environment in different populations; further definition of prevalence differences would be useful in identifying patients at risk and in public health policy decisions. Better definition of the clinical consequences of snoring, and specific comparisons between patients with PS and those with UARS, are needed. Given the current, but limited, evidence of the long-term sequelae of snoring in children, more prospective studies are necessary to better identify and treat at-risk children.

Clinical Pearls

- Snoring is the most common presenting symptom of sleep-disordered breathing in children.
- A spectrum of snoring exists, ranging from primary snoring to upper airway resistance syndrome to obstructive sleep apnea syndrome.
- History alone cannot distinguish primary snoring from obstructive sleep apnea syndrome.
- Careful evaluation and treatment of snoring in children is necessary to avoid long-term sequelae.

References

1. Schechter MS; Pediatric Pulmonology Subcommittee on Obstructive Sleep Apnea Syndrome. Technical report: diagnosis and management of childhood obstructive sleep apnea syndrome. Pediatrics 2002;109:e69.
2. Carroll JL, McColley SA, Marcus CL, et al. Inability of clinical history to distinguish primary snoring from obstructive sleep apnea syndrome in children. Chest 1995;108:610–18.
3. Suen JS, Arnold JE, Brooks LJ. Adenotonsillectomy for treatment of obstructive sleep apnea in children. Arch Otolaryngol Head Neck Surg 1995;121:525–30.
4. Nieminen P, Tolonen U, Lopponen H, et al. Snoring children: factors predicting sleep apnea. Acta Otolaryngol Suppl 1997 529:190–4.
5. Leach J, Olson J, Hermann J et al. Polysomnographic and clinical findings in children with obstructive sleep apnea. Arch Otolaryngol Head Neck Surg 1992;118(7):741–4.
6. Wang RC, Elkins TP, Keech D, et al. Accuracy of clinical evaluation in pediatric obstructive sleep apnea. Otolaryngol Head Neck Surg 1998;118:69–73.
7. Goldstein NA, Abramowitz T, Weedon J, et al. Racial/ethnic differences in the prevalence of snoring and sleep disordered breathing in young children. J Clin Sleep Med 2011;7(2):163–71.
8. Spruyt K, Gozal D. Screening of pediatric sleep-disordered breathing: a proposed unbiased discriminative set of questions using clinical severity scales. Chest 2012;142(6):1508–15.
9. Lumeng JC, Chervin RD. Epidemiology of pediatric obstructive sleep apnea. Proc Am Thorac Soc 2008;5:242–52.
10. Gold AR, Marcus CL, et al. Upper airway collapsibility during sleep in upper airway resistance syndrome. Chest 2002;121:1531–40.
11. Guilleminault C, Winkle R, Korobkin K, et al. Children and nocturnal snoring: Evaluation of the effects of sleep related respiratory resistive load and daytime functioning. Eur J Pediar 1982;139:165–71.
12. Exar EN, Collop NA. The upper airway resistance syndrome. Chest 1999;115:1127–39.
13. Chervin R, DIllon J, Bassetti C, et al. Symptoms of sleep disorders, inattention, and hyperactivity in children. Sleep 1997 20:1185–92.
14. Gozal, D. Sleep-disordered breathing and school performance in children. Pediatrics 1998;102:616–20.
15. Gozal D, Pope DW Jr. Snoring during early childhood and academic performance at ages 13–14 years. Pediatrics 2001;107 1394–9.
16. Blunden S, Lushington K, Kennedy D, et al. Behavior and neurocognitive performance in children aged 5–10 years who snore compared to controls. J Clin Exp Neuropsychol 2000;22(5):554–68.
17. O'Brien LM, Mervis CB, Holbrook CR, et al. Neurobehavioral implications of habitual snoring in children. Pediatrics 2004;114:44–9.
18. Ng DK, Chow PY, Kwok KL, et al. An update on childhood snoring. Acta Paediatr 2006;95(9):1029–35.
19. Urschitz MS, Guenther A, Eitner S, et al. Risk factors and natural history of habitual snoring. Chest 2004;126:790–800.
20. Rosen CL. Clinical features of obstructive sleep apnea in otherwise healthy children. Pediatr Pulmonol 1999;27:403–9.
21. Marcus CL, Hamer A, Loughlin GM. Natural history of primary snoring in children. Pediatr Pulmonol 1998;26:6–11.
22. Topol HI, Brooks LJ. Follow-up of primary snoring in children. J Pediatr 2001;138:291–3.
23. Kwok KL, Ng DK, Cheung YF. BP and arterial distensibility in children with primary snoring. Chest 2003;123:1561–6.
24. Enright PL, Goodwin JL, Sherrill DL, et al. Blood pressure elevation associated with sleep-related breathing disorder in a community sample of white and Hispanic children: the Tucson Children's Assessment of Sleep Apnea Study. Arch Pediatr Adolesc Med 2003;157:901–4.
25. Kaditis AG, Alexopoulos EI, Kostadima E, et al. Comparison of blood pressure measurements in children with and without habitual snoring. Pediatr Pulmonol 2005;39:408–14.
26. Amin RS, Carroll JL, Jeffries JL, et al. Twenty-four-hour ambulatory blood pressure in children with sleep-disordered breathing. Am J Respir Crit Care Med 2004;169:950–6.
27. Li AM, Au CT, Ho C, et al. Blood pressure is elevated in children with primary snoring. J Pediatr 2009;155:362–8.
28. Nieminen P, Löppönen T, Tolonen U, et al. Growth and biochemical markers of growth in children with snoring and obstructive sleep apnea. Pediatrics 2002;109:e55.
29. Guilleminault C, Lee JH. Does benign 'primary snoring' ever exist in children? Chest 2004;126:1396–8.
30. Subcommittee on Obstructive Sleep Apnea Syndrome. American Academy of Pediatrics. Clinical practice guideline: diagnosis and

management of childhood obstructive sleep apnea syndrome. section on pediatric pulmonology. Pediatrics 2002;109:4 704–12.

31. Gozal D, Kheirandish-Gozal L, Capdevila OS, et al. Prevalence of recurrent otitis media in habitually snoring school-aged children. Sleep Med 2008;9:549–54.

32. Corbo GM, Fuciarelli F, Foresi A, et al. Snoring in children: association with respiratory symptoms and passive smoking. BMJ 1989;299:1491–4.

33. Kalra M, LeMasters G, Bernstein D, et al. Atopy as a risk factor for habitual snoring at age 1 year. Chest 2006;129:942–6.

34. Johnson P, Edwards N, Burgess K, et al. Detection of increased upper airway resistance during overnight polysomnography. Sleep 2005;28(1):85–90.

35. Bandla HP, Gozal D. Dynamic changes in EEG spectra during obstructive apnea in children. Pediatr Pulmonol 2000;29(5):359–65.

36. Chervin RD, Shelgikar AV, Burns JW. Respiratory cycle-related EEG changes: response to CPAP. Sleep 2012;35(2):203–9.

37. Tauman R, O'Brien LM, Mast BT, et al. Peripheral arterial tonometry events and electroencephalographic arousals in children. Sleep 2004; 27(3):502–6.

38. Zhang G, Spickett J, Rumchev K, et al. Snoring in primary school children and domestic environment: a Perth school based study. Respir Res 2004;5:19.

39. Tecculescu D, Caillier I, Perrin P, et al. Snoring in French preschool children. Pediatr Pulmonol 1992;13:239–44.

40. Ali NJ, Pitson DJ, Stradling JR. Snoring, sleep disturbance, and behavior in 4–5-year-olds. Arch Dis Child 1993;68:360–6.

41. Ali NJ, Pitson D, Stradling JR. Natural history of snoring and related behaviour problems between the ages of 4 and 7 years. Arch Dis Child 1994;71:74–6.

42. Gislason T, Benediktsdottir B. Snoring apneic episodes and nocturnal hypoxemia among children 6 months to 6 years old. Chest 1995;107:963–6.

43. Hultcrantz E, Lofstrand-Tidestrom B, Ahlquit-Rastad J. The epidemiology of sleep related breathing disorder in children. Int J Pediatr Otorhinolaryngol 1995;32(Suppl.):S63–6.

44. Smedje H, Broman J-E, Hetta J. Parents' reports of disturbed sleep in 5–7 year old Swedish children. Acta Paediatr 1999;88:858–65.

45. Ferreira AM, Clemente V, Gozal D, et al. Snoring in Portuguese primary school children. Pediatrics 2000;106:E64.

46. Corbo GM, Forastiere F, Agabiti N, et al. Snoring in 9- to 15-year-old children: risk factors and clinical relevance. Pediatrics 2001;108:1149–54.

47. Anuntaseree W, Rookkapan K, Kuasirikul S, et al. Snoring and obstructive sleep apnea in Thai school-age children: prevalence and predisposing factors. Pediatr Pulmonol 2001;32:222–7.

48. Tafur A, Chérrez-Ojeda I, Patiño C, et al. Rhinitis symptoms and habitual snoring in Ecuadorian children. Sleep Med 2009;10:1035–9.

49. Li AM, Au CT, So HK, et al. Prevalence and risk factors of habitual snoring in primary school children. Chest 2010;138:519–27.

Obstructive Sleep Apnea Syndrome: Pathophysiology and Clinical Characteristics

Asher Tal

INTRODUCTION

Sleep-disordered breathing (SDB) represents a spectrum of breathing disorders ranging from habitual snoring to obstructive sleep apnea that disrupt nocturnal respiration and sleep architecture.

DEFINITIONS

The spectrum of obstructive sleep-disordered breathing (SDB) ranges from habitual snoring to upper airway resistance syndrome (UARS), obstructive hypoventilation to intermittent occlusion of the upper airway as seen in obstructive sleep apnea syndrome (OSAS). Habitual snoring ('always,' 'frequently,' or ≥3 nights per week) may be associated with increased respiratory effort, without apnea, sleep disruption, or gas exchange alteration. The upper airway resistance syndrome (UARS) is characterized by increasingly negative intrathoracic pressures during inspiration that lead to arousals and sleep fragmentation, in the absence of readily perceived apneas, hypopneas, or oxygen desaturations. Obstructive hypoventilation is a pattern of persistent partial upper airway obstruction associated with hypercapnia and/or hypoxemia rather than cyclic discrete obstructive apneas.

Obstructive sleep apnea syndrome (OSA) is defined by the American Thoracic Society (ATS)[1] as 'a disorder of breathing during sleep characterized by prolonged partial upper airway obstruction and/or intermittent complete obstruction (obstructive apnea) that disrupts normal ventilation during sleep and normal sleep patterns.'

Sleep apnea in children was well described as early as 1976 by Guilleminault et al.[2,3] Sleep-disordered breathing occurs in children of all ages, from neonates to adolescents, with a peak prevalence between 2 and 8 years of age. Habitual snoring occurs in 5% to 12% of children; the prevalence of SDB is estimated at 4% to 11%,[4] and the prevalence of OSA is estimated at 1% to 4%.[5-7] SDB is more common among boys and among children who are heavier.[4]

PATHOPHYSIOLOGY

Transition to the sleep state normally results in elevation of upper airway resistance, mainly due to reduction in airway diameter, resulting from the reduced tone of the pharyngeal dilator and constrictor muscles. Normal sleep is characterized by relative hypoxemia and hypercapnia, particularly during REM sleep, when compared to wakefulness. This normal phenomenon is magnified in patients with underlying pulmonary (such as nocturnal asthma) or upper airway (such as OSA) disease. This is the result of the following physiologic factors:[8]

- Functional residual capacity is reduced during sleep mainly during rapid eye movement (REM) sleep, leading to more rapid hypoxemia with apnea. This is due to decreased intercostal and upper airway muscle tone, particularly during REM sleep.
- Central ventilatory drive regulating upper airway tone and ventilatory response to hypoxia and hypercapnia decrease during normal sleep.
- Upper airway resistance increases during sleep, as a result of the decrease in upper airway tone. Small increases in upper airway resistance can have a significant impact on breathing.

Children with OSA tend to have a narrow upper airway. The patency of the upper airway is determined by both anatomic and physiologic factors. The site of obstruction in children tends to be more distal than in adults, typically involving the oropharynx and hypopharynx. Magnetic resonance imaging of upper airway structures confirmed that children with OSA have significantly larger adenoids and tonsils than those of controls.[9] Arens et al. described the region in which these two lymphoid tissues overlap to constitute the site with the smallest airway diameter as the 'overlap region.' The upper airway is rich in neural receptors, which play a part in controlling baseline muscle tone. Any loss in this tone, as occurs at sleep onset, contributes to increased pharyngeal resistance. During inspiration, many dilator upper airway muscles exhibit phasic respiratory activity. This phasic activation of the muscles of the nose, pharynx, and larynx occurs before diaphragm and intercostal muscle activity, suggesting pre-activation of the upper airway muscles in preparation for the development of negative pressure.

The Starling Resistor Theory

Under conditions of negative inter-luminal pressure, collapse of the upper airway occurs variably during inspiration. The pattern of flow on the driving pressure occurs in 'Starling resistors,' which are a specific model of 'collapsible tube' behavior (Figure 27-1).[8] The model predicts that, under conditions of flow limitation, maximal inspiratory airflow is determined by the pressure changes upstream (nasal) from the collapsible site of the upper airway and is independent of the downstream (hypopharyngeal and tracheal) pressure generated by the diaphragm. The upper airway can be represented

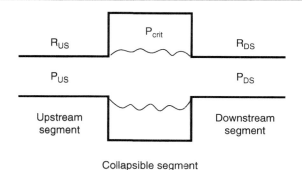

FIGURE 27-1 **Starling resistor model of the upper airway.** The upper airway is represented as a tube with a collapsible segment. The upstream (nasal) and downstream (trachea) segments have fixed diameters and resistance (R_{US}, R_{DS}) and pressures (P_{US}, P_{DS}). Collapse occurs when the pressure surrounding the airway (P_{crit}) is greater than that within the airway. *Redrawn with permission from Marcus CL. Pathophysiology of OSAS in children. In: Loughlin GM, Carrol JL, Marcus CL editors. Sleep and breathing in children, A developmental approach. Marcel Dekker Inc. NY; 2000. p. 601–24.*

as a tube with a collapsible segment, the resistance of which is zero. The segments upstream and downstream from the collapsible segment each have a fixed diameter, resistance, and pressure. The upstream pressure can be approximated by the nasal pressure and the downstream pressure can be approximated by the hypopharyngeal pressure. In this model of the upper airway, inflow pressure at the airway opening (the nares) is atmospheric, and downstream pressure is equal to tracheal pressure. Collapse occurs when the pressure surrounding the collapsible segment of the upper airway (critical tissue pressure = P_{crit}) becomes greater than the pressure within the collapsible segment of the airway. In normal subjects with low upstream resistance or sub-atmospheric critical tissue pressure, hypopharyngeal pressure never drops to critical pressure; thus, airflow is not limited and is largely determined by negative tracheal pressure. However, if hypopharyngeal pressure falls below critical pressure, maximal inspiratory flow reaches its maximum limitation, and becomes independent of downstream pressure swings. Under these circumstances, nasal resistance and critical pressure determine maximal inspiratory flow as described by the following equation:

$$VI_{max} = (P_N - P_{crit})/R_N$$

where VI_{max} is maximal inspiratory flow; P_N is nasal pressure; P_{crit} is critical tissue pressure; R_N is nasal resistance. Airflow will become zero (i.e., the airway will occlude) when nasal pressure falls below critical pressure.

Normal infants and children have a narrower upper airway than adults. Nevertheless, they snore less and have fewer obstructive apneas. This could be due to either structural differences or differences in neuromotor regulation of the upper airway. It is difficult to determine critical pressure in normal children, as their upper airway is very resistant to collapse. Marcus et al. have shown that P_{crit} in children correlated with the severity of OSA.[10]

The upper airway in children with OSA is more collapsible compared with control subjects during wakefulness and sleep, and under general anesthesia. Several mechanisms might lead

to more airway collapse in these subjects, including: decreased motor tone, increased airway compliance, and excessive inspiratory driving pressures caused by proximal airway narrowing. This increased propensity of the airway to collapse should be reflected by increased motion of airway boundary during respiration as negative upper airway intraluminal pressure is increased. Using respiratory-gated magnetic resonance imaging to quantify changes in shape and airway cross-section area during tidal breathing in children with OSA, compared with control subjects, it has been shown that fluctuations in airway area during tidal breathing are significantly greater in subjects with OSA compared with control subjects.[11]

Resistive pressure loading is a probable explanation, although increased airway compliance may be a contributing factor. Studies using denervated upper airways have shown that when upper airway muscle function is decreased or absent, the airway is more prone to collapse.[12,13] Children have active upper airway dynamic responses to both negative pressure pulses and hypercapnia during sleep.[14] Normal children compensate for their smaller upper airway by increasing the ventilatory drive to their upper airway muscles. This compensatory mechanism may be absent or diminished in children with OSA.

PHYSIOLOGICAL CONSEQUENCES OF OSA

Intermittent hypoxemia during sleep is common in children with OSA. Intermittent hypoxemia may contribute to the increase in pulmonary pressure and the development of *cor pulmonale*; however, this effect will probably be more prominent with chronic hypoxemia. The more potentially serious consequence of intermittent hypoxemia is the behavioral and cognitive adverse effect on the brain. The relationship between the degree and duration of hypoxemia and neurological and cardiopulmonary outcome is not yet known.

Sleep fragmentation is a well-established consequence of OSA in adults, but is much less determined in children. While arousal from sleep is a protective reflex mechanism that restores breathing, an increase in the number of arousals per hour of sleep (arousal index) may cause sleep fragmentation and sympathetic activation.

Alveolar hypoventilation or 'obstructive hypoventilation' is the result of long periods of increased upper airway resistance and hypercapnia, with or without hypoxemia. Intermittent elevations in PCO_2 can exacerbate the effect of intermittent hypoxemia on neural tissue, and can affect cerebral circulation and vasomotor activity.

THE ETIOLOGY OF OSA

The etiology of OSA in children is multifactorial, and is probably a combination of abnormal airway structure, decreased neuromuscular control, and other factors such as genetic, hormonal, and metabolic (Figure 27-2).

Airway structure is an important factor in pediatric OSA. Bony structure and soft tissue are two major contributing factors in determining upper airway patency.

Genetic syndromes that are associated with OSA include those producing micrognathia and those producing midfacial hypoplasia.

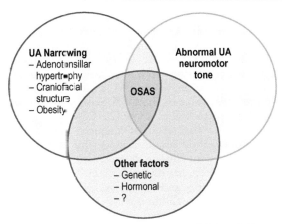

FIGURE 27-2 Obstructive sleep apnea syndrome (OSA) in children may result from a combination of factors. *With permission from Marcus CL. Pathophysiology of OSAS in children. In: Loughlin GM, Carrol JL, Marcus CL editors. Sleep and breathing in children, A developmental approach. Marcel Dekker Inc. NY; 2000. p. 601–24.*

Pierre Robin sequence, consisting of micrognathia and posterior displacement of the tongue and soft palate, is frequently associated with sleep-disordered breathing, presenting in early infancy, in the first few weeks of life.

Treacher Collins syndrome, caused by mutations in the region of 5q32-32.2 that codes for the treacle protein, is characterized by mandibular hypoplasia, malar hypoplasia, antimongoloid slanting palpebral fissures, malformation of the auricles, and coloboma of the eyelid.

Midfacial hypoplasia syndromes include *Crouzon syndrome*, *Apert syndrome*, and *Pfeiffer syndrome*.

Achondroplasia an autosomal dominant skeletal dysplasia, is associated with OSA as the most common respiratory complication. About two-thirds of patients with achondroplasia present OSA.

Children with *Down syndrome* frequently present OSA because of their craniofacial structure: maxillary hypoplasia and small nose with low nasal bridge. In addition, recurrent upper airway infections result in adenotonsillar hypertrophy.[15] Children with *Arnold–Chiari malformation* may be at risk for developing both central and obstructive sleep apnea due to brainstem compression affecting respiratory drive, and/or activation of the pharyngeal and laryngeal muscles that are enervated by the ninth and tenth cranial nerves.

Children with *Prader–Willi syndrome*, consisting of hypotonia, obesity, hypogonadism, and mental retardation, might also present OSA. In children with *mucopolysaccharidoses*, OSA is caused as a result of deposition of mucopolysaccharides in the airways, including the tongue, pharynx, trachea, and bronchi.

The high prevalence of habitual snoring in first-degree relatives of children with OSA, and documented familial aggregation of OSA, suggest a familial predisposition to this condition.[16,17] African-Americans are at greater risk than Caucasians when controlling for age, sex, and BMI, indicating *ethnicity* as another risk factor for OSA.[18]

Prematurity was also identified as a risk factor for OSA.[5,19] Former preterm infants are at increased risk to develop OSA in early infancy, possibly due to facial asymmetry, greater incidence of muscle hypotonia, or nasal obstruction following prolonged intubation.[20]

Adenotonsillar hypertrophy is the most common etiology of OSA in children, making adenotonsillectomy the first-line treatment at this age. The fact that most children significantly improve following surgery[21] proves their role in the etiology of OSA in children. However, the fact that cure is not achieved in all children[22] indicates that other factors are involved. The tonsils and adenoids increase in size from birth to about 12 years of age, and are largest in relation to the underlying upper airway size between 3 and 6 years of age.[23] The correlation between adenotonsillar size and OSA is not strong. While the severity of obstructive events was related to the size of the adenoids in one study,[24] other studies have failed to show a correlation between adenotonsillar size and OSA severity.[25]

OSA AND OBESITY

The steadily increasing incidence of childhood obesity in Western countries dictates the need to distinguish between obese and non-obese children. The presence of obesity in children significantly increases the risk of developing OSA.[26] The risk for residual OSA after adenotonsillectomy is markedly greater in obese children.[27] In addition, obesity-induced childhood OSA is different from OSA in otherwise healthy children with adenotonsillar hypertrophy. These observations resulted in a proposed differentiation between type I OSA associated with marked lymphadenoid hypertrophy without obesity, and type II OSA associated with obesity with only mild lymphadenoid hypertrophy.[28]

OSA AND ASTHMA

Obstructive sleep apnea has been identified as a risk factor for severe asthma in adults.[29] Asthma and obstructive sleep apnea (OSA) in children share multiple epidemiological risk factors and the prevalence of snoring is greater in asthmatic children. Asthma and OSA may coexist in children due to a shared relationship with atopy. Sleep-disordered breathing was recently reported as a modifiable risk factor for severe asthma in children.[30,31] The treatment of OSA appeared to be associated with substantial improvements in the severity of the underlying asthmatic condition.[32]

OSA AND INFLAMMATION

Recent research indicates that adults and children with SDB present with local (upper airway apparatus) inflammatory changes and systemic correlates.[33] The measured inflammatory changes reflect activation of specific pathways such as the lipoxygenase pathway, which is involved in other inflammatory conditions that affect children and adults, such as asthma and allergic rhinitis. Golbart et al.[34] suggested that an inflammatory process involving leukotrienes (LT) expression and regulation occurs in children with OSA.[34–36] The main evidence of systemic inflammation associated with childhood OSA was the finding of elevated C-reactive protein (CRP) plasma levels. Tauman and others reported on increases in plasma CRP levels among American children with SDB, which correlated with apnea hypopnea index, arterial oxygen saturation nadir, and arousal index measures.[37]

Several other inflammatory biomarkers were reported in children with OSA: interleukin-6,[38] interferon-gamma and IL-8 levels, TNF-alpha, and fibrinogen.[39,40] The distinction between inflammatory mechanisms leading to SDB as opposed to the systemic/local inflammation resulting from the presence of SDB is difficult. The importance of understanding the inflammatory mechanisms involved in the etiology of OSA is recognizing the potential role of anti-inflammatory drugs as an alternative, non-surgical treatment of OSA in children: intranasal corticosteroid spray, and leukotriene modifiers.[41,42]

CLINICAL CHARACTERISTICS

OSA may present with nocturnal and/or diurnal symptoms (Box 27-1).

Nocturnal Symptoms

Snoring is the most characteristic presenting symptom of OSA in children.[43,44] Worsening is usually reported with upper respiratory tract infections. In young children, compared with adults, snoring occurs in any position, and is not necessarily worse in the supine position. Habitual snoring alone is not a specific symptom of OSA. Most children with habitual snoring do not progress to having OSA, and those who do so have only mild OSA. Several recent reports have indicated a significant impact of habitual snoring on behavioral and cognitive functions, even without polysomnographic evidence of OSA.

Difficulty in breathing during sleep: Parents usually describe paradoxical respiratory movements with 'the abdomen going down when the thorax goes up.'

Witnessed apnea is described either spontaneously or after a direct question. The prevalence of parent-reported apneic events during sleep is in the range of 0.2% to 4%.[4] Many parents describe the acoustic result of the sudden disappearance of snoring ending with a snort or gasp.

Box 27-1 Symptoms of Obstructive Sleep Apnea Syndrome in Children

Nocturnal
- Snoring
- Difficulty in breathing during sleep
- Witnessed apnea
- Restless sleep
- Frequent awakenings
- Night sweating
- Nocturnal enuresis

Diurnal
- Behavior problems
  - Irritability
  - Aggressiveness
- Impaired cognitive function
  - Poor school performance
- Poor appetite
- Daytime sleepiness

These first three symptoms are the most sensitive and specific for children with OSA. In the early 1980s, Brouillette et al.[45] used these to create an 'OSA Score' that practically showed that a child who snores every night, presents difficulties in breathing during sleep, and whose parent reported witnessing apneas suffers from OSA. Unfortunately, while the positive predicted value of the OSA Score is high (50–75%), its negative predicted value is low (25–80%).

Restless sleep is the result of frequent arousals. Parents usually describe a child who disarranges his or her sheets and blankets, moves a lot during sleep, and is found in strange postures during sleep, mainly with the neck hyperextended.

Frequent awakening and *night sweating* are also common parental complaints in children with OSA.

Nocturnal enuresis is reported in 8–47% of children with OSAS.[46] A recent study reported two-thirds of children with OSA with primary enuresis, and one-third with secondary enuresis. The findings of a high prevalence of nocturnal enuresis in children with mild OSA indicate an increased risk of enuresis in children with sleep-disordered breathing, even without OSA. Retrospective data indicated a remarkable decrease in enuresis soon after adenotonsillectomy.[47–49]

Daytime Symptoms

In many children with OSA, the presenting symptoms may be the result of disrupted sleep, namely *abnormal daytime functioning*. While daytime sleepiness is a common symptom of OSA in adults, only the minority of pediatric OSA patients (<15%) present it. In fact, sleepiness and fatigue may present in young children as irritability, nervousness, and aggressiveness, as well as attention deficit hyperactivity disorder and poor school performance. This aspect of the impact of OSA in children is discussed in detail in Chapter 32.

Children with hypertrophied adenoids and tonsils may present with mouth breathing, recurrent upper respiratory infections, and hearing and speech problems. Morning headaches, a common complaint in adult patients with OSA, are much less common in children.

CLINICAL CONSEQUENCES OF OSA

The clinical consequences of OSA are probably the result of a combination of intermittent hypoxia, sleep fragmentation, and inflammation that are associated with the sleep-disordered breathing. There is increasing evidence to support the association between OSA, SDB, and habitual snoring and *attention deficit hyperactivity disorder* (ADHA) in children.[50] Neurocognitive consequences associated with OSA are described in detail in Chapter 32.

Pulmonary hypertension is the most common cardiovascular complication in children with OSA. Initial case reports in the early 1960s indicated that in untreated cases of chronic nasopharyngeal obstruction, cardiomegaly, *cor pulmonale*, and pulmonary edema may develop.[51] Right ventricular dysfunction in children with OSA is reversible soon after adenotonsillectomy.[52] Cardiovascular consequences of OSA are described in Chapter 33.

Failure to thrive and *growth retardation* have been known as complications of OSA since the very first publications on this syndrome.[3] Three main factors contribute to the growth retardation: (1) low caloric intake: children with hypertrophied tonsils often present with poor appetite and dysphagia, resulting in poor caloric intake; (2) high energy expenditure due to increased work of breathing during sleep;[10,53] (3) growth hormone (GH) secretion is impaired in children with OSA. Insulin growth factor-I (IGF-I) was found to be low in children with OSA. Respiratory improvement after adenotonsillectomy results in weight gain and restores IGF-I and GH secretion.[54,55]

Children with OSA are heavy users of healthcare services, indicating higher morbidity.[56] Children with OSA who were diagnosed at the age of 4 years have *greater respiratory morbidity and healthcare costs*, starting from the first year of life.[57] After adenotonsillectomy, healthcare cost significantly decreases as a result of reduced morbidity.[58] The reasons for higher costs before treatment are the result of an increase in the rates of hospitalization, emergency room referrals, and use of medications. Respiratory tract infections (upper and lower respiratory infection) are the most common causes of morbidity in children with OSA. We have recently reported that OSA represents a predisposing risk for community-acquired alveolar pneumonia in children <5 years old.[59]

SUMMARY

Obstructive Sleep Apnea Syndrome (OSA) is a common disorder in children. Children with OSA tend to have a narrow upper airway caused by both anatomic and physiologic factors. The consequences are increased work of breathing, intermittent hypoxemia, sleep fragmentation and alveolar hypoventilation. In addition, OSA may be associated with local and systemic inflammation, obesity and asthma. Risk factors for OSA include adenotonsillar hypertrophy, craniofacial anomalies, familial predisposition, ethnicity and prematurity. OSA is associated with substantial morbidities, such as behavioral and cognitive impairment, growth retardation, and cardiovascular involvement. The significant improvement following treatment emphasizes the need for early diagnosis and treatment. Understanding the pathophysiology, risk factors, daytime and nocturnal symptoms and clinical implications of OSA in children is essential in order to early diagnose and treat this common disorder.

Clinical Pearls

- Obstructive sleep apnea in children is caused by a combination of abnormal airway structure, decreased neuromuscular control, and other factors such as genetic, hormonal, and metabolic.
- Physiological consequences of OSA include increased work of breathing, intermittent hypoxemia, sleep fragmentation, and alveolar hypoventilation.
- Clinical characteristics include nocturnal symptoms (most specific are snoring, labored breathing during sleep, and witnessed apnea) and daytime symptoms (hyperactivity, attention deficit, and learning problems).
- Children who snore on a regular basis and present any of the characteristic symptoms need further investigation to rule out OSA, especially if one of the clinical consequences is reported (behavior and/or cognitive impairment, failure to thrive, obesity, hypertension).

References

1. American Thoracic Society. Standards and indications for cardiopulmonary sleep studies in children. Am J Respir Crit Care Med 1996;153:866–78.
2. Guilleminault C, Eldridge F, Simmons FB, et al. Sleep apnea in eight children. Pediatrics 1976;58:28–31.
3. Guilleminault C, Korobkin E, Winkle R. A review of 50 children with obstructive sleep apnea syndrome. Lung 1981;159:275–87.
4. Lumeng JC, Chervin RD. Epidemiology of pediatric obstructive sleep apnea. Proc Am Thorac Soc 2008;5:242–52.
5. Rosen CL, Larkin EK, Kirchner HL, et al. Prevalence and risk factors for sleep-disordered breathing in 8- to 11-year-old children: association with race and prematurity. J Pediatr 2003;142:383–9.
6. Corbo GM, Forastier F, Agabiti N, et al. Snoring in 9- to 15-year-old children: risk factors and clinical relevance. Pediatrics 2001;108:1149–54.
7. Tang JP, Rosen CL, Larkinn EK, et al. Identification of sleep-disordered breathing in children: variation with event definition. Sleep 2002;25:72–9.
8. Marcus CL. Pathophysiology of OSAS in children. In: Loughlin GM, Carrol JL, Marcus CL, editors. Sleep and breathing in children, A developmental approach. New York: Marcel Dekker; 2000. p. 601–24.
9. Arens R, McDonough JM, Costarino AT, et al. Magnetic resonance imaging of the upper airway structure of children with obstructive sleep apnea syndrome. Am J Respir Crit Care Med 2001;164:698–703.
10. Marcus CL, Carrol JL, Koerner CB, et al. Determinants of growth in children with obstructive sleep apnea syndrome. J Pediatr 1994;125:556–62.
11. Arens R, Sin S, McDonough JM. Changes in upper airway size during tidal breathing in children with obstructive sleep apnea syndrome. Am J Respir Crit Care Med 2005;171:1298–304.
12. Smith PL, Schwartz AR, Gauda E, et al. The modulation of upper airway critical pressure during sleep. Prog Clin Biol Res 1990;345:253–8.
13. Brouillette RT, Tach BT. A neuromuscular mechanism maintaining extrathoracic airway patency. J Appl Physiol 1979;46:772–9.
14. Marcus, CL, Fernandes Do Prado LB, Lutz J, et al. Dynamic responses to both negative pressure pulses and hypercapnia during sleep. J Appl Physiol 2004;97:98–108.
15. Marcus CL, Keens TG, Bautsta DB, et al. Obstructive sleep apnea in children with Down syndrome. Pediatrics 1991;88:132–9.
16. Pillar G, Lavie P. Assessment of the role of inheritance in sleep apnea syndrome. Am J Respir Crit Car Med 1995;151:688–91.
17. Redline S, Tishler PV, Schluchter M, et al. Risk factors for sleep-disordered breathing in children: association with obesity, race, and respiratory problems. Am J Respir Crit Care Med 1999;159:1527–32.
18. Palmer LJ, Buxbaum SG, Larkin EK, et al. Whole genome scan for obstructive sleep apnea and obesity in African-American families. Am J Respir Crit Care Med 2004;169:1314–21.
19. Greenfeld M, Tauman R, DeRow A, et al. Obstructive sleep apnea syndrome due to adenotonsillar hypertrophy in infants. Int J Pediatr Otorhinolaryngol 2003;67:1055–60.
20. Sharma PB, Baroody F, Gozal D, et al. Obstructive sleep apnea in the formerly preterm infant: an overlooked diagnosis. Front in Neurol 2011;2:75.
21. Tal A, Bar A, Leiberman A, et al. Sleep characteristics following adenotonsillectomy in children with obstructive sleep apnea syndrome. Chest 2003;124:948–53.
22. Tauman R, Gulliver TE, Krishna J, et al. Persistence of obstructive sleep apnea syndrome in children after adenotonsillectomy. J Pediatr 2006;149:803–8.
23. Jeans WD, Fernando DCJ, Maw AR, et al. A longitudinal study of the growth of the nasophaynx and its content in normal children. Br J Radiol 1981;54:117–21.
24. Brooks LJ, Stephens B, Bacevic AM. Adenoid size is related to severity but not the number of obstructive apnea in children. J Pediatr 1998;132:682–6.
25. Lam YY, Chan EY, Ng DK, et al. The correlation among obesity, apnea–hypopnea index, and tonsil size in children. Chest 2006;130:1751–6.
26. Verhulst SL, Schrauwen N, Haentiens D, et al. Sleep-disordered breathing in overweight and obese children and adolescents: prevalence, characteristics and the role of fat distribution. Arch Dis Child 2007;92:205–8.
27. Bhattacharjee R, Kheirandish-Gozal L, Spruyt K, et al. Adenotonsillectomy outcomes in treatment of obstructive sleep apnea in children: a multicenter retrospective study. Am J Respir Crit Care Med 2010;182:676–83.

28. Dayyat E, Kheirandish-Gozal L, Gozal D. Childhood obstructive sleep apnea: one or two distinct disease entity? Sleep Med Clin 2007;2: 433–44.

29. ten Brinke A, Sterk PJ, Masclee AA, et al. Risk factors of frequent exacerbations in difficult-to-treat asthma. Eur Respir J 2005;26:812–18.

30. Ramagopal M, Scharf SM, Roberts DW, et al. Obstructive sleep apnea and history of asthma in snoring children. Sleep Breath 2008;12(4): 381–92.

31. Ross KR, Storfer-Isser A, Hart MA, et al. Sleep-disordered breathing is associated with asthma severity in children. J Pediatr 2011. [Epub ahead of print].

32. Kheirandish-Gozal L, Dayyat EA, Eid NS, et al. Obstructive sleep apnea in poorly controlled asthmatic children: effect of adenotonsillectomy. Pediatr Pulmonol 2011;46:913–18.

33. Goldbart AD, Tal A. Inflammation and sleep-disordered breathing in children: A state of the art review. Pediatr Pulmonol 2008;43:1151–60.

34. Goldbart AD, Goldman JL, Li RC, et al. Differential expression of cysteinil leukotriene receptors 1 and 2 in tonsils of children with obstructive sleep apnea syndrome or recurrent infection. Chest 2004;126: 13–18.

35. Goldbart AD, Goldman JL, Veling MC, et al. Leukotriene modifier therapy for mild sleep-disordered breathing in children. Am J Respir Crit Care Med 2005;172:364–70.

36. Goldbart AD, Krishna J, Li RC, et al. Inflammatory mediators in exhaled breath condensate of children with obstructive sleep apnea syndrome. Chest 2006;130:143–8.

37. Tauman R, Ivanenko A, O'Brien LM, et al. Plasma C-reactive protein levels among children with sleep-disordered breathing. Pediatrics 2004;113:e564–9.

38. Gozal D, Kheirandish-Gozal L, Sans Capdevila O, et al. TNF-alpha plasma levels are increased excessively in sleepy school-aged children with obstructive sleep apnea. Sleep 2008;31:186.

39. Tam CS, Wong M, McBain R, et al. Inflammatory measures in children with obstructive sleep apnoea. J Pediatr Child Health 2006;42:277–82.

40. Kaditis AG, Alexopoulos EI, Kalampouka E, et al. Morning levels of fibrinogen in children with sleep-disordered breathing. Eur Respir J 2004;24:790–7.

41. Brouillette RT, Manoukian JJ, Ducharme FM, et al. Efficacy of fluticasone nasal spray for pediatric obstructive sleep apnea. J Pediatr 2001; 138:838–44.

42. Goldbart AD, Greenberg-Dotan S, Tal A. Montelukast for children with obstructive sleep apnea. a double-blind placebo-controlled study. Pediatrics 2012;130(3):e575–80.

43. Ali NJ, Piterson DJ, Stradling JR. Snoring, sleep disturbance, and behaviour in 4–5 year olds. Arch Dis Child 1993;68:360–6.

44. Gisalson T, Benediktsdottir B. Snoring, apneic episodes, and nocturnal hypoxemia among children 6 months to 6 years old. Chest 1995;107: 963–6.

45. Broullette R, Hanson D, David R, et al. A diagnostic approach to suspected obstructive sleep apnea in children. J Pediatr 1984;105:10–14.

46. Brooks LJ, Topol HI. Enuresis in children with sleep apnea. J Pediatr 2003;142:515–18.

47. Weider DJ, Sateia MJ, West RP. Nocturnal enuresis in children with upper airway obstruction. Otolaryngol Head Neck Surg 1991;105: 427–32.

48. Weissbach A, Leiberman A, Tarasiuk A, et al. Adenotonsillectomy improves enuresis in children with OSAS. Int J Pediatr Otolaryngol 2006;80:1351–6.

49. Jeyakumar A, Rahman SI, Armbrecht ES, et al. The association between sleep-disordered breathing and enuresis in children. Laryngoscope 2012. doi: 10.1002/lary.23323. [Epub ahead of print].

50. Chervin RD, Ruzicka DL, Giordani BJ, et al. Sleep-disordered breathing, behavior, and cognition in children before and after adenotonsillectomy. Pediatrics 2006;117:e769–78.

51. Sofer S, Weinhouse E, Tal A, et al. Cor pulmonale due to adenoid or tonsillar hypertrophy or both in children. Chest 1988;93:119–22.

52. Tal A, Leiberman A, Margulis G, et al. Ventricular dysfunction in children with obstructive sleep apnea: Radionuclide assessment. Pediatr Pulmonol 1988;4:139–43.

53. Bonuck K, Parikh S, Bassila M. Growth failure and sleep disordered breathing: a review of the literature. Int J Pediatr Otorhinolaryngol 2006;70(5):769–78.

54. Bar A, Tarasiuk A, Segev M, et al. The effect of adenotonsillectomy on serum insulin-like growth factor-1 and growth in children with obstructive sleep apnea syndrome. J Pediatr 1999;135:76–80.

55. Nieminen P, Lopponen T, Tolonen U, et al. Growth and biochemical markers of growth in children with snoring and obstructive sleep apnea. Pediatrics 2002;109:e55.

56. Tarasiuk A, Greenberg-Dotan S, Simon-Tuval C, et al. Elevated Morbidity and Health Care Utilization in Children with Obstructive Sleep Apnea Syndrome. Am J Respir Crit Care Med 2007;175:55–61.

57. Tarasiuk A, Greenberg-Dotan S, Simon-Tuval T, et al. Elevated morbidity and health care utilization in children with obstructive sleep apnea syndrome. Am J Respir Crit Care Med 2007;175:55–61.

58. Tarasiuk A, Simon T, Tal A, et al. Adenotonsillectomy in children with obstructive sleep apnea syndrome reduces health care utilization. Pediatrics 2004;113:351–6.

59. Goldbart AD, Tal A, Givon-Lavi N, et al. Sleep-disordered breathing is a risk factor for community-acquired alveolar pneumonia in early childhood. Chest 2012;141(5):1210–15.

Chapter 28

Diagnosis of Obstructive Sleep Apnea

Eliot S. Katz and Carole L. Marcus

INTRODUCTION

Sleep-disordered breathing (SDB) is a common and serious cause of morbidity during childhood. This chapter is concerned with diagnosing the spectrum of obstructive SDB, ranging from the frank, intermittent occlusion seen in *obstructive sleep apnea syndrome* (OSAS), to persistent, *primary snoring* (PS). OSAS is characterized by recurrent episodes of partial or complete airway obstruction resulting in hypoxemia, hypercapnia, and/or respiratory arousal (Figure 28-1). The sleep fragmentation and gas exchange abnormalities observed with OSAS may produce serious cardiovascular and neurobehavioral impairment. The *upper airway resistance syndrome* (UARS) is characterized by brief, repetitive respiratory effort-related arousals (RERA) during sleep in the absence of overt apnea, hypopnea or gas exchange abnormalities.[1] It has been linked to significant cognitive and behavioral sequelae in children including learning disabilities, attention deficit, hyperactivity, and aggressive behavior.[2] *Obstructive hypoventilation* (OH) features prolonged increased upper airway resistance accompanied by gas exchange abnormalities, but not frank apnea or hypopnea.[3] Children with PS may have increased respiratory effort, but lack identifiable arousals, including respiratory-effort-related, EEG and subcortical arousals.[4] Though PS has been traditionally defined as a benign condition, without polysomnographic abnormalities,[5] recent evidence suggests that the increased respiratory effort in PS *per se* may be associated with untoward neurobehavioral consequences.[6–9]

Habitual snoring has been reported in 3–12% of the general pediatric population, although only 1–3% will have OSAS.[10–12] Early recognition of SDB is important insofar as treatment with adenotonsillectomy or continuous positive airway pressure is effective. Establishing strict criteria for OSAS diagnosis and severity is the basis for optimizing the surgical and medical management of this condition.[13] The diagnosis and management of pediatric OSAS continues to evolve as more precise measures of flow limitation and sleep fragmentation are introduced. Both the intermittent hypoxemia and sleep fragmentation characteristic of OSAS pose a risk to the vulnerable developing brain. The increased recognition of subtle neurocognitive impairments in children with SDB has forced clinicians to rethink the threshold level of disease requiring intervention.

The optimal methodology and criteria for the diagnosis of OSAS in children has not been validated with outcomes data. Categorizing OSAS severity with threshold levels of the apnea–hypopnea index, gas exchange abnormalities, or sleep fragmentation have proven unsatisfactory, since they fail to account for the individual trait susceptibility to the neurocognitive, cardiovascular, and metabolic sequelae of OSAS. That is, the threshold amount of OSAS associated with adverse consequences varies widely among children.

HISTORY AND PHYSICAL EXAMINATION

The high incidence of OSAS in children mandates that screening inquiries about sleep disturbances should be a routine part of the primary care interview[14] (Table 28.1). Particular attention should be given to conditions known to exacerbate SDB such as craniofacial abnormalities, neuromuscular weakness, and genetic conditions. A parent typically provides the clinical history, with the patient oblivious to their condition, other than sometimes the complaint of excessive daytime sleepiness. Nightly snoring is observed in most children with OSAS. However, snoring may be absent in the setting of craniofacial abnormalities in infants.[15] A parental report of a snoring child is an accurate predictor of polysomnographic snoring, but not of OSAS.[16] In addition, a population-based study using home-based polysomnography found that loud snoring one to two times per week during the last month was absent in at least 25% of children with documented OSAS.[17] Snoring is often accompanied by labored breathing, hyperextension of the neck, and witnessed apneic pauses. Subjective reports of excessive daytime sleepiness are less common in young children with OSAS, although they are often present in adolescents. A recent study reported that only 7.5% of children with polysomnographically proven OSAS had a history of EDS.[18] Using an objective measure of sleepiness, such as the multiple sleep latency test, reveals that only 13% of children with OSAS have a sleep latency <10 minutes.[18] However, the incidence of objective sleepiness is higher in obese children with OSAS.[19,20] Also, although not considered sleepy by adult standards, children with SDB may be relatively sleepier than normal children.[21] Increasing BMI and apnea index (usually greater than 15–20 events/hour) have been independently correlated with shorter sleep latencies.[18]

The use of standardized screening questionnaires for OSAS has been disappointing. Brouillette et al. presented a questionnaire aimed at distinguishing children with OSAS from normal controls.[22] However, subsequent application of this and other questionnaires to a population of snoring children demonstrated a wide-ranging positive predictive value, 48.3–76.9%, and negative predictive value, 26.9–93%.[22–25] Although children with OSAS are statistically more likely to have reported symptoms such as witnessed apnea, cyanosis, and/or labored breathing, no questionnaire has a sufficiently high positive predictive value and negative predictive value to be used as a primary diagnostic tool.[25,26] Thus, the clinical history alone is insufficient to diagnose OSAS amongst a population

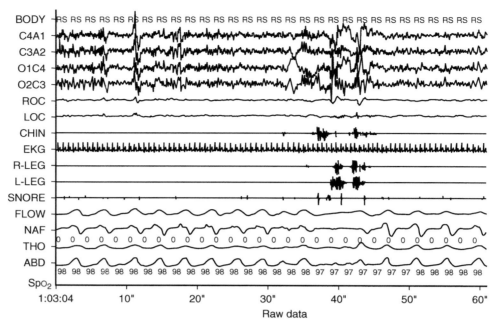

FIGURE 28-1 A 60-second epoch from a 16-year-old with snoring and excessive daytime sleepiness. Note flow limitation and reduction in the amplitude of the nasal pressure tracing leading to an EEG arousal. Inspiration is upward. Flow, thermistor; NAF, nasal pressure; Tho, thorax; Abd, abdomen; Body, body position; RS, right side; SpO2, pulse oximetry.

TABLE 28.1	Clinical History in OSAS
SLEEP	**WAKEFULNESS**
Snoring	Poor school performance
Witnessed apnea	Aggressive behavior
Choking noises	Hyperactivity
Increased work of breathing	Attention deficit disorder
Paradoxical breathing	Excessive daytime sleepiness
Enuresis	Morning headaches
Mouth breathing	Age-inappropriate napping
Restless sleep	Difficult to arouse from sleep
Diaphoresis	Depression
Hyperextended neck	
Frequent awakenings	
Dry mouth	

BOX 28-1   Physical Examination in OSAS

General
- Sleepiness
- Obesity
- Failure to thrive

Head
- Swollen mucous membranes
- Deviated septum
- Adenoidal facies
  - Infraorbital darkening
  - Elongated midface
  - Mouth-breathing
- Tonsillar hypertrophy
- High arched palate
- Overjet

- Posterior buccal cross-bite
- Crowded oropharynx
- Macroglossia
- Glossoptosis
- Midfacial hypoplasia
- Micrognathia/retrognathia
- Increased neck circumference

Cardiovascular
- Hypertension
- Loud P2

Extremities
- Edema
- Clubbing (rare)

of snoring children. Questionnaires have also been developed that incorporate questions relating to the consequences of OSA, including hyperactivity and behavior. An affirmative response to at least one-third of these questions on the 22-question Pediatric Sleep Questionnaire had a sensitivity of 0.85 and a specificity of 0.87.[27,28]

Physical examination of children with OSAS is most often normal, with the exception of adenotonsillar hypertrophy or craniofacial abnormalities (Box 28-1). The majority of children with OSAS are of normal height and weight, although both obesity and failure to thrive may occur. Cardiovascular sequelae of SDB such as cor pulmonale and congestive heart failure are infrequently observed in current clinical practice, as heightened awareness has facilitated earlier diagnosis.

Although blood pressure is statistically elevated in children with OSAS, the wide range of normal makes this measurement a poor screening tool.[29] The neurocognitive consequences of OSAS are non-specific, such as poor school performance,[30] aggressive behavior, and hyperactivity.[31]

IMAGING AND LABORATORY EVALUATION

The diagnosis of SDB is firmly established using polysomnography, and ancillary testing is rarely indicated. Further screening may be useful to facilitate the perioperative care and to exclude underlying conditions (Box 28-2). For example, concern regarding right ventricular dysfunction may

Box 28-2   Ancillary Diagnostic Studies in OSAS

Serum Markers
- Hematocrit
- Serum bicarbonate

Imaging
- Brain MRI
- Anteroposterior and lateral neck radiograph
- Upper airway CT/MRI (craniofacial)
- Cine MRI
- Dynamic fluoroscopy

Sleep Monitoring
- MSLT

Miscellaneous
- Echocardiogram
- Neurocognitive testing
- Electrocardiogram
- Flow–volume loop

Box 28-3   Example of Polysomnogram Montage

Electroencephalography (C_4-M_1, O_2-M_1, F_4-M_1)
Electromyogram (chin, both legs)
Electrooculogram (right/left)
Electrocardiogram
Abdominal and thoracic excursion
Oximetry (3 second averaging), pulse waveform
End-tidal PCO_2 (peak value, waveform)
Flow: nasal pressure, oronasal thermistor
Snore volume
Body position sensor
Esophageal pressure (in special circumstances)
Video and audio taping

necessitate an EKG or echocardiogram. Occasionally, chronic intermittent hypoxemia may induce polycythemia, while persistent hypercarbia can elevate serum bicarbonate. Routine pulmonary function testing is not indicated in children suspected of having OSAS unless restrictive or obstructive lung disease is suspected. A fluttering pattern in the flow volume loop has been described in adults with OSAS.[32] Magnetic resonance imaging (MRI) of the upper airway in children with OSAS compared to normal controls reveals a statistically smaller upper airway luminal volume and elongation of the soft palate, as well as enlarged tonsils and adenoids.[33] However, there is considerable overlap between the groups, rendering MRI a poor screening tool. The measurement of the ratio of the width of the tonsil to the depth of the pharyngeal space on a lateral neck radiograph was reported to have a good sensitivity and specificity for distinguishing mild from moderate/severe OSAS in a small number of patients.[34] Adenoidal enlargement measured by cephalometry was present in over 80% of children with OSAS but also in 42% with primary snoring.[35] Though neck radiographs may be suggestive of adenoidal hypertrophy, direct visualization of the adenoids remains the diagnostic standard.[36] Dynamic fluoroscopy under sedation may demonstrate glossoptosis, particularly in children with macroglossia, micrognathia, or neuromuscular weakness.[37] Anatomical localization of the site of obstruction with cine MRI may alter the therapeutic approach in some children with residual OSAS following adenotonsillectomy or craniofacial anomalies.[38] Other promising but understudied tools for identifying OSAS in children include nasal rhinometry[39] and acoustic pharyngometry.[40]

Video/Audio Recordings

Diagnosing OSAS using home audio recordings, in addition to a standard clinical history and physical examination, revealed a sensitivity of 71–92% and a specificity of 29–80%.[41,42] Subtle forms of SDB are particularly difficult to evaluate using this technique. However, computer-aided processing of audio signals for regularity may improve predictive value.[43] Frequency domain analysis of the snoring signal has also shown promise in distinguishing OSAS from PS.[44] Video

recordings can also yield a noninvasive measure of movement and therefore arousal.[45–47] Video is also a useful adjunct to a comprehensive polysomnogram to evaluate body and head positioning, paradoxing, snoring, and mouth breathing. Studies correlating video scoring systems to standard polysomnography have been encouraging.[47] Future research will be necessary to validate the utility of a particular domiciliary video/audio study in a population with a well-characterized symptomatology.

Overnight Polysomnography

Polysomnography represents the gold standard for establishing the presence and severity of SDB in children, and can be performed in children of all ages. An expert consensus panel from the American Academy of Pediatrics has recommended overnight polysomnography as the diagnostic test of choice in evaluating children with suspected SBD.[14] Guidelines for performing laboratory-based polysomnography in children have been established.[48,49] The sleep laboratory should be a non-threatening environment that comfortably accommodates a parent during the study. Personnel with pediatric training should record, score, and interpret the study. The use of sedatives[50] and sleep deprivation[51] may worsen SDB, and is therefore not recommended. To the extent possible, sleep studies should conform to the child's usual sleep period. Infants may reasonably be studied during the day, while adolescent studies should generally start later at night. The polysomnographic montage will vary with the patient's suspected disorder (Box 28-3).

Electroencephalogram

Consensus guidelines for analyzing sleep architecture have been established in infants,[48,52,53] children,[48,52] and adults.[48] Standard practice is to apply adult EEG criteria to children older than 2–3 months of age. Sleep staging establishes that an adequate amount of total sleep time (TST) and sufficient REM sleep was obtained on the night of the study, and demonstrates the presence or absence of sleep fragmentation. In addition to sleep staging, the EEG tracing is useful for scoring cortical arousals and detecting epileptiform discharges. By consensus, an electrocortical (EEG) arousal is defined in adults as an abrupt 3-second shift in EEG frequency.[48] These criteria appear to be appropriate for use in children as well.[54] However, visible EEG arousals are present in only 51% of obstructive events in children,[55] complicating the diagnosis of

UARS in children. Frequency domain analysis of the EEG tracing may further enhance the sensitivity of detecting respiratory events or arousal.[56,57] Initial reports indicated that children with snoring[58] or even severe OSAS may have normal sleep state distribution.[59] However, a large cohort (n=559) comparing normal children to children with OSAS revealed that OSAS patients have increases in slow-wave sleep (23.5 vs. 28.8% TST) and decreases in REM sleep (22.3 vs. 17.3% TST).[60] Furthermore, these authors observed a decline in the spontaneous arousal index in OSAS patients versus controls (8.4 vs. 5.3), suggesting a homeostatic elevation in the arousal threshold.[60]

Arousal

Arousal from sleep is a protective reflex mechanism that restores airway patency through dilator muscle activation. Both mechano- and chemoreceptors have a role in initiating the arousal response. Though arousals reverse the airway obstruction, they result in the untoward consequences of sleep fragmentation and sympathetic activation.[61] Polysomnographically, arousal may be associated with EEG changes,[57] increased airflow, elimination of airflow limitation, cessation of paradoxical breathing, tachycardia, movement,[45] blood pressure elevation,[62] and autonomic activation. In children, however, approximately 50% of obstructive events do not result in an EEG arousal.[55] In infants, EEG arousals are even less common.[55] Thus, depending on the EEG arousal index for the diagnosis of UARS is unreliable. Frequency domain analysis may reveal evidence of EEG arousal not readily visible, and may be a clinically useful tool in the future.[56,57] Obstructive events that terminate with autonomic activation are termed subcortical arousals. Autonomic measures include heart rate variability,[63] blood pressure elevations,[62] pulse transit time,[4] and peripheral arterial tonometry.[64] The pulse transit time was reported to be a more sensitive measure of respiratory arousal compared to 3-second EEG arousals.[4] As a screening tool for OSAS, the pulse transit time had a sensitivity of 81% and a specificity of 76%.[65] Subcortical arousals alone have been demonstrated to result in neurocognitive impairment in adults.[66]

Measures of Respiratory Movements

A variety of methodologies to categorize central and obstructive respiratory events is amenable to overnight polysomnography. Thoracic and abdominal excursion is measured most commonly with respiratory inductive plethysmography (RIP). The classification of central and obstructive apneas is achieved by determining whether respiratory efforts are present during intervals of reduced flow. Uncalibrated RIP tracings may also be used as an index of thoraco-abdominal asynchrony. The highly compliant chest wall in children results in asynchronous motion between the thoracic and abdominal tracings, termed paradoxical breathing. This disparity may be quantified using phase angle analysis that is independent of the relative contribution of the two compartments.[67] Thoraco-abdominal asynchrony has been demonstrated in children with increased respiratory effort due to upper airway obstruction and OSAS.[67,68] Paradoxical breathing is normally seen in infants due to the high compliance of their chest wall, particularly during REM sleep, but is rare after 3 years of age.[69]

Esophageal manometry (P_{es}) represents the gold standard for quantifying respiratory effort and permits the detection of subtle, partially obstructive events that may produce sleep fragmentation.[70] However, P_{es} monitoring is uncomfortable and may itself alter the frequency of respiratory events.[71] The introduction of non-invasive, nasal pressure measurements has largely supplanted P_{es} in establishing the diagnosis of UARS (see Figure 28-1). Nevertheless, esophageal manometry peak amplitude and percent of time spent lower than -10 cmH$_2$O has been reported to have a better correlation with behavioral outcomes than the traditional apnea–hypopnea index with or without respiratory-effort-related arousals.[72] Current practice is to reserve P_{es} monitoring for rare cases of children with diagnostic uncertainty even after standard overnight polysomnography.

Measures of Airflow

Airflow can be quantitatively measured using an oronasal mask and pneumotachograph. However, mask breathing is uncomfortable and has been shown to alter respiratory mechanics. Practically speaking, this methodology is restricted to research settings and continuous positive airway pressure (CPAP) titration studies. Thermistors provide qualitative measures of oronasal airflow by measuring the temperature of expired air. Though thermistors accurately indicate complete cessation of flow, they are not an accurate measure of tidal volume and therefore hypopnea.[73] Another drawback of the thermistor is its long time constant that obscures the nuance of the flow profile, making the evaluation of flow limitation impossible.[73]

Nasal cannula pressure recordings provide a minimally invasive, semi-quantitative measure of airflow.[74,75] The resulting signal has been shown to be proportional to flow squared. Since nasal pressure measurements have a fast time constant, it is possible to detect flattening of the inspiratory nasal pressure signal, termed flow limitation, that occurs in a collapsible tube when flow becomes independent of driving pressure (Figure 28-2). Limitations of the nasal cannula pressure recordings include obstruction of the tubing with secretions, mouth breathing (especially in children with adenoidal hypertrophy), and the possible increase in nasal resistance due to obstruction of the nares. In children, the reported signal quality has varied in laboratory-based studies. Trang et al. reported an overall uninterpretable nasal cannula signal during only 4% of total sleep time.[76] However, 17% of subjects had uninterpretable signals for more than 20% of total sleep time. In contrast, Serebrisky et al. reported adequate nasal cannula flow signals (>50% of total sleep time) during sleep in only 71.8% of patients.[77] In a domiciliary study, the nasal cannula channel was not available overall for more than 50% of the night.[78] Verginis et al. compared the combination of the thermistor and nasal pressure measurement with either modality alone and found the combination significantly lowered the scoring of false-negative and false-positive obstructive events.[79]

Airflow may be approximated using RIP by considering that lung volume can be approximated by a two-compartment model (thoracic and abdomen excursion). RIP may be calibrated using an isovolume maneuver or a statistical technique and used to derive a 'sum' channel proportional to tidal volume.[80,81] Thus, the time derivative of the sum channel is proportional to flow. The RIP signal may therefore be analyzed for apnea, hypopnea, and flow limitation.[82] Our current practice is to combine RIP, nasal cannula pressure,

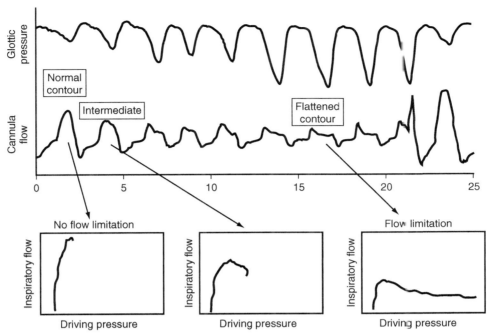

FIGURE 28-2 Nasal cannula pressure tracing demonstrating that flow becomes independent of driving pressure during flow-limited breaths *(Reproduced with permission from Hosselet JJ, Norman RG, Ayappa I, Rapoport DM. Detection of flow limitation with a nasal cannula/pressure transducer system. Am J Respir Crit Care Med. 1998;157:1461–1467).*

capnometry, and an oronasal thermistor in our laboratory-based studies to ensure that a flow signal is likely to be available throughout the night.

Gas Exchange

Pulse oximetry, which is based on the absorption spectra of hemoglobin, is the standard polysomnographic measure of hypoxemia. The relationship between the arterial oxygen tension and the SpO_2, the oxyhemoglobin curve, is sigmoidal. Patients with normal pulmonary function, whose baseline SpO_2 is on the flat portion of the curve, require large changes in PaO_2 to affect their SpO_2. By contrast, patients with parenchymal lung disease may be operating on the steep portion of the oxyhemoglobin curve, thereby experiencing a profound decline in SpO_2 with small decrements in PaO_2. In sickle cell disease, the oxyhemoglobin curve is variably shifted, thus limiting the utility of SpO_2 measurements in some patients.[83]

The adequacy of ventilation can be assessed non-invasively during sleep by sampling CO_2 tension in respired air, termed capnography. Expired gas initially consists of dead space ventilation in the measuring apparatus as well as the physiologic dead space. In the setting of normal lungs, the terminal expired concentration of CO_2 reaches a plateau and reflects alveolar gas. The concentration of CO_2 in a given alveolus is predicated on the ventilation–perfusion relationship. In subjects with normal lung mechanics, end-tidal PCO_2 ($P_{ET}CO_2$) is approximately 2–5 mmHg below the arterial $PaCO_2$ level.[84] However, in diseases with uneven ventilation–perfusion or altered alveolar time constants, such as cystic fibrosis, the $P_{ET}CO_2$ will not be an accurate measure of $PaCO_2$. Also, the rapid respiratory rates characteristic of infants may not permit the alveolar CO_2 to plateau, and therefore may underestimate the true CO_2 value.[85] The capnometry signal is prone to artifact due to nasal secretions obstructing the sampling cannula. Morielli et al. reported that 27% of polysomnographic epochs in their laboratory had a poor $P_{ET}CO_2$ waveform, stressing the importance of careful attention to technique.[85] Transcutaneous CO_2 ($TcCO_2$) monitors might be valuable in patients in whom $P_{ET}CO_2$ is not accurate, such as infants or patients with parenchymal lung disease.[85] Though absolute values of $TcCO_2$ are variable, the trend is proportional to the $PaCO_2$ with a lag of several minutes. Sleep is normally associated with a 4–6 mmHg increase in $TcCO_2$.

Normative Polysomnographic Data

Normative data for the EEG and respiratory parameters of sleeping children are shown in Table 28.2.[59,60,86–83] In infants, longitudinal arterial oxygen saturation monitoring revealed a median SpO_2 baseline of 98%, but the SpO_2 was <90% during 0.51% of epochs.[89] Marcus et al. presented the respiratory data of 50 normal, non-obese children between 1 and 18 years of age (mean 9.7±4.6), using a thermistor and $P_{ET}CO_2$ monitoring.[88] Nine subjects had at least one obstructive apneic event. One 'normal' child had an apnea index of 3.1/h, though he had a sibling with OSAS. Including this outlier, an obstructive apnea index >1/h was determined to be statistically abnormal. However, the threshold level at which the apnea index becomes clinically significant has not been established. Only 15% of normal children had any hypopneas, with the mean hypopnea index being 0.1±0.1 (range 0.1–0.7).[90] Acebo et al. also reported that hypopneas were rare in older children and adolescents.[87] Normative data using nasal pressure during sleep have not been presented in children. Experience from our laboratory indicates that hypopneas and respiratory-effort-related arousals occur infrequently in normal young children (<1.5/hour).

TABLE 28.2   Polysomnographic Data in Normal 5–10-year-old Children

SLEEP		RESPIRATORY	
EEG arousal index, n/h	7±22	Obstructive apnea Index, n/h TST	0.0±20.1
Sleep efficiency, %	84±213	Obstructive hypopnea Index, n/h TST	0.1±20.1
Stage 1, %TST	5±23	Central apneas with desaturation n/hr TST	0.0±20.1
Stage 2, %TST			
Slow wave sleep, %TST	51±29		
	25±28	Duration of Hypoventilation ($P_{ET}CO_2 \geq 45$ mmHg), %TST	1.6±20.8
REM sleep, %TST	19±26	Peak $P_{ET}CO_2$, mmHg	46±23
REM cycles, n	4±21	S_pO_2 Nadir, %	95±21

Data, Mean ± 2 SD; see references[47,48,70,72]

Normative data for esophageal manometry (ΔP_{es}) from 10 normal subjects in our laboratory, aged 2–11 years, showed that control subjects had a mean ΔP_{es} of -8 ± 2 cmH$_2$O (range -6 to -12), a peak ΔP_{es} of -12 ± 3 cmH$_2$O (range -9 to -19 cmH$_2$O), and had a $\Delta P_{es} \geq -10$ cmH$_2$O for $8\pm12\%$ of breaths (range 3–61%).[4] Other investigators have considered ΔP_{es} swings of -8 to -14 cmH$_2$O as normal,[91] and suggested that normal children spend $\leq10\%$ of the night with inspiratory esophageal pressure swings ≤-10 cmH$_2$O.[70] However, our data showed that two control patients spent 21% and 61% of the night with a $\Delta P_{es} \leq -10$ cmH$_2$O. Thus, normative data from non-snoring controls reveal considerable variability in respiratory effort. ΔP_{es} is lower in normal infants, 5–6 cmH$_2$O.[92]

Domiciliary and Nap Studies

Attended overnight polysomnography in a designated pediatric sleep laboratory represents the gold standard for the diagnosis of SDB in children.[49] However, such comprehensive testing is expensive, labor-intensive, and not widely available. Recognizing that only 10–20% of children who snore will have OSAS[10,11] has prompted considerable interest in limited, nap or unattended domiciliary studies. Choosing the most appropriate evaluation is predicated on understanding the relative risks of OSAS and its treatments. Testing is indicated to determine the presence and severity of SDB, the type of treatment, the perioperative care, and necessary follow-up.

Polysomnography during a daytime nap may underestimate the degree of SDB.[93,94] REM sleep often does not occur during naps. Furthermore, obstructive respiratory events worsen as sleep progresses.[59] Thus, although the positive predictive value of an abnormal nap study is 100%, the negative predictive value is only 20%.[93,94] Home study devices may range in complexity from oximetry alone[95,96] to multi-channel recordings.[97] Ambulatory studies may be used to evaluate oxygenation in infants with chronic lung disease, cystic fibrosis, restrictive lung diseases, and neuromuscular conditions. Jacob et al. compared laboratory and domiciliary studies in a population of symptomatic children with adenotonsillar hypertrophy.[98] The multi-channel monitor used in that study included saturation, waveform, electrocardiogram, RIP, and video recording, and therefore cannot be compared to commercially available ambulatory systems.[98] Similar indices of apnea–hypopnea, desaturation and arousal were observed during attended laboratory-based polysomnograms and domiciliary studies.[98] Goodwin et al. performed a home-based

study that was set up by a technician and then was completed unattended, with an excellent success rate of 91%.[99] Similarly, Rosen et al. performed 850 abbreviated home studies with 94% yielding technically satisfactory data.[17] A subset of 55 children also underwent laboratory-based polysomnography and the sensitivity and specificity of the home study to detect OSAS as defined by an AHI >5/hour on the laboratory study were 88% and 98%, respectively.[17] Overall, the utility of ambulatory studies depends on the age group and channels acquired.

Documenting oximeters should include an algorithm for artifact reduction such as a plethysmograph waveform or heart rate detected by the oximeter. The oximetry channel alone has been compared to full polysomnography in a population of snoring children with adenotonsillar hypertrophy suspected to have SDB with adenotonsillar hypertrophy.[100] One study reported that oximetry demonstrated an excellent positive predictive value, 97%, but a poor negative predictive ability, 53%.[100] By contrast, Kirk reported that overnight oximetry alone has a poor correlation with laboratory-based polysomnography.[101] Many children with SDB and clinically significant respiratory-effort-related arousals will not demonstrate oxygen desaturation.[1,70] Similar observations have been made regarding the limitations of using oximetry as a screening tool for adult OSAS.[95,96] Oximetry is inadequate to diagnose a considerable percentage of pediatric SDB in which arousal or hypoventilation, rather than hypoxemia, predominate.[1]

Night-to-Night Polysomnographic Variability

A single overnight polysomnogram is a well-recognized diagnostic tool used to determine the presence and severity of OSAS in symptomatic children.[49] However, in adults an adaptation effect of the sleep laboratory environment, termed the 'first night effect,' has been reported to disrupt sleep architecture[102] and perhaps underestimate respiratory disturbance.[103,104] There are several pediatric studies that have documented the excellent consistency in the diagnosis of OSAS from night to night.[102,105–107] In children, the clinical diagnosis of either OSAS or primary snoring remained the same in two polysomnogram studies 1–4 weeks apart.[105] Although the overall classification of subjects was unchanged, there were minimal changes in OSAS severity between nights. This supports the view that a single polysomnographic night is sufficient for the diagnosis of OSAS in otherwise normal, snoring children with adenotonsillar hypertrophy. No night-to-night systematic bias has been observed in any of the mean intersubject respiratory parameters.[102,105] The intrasubject respiratory parameters, however, demonstrated considerable variability, particularly in children with severe disease. The variability in respiratory parameters could not be accounted for by changes in body position or percentage REM time. Among the sleep variables, a first night effect including increased wakefulness and a reduction of REM sleep was observed as the result of adaptation to the sleep laboratory environment.[102] Circumstances in which a single study night may not be sufficient include studies with inadequate REM time, technical limitations in acquiring key channels, or if the parents report that the particular study night did not reflect a typical night's sleep. However, studies primarily performed to assess sleep architecture (usually only in a research context) require adaptation nights in the sleep laboratory.

Diagnostic and Event Classification

The optimal definition for respiratory events and clinical classification has not been established in children. There are few clinical studies evaluating the relative merit of specific event definitions in relation to clinical outcomes. The polysomnographic criteria for event scoring and clinical diagnosis, based on our clinical experience, are summarized in Tables 28.3 and

28.4. However, well-designed outcomes studies are desperately needed to validate these criteria. Additional abnormal breathing patterns, including tachypnea and increased respiratory effort have been described in children with OSAS.[108] Normative data for respiratory-effort-related arousals and flow limitation are scant in children, but these events appear to be uncommon. Nevertheless, the clinical classification of symptomatic children cannot be exclusively based on the apnea–hypopnea index alone. Consideration of the AHI, flow limitation, S_pO_2, $P_{ET}CO_2$, work of breathing, and arousal indices, in conjunction with the clinical picture, also contribute to the diagnosis of OSAS. Thus, diagnostic interpretation of pediatric PSG will continue to require consideration of all respiratory parameters.

Special Considerations in Infants

The pathophysiology of OSAS in infants frequently differs from that observed in older children, with infants having a higher likelihood of congenital anomalies of the upper airway including laryngomalacia, choanal atresia, laryngeal webs, and pyriform aperature stenosis, in addition to gastroesophageal reflux, hypotonia and other issues.[109] Therefore, direct endoscopic visualization of the upper airway is a helpful part of the

TABLE 28.3   Respiratory Pattern Scoring

Obstructive

Apnea	Reduction of oronasal thermal airflow by ≥90% lasting at least 2 missed breaths with persistent respiratory effort
Hypopnea	Fall in the nasal pressure amplitude >50% for at least a 2-breath duration with persistent respiratory effort accompanied by a desaturation ≥3%, awakening, or arousal
Respiratory effort-related arousal	Discernible fall in the amplitude of the nasal pressure signal <50% of baseline or flattening of the signal contour lasting at least 2 breaths duration. Evidence of increased work of breathing, snoring or elevation of CO_2
Flow limitation	Flattening of the inspiratory limb of nasal pressure channel
Snoring	Coarse, low-pitched inspiratory sound
Hypoventilation	End-tidal or transcutaneous CO_2 >50 mmHg for >25% TST

Central

Apnea	Absence of oronasal airflow for ≥20 seconds duration without respiratory effort. Alternatively, the event lasts at least 2 missed breaths duration and is associated with arousal, awakening or ≥3% desaturation
Periodic breathing	Succession of >3 central apneas of >3-second duration separated by <20 seconds of normal breathing
Mixed apneas	Reduction of oronasal thermal airflow by ≥90% lasting at least 2 missed breaths. Absent respiratory effort during the initial portion only

TABLE 28.4   Diagnostic Classification and Severity of SDB

	APNEA INDEX (Events/h)	**SpO₂ NADIR (%)**	**P$_{ET}$CO₂ PEAK (Torr)**	**P$_{ET}$CO₂ > 50 Torr (%TST)**	**AROUSALS (Events/h)**
		(ONE OR MORE OF THE FOLLOWING)			
Primary Snoring	≤1	>92	<53	<10%	EEG <11
Upper Airway Resistance Syndrome	≤1	>92	<53	<10%	RERA >1 EEG >11
Mild OSAS	1–4	86–91	>53	10–24%	EEG >11
Moderate OSAS	5–10	76–85	>60	25–49%	EEG >11
Severe OSAS	10	≤75	>65	≥50%	EEG >11

Arterial oxygen saturation, SpO₂; End tidal Pco₂, P$_{ET}$CO₂; EEG, electrocortical; RERA, respiratory effort related arousal; Total sleep time, TST diagnostic work-up to establish nasal size, adenoidal volume, laryngeal stability/anatomy, mucosal swelling, and vocal cord function. Infants with OSA may not snore,[15] and many snoring infants do not have OSA.[110] Therefore polysomnography should be performed to confirm the diagnosis and establish the severity. Polysomnographically, normative data are different in infants with respect to REM sleep percentage, respiratory rate, oximetry, and the arousal index compared to older children.[109] A few scored obstructive apneas and hypopneas may be observed in otherwise normal infants.

Clinical Pearls

- Obstructive sleep-disordered breathing in children includes non-apneic and non-hypopneic patterns including sustained increased respiratory effort and respiratory-effort-related arousals.
- The threshold level of OSAS severity that necessitates treatment varies widely among children.
- Subjective reports of sleepiness are most often not present in pre-pubescent children with OSAS.
- Direct endoscopic visualization of the airway is an essential part of the work-up in infants with OSAS.

References

1. Guilleminault C, Stoohs R, Clerk A, et al. A cause of excessive daytime sleepiness. The upper airway resistance syndrome. Chest 1993;104: 781–7.
2. Guilleminault C, Korobkin R, Winkle R. A review of 50 children with obstructive sleep apnea syndrome. Lung 1981;159:275–87.
3. Rosen CL, D'Andrea L, Haddad GG. Adult criteria for obstructive sleep apnea do not identify children with serious obstruction. Am Rev Respir Dis 1992;146:1231–4.
4. Katz ES, Lutz J, Black C, et al. Pulse transit time as a measure of arousal and respiratory effort in children with sleep-disordered breathing. Pediatr Res 2003;53:580–8.
5. International Classification of Sleep Disorders, Diagnostic and Coding Manuel. Westchester, IL: American Academy of Sleep Medicine; 2005.
6. Bourke R, Anderson V, Yang JS, et al. Cognitive and academic functions are impaired in children with all severities of sleep-disordered breathing. Sleep Med 2011;12:489–96.
7. Brockmann PE, Urschitz MS, Schlaud M, et al. Primary snoring in school children: prevalence and neurocognitive impairments. Sleep Breath 2012;16:23–9.
8. O'Brien LM, Mervis CB, Holbrook CR, et al. Neurobehavioral implications of habitual snoring in children. Pediatrics 2004;114:44–9.
9. Urschitz MS, Guenther A, Eggebrecht E, et al. Snoring, intermittent hypoxia and academic performance in primary school children. Am J Respir Crit Care Med 2003;168:464–8.
10. Ali J, Pitson J, Stradling R. Snoring, sleep disturbance, and behaviour in 4–5 year olds. Arch Dis Child 1993;68:360–6.
11. Gislason T, Benediktsdóttir B. Snoring, apneic episodes, and nocturnal hypoxemia among children 6 months to 6 years old. Chest 1995;107:963.
12. Redline S, Tishler PV, Schluchter M, et al. Risk factors for sleep-disordered breathing in children. Associations with obesity, race, and respiratory problems. Am J Respir Crit Care Med 1999;159:1527–532.
13. Wilson K, Lakheeram I, Morielli A, et al. Can assessment for obstructive sleep apnea help predict postadenotonsillectomy respiratory complications? Anesthesiology 2002;96:313–22.
14. Section on Pediatric Pulmonology, Subcommittee on Obstructive Sleep Apnea Syndrome. American Academy of Pediatrics. Clinical practice guideline: diagnosis and management of childhood obstructive sleep apnea syndrome. Pediatrics 2002;109:704–12.
15. Anderson IC, Sedaghat A, McGinley B, et al. Prevalence and severity of obstructive sleep apnea and snoring in infants with Pierre Robin sequence. Cleft Palate Craniofac J 2011;48(5):614–18.

16. Preutthipan A, Chantarojanasiri T, Suwanjutha S, et al. Can parents predict the severity of childhood obstructive sleep apnoea? Acta Paediatr 2000;89:708–12.
17. Rosen CL, Larkin EK, Kirchner HL, et al. Prevalence and risk factors for sleep-disordered breathing in 8- to 11-year-old children: association with race and prematurity. J Pediatr 2003;142:383–9.
18. Gozal D, Wang M, Pope DW Jr. Objective sleepiness measures in pediatric obstructive sleep apnea. Pediatrics 2001;108:693.
19. Gozal D, Kheirandish-Gozal L. Obesity and excessive daytime sleepiness in prepubertal children with obstructive sleep apnea. Pediatrics 2009;123:13–18.
20. Marcus CL, Curtis S, Koerner CB, et al. Evaluation of pulmonary function and polysomnography in obese children and adolescents. Pediatr Pulmonol 1996;21:176–83.
21. Melendres MC, Lutz JM, Rubin ED, et al. Daytime sleepiness and hyperactivity in children with suspected sleep-disordered breathing. Pediatrics 2004;114:768–75.
22. Brouilette R, Hanson D, David R, et al. A diagnostic approach to suspected obstructive sleep apnea in children. J Pediatr 1984;105: 10–14.
23. Carroll L, McColley A, Marcus L, et al. Inability of clinical history to distinguish primary snoring from obstructive sleep apnea syndrome in children. Chest 1995;108:610–18.
24. Rosen CL. Clinical features of obstructive sleep apnea hypoventilation syndrome in otherwise healthy children. Pediatr Pulmonol 1999;27: 403–9.
25. Spruyt K, Gozal D. Screening of pediatric sleep-disordered breathing: a proposed unbiased discriminative set of questions using clinical severity scales. Chest 2012;142:1508–15.
26. Suen JS, Arnold JE, Brooks LJ. Adenotonsillectomy for treatment of obstructive sleep apnea in children. Arch Otolaryngol Head Neck Surg 1995;121:525–30.
27. Chervin RD, Hedger K, Dillon JE, et al. Pediatric sleep questionnaire (PSQ): validity and reliability of scales for sleep-disordered breathing, snoring, sleepiness, and behavioral problems. Sleep Med 2000;1: 21–32.
28. Chervin RD, Weatherly RA, Garetz SL, et al. Pediatric sleep questionnaire: prediction of sleep apnea and outcomes. Arch Otolaryngol Head Neck Surg 2007;133:216–22.
29. Marcus CL, Greene MG, Carroll JL. Blood pressure in children with obstructive sleep apnea. Am J Respir Crit Care Med 1998;157: 1098–103.
30. Gozal D. Sleep-disordered breathing and school performance in children. Pediatrics 1998;102:616–20.
31. Guilleminault C, Winkle R, Korobkin R, et al. Children and nocturnal snoring: evaluation of the effects of sleep related respiratory resistive load and daytime functioning. Eur J Pediatr 1982;139:165–71.
32. Haponik F, Smith L, Kaplan J, et al. Flow-volume curves and sleep-disordered breathing: therapeutic implications. Thorax 1983;38:609–15.
33. Arens R, McDonough JM, Costarino AT, et al. Magnetic resonance imaging of the upper airway structure of children with obstructive sleep apnea syndrome. Am J Respir Crit Care Med 2001;164:698–703.
34. Li AM, Wong E, Kew J, et al. Use of tonsil size in the evaluation of obstructive sleep apnoea. Arch Dis Child 2002;87:156–9.
35. Xu Z, Cheuk DK, Lee SL. Clinical evaluation in predicting childhood obstructive sleep apnea. Chest 2006;130:1765–71.
36. Mlynarek A, Tewfik MA, Hagr A, et al. Lateral neck radiography versus direct video rhinoscopy in assessing adenoid size. J Otolaryngol 2004;33:360–5.
37. Donnelly LF, Strife JL, Myer CM. Glossoptosis (posterior displacement of the tongue) during sleep: a frequent cause of sleep apnea in pediatric patients referred for dynamic sleep fluoroscopy. AJR Am J Roentgenol 2000;175:1557–60.
38. Donnelly LF, Shott SR, LaRose CR, et al. Causes of persistent obstructive sleep apnea despite previous tonsillectomy and adenoidectomy in children with Down syndrome as depicted on static and dynamic cine MRI. AJR Am J Roentgenol 2004;183:175–81.
39. Rizzi M, Onorato J, Andreoli A, et al. Nasal resistances are useful in identifying children with severe obstructive sleep apnea before polysomnography. Int J Pediatr Otorhinolaryngol 2002;65:7–13.
40. Monahan J. Utility of noninvasive pharyngometry in epidemiologic studies of childhood sleep-disordered breathing. Am J Respir Crit Care Med 2002;165:1499–503.
41. Lamm C, Mandeli J, Kattan M. Evaluation of home audiotapes as an abbreviated test for obstructive sleep apnea syndrome (OSAS) in children. Pediatr Pulmonol 1999;27:267–72.

42. Goldstein NA, Sculerati N, Walsleben JA, et al. Clinical diagnosis of pediatric obstructive sleep apnea validated by polysomnography. Otolaryngology Head Neck Surg 1994;111:611.

43. Potsic WP. Comparison of polysomnography and sonography for assessing regularity of respiration during sleep in adenotonsillar hypertrophy. Laryngoscope 1987;97:1430–7.

44. McCombe AW, Kwok V, Hawke WM. An acoustic screening test for obstructive sleep apnoea. Clin Otolaryngol Allied Sci 1995;20:348–51.

45. Mograss MA, Ducharme FM, Brouillette RT. Movement/arousals. Description, classification, and relationship to sleep apnea in children. Am J Respir Crit Care Med 1994;150:1690–6.

46. Morielli A, Ladan S, Ducharme M, et al. Can sleep and wakefulness be distinguished in children by cardiorespiratory and videotape recordings? Chest 1996;109:680–7.

47. Sivan Y, Kornecki A, Schonfeld T. Screening obstructive sleep apnoea syndrome by home videotape recording in children. Eur Resp J 1996;9:2127–31.

48. Iber C, Ancoli-Israel S, Chesson A, Quan SF, editors. The AASM manual for the scoring of sleep and associated events: Rules, terminology and technical specifications. 1st ed. Westchester, IL: American Academy of Sleep Medicine; 2007.

49 Aurora RN, Zak RS, Karippot A, et al. Practice parameters for the respiratory indications for polysomnography in children. Sleep 2011;34:379–88.

50. Hershenson M, Brouillette RT, Olsen E, et al. The effect of chloral hydrate on genioglossus and diaphragmatic activity. Pediatr Res 1984;18:516–19.

51. Canet E, Gaultier C, D'Allest AM, et al. Effects of sleep deprivation on respiratory events during sleep in healthy infants. J Appl Physiol 1989;66:1158.

52. Grigg-Damberger M, Gozal D, Marcus CL, et al. The visual scoring of sleep and arousal in infants and children. J Clin Sleep Med 2007;3:201–40.

53. Anders T, Emde R, Parmelee A. A manual of standardized terminology, technique, and criteria for scoring of states of sleep and wakefulness in newborn infants. UCLA Brain Information Service, NINDS, Neurological Information Network, Los Angeles, USA, 1971.

54. Wong TK, Galster P, Lau TS, et al. Reliability of scoring arousals in normal children and children with obstructive sleep apnea syndrome. Sleep 2004;27:1139–45.

55. McNamara F, Issa FG, Sullivan CE. Arousal pattern following central and obstructive breathing abnormalities in infants and children. J Appl Physiol 1996;81:2651–7.

56. Bandla HP, Gozal D. Dynamic changes in EEG spectra during obstructive apnea in children. Pediatr Pulmonol 2000;29:359–65.

57. Black JE, Guilleminault C, Colrain IM, et al. Upper airway resistance syndrome. Central electroencephalographic power and changes in breathing effort. Am J Respir Crit Care Med 2000;162:406–11.

58. Fuentes-Pradera MA, Botebol G, Sánchez-Armengol A, et al. Effect of snoring and obstructive respiratory events on sleep architecture in adolescents. Arch Pediatr Adolesc Med 2003;157:649–54.

59. Goh DY, Galster P, Marcus CL. Sleep architecture and respiratory disturbances in children with obstructive sleep apnea. Am J Respir Crit Care Med 2000;162:682–6.

60. Tauman R, O'Brien LM, Holbrook CR, et al. Sleep pressure score: a new index of sleep disruption in snoring children. Sleep 2004;27:274–8.

61. Somers VK, Dyken ME, Clary MP, et al. Sympathetic neural mechanisms in obstructive sleep apnea. J Clin Invest 1995;96:1897–904.

62. Davies J, Vardi-Visy K, Clarke M, et al. Identification of sleep disruption and sleep disordered breathing from the systolic blood pressure profile. Thorax 1993;48:1242–7.

63. Aljadeff G, Gozal D, Schechtman VL, et al. Heart rate variability in children with obstructive sleep apnea. Sleep 1997;20:151.

64. Schnall RP, Shlitner A, Sheffy J, et al. Periodic, profound peripheral vasoconstriction – a new marker of obstructive sleep apnea. Sleep 1999;22:939–46.

65. Brietzke SE, Katz ES, Roberson DW. Pulse transit time as a screening test for pediatric sleep-related breathing disorders. Arch Otolaryngol Head Neck Surg 2007;133:980–4.

66. Martin SE, Wraith PK, Deary IJ, et al. The effect of nonvisible sleep fragmentation on daytime function. Am J Respir Crit Care Med 1997;155:1596–601.

67. Sivan Y, Ward SD, Deakers T, et al. Rib cage to abdominal asynchrony in children undergoing polygraphic sleep studies. Pediatr Pulmonol 1991;11:141–6.

68. Kohyama J. Asynchronous breathing during sleep. Arch Dis Child 2001;84:174–7.

69. Gaultier C, Praud JP, Canet E, et al. Paradoxical inward rib cage motion during rapid eye movement sleep in infants and young children. J Dev Physiol 1987;9:391–7.

70. Guilleminault C, Pelayo R, Leger D, et al. Recognition of sleep-disordered breathing in children. Pediatrics 1996;98:371–82.

71. Groswasser J, Scaillon M, Rebuffat E, et al. Naso-oesophageal probes decrease the frequency of sleep apnoeas in infants. J Sleep Res 2000;9:193–6.

72. Chervin RD, Ruzicka DL, Hoban TF, et al. Esophageal pressures, polysomnography, and neurobehavioral outcomes of adenotonsillectomy in children. Chest 2012;142(1):101–10.

73. Farré R, Montserrat JM, Rotger M, et al. Accuracy of thermistors and thermocouples as flow-measuring devices for detecting hypopnoeas. Eur Resp J 1998;11:179–82.

74. Norman RG, Ahmed MM, Walsleben JA, et al. Detection of respiratory events during NPSG: nasal cannula/pressure sensor versus thermistor. Sleep 1997;20:1175–84.

75. Hosselet JJ, Norman RG, Arappa I, et al. Detection of flow limitation with a nasal cannula/pressure transducer system. Am J Respir Crit Care Med 1998;157:1461–7.

76. Trang H, Leske V, Gaultier C. Use of nasal cannula for detecting sleep apneas and hypopneas in infants and children. Am J Respir Crit Care Med 2002;166:464.

77. Serebrisky D, Cordero R, Mandeli J, et al. Assessment of inspiratory flow limitation in children with sleep-disordered breathing by a nasal cannula pressure transducer system. Pediatr Pulmonol 2002;33:380–7.

78. Poels PJ, Schilder AG, van den Berg S, et al. Evaluation of a new device for home cardiorespiratory recording in children. Arch Otolaryngol Head Neck Surg 2003;129:1281–4.

79. Verginis N, Davey MJ, Horne RS. Scoring respiratory events in paediatric patients: evaluation of nasal pressure and thermistor recordings separately and in combination. Sleep Med 2010;11:400–5.

80. Sackner MA, Watson H, Belsito AS, et al. Calibration of respiratory inductive plethysmograph during natural breathing. J Appl Physiol 1989;66:410–20.

81. Adams JA, Zabaleta IA, Stroh D, et al. Measurement of breath amplitudes: comparison of three noninvasive respiratory monitors to integrated pneumotachograph. Pediatr Pulmonol 1993;16:254–8.

82. Griffiths A, Maul J, Wilson A, et al. Improved detection of obstructive events in childhood sleep apnoea with the use of the nasal cannula and the differentiated sum signal. J Sleep Res 2005;14:431–6.

83. Seakins M, Gibbs WN, Milner PF, et al. Erythrocyte Hb-S concentration. An important factor in the low oxygen affinity of blood in sickle cell anemia. J Clin Invest 1973;52:422–32.

84. Bhavani-Shankar K, Moseley H, Kumar AY, et al. Capnometry and anaesthesia. Can J Anaesth 1992;39:617–32.

85. Morielli A, Desjardins D, Brouillette RT. Transcutaneous and end-tidal carbon dioxide pressures should be measured during pediatric polysomnography. Am Rev Respir Dis 1993;148:1599–604.

86. Uliel S, Tauman R, Greenfeld M, et al. Normal polysomnographic respiratory values in children and adolescents. Chest 2004;125:872.

87. Acebo C, Millman RP, Rosenberg C, et al. Sleep, breathing, and cephalometrics in older children and young adults. Part I – Normative values. Chest 1996;109:664–72.

88. Marcus CL, Omlin KJ, Basinki DJ, et al. Normal polysomnographic values for children and adolescents. Am Rev Respir Dis 1992;146:1235–9.

89. Hunt CE, Corwin MJ, Lister G, et al. Longitudinal assessment of hemoglobin oxygen saturation in healthy infants during the first 6 months of age. Collaborative Home Infant Monitoring Evaluation (CHIME) Study Group. J Pediatr 1999;135:580–6.

90. Witmans MB, Keens TG, Davidson Ward SL, et al. Obstructive hypopneas in children and adolescents: normal values. Am J Respir Crit Care Med 2003;168:1540.

91. Miyazaki S, Itasaka Y, Yamakawa K, et al. Respiratory disturbance during sleep due to adenoid-tonsillar hypertrophy. Am J Otolaryngol 1989;10:143–9.

92. Skatvedt O, Grogaard J. Infant sleeping position and inspiratory pressures in the upper airways and oesophagus. Arch Dis Child 1994;71:138–40.

93. Marcus CL, Keens TG, Ward SL. Comparison of nap and overnight polysomnography in children. Pediatr Pulmonol 1992;13:16–21.

94. Saeed M. Should children with suspected obstructive sleep apnea syndrome and normal nap sleep studies have overnight sleep studies? Chest 2000;118:360–5.

95. Cooper G, Veale D, Griffiths J, et al. Value of nocturnal oxygen saturation as a screening test for sleep apnoea. Thorax 1991;46:586–8.

96. Ryan J, Hilton F, Boldy A, et al. Validation of British Thoracic Society guidelines for the diagnosis of the sleep apnoea/hypopnoea syndrome: can polysomnography be avoided? Thorax 1995;50:972–5.

97. Redline S, Tosteson T, Boucher M, et al. Measurement of sleep-related breathing disturbances in epidemiologic studies. Assessment of the validity and reproducibility of a portable monitoring device. Chest 1991;100:1281–6.

98. Jacob SV, Morielli A, Mograss MA, et al. Home testing for pediatric obstructive sleep apnea syndrome secondary to adenotonsillar hypertrophy. Pediatr Pulmonol 1995;20:241–52.

99. Goodwin JL, Enright PL, Kaemingk KL, et al. Feasibility of using unattended polysomnography in children for research – report of the Tucson Children's Assessment of Sleep Apnea study (TuCASA). Sleep 2001;24:937–44.

100. Brouillette T, Morielli A, Leimanis A, et al. Nocturnal pulse oximetry as an abbreviated testing modality for pediatric obstructive sleep apnea. Pediatrics 2000;105:405–12.

101. Kirk G. Comparison of home oximetry monitoring with laboratory polysomnography in children. Chest 2003;124:1702–8.

102. Scholle S, Scholle HC, Kemper A, et al. First night effect in children and adolescents undergoing polysomnography for sleep-disordered breathing. Clin Neurophysiol 2003;114:2138–145.

103. Le Bon O, Hoffmann G, Tecco J, et al. Mild to moderate sleep respiratory events: one negative night may not be enough. Chest 2000;118:353–9.

104. Bliwise DL, Carey E, Dement WC. Nightly variation in sleep-related respiratory disturbance in older adults. Exp Aging Res 1983;9:77–81.

105. Katz ES, Greene MG, Carson KA, et al. Night-to-night variability of polysomnography in children with suspected obstructive sleep apnea. J Pediatr 2002;140:589–94.

106. Verhulst SL, Schrauwen N, De Backer WA, et al. First night effect for polysomnographic data in children and adolescents with suspected sleep disordered breathing. Arch Dis Child 2006;91:233–7.

107. Li AM, Wing YK, Cheung A, et al. Is a 2-night polysomnographic study necessary in childhood sleep-related disordered breathing? Chest 2004;126:1467–72.

108. Guilleminault C, Li K, Khramtsov A, et al. Breathing patterns in prepubertal children with sleep-related breathing disorders. Arch Pediatr Adolesc Med 2004;158:153–61.

109. Katz ES, Mitchell RB, D'Ambrosio CM. Obstructive sleep apnea in infants. Am J Respir Crit Care Med 2012;185:805–16.

110. Kahn A, Groswasser J, Sottiaux M, et al. Clinical symptoms associated with brief obstructive sleep apnea in normal infants. Sleep 1993;16:409–13.

Cognitive and Behavioral Consequences of Obstructive Sleep Apnea

Louise M. O'Brien

INTRODUCTION

Sleep-disordered breathing (SDB) describes a range of breathing problems during sleep from habitual snoring to obstructive sleep apnea (OSA). It is a frequent condition characterized by repeated events of partial or complete upper airway obstruction during sleep, resulting in disruption of normal ventilation, hypoxemia, and sleep. A recent systematic review found that the estimated population prevalence for SDB by varying constellations of parent-reported symptoms on questionnaire is ~11% while OSA diagnosed by varying criteria on diagnostic studies, is approximately 1–4%.[1] Although OSA was first described by McKenzie over a century ago,[2] it was not until the mid 1970s that it was recognized in children.[3] Using polysomnography in 8 children aged 5–14 years Guilleminault et al. published the first detailed report of children with adenotonsillar hypertrophy and OSA and suggested that surgery may eliminate their clinical symptoms.[3] Since this initial report there has been considerable research effort in this area and it is now clear that OSA in children is a distinct disorder from the OSA that occurs in adults, in particular with respect to gender distribution, clinical manifestations, polysomnographic findings, and treatment.[4,5] OSA is frequently diagnosed in association with adenotonsillar hypertrophy, and is also common in children with craniofacial abnormalities and neurological disorders affecting upper airway patency.

Snoring is the primary symptom of OSA and while snoring is not normal, as it indicates the presence of heightened upper airway resistance, many snoring children may have primary snoring, i.e., habitual snoring without alterations in sleep architecture, alveolar ventilation and oxygenation. Nonetheless, definitive criteria that allow for reliable distinction between primary snoring and OSA and the threshold at which morbidity occurs remain elusive. Polysomnography remains the gold standard for the definitive diagnosis of OSA, since clinical history and physical examination are insufficient to confirm its presence or severity.[6] However, alternative screening methods and novel technological advances may improve diagnostic accuracy in the future.[7–13]

The implications of SDB in children are multifaceted and potentially complex. If left untreated or, alternatively, if treated late, pediatric SDB may lead to substantial morbidity that affects multiple target organs and systems, and that may not be completely reversed with appropriate treatment. There is now a wealth of literature showing strong and significant associations between parental report and/or objective measures of SDB with a range of neurobehavioral, cognitive, and psychiatric problems. The potential consequences of SDB in children include behavioral disturbances and learning deficits,[14–24] psychiatric symptoms,[25–28] autonomic dysfunction,[29,30] and hypertension.[31,32] This chapter will focus on behavioral and cognitive consequences of SDB.

BEHAVIOR

Behavioral dysregulation is the most commonly encountered comorbidity of SDB, and the vast majority of studies consistently report, mostly robust, associations between SDB symptoms, or objective measures of SDB, and hyperactivity, impulsivity, and ADHD-like symptoms.[15,33–35]

Hyperactivity

Hyperactivity is frequently reported in both children with habitual snoring,[14,15,18,21,33,36–41] as well as those in whom SDB was formally diagnosed by polysomnography (PSG).[17,20,35,42–47] Despite differences in definition of snoring or PSG-confirmed SDB, many studies support the relationship between snoring/SDB and hyperactive behaviors even when hyperactivity is measured with a range of parent-report tools, including the Conners' Parent Rating Scales,[15,42,43,45] the Child Behavior Checklist,[20,35,42,44,47] or the Behavioral Assessment Scale for Children.[23,46] In a survey of over 800 families using validated instruments,[15] symptoms of SDB were associated with hyperactive behaviors with a trend toward a dose–response relationship between reported snoring frequency and behavior. Only a small number of studies have failed to find associations with SDB and hyperactive behaviors.[48–50]

Inattention

Attention, which is a prerequisite to optimal learning, is a critical behavior arising from brain mechanisms and can be categorized as sustained, selective, and divided attention, thus representing a cluster of variables, each of which contributes to learning and memory. Inattentive behaviors identified by parental report have been observed in children with habitual snoring[15,21,37,51] and PSG-defined SDB[20,23,46–49] although this finding is not as robust as the associations with hyperactivity. Different categories of attention, for example, selective and sustained attention, can also be measured using objective assessments such as auditory or visual continuous performance tests (CPT) and therefore may provide more robust assessment than parental report. Such studies have shown that even children with mild SDB exhibit some deficits in attention compared to controls.[52–54]

A small study of Australian children found that both selective and sustained attention measured objectively using the auditory CPT were found to be impaired in children with habitual snoring compared to controls.[55] Similarly, in New Zealand, Galland et al.[56] found that in comparison to a normal population, children with objectively confirmed SDB, compared to those without, had significantly higher scores on a visual CPT for inattention and impulsivity albeit within the average range of a normal non-clinical score.

Impaired auditory and visual attention has also been reported in children with objectively confirmed SDB compared to standardized norms.[57] Recently, event-related potential (ERP) recordings using a high-density array during an oddball attention task have shown objective evidence of impaired attention in children with SDB.[58] Since ERP patterns strongly correlate with learning, reading and school performance, the authors postulated that their findings suggest that brain changes associated with pediatric SDB have the potential to be used to determine which children might require earlier diagnosis or treatment. Nonetheless, some studies fail to observe differences in visual attention.[46,59] Emancipator et al.[60] proposed that the CPT might either not be sufficiently sensitive in children who are not obviously sleepy or possibly, with the increase in time children now spend playing video games, such CPT tools might be less discriminating.

Aggressive Behaviors

In addition to hyperactivity and inattention, aggressive and bullying behaviors are beginning to receive more attention in the SDB literature. Estimates suggest that up to 25% of children in elementary schools are affected,[61] with a higher prevalence in boys.[62] Aggressive behaviors present a major challenge not only for schools, which often have local, state, and national programs to address this issue, but also for society, as aggressive children are at high risk for future psychiatric symptoms, violence, substance abuse, and criminality,[63] while the victims of bullying also suffer. Clearly, the causes of aggressive behaviors are complex and include social, biological, and cultural factors; however, there is now emerging evidence that sleep problems might play a role.

In a large population-based study of over 3000 5-year-old children, those with symptoms of SDB were twice as likely to have parentally reported aggressive behaviors,[33] which is similar to a study that also adjusted for comorbid hyperactivity and stimulant use.[64] A recent report from our group, the first specifically designed to query parents of aggressive elementary school children as well as non-aggressive controls about symptoms of SDB, found that aggressive children were twice as likely to have SDB symptoms compared to non-aggressive children.[22] Notably, daytime sleepiness rather than snoring appeared to drive the relationship with aggressive behavior, which suggests that other causes of daytime sleepiness, such as poor sleep hygiene, are also important.

Of note, short sleep duration – which perhaps might partially explain sleepiness – and sleep difficulties have been found to be associated with aggressive behaviors in young children[65,66] and suicidal ideation in adolescents.[67] In children with objectively confirmed SDB, aggressive behaviors are more frequent than in children without SDB[48] even when SDB is mild.[20] Children with aggressive behaviors also have EEG slowing during wakefulness,[68] which might reflect deficient levels of arousal or excessive daytime sleepiness, likely mediated via the prefrontal cortex.[69]

Parent versus Teacher Report of Behavior

There are conflicting findings on the association between SDB and behavior depending on whether behavioral reports are provided by parents or teachers. The literature regarding teacher reports is small compared to parental reports. Some studies report elevated hyperactive behaviors on both parent and teacher scales,[14,17,46] while others found only elevated hyperactive behaviors on parent scales.[23,37] Our own data have shown that teacher-reported bullying behaviors did not show associations with symptoms of SDB but parent reports did.[22]

Recently, Kohler et al.[70] performed a direct comparison of parent and teacher reports in children with SDB. They found that both parents and teachers report more problematic behavior, which is predominantly internalizing such as anxious and withdrawn behavior, somatic complaints, and social and affective problems. In addition, parents reported a greater severity and range of behaviors. Overall, the concordance for individual children was poor. The limited number of studies that have collected teacher reports, the different tools used, and the sample sizes involved make it difficult to reach conclusions regarding classroom behavior. However, despite the inconsistencies, the teacher-report studies published to date appear to support a role for SDB in at least some areas of behavioral regulation.

SDB and ADHD

Attention deficit hyperactivity disorder (ADHD) is the most commonly diagnosed pediatric mental health disorder in North America, and sleep problems are one of the most frequently reported comorbidities in these children. The major features of ADHD (e.g., inattention, hyperactivity, and impulsivity) are also frequent manifestations of childhood SDB and, conversely, comorbid sleep problems are highly prevalent in ADHD. Therefore it is unsurprising that the relationship between SDB and ADHD is of great interest. Multiple studies have shown that children with ADHD demonstrate a number of parentally reported sleep problems,[71-74] with a frequency up to five times greater than that of otherwise healthy children.[75] Children with ADHD have been reported to snore more than their peers,[76,77] with some studies suggesting that snoring is more common in those with the hyperactive/impulsive subtype of ADHD.[78] However, polysomnographic data are less clear in terms of an association between SDB and ADHD.[79]

Methodological issues may be at least in part related to such inconsistencies, particularly since the majority of studies did not use criteria from the diagnostic and statistical manual of mental disorders (DSM) for ADHD but instead relied on parental report of hyperactivity symptoms. In one study of school-aged children that did use formal criteria, diagnoses of ADHD were found in almost a third of children.[53] However, a recent meta-analysis,[25] which included studies utilizing rigorous criteria for ADHD, suggested that the apnea–hypopnea index (AHI) in the three objective studies retained in the meta-analysis[80-82] were not very elevated (1.0, 5.8, and 3.57, respectively). Nonetheless, using a pediatric AHI threshold of 1,[83] these values suggest that SDB may indeed be more frequent in children with ADHD compared to controls. Interestingly, children with ADHD and an AHI between 1 and 5 have been reported to improve more following adenotonsillectomy than after stimulant treatment.[26,84] This raises questions about appropriate screening and intervention in these children. A recent working group report has suggested key areas for future research in this field.[85]

COGNITION

Studies of the associations between SDB and behavioral deficits are vast and demonstrate robust associations[86,87] but the cognitive impact of SDB is less well understood. Cognition is a mental act or process by which knowledge is acquired, including awareness, perception, intuition, and reasoning. It is often used interchangeably with intelligence; however, cognitive processes can be influenced by intelligence and generally show an age-dependent performance increase whereas intelligence typically refers to developmental differences between individuals.[88] Lower-order cognitive processes, which include perceptual motor learning, visual short-term memory, and selective attention, can be measured by tasks such as reaction times or problem solving. Intelligence, on the other hand, is indirectly inferred typically via psychometric testing. A detailed discussion of the associations between sleep, cognition, and intelligence can be found in a recent article.[89]

One of the fundamental roles of sleep is believed to involve learning, memory consolidation, and brain plasticity;[90] thus, sleep disruption has the potential to impair cognition during wake. Indeed several studies – but not all[91] – find differences in cognition of children with and without SDB. Of note, however, the vast majority of studies in this area are from a limited age range, often elementary school age, thus limiting the conclusions that can be drawn.

Intelligence

The intelligence quotient (IQ) is often reported in studies of SDB although findings are not consistent. Lower IQ scores have been reported in children with SDB compared to controls, although these scores are typically still within the normal range.[19,21,49,50,55,59,92–96] One study in children awaiting adenotonsillectomy found that compared to healthy non-snoring children, the snoring children had a 10-point reduction in IQ.[95] Of course, the clinical significance of this remains to be shown for a high-functioning child, but a 10-point IQ difference could be rather significant in children performing at a lower level. Several studies fail to support findings of differences in full-scale IQ,[44,91,97,98] although some have found lower scores for verbal IQ (language skills) in children with SDB.[44,97]

Lack of robust findings between SDB and IQ is perhaps not surprising given that measurement of IQ is complex and, in essence, measures performance across several tasks rather than a focus on a particular area of cognition. Standardized vocabulary tests, as a proxy measure of IQ and an excellent predictor of cognition and academic success,[99] have demonstrated that the difference in scores between children with and without SDB may be equivalent to the impact of lead exposure.[100] These findings clearly have great clinical significance for a child's future if indeed they are supported by additional studies. Nonetheless, there are many other factors which clearly impact a child's IQ and which require consideration in studies of SDB, including genetics, parental education level, as well as biological and environmental factors.[23,101,102]

Memory

Multiple studies have failed to find evidence for memory impairment in children with SDB.[21,49,103] In those that have reported memory deficits[50,55,104] only one has reported a dose-response effect.[105] Inconsistencies in memory findings are likely related to the type of memory measured (such as verbal memory or working memory). In addition, many reports provide only a cumulative memory score rather than address specific processes involved in memory acquisition.

A recent study of memory recall in children with and without SDB[104] found that memory recall to a picture was impaired in children at both an immediate memory assessment as well as a follow-up assessment the following day. Notably, the children with SDB also demonstrated declines in recall performance, which suggests that children with SDB require more time and additional learning opportunities to reach immediate and longer-term recall performance and that these children may have slower information processing and/or secondary memory problems perhaps due to inefficient encoding.[106] Indeed, changes in basic perceptual processes that underlie higher-order functions have been shown to be impaired in pediatric SDB even when performance is not altered on standard measures of memory.[107]

Academic Performance

Good academic performance is often essential for future career success and many studies have reported on deficits in academic performance in children with SDB. The term 'academic performance' encompasses a range of achievements/abilities and it can be assessed by various means including mathematical abilities, spelling, reading, writing, and overall school grade. In a landmark study of first-grade children, Gozal[16] found a 6–9-fold increase in gas-exchange abnormalities in the lowest-performing tenth percentile.

Several studies have reported lower grades in mathematics, spelling, reading, and science[51,108,109] in children with SDB compared to controls, even when intermittent hypoxemia is absent,[110] which suggests that primary snoring may impact academic achievement. It is also possible that the presence of hypoxemia may affect the threshold of respiratory events associated with performance deficits, as the threshold for respiratory disturbances associated with learning problems may be lower in the presence of hypoxemia.[111] For example, in the absence of hypoxemia, a respiratory disturbance index >5 has been associated with parent-report of learning problems in young children; however, when the presence of hypoxemia was used to define the respiratory event, a respiratory disturbance index >1 was associated with learning problems.[111] Children with SDB have also been found to perform lower than controls on a phonological processing test,[49,112] which measures phonological awareness, a skill that is critical for learning to read. In addition, processes mentioned earlier[106,107] that may underlie memory encoding and storage will also impact academic performance.

We should also be reminded that the vast majority of current literature focuses on young school-aged children and does not include adolescents, a unique developmental stage where challenges differ considerably from young children and where any SDB-associated behavioral difficulties may result in significant impairment in school performance at a critical time for future success.[23] In addition to verbal problems, poor academic achievement may also be affected by inattention difficulties due to the complex brain associations involved. Measurement of school performance is inherently difficult, and the role of SDB difficult to tease out, as it really represents a number of factors, which include age, SES, home environment, genetics, behavior, and cognition.[23] Unsurprisingly, when some of the latter variables are accounted for, a number of studies fail to find evidence of an association between SDB and academic performance.[50,60,113,114]

Executive Functions

Executive function encompasses cognitive processes, including memory, planning, problem solving, verbal reasoning, inhibition, mental flexibility, and multi-tasking that are crucial for normal psychological and social development. Executive function is complex and it is difficult to isolate certain executive functions from other cognitive abilities; despite this, executive dysfunction is often reported in children with SDB compared to controls.[44,46,57,93] A recent study in snoring preschool children found substantially lower performance on executive function dimensions such as inhibition, working memory, and planning compared to controls,[115] which highlights the need to identify SDB risk in very young children.

CAUSALITY

The vast majority of studies to date provide cross-sectional data on associations between SDB and learning and behavior. Clearly such cross-sectional data cannot prove that SDB causes the observed deficits. Evidence for causality can only be provided by data from randomized, controlled intervention trials. To date, none have been published although a multi-center randomized, controlled trial is currently underway.[116] However, a number of longitudinal and treatment intervention studies have been published, which are described in the following paragraphs.

Longitudinal Evidence
The vast majority of published studies report cross-sectional findings, which while important, provide no information on the direction of the proposed relationships. Data from a case-control study of seventh- and eighth-grade children with poor school performance have demonstrated that these children were more likely than others in their grades to have snored frequently and loudly during their early childhood.[117] In a prospective 4-year follow-up study, snoring and symptoms of SDB were strong risk factors for the future development or exacerbation of hyperactive behaviors, with habitual snoring at baseline increasing the risk for hyperactivity at follow-up by more than fourfold, especially in boys. Results were independent of hyperactivity at baseline and stimulant use as well as SDB symptoms at follow-up.

In support of these findings, a recent study from the Avon Longitudinal Study of Parents and Children[118] examined the effects of snoring, apnea, and mouth-breathing patterns on behavior, from infancy through 7 years in more than 11 000 children. By 4 years, symptomatic children were 20–60% more likely to exhibit behavioral difficulties consistent with a clinical diagnosis; by 7 years, they were 40–100% more likely, even after controlling for 15 major confounders.[41] Furthermore, SDB effects at 4 years were as predictive of behavioral difficulties at 7 years, and the worst symptoms were associated with the worst behavioral outcomes, with hyperactivity being most affected. Taken together, these findings suggest that damage done years earlier may be visible as a behavioral phenotype only years later, and alludes to the belief that there may be a 'window of vulnerability' in developing humans.

Treatment Interventions
In one of the first intervention studies, first-grade children in the lowest tenth percentile were screened for SDB and parents were advised to seek treatment if their child had gas-exchange abnormalities.[16] Children's school grades were obtained in first grade and also during follow-up in second grade; children who had evidence of SDB and had received treatment had significantly improved school grades, whereas those who had declined treatment did not have significant improvement. The same group[117] showed that middle-school children with academic performance in the lowest 25% of their class were more likely to have snored during their preschool years and to have required adenotonsillectomy for snoring compared with schoolmates in the top 25% of class.

In the past decade, there have been a number of treatment intervention studies, typically adenotonsillectomy, showing that cognitive function appears to improve at follow-up, approximately 6–12 months later on multiple subtests including general conceptual ability, verbal and non-verbal ability, phonological processing and naming,[119] IQ,[120] attention, as measured by continuous performance assessment,[53,17] visual attention and processing speed,[121] matrix analogies, sequential and simultaneous processing scales, and mental processing scales,[122] with medium to large effect sizes.[122]

However, not all studies report significant improvement in cognitive measures following treatment.[56,123] A recent study from Australia showed a wide range of cognitive deficits in 3–12-year-old children at baseline, including IQ, language and executive function which did not improve to control levels following adenotonsillectomy.[95] The magnitude of the deficits persisted at the 6-month follow-up with a mean full-scale IQ difference of 10 points between children with SDB and controls. Of particular note, the fluid reasoning, knowledge, quantitative reasoning, visuospatial and working memory composite scores, as well as corresponding verbal and nonverbal subtest scores, were all significantly reduced in children with SDB compared to controls at both baseline and follow-up. In addition, composite scores for attention/executive function (specifically planning, inhibition, auditory and visual attention), language (phonological processing), sensorimotor function and memory (especially narrative memory) were significantly reduced in children with SDB at both baseline and follow-up. The finding that measures of executive function remain significantly lower in children with SDB following adenotonsillectomy is supported by another study,[121] although mean postoperative scores in the latter study were lower than preoperative scores.

Lack of improvement post adenotonsillectomy may be somewhat unexpected given the increasing number of studies showing improvement towards control levels. However, it should be noted that children undergoing adenotonsillectomy for non-SDB reasons as well as SDB perform worse on specific cognitive measures such as short-term attention, visuospatial ability, memory, and arithmetic academic achievement compared to control children.[124] Interestingly, children without SDB had more consistent as well as larger deficits compared to those with SDB. At 12-month follow-up measures of verbal abstraction ability, arithmetic calculations, visual and verbal learning, verbal delayed recall, sustained attention, and another measure of visual delayed recall demonstrated declines in ability, measures of executive function and academic performance improved, while other measures did not improve over time.[125] The authors suggested that their findings question the expectation that adenotonsillectomy resolves the majority of deficits in children with SDB, which has the potential to translate into significant life-time impact later in life.

Despite the persuasive arguments above, it should be noted that there are some arguments against a causal relationship between SDB, behavior and cognition. Importantly, as discussed earlier, there is no consistent phenotype, there is a lack of expected relationships as well as dose–response across studies, and the response to treatment is not entirely clear. In addition, there is added complexity that arises from the developmental context in which these studies are conducted, as compensatory mechanisms to an insult may occur in these children.

POTENTIAL MECHANISMS

The most plausible mechanisms of behavioral and cognitive deficits in children with SDB include intermittent hypoxia and sleep fragmentation, the two main components of SDB which likely impact the prefrontal cortex. The importance of executive dysfunction and the involvement of the prefrontal cortex in SDB have been reviewed[126] and a model linking sleep disruption, hypoxemia, and disruption of the prefrontal cortex was proposed. The prefrontal cortex is believed to play a critical role in the regulation of arousal, sleep, affect, and attention in children.[127] Indeed, disturbances of prefrontal inhibitory functions have been implicated in deficits observed in children with ADHD,[128] and neuroimaging studies in ADHD have supported specific impairments in prefrontal cortical functioning.[129,130]

Hypoxemia even in the absence of SDB is known to impact cognition.[131] Animal models demonstrate that intermittent hypoxia during sleep induces neuronal cell loss and impairs spatial memory[132–134] and that early development might be a particularly vulnerable time.[135] Interestingly, data from a brain imaging study have shown that neuronal metabolites are altered in children with SDB in the hippocampal and right frontal cortical regions,[93] the very areas that are implicated in executive function and cognition.

Similarly, sleep fragmentation or deprivation does not only affect those with SDB and such disruption in the absence of SDB has also been shown to impact behavior and cognition in several adult studies.[136–139] In a recent pediatric study, children with daytime sleepiness were significantly more likely to have hyperactivity, inattention, and conduct problems as well as worse measures of processing speed and working memory.[140] In addition, we have shown that aggressive elementary school children were more likely to have daytime sleepiness than their peers.[22] Sleep disruption has been associated with inflammatory markers,[141–143] and rodent models have shown associations with sleep deprivation and oxidative stress,[144] hippocampal-dependent learning,[145,146] and dysfunction of systems that are involved in learning, goal direction, and attention.[147]

SUMMARY

There is now a wealth of robust data that supports a role for SDB in behavioral deficits in children, as well as less consistent evidence to support its role in cognitive deficits. Current data are mixed with regards to the reversibility of such dysfunction with treatment, perhaps due to brain plasticity or genetic/environmental interactions. Despite the current lack of definitive data in the form of randomized, controlled trials, in light of increasing cross-sectional and intervention studies, it would appear pertinent to ensure that education and awareness regarding SDB reaches healthcare providers, parents, and indeed, children themselves.

Clinical Pearls

- Habitual snoring and obstructive sleep apnea are associated with neurobehavioral morbidity in children.
- Insults may manifest phenotypically years later suggestive of a window of vulnerability in developing children.
- Treatment interventions such as adenotonsillectomy may at least partially reverse some of the neurobehavioral deficits.

References

1. Lumeng JC, Chervin RD. Epidemiology of pediatric obstructive sleep apnea. Proc Am Thorac Soc 2008;5(2):242–52.
2. McKenzie M. A manual of diseases of the throat and nose, including the pharynx, larynx, trachea oesophagus, nasal cavities, and neck. London: Churchill; 1880.
3. Guilleminault C, Eldridge FL, Simmons FB, et al. Sleep apnea in eight children. Pediatrics 1976;58(1):23–30.
4. Rosen CL, D'Andrea L, Haddad GG. Adult criteria for obstructive sleep apnea do not identify children with serious obstruction. Am Rev Respir Dis 1992;146(5 Pt 1):1231–4.
5. Carroll JL, Loughlin GM. Diagnostic criteria for obstructive sleep apnea syndrome in children. Pediatr Pulmonol 1992;14(2):71–4.
6. Carroll JL, McColley SA, Marcus CL, et al. Inability of clinical history to distinguish primary snoring from obstructive sleep apnea syndrome in children. Chest 1995;108(3):610–18.
7. Brouillette RT, Morielli A, Leimanis A, et al. Nocturnal pulse oximetry as an abbreviated testing modality for pediatric obstructive sleep apnea. Pediatrics 2000;105(2):405–12.
8. Sivan Y, Kornecki A, Schonfeld T. Screening obstructive sleep apnoea syndrome by home videotape recording in children. Eur Respir J 1996;9(10):2127–31.
9. Lamm C, Mandeli J, Kattan M. Evaluation of home audiotapes as an abbreviated test for obstructive sleep apnea syndrome (OSAS) in children. Pediatr Pulmonol 1999;27(4):267–72.
10. O'Brien LM, Gozal D. Potential usefulness of noninvasive autonomic monitoring in recognition of arousals in normal healthy children. J Clin Sleep Med 2007;3(1):41–7.
11. Schnall RP, Shlitner A, Sheffy J, et al. Periodic, profound peripheral vasoconstriction – a new marker of obstructive sleep apnea. Sleep 1999;22(7):939–46.
12. Chervin RD, Burns JW, Subotic NS, et al. Method for detection of respiratory cycle-related EEG changes in sleep-disordered breathing. Sleep 2004;27(1):110–15.
13. Foo JY. Pulse transit time in paediatric respiratory sleep studies. Med Eng Phys 2007;29(1):17–25
14. Ali NJ, Pitson DJ, Stradling JR. Snoring, sleep disturbance, and behaviour in 4–5 year olds. Arch Dis Child 1993;68(3):360–6.
15. Chervin RD, Archbold KH, Dillon JE, et al. Inattention, hyperactivity, and symptoms of sleep-disordered breathing. Pediatrics 2002;109(3):449–56.
16. Gozal D. Sleep-disordered breathing and school performance in children. Pediatrics 1998;102(3 Pt 1):616–20.
17. Landau YE, Bar-Yishay O, Greenberg-Dotan S, et al. Impaired behavioral and neurocognitive function in preschool children with obstructive sleep apnea. Pediatr Pulmonol 2012;47(2):180–8.
18. Scullin MH, Ornelas C, Montgomery-Downs HE. Risk for sleep-disordered breathing and home and classroom behavior in Hispanic preschoolers. Behav Sleep Med 2011;9(3):194–207.
19. Bourke R, Anderson V, Yang JS, et al. Cognitive and academic functions are impaired in children with all severities of sleep-disordered breathing. Sleep Med 2011;12(5):489–96.
20. Bourke RS, Anderson V, Yang JS, et al. Neurobehavioral function is impaired in children with all severities of sleep disordered breathing. Sleep Med 2011;12(3):222–9.

21. O'Brien LM, Mervis CB, Holbrook CR, et al. Neurobehavioral implications of habitual snoring in children. Pediatrics 2004;114(1):44–9.
22. O'Brien LM, Lucas NH, Felt BT, et al. Aggressive behavior, bullying, snoring, and sleepiness in schoolchildren. Sleep Med 2011;12(7):652–8.
23. Beebe DW, Ris MD, Kramer ME, et al. The association between sleep disordered breathing, academic grades, and cognitive and behavioral functioning among overweight subjects during middle to late childhood. Sleep 2010;33(11):1447–56.
24. Owens JA. Neurocognitive and behavioral impact of sleep disordered breathing in children. Pediatr Pulmonol 2009;44(5):417–22.
25. Cortese S, Faraone SV, Konofal E, et al. Sleep in children with attention-deficit/hyperactivity disorder: meta-analysis of subjective and objective studies. J Am Acad Child Adolesc Psychiatry 2009;48(9):894–908.
26. Dillon JE, Blunden S, Ruzicka DL, et al. DSM-IV diagnoses and obstructive sleep apnea in children before and 1 year after adenotonsillectomy. J Am Acad Child Adolesc Psychiatry 2007;46(11):1425–36.
27. Crabtree VM, Varni JW, Gozal D. Health-related quality of life and depressive symptoms in children with suspected sleep-disordered breathing. Sleep 2004;27(6):1131–8.
28. Aronen ET, Paavonen EJ, Fjallberg M, et al. Sleep and psychiatric symptoms in school-age children. J Am Acad Child Adolesc Psychiatry 2000;39(4):502–8.
29. O'Brien LM, Gozal D. Autonomic dysfunction in children with sleep-disordered breathing. Sleep 2005;28(6):747–52.
30. Gozal D, Kheirandish-Gozal L, Bhattacharjee R, et al. Neurocognitive and endothelial dysfunction in children with obstructive sleep apnea. Pediatrics 2010;126(5):e1161–7.
31. Bixler EO, Vgontzas AN, Lin HM, et al. Blood pressure associated with sleep-disordered breathing in a population sample of children. Hypertension 2008;52(5):841–6.
32. Horne RS, Yang JS, Walter LM, et al. Elevated blood pressure during sleep and wake in children with sleep-disordered breathing. Pediatrics 2011;128(1):e85–92.
33. Gottlieb DJ, Vezina RM, Chase C, et al. Symptoms of sleep-disordered breathing in 5-year-old children are associated with sleepiness and problem behaviors. Pediatrics 2003;112(4):870–7.
34. Beebe DW, Wells CT, Jeffries J, et al. Neuropsychological effects of pediatric obstructive sleep apnea. J Int Neuropsychol Soc 2004;10(7):962–75.
35. Rosen CL, Storfer-Isser A, Taylor HG, et al. Increased behavioral morbidity in school-aged children with sleep-disordered breathing. Pediatrics 2004;114(6):1640–8.
36. Brockmann PE, Urschitz MS, Schlaud M, et al. Primary snoring in school children: prevalence and neurocognitive impairments. Sleep Breath 2012;16(1):23–9.
37. Arman AR, Ersu R, Save D, et al. Symptoms of inattention and hyperactivity in children with habitual snoring: evidence from a community-based study in Istanbul. Child Care Health Dev 2005;31(6):707–17.
38. Urschitz MS, Eitner S, Guenther A, et al. Habitual snoring, intermittent hypoxia, and impaired behavior in primary school children. Pediatrics 2004;114(4):1041–8.
39. Fagnano M, van Wijngaarden E, Connolly HV, et al. Sleep-disordered breathing and behaviors of inner-city children with asthma. Pediatrics 2009;124(1):218–25.
40. Chervin RD, Dillon JE, Bassetti C, et al. Symptoms of sleep disorders, inattention, and hyperactivity in children. Sleep 1997;20(12):1185–92.
41. Bonuck K, Freeman K, Chervin RD, et al. Sleep-disordered breathing in a population-based cohort: behavioral outcomes at 4 and 7 years. Pediatrics 2012;129(4):e857–65.
42. Zhao Q, Sherrill DL, Goodwin JL, et al. Association between sleep disordered breathing and behavior in school-aged children: The Tucson Children's Assessment of Sleep Apnea Study. Open Epidemiol J 2008;1:1–9.
43. Melendres MC, Lutz JM, Rubin ED, et al. Daytime sleepiness and hyperactivity in children with suspected sleep-disordered breathing. Pediatrics 2004;114(3):768–75.
44. Lewin DS, Rosen RC, England SJ, et al. Preliminary evidence of behavioral and cognitive sequelae of obstructive sleep apnea in children. Sleep Med 2002;3(1):5–13.
45. O'Brien LM, Holbrook CR, Mervis CB, et al. Sleep and neurobehavioral characteristics of 5- to 7-year-old children with parentally reported symptoms of attention-deficit/hyperactivity disorder. Pediatrics 2003;111(3):554–63.
46. Beebe DW, Wells CT, Jeffries J, et al. Neuropsychological effects of pediatric obstructive sleep apnea. J Int Neuropsychol Soc 2004;10(7):962–75.
47. Ting H, Wong RH, Yang HJ, et al. Sleep-disordered breathing, behavior, and academic performance in Taiwan schoolchildren. Sleep Breath 2011;15(1):91–8.
48. Mulvaney SA, Goodwin JL, Morgan WJ, et al. Behavior problems associated with sleep disordered breathing in school-aged children – the Tucson children's assessment of sleep apnea study. J Pediatr Psychol 2006;31(3):322–30.
49. O'Brien LM, Mervis CB, Holbrook CR, et al. Neurobehavioral correlates of sleep-disordered breathing in children. J Sleep Res 2004;13(2):165–72.
50. Kaemingk KL, Pasvogel AE, Goodwin JL, et al. Learning in children and sleep disordered breathing: findings of the Tucson Children's Assessment of Sleep Apnea (tuCASA) prospective cohort study. J Int Neuropsychol Soc 2003;9(7):1016–26.
51. Kim JK, Lee JH, Lee SH, et al. School performance and behavior of Korean elementary school students with sleep-disordered breathing. Ann Otol Rhinol Laryngol 2011;120(4):268–72.
52. Blunden S, Lushington K, Kennedy D, et al. Behavior and neurocognitive performance in children aged 5–10 years who snore compared to controls. J Clin Exp Neuropsychol 2000;22(5):554–68.
53. Chervin RD, Ruzicka DL, Giordani BJ, et al. Sleep-disordered breathing, behavior, and cognition in children before and after adenotonsillectomy. Pediatrics 2006;117(4):e769–78.
54. Galland BC, Dawes PJ, Tripp EG, et al. Changes in behavior and attentional capacity after adenotonsillectomy. Pediatr Res 2006;59(5):711–16.
55. Kennedy JD, Blunden S, Hirte C, et al. Reduced neurocognition in children who snore. Pediatr Pulmonol 2004;37(4):330–7.
56. Galland BC, Dawes PJ, Tripp EG, et al. Changes in behavior and attentional capacity after adenotonsillectomy. Pediatr Res 2006;59(5):711–16.
57. Archbold KH, Giordani B, Ruzicka DL, et al. Cognitive executive dysfunction in children with mild sleep-disordered breathing. Biol Res Nurs 2004;5(3):168–76.
58. Barnes ME, Gozal D, Molfese DL. Attention in children with obstructive sleep apnoea: an event-related potentials study. Sleep Med 2012;13(4):368–77.
59. Gottlieb DJ, Chase C, Vezina RM, et al. Sleep-disordered breathing symptoms are associated with poorer cognitive function in 5-year-old children. J Pediatr 2004;145(4):458–64.
60. Emancipator JL, Storfer-Isser A, Taylor HG, et al. Variation of cognition and achievement with sleep-disordered breathing in full-term and preterm children. Arch Pediatr Adolesc Med 2006;160(2):203–10.
61. Nansel TR, Overpeck M, Pilla RS, et al. Bullying behaviors among US youth: prevalence and association with psychosocial adjustment. JAMA 2001;285(16):2094–100.
62. Boulton MJ, Underwood K. Bully/victim problems among middle school children. Br J Educ Psychol 1992;62(Pt 1):73–87.
63. Kumpulainen K, Rasanen E. Children involved in bullying at elementary school age: their psychiatric symptoms and deviance in adolescence. An epidemiological sample. Child Abuse Negl 2000;24(12):1567–77.
64. Chervin RD, Dillon JE, Archbold KH, et al. Conduct problems and symptoms of sleep disorders in children. J Am Acad Child Adolesc Psychiatry 2003;42(2):201–8.
65. Komada Y, Abe T, Okajima I, et al. Short sleep duration and irregular bedtime are associated with increased behavioral problems among Japanese preschool-age children. Tohoku J Exp Med 2011;224(2):127–36.
66. Ivanenko A, Crabtree VM, Obrien LM, et al. Sleep complaints and psychiatric symptoms in children evaluated at a pediatric mental health clinic. J Clin Sleep Med 2006;2(1):42–8.
67. Wong MM, Brower KJ, Zucker RA. Sleep problems, suicidal ideation, and self-harm behaviors in adolescence. J Psychiatr Res 2011;45(4):505–11.
68. Forssman H. Electroencephalograms of boys with behavior disorders. Acta Psychiatr Neurol Scand 1953;28:61–73.
69. Thomas M, Belenky G, Holcomb H, et al. Neural basis of alertness and cognitive performance impairments during sleepiness. I. Effects of 24 h of sleep deprivation on waking human regional brain activity. J Sleep Res 2000;9(4):335–52.
70. Kohler MJ, Kennedy JD, Martin AJ, et al. Parent versus teacher report of daytime behavior in snoring children. Sleep Breath 2013;17(2):637–45.
71. Gaultney JF, Terrell DF, Gingras JL. Parent-reported periodic limb movement, sleep disordered breathing, bedtime resistance behaviors, and ADHD. Behav Sleep Med 2005;3(1):32–43.
72. Corkum P, Tannock R, Moldofsky H. Sleep disturbances in children with attention-deficit/hyperactivity disorder. J Am Acad Child Adolesc Psychiatry 1998;37(6):637–46.

73. Sung V, Hiscock H, Sciberras E, et al. Sleep problems in children with attention-deficit/hyperactivity disorder: prevalence and the effect on the child and family. Arch Pediatr Adolesc Med 2008;162(4):336–42.

74. Owens JA, Maxim R, Nobile C, et al. Parental and self-report of sleep in children with attention-deficit/hyperactivity disorder. Arch Pediatr Adolesc Med 2000;154(6):549–55.

75. Corkum P, Tannock R, Moldofsky H. Sleep disturbances in children with attention-deficit/hyperactivity disorder. J Am Acad Child Adolesc Psychiatry 1998;37(6):637–46.

76. Rodopman-Arman A, Perdahli-Fis N, Ekinci O, et al. Sleep habits, parasomnias and associated behaviors in school children with attention deficit hyperactivity disorder (ADHD). Turk J Pediatr 2011;53(4): 397–403.

77. Gau SS, Chiang HL. Sleep problems and disorders among adolescents with persistent and subthreshold attention-deficit/hyperactivity disorders. Sleep 2009;32(5):671–9.

78. LeBourgeois MK, Avis K, Mixon M, et al. Snoring, sleep quality, and sleepiness across attention-deficit/hyperactivity disorder subtypes. Sleep 2004;27(3):520–5.

79. Sadeh A, Pergamin L, Bar-Haim Y. Sleep in children with attention-deficit/hyperactivity disorder: a meta-analysis of polysomnographic studies. Sleep Med Rev 2006;10(6):381–98.

80. Huang YS, Chen NH, Li HY, et al. Sleep disorders in Taiwanese children with attention deficit/hyperactivity disorder. J Sleep Res 2004;13(3):269–77.

81. Cooper J, Tyler L, Wallace I, et al. No evidence of sleep apnea in children with attention deficit hyperactivity disorder. Clin Pediatr (Phila) 2004;43(7):609–14.

82. Golan N, Pillar G. [The relationship between attention deficit hyperactivity disorder and sleep-alertness problems]. Harefuah 2004;143(9):675–80, 693.

83. Chervin RD. How many children with ADHD have sleep apnea or periodic leg movements on polysomnography? Sleep 2005;28(9): 1041–2.

84. Huang YS, Guilleminault C, Li HY, et al. Attention-deficit/hyperactivity disorder with obstructive sleep apnea: a treatment outcome study. Sleep Med 2007;8(1):18–30.

85. Owens J, Gruber R, Brown T, et al. Future research directions in sleep and ADHD: report of a consensus working group. J Atten Disord 2013;17(7):550–64.

86. Beebe DW. Neurobehavioral morbidity associated with disordered breathing during sleep in children: a comprehensive review. Sleep 2006;29(9):1115–34.

87. O'Brien L. Neurocognitive and behavioral consequences of sleep disordered breathing in children. In: Ivanenko A, editor. Sleep and psychiatric disorders in children and adolescents. New York: Informa Healthcare USA, Inc.; 2008. p. 149–61.

88. Anderson M. Marrying intelligence and cognition – a developmental view. New York: Cambridge University Press; 2005.

89. Geiger A, Achermann P, Jenni OG. Sleep, intelligence and cognition in a developmental context: differentiation between traits and state-dependent aspects. Prog Brain Res 2010;185:167–79.

90. Walker MP. The role of sleep in cognition and emotion. Ann NY Acad Sci 2009;1156:168–97.

91. Calhoun SL, Mayes SD, Vgontzas AN, et al. No relationship between neurocognitive functioning and mild sleep disordered breathing in a community sample of children. J Clin Sleep Med 2009;5(3):228–34.

92. Blunden S, Lushington K, Kennedy D, et al. Behavior and neurocognitive performance in children aged 5–10 years who snore compared to controls. J Clin Exp Neuropsychol 2000;22(5):554–68.

93. Halbower AC, Degaonkar M, Barker PB, et al. Childhood obstructive sleep apnea associates with neuropsychological deficits and neuronal brain injury. PLoS Med 2006;3(8):e301.

94. Suratt PM, Peruggia M, D'Andrea L, et al. Cognitive function and behavior of children with adenotonsillar hypertrophy suspected of having obstructive sleep-disordered breathing. Pediatrics 2006;118(3): e771–81.

95. Kohler MJ, Lushington K, van den Heuvel CJ, et al. Adenotonsillectomy and neurocognitive deficits in children with sleep disordered breathing. PLoS One 2009;4(10):e7343.

96. Miano S, Paolino MC, Urbano A, et al. Neurocognitive assessment and sleep analysis in children with sleep-disordered breathing. Clin Neurophysiol 2011;122(2):311–19.

97. Aronen ET, Liukkonen K, Simola P, et al. Mood is associated with snoring in preschool-aged children. J Dev Behav Pediatr 2009;30(2): 107–14.

98. Hill CM, Hogan AM, Onugha N, et al. Increased cerebral blood flow velocity in children with mild sleep-disordered breathing: a possible association with abnormal neuropsychological function. Pediatrics 2006;118(4):e1100–8.

99. Lezak MD, Howieson DB, Loring DW. Neuropsychological assessment. 4th ed. New York: Oxford University Press; 2004.

100. Suratt PM, Barth JT, Diamond R, et al. Reduced time in bed and obstructive sleep-disordered breathing in children are associated with cognitive impairment. Pediatrics 2007;119(2):320–9.

101. Montgomery-Downs HE, Jones VF, Molfese VJ, et al. Snoring in preschoolers: associations with sleepiness, ethnicity, and learning. Clin Pediatr (Phila) 2003;42(8):719–26.

102. Spruyt K, Gozal D. A mediation model linking body weight, cognition, and sleep disordered breathing. Am J Respir Crit Care Med 2012; 185(2):199–205.

103. Blunden S, Lushington K, Lorenzen B, et al. Neuropsychological and psychosocial function in children with a history of snoring or behavioral sleep problems. J Pediatr 2005;146(6):780–6.

104. Kheirandish-Gozal L, De Jong MR, Spruyt K, et al. Obstructive sleep apnoea is associated with impaired pictorial memory task acquisition and retention in children. Eur Respir J 2010;36(1):164–9.

105. Rhodes SK, Shimoda KC, Waid LR, et al. Neurocognitive deficits in morbidly obese children with obstructive sleep apnea. J Pediatr 1995;127(5):741–4.

106. Spruyt K, Capdevila OS, Kheirandish-Gozal L, et al. Inefficient or insufficient encoding as potential primary deficit in neurodevelopmental performance among children with OSA. Dev Neuropsychol 2009;34(5): 601–14.

107. Key AP, Molfese DL, O'Brien L, et al. Sleep-disordered breathing affects auditory processing in 5–7-year-old children: evidence from brain recordings. Dev Neuropsychol 2009;34(5):615–28.

108. Urschitz MS, Wolff J, Sokollik C, et al. Nocturnal arterial oxygen saturation and academic performance in a community sample of children. Pediatrics 2005;115(2):e204–9.

109. Ravid S, Afek I, Suraiya S, et al. Sleep disturbances are associated with reduced school achievements in first-grade pupils. Dev Neuropsychol 2009;34(5):574–87.

110. Urschitz MS, Guenther A, Eggebrecht E, et al. Snoring, intermittent hypoxia and academic performance in primary school children. Am J Respir Crit Care Med 2003;168(4):464–8.

111. Goodwin JL, Kaemingk KL, Fregosi RF, et al. Clinical outcomes associated with sleep-disordered breathing in Caucasian and Hispanic children – the Tucson Children's Assessment of Sleep Apnea study (TuCASA). Sleep 2003;26(5):587–91.

112. Lundeborg I, McAllister A, Samuelsson C, et al. Phonological development in children with obstructive sleep-disordered breathing. Clin Linguist Phon 2009;23(10):751–61.

113. Mayes SD, Calhoun SL, Bixler EO, et al. Nonsignificance of sleep relative to IQ and neuropsychological scores in predicting academic achievement. J Dev Behav Pediatr 2008;29(3):206–12.

114. Chervin RD, Clarke DF, Huffman JL, et al. School performance, race, and other correlates of sleep-disordered breathing in children. Sleep Med 2003;4(1):21–7.

115. Karpinski AC, Scullin MH, Montgomery-Downs HE. Risk for sleep-disordered breathing and executive function in preschoolers. Sleep Med 2008;9(4):418–24.

116. Redline S, Amin R, Beebe D, et al. The Childhood Adenotonsillectomy Trial (CHAT): rationale, design, and challenges of a randomized controlled trial evaluating a standard surgical procedure in a pediatric population. Sleep 2011;34(11):1509–17.

117. Gozal D, Pope DW Jr. Snoring during early childhood and academic performance at ages thirteen to fourteen years. Pediatrics 2001; 107(6):1394–9.

118. Golding J, Pembrey M, Jones R. ALSPAC – the Avon Longitudinal Study of Parents and Children. I. Study methodology. Paediatr Perinat Epidemiol 2001;15(1):74–87.

119. Montgomery-Downs HE, Crabtree VM, Gozal D. Cognition, sleep and respiration in at-risk children treated for obstructive sleep apnoea. Eur Respir J 2005;25(2):336–42.

120. Ezzat WF, Fawaz S, Abdelrazek Y. To what degree does adenotonsillectomy affect neurocognitive performance in children with obstructive sleep apnea hypopnea syndrome due to adenotonsillar enlargement? ORL J Otorhinolaryngol Relat Spec 2010;72(4):215–19.

121. Hogan AM, Hill CM, Harrison D, et al. Cerebral blood flow velocity and cognition in children before and after adenotonsillectomy. Pediatrics 2008;122(1):75–82.

122. Friedman BC, Hendeles-Amitai A, Kozminsky E, et al. Adenotonsillectomy improves neurocognitive function in children with obstructive sleep apnea syndrome. Sleep 15 2003;26(8):999–1005.
123. Li HY, Huang YS, Chen NH, et al. Impact of adenotonsillectomy on behavior in children with sleep-disordered breathing. Laryngoscope 2006;116(7):1142–7.
124. Giordani B, Hodges EK, Guire KE, et al. Neuropsychological and behavioral functioning in children with and without obstructive sleep apnea referred for tonsillectomy. J Int Neuropsychol Soc 2008;14(4):571–81.
125. Giordani B, Hodges EK, Guire KE, et al. Changes in neuropsychological and behavioral functioning in children with and without obstructive sleep apnea following tonsillectomy. J Int Neuropsychol Soc 25 2012: 1–11.
126. Beebe DW, Gozal D. Obstructive sleep apnea and the prefrontal cortex: towards a comprehensive model linking nocturnal upper airway obstruction to daytime cognitive and behavioral deficits. J Sleep Res 2002; 11(1):1–16.
127. Dahl RE. The impact of inadequate sleep on children's daytime cognitive function. Semin Pediatr Neurol 1996;3(1):44–50.
128. Chelune GJ, Ferguson W, Koon R, et al. Frontal lobe disinhibition in attention deficit disorder. Child Psychiatry Hum Dev 1986;16(4): 221–34.
129. Arnsten AF, Rubia K. Neurobiological circuits regulating attention, cognitive control, motivation, and emotion: disruptions in neurodevelopmental psychiatric disorders. J Am Acad Child Adolesc Psychiatry 2012;51(4):356–67.
130. Cortese S, Castellanos FX. Neuroimaging of attention-deficit/hyperactivity disorder: current neuroscience-informed perspectives for clinicians. Curr Psychiatry Rep 2012;14(5):568–78.
131. Bass JL, Corwin M, Gozal D, et al. The effect of chronic or intermittent hypoxia on cognition in childhood: a review of the evidence. Pediatrics 2004;114(3):805–16.
132. Gozal D, Daniel JM, Dohanich GP. Behavioral and anatomical correlates of chronic episodic hypoxia during sleep in the rat. J Neurosci 2001;21(7):2442–50.
133. Nair D, Dayyat EA, Zhang SX, et al. Intermittent hypoxia-induced cognitive deficits are mediated by NADPH oxidase activity in a murine model of sleep apnea. PLoS One 2011;6(5):e19847.
134. Row BW. Intermittent hypoxia and cognitive function: implications from chronic animal models. Adv Exp Med Biol 2007;618:51–67.
135. Row BW, Kheirandish L, Neville JJ, et al. Impaired spatial learning and hyperactivity in developing rats exposed to intermittent hypoxia. Pediatr Res 2002;52(3):449–53.
136. Steenari MR, Vuontela V, Paavonen EJ, et al. Working memory and sleep in 6- to 13-year-old schoolchildren. J Am Acad Child Adolesc Psychiatry 2003;42(1):85–92.
137. Sadeh A, Gruber R, Raviv A. The effects of sleep restriction and extension on school-age children: what a difference an hour makes. Child Dev 2003;74(2):444–55.
138. Sadeh A, Gruber R, Raviv A. Sleep, neurobehavioral functioning, and behavior problems in school-age children. Child Dev 2002;73(2): 405–17.
139. Randazzo AC, Muehlbach MJ, Schweitzer PK, et al. Cognitive function following acute sleep restriction in children ages 10–14. Sleep 1998;21(8):861–8.
140. Calhoun SL, Fernandez-Mendoza J, Vgontzas AN, et al. Learning, attention/hyperactivity, and conduct problems as sequelae of excessive daytime sleepiness in a general population study of young children. Sleep 2012;35(5):627–32.
141. Meier-Ewert HK, Ridker PM, Rifai N, et al. Effect of sleep loss on C-reactive protein, an inflammatory marker of cardiovascular risk. J Am Coll Cardiol 2004;43(4):678–83.
142. Vgontzas AN, Zoumakis E, Bixler EO, et al. Adverse effects of modest sleep restriction on sleepiness, performance, and inflammatory cytokines. J Clin Endocrinol Metab 2004;89(5):2119–26.
143. Clinton JM, Davis CJ, Zielinski MR, et al. Biochemical regulation of sleep and sleep biomarkers. J Clin Sleep Med 2011;7(5 Suppl):S38–42.
144. Silva RH, Abilio VC, Takatsu AL, et al. Role of hippocampal oxidative stress in memory deficits induced by sleep deprivation in mice. Neuropharmacology 2004;46(6):895–903.
145. Hairston IS, Little MT, Scanlon MD, et al. Sleep restriction suppresses neurogenesis induced by hippocampus-dependent learning. J Neurophysiol 2005;94(6):4224–33.
146. Nair D, Zhang SX, Ramesh V, et al. Sleep fragmentation induces cognitive deficits via nicotinamide adenine dinucleotide phosphate oxidase-dependent pathways in mouse. Am J Respir Crit Care Med 2011; 184(11):1305–12.
147. Hanlon EC, Andrzejewski ME, Harder BK, et al. The effect of REM sleep deprivation on motivation for food reward. Behav Brain Res 2005;163(1):58–69.

Cardiovascular Consequences of Obstructive Sleep Apnea

Abu Shamsuzzaman and Raouf Amin

INTRODUCTION

Our knowledge about the link between sleep-disordered breathing (SDB) and cardiovascular dysfunction in children has grown significantly in the last three decades.[1-4] Cardiovascular research in children with SDB has primarily focused on disease mechanisms and has been relatively limited on defining the end points that provide unequivocal evidence of cardiovascular morbidity. Nevertheless, small differences in cardiovascular functions between children with SDB and healthy controls have been described in more recent years. The clinical significance of these observations in terms of cardiovascular morbidity either during childhood or in adult life has yet to be delineated. It is also worth noting that the changes in structure and functions of the cardiovascular system are not universally observed across affected populations, with substantial variance occurring in the context of ethnic background, socioeconomic status and body habitus. Therefore, future research that focuses on better understanding the putative contributions of environmental factors, genetic variance, and socioeconomic conditions will be critical to reinforce and explain the observations made to date. This chapter will describe the most recent evidence-based understanding of cardiovascular dysfunction in children with SDB. Proposed hypothetical mechanisms of cardiovascular disease in SDB and evidence of end-organ damage in childhood SDB that have been investigated to date will be discussed (Figure 30-1).

NORMAL SLEEP AND CARDIOVASCULAR SYSTEM

Normal sleep is associated with cardiovascular and autonomic changes that exhibit sleep stage dependency.[5,6] Progressive reduction of heart rate (HR), blood pressure (BP) and stroke volume during non-rapid eye movement (NREM) sleep occurs synchronously with reduced sympathetic nervous system activity (SNA).[7] During REM sleep, sympathetic drive increases markedly with consequent increases in vascular resistance, resulting in elevations of BP and HR.[7] Although the exact significance of cyclical and rhythmic alterations in cardiovascular functions during NREM and REM sleep cycle remains unclear, it is believed to be critical for normal cardiovascular health.

Sleep-Disordered Breathing and the Cardiovascular System

Repetitive apneas during sleep disrupt the homeostatic balance of the cardiovascular and autonomic nervous systems.[8-10] Increased SNA during episodes of apnea is associated with increased systemic BP, pulmonary arterial pressure and left ventricular (LV) afterload (Figure 30-2).[9,11] Hypoxemia and

hypercapnia during SDB events are major contributors for chemoreflex-mediated increases in SNA and cardiovascular changes.[9] Negative intrathoracic pressures during upper airway obstruction in SDB events affect intrathoracic hemodynamics including LV transmural pressure and LV afterload.[12] LV relaxation and LV filling might also be affected by the exaggerated negative intrathoracic pressure swings.[13,14] In addition, negative intrathoracic pressure alters aortic pressure, inducing stretch of the aortic wall, activating aortic baroreceptors, and thus buffering sympathetic activation during obstructive apnea.[15,16] Upon resumption of breathing, increased venous return distends the right ventricle, reduces LV compliance due to leftward shift of the interventricular septum and thus alters LV diastolic filling.[12] Increased stroke volume upon resumption of breathing, at a time when systemic vascular resistance is highest, elicits further increases of BP. SDB events are commonly associated with arousals from sleep, although such might not be as frequent in young children. Nevertheless, arousal may also contribute to the acute increases in BP at termination of SDB events.[17] Repetitive nocturnal arousals cause sleep fragmentation that might also be associated with daytime cardiovascular dysfunction.

Mechanisms of Cardiovascular Diseases in SDB

A number of neural, inflammatory and hormonal abnormalities are evident in children with SDB. These are implicated in the initiation and progression of cardiac and vascular disease conditions.

Neural Mechanisms

Neural control of the circulation represents the integrated response to diverse reflexes including baroreflex, chemoreflex and low-pressure cardiopulmonary reflexes. The interaction between cardiovascular and respiratory variables constitutes an important influence on neurally mediated changes in cardiac and vascular control (Figure 30-3). Interactions between these reflexes in conditions of hypoxemia and hypercapnia during episodes of OSA are implicated as the primary mechanisms of cardiovascular dysfunction in children with SDB.

Chemoreflex and Cardiovascular System

The chemoreflexes exert profound effects on respiratory, autonomic and cardiovascular functions during apnea events.[18] The central chemoreceptors are widely distributed across the central nervous system, are preferentially situated in brainstem regions, and are vital for cardiorespiratory control.[19,20] The peripheral chemoreceptors are located within the carotid bodies that respond primarily to hypoxemia and hypercapnia to elicit hyperventilation, tachycardia, and increased sympathetic vasoconstrictor activity.[21,22] Activation of peripheral chemoreceptors as a result of cessation of airflow during OSA

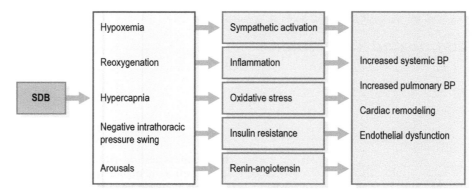

FIGURE 30-1 Mechanisms of Cardiovascular Disease in SDB. The schematic showing hypothetical mechanisms of cardiovascular diseases in SDB and cardiovascular dysfunction in children with SDB.

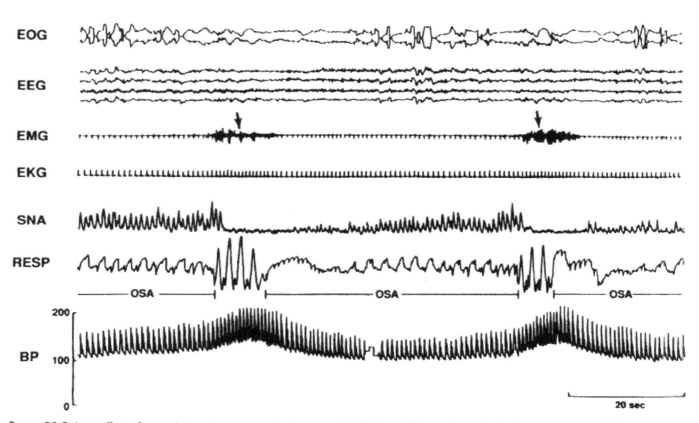

FIGURE 30-2 Acute effects of apnea during sleep on sympathetic nerve activity (SNA) and BP. Apnea is associated with progressive arterial deoxygenation and sympathetic activation. Resumption of breathing and arousal at the end apnea increases stroke volume and HR and consequent increase in arterial pressure. *From Somers VK, Dyken ME, Clary MP, Abboud FM. Sympathetic neural mechanisms in obstructive sleep apnea. J Clin Invest 1995;96(4):1897–904.*

elicits simultaneous activation of vascular sympathetic and cardiac vagal drives with consequent cardiac slowing and increased BP. Hypercapnia primarily acts through the central chemoreceptors in the brainstem, but also in part through the peripheral chemoreceptors, to produce hyperventilation and increased sympathetic traffic to peripheral blood vessels.[23] Interestingly, hypercapnia does not induce vagally mediated bradycardia as seen during hypoxia. Hypoxemia and hypercapnia administered simultaneously induce synergistic increases in minute ventilation.[24] Sympathetic activation is also greater during combined hypoxia and hypercapnia than the magnitude of the responses induced by either of the stimuli alone. During OSA, combined hypoxemic–hypercapnic stimuli potentiate the chemoreflex-mediated neural and circulatory responses. Hyperactivity of the peripheral chemoreceptors significantly contributes to the pathogenesis of hypertension in adult patients with OSA.[25] In addition, the peripheral chemoreceptors have a greater role in hypoxic responses in young children compared to adults, suggesting that attenuation of peripheral chemoreceptor function

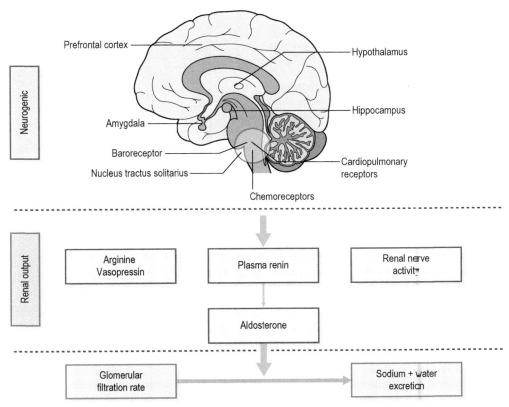

FIGURE 30-3 Interaction of baro- and chemoreflex for central nervous system control of the cardiovascular and renal system.

develops during maturation.[26] Thus, alterations in chemoreceptor-mediated responses in children with SDB and the effects of gas-exchange abnormalities on the developing brain, heart and kidney might be associated with increased risk of cardiovascular morbidity.

Baroreflex and Cardiovascular System

The baroreflex provides critical negative feedback control of arterial pressure.[18] Arterial baroreceptors are nerve endings innervating large arteries. Changes in arterial pressure in the aorta and carotid arteries alter the stretch status of the vessels, and result in changes in the frequency of baroreceptor inhibitory impulses to the brainstem cardiovascular centers. Increased baroreceptor activity during a rise in BP triggers reflex inhibition of sympathetic activity, parasympathetic activation, and subsequent decrease in vascular resistance and HR.[27,28] Conversely, a decrease in arterial pressure reduces baroreceptor afferent discharge and triggers a reflex increase in sympathetic activity, parasympathetic inhibition and increase in vascular resistance and HR. Thus, reduced baroreflex function may be associated with abnormal control of autonomic and circulatory functions.

Baroreflex and Chemoreflex Interactions

Baroreflex activation inhibits both ventilatory and vasoconstrictor responses to peripheral chemoreflex stimulation.[29] Increased BP activates arterial baroreceptors and causes bradycardia.[30] Chemoreflex activation in the setting of apnea also elicits bradycardia. The bradycardic response is

attenuated when chemoreflex activation and apnea occur in a setting of increased baroreflex activation. Thus, the arterial baroreflex inhibits not only the chemoreflex-mediated sympathetic vasoconstrictor response, but also the vagal bradycardic response.[30] The normal buffering influence of the baroreflex may be diminished in patients with SDB,[30] resulting in excessive potentiation of chemoreflex sensitivity with consequent exaggerated sympathetic activation and/or brady-dysrhythmias during hypoxemia and apnea. Interaction of chemoreceptor and baroreceptor reflexes during repeated episodes of OSA could be a mechanism for increased BP and promoting hypertension in OSA.[31] Decreased baroreflex sensitivity is a potential mechanism of BP elevation in children with SDB.[32] Evidence of abnormal baroreflex function in children with SDB will be discussed in the section on SDB-related cardiac dysfunction.

Cortical Modulation of Baroreflex and Chemoreflex

Central command continuously modulates the baroreflex- and chemoreflex-mediated cardiovascular and autonomic functions.[33,34] This modulation is important for BP variability during sleep and daytime activities. Several cortical and subcortical brain sites have direct neural projections to the autonomic centers located in the brainstem and modulate their functions. These specific regions in the hypothalamus, amygdala, periaqueductal gray matter and parabranchial nucleus primarily modulate the autonomic drive to the heart and blood vessels to control HR and BP (see Figure 30-3). The interactions between cortical and subcortical brain areas and the brainstem autonomic centers are important for the control of circulatory functions. Intermittent hypoxemia in SDB might affect the CNS integration of baroreflex function, especially in the developing brain of children.

Renin–Angiotensin–Aldosterone System (RAS) Activation

The RAS is important for the regulation of extracellular fluid volume and thus BP (see Figure 30-3).[35] Angiotensin II (ANG-II) is a potent vasoconstrictor which acts directly on vascular smooth muscle cells, causing vasoconstriction. ANG-II also regulates blood volume by increasing aldosterone production. Combined effects of ANG-II on vascular resistance and extracellular fluid volume play an important role on BP regulation. Renin released from the kidney is regulated by renal sympathetic nerves. Hypoxia is associated with an increased level of sympathetic nerve and angiotensin II.[36,37] OSA patients have higher angiotensin II concentrations compared to healthy subjects.[38] Recent studies suggest that resistant hypertension in adults with OSA is associated with activation of the RAS system.[39,40] The RAS system also affects 24-hour ambulatory BP in children.[35] The role of RAS for BP regulation in children with OSA is poorly understood.

Systemic and Local Inflammation in Sleep-Disordered Breathing

The evidence of increased systemic inflammatory markers in children with SDB is emerging.[41] Chronic low-grade inflammation has been linked to the pathophysiology of cardiovascular diseases in SDB.[42,43] Patients with OSA have increased levels of interleukin-6, TNF-alpha and C-reactive protein.[44] The combination of hypoxemia and sleep deprivation/fragmentation in patients with SDB might lead to increased levels of inflammatory markers. C-reactive protein might itself contribute to vascular disease by inhibiting nitric oxide synthase and increasing cell adhesion molecule expression.[45,46] P-selectin, C-reactive protein, fibrinogen, interleukin-8, and interferon levels were found to be higher in children with snoring and/or SDB compared with control subjects. Levels of these cytokines and of circulating adhesion molecules may be reduced by CPAP. A recent study in 143 adolescents reported an elevated level of C-reactive protein in SDB and the levels were directly related to the severity of nocturnal hypoxemia independent of BMI (Figure 30-4).[47] Although the majority of the available studies reported significant associations between C-reactive protein serum levels and SDB severity,[48] not all studies demonstrated such a relationship.[49,50] The conflicting results were in part attributed to the difference in the degree of adiposity and to genetic variance between the study populations.

Local inflammation of the upper airway has an important role in modulating airway patency.[51] Sputum in children with SDB showed increased neutrophils compared to controls and the level of neutrophil density correlated significantly and positively with the severity of SDB.[52] Infiltration of inflammatory cells in the muscular layer of the pharynx has also been described in patients with SDB.[53] Active processes of nerve degeneration and regeneration and muscular damage in patients with SDB suggest that inflammation might negatively impact the function of upper airway tissues. However, its role in modulating upper airway collapsibility in patients with SDB has not been fully investigated. Local inflammatory response in the upper airway might be associated with

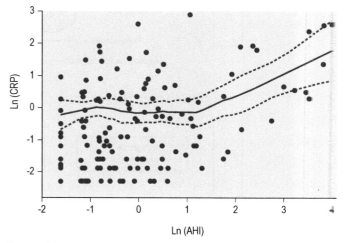

Geometric Mean Values of CRP, mg/L*			
	Unadjusted	Partially Adjusted†	Fully Adjusted‡
AHI <1	0.42 (0.33–0.54)	0.43 (0.33–0.56)	0.50 (0.40–0.63)
AHI 1–4.9	0.56 (0.36–0.88)	0.54 (0.34–0.86)	0.43 (0.29–0.66)
AHI 5–14.9	1.48 (0.62–3.53)	1.37 (0.56–3.34)	0.97 (0.43–2.16)
AHI ≥15	3.11 (1.38–7.03)	2.73 (1.17–6.37)	1.66 (0.76–3.60)

FIGURE 30-4 Plasma CRP levels in adolescents with OSA and normal controls. Adolescents with OSA, particularly with severe OSA (AHI >5 events/hour) have significantly higher CRP levels. Elevated CRP levels in these patients are directly proportional to the severity of OSA as measured by AHI. *Values are geometric means (95% confidence limits) of CRP (mg/L) values in unadjusted and adjusted models. †Adjusted for age, sex, race. ‡Adjusted for age, sex, race, BMI percentile, (BMI percentile²). *From Larkin EK, Rosen CL, Kirchner HL, et al. Variation of C-reactive protein levels in adolescents: association with sleep-disordered breathing and sleep duration. Circulation 2005;111(15):1978–84.*

mechanical trauma induced by large intraluminal pharyngeal pressure swings, tissue vibration, and eccentric muscle contraction. Recent studies on the relationship between local inflammation and airway collapsibility suggest an important role of surface tension of upper airway lining fluid for generation of a force which hinders airway opening.[54,55] However, the exact mechanisms underlying the up-regulation of inflammatory processes within the upper airway are not clear.

Oxidative Stress and Coagulation in Sleep-Disordered Breathing

Hypoxemia and reperfusion during repetitive nocturnal apneas may generate highly reactive free oxygen radicals.[56] Ischemia–reperfusion injury to the vascular wall may result in increased risk for atherosclerosis.[57] Low oxygen tension is a trigger for activation of polymorphonuclear neutrophils and monocytes, and increases the production and release of free oxygen radicals. In SDB, repeated cycles of arterial oxygen desaturation and reoxygenation occur in response to apneas followed by hyperventilation. Treatment of OSA reduces production of free radicals.[58] Increased platelet and platelet aggregability occurs in patients with OSA and is reduced after treatment of SDB.[59,60] Increased hematocrit, nocturnal and daytime fibrinogen levels and blood viscosity in SDB might also contribute to any predisposition to clot formation and cardiovascular morbidity.[61] Treatment of SDB reduces factor

VII clotting activity suggesting that SDB may indeed be causally related to increased coagulability.[62] Oxidative stress and inflammatory markers in the exhaled breath condensate are increased in children with SDB.[63] Oxidant and antioxidant defense mechanisms are altered in children with obstructive adenotonsillar hypertrophy, and this alteration improves after tonsillectomy.[64]

SDB-RELATED CARDIAC AND VASCULAR DYSFUNCTION

Unlike adults, children with SDB exhibit much more subtle evidence of cardiovascular dysfunction, and such manifestations primarily include abnormalities in BP regulation and changes in cardiac structure and endothelial function.

Elevated Systemic Arterial Pressure and Hypertension in Sleep-Disordered Breathing

Children with SDB are at higher risk of developing elevated BP compared to healthy children during nighttime sleep and even during the daytime when awake in resting conditions (Figure 30-5).[65-69] Habitual snoring in children without SDB is also associated with a higher risk for increased daytime resting BP. The degree of increased systolic and diastolic BP in these patients is associated with the respiratory disturbance index.[68] Increased 24-hour BP variability during wakefulness and sleep is also associated with the presence of SDB in children.[66] In addition, SDB severity measured by desaturation indices during sleep and the AHI are also associated with increased daytime and nocturnal BP variability.[66] It is very important to note that the level of BP in children with SDB reported in several cross-sectional studies did not reach the

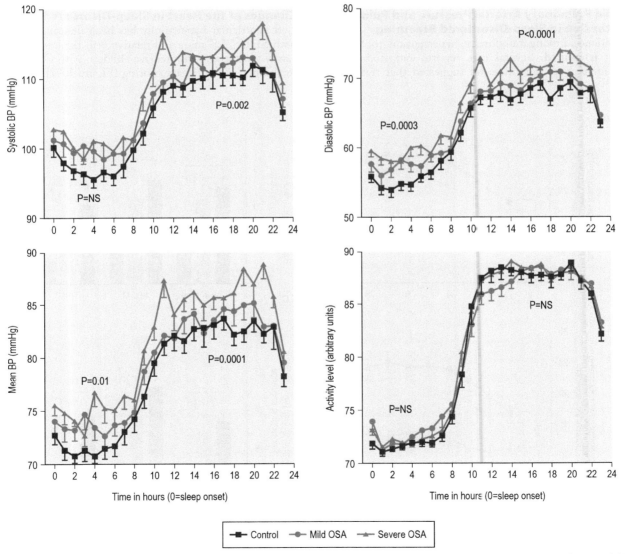

FIGURE 30-5 Elevated BP during 24-hour activated adjusted ambulatory BP monitoring in children with mild and severe SDB. Children with severe OSA have significantly higher BP compared to control during nighttime sleep and daytime activity. *From Amin R, Somers VK, McConnell K, et al. Activity-adjusted 24-hour ambulatory blood pressure and cardiac remodeling in children with sleep disordered breathing. Hypertension 2008;51(1):84–91.*

level that is considered compatible with the current definitions of clinically significant hypertension.[70] Unlike adult patients with SDB, hypertension in children and adolescents is not independently associated with SDB. However, severe SDB may be associated with hypertension in children. The BP load is a measure of hypertension and is defined as the percentage of BP measurements that exceed the 95th percentile during 24-hour BP monitoring.[66] A recent study in 140 children with AHI >5 events/h, nightly snoring and tonsillar hypertrophy reported increases in BP load and morning BP surges.[66] Significant reductions in 24-hour ambulatory BP are observed after treatment of SDB with adenotonsillectomy.[71] Although the exact mechanisms of increased BP in children with SDB are not clear, reduced baroreflex during nighttime and daytime is a likely contributing factor (Figure 30-6).[32] It is unlikely that the relatively modest increases in BP and BP variability in children with SDB will lead to significant cardiac dysfunction during childhood. However, it remains unclear whether early childhood SDB may predispose to BP deregulation later in life.

Elevated Pulmonary Arterial Pressure and Pulmonary Hypertension in Sleep-Disordered Breathing

The evidence linking pulmonary hypertension to SDB in children is limited. Several case reports and studies with small sample sizes have thus far suggested that statistically significant increases in pulmonary arterial pressures occur in SDB.[72,73] However, these studies are further limited by either the procedures employed for the diagnosis of SDB or by the techniques utilized in the measurements of pulmonary arterial pressures. Increased prevalence of echocardiographic diagnosis of cor pulmonale has been reported in children with adenotonsillar hypertrophy and snoring.[73] Presence of comorbid conditions, such as congenital heart diseases, in these children might be linked to the presence of SDB. Although both the absence[74] and presence[75] of pulmonary hypertension in children with adenotonsillar hypertrophy and OSA have been reported, improvements in pulmonary hypertension after treatment of SDB occur.[72,76] Direct measurements of pulmonary artery pressure by cardiac catheterization reported the presence of pulmonary hypertension in children with SDB who also suffered from underlying genetic disorders and heart failure. A recent study demonstrated decreases in pulmonary artery pressure measured by echocardiography after treatment of SDB.[77]

Cardiac Remodeling: Structural and Functional Changes of the Heart in Sleep-Disordered Breathing

Left ventricular hypertrophy has been described in children with SDB.[78] LV mass and relative wall thickness are significantly greater in normotensive children with OSA compared to children with primary snoring (Figure 30-7).[78] An AHI of

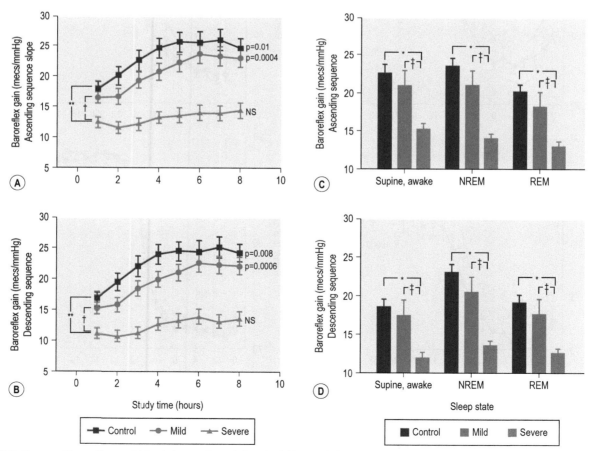

FIGURE 30-6 Decreased baroreflex sensitivity during awake and sleep in children with SDB, particularly in children with severe SDB. *From McConnell K, Somers VK, Kimball T, et al. Baroreflex gain in children with obstructive sleep apnea. Am J Respir Crit Care Med 2009;180(1):42–8.*

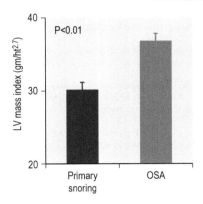
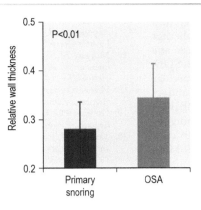

FIGURE 30-7 Cardiac modeling in children with SDB. Children with OSA have significantly elevated LV mass and relative wall thickness compared to matched children with primary snoring. *From Amin RS, Kimball TR, Bean JA, et al. Left ventricular hypertrophy and abnormal ventricular geometry in children and adolescents with obstructive sleep apnea. Am J Respir Crit Care Med 2002;165(10):1395–9.*

10 is associated with a sixfold increased risk for hypertrophy. LV posterior wall thickness is also correlated with the severity of SDB as measured by respiratory disturbance index, with the severity of SDB being directly related to the decrease in LV diastolic function.[79] Recently, impaired right ventricular function has also been reported in children with adenotonsillar hypertrophy.[80] Brain natriuretic peptide, a hormone released by ventricular myocytes in response to pressure and volume overload, was increased in children with snoring and correlated with severity of SDB.[81,82] In otherwise healthy children, those with more severe SDB (AHI >5 events/h) had echocardiographic evidence of increased LV wall thickness. LV end-diastolic dimension and thickness of interventricular septum are significantly greater in children with SDB compared to control children. Adenotonsillectomy was associated with a reduction in LV dimension and posterior wall and septal thickness. However, pre- and post-adenotonsillectomy differences for LV dimension and ventricular septal thickness were significantly different.[83] Improvement of LV ejection fraction after treatment of OSA was also described recently.[79] The mechanism of LV hypertrophy in children with OSA is not well understood. Hypoxia-induced activation of the renin–angiotensin–aldosterone system might be linked to the cardiac remodeling that develops in some patients with SDB.[84] Similarly, the degree of reversibility of abnormal LV geometry after treatment has not been comprehensively examined.

Endothelial Dysfunction in Sleep-Disordered Breathing

Endothelial dysfunction is associated with cardiovascular morbidity in SDB.[85] Flow-mediated dilatation of the brachial artery is an indirect measure of endothelial dysfunction that is altered in SDB and normalizes after treatment with CPAP. The hypoxia, hypercapnia and pressor surges accompanying obstructive apneic events may serve as potent stimuli for the release of vasoactive substances and an impairment of endothelial function. Endothelin, a marker of endothelial dysfunction, is increased in SDB.[86,87] Elevated levels of endothelin in response to the hypoxemia of SDB may contribute to sustained vasoconstriction and other cardiac and vascular changes.[88] In a recent study in children with SDB, both obesity and OSA were shown to independently and additively increase the risk for endothelial dysfunction (Figure 30-8).[89,90] Although the mechanisms of endothelial dysfunction in children are not clear, it is highly likely that both oxidative stress and inflammatory mediators play an important role in vascular

Percentage of subjects with Tmax>45 sec			
	OAHI<2	2<OAHI<5	OAHI>5
Non-obese	0.0%	15.4%	20.0%
Obese	35.7%	40.0%	62.5%

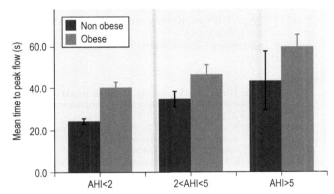

FIGURE 30-8 Endothelial function in obese and non-obese children with and without OSA. Obesity alone, OSA alone, and combination of both obesity and OSA in children is associated with significant endothelial dysfunction. *From Bhattacharjee R, Kim J, Alotaibi WH, Kheirandish-Gozal L, Capdevila OS, Gozal D. Endothelial dysfunction in children without hypertension: potential contributions of obesity and obstructive sleep apnea. Chest 2012;141(3):682–91.*

injury.[91] Thus, elevated inflammatory mediators in children with SDB might contribute to endothelial dysfunction and also serve as reliable reporters of endothelial damage in the context of pediatric SDB.

CONCLUSION

The existence of significant cardiovascular dysfunction in the pediatric SDB population has been recognized in recent years. Most of the research efforts in these patients have, however, primarily focused on the comparison of cardiovascular risk factors between children with SDB and controls, and the cumulative evidence suggests an increase in several established risk factors for CVD in the context of pediatric SDB. Nevertheless, whether alterations in cardiovascular biomarkers are indeed present and whether treatment of SDB will reverse the cardiovascular risk remains controversial. The confounder effects of age, ethnicity, body habitus, as well as genetic and environmental factors, further add to the complexity and uncertainty of these issues. In addition, it is not clear whether abnormalities in cardiovascular biomarkers will cause any long-term cardiovascular morbidity in children with SDB, and longitudinal studies on effects of SDB on cardiovascular outcomes in children are clearly needed. Improved understanding of cardiovascular disease mechanisms in SDB may provide a rationale for early intervention trials aiming to prevent cardiovascular morbidity later in life. In the absence of any conclusive evidence of cardiovascular risk in children with SDB, generalized therapeutic interventions solely aimed at improving cardiovascular outcomes are premature, and therefore the risk:benefit ratio of treating SDB in children should be considered on an individualized basis.

Clinical Pearls

- Neurogenic factors that contribute to abnormal cardiovascular control; chemoreceptors, baroreceptors and cortex.
- Central role of sympathetic nerve activity in mediating chronic inflammation, vascular dysfunction and activation of the renin–angiotensin–aldosterone system.
- Effect of OSA on left ventricular structure and function and on blood pressure control.
- How rare pulmonary hypertension is in pediatric OSA.

References

1. O'Driscoll DM, Horne RS, Davey MJ, et al. Increased sympathetic activity in children with obstructive sleep apnea: cardiovascular implications. Sleep Med 2011;12(5):483–8.
2. Bhattacharjee R, Kheirandish-Gozal L, Pillar G, et al. Cardiovascular complications of obstructive sleep apnea syndrome: evidence from children. Prog Cardiovasc Dis 2009;51(5):416–33.
3. Kwok KL, Ng DK, Chan CH. Cardiovascular changes in children with snoring and obstructive sleep apnoea. Ann Acad Med Singapore 2008;37(8):715–21.
4. Baharav A, Kotagal S, Rubin BK, et al. Autonomic cardiovascular control in children with obstructive sleep apnea. Clin Auton Res 1999;9(6):345–51.
5. Monti A, Medigue C, Nedelcoux H, et al. Autonomic control of the cardiovascular system during sleep in normal subjects. Eur J Appl Physiol 2002;87(2):174–81.
6. Penzel T, Wessel N, Riedl M, et al. Cardiovascular and respiratory dynamics during normal and pathological sleep. Chaos 2007;17(1):115–16.
7. Somers VK, Dyken ME, Mark AL, et al. Sympathetic-nerve activity during sleep in normal subjects [see comments]. N Engl J Med 1993;328(5):303–7.
8. Tilkian AG, Guilleminault C, Schroeder JS, et al. Hemodynamics in sleep-induced apnea. Studies during wakefulness and sleep. Ann Intern Med 1976;85(6):714–19.
9. Somers VK, Dyken ME, Clary MP, et al. Sympathetic neural mechanisms in obstructive sleep apnea. J Clin Invest 1995;96(4):1897–904.
10. Morgan BJ. Acute and chronic cardiovascular responses to sleep disordered breathing. Sleep 1996;19(Suppl. 10):S206–9.
11. Sajkov D, Cowie RJ, Thornton AT, et al. Pulmonary hypertension and hypoxemia in obstructive sleep apnea syndrome. Am J Resp Critl Care Med 1994;149(2 Pt 1):416–22.
12. Shiomi T, Guilleminault C, Stoohs R, et al. Leftward shift of the interventricular septum and pulsus paradoxus in obstructive sleep apnea syndrome. Chest 1991;100(4):894–902.
13. Stoohs R, Guilleminault C. Cardiovascular changes associated with obstructive sleep apnea syndrome. J Appl Physiol 1992;72(2):583–9.
14. Virolainen J, Ventila M, Turto H, et al. Effect of negative intrathoracic pressure on left ventricular pressure dynamics and relaxation. J Appl Physiol 1995;79(2):455–60.
15. Morgan BJ, Denahan T, Ebert TJ. Neurocirculatory consequences of negative intrathoracic pressure vs. asphyxia during voluntary apnea. J Appl Physiol 1993;74(6):2969–75.
16. Somers VK, Dyken ME, Skinner JL. Autonomic and hemodynamic responses and interactions during the Mueller maneuver in humans. J Auton Nerv Syst 1993;44(2-3):253–9.
17. Morgan BJ, Crabtree DC, Puleo DS, et al. Neurocirculatory consequences of abrupt change in sleep state in humans. J Appl Physiol 1996;80(5):1627–36.
18. Shamsuzzaman AS, Somers VK. Cardiorespiratory interactions in neural circulatory control in humans. Ann NY Acad Sci 2001;940:488–99.
19. Guyenet PG. Neural structures that mediate sympathoexcitation during hypoxia. Respir Physiol 2000;121(2-3):147–62.
20. Taylor EW, Jordan D, Coote JH. Central control of the cardiovascular and respiratory systems and their interactions in vertebrates. Physiol Rev 1999;79(3):855–916.
21. Wade JG, Larson CP Jr, Hickey RF, et al. Effect of carotid endarterectomy on carotid chemoreceptor and baroreceptor function in man. N Engl J Med 1970;282(15):823–9.
22. Somers VK, Mark AL, Zavala DC, et al. Influence of ventilation and hypocapnia on sympathetic nerve responses to hypoxia in normal humans. J Appl Physiol 1989;67(5):2095–100.
23. Gelfand R, Lambertsen CJ. Dynamic respiratory response to abrupt change of inspired CO_2 at normal and high PO_2. J Appl Physiol 1973;35(6):903–13.
24. Somers VK, Mark AL, Zavala DC, et al. Contrasting effects of hypoxia and hypercapnia on ventilation and sympathetic activity in humans. J Appl Physiol 1989;67(5):2101–6.
25. Loredo JS, Clausen JL, Nelesen RA, et al. Obstructive sleep apnea and hypertension: are peripheral chemoreceptors involved? Med Hypotheses 2001;56(1):17–9.
26. Springer C, Cooper DM, Wasserman K. Evidence that maturation of the peripheral chemoreceptors is not complete in childhood. Respir Physiol 1988;74(1):55–64.
27. Cooper VL, Bowker CM, Pearson SB, et al. Effects of simulated obstructive sleep apnoea on the human carotid baroreceptor-vascular resistance reflex. J Physiol 2004;557(Pt 3):1055–65.
28. Narkiewicz K, Pesek CA, Kato M, et al. Baroreflex control of sympathetic nerve activity and heart rate in obstructive sleep apnea. Hypertension 1998;32(6):1039–43.
29. Heistad DD, Abboud FM, Mark AL, et al. Interaction of baroreceptor and chemoreceptor reflexes. Modulation of the chemoreceptor reflex by changes in baroreceptor activity. J Clin Invest 1974;53(5):1226–36.
30. Somers VK, Dyken ME, Mark AL, et al. Parasympathetic hyperresponsiveness and bradyarrhythmias during apnoea in hypertension. Clin Auto Res 1992;2(3):171–6.
31. Cooper VL, Pearson SB, Bowker CM, et al. Interaction of chemoreceptor and baroreceptor reflexes by hypoxia and hypercapnia – a mechanism for promoting hypertension in obstructive sleep apnoea. J Physiol 2005;568(Pt 2):677–87.
32. McConnell K, Somers VK, Kimball T, et al. Baroreflex gain in children with obstructive sleep apnea. Am J Respir Crit Care Med 2009;180(1):42–8.
33. Gianaros PJ, Onyewuenyi IC, Sheu LK, et al. Brain systems for baroreflex suppression during stress in humans. Hum Brain Mapp 2012;33(7):1700–16.
34. Netzer F, Bernard JF, Verberne AJ, et al. Brain circuits mediating baroreflex bradycardia inhibition in rats: an anatomical and functional link between the cuneiform nucleus and the periaqueductal grey. J Physiol 2011;589(Pt 8):2079–91.
35. Harshfield GA, Pulliam DA, Alpert BS, et al. Ambulatory blood pressure patterns in children and adolescents: influence of renin–sodium profiles. Pediatrics 1991;87(1):94–100.
36. Foster GE, Hanly PJ, Ahmed SB, et al. Intermittent hypoxia increases arterial blood pressure in humans through a renin–angiotensin system-dependent mechanism. Hypertension 2010;56(3):369–77.
37. Ip SP, Chan YW, Leung PS. Effects of chronic hypoxia on the circulating and pancreatic renin–angiotensin system. Pancreas 2002;25(3):296–300.
38. Barcelo A, Elorza MA, Barbe F, et al. Angiotensin converting enzyme in patients with sleep apnoea syndrome: plasma activity and gene polymorphisms. Eur Respir J 2001;17(4):728–32.
39. Dudenbostel T, Calhoun DA. Resistant hypertension, obstructive sleep apnoea and aldosterone. J Hum Hypertens 2012;26(5):281–7.
40. Di Murro A, Petramala L, Cotesta D, et al. Renin–angiotensin–aldosterone system in patients with sleep apnoea: prevalence of primary aldosteronism. J Renin Angiotensin Aldosterone Syst 2010;11(3):165–72.
41. Gozal D, Kheirandish-Gozal L. Cardiovascular morbidity in obstructive sleep apnea: oxidative stress, inflammation, and much more. Am J Respir Crit Care Med 2008;177(4):369–75.

42. Danesh J, Whincup P, Walker M, et al. Low grade inflammation and coronary heart disease: prospective study and updated meta-analyses. BMJ 2000;321(7255):199–204.

43. Smith SC Jr, Anderson JL, Cannon RO 3rd, et al. CDC/AHA Workshop on Markers of Inflammation and Cardiovascular Disease: Application to Clinical and Public Health Practice: report from the clinical practice discussion group. Circulation 2004;110(25):e550–3.

44. Dyugovskaya L, Lavie P, Hirsh M, et al. Activated CD8+ T-lymphocytes in obstructive sleep apnoea. Eur Respir J 2005;25(5):820–8.

45. Venugopal SK, Devaraj S, Yuhanna I, et al. Demonstration that C-reactive protein decrease eNOS expression and bioactivity in human aortic endothelial cells. Circulation 2002;106(12):1439–41.

46. Woollard KJ, Phillips DC, Griffiths HR. Direct modulatory effect of C-reactive protein on primary human monocyte adhesion to human endothelial cells. Clin Exp Immunol 2002;130(2):256–62.

47. Larkin EK, Rosen CL, Kirchner HL, et al. Variation of C-reactive protein levels in adolescents: association with sleep-disordered breathing and sleep duration. Circulation 2005;111(15):1978–84.

48. Gozal D, Kheirandish-Gozal L, Bhattacharjee R, et al. C-Reactive protein and obstructive sleep apnea syndrome in children. Frontiers Bio 2012;4:2410–22.

49. Guilleminault C, Li KK, Khramtsov A, et al. Sleep disordered breathing: surgical outcomes in prepubertal children. Laryngoscope 2004;114(1):132–7.

50. Kaditis AG, Alexopoulos EI, Kalampouka E, et al. Morning levels of C-reactive protein in children with obstructive sleep-disordered breathing. Am J Respir Crit Care Med 2005;171(3):282–6.

51. Dusser DJ, Djokic TD, Borson DB, et al. Cigarette smoke induces bronchoconstrictor hyperresponsiveness to substance P and inactivates airway neutral endopeptidase in the guinea pig. Possible role of free radicals. J Clin Invest 1989;84(3):900–6.

52. Li AM, Hung E, Tsang T, et al. Induced sputum inflammatory measures correlate with disease severity in children with obstructive sleep apnoea. Thorax 2007;62(1):75–9.

53. Boyd JH, Petrof BJ, Hamid Q, et al. Upper airway muscle inflammation and denervation changes in obstructive sleep apnea. Am J Respir Crit Care Med 2004;170(5):541–6.

54. Kirkness JP, Macronio M, Stavrinou R, et al. Surface tension of upper airway mucosal lining liquid in obstructive sleep apnea/hypopnea syndrome. Sleep 2005;28(4):457–63.

55. Kirkness JP, Madronio M, Stavrinou R, et al. Relationship between surface tension of upper airway lining liquid and upper airway collapsibility during sleep in obstructive sleep apnea hypopnea syndrome. J Appl Physiol 2003;95(5):1761–6.

56. Dean RT, Wilcox I. Possible atherogenic effects of hypoxia during obstructive sleep apnea. Sleep 1993;16(Suppl. 8):S15–21; discussion S22.

57. Halliwell B. The role of oxygen radicals in human disease, with particular reference to the vascular system. Haemostasis 1993;23(Suppl. 1):118–26.

58. Schulz R, Mahmoudi S, Hattar K, et al. Enhanced release of superoxide from polymorph-nuclear neutrophils in obstructive sleep apnea. Impact of continuous positive airway pressure therapy. Am J Respir Crit Care Med 2000;162(2 Pt 1):566–70.

59. Kim J, Bhattacharjee R, Kheirandish-Gozal L, et al. Circulating microparticles in children with sleep disordered breathing. Chest 2011;140(2):408–17.

60. Sanner BM, Kortermann M, Tepel M, et al. Platelet function in patients with obstructive sleep apnoea syndrome. Eur Respir J 2000;16(4):648–52.

61. Kaditis AG, Alexopoulos EI, Kalampouka E, et al. Morning levels of fibrinogen in children with sleep-disordered breathing. Eur Respir J 2004;24(5):790–7.

62. Chin K, Ohi M, Kita H, et al. Effects of NCPAP therapy on fibrinogen levels in obstructive sleep apnea syndrome. Am J Resp Crit Care Med 1996;153(6 Pt 1):1972–6.

63. Malakasioti G, Alexopoulos E, Befani C, et al. Oxidative stress and inflammatory markers in the exhaled breath condensate of children with OSA. Sleep Breath 2012;16(3):703–8.

64. Dogruer ZN, Ural M, Eskandari G, et al. Malondialdehyde and antioxidant enzymes in children with obstructive adenotonsillar hypertrophy. Clin Biochem 2004;37(8):718–21.

65. Weber SA, Santos VJ, Semenzati G de O, et al. Ambulatory blood pressure monitoring in children with obstructive sleep apnea and primary snoring. Int J Pediatr Otorhinolaryngol 2012;76(6):787–90.

66. Amin R, Somers VK, McConnell K, et al. Activity-adjusted 24-hour ambulatory blood pressure and cardiac remodeling in children with sleep disordered breathing. Hypertension 2008;51(1):84–91.

67. Xu Z, Li B, Shen K. Ambulatory blood pressure monitoring in Chinese children with obstructive sleep apnea/hypopnea syndrome. Pediatr Pulmonol 2013;48(3):274–9.

68. Leung LC, Ng DK, Lau MW, et al. Twenty-four-hour ambulatory BP in snoring children with obstructive sleep apnea syndrome. Chest 2006;130(4):1009–17.

69. Ng DK, Leung LC, Chan CH. Blood pressure in children with sleep-disordered breathing. Am J Respir Crit Care Med 2004;170(4):467; author reply 468.

70. Zintzaras E, Kaditis AG. Sleep-disordered breathing and blood pressure in children: a meta-analysis. Arch Pediatr Adolesc Med 2007;161(2):172–8.

71. Ng DK, Wong JC, Chan CH, et al. Ambulatory blood pressure before and after adenotonsillectomy in children with obstructive sleep apnea. Sleep Med 2010;11(7):721–5.

72. Brown OE, Manning SC, Ridenour B. Cor pulmonale secondary to tonsillar and adenoidal hypertrophy: management considerations. Int J Pediatr Otorhinolaryngol 1988;16(2):131–9.

73. Wilkinson AR, McCormick MS, Freeland AP, et al. Electrocardiographic signs of pulmonary hypertension in children who snore. Br Med J (Clin Res Ed) 1981;282(6276):1579–81.

74. Li AM, Hui S, Wong E, et al. Obstructive sleep apnoea in children with adenotonsillar hypertrophy: prospective study. Hong Kong Med J 2001;7(3):236–40.

75. Miman MC, Kirazli T, Ozyurek R. Doppler echocardiography in adenotonsillar hypertrophy. Int J Pediatr Otorhinolaryngol 2000;54(1):21–6.

76. Hunt CE, Brouillette RT. Abnormalities of breathing control and airway maintenance in infants and children as a cause of cor pulmonale. Pediatr Cardiol 1982;3(3):249–56.

77. Arias MA, Garcia-Rio F, Alonso-Fernandez A, et al. Pulmonary hypertension in obstructive sleep apnoea: effects of continuous positive airway pressure: a randomized, controlled cross-over study. Eur Heart J 2006;27(9):1106–13.

78. Amin RS, Kimball TR, Bean JA, et al. Left ventricular hypertrophy and abnormal ventricular geometry in children and adolescents with obstructive sleep apnea. Am J Respir Crit Care Med 2002;165(10):1395–9.

79. Amin RS, Kimball TR, Kalra M, et al. Left ventricular function in children with sleep-disordered breathing. Am J Cardiol 2005;95(6):801–4.

80. Duman D, Naiboglu B, Esen HS, et al. Impaired right ventricular function in adenotonsillar hypertrophy. Int J Cardiovasc Imaging 2008;24(3):261–7.

81. Kaditis AG, Alexopoulos EI, Hatzi F, et al. Overnight change in brain natriuretic peptide levels in children with sleep-disordered breathing. Chest 2006;130(5):1377–84.

82. Sans Capdevila O, Crabtree VM, Kheirandish-Gozal L, et al. Increased morning brain natriuretic peptide levels in children with nocturnal enuresis and sleep-disordered breathing: a community-based study. Pediatrics 2008;121(5):e1208–14.

83. Gorur K, Doven O, Unal M, et al. Preoperative and postoperative cardiac and clinical findings of patients with adenotonsillar hypertrophy. Int J Pediatr Otorhinolaryngol 2001;59(1):41–6.

84. Miwa Y, Sasaguri T. Hypoxia-induced cardiac remodeling in sleep apnea syndrome: involvement of the renin-angiotensin-aldosterone system. Hypertens Res 2007;30(12):1147–9.

85. Lavie L. Sleep apnea syndrome, endothelial dysfunction, and cardiovascular morbidity. Sleep 2004;27(6):1053–5.

86. Phillips BG, Narkiewicz K, Pesek CA, et al. Effects of obstructive sleep apnea on endothelin-1 and blood pressure. J Hypertens 1999;17(1):61–6.

87. Grimpen F, Kanne P, Schulz E, et al. Endothelin-1 plasma levels are not elevated in patients with obstructive sleep apnoea. Eur Respir J 2000;15(2):320–5.

88. Allen SW, Chatfield BA, Koppenhafer SA, et al. Circulating immunoreactive endothelin-1 in children with pulmonary hypertension. Association with acute hypoxic pulmonary vasoreactivity. Am Rev Respir Dis 1993;148(2):519–22.

89. Bhattacharjee R, Alotaibi WH, Kheirandish-Gozal L, et al. Endothelial dysfunction in obese non-hypertensive children without evidence of sleep disordered breathing. BMC Pediatr 2010;10:8.

90. Bhattacharjee R, Kim J, Alotaibi WH, et al. Endothelial dysfunction in children without hypertension: potential contributions of obesity and obstructive sleep apnea. Chest 2012;141(3):682–91.

91. Gozal D, Kheirandish-Gozal L, Serpero LD, et al. Obstructive sleep apnea and endothelial function in school-aged nonobese children: effect of adenotonsillectomy. Circulation 2007;116(20):2307–14.

Metabolic Consequences of Sleep Disordered Breathing

David Gozal

INTRODUCTION

Epidemiological studies over the last several decades have conclusively demonstrated that both the prevalence and severity of overweight and obesity in children and adolescents have clearly been increasing worldwide, even if some deceleration in such trends has emerged more recently, possibly as the result of public health campaigns aiming to curb the alarming rates of obesity in childhood.[1-4] Nonetheless, reported prevalences of overweight hovering around 10.4% among toddlers, 15.3% among school-aged children and 15.5% among adolescents are now frequently exceeded in many of the underserved communities across the USA and the world.[5-8] A major consequence of this epidemic of obesity has been the concomitant increase in the prevalence of obesity-associated morbidities, such that previously infrequent conditions such as the metabolic syndrome, cardiovascular disease, non-alcoholic liver steatosis, depression, and decreased quality of life have all begun to emerge even among the youngest of the children.[9-12]

SLEEP CURTAILMENT, IRREGULAR SLEEP, AND OBESITY

The increasingly demanding life pace of technology-driven societies has radically changed the way we sleep, as well as the way our children sleep. Over a period of 100 years or so, the overall duration of sleep in children has steadily declined.[13-15] Although the reasons underlying these trends in sleep curtailment are multifactorial,[16-18] reductions in sleep duration have also been accompanied by increased irregularity in sleep schedules. There is now compelling evidence linking the progressive decrements in sleep duration and sleep regularity to the reciprocal increases observed in the prevalence of childhood obesity.[19-2] However, the associations between obesity and sleep have not been consistently reported by all studies,[29] raising the possibility that the current definitions of short sleep and insufficient sleep are quite arbitrary, and therefore operate as a confounder rather than a true causal pathway.[30-32] Furthermore, additional confounding factors that play a role in the propensity for obesity may begin in early life,[33] such that extrication of the role of sleep may not be trivial. In a cross-sectional and longitudinal study, Chaput and collaborators reported that only those subjects who exhibited the combination of short sleep duration, high disinhibition eating behavior, and low dietary calcium intake had significantly higher BMI.[34] Based on the aforementioned considerations, it is clear that intervention trials aiming to establish whether restoration of sleep quality and quantity will ameliorate metabolic and ponderal indices in children are needed.[35] It is also noteworthy that sleep-associated changes in BMI appear to be primarily affecting those children whose BMI is already elevated.[36]

Some of the putative biological pathways linking sleep duration and regularity to obesity clearly involve alterations in some of the neuropeptides that regulate appetite both peripherally and centrally. In addition, the contribution of perturbations in circadian timing cannot be overlooked.[37] For example, increased levels of ghrelin, reduced levels of leptin, and reduced central biological activity of orexin have all been identified in experimental sleep restriction paradigms, and will lead to increased food intake.[38,39] Furthermore, disruptions of the circadian clock have been implicated in perturbations within a complex network of metabolic pathways that not only affect regulatory CNS regions such as in the hypothalamus, but also alter metabolic processes in peripheral tissues.[40,41]

Unfortunately, in-depth exploration of these pathways in the context of childhood is almost completely lacking; furthermore, we should keep in mind that both sleep duration and body weight trajectory are determined by a multitude of factors, such as sociodemographic, socioeconomic, familial (e.g., family structure, overweight parent) and individual (e.g., health behavior, physical activity, health status, stress levels) factors (Figure 31-1).[42-44] Regardless, we need to be cognizant that obese children are 1.5- to 2-fold (odds ratios ranging from 1.15 to 11) more likely of being short sleepers,[45,46] and that any interventions seeking to modify sleep patterns in children are less likely to succeed if implemented later in childhood, since both sleep regularity and sleep duration are consistently preserved across long periods of time even in children.[47] Thus, sleep interventions need to be implemented early in life, and therefore identification of children at risk during infancy and early childhood and prospective interventions to prolong and regularize sleep are required to delineate the role of sleep in the context of BMI regulation and metabolic homeostasis.

OBESITY AS A RISK FACTOR OF OBSTRUCTIVE SLEEP APNEA

Since the early descriptions of obstructive sleep apnea (OSA) in the pediatric age range, a clear change has occurred, with a majority of the patients being evaluated in most pediatric sleep centers fulfilling the criteria for either overweight or obese.[48] This is not surprising, considering that the risk of OSA in obese children is markedly increased.[49] In a case-control study design, Redline and colleagues examined risk factors for sleep-disordered breathing in children aged 2–18 years, and found that the risk among obese children was increased 4–5-fold.[50] In fact, for every increment in BMI by 1 kg/m^2 beyond the mean BMI for age and gender, the risk of OSAS increased by 12%. Similar trends demonstrating increased risk of OSA among obese and overweight children have been consistently reported in many countries.[51-60]

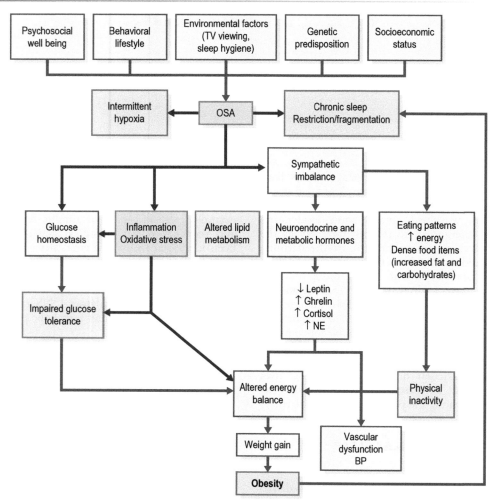

FIGURE 31-1 Schematic diagram illustrating the potential interactions between sleep, obstructive sleep apnea, obesity, and metabolic dysfunction in children.

Upper airway narrowing in obese children could result from fatty infiltration of upper airway structures and tongue, while subcutaneous fat deposits in the anterior neck region and other cervical structures will undoubtedly contribute and exert collapsing forces promoting increased pharyngeal collapsibility.[61,62] Interestingly, Arens and collaborators have recently shown that obese children exhibit enlarged lymphadenoid tissues in the upper airway, the latter potentially reflecting the result of systemic low-grade inflammatory processes that accompany the obese state.[63,64] Obesity may also affect lung volumes through mass loading of the respiratory system,[65] and increased adipose tissue deposition in the abdominal and thoracic walls and around the viscera will increase the overall respiratory load, and reduce intrathoracic volumes and diaphragmatic excursion, particularly when in the supine position. Thus, obesity will lead to decreased lung volumes and oxygen reserve, and will augment the work of breathing during sleep.

Obesity is also associated with peripheral and central leptin tissue resistance, resulting in reduced biological effectiveness despite elevation of circulating leptin levels.[66–68] The unique properties of leptin as a potent respiratory stimulant with both central and peripheral chemoreceptor modulatory properties are therefore markedly dampened by the emergence of leptin resistance, and may precipitate the gradual onset of attenuated respiratory reflexes, particularly during sleep.[69,70] Obesity can be accompanied by fragmented sleep that will progressively increase the arousal threshold, thereby potentially aggravating the duration of upper airway obstruction events.[71]

OSA MAY PROMOTE OBESITY AND ITS CONSEQUENCES

Although there is currently only incipient evidence, it is plausible to assume that the presence of OSA could promote or aggravate obesity or its consequences (see Figure 31-1). This concept has developed in recent years whereby the presence of OSA would promote weight gain and obesity, via sleep fragmentation and associated daytime sleepiness.[72–75] The presence of sleepiness is likely to reduce overall daily physical activity,[76] particularly in those children at risk for obesity. In addition, the degree of daytime sleepiness resulting from OSA is amplified in obese children.[77]

Similar to obesity, OSA should nowadays be viewed as a low-grade systemic inflammatory disease, and the coexistence of obesity and OSA further exacerbates the magnitude of the inflammatory responses.[78-83] Thus, OSA is viewed as a major risk factor for development of the metabolic syndrome in children (see also Chapter 18).

OSA Potentiates Alterations in Serum Lipids in Children

In a large series of studies in adult patients, OSA has been identified as a risk factor for dyslipidemia and insulin resistance.[84-86] However, since most adult OSA patients are obese, it is nearly impossible to determine the exact contribution of OSA on lipid metabolism.

The evidence in children linking OSA to lipid alterations is relatively scarce. In a study of 135 children (many of them being obese), no associations emerged between polysomnographic indices of OSA severity and fasting serum lipids, even though strong association was apparent between BMI and lipid levels.[87] Verhulst et al.[88] showed significant correlations between the degree of oxyhemoglobin desaturation (but not the respiratory disturbance index) and serum lipid and cholesterol levels among 104 relatively older obese children (42% post pubertal), even when controlling for gender, puberty and body mass index. In a retrospective study of Greek children being evaluated for suspected OSA, Alexopoulos and colleagues[89] reported that the risk of low HDL cholesterol was 3-fold higher in non-obese children with moderate to severe OSA compared to those children with mild OSA or primary snoring. In a prospective cohort study of adolescents recruited from the general community, Redline et al.[90] reported a 6-fold increase in the risk for developing the metabolic syndrome in those individuals with OSA. Furthermore, OSA in these adolescent subjects was closely associated with serum LDL concentrations. In a more recent study, Zong and collaborators further confirmed the existence of putative inverse associations between HDL cholesterol and AHI in a small cohort of 44 children in China.[91]

In a prospective study of 62 consecutive pre-pubertal obese and non-obese children with OSA, surgical adenotonsillectomy resulted in improvements of OSA in all children, but normalization of the respiratory disturbances during sleep occurred only in a fraction of these children. In non-obese children, surgical removal of adenoids and tonsils led to significant improvements in LDL, HDL, and LDL/HDH levels, and overall similar findings occurred in obese children with OSA after treatment, in the absence of any significant changes in BMI. These findings suggest that the improvements in serum lipids can be ascribed to OSA rather than obesity. Apolipoprotein B serum levels were improved in both non-obese and obese groups following surgery, and all lipids were correlated with measures of OSA severity.[92] Taken together, these findings strongly support that disrupted sleep and episodic hypoxia in the context of OSAS impose substantial changes in lipid regulatory mechanisms in children.

Since not every child with OSA will manifest alterations in serum lipids, it is possible that genetic factors may contribute. To examine this issue, Bhushan and colleagues[93] assessed gene variants in the fatty-acid-binding protein 4 (FABP4) gene, a gene that plays a major role in inflammation and metabolism, particularly in the regulation of the intracellular processing of lipids in critical tissues such as adipose tissues and macrophages. Children with OSA had elevated concentrations of FABP4 in plasma, and the presence of the rs1054135 polymorphism in the FABP4 gene was associated with elevated levels of FABP4 and serum lipids, even after adjustment of BMI, suggesting that genetic predisposition may contribute to impaired lipid homeostasis in children with OSA.

OSA Adversely Affects Insulin Sensitivity

In 110 non-obese children, Kaditis et al.[94] found no correlations between the severity of OSAS and fasting insulin or HOMA levels, with serum lipids not being reported. However, most other studies have found that OSA imposes independent alterations on insulin sensitivity, particularly if obesity is present.[92] In a small cohort of obese Latino males, the presence of OSA with corresponding sleep fragmentation and intermittent hypoxemia was associated with metabolic impairments manifesting as increased insulin resistance.[95] Similar results were reported by Canapari et al. who also pointed out the importance of visceral fat mass in the associations between OSA and insulin resistance.[96]

OSA Imposes Increased Risk for Systemic Blood Pressure Elevations

See Chapter 30, by Shamsuzzaman and Amin.

OSA and Non-Alcoholic Hepatic Steatosis

The potential adverse effects of OSA on liver function, particularly when underlying obesity is present, have been critically explored by Polotsky and collaborators in a murine model.[97] In a study from our laboratory, we showed that the prevalence of elevated liver enzymes in serum of obese patients was significantly higher if OSA was concurrently present, and that effective treatment of OSA ameliorated liver function tests, indicating that sleep-disordered breathing may serve as a catalyst of non-alcoholic hepatic steatosis via its oxidant stress and inflammatory effects.[98] Similar findings were subsequently reported in another study.[99]

OSA and the Metabolic Syndrome

From the individually analyzed effects of OSA described above, it becomes apparent that when obesity is present, the risk for developing the metabolic syndrome is markedly exacerbated by the concurrent presence of OSA.[92,100,101] However, although the bidirectional interactions between OSAS and obesity appear to be irrefutable, well-controlled interventional trials aiming to assess the implications of treating one of the disorders to ameliorate the other have yet to be conducted. There is now little doubt that the usual treatment of OSA, i.e., surgical adenotonsillectomy, is associated with a much higher failure rate in obese children,[102,103] and initial encouraging studies would suggest that weight loss promotes beneficial effects on OSA severity as well as on metabolic function.[104]

Taken together, the deleterious interplay between obesity and OSA on metabolic function needs to be viewed as an extremely concerning consequence of these two conditions, particularly in the context of the potentially long-term effects that can ensue.

Clinical Pearls

- Alterations in sleep patterns and duration may contribute to the increased prevalence and severity of obesity in children and adolescents.
- Obstructive sleep apnea and obesity interact to increase the severity and morbid consequences of each other, possibly via their shared effects on the recruitment and potentiation of inflammatory pathways.
- Not every child with OSA will manifest metabolic dysfunction, suggesting that genetic and environmental factors may also play a role.
- Randomized, controlled intervention trials are urgently needed to more conclusively delineate the causative roles played by sleep and OSA in metabolic function.

References

1. Magarey AM, Daniels LA, Boulton TJ. Prevalence of overweight and obesity in Australian children and adolescents: reassessment of 1985 and 1995 data against new standard international definitions. Med J Aust 2001;174:561–4.
2. Lobstein T, Baur L, Uauy R; IASO International Obesity Task Force. Obesity in children and young people: a crisis in public health. Obes Rev 2004;(Suppl. 1):1–4.
3. Oza-Frank R, Hade EM, Norton A, et al. Trends in body mass index among Ohio's third-grade children: 2004–2005 to 2009–2010. J Acad Nutr Diet 2013;113(3):440–6.
4. Smith SM, Craig LC, Raja AE, et al. Growing up before growing out: secular trends in height, weight and obesity in 5–6-year-old children born between 1970 and 2006. Arch Dis Child 2013 [Epub ahead of print]
5. Ogden CL, Flegal KM, Carroll MD, et al. Prevalence and trends in overweight among US children and adolescents, 1999–2000. JAMA 2002;288:1728–32.
6. Edwards KL, Clarke GP, Ransley JK, et al. Serial cross-sectional analysis of prevalence of overweight and obese children between 1998 and 2003 in Leeds, UK, using routinely measured data. Public Health Nutr 2010;25:1–6.
7. Broyles S, Katzmarzyk PT, Srinivasan SR, et al. The pediatric obesity epidemic continues unabated in Bogalusa, Louisiana. Pediatrics 2010;125(5):900–5.
8. Wang YC, Gortmaker SL, Taveras EM. Trends and racial/ethnic disparities in severe obesity among US children and adolescents, 1976–2006. Int J Pediatr Obes 2010. [Epub ahead of print]
9. Luepker RV, Jacobs DR, Prineas RJ, et al. Secular trends of blood pressure and body size in a multi-ethnic adolescent population: 1986 to 1996. J Pediatr 1999;134:668–74.
10. Daniels SR, Arnett DK, Eckel RH, et al. Overweight in children and adolescents: pathophysiology, consequences, prevention, and treatment. Circulation 2005;111:1999–2012.
11. Barlow SE, Dietz WH. Obesity evaluation and treatment: Expert Committee recommendations. The Maternal and Child Health Bureau, Health Resources and Services Administration and the Department of Health and Human Services. Pediatrics 1998;102:e29.
12. Biro FM, Wien M. Childhood obesity and adult morbidities. Am J Clin Nutr 2010;91(5):1499S–505S.
13. Matricciani LA, Olds TS, Blunden S, et al. Never enough sleep: a brief history of sleep recommendations for children. Pediatrics 2012;129(3):548–56.
14. Krueger PM, Friedman EM. Sleep duration in the United States: a cross-sectional population-based study. Am J Epidemiol 2009;169(9):1052–63.
15. National Sleep Foundation. Sleep in America Poll – sleep in children survey. http://www.sleepfoundation.org/article/sleep-america-polls/2004-children-and-sleep2004.
16. Jones CH, Ball HL. Napping in English preschool children and the association with parents' attitudes. Sleep Med 2013. [Epub ahead of print]
17. Foley LS, Maddison R, Jiang Y, et al. Presleep activities and time of sleep onset in children. Pediatrics 2013;131(2):276–82.
18. Koulouglioti C, Cole R, Moskow M, et al. The longitudinal association of young children's everyday routines to sleep duration. J Pediatr Health Care 2013. [Epub ahead of print]
19. Wang Y, Beydoun MA. The obesity epidemic in the United States – gender, age, socioeconomic, racial/ethnic, and geographic characteristics: a systematic review and meta-regression analysis. Epidemiol Rev 2007;29:6–28.
20. Chen X, Beydoun MA, Wang Y. Is sleep duration associated with childhood obesity? A systematic review and meta-analysis. Obesity (Silver Spring) 2008;16(2):265–74.
21. Marshall NS, Glozier N, Grunstein RR. Is sleep duration related to obesity? A critical review of the epidemiological evidence. Sleep Med Rev 2008;12(4):289–98.
22. Taheri S, Thomas GN. Is sleep duration associated with obesity – Where do U stand? Sleep Medicine Reviews 2008;12(4):299–302.
23. Spruyt K, Gozal D. The underlying interactome of childhood obesity: the potential role of sleep. Child Obes 2012;8(1):38–42.
24. Spruyt K, Molfese DL, Gozal D. Sleep duration, sleep regularity, body weight, and metabolic homeostasis in school-aged children. Pediatrics 2011;127(2):e345–52.
25. Golley RK, Maher CA, Matricciani L, et al. Sleep duration or bedtime? Exploring the association between sleep timing behaviour, diet and BMI in children and adolescents. Int J Obes (Lond) 2013. [Epub ahead of print]
26. Jarrin DC, McGrath JJ, Drake CL. Beyond sleep duration: distinct sleep dimensions are associated with obesity in children and adolescents. Int J Obes (Lond) 2013. [Epub ahead of print]
27. Chahal H, Fung C, Kuhle S, et al. Availability and night-time use of electronic entertainment and communication devices are associated with short sleep duration and obesity among Canadian children. Pediatr Obes 2013;8(1):42–51.
28. O'Dea JA, Dibley MJ, Rankin NM. Low sleep and low socioeconomic status predict high body mass index: a 4-year longitudinal study of Australian schoolchildren. Pediatr Obes 2012;7(4):295–303.
29. Nielsen LS, Danielsen KV, Sørensen TI. Short sleep duration as a possible cause of obesity: critical analysis of the epidemiological evidence. Obes Rev 2010. [Epub ahead of print]
30. Calamaro CJ, Park S, Mason TB, et al. Shortened sleep duration does not predict obesity in adolescents. J Sleep Res 2010. [Epub ahead of print]
31. Sun Y, Sekine M, Kagamimori S. Lifestyle and overweight among Japanese adolescents: the Toyama Birth Cohort Study. J Epidemiol 2009;19(6):303–10.
32. Grandner MA, Patel NP, Gehrman PR, et al. Problems associated with short sleep: bridging the gap between laboratory and epidemiological studies. Sleep Med Rev 2010;14(4):239–47.
33. Monasta L, Batty GD, Cattaneo A, et al. Early-life determinants of overweight and obesity: a review of systematic reviews. Obes Rev 2010. [Epub ahead of print]
34. Chaput JP, Leblanc C, Pérusse L, et al. Risk factors for adult overweight and obesity in the Quebec Family Study: have we been barking up the wrong tree? Obesity (Silver Spring) 2009;17(10):1964–70.
35. Cizza G, Marincola P, Mattingly M, et al. Treatment of obesity with extension of sleep duration: a randomized, prospective, controlled trial. Clin Trials 2010;7(3):274–85.
36. Bayer O, Rosario AS, Wabitsch M, et al. Sleep duration and obesity in children: is the association dependent on age and choice of the outcome parameter? Sleep 2009;32(9):1183–9.
37. Bass J, Takahashi JS. Circadian integration of metabolism and energetics. Science 2010;330(6009):1349–54.
38. Zheng H, Berthoud H-R. Neural systems controlling the drive to eat: mind versus metabolism. Physiology 2008;23(2):75–83.
39. Mavanji V, Teske JA, Billington CJ, et al. Elevated sleep quality and orexin receptor mRNA in obesity-resistant rats. Int J Obes (Lond) 2010. [Epub ahead of print]
40. Maury E, Ramsey KM, Bass J. Circadian rhythms and metabolic syndrome: from experimental genetics to human disease. Circ Res 2010;106(3):447–62.
41. Eckel-Mahan KL, Patel VR, Mohney RP, et al. Coordination of the transcriptome and metabolome by the circadian clock. Proc Natl Acad Sci USA 2012;109(14):5541–6.
42. Reilly JJ, Armstrong J, Dorosty AR, et al. Early life risk factors for obesity in childhood: cohort study. BMJ 2005;330(7504):1357.
43. Flynn MA, McNeil DA, Maloff B, et al. Reducing obesity and related chronic disease risk in children and youth: a synthesis of evidence with 'best practice' recommendations. Obes Rev 2006;7(Suppl. 1):7–66.

44. Sekine M, Yamagami T, Handa K, et al. A dose–response relationship between short sleeping hours and childhood obesity: Results of the Toyama birth cohort study. Child: Care, Health and Development 2002;28(2):163–70.

45. Padez C, Mourao I, Moreira P, et al. Long sleep duration and childhood overweight/obesity and body fat. Am J Hum Biol 2009;21(3):371–6.

46. Taveras EM, Rifas-Shiman SL, Oken E, et al. Short sleep duration in infancy and risk of childhood overweight. Arch Pediatr Adol Med 2008;162(4):305–11.

47. Touchette A, Petit D, Tremblay RE, et al. Associations between sleep duration patterns and overweight/obesity at age 6. Sleep 2008;31(11): 1507–14.

48. Dayyat E, Kheirandish-Gozal L, Gozal D. Childhood obstructive sleep apnea: one or two distinct disease entities? Sleep Med Clin 2007; 2(3):433–44.

49. Arens R, Muzumdar H. Childhood obesity and obstructive sleep apnea syndrome. J Appl Physiol 2010;108(2):436–44.

50. Redline S, Tishler PV, Schluchter M, et al. Risk factors for sleep-disordered breathing in children. Associations with obesity, race, and respiratory problems. Am J Respir Crit Care Med 1999;159(5 Pt 1): 1527–32.

51. Wing YK, Hui SH, Pak WM, et al. A controlled study of sleep related disordered breathing in obese children. Arch Dis Child 2003;88: 1043–7.

52. Kalra M, Inge T, Garcia V, et al. Obstructive sleep apnea in extremely overweight adolescents undergoing bariatric surgery. Obes Res 2005; 13:1175–9.

53. Kahn A, Mozin MJ, Rebuffat E, et al. Sleep pattern alterations and brief airway obstructions in overweight infants. Sleep 1989;12:430–8.

54. Shine NP, Coates HL, Lannigan FJ. Obstructive sleep apnea, morbid obesity, and adenotonsillar surgery: a review of the literature. Int J Ped Otolaryngol 2005;69:1475–82.

55. Bixler EO, Vgontzas AN, Lin HM, et al. Sleep disordered breathing in children in a general population sample: prevalence and risk factors. Sleep 2009;32(6):731–6.

56. Verhulst SL, Franckx H, Van Gaal L, et al. The effect of weight loss on sleep-disordered breathing in obese teenagers. Obesity (Silver Spring) 2009;17(6):1178–83.

57. Dayyat E, Kheirandish-Gozal L, Sans Capdevila O, et al. Obstructive sleep apnea in children: relative contributions of body mass index and adenotonsillar hypertrophy. Chest 2009;136(1):137–44.

58. Brunetti L, Tesse R, Miniello VL, et al. Sleep-disordered breathing in obese children: the southern Italy experience. Chest 2010;137(5): 1085–90.

59. Kohler MJ, Thormaehlen S, Kennedy JD, et al. Differences in the association between obesity and obstructive sleep apnea among children and adolescents. J Clin Sleep Med 2009;5(6):506–11.

60. Mitchell RB, Boss EF. Pediatric obstructive sleep apnea in obese and normal-weight children: impact of adenotonsillectomy on quality-of-life and behavior. Dev Neuropsychol 2009;34(5):650–61.

61. White DP, Lombard RM, Cadieux RJ, et al. Pharyngeal resistance in normal humans: influence of gender, age, and obesity. J Appl Physiol 1985;58:365–71.

62. Horner RL, Mohiaddin RH, Lowell DG, et al. Sites and sizes of fat deposits around the pharynx in obese patients with obstructive sleep apnoea and weight matched controls. Eur Respir J 1989;2:613–22.

63. Arens R, Sin S, Nandalike K, et al. Upper airway structure and body fat composition in obese children with obstructive sleep apnea syndrome. Am J Respir Crit Care Med 2011;183(6):782–7.

64. Kheirandish-Gozal L. Fat and lymphadenoid tissues: a mutually obstructive combination. Am J Respir Crit Care Med 2011;183(6): 694–5.

65. Naimark A, Cherniack RM. Compliance of the respiratory system and its components in health and obesity. J Appl Physiol 1960;15:377–82.

66. Aygun AD, Gungor S, Ustundag B, et al. Proinflammatory cytokines and leptin are increased in serum of prepubertal obese children. Mediators Inflamm 2005;2005(3):180–3.

67. Reinehr T, Kratzsch J, Kiess W, et al. Circulating soluble leptin receptor, leptin, and insulin resistance before and after weight loss in obese children. Int J Obes (Lond) 2005;29:1230–5.

68. Celi F, Bini V, Papi F, et al. Leptin serum levels are involved in the relapse after weight excess reduction in obese children and adolescents. Diabetes Nutr Metab 2003;16:306–11.

69. Polotsky VY, Smaldone MC, Scharf MT, et al. Impact of interrupted leptin pathways on ventilatory control. J Appl Physiol 2004;96:991–8.

70. Arens R, Marcus CL. Pathophysiology of upper airway obstruction: a developmental perspective. Sleep 2004;27(5):997–1019.

71. Beebe DW, Lewin D, Zeller M, et al. Sleep in overweight adolescents: shorter sleep, poorer sleep quality, sleepiness, and sleep-disordered breathing. J Pediatr Psychol 2007;32(1):69–79.

72. Gozal D, Wang M, Pope DW Jr. Objective sleepiness measures in pediatric obstructive sleep apnea. Pediatrics 2001;108(3):693–7.

73. Tauman R, O'Brien LM, Holbrook CR, et al. Sleep pressure score: a new index of sleep disruption in snoring children. Sleep 2004;27(2): 274–8.

74. Melendres MC, Lutz JM, Rubin ED, et al. Daytime sleepiness and hyperactivity in children with suspected sleep-disordered breathing. Pediatrics 2004;114(3):768–75.

75. Chervin RD, Weatherly RA, Ruzicka DL, et al. Subjective sleepiness and polysomnographic correlates in children scheduled for adenotonsillectomy vs other surgical care. Sleep 2006;29(4):495–503.

76. Spruyt K, Sans Capdevila O, Serpero LD, et al. Dietary and physical activity patterns in children with obstructive sleep apnea. J Pediatr 2010;156(5):724–30, 730.e1–730.e3.

77. Gozal D, Kheirandish-Gozal L. Obesity and excessive daytime sleepiness in prepubertal children with obstructive sleep apnea. Pediatrics 2009;123(1):13–18.

78. Gozal D, Serpero LD, Sans Capdevila O, et al. Systemic inflammation in non-obese children with obstructive sleep apnea. Sleep Med 2008;9(3):254–9.

79. Tauman R, Ivanenko A, O'Brien LM, et al. Plasma C-reactive protein levels among children with sleep-disordered breathing. Pediatrics 2004;113(6):e564–9.

80. Gozal D. Sleep, sleep disorders and inflammation in children. Sleep Med 2009;10(Suppl. 1):S12–16.

81. Khalyfa A, Capdevila OS, Buazza MO, et al. Genome-wide gene expression profiling in children with non-obese obstructive sleep apnea. Sleep Med 2009;10(1):75–86.

82. Kim J, Bhattacharjee R, Snow AB, et al. Myeloid-related protein 8/14 levels in children with obstructive sleep apnoea. Eur Respir J 2010;35(4):843–50.

83. Gozal D, Serpero LD, Kheirandish-Gozal L, et al R. Sleep measures and morning plasma TNF-alpha levels in children with sleep-disordered breathing. Sleep 2010;33(3):319–25.

84. Davies RJ, Turner R, Crosby J, et al. Plasma insulin and lipid levels in untreated obstructive sleep apnoea and snoring; their comparison with matched controls and response to treatment. J Sleep Res 1994; 3(3):180–5.

85. Punjabi NM, Sorkin JD, Katzel LI, et al. Sleep-disordered breathing and insulin resistance in middle-aged and overweight men. Am J Respir Crit Care Med 2002;165(5):677–82.

86. Ip MS, Lam B, Ng MM, Lam WK, Tsang KW, Lam KS. Obstructive sleep apnea is independently associated with insulin resistance. Am J Respir Crit Care Med 2002;165(5):670–6.

87. Tauman R, O'Brien LM, Ivanenko A, et al. Obesity rather than severity of sleep-disordered breathing as the major determinant of insulin resistance and altered lipidemia in snoring children. Pediatrics 2005;116(1): e66–73.

88. Verhulst SL, Schrauwen N, Haentjens D, et al. Sleep-disordered breathing and the metabolic syndrome in overweight and obese children and adolescents. J Pediatr 2007;150(6):608–12.

89. Alexopoulos EI, Gletsou E, Kostadima E, et al. Effects of obstructive sleep apnea severity on serum lipid levels in Greek children with snoring. Sleep Breath 2011;15(4):625–31.

90. Redline S, Storfer-Isser A, Rosen CL, et al. Association between metabolic syndrome and sleep-disordered breathing in adolescents. Am J Respir Crit Care Med 2007;176(4):401–8.

91. Zong J, Liu Y, Huang Y, et al. Serum lipids alterations in adenoid hypertrophy or adenotonsillar hypertrophy children with sleep disordered breathing. Int J Pediatr Otorhinolaryngol 2013; in press

92. Gozal D, Capdevila OS, Kheirandish-Gozal L. Metabolic alterations and systemic inflammation in obstructive sleep apnea among nonobese and obese prepubertal children. Am J Respir Crit Care Med 2008; 177(10):1142–9.

93. Bhushan B, Khalyfa A, Spruyt K, et al. Fatty-acid binding protein 4 gene polymorphisms and plasma levels in children with obstructive sleep apnea. Sleep Med 2011;12(7):666–71.

94. Kaditis AG, Alexopoulos EI, Damani E, et al. Obstructive sleep-disordered breathing and fasting insulin levels in nonobese children. Pediatr Pulmonol 2005;40(6):515–23.

95. Lesser DJ, Bhatia R, Tran WH, et al. Sleep fragmentation and intermittent hypoxemia are associated with decreased insulin sensitivity in obese adolescent Latino males. Pediatr Res 2012;72(3):293–8.

96. Canapari CA, Hoppin AG, Kinane TB, et al. Relationship between sleep apnea, fat distribution, and insulin resistance in obese children. J Clin Sleep Med 2011;7(3):268–73.

97. Mirrakhimov AE, Polotsky VY. Obstructive sleep apnea and non-alcoholic fatty liver disease: is the liver another target? Front Neurol 2012;3:149.

98. Kheirandish-Gozal L, Sans Capdevila O, Kheirandish E, et al. Elevated serum aminotransferase levels in children at risk for obstructive sleep apnea. Chest 2008;133(1):92–9.

99. Verhulst SL, Jacobs S, Aerts L, et al. Sleep-disordered breathing: a new risk factor of suspected fatty liver disease in overweight children and adolescents? Sleep Breath 2009;13(2):207–10.

100. Verhulst SL, Rooman R, Van Gaal L, et al. Is sleep-disordered breathing an additional risk factor for the metabolic syndrome in obese children and adolescents? Int J Obes (Lond) 2009;33(1):8–13.

101. Tsaoussoglou M, Bixler EO, Calhoun S, et al. Sleep-disordered breathing in obese children is associated with prevalent excessive daytime sleepiness, inflammation, and metabolic abnormalities. J Clin Endocrinol Metab 2010;95(1):143–50.

102. Tauman R, Gulliver TE, Krishna J, et al. Persistence of obstructive sleep apnea syndrome in children after adenotonsillectomy. J Pediatr 2006; 149(6):803–8.

103. Bhattacharjee R, Kheirandish-Gozal L, Spruyt K, et al. Adenotonsillectomy outcomes in treatment of OSA in children: a multicenter retrospective study. Am J Respir Crit Care Med 2010;182(5):676–83.

104. Verhulst SL, Franckx H, Van Gaal L, et al. The effect of weight loss on sleep-disordered breathing in obese teenagers. Obesity (Silver Spring) 2009;17(6):1178–83.

Treatment Options in Obstructive Sleep Apnea

Sally L. Davidson Ward and Iris A. Perez

Chapter

32

INTRODUCTION

Obstructive sleep apnea syndrome (OSAS) is a common childhood sleep-related disorder resulting from an anatomically or functionally narrowed upper airway. The most common etiologies include adenotonsillar hypertrophy, obesity, craniofacial malformations, Down syndrome, and cerebral palsy.[1-3] When left untreated, childhood OSA can lead to significant morbidity[4-8] and may lay the foundation for adult cardiovascular and metabolic disease; thus, effective treatment may confer a life-long benefit. In this chapter, we review the different treatment options, their indications, efficacy and limitations for OSA in the pediatric population.

TREATMENT OPTIONS

Adenotonsillectomy

Most children with OSA will be treated with adenotonsillectomy (AT) as the first-line therapy.

Isolated adenoidectomy is commonly performed in children 5 years of age and younger.[9,10] Tonsillectomy involves the complete removal of the palatine tonsils with dissection. The capsule of the tonsil is also removed with the tonsil and muscle disrupted. A frequently used method in pediatrics is electrocautery dissection, which involves the application of electric energy-generating temperatures of 400–600°C directly to the tonsillar tissue, separating the muscle and simultaneously coagulating the blood vessels. Coblation tonsillectomy is performed using a device that delivers a bipolar frequency current through a conductive saline medium, converting it to an ionized plasma layer with effective energy to break molecular bonds between the tissues. The heat produced is limited to 40–70°C. It is associated with less postoperative pain and shorter recovery time.[11] Other surgical techniques involve the use of harmonic scalpel (ultrasonic dissector), coagulator,[12,13] and bipolar scissors.[13]

Recently, tonsillotomy (TT) or partial removal of the hypertrophied tonsils, has gained favor over total tonsillectomy. In tonsillotomy, the capsule is not breached and the muscle is protected. Different surgical techniques used include use of a CO_2 laser,[14,15] intracapsular microdebrider,[16] coblation,[17] electrocautery,[18] or radiofrequency.[19,20] Tonsillotomy with or without adenoidectomy results in resolution of symptoms of OSA with less postoperative pain, faster recovery, and lower rate of secondary postoperative hemorrhage compared to total tonsillectomy.[14-18] One study of children with a mean age of 4 years showed improvement of apnea-hypopnea index (AHI) to normal and increased oxygen saturation 3–12 months following CO_2 laser tonsillotomy in combination with adenoidectomy.[21] Following microdebrider technique there

was complete resolution of OSA by polysomnography in 50% of patients.[22] The major disadvantage of tonsillotomy is regrowth of tonsils with recurrence of snoring and obstructive symptoms. The rate of regrowth following tonsillotomy varies from 4% to 16%.[19,20,23] Celenk et al. reported that the majority of the children affected were younger than 4 years and had acute tonsillitis prior to tonsillar regrowth.[19] However, in a 10-year post surgery follow-up study of children who underwent tonsillotomy by electrocautery versus conventional tonsillectomy, no difference in tonsillar regrowth was noted.[18] Thus it is possible that factors affecting regrowth following tonsillotomy may include young age, inflammation, and surgical technique (radiofrequency).

AT results in improvements not only in symptoms, but also in sleep quality[24,25] and homeostasis.[26] There are also improvements in daytime behavior,[27,28] academic performance,[29] neurocognitive functioning[27,30] and quality of life.[25,27,28] These improvements can persist up to 1 year after AT in preschool children with OSA.[5] AT can also lead to weight gain with associated increase in growth markers (IGF-1 and IGFBP-3).[31-33] Children may have improved right ventricular function,[34] resolution of tachycardia and decreased pulse rate variability,[35] and significant decreases in diastolic blood pressure to near normal values.[36]

Unfortunately, up to 27% of children will have persistence of OSAS following AT.[37] Factors that contribute to persistent OSA include obesity,[37-40] asthma,[37] Down syndrome,[41] cerebral palsy,[39] gastroesophageal reflux disease,[42] and high preoperative apnea–hypopnea index (AHI).[37,38,43] In this group of patients, postoperative polysomnography will help identify the response to AT and additional treatments needed for residual OSA.[44]

Patients with mild OSAS may do well postoperatively from a respiratory standpoint, irrespective of the use of opiates for analgesia.[45] Complications following AT include postoperative bleeding, infection, upper airway obstruction secondary to airway edema, pulmonary edema, oxygen desaturation or respiratory failure requiring admission to the intensive care unit.[46,47] Pulmonary complication rates range between 5% and 38%.[48-51] Risk factors for pulmonary complications following AT are listed in Box 32-1.[48-52] These are the children who will benefit from overnight hospitalization for observation and monitoring following AT. One study reported an intensive care admission rate of 2.4% in a group of children with known risk factors for respiratory complications. Of these patients, about 1% required unanticipated transfer to the PICU.[47]

Polysomnography Prior to Adenotonsillectomy

Preoperative PSG is important to identify the presence and severity of OSA because symptoms, physical examination and certain laboratory tests do not predict PSG findings in

Box 32-1 Risk Factors for Pulmonary Complications Following Adenotonsillectomy

- Age less than 3 years
- Severe OSAS (profound hypoxemia (S_{PO2} <80%, AHI >10, significant hypoventilation)
- Morbid obesity
- Neuromuscular disease
- Pulmonary hypertension
- Down syndrome
- Craniofacial anomalies
- Asthma
- Sickle cell disease
- Failure to thrive
- History of respiratory compromise or anesthesia complications
- Congenital heart disease

children. PSG findings will help determine the type of therapy for the patient. PSG evidence of minimal respiratory disturbance is associated with low risk for perioperative complications supporting the decision to perform AT in an ambulatory center. Because increased preoperative obstructive apnea–hypopnea index and low SpO2 nadir are highly predictive of pulmonary complication post surgery, performing AT without the guidance of a polysomnogram can place children at risk for unexpected postoperative complications. Furthermore, since elevated preoperative AHI is predictive of residual OSA, PSG prior to AT will help identify those patients who will need close follow-up and further evaluation.[37]

Inpatient versus Outpatient
Many procedures are completed in the ambulatory center or with one night of observation postoperatively on pediatric inpatient units.[47] The decision to perform surgery in the ambulatory setting is not straightforward. Professional societies with vested interest in the safety of children undergoing AT recommend inpatient monitoring for high-risk patients,[53] children younger than age 3 or those who have severe obstructive sleep apnea, oxygen saturation nadir less than 80%, or both,[54] and patients with a score of ≥5 on a scoring system used to estimate increased perioperative risk for OSA complications.[55] In summary, patients who are at higher risk for postoperative complications will require a higher level of care and should be admitted for overnight observation and may even require the intensive cardiorespiratory monitoring afforded by a PICU.

Some children with associated neuromuscular disability, e.g., cerebral palsy or Down syndrome, might benefit from more extensive surgical procedures such as uvulopalatopharyngoplasty.[39,56–58] These patients require careful monitoring, as they are at risk for residual OSA. One study of UPPP with tonsillectomy in children reported relapse of OSA and need for tracheostomy in 23% of patients undergoing a 5-year follow-up period.[56]

Skeletal Advancement Procedures in Children with Craniofacial Abnormalities
Infants and children with craniofacial abnormalities and severe OSA can benefit from skeletal advancement procedures to prevent tracheostomy or to facilitate decannulation. Two

procedures performed in children include mandibular distraction osteogenesis and rapid maxillary expansion.

Mandibular Distraction Osteogenesis
Patients with micrognathia or retrognathia have upper airway obstruction from retro-positioning of the base of the tongue, compromising the hypopharyngeal space. Mandibular distraction osteogenesis has been shown to be successful in patients with micro- and retrognathia with more severe disease. This procedure improves the position of the tongue in the posterior pharynx by lengthening the mandible and bringing its muscular insertions forward, thus increasing the antero-posterior dimension of the airway. This has allowed relief of symptoms and avoidance of a tracheostomy in infants or children with OSA[59–61] and allowed decannulation in those who are already tracheostomy-dependent.[62,63]

Rapid Maxillary Expansion
Some patients with OSA and maxillofacial malformation and dental malocclusion may benefit from rapid maxillary expansion (RME). RME is an orthodontic procedure that widers the maxillary bone by gradual distraction osteogenesis. Bone distraction at the mid-palatal suture widens the maxilla and increases the volume of the nasal cavity and thus decreases nasal resistance. Following this procedure, patients have shown improvement in symptoms, apnea–hypopnea index, arousal index, and with almost normalized sleep architecture up to 24 months after the completion of treatment.[64–65]

Other surgical procedures include maxilla–mandibular advancement for mid-face hypoplasia, as well as tongue reduction, genioglossal advancement, or hyoid myotomy and suspension, which are aimed at relieving retroglossal obstruction. These are infrequently performed in children and are generally only indicated in those with craniofacial malformations or specific genetic syndromes. Ultimately, in children with severe OSA who have failed standard therapies, positive pressure therapy or tracheostomy may be required.

Positive Pressure Therapy
See also Chapter 35 by Sivan and Gut.

Positive airway pressure therapy (PAP), i.e., continuous positive airway pressure (CPAP) or bi-level positive airway pressure (BPAP), can be a highly effective means of treatment for OSAS. PAP is the treatment of choice for patients who do not improve sufficiently following AT or when surgery is not possible or indicated. It is often used for patients with OSA related to obesity, Down syndrome, craniofacial disorders, and neuromuscular disorders such as cerebral palsy. Positive pressure therapy has been shown to be effective in children for the treatment of OSA. It is less invasive than surgery and offers temporary treatment for conditions such as postoperative airway obstruction.[53]

AT remains the first line of treatment for OSA in most situations; however, residual symptoms may persist in up to 20% of children[43] with some studies reporting an even higher failure rate.[38,67] When a PSG reveals an AHI of more than 5 events per hour following AT, then PAP should be considered.[68] A titration study should be performed in the sleep laboratory with a technician in attendance. At this time, insufficient evidence and lack of FDA approval preclude the recommendation of auto-titrating devices in children. Practice guidelines for detailed, step-by-step titration strategies for positive pressure therapy in adults and children have been proposed in the Clinical Guidelines for the Manual Titration of Positive Airway Pressure in Patients with OSA sponsored by the American Academy of Sleep Medicine.[69] Four separate algorithms for CPAP and BPAP titrations for patients less than and greater than 12 years of age, respectively, are presented. These can be adapted for use in the sleep laboratory to guide technicians in decision making throughout the night. The goal for an optimal titration is to reduce the respiratory disturbance index to less than 5 events per hour with supine REM sleep recorded at the selected pressure. Evidence-based guidelines for the selection of continuous versus bi-level positive pressure therapy are lacking. Studies have not found an advantage in adherence or outcome in either adults or children.[70] The practice of the authors is to use bi-level therapy when high pressures (>14 CWP) are needed to relieve airway obstruction or the patient complains of intolerably high pressure during the study. Bi-level therapy is also utilized for OSA in the face of hypoventilation ($P_{ET}CO_2$ >50 mmHg), with coexisting muscle weakness, or with extreme obesity. A back-up rate can be provided with prolonged central apneas. Supplemental oxygen may be required with coexisting pulmonary disease when hypoxemia persists despite control of obstructive events and respiratory-related arousals.

The most important consideration in selecting the PAP interface is patient comfort. Generally, nasal masks are preferred over nasal–oral (full-face) masks in the pediatric population as there is less chance for gaseous distension of the stomach or aspiration if emesis occurs. However, some patients have marked nasal occlusion and a nasal–oral mask is the only route available. Some patients will prefer nasal prongs or 'pillows,' especially if they have a strong preference to sleep on their side. The headgear should be snug but not tight. Some redness of the skin in the morning that fades during the day is acceptable, but persistent tenderness or erythema over the nasal bridge is not, as it can lead to painful skin breakdown and thus must be addressed quickly. Covering the site with a hydrocolloid gel dressing is helpful as an interim solution. Masks should fit such that air leak, or the mask itself, does not irritate the eyes.

At each follow-up, potential problems with the interface and other complications associated with the therapy that might interfere with usage are discussed. Complications such as nasal dryness or congestion, epistaxis, eye irritation, skin compromise, gastric distension, emesis in those patients using full-face mask, and mouth breathing with excessive leak in those using nasal mask or prongs are addressed. Nasal steroids and/or warm humidification can help relieve nasal obstruction and improve adherence. Skin complications can be avoided by regular follow-up to assess mask fit and by changing the interface from time to time. Monitoring of facial growth for the development of mid-face hypoplasia related to nightly pressure from the mask interface has been suggested. At this time, in the United States, FDA-approved interfaces for PAP are only available for children age 7 years and older. Some countries have interfaces available for younger children and infants; however, in the USA these devices are used 'off label' at the discretion of the prescribing physician and this information should be shared with parents.

When the decision has been made to institute PAP, one of the most important considerations is preparing the child and family for the use of the therapy on a nightly basis. This approach varies with the age and developmental level of the child. The patient and family should be educated about the titration study, the PAP equipment, and the interface, with verbal and written material in advance.[70] The medical care team must convey a high level of confidence and trust in the parents' abilities to master the techniques, and more importantly in their ability to work with their child to use the therapy each night. A parental approach that is consistent, committed, and calm should be emphasized. Patients ideally should be fitted with and given an appropriate interface to wear at home at bedtime for practice and desensitization prior to the study. The interface is worn without being attached to the tubing or positive pressure device so there is no flow or pressure. Parents are encouraged to build this into the child's usual bedtime routine. If the child is to sleep with the practice mask in place, care must be taken to avoid re-breathing by modifying the mask. An age-appropriate reward system (behavior modification) for wearing the interface is often helpful. Child developmental psychologists with expertise in sleep medicine can guide desensitization in difficult cases. In this way, when the patient arrives for the titration study, the focus can be on identifying the correct settings to achieve adequate gas exchange, normal respiratory pattern, and optimal sleep quality. Similar to adults, split studies are possible with typically developing adolescents; the educational session need not be extensive and can be accomplished with pre-study explanation or video.[71]

Pressure titration is affected by the age of the child. Younger children generally do not tolerate pressures at the higher range (>15 CWP) and, in general, OSA can be managed with pressures lower than this. Children are also poorly tolerant of painful procedures, thus non-invasive monitoring of gas exchange is used rather than blood gases. The use of end-tidal CO_2 monitoring during the titration study can provide an accurate measure of ventilation and avoid the use of arterial or capillary blood gas collection. To this effect, a small end-tidal CO_2 catheter is placed at one of the nares under the mask interface. Readings are deemed accurate when a plateau is present in the waveform. If the plateau is lost the catheter can be repositioned at the first wakefulness opportunity. Because the catheter is small, the interface seal is not disrupted. However, subjects who use nasal prongs or pillows as their preferred interface cannot be monitored in this way and gas exchange must be inferred from SpO_2 measurements or transcutaneous CO_2 measurements. Blood gas sampling is not needed for sleep lab titration of PAP for OSA in children, but is useful for patients with severe, obesity-related OSA with hypoventilation who have been hospitalized for initiation of treatment.

Some children with OSA are very young or have developmental disabilities and thus cannot communicate with the polysomnographic technician or respiratory therapist to express discomfort with the interface or the pressures. Technicians and therapists who are skilled in working with children of all ages and abilities are required for a successful PAP titration in the pediatric sleep lab. Understanding that a patient's discomfort can have different origins and working carefully with the child and parent to minimize fear and maximize comfort require patience and skills that develop over years of experience. Reducing pressures, selecting a different interface, and changing the patient's position should all be tried. However, there are occasions, despite advance preparation, when the child's inability to cooperate prevents completion of an adequate titration. If OSA is not severe, a further period of time acclimating in the home setting can be tried. The PAP interface and device can be used for a short time each night in the home on the best-tolerated pressure levels identified during the study with a gradual increase in the time used each night. When use has increased to more than 4–6 hours per night the laboratory titration can be repeated to identify optimal pressures. If the clinical situation dictates a more rapid initiation of therapy, then hospitalization would be indicated.

Expert opinion recommends periodic re-titration studies for children treated with PAP. This is logically based on the notion that children are growing and developing and that these changes may interact with upper airway anatomy and neuromuscular function such that positive pressure needs may increase or decrease. Thus, younger patients would need more frequent re-evaluations than older children. Repeat titration should be performed after surgeries of the upper airway, significant change in weight, and certainly if new symptoms indicating poor control of OSA or tolerance of PAP arise. Very limited data are available to guide the frequency of routine repeat titration studies in children.

Perioperative Use
Obstructive sleep apnea increases the risk of poor outcomes with surgery requiring general anesthesia.[72] PAP has been proposed as a strategy for stabilization of patients with severe OSA in the perioperative period prior to AT and prior to other elective surgical procedures.[73–76] A case series of 48 children with severe OSA (respiratory disturbance index ranged from 50 to 80/hour of sleep) treated with this approach prior to AT found that mean nightly use was just 4.5 hours, with 73% of subjects using the device for more than 3 hours per night; data regarding postoperative course were not presented.[76] Data are lacking regarding the cost effectiveness and efficacy of this approach, but there is some evidence in the adult literature documenting decreased surgical risk in patients with OSA treated with preoperative PAP in preparation for elective surgery.[65] Use of PAP for 4–6 weeks prior to surgery has been recommended.[72,77] As is typical for any indication for PAP, strategies and technologies to improve adherence remain critical needs.

Adherence
Adherence to PAP is a major problem in patients with OSA, both in children and adults. Ideally, adherence should be determined objectively via machine download information. Information regarding patient use rather than the time the unit is simply turned on is more useful. In one study, treatment with PAP was associated with a high drop-out rate (one-third of children) before 6 months and with mean nightly use of only 5.3 hours in those who were adherent. This is brief, considering the long sleep hours in children.[70] Behavioral therapy, in conjunction with ongoing support and close follow-up, increased adherence to PAP in children.[78,79] Uong and co-workers identified 70% PAP adherence in a retrospective study of 27 cognitively intact children with residual OSA post AT (adherence defined as more than 4 hours nightly use at least 5 nights per week determined objectively by machine counter clock/meter). They found that adherence in terms of days of use was better in patients with more severe OSA and

in those with the greatest decrease in AHI with PAP. Age, gender, race, BMI, and PAP mode did not affect adherence. Parental report of adherence correlated with the meter readings.[80] The initial use of PAP during the first week of use was a predictor of subsequent use in a prospective study of 30 children, including those with developmental disability. This emphasizes the importance of starting out on the 'right foot,' as outlined above. The authors commented that using PAP at low, perhaps sub-therapeutic pressures, during sleep prior to formal titration may interfere with subsequent adherence.[81] Demographic factors impacting adherence were found by DiFeo and co-workers, with maternal education being the greatest predictor of higher use, whereas African-American race and older patient age predicted poorer adherence. The children studied had a number of underlying conditions, and 23% had developmental disabilities. In general, adherence was rated suboptimal for the group as a whole with an average use of 3 hours per night and 22 days per month.[82] Designing effective strategies to enhance PAP adherence would be facilitated by an understanding of perceived barriers on the part of parents and patients. Simon et al. devised a questionnaire evaluating barriers to PAP use and identified a number of psychosocial issues including embarrassment, forgetfulness and denial as frequently playing a role.[83] A reasonable hypothesis has been that patients would find BPAP to be more comfortable than CPAP, with greater ease of exhalation and synchrony with natural breathing patterns, and furthermore that increased comfort would improve adherence. Marcus and co-workers examined this relationship in two studies, the first comparing BPAP and CPAP and the second comparing CPAP with a bi-level technology that includes pressure relief. Neither study identified better adherence in the bi-level group and adherence was suboptimal in both groups despite efficacy.[70,84]

PAP desensitization can be considered for patients who are simply unable to wear the equipment, a scenario common in very young patients or those with developmental disability. Harford et al. describe a multidisciplinary in-patient approach to desensitization in a case report of two children. The centerpiece of desensitization therapy is a child psychologist who can identify both motivating factors and barriers to acceptance for the child and family and design an individualized plan of gradual acclimatization to the mask, headgear, and PAP flow. Close follow-up is needed to reinforce adherence.[85] Clearly, a major challenge for the pediatric sleep medicine community is to refine methods of increasing adherence to PAP therapy. The therapy itself is safe and effective, and the potential to reduce both childhood comorbidities and the early development of adult cardiovascular disease is of extraordinary value to the individual child and society.

Supplemental Oxygen
Supplemental oxygen can relieve hypoxemia in patients with OSA while awaiting definitive therapy or in patients in whom no other treatment option is available.[86,87] In those with long-term hypercapnia, oxygen must be used with caution and preferably started during the polysomnogram when gas exchange is carefully monitored, or during hospitalization with blood gas monitoring.

Anti-Inflammatory Therapies
There are increasing data on the efficacy of anti-inflammatory therapies, i.e., nasal steroids[88–90] and montelukast,[91] in the

management of mild OSA, with improvement in symptoms and reduction in adenoid size.[89,92] A recent randomized, controlled trial in a small number of children appears to support the use of this pharmacological agent in young children with mild OSA.[93] Combined montelukast and intranasal budesonide may help children with residual mild OSA following AT.[94] In children treated with nasal steroids, clinical improvement might persist up to 9 months after the completion of treatment,[90] and reduction in adenoid size may continue 8 weeks after discontinuation of therapy.[92] In a prospective study of subjects scheduled for surgery, intranasal fluticasone resulted in significant improvement such that 76% of the patients no longer required surgery and were removed from the surgical waiting list.[95] Goldbart et al. demonstrated the expression of glucocorticoid receptor in the adenotonsillar tissue of children with OSAS.[96,97] There is reduction in proliferative responses, increased cellular apoptosis, and decreased release of pro-inflammatory cytokines (TNF-α, IL-8, and IL-6) in tonsils or adenoids from children with OSA treated with intranasal steroids[98,99] and leukotriene receptor antagonists.[100]

Oral Appliances

Oral appliances enlarge the upper airway by positioning the mandible and tongue forward. The two types of oral appliances are the mandibular repositioning and tongue retaining devices. Two small 6-month trials in children with coexisting malocclusion and OSA showed improvement in AHI by 50% without return to normal pediatric values. The side effects included brief excessive salivation[101,102] and discomfort on awakening[102] that improved after a few days. A 3-year-old boy with severe OSA and laryngomalacia but without malocclusion who had undergone adenoidectomy at 2 years of age treated with oral appliance for 14 months reportedly showed significant clinical improvement without observed dental or skeletal changes.[103] Although frequently used in the adult population with snoring or mild to moderate OSAS,[104] there are insufficient data at present to state that it is effective in children. Furthermore, there are no long-term data to support the use of oral appliances before full maturation of the jaw and teeth.

Specific Populations
Obesity

The prevalence of OSA is estimated at 13–59% in obese children. OSA can be severe with frequent obstructive events, profound hypoxemia and significant hypoventilation. In this higher-risk group, adenotonsillectomy remains the first line of treatment. These patients are at risk for hypoventilation; thus, oxygen and narcotics should be used judiciously postoperatively. Obese children are at risk for residual OSA following adenotonsillectomy[40] and frequently require treatment with positive airway pressure therapy even after AT. Weight loss should be a part of the treatment plan.[53]

Weight Loss/Role of Bariatric Surgery

Weight loss and lifestyle intervention can be an effective treatment for mild OSA,[105,106] although there is significant rate of relapse even in the most aggressive weight loss therapy, including use of pharmacotherapy. For this reason, bariatric surgery may play a role. Few studies of bariatric surgery in adolescents show promising short-term outcome with early weight loss and improvement of medical comorbidities, i.e., hypertension and metabolic syndrome, improvement in quality of life,[107] and near complete resolution of OSA.[108] One study of obese children and adolescents with median BMI of 47.4 kg/m² who underwent laparoscopic sleeve gastrectomy showed short-term weight loss in more than 90% of the patients. Of these patients 20 of 22 patients with OSA had resolution of symptoms.[109] With these results, it can be assumed that if bariatric surgery can provide a long-term effective reduction of body weight, it can also lead to successful improvement of OSA. However, adult studies showed that despite remarkable weight loss, many patients had residual OSA following bariatric surgery.[110,111]

Adolescents being considered for bariatric surgery must meet stringent criteria: (1) BMI of 40 kg/m² with mild comorbidities or >35 kg/m² with severe comorbidities (diabetes, moderate to severe OSA, pseudotumor cerebri), (2) failure to attain healthy weight with nonsurgical measures, (3) have attained 95% of adult stature, (4) have achieved or nearly achieved physiologic maturity, (5) commitment to psychological evaluation in the perioperative period, (6) completed comprehensive psychological assessment, and (7) will adhere to postoperative nutritional guidelines, have decisional capacity, and will provide informed consent.[112,113]

Down Syndrome

Patients with Down syndrome develop OSA due to a combination of mid-face hypoplasia, relatively large tongue,[114] hypotonia, frequent obesity, and occasionally hypothyroidism.[115] The primary treatment is AT. However, persistent OSA with recurrent adenoidal hypertrophy, enlargement of lingual tonsils, or obesity is common.[116] Therefore, children with Down syndrome should be followed closely for recurrent OSA. Some patients benefit at least temporarily with UPPP in addition to AT.[28,44,45] One study reported improvement in airway obstruction in children with Down syndrome treated with rapid maxillary expansion.[117] PAP can provide successful therapy in those with residual OSA or with persistent hypoventilation. Periodic evaluation of thyroid function is indicated in Down syndrome because hypothyroidism can worsen OSA.[118–120]

Infancy

Infants can have OSA from nasal obstruction, craniofacial abnormalities, laryngomalacia, subglottic stenosis, cleft palate, or gastroesophageal reflux disease.[121] Therapy is directed to the underlying cause. Those who are not stable or are not candidates for surgery can be placed on supplemental oxygen, if hypoxemia is present. PAP therapy is limited in this age group as it is not well tolerated and there is not an array of appropriate nasal interfaces. Adenoidectomy has been found to relieve OSA and failure to thrive.[122] Tongue lip adhesion, mandibular distraction osteogenesis or nasopharyngeal tube may relieve OSA in infants with micrognathia or retrognathia.[59–61,123–125] Infants with laryngomalacia and mild symptoms may be observed as this usually improves with maturation. However, those with associated feeding difficulties and poor growth will require supratoglottoplasty.[126,127] Surgical repair or tracheostomy is necessary in those with severe subglottic stenosis and OSA. GERD is common in infants and worsens OSA via increased inflammation of the upper airway. Most often, medical management with acid suppression is sufficient. However, when GERD is not improved with medical therapy, antireflux surgical procedure with or without gastrostomy tube placement may be necessary.

Clinical Pearls

- Careful attention to risk factors for perioperative complications of adenotonsillectomy with plans for hospital observation of high-risk patients is key to minimizing adverse outcomes.
- Parental and patient education regarding PAP therapy well in advance of the initial titration study is very important in subsequent adherence.
- Not all patients will be cured following adenotonsillectomy, and follow-up directed at persistent symptoms or complications of OSA is indicated.
- A very high index of suspicion for OSA is needed in overweight and obese children; OSA may represent a modifiable risk factor in this population for the reduction of risk for serious cardiovascular and metabolic disease in later life.

References

1. Lumeng JC, Chervin RD. Epidemiology of pediatric obstructive sleep apnea. Proc Am Thorac Soc 2008;5(2):242–52.
2. Redline S, Tishler PV, Schluchter M, et al. Risk factors for sleep-disordered breathing in children. Associations with obesity, race, and respiratory problems. Am J Respir Crit Care Med 1999;159(5 Pt 1):1527–32.
3. Rosen CL, Larkin EK, Kirchner HL, et al. Prevalence and risk factors for sleep-disordered breathing in 8- to 11-year-old children: association with race and prematurity. J Pediatr 2003;142(4):383–9.
4. Melendres MC, Lutz JM, Rubin ED, et al. Daytime sleepiness and hyperactivity in children with suspected sleep-disordered breathing. Pediatrics 2004;114(3):768–75.
5. Landau YE, Bar-Yishay O, Greenberg-Dotan S, et al. Impaired behavioral and neurocognitive function in preschool children with obstructive sleep apnea. Pediatr Pulmonol 2012;47(2):180–8.
6. Leung LC, Ng DK, Lau MW, et al. Twenty-four-hour ambulatory BP in snoring children with obstructive sleep apnea syndrome. Chest 2006;130(4):1009–17.
7. Redline S, Storfer-Isser A, Rosen CL, et al. Association between metabolic syndrome and sleep-disordered breathing in adolescents. Am J Respir Crit Care Med 2007;176(4):401–8.
8. Everett AD, Koch WC, Saulsbury FT. Failure to thrive due to obstructive sleep apnea. Clin Pediatr (Phila) 1987;26(2):90–2.
9. Tomkinson A, Harrison W, Owens D, et al. Postoperative hemorrhage following adenoidectomy. Laryngoscope 2012;122(6):1246–53.
10. Leonardis RL, Robison JG, Otteson TD. Evaluating the management of obstructive sleep apnea in neonates and infants. JAMA Otolaryngol Head Neck Surg 2013;139(2):139–46.
11. Benninger M, Walner D. Coblation: improving outcomes for children following adenotonsillectomy. Clin Cornerstone 2007;9(Suppl. 1):S13–23.
12. Willging JP, Wiatrak BJ. Harmonic scalpel tonsillectomy in children: a randomized prospective study. Otolaryngol Head Neck Surg 2003;128(3):318–25.
13. Isaacson G, Szeremeta W. Pediatric tonsillectomy with bipolar electro-surgical scissors. Am J Otolaryngol 1998;19(5):291–5.
14. Densert O, Desai H, Eliasson Å, et al. Tonsillotomy in children with tonsillar hypertrophy. Acta Otolaryngol 2001;121(7):854–8.
15. Hultcrantz E, Linder A, Markstrom A. Tonsillectomy or tonsillotomy? – A randomized study comparing postoperative pain and long-term effects. Int J Pediatr Otorhinolaryngol 1999;51(3):171–6.
16. Koltai PJ, Solares CA, Koempel JA, et al. Intracapsular tonsillar reduction (partial tonsillectomy): reviving a historical procedure for obstructive sleep disordered breathing in children. Otolaryngol Head Neck Surg 2003;129(5):532–8.

17. Arya AK, Donne A, Nigam A. Double-blind randomized controlled study of coblation tonsillotomy versus coblation tonsillectomy or postoperative pain in children. Clin Otolaryngol 2005;30(3):226–9.
18. Eviatar E, Kessler A, Shlamkovitch N, et al. Tonsillectomy vs. partial tonsillectomy for OSAS in children – 10 years post-surgery follow-up. Int J Pediatr Otorhinolaryngol 2009;73(5):637–40.
19. Celenk F, Bayazit YA, Yilmaz M, et al. Tonsillar regrowth following partial tonsillectomy with radiofrequency. Int J Pediatr Otorhinolaryngol 2008;72(1):19–22.
20. Moriniere S, Roux A, Bakhos D, et al. Radiofrequency tonsillotomy versus bipolar scissors tonsillectomy for the treatment of OSAS in children: A prospective study. Eur Ann Otorhinolaryngol Head Neck Dis 2013;130(2):67–72.
21. de la Chaux R, Klemens C, Patscheider M, et al. Tonsillotomy in the treatment of obstructive sleep apnea syndrome in children: polysomnographic results. Int J Pediatr Otorhinolaryngol 2008;72(9):1411–17.
22. Reilly BK, Levin J, Sheldon S, et al. Efficacy of microdebrider intracapsular adenotonsillectomy as validated by polysomnography. Laryngoscope 2009;119(7):1391–3.
23. Ericsson E, Lundeborg I, Hultcrantz E. Child behavior and quality of life before and after tonsillotomy versus tonsillectomy. Int J Pediatr Otorhinolaryngol 2009;73(9):1254–62.
24. Lee SH, Choi JH, Park IH, et al. Measuring sleep quality after adenotonsillectomy in pediatric sleep apnea. Laryngoscope 2012;122(9):2115–21.
25. Constantin E, Kermack A, Nixon GM, et al. Adenotonsillectomy improves sleep, breathing, and quality of life but not behavior. J Pediatr 2007;150(5):540–6, 546 e1.
26. Ben-Israel N, Zigel Y, Tal A, et al. Adenotonsillectomy improves slow-wave activity in children with obstructive sleep apnoea. Eur Respir J 2011;37(5):1144–50.
27. Mitchell RB, Kelly J. Outcomes and quality of life following adenotonsillectomy for sleep-disordered breathing in children. ORL J Otorhinolaryngol Relat Spec 2007;69(6):345–8.
28. Ye J, Liu H, Zhang GH, et al. Outcome of adenotonsillectomy for obstructive sleep apnea syndrome in children. Ann Otol Rhinol Laryngol 2010;119(8):506–13.
29. Gozal D, Pope DW Jr. Snoring during early childhood and academic performance at ages thirteen to fourteen years. Pediatrics 2001;107(6):1394–9.
30. Friedman BC, Hendeles-Amitai A, Kozminsky E, et al. Adenotonsillectomy improves neurocognitive function in children with obstructive sleep apnea syndrome. Sleep 2003;26(8):999–1005.
31. Kiris M, Muderris T, Celebi S, et al. Changes in serum IGF-1 and IGFBP-3 levels and growth in children following adenoidectomy, tonsillectomy or adenotonsillectomy. Int J Pediatr Otorhinolaryngol 2010;74(5):528–31.
32. Bonuck KA, Freeman K, Henderson J. Growth and growth biomarker changes after adenotonsillectomy: systematic review and meta-analysis. Arch Dis Child 2009;94(2):83–91.
33. Bar A, Tarasiuk A, Segev Y, et al. The effect of adenotonsillectomy on serum insulin-like growth factor-I and growth in children with obstructive sleep apnea syndrome. J Pediatr 1999;135(1):76–80.
34. Koc S, Aytekin M, Kalay N, et al. The effect of adenotonsillectomy on right ventricle function and pulmonary artery pressure in children with adenotonsillar hypertrophy. Int J Pediatr Otorhinolaryngol 2012;76(1):45–8.
35. Constantin E, McGregor CD, Cote V, et al. Pulse rate and pulse rate variability decrease after adenotonsillectomy for obstructive sleep apnea. Pediatr Pulmonol 2008;43(5):498–504.
36. Ng DK, Wong JC, Chan CH, et al. Ambulatory blood pressure before and after adenotonsillectomy in children with obstructive sleep apnea. Sleep Med 2010;11(7):721–5.
37. Bhattacharjee R, Kheirandish-Gozal L, Spruyt K, et al. Adenotonsillectomy outcomes in treatment of obstructive sleep apnea in children: a multicenter retrospective study. Am J Respir Crit Care Med 2010;182(5):676–83.
38. Tauman R, Gulliver TE, Krishna J, et al. Persistence of obstructive sleep apnea syndrome in children after adenotonsillectomy. J Pediatr 2006;149(5):803–8.
39. Wiet GJ, Bower C, Seibert R, et al. Surgical correction of obstructive sleep apnea in the complicated pediatric patient documented by polysomnography. Int J Pediatr Otorhinolaryngol 1997;41(2):133–43.
40. Amin R, Anthony L, Somers V, et al. Growth velocity predicts recurrence of sleep-disordered breathing 1 year after adenotonsillectomy. Am J Respir Crit Care Med 2008;177(6):654–9.

41. Marcus CL, Keens TG, Bautista DB, et al. Obstructive sleep apnea in children with Down syndrome. Pediatrics 1991;88(1):132–9.

42. Wasilewska J, Kaczmarski M, Debkowska K. Obstructive hypopnea and gastroesophageal reflux as factors associated with residual obstructive sleep apnea syndrome. Int J Pediatr Otorhinolaryngol 2011. E-pub ahead of print

43. Mitchell RB. Adenotonsillectomy for obstructive sleep apnea in children: outcome evaluated by pre- and postoperative polysomnography. Laryngoscope 2007;117(10):1844–54.

44. Wise MS, Nichols CD, Grigg-Damberger MM, et al. Executive summary of respiratory indications for polysomnography in children: an evidence-based review. Sleep 2011;34(3):389–98.

45. Kalantar N, Takehana CS, Shapiro NL. Outcomes of reduced postoperative stay following outpatient pediatric tonsillectomy. Int J Pediatr Otorhinolaryngol 2006;70(12):2103–7.

46. Sanders JC, King MA, Mitchell RB, et al. Perioperative complications of adenotonsillectomy in children with obstructive sleep apnea syndrome. Anesth Analg 2006;103(5):1115–21.

47. Tweedie DJ, Bajaj Y, Ifeacho SN, et al. Peri-operative complications after adenotonsillectomy in a UK pediatric tertiary referral centre. Int J Pediatr Otorhinolaryngol 2012;76(6):809–15.

48. Ye J, Liu H, Zhang G, et al. Postoperative respiratory complications of adenotonsillectomy for obstructive sleep apnea syndrome in older children: prevalence, risk factors, and impact on clinical outcome. J Otolaryngol Head Neck Surg 2009;38(1):49–58.

49. Spencer DJ, Jones JE. Complications of adenotonsillectomy in patients younger than 3 years. Arch Otolaryngol Head Neck Surg 2012;138(4):335–9.

50. Hill CA, Litvak A, Canapari C, et al. A pilot study to identify pre- and peri-operative risk factors for airway complications following adenotonsillectomy for treatment of severe pediatric OSA. Int J Pediatr Otorhinolaryngol 2011;75(11):1385–90.

51. McColley SA, April MM, Carroll JL, et al. Respiratory compromise after adenotonsillectomy in children with obstructive sleep apnea. Arch Otolaryngol Head Neck Surg 1992;118(9):940–3.

52. Wilson K, Lakheeram I, Morielli A, et al. Can assessment for obstructive sleep apnea help predict postadenotonsillectomy respiratory complications? Anesthesiology 2002;96(2):313–22.

53. Marcus CL, Brooks LJ, Draper KA, et al. Diagnosis and management of childhood obstructive sleep apnea syndrome. Pediatrics 2012;130(3):576–84.

54. Roland PS, Rosenfeld RM, Brooks LJ, et al. Clinical practice guideline: Polysomnography for sleep-disordered breathing prior to tonsillectomy in children. Otolaryngol Head Neck Surg 2011;145(Suppl. 1):S1–15.

55. Gross JB, Bachenberg KL, Benumof JL, et al. Practice guidelines for the perioperative management of patients with obstructive sleep apnea: a report by the American Society of Anesthesiologists Task Force on Perioperative Management of patients with obstructive sleep apnea. Anesthesiology 2006;104(5):1081–93; quiz 1117–18.

56. Kerschner JE, Lynch JB, Kleiner H, et al. Uvulopalatopharyngoplasty with tonsillectomy and adenoidectomy as a treatment for obstructive sleep apnea in neurologically impaired children. Int J Pediatr Otorhinolaryngol 2002;62(3):229–35.

57. Jacobs IN, Gray RF, Todd NW. Upper airway obstruction in children with Down syndrome. Arch Otolaryngol Head Neck Surg 1996;122(9):945–50.

58. Kosko JR, Derkay CS. Uvulopalatopharyngoplasty: treatment of obstructive sleep apnea in neurologically impaired pediatric patients. Int J Pediatr Otorhinolaryngol 1995;32(3):241–6.

59. Lin SY, Halbower AC, Tunkel DE, et al. Relief of upper airway obstruction with mandibular distraction surgery: Long-term quantitative results in young children. Arch Otolaryngol Head Neck Surg 2006;132(4):437–41.

60. Wittenborn W, Panchal J, Marsh JL, et al. Neonatal distraction surgery for micrognathia reduces obstructive apnea and the need for tracheotomy. J Craniofac Surg 2004;15(4):623–30.

61. Scott AR, Tibesar RJ, Lander TA, et al. Mandibular distraction osteogenesis in infants younger than 3 months. Arch Facial Plast Surg 2011;13(3):173–9.

62. Rachmiel A, Srouji S, Emodi O, et al. Distraction osteogenesis for tracheostomy dependent children with severe micrognathia. J Craniofac Surg 2012;23(2):459–63.

63. Williams JK, Maull D, Grayson BH, et al. Early decannulation with bilateral mandibular distraction for tracheostomy-dependent patients. Plast Reconstr Surg 1999;103(1):48–57; discussion 58–9.

64. Villa MP, Rizzoli A, Miano S, et al. Efficacy of rapid maxillary expansion in children with obstructive sleep apnea syndrome: 36 months of follow-up. Sleep Breath 2011;15(2):179–84.

65. Villa MP, Malagola C, Pagani J, et al. Rapid maxillary expansion in children with obstructive sleep apnea syndrome: 12-month follow-up. Sleep Med 2007;8(2):128–34.

66. Monini S, Malagola C, Villa MP, et al. Rapid maxillary expansion for the treatment of nasal obstruction in children younger than 12 years. Arch Otolaryngol Head Neck Surg 2009;135(1):22–7.

67. Guilleminault C, Huang YS, Glamann C, et al. Adenotonsillectomy and obstructive sleep apnea in children: a prospective survey. Otolaryngol Head Neck Surg 2007;136(2):169–75.

68. Capdevila OS, Kheirandish-Gozal L, Dayyat E, et al. Pediatric obstructive sleep apnea: complications, management, and long-term outcomes. Proc Am Thorac Soc 2008;5(2):274–82.

69. Kushida CA, Chediak A, Berry RB, et al. Clinical guidelines for the manual titration of positive airway pressure in patients with obstructive sleep apnea. J Clin Sleep Med 2008;4(2):157–71.

70. Marcus CL, Rosen G, Ward SL, et al. Adherence to and effectiveness of positive airway pressure therapy in children with obstructive sleep apnea. Pediatrics 2006;117(3):e442–51.

71. Waters K. Interventions in the paediatric sleep laboratory: the use and titration of respiratory support therapies. Paediatr Respir Rev 2008;9(3):181–91; quiz 191–2.

72. Jain SS, Dhand R. Perioperative treatment of patients with obstructive sleep apnea. Curr Opin Pulm Med 2004;10(6):482–8.

73. Rosen GM, Muckle RP, Mahowald MW, et al. Postoperative respiratory compromise in children with obstructive sleep apnea syndrome: can it be anticipated? Pediatrics 1994;93(5):784–8.

74. Waters KA, Everett F, Bruderer J, et al. The use of nasal CPAP in children. Pediatr Pulmonol Suppl 1995;11:91–3.

75. Waters KA, Everett FM, Bruderer JW, et al. Obstructive sleep apnea: the use of nasal CPAP in 80 children. Am J Respir Crit Care Med 1995;152(2):780–5.

76. Castorena-Maldonado A, Torre-Bouscoulet L, Meza-Vargas S, et al. Preoperative continuous positive airway pressure compliance in children with obstructive sleep apnea syndrome: assessed by a simplified approach. Int J Pediatr Otorhinolaryngol 2008;72(12):1795–800.

77. Mehta Y, Manikappa S, Juneja R, et al. Obstructive sleep apnea syndrome: anesthetic implications in the cardiac surgical patient. J Cardiothorac Vasc Anesth 2000;14(4):449–53.

78. O'Donnell AR, Bjornson CL, Bohn SG, et al. Compliance rates in children using noninvasive continuous positive airway pressure. Sleep 2006;29(5):651–8.

79. Koontz KL, Slifer KJ, Cataldo MD, et al. Improving pediatric compliance with positive airway pressure therapy: the impact of behavioral intervention. Sleep 2003;26(8):1010–15.

80. Uong EC, Epperson M, Bathon SA, et al. Adherence to nasal positive airway pressure therapy among school-aged children and adolescents with obstructive sleep apnea syndrome. Pediatrics 2007;120(5):e1203–11.

81. Nixon GM, Mihai R, Verginis N, et al. Patterns of continuous positive airway pressure adherence during the first 3 months of treatment in children. J Pediatr 2011;159(5):802–7.

82. DiFeo N, Meltzer LJ, Beck SE, et al. Predictors of positive airway pressure therapy adherence in children: a prospective study. J Clin Sleep Med 2012;8(3):279–86.

83. Simon SL, Duncan CL, Janicke DM, et al. Barriers to treatment of paediatric obstructive sleep apnoea: Development of the adherence barriers to continuous positive airway pressure (CPAP) questionnaire. Sleep Med 2012;13(2):172–7.

84. Marcus CL, Beck SE, Traylor J, et al. Randomized, double-blind clinical trial of two different modes of positive airway pressure therapy on adherence and efficacy in children. J Clin Sleep Med 2012;8(1):37–42.

85. Harford KL, Jambhekar S, Com G, et al. An in-patient model for positive airway pressure desensitization: a report of 2 pediatric cases. Respir Care 2012;57(5):802–7.

86. Aljadeff G, Gozal D, Bailey-Wahl SL, et al. Effects of overnight supplemental oxygen in obstructive sleep apnea in children. Am J Respir Crit Care Med 1996;153(1):51–5.

87. Brouillette RT, Waters K. Oxygen therapy for pediatric obstructive sleep apnea syndrome: how safe? How effective? Am J Respir Crit Care Med 1996;153(1):1–2.

88. Brouillette RT, Manoukian J, Ducharme FM, et al. Efficacy of fluticasone nasal spray for pediatric obstructive sleep apnea. J Pediatr 2001;138(6):838–44.

89. Demain JG, Goetz DW. Pediatric adenoidal hypertrophy and nasal airway obstruction: reduction with aqueous nasal beclomethasone. Pediatrics 1995;95(3):355–64.

90. Alexopoulos EI, Kaditis AG, Kalampouka E, et al. Nasal corticosteroids for children with snoring. Pediatr Pulmonol 2004;38(2):161–7.

91. Goldbart AD, Goldman JL, Veling MC, et al. Leukotriene modifier therapy for mild sleep-disordered breathing in children. Am J Respir Crit Care Med 2005;172(3):364–70.

92. Kheirandish-Gozal L, Gozal D. Intranasal budesonide treatment for children with mild obstructive sleep apnea syndrome. Pediatrics 2008;122(1):e149–55.

93. Goldbart AD, Greenberg-Dotan S, Tal A. Montelukast for children with obstructive sleep apnea: a double-blind, placebo-controlled study. Pediatrics 2012;130(3):e575–80.

94. Kheirandish L, Goldbart AD, Gozal D. Intranasal steroids and oral leukotriene modifier therapy in residual sleep-disordered breathing after tonsillectomy and adenoidectomy in children. Pediatrics 2006;117(1): e61–6.

95. Demirhan H, Aksoy F, Ozturan O, et al. Medical treatment of adenoid hypertrophy with 'fluticasone propionate nasal drops'. Int J Pediatr Otorhinolaryngol 2010;74(7):773–6.

96. Goldbart AD, Goldman JL, Li RC, et al. Differential expression of cysteinyl leukotriene receptors 1 and 2 in tonsils of children with obstructive sleep apnea syndrome or recurrent infection. Chest 2004; 126(1):13–18.

97. Goldbart AD, Veling MC, Goldman JL, et al. Glucocorticoid receptor subunit expression in adenotonsillar tissue of children with obstructive sleep apnea. Pediatr Res 2005;57(2):232–6.

98. Kheirandish-Gozal L, Serpero LD, Dayyat E, et al. Corticosteroids suppress in vitro tonsillar proliferation in children with obstructive sleep apnoea. Eur Respir J 2009;33(5):1077–84.

99. Esteitie R, Emani J, Sharma S, et al. Effect of fluticasone furoate on interleukin 6 secretion from adenoid tissues in children with obstructive sleep apnea. Arch Otolaryngol Head Neck Surg 2011;137(6):576–82.

100. Dayyat E, Serpero LD, Kheirandish-Gozal L, et al. Leukotriene pathways and in vitro adenotonsillar cell proliferation in children with obstructive sleep apnea. Chest 2009;135(5):1142–9.

101. Villa MP, Bernkopf E, Pagani J, et al. Randomized controlled study of an oral jaw-positioning appliance for the treatment of obstructive sleep apnea in children with malocclusion. Am J Respir Crit Care Med 2002;165(1):123–7.

102. Cozza P, Ballanti F, Prete L. A modified monobloc for treatment of young children with obstructive sleep apnea. J Clin Orthod 2004;38(4): 241–7.

103. Schessl J, Rose E, Korinthenberg R, et al. Severe obstructive sleep apnea alleviated by oral appliance in a three-year-old boy. Respiration 2008;76(1):112–16.

104. Ferguson KA. The role of oral appliance therapy in the treatment of obstructive sleep apnea. Clin Chest Med 2003;24(2):355–64.

105. Verhulst SL, Franckx H, Van Gaal L, et al. The effect of weight loss on sleep-disordered breathing in obese teenagers. Obesity (Silver Spring) 2009;17(6):1178–83.

106. Tuomilehto HP, Seppa JM, Partinen MM, et al. Lifestyle intervention with weight reduction: first-line treatment in mild obstructive sleep apnea. Am J Respir Crit Care Med 2009;179(4):320–7.

107. Holterman AX, Browne A, Dillard BE 3rd, et al. Short-term outcome in the first 10 morbidly obese adolescent patients in the FDA-approved trial for laparoscopic adjustable gastric banding. J Pediatr Gastroenterol Nutr 2007;45(4):465–73.

108. Kalra M, Inge T, Garcia V, et al. Obstructive sleep apnea in extremely overweight adolescents undergoing bariatric surgery. Obes Res 2005;13(7):1175–9.

109. Alqahtani AR, Antonisamy B, Alamri H, et al. Laparoscopic sleeve gastrectomy in 108 obese children and adolescents aged 5 to 21 years. Ann Surg 2012;256(2):266–73.

110. Greenburg DL, Lettieri CJ, Eliasson AH. Effects of surgical weight loss on measures of obstructive sleep apnea: a meta-analysis. Am J Med 2009;122(6):535–42.

111. Lettieri CJ, Eliasson AH, Greenburg DL. Persistence of obstructive sleep apnea after surgical weight loss. J Clin Sleep Med 2008;4(4): 333–8.

112. Hsia DS, Fallon SC, Brandt ML. Adolescent bariatric surgery. Arch Pediatr Adolesc Med 2012;166(8):757–66.

113. Shield JP, Crowne E, Morgan J. Is there a place for bariatric surgery in treating childhood obesity? Arch Dis Child 2008;93(5):369–72.

114. Guimaraes CV, Donnelly LF, Shott SR, et al. Relative rather than absolute macroglossia in patients with Down syndrome: implications for treatment of obstructive sleep apnea. Pediatr Radiol 2008;38(10): 1062–7.

115. Mitchell C, Blachford J, Carlyle MJ, et al. Hypothyroidism in patients with Down syndrome. Arch Pediatr Adolesc Med 1994;148(4):441–2.

116. Mitchell RB, Call E, Kelly J. Ear, nose and throat disorders in children with Down syndrome. Laryngoscope 2003;113(2):259–63.

117. de Moura CP, Andrade D, Cunha LM, et al. Down syndrome: otolaryngological effects of rapid maxillary expansion. J Laryngol Otol 2008;122(12):1318–24.

118. Carroll KN, Arbogast PG, Dudley JA, et al. Increase in incidence of medically treated thyroid disease in children with Down syndrome after rerelease of American Academy of Pediatrics Health Supervision guidelines. Pediatrics 2008;122(2):e493–8.

119. Rosen D. Severe hypothyroidism presenting as obstructive sleep apnea. Clin Pediatr (Phila) 2010;49(4):381–3.

120. Kapur VK, Koepsell TD, deMaine J, et al. Association of hypothyroidism and obstructive sleep apnea. Am J Respir Crit Care Med 1998;158(5 Pt 1):1379–83.

121. Katz ES, Mitchell RB, D'Ambrosio CM. Obstructive sleep apnea in infants. Am J Respir Crit Care Med 2012;185(8):805–16.

122. Shatz A. Indications and outcomes of adenoidectomy in infancy. Ann Otol Rhinol Laryngol 2004;113(10):835–8.

123. Chigurupati R, Massie J, Dargaville P, et al. Internal mandibular distraction to relieve airway obstruction in infants and young children with micrognathia. Pediatr Pulmonol 2004;37(3):230–5.

124. Sedaghat AR, Anderson IC, McGinley BM, et al. Characterization of obstructive sleep apnea before and after tongue-lip adhesion in children with micrognathia. Cleft Palate Craniofac J 2012;49(1):21–6.

125. Whitaker IS, Koron S, Oliver DW, et al. Effective management of the airway in the Pierre Robin syndrome using a modified nasopharyngeal tube and pulse oximetry. Br J Oral Maxillofac Surg 2003;41(4): 272–4.

126. Landry AM, Thompson DM. Laryngomalacia: disease presentation, spectrum, and management. Int J Pediatr 2012;2012:753526.

127. Chan DK, Truong MT, Koltai PJ. Supraglottoplasty for occult laryngomalacia to improve obstructive sleep apnea syndrome. Arch Otolaryngol Head Neck Surg 2012;138(1):50–4.

The Otolaryngologist Approach to Obstructive Sleep Apnea

Cecille G. Sulman and B. Tucker Woodson

INTRODUCTION

Pediatric obstructive sleep apnea (OSA) often presents in the pediatric population with loud snoring, respiratory pauses and mouth-breathing OSA is caused by anatomic variations and is complicated by the diminished pharyngeal muscle tone and neurophysiologic changes that typically accompany sleep. Tonsil and adenoid hyperplasia is the most common cause, but craniofacial abnormalities, palate, base of tongue, supraglottic, and glottis may also be contributory sites. Successful management in children depends on the accurate identification of the site of obstruction and the assessment of the severity, with polysomnogram as an important adjunct. This enables decision-making for the appropriate surgical and nonsurgical interventions.[1]

EVALUATION OF THE PATIENT WITH OSA

History

Snoring is the primary complaint of children presenting to the otolaryngologist; the prevalence has been reported as 3–12% in children,[2] although some studies suggest that the rate may be as high as 27%.[3] Primary snoring has implications with associated morbidity of elevated blood pressure and reduced arterial distensibility.[4] Approximately 40% of children who snore have more significant manifestations with obstructive sleep apnea (OSA). Additional complaints may include mouth-breathing, breath-holding, and gasping.[5] Sleep is disrupted by episodic arousals resulting from partial obstruction of the upper airway. Manifestations include morning headache, dry mouth, halitosis, and behavioral and neurocognitive disorders less commonly sleepwalking, parasomniloquy, enuresis, night terrors, or bruxism.[5,6] Dysphagia may occur with significant tonsil enlargement. Children may avoid certain foods that are more difficult to swallow. Major predisposing factors identified in upper airway obstruction include: anatomic narrowing, abnormal mechanical linkage between airway dilating muscles and airway walls, muscle weakness, and abnormal neural regulation.[7] Complications related to severe OSA include cor pulmonale, right ventricular hypertrophy, congestive heart failure, hypoventilation, pulmonary hypertension, pulmonary edema, and failure to thrive.[8] History alone is insufficient to diagnose OSA. Symptoms often worsen during REM sleep when parental observation is absent.[9] A polysomnogram (PSG) is the gold standard in differentiating between the spectrum of snoring, increased upper airway resistance, and OSA.

Infants with upper airway obstruction can present with stridor. This worsens with activity or feeding. Inspiratory or biphasic stridor may indicate laryngomalacia, vocal fold dysfunction (VCD), or supraglottic lesions.[10] Biphasic or expiratory stridor may indicate VDC, a lower airway lesion such as subglottic stenosis or tracheobronchomalacia.[10] Concerning symptoms include retractions observed apneic episodes, cyanosis, and failure to thrive. Previous history of intubation and prematurity are specific risk factors for obstructive airway lesions.[11]

Other factors may place a child at risk (Table 33.1). Obesity is a risk factor that may cause fatty infiltration of the pharyngeal soft tissues, which narrows the upper airway and contributes to airway resistance and reduced lung volume.[12,13] The prevalence of OSA in children with Down syndrome ranges between 31% and 100%,[14] and may be related to hypotonia, relative macroglossia, midfacial and mandibular hypoplasia, a narrow nasopharynx, and a shortened (high-arched) palate.[15] Children with other craniofacial syndromes and abnormalities also have a higher prevalence of OSA. Robison and Otteson[16] found that 172 out of 459 (37.5%) children with nonsyndromic cleft palate had symptoms of OSA, and that 39 (8.5%) had a positive PSG. Children with Apert, Crouzon, Nager, and Pfeiffer syndromes have a high rate of OSA.[17,18] Other medical conditions with a high risk for the development of OSA include mucopolysaccharide disease, vascular malformations of the head and neck, and children with neuromuscular disorders.

OSA may exacerbate underlying medical conditions such as congenital heart disease, pulmonary disease, and sickle cell disease (SCD). In SCD, adenotonsillar hypertrophy or recurrent tonsillitis is frequently linked with an increased risk of OSA, cerebrovascular ischemia, or frequent pain episodes, and often require an adenoidectomy and/or tonsillectomy.[19] Adenotonsillectomy has been demonstrated to be cost-effective for treating obstructive sleep apnea and preventing cerebrovascular ischemia without increasing vaso-occlusive pain episodes or long-term acute service costs in routine clinical practice settings.

Physical Examination

The general appearance of the child provides a great deal of information. An open mouth posture and stertorous or sonorous breathing may indicate upper airway resistance. Examination of the craniofacial skeleton may reveal deformities such as midface hypoplasia or mandibular hypoplasia. Some children present with failure to thrive due to difficulty in coordinating feeding and breathing or dysphagia related to tonsillar hypertrophy.

On routine examination, nasal mucosa, turbinates, septum, and nasal cavity may demonstrate septal deviation, inflamed, edematous mucosa, and inferior turbinate hypertrophy. The nasal passages should be inspected for masses or polyps. No single feature defines OSA in children.

TABLE 33.1	Risk factors for Sleep Disordered Breathing	
Anatomic factors	Lingual tonsil hypertrophy	Adenotonsillar hypertrophy
	Airway lesions:	Laryngomalacia
		Tracheobronchomalacia
		Vocal fold paralysis
		Subglottic stenosis
	Craniofacial abnormalities:	Down syndrome
		Pierre–Robin sequence
		Apert
		Crouzon
		Pfeiffer
		Hallerman-Strief
	Vascular anomalies	
Systemic factors	Obesity	
	Neurologic impairment	
	Mucopolysaccharide diseases	

Oral cavity examination should include evaluation of the tonsils, tongue and palate. Tonsil grading is typically on a scale of 0 (surgically absent) to 4 (tonsils touching each other) (Figure 33-1). The static pressure and/or area relationships of the passive pharynx were endoscopically measured in 14 children with obstructive sleep apnea and in 13 healthy children under general anesthesia with complete paralysis; it was determined that children with obstructive sleep apnea closed their airways at the level of enlarged adenoids and tonsils at low positive pressures, whereas healthy children required subatmospheric pressures to induce upper airway closure.[20] The cross-sectional area of the narrowest segment was significantly smaller in children with obstructive sleep apnea and particularly in the retropalatal and retroglossal segments. Thus, both congenital and acquired anatomic factors clearly play a significant role in the pathogenesis of pediatric obstructive sleep apnea. Macroglossia, such as in the case of Down syndrome or Beckwith–Wiedermann, may be contributory to upper airway obstruction. The appearance of the palate should be noted, as an elongated palate may also play an important role in obstruction, particularly after adenotonsillectomy (Figure 33-2).

Flexible endoscopy is an important tool that can allow for comprehensive evaluation of the upper airway in infants and children. This may be performed in the office in an awake child or with anesthesia. Lidocaine is used for topical anesthesia and oxymetazolone for decongestion to increase the comfort for this examination. Sites of obstruction may occur anywhere from the tip of the nose to the glottis. Therefore endoscopy can be used to visualize the nasal passages, nasopharynx, oropharynx, hypopharynx, and larynx. Nasal patency is assessed for nasal septal deviation, turbinate

hypertrophy, polyps, or masses. Choanae are evaluated for stenosis or atresia. Adenoids may be visualized for hypertrophy. Oropharyngeal and hypopharyngeal examination provides a view of the posterior aspect of the tonsils and base of tongue. Tonsils may appear normal during an oral cavity exam. However, the tonsil pole may be elongated or posteriorly displaced and occupy a significant portion of the hypopharynx. Base of tongue enlargement may result in effacement of the vallecular with compression and displacement of the epiglottis posteriorly. Enlargement of the lingual tonsils at the tongue base is increasingly recognized as a treatable cause of OSA. Obese children have a high frequency of enlargement of the lingual tonsils with a significantly higher prevalence in those with previous tonsillectomy,[21] as demonstrated by MRI. Flexible endoscopy with the child in a supine position may further highlight narrowing at the level of the hypopharynx. Collapse of the lateral pharyngeal walls during inspiration with a closed airway (mouth shut and nostrils occluded) may be noted. The supraglottic structures are evaluated for laryngomalacia, as identified with epiglottis and/or arytenoids prolapse over the glottis. The vocal folds are assessed for mobility and masses.

Polysomnogram

Although history, physical examination, and flexible endoscopy of the airway are important tools, these cannot fully simulate the complexity of airway dynamics during sleep. Polysomnogram (PSG) is a valuable asset in assessing breathing. Indications for PSG have been outlined in the Clinical Practice Guideline developed by the American Academy of Otolaryngology-Head and Neck Surgery (AAO-HNS).[22] Children with complex medical conditions such as obesity, Down syndrome, craniofacial abnormalities, neuromuscular disorders, sickle cell disease, or mucopolysaccharidoses may benefit from preoperative PSG. PSG may be indicated in children for whom the need for surgery is uncertain, such as in the case of tonsillar hypertrophy and lack of sufficient history or when significant symptoms are present in the face of a negative physical examination.[22] Prior to surgical intervention and anesthesia induction, the results of the study should be relayed to the anesthesia team. Inpatient admission after surgery should be considered for children under the age of 3 years or with severe OSA by PSG (apnea–hypopnea index of 10 or more obstructive events/hour, oxygen saturation nadir less than 80%, or both).[23,24] Intensive care unit monitoring may be warranted in a child with very severe OSA, medical comorbidities that cannot be managed on the floor, and those who demonstrate significant airway obstruction and desaturation in the initial postoperative period that requires interventions beyond repositioning and/or oxygen supplementation.[22]

Imaging

Plain radiography with a high-kilovoltage lateral neck film may be used to evaluate for adenotonsillar hypertrophy in a child who is difficult to examine or when a caregiver defers flexible endoscopy. Adenoid hypertrophy visualized by lateral neck radiograph correlates well with flexible nasopharyngoscopy.[25] Most techniques focus on the size of the nasopharyngeal stripe, which indicates the amount of airflow through the nasopharynx. When the nasopharyngeal stripe is half the size of the soft palate, significant obstruction occurs. However, the

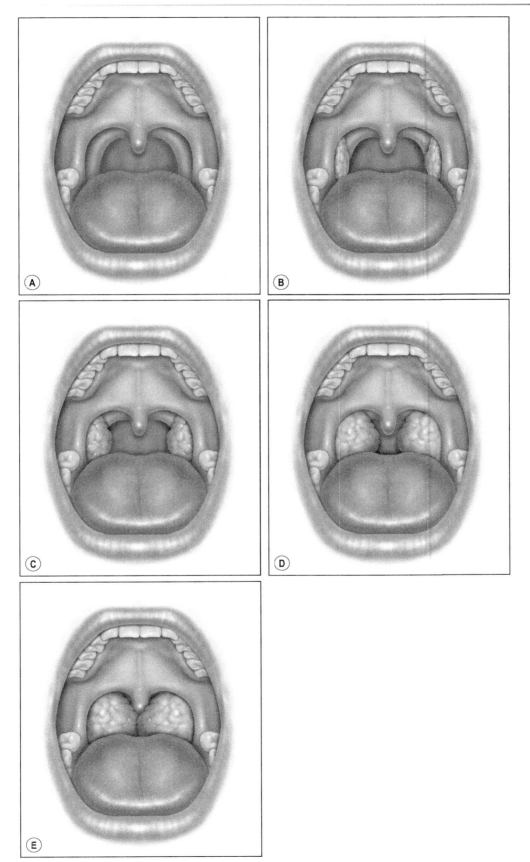

FIGURE 33-1 **Tonsil Staging.** *Friedman M. Friedman tongue position and the staging of obstructive sleep apnea/hypopnea syndrome. In: Friedman, editor. Sleep Apnea and Snoring. Surgical and Nonsurgical Therapy. China: Saunders, Elsevier; 2009. Fig 16.2, p 108.*

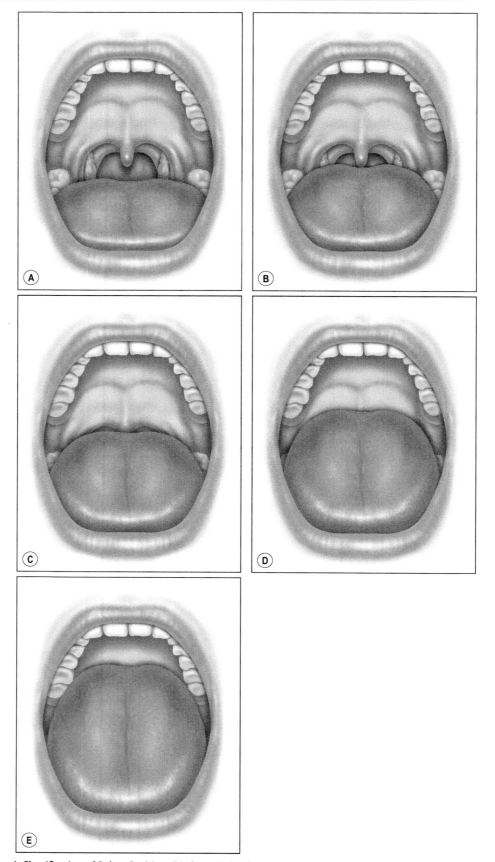

FIGURE 33-2 Friedman's Classification of Palate Position. *Friedman M. Friedman tongue position and the staging of obstructive sleep apnea/hypopnea syndrome. In: Friedman, editor. Sleep Apnea and Snoring. Surgical and Nonsurgical Therapy. China: Saunders, Elsevier; 2009. Fig 16.1, p 106.*

actual size of the adenoid pad is not as relevant as the amount of obstruction caused by hypertrophy.

Anterior–posterior high-kilovoltage neck films evaluate the laryngeal suprastructure and subglottis. Cephalometry and computed tomography are useful in evaluating children with craniofacial disorders. Research suggest that there are evident and early changes in facial growth and development among children with OSA, characterized by increased total and inferior anterior heights of the face, as well as a more anterior and inferior position of the hyoid bone.[26] Chest radiography may help identify evidence of pulmonary hypertension or right ventricular hypertrophy in a child with severe OSA.[27]

Cine magnetic resonance imaging is a useful radiographic adjunct to the physical examination because it allows the clinician to screen for and to observe airway collapse in three planes (axial, coronal and sagittal).[28,29] This is particularly helpful in isolating anatomic sites of airway obstruction in children who have persistent apnea after adenotonsillectomy (Tonsillectomy and Adenoidectomy).

Additional Testing

Patients with severe OSA or abnormal electrocardiogram findings on PSG warrant a complete electrocardiogram. Electrocardiographic findings are not specific for pulmonary hypertension or right ventricular hypertrophy but may include voltage or axis abnormalities, a t-wave pattern (strain pattern), or mixed criteria. On occasion, a normal electrocardiogram may occur even with echocardiographic findings of pulmonary hypertension.[27] Laboratories are not routinely ordered prior to Tonsillectomy and Adenoidectomy unless a history is concerning for a bleeding disorder.[30] Patients who have a history of easy bruising and prolonged bleeding warrant a CBC/PT/T. Arterial blood gas analysis in conjunction with PSG may demonstrate hypoxemia or hypercarbia. Chronic hypercarbia may be associated with a compensatory metabolic alkalosis.[27]

MEDICAL INTERVENTION

Antibiotics are not beneficial in long-term reduction of tonsil hypertrophy, although during acute inflammation broad-spectrum antibiotics may provide a short-term decrease in tonsil size; one study reported only 15% of patients avoided surgery in long-term follow-up.[31]

Intranasal Steroids

Intranasal steroids may be helpful if adenoid hypertrophy is the predominant cause of mild OSA in children. Decreases of 29% in adenoid size and 82% in symptom scores were noted in one study.[32] Another study assessed a 6-week course of intranasal steroids,[33] reporting a significant improvement of the AHI post-treatment compared to the placebo group. Results may be maintained 8 weeks after completion of active treatment.[34] Intranasal steroids have not been found to impact tonsil size.[33]

Twenty-four children with residual OSA (AHI >1 and <5/hour) were treated with montelukast and intranasal budesonide aqueous solution for 12 weeks.[35] This combined anti-inflammatory therapy effectively improved and/or normalized respiratory and sleep disturbances in children with residual SDB after adenotonsillectomy.

Systemic steroids have been tried in non-acute adenotonsillar hypertrophy. A short-term decrease in tonsil size has been noted, but long-term improvement and avoidance of surgery are usually not seen.[36] Although there is indication that intranasal steroids and montelukast may be helpful in mild OSA, pharmacologic agents have no significant and persistent effect in the treatment of moderate to severe OSA in children.

Oral Appliances

Villa et al. randomized children with OSA and dysgnathia to either a personalized jaw-positioning oral appliance for 6 months or no intervention.[37] The authors reported that the AHI in the intervention group decreased significantly from 7.1 to 2.6/h. The oral appliance significantly lowered parent-reported snoring and apnea. A few of the patients had excessive salivation that subsided spontaneously. A Cochrane review (2007) on oral appliances and functional orthopedic appliances for OSA in children 15 years old or younger reported that there is insufficient evidence to state that oral appliances or functional orthopedic appliances are effective in the treatment of OSA in the majority of children. However, they may be helpful in the treatment of children with craniofacial anomalies that are risk factors of apnea.[38]

ADENOTONSILLECTOMY

If OSA is present, tonsillectomy alone or adenoidectomy alone is not sufficient, and adenotonsillectomy should be performed together. Fortunately, because most pediatric OSA is caused by adenotonsillar hypertrophy, T&A alone is an effective and durable treatment for most children[39] and is the first choice for children with OSA.[40-42] There is an indication that children older than 3 years of age, in the absence of comorbidities, can safely undergo adenotonsillectomy without undergoing preoperative PSG, provided those patients have close postoperative monitoring.[43]

The preoperative evaluation of children scheduled for adenotonsillectomy should include careful assessment for evidence of upper airway obstruction, pulmonary hypertension, and right heart dysfunction. The anesthesiologist will screen for symptoms of upper airway obstruction and congenital or acquired disorders associated with abnormal facial structure, decreased muscle tone or development, developmental delay and/or cardiopulmonary disease.[44] Other clinical findings in patients with pulmonary hypertension and right ventricular dysfunction can include jugular venous distension, hepatomegaly, loud pulmonic component of the second heart sound, right ventricular heave and peripheral edema, failure to thrive, developmental delay, and altered mental status.[44]

T&A may be performed safely in an outpatient setting in appropriate selected patients. The AAO-HNS society recommends that patients be greater than 3 years of age, not have OSA, and be American Society for Anesthesia (ASA) Class I/II (low anesthesia risk).[45] Parents must be advised that a low threshold for readmission exists.[45] The postoperative complication rate is higher in children with craniofacial disorders, failure to thrive, neurological impairment, Down syndrome, obstructive sleep apnea, and in children age 3 years or less.[24] Children who are at risk for perioperative complications should remain overnight for observation.

The most common complications of adenotonsillectomy are anesthesia risks, pain, otalgia, and bleeding.[46] Dehydration may occur due to poorly controlled pain, refusal of oral intake, nausea and vomiting secondary to narcotic use.[46] Rare complications of tonsillectomy include subcutaneous emphysema, pneumomediastinum, and taste disturbance due to damage to the lingual branch of the glossopharyngeal nerve.[47,48] Nasopharyngeal stenosis, also an uncommon outcome, results from approximation of raw mucosal surfaces during the healing process.[46]

Multiple techniques and tools may be used to perform tonsillectomy. The literature presents a variety of evidence regarding outcomes related to device usage, but consensus has not been reached regarding the optimal technique with the lowest morbidity.[49,50] Device choice may be influenced by exposure in training programs as well as operator experience. Patient recovery times, postoperative morbidities, as well as cost related to the device are also important factors that may drive device choice.

The most common techniques used include cold steel dissection and electrosurgical dissection. Cold steel dissection is the oldest proven technique, and the basic approach has not changed significantly in the past 100 years.[51] Electrocautery is typically used for hemostasis. Electrosurgical dissection uses thermal energy to dissect tissues with either a monopolar or bipolar tip; little blood loss occurs with this technique.[52] Postoperative morbidities for these techniques are similar, and include hemorrhage (1.2–2.1%), dysphagia, and otalgia.[52]

Plasma surgical dissection is a technique that ablates and coagulates soft tissue by generating a field of ionized sodium molecules. Many studies have shown that plasma surgical dissection tonsillectomy causes less pain, has a shorter recovery period and requires less postoperative narcotics than other methods of tonsillectomy.[53]

The Harmonic scalpel (vessel sealing system) uses ultrasonic energy to vibrate its blade at 55 kHz, providing simultaneous cutting and coagulation of the tissue with less trauma.[54] Postoperative hemorrhage and intraoperative blood loss are low. Some studies have variably found decreased postoperative pain compared to electrosurgical dissection.[54]

Adenoidectomy may also be performed with a variety of devices, with either a transnasal or transoral approach. Revision adenoidectomy occurs at a rate of 1.3%.[55] Reasons for revision include persistent symptoms ranging from adenoiditis to recurrent otitis to OSA. Device choice for T&A is driven by surgeon experience and attempts to decrease postoperative morbidity.

Partial tonsillectomy, also known as tonsillotomy or intracapsular tonsillectomy, may be performed for tonsil hypertrophy with UAO, but is contraindicated for chronic tonsillitis. The premise of partial tonsillectomy is reduction of obstructive tonsillar tissue while sparing the tonsillar capsule, thus preventing exposure of the underlying pharyngeal muscles. Technology utilized for partial tonsillectomy includes microdebrider techniques or radiofrequency devices. Eviatar et al.,[56] in a small retrospective study of partial tonsillectomy compared to complete tonsillectomy, observed no difference in all parameters compared: non-obstructing tonsils recurred (97% vs 87%); snoring (3% vs 12.5%); recurrent tonsillitis (6% vs 6.25%); and recurrent obstruction and unilateral enlargement (3% vs 12.5%) at 8 to 10 years. An advantage of partial tonsillectomy includes decreased hemorrhage rates; however, intraoperative bleeding is increased, and may impede visualization at times.[57]

Success rates have been reported for T&A ranging from 59.8% to 85%, with a significant improvement in AHI from preoperative levels[41] as well as an overall improvement in quality of life.[58–60] However, the correlation between improvements in respiratory parameters and improvements in quality of life is poor.[39] Mitchell[39] evaluated outcomes in a prospective cohort study of children (ages 3–14, mean 6.3, included 79 healthy children, 40 of who were male) undergoing T&A for obstructive sleep apnea in children. Measures included PSG and OSA-18. Patients with an AHI of 5 or greater underwent adenotonsillectomy. OSA was classified as mild (AHI≥5<10), moderate (AHI≥10<20), or severe (AHI≥20). For all children, the preoperative AHI value was higher than the postoperative value. The mean preoperative AHI for the study population was 27.5, whereas the mean postoperative AHI was 3.5 ($P<0.001$). The percentage of children with normal polysomnography parameters after adenotonsillectomy ranged from 71% to 90%. Overnight respiratory parameters after adenotonsillectomy were normal for all children with mild OSA. Three (12%) children with moderate preoperative OSA, and 13 (36%) children with severe preoperative OSA had persistent OSA after adenotonsillectomy. Resolution of OSA occurred in all children with a preoperative AHI≤10 and in 73% of children with a preoperative AHI<10. The mean total OSA-18 score and the mean scores for all domains showed significant improvement after surgery ($P<0.001$). The preoperative AHI values had a fair correlation with the preoperative total OSA-18 scores (r =0.28), but postoperative AHI values had a poor correlation with the postoperative total OSA-18 scores (r=0.16). Caregivers reported snoring some, most, or all of the time in 22 (28%) children; this group included all children with persistent OSA. T&A for OSA results in a dramatic improvement in respiratory parameters and the quality of life in the majority of healthy children with OSA.

However, children with severe preoperative OSA, asthma, age greater than 7, or obesity are at risk for persistence of OSA after T&A.[61–63] T&A outcomes may not be favorable in patients with severe preoperative OSA or when obesity is present;[64,65] however, it remains the currently recommended initial treatment for OSA in obese patients. Increasing rates of residual obstructive sleep apnea indicate a future role for adjunct medical as well as surgical interventions. Postoperative polysomnograms are recommended 6–8 weeks following surgery for those with additional risk factors for OSA: age < 3 years, severe OSA present on pre-operative PSG (a respiratory disturbance index of 19 or greater), cardiac complications of OSA (e.g., right ventricular hypertrophy), failure to thrive, obesity, prematurity, recent respiratory infection, craniofacial anomalies, neuromuscular disorders, or those with a high apnea index to ensure that OSA is resolved.[66] Patients with mild to moderate OSA who have complete resolution of signs and symptoms require follow-up clinical evaluations but do not require repeat PSG.[67] Postoperative reports of symptoms such as snoring and witnessed apneas correlate well with persistence of OSA after T&A.[39]

SURGERY FOR MULTILEVEL OBSTRUCTION

Multilevel obstruction involving any combination of the nasal, nasopharyngeal, retropalatal, retroglossal, and hypopharyngeal anatomy may be found in otherwise healthy children.[68] However, certain populations are predisposed to multilevel airway collapse, including those with obesity, nasal obstruction, neurological impairments, laryngotracheomalacia, laryngotracheal or bronchial stenosis, and craniofacial anomalies, such as Pierre Robin sequence and Down syndrome.[67] The exact nature of dynamic airway collapse may not be appreciated by a detailed history and physical examination; therefore, cine MRI and flexible endoscopy performed in the office and the operating room may help identify the anatomic level(s) of obstruction.[69]

There is limited evidence available regarding surgical techniques for multilevel OSA. Lack of objective PSG criteria for comparison between surgical treatment options as well as the nature of surgical intervention makes it difficult to conduct blinded studies.[70] A staged approach should be considered in children.[71,72]

Nasal Passages

A deviated septum or turbinate hypertrophy may be contributory to nasal airway obstruction. Both are readily visualized by anterior rhinoscopy as well as by flexible endoscopy. An adequate course of medical therapy including nasal steroids and allergy therapy (if indicated) should be trialed prior to considering surgery. A limited septoplasty may be performed with careful patient selection. Complications include persistent septal deviation, bleeding, and septal perforation. Septoplasty may be useful in improving CPAP tolerance, particularly in older children.

Two main techniques exist for turbinate volume reduction: radiofrequency ablation and microdebrider-assisted reduction. A review of turbinate surgery in children comparing both techniques demonstrated that both are effective.[73] Six-month outcomes are equivalent for both techniques; however, maintenance of improvement at 3 years was better with the microdebrider-assisted technique. Mild-to-moderate edema with subsequent nasal obstruction and thick mucus formation can be expected for the first week after the procedure.[74] If mucosal erosion is present, the risk of postoperative bleeding and adherent crust formation increases with radiofrequency ablation.[75]

Oropharynx

Patients with an elongated palate may benefit from techniques to widen or stabilize the palate, including lateral pharyngoplasty, expansion sphincter pharyngoplasty, and uvulopalatopharyngoplasty. Palatal procedures may be performed with or without adenotonsillectomy.

Lateral pharyngoplasty is a minimally invasive procedure that is performed concurrently with tonsillectomy. After removal of the tonsils, the tonsillar pillars are sutured together over the tonsillar fossa to reduce the collapsibility of the pharynx.[76] Outcomes in healthy children have not been studied, but retrospective analysis did not demonstrate a difference in Down syndrome patients who underwent T&A alone or T&A plus lateral pharyngoplasty.[77]

Expansion sphincter pharyngoplasty is a more technically involved approach, with rotation and suspension of the palatopharyngeus muscle onto the soft palate, sparing the uvula. This technique provides stabilization of the palate and an improved airway diameter. This may be incorporated into the initial surgical approach with tonsillectomy or as a secondary procedure in patients who have persistent OSA after T&A. Pang and Woodson demonstrated an improvement in AHI

from 44.2 ± 10.2 to 12.0 ± 6.6 ($P < 0.005$) following expansion sphincter pharyngoplasty in select patients with small tonsils and an elongated palate.[78] Long-term outcomes in children for both lateral pharyngoplasty and expansion sphincter pharyngoplasty are yet to be determined.

Uvulopalatopharyngoplasty (UPPP) involves removal of the soft palate and uvula, widening the oropharyngeal airway. UPPP has been reported to be successful in children with cerebral palsy and hypotonic upper airway muscles.[79] Although an initial report of UPPP in an otherwise normal child was promising,[80] UPPP is not commonly performed in children. Significant complications such as nasopharyngeal stenosis, palatal incompetence, and speech difficulties may occur with this technique.[81]

Base of Tongue

Surgical procedures to increase the volume of the retrolingual airway include lingual tonsillectomy, glossectomy, and advancement and suspension procedures. Comparison of preoperative and postoperative PSG demonstrated statistically significant reductions in the respiratory distress index (RDI) (mean, 14.7 vs 8.1).[82] There were similar reductions in the number of obstructive apneas and hypopneas. The mean minimum O_2 saturation did not change. Complications related to lingual tonsillectomy include edema[82] and adhesions between the epiglottis and tongue base.[83]

Glossectomy or tissue volume reduction procedures decrease tongue volume and proportionally increase airway size. Glossectomy involving a wedge of tongue muscle is an effective technique[84] that may be applied to children with significant tongue hypertrophy as in Beckwith–Wiedemann or Down syndrome. Midline glossectomy is performed open or via a minimally invasive technique submucosally.[85] Success rates for the submucosal minimally invasive lingual excision are reported to be 60%.[85] Risks include airway edema, hematoma, abscess formation, and permanent hypoglossal injury.[86]

Other procedures to improve the retroglossal airway include genioglossus advancement and tongue base stabilization (Repose). Genioglossus advancement was initially described with a midline osteotomy of the mandible with advancement of the tongue,[87] which is not amenable in children due to the presence of tooth buds.[69] A minimally invasive approach (Repose) involves placement of a suture through the tongue which is stabilized to the medial aspect of the mandible.[88]

Woodson et al.[89] retrospectively evaluated 31 operations involving a combination of genioglossus advancement and radiofrequency ablation utilizing preoperative and postoperative PSG data for each patient. Success of surgery was determined using the criteria of a postoperative AHI of 5 or fewer events per hour, without evidence of hypoxemia and without prolonged hypercarbia. Thirty-one patients who underwent genioglossus advancement were analyzed. Nineteen (61%) had Down syndrome. The overall success rate was 61%. The success rate was lower in children with Down syndrome versus children without Down syndrome (58% vs 66%).

Radiofrequency ablation described by Powell et al.[90] involves insertion of a two-pronged probe at the vertex of the circumvallate papillae, creating thermal damage. Subsequent lesions are created 1 cm anterior to the first treatment site, and additional lesions as indicated 1 cm anterior to the second treatment site. Tongue bulk and flaccidity of the tongue base is reduced through fibrosis.[69] A low rate of complications (3.4%) is reported, ranging from mucosal ulceration, to superficial infection, and transient parasthesia of the hypoglossal nerve.[91]

Larynx

Laryngomalacia, or obstruction of the glottis secondary to collapse of supraglottic structures, is diagnosed with flexible laryngoscopy. This condition is primarily seen in infancy, but may present in older children (non-congenital laryngomalacia). For the majority of patients, laryngomalacia may be managed expectantly without intervention. Infants and children who have laryngomalacia that results in OSA, failure to thrive, or feeding difficulties may be managed with a supraglottoplasty. Sharp dissection or laser techniques are used to reduce redundant mucosa or incise shortened aryepiglottic folds.[10] Chen et al. evaluated supraglottoplasty in children with non-congenital laryngomalacia (occult laryngomalacia) with obstructive sleep apnea.[92] Twenty-two patients aged 2 to 17 years underwent carbon dioxide laser supraglottoplasty either alone or in conjunction with other operations for OSA. There was a statistically significant reduction in the AHI from 15.4 to 5.4 events per hour. Medical comorbidities were associated with worsened postoperative outcomes. Overall, 91% of children had an improvement in AHI, and 64% had only mild or no residual OSA after supraglottoplasty.

Craniofacial

Distraction osteogenesis is used to expand the facial skeleton in children with congenital micrognathia or midface hypoplasia.[93] Distraction osteogenesis allows large advancements without the need for bone grafting and with less risk of relapse. In a meta-analysis of mandibular distraction osteogenesis (DOG), Ow and Cheung[94] concluded that mandibular DOG is effective in treating craniofacial deformities. Mandell[95] performed a retrospective analysis of patients with mandibular hypoplasia and severe OSA. Seven out of eight patients with Pierre Robin sequence (88%) avoided tracheostomy. Only two of seventeen patients (17%) with a complex congenital syndrome (17%) were decannulated. Complications included premature callus consolidation requiring another DOG procedure, cheek abscess requiring incision and drainage, minor lip erosion from pin contact, facial cellulitis, unilateral facial paralysis, and temporal mandibular joint ankylosis.[95] Distraction osteogenesis of both the maxilla and mandible can correct micrognathia accompanying OSA, lower AHI to less than 5 events per hour, and increase SaO_2 to more than 90%.[96]

Rapid maxillary expansion (RME) involves the use of an oral appliance that is adjusted daily to increase palatal width. RME presents another option of treatment for children with high-arched palates with associated increased nasal resistance and mild OSA. A high-arched palate may also be associated with a posterior tongue posture, which contributes to retroglossal airway narrowing.[97] RME is most effective in prepubertal children prior to palatal suture closure. Villa et al. evaluated 10 patients after 24 months of follow-up.[98] After treatment, the apnea AHI decreased and clinical symptoms resolved by the end of the treatment period. RME may be used in combination with T&A to improve the nasal and oral airway.

Guilleminault et al. randomized children with OSA and narrow maxilla to either T&A or maxillary distraction.[99] PSG after 3 months showed residual events severe enough to warrant the complementary intervention in all children. In combination with T&A, maxillary distraction has a cure rate of 87.5% in children with sleep apnea.[100]

Tracheostomy

Patients who are refractory to surgical therapy or CPAP and have persistent severe OSA are appropriate candidates for tracheostomy. Tracheostomy allows the obstructive airway to be bypassed. A significant degree of counseling is involved in preparation for surgery due to the life-altering changes a family will experience managing a child with a tracheostomy. Drawbacks of tracheostomy include further impairment to already rudimentary communication skills, increased need for specialized and institutionalized care, and decreased quality of life. Long-term, tracheostomy-specific complications have decreased with improvements in technique, nursing care, and monitoring.[101] Complications associated with tracheostomy include subglottic stenosis, airway obstruction, granulation tissue, bleeding, and death.[102]

ANESTHETIC IMPLICATIONS

Preoperative sedation should be used with caution in patients with severe OSA. During induction of anesthesia, these patients are at high risk for airway obstruction, desaturation and laryngospasm.[44] Pulmonary edema can develop from either severe exacerbation of upper airway obstruction and/or following intubation and relief of the obstruction. Patients with severe OSA have an abnormal ventilator response to carbon dioxide and are likely to also have greater respiratory depression in response to sedatives, narcotics, and general anesthetics, and can have significant delay in the return to spontaneous ventilation and emergence from general anesthesia.[44] The presence of trace volatile anesthetics will further reduce a pre-existing abnormal ventilatory drive and potentiate airway obstruction because of reduced function of the genioglossus and other airway muscles.[103] After extubation patients are at risk for post-extubation obstruction, laryngospasm, desaturation, pulmonary edema, and respiratory arrest.[104]

Sanders and King[105] evaluated the rate of complications experienced by children who undergo T&A for OSA, the safety of a standard anesthetic protocol for these children, and preoperative predictors of complications. The numbers of complications and medical interventions in the perioperative period were recorded and correlated with the presence and severity of OSA for 61 children with OSA, confirmed by polysomnography, and 21 children with recurrent tonsillitis. Children with OSA had more respiratory complications per operation than non-OSA children (5.7 vs 2.9, $P<0.0001$). Supraglottic obstruction, breath holding, and desaturation on anesthetic induction and emergence were the most common complications. Increased severity of OSA, low weight and young age are correlated with an increased rate of complications. Medical intervention was necessary in more children with OSA during recovery and emergence than in the non-OSA group (17/61 vs 1/21, $P<0.05$). Children with OSA are at risk for respiratory compromise postoperatively due to upper airway edema, increased secretions, respiratory depression secondary to analgesic and anesthetic agents, and post-obstructive pulmonary edema.[106] Postoperative respiratory compromise has been reported to occur in 16–27% of children with OSA.[107,108] Despite an increased risk for complications, it is advantageous to extubate patients immediately after surgery if criteria are met. A retrospective study showed that children who remained electively intubated had a higher complication rate (47%) than those who did not (2%).[109] Children who remained intubated were younger and had a higher American Society of Anesthesiologists (ASA) classification and had a longer PICU and hospital stay. Both groups of children had similar opioid requirements and time to discharge from the recovery room. These findings suggest that children with OSA are at risk for respiratory complications after adenotonsillectomy, but that these complications do not prolong the time to discharge.

Another special population to consider is the child with the neurologically impaired (NI) swallow. Conley et al.[110] compared 45 children with documented dysphagia to age- and procedure-matched normal children for operating room and clinical experience. No intraoperative complications, early post-tonsillectomy hemorrhage, hospital readmission, or mortality occurred in either group. Three NI children each had an episode of aspiration pneumonia (early or late) without sequelae. Of the 32, videoflouroscopic swallow study (VFSS) available for review, postoperative aspiration incidence was significantly improved, but with new-onset aspiration occurring in five children. Of available matched pre- and postoperative PSG, 91% confirmed resolution of identified preoperative obstructive sleep apnea. Long-term telephone follow-up of 20 NI children revealed improved breathing (95%), communication (90%), and feeding efficiency (55%). This study suggests tonsillectomy in NI children can be performed safely with appropriate monitoring and precautions with a 48-hour hospital postoperative stay recommended. Swallowing safety appears to improve both objectively and subjectively in most NI children following tonsillectomy. Both preoperative and postoperative VFSS are recommended for any NI child undergoing tonsillectomy.

CPAP

Nasal CPAP has been reported to be both effective and well-tolerated in children.[111–113] This is discussed in depth in Chapter 32.

CONCLUSION

The evaluation of the patient of upper airway obstruction includes a thorough history and physical examination. Risk factors including obesity, Down syndrome, craniofacial disorders, or neurologically impaired may indicate the need for preoperative PSG. Adenotonsillectomy is effective in the majority of children, but increasing rates of residual OSA are seen, particularly in obese patients and those with Down syndrome. For patients with residual OSA, multiple-level surgery may be undertaken after evaluation with flexible endoscopy and/or imaging studies to identify the levels of obstruction. Children with OSA are at increased risk for perioperative complications and should be monitored accordingly postoperatively.

Clinical Pearls

- Tonsil and adenoid hyperplasia is the most common cause of OSA.
- Craniofacial abnormalities, the nose, palate, base of tongue, hypopharynx, supraglottis and glottis may be contributory sites.
- Successful management of OSA in children depends on the accurate identification of the site of obstruction and the assessment of the severity with polysomnogram as an important adjunct.

References

1. Darrow DH, Johnson KE. Management of sleep-related breathing disorders in children. In: Friedman M, editor. Sleep Apnea and snoring: surgical and non-surgical therapy. China: Saunders, Elsevier; 2009. p. 398–413.
2. Schecher MS, Section on Pediatric Pulmonology, Subcommittee on Obstructive Sleep Apnea Syndrome. Technical report: diagnosis and management of childhood obstructive sleep apnea syndrome. Pediatrics 2002;109:e69.
3. Owen GO, Canter RJ, Robirson A. Snoring, apnoea, and ENT symptoms in the paediatric community. Clin Otolaryngol 1996;21:130–4.
4. Kwok KL, Ng DK, Cheung YF. BP and arterial distensibility in children with primary snoring. Chest 2003;123:1561–6.
5. Owens J, Spirito A, Nobile C, et al. Incidence of parasomnias in children with obstructive sleep apnea. Sleep 1997;20(12):1193–6.
6. Gozal D. Sleep disordered breathing and school performance in children. Pediatrics 1998;102:616–20.
7. Kirknessa JP, Krishnana V, Patila SP, et al. Upper airway obstruction in snoring and upper airway resistance syndrome. In: Sanner BM, Somers VK, Randerath WJ, editors. Sleep apnea progress in respiratory research, Vol. 35. Basel: Karger; 2006. p. 79–89.
8. Brouillette RT, Fernbach SK, Hunt CE. Obstructive sleep apnea in infants and children. Pediatrics 1982;100(1):31–40.
9. Goh DY, Galster P, Marcus CL. Sleep architecture and respiratory disturbances in children with obstructive sleep apnea. Crit Care Med 2000;162:682–6.
10. Sulman CS, Holinger LD. Stridor. In: Bailey BJ, Johnson JT, editors. Head and neck surgery – otolaryngology. 4th ed. Philadelphia: Lippincott Williams & Wilkins; 2006. p. 1095–118.
11. Parkin JL, Stevens MH, Jung AL. Acquired and congenital subglottic stenosis in the infant. Ann Otol Rhinol Laryngol 1976;85(5 pt1):573–81.
12. O'Brien LM, Sitha S, Bau LA, et al. Obesity increases the risk for persisting obstructive sleep apnea after treatment in children. Int J Pediatr Otorhinolaryngol 2006;70:1555–60.
13. Verhulst SL, Van Gaal L, De Backer W, et al. The prevalence, anatomical correlates and treatment of sleep-disordered breathing in obese children and adolescents. Sleep Med Rev 2008;12(5):339–46.
14. Dahlquist A, Rask E, Rosenquist CJ. Sleep apnea and Down's syndrome. Acta Otolaryngol 2003;123:1094–7.
15. Levanon A, Tarasuik A, Tal A. Sleep characteristics in children with Down syndrome. J Pediatrics 1999;134(6):755–60.
16. Robison JG, Otteson TD. Increased prevalence of obstructive sleep apnea in patients with cleft palate. Arch Otol Head Neck Surg 2011;137:269–74.
17. Lo LI, Chen YR. Airway obstruction in severe syndromic craniosynostosis. Ann Plast Surg 1999;43:258–64.
18. de Jong T, Bannink N, Bredero-Boelhouwer HH, et al. Long-term functional outcome in 167 patients with syndromic craniosynostosis: designing a syndrome-specific risk profile. J Plast Reconstr Aesthet Surg 2010;63:1635–41.
19. Tripathi A, Jerrell JM, Stallworth JR. Clinical complications in severe pediatric sickle cell disease and the impact of hydroxyurea. Ann Hematol 2011;90(2):145–50.
20. Isono S, Shimada A, Utsigi M, et al. Comparison of static mechanical properties of the passive pharynx between normal children and children with sleep-disordered breathing. Am J Resp Crit Care Med 1998;157(4 pt 1):1204–12.

21. Guimaraes CVA, Kalra M, Donnelly L et al. The frequency of lingual tonsil enlargement in obese children. Am J Roentgenol 2008;190(4): 973–5.

22. Roland PS, Rosenfeld RM, Brooks LJ, et al. Clinical practice guideline: polysomnography for sleep-disordered breathing prior to tonsillectomy in children. Otolaryngol Head Neck Surg 2011;145:S1–15.

23. McColley SA, April MM, Carroll JL, et al. Respiratory compromise after adenotonsillectomy in children with obstructive sleep apnea. Arch Otolaryngol Head Neck Surg 1992;118:940–3.

24. Biavati MJ, Manning SC, Phillips DL. Predictive factors for respiratory complications after tonsillectomy and adenoidectomy in children. Arch Otolaryngol Head Neck Surg 2007;123:517–21.

25. Lertsburapa K, Schroeder JW, Sullivan C. Assessment of adenoid size: A comparison of lateral radiographic measurements, radiologist assessment, and nasal endoscopy. Int J Pediatr Otorhinolaryngol 2011; 74(12):1281–5.

26. Vieira BB, Itikawa CE, de Almeida LA, et al. Cephalometric evaluation of facial pattern and hyoid bone position in children with obstructive sleep apnea syndrome. Int J Pediatr Otorhinolaryngol 2011;75: 383–6.

27. Brown OE, Manning SC, Ridenour B. Cor pulmonale secondary to tonsillar and adenoidal hypertrophy: management considerations. Int J Pediatr Otorhinolaryngol 1998;16:131–9.

28. Donnelly LF, Shott SR, LaCrosse CR, et al. Causes of persistent obstructive sleep apnea despite previous tonsillectomy and adenoidectomy in children with Down syndrome as depicted on static and dynamic cine MRI. Am J Roentgenol 2004;183(1):175–81.

29. Shott SR, Donnelly LF. Cine magnetic resonance imaging evaluation of persistent airway obstruction after tonsil and adenoidectomy in children with Down syndrome. Laryngoscope 2004;(114):1724–9.

30. Burk CD, Miller L, Handler SD, et al. Preoperative history and coagulation screening in children undergoing tonsillectomy. Pediatrics 1992;89(4 pt 2):691–5.

31. Brodsky L. Tonsil and adenoid disorders. In: Gates G, editor. Current therapy in otolaryngology-head neck surgery. St. Louis: Mosby; 1998. p. 414–17.

32. Demain JG, Goetz DW. Pediatric adenoidal hypertrophy and nasal airway obstruction: reduction with aqueous nasal beclomethasone. Pediatrics 1995;95:355–64.

33. Broullette RT, Manoukian JJ, Ducharme FM, et al. Efficacy of fluiticasone nasal spray for pediatric obstructive sleep apnea. J Pediatr 2001;138:838–44.

34. Kheirandish-Gozal L, Gozal D. Intranasal budesonide treatment for children with mild obstructive sleep apnea syndrome. Pediatrics 2008;122:149–55.

35. Kheirandish L, Goldbart AD, Gozal D. Intranasal steroids and oral leukotriene modifier therapy in residual sleep-disordered breathing after tonsillectomy and adenoidectomy in children. Pediatrics 2006;117(1): e61–6.

36. Al-Ghamadi SA, Manoukian JJ, Morielle A, et al. Do systemic corticosteroids effectively treat obstructive sleep apnea secondary to adenotonsillar hypertrophy. Laryngoscope 1997;107(10):1382–7.

37. Villa MP, Bernkopf E, Pagani J, et al. Randomized controlled study of an oral jaw-positioning appliance for the treatment of obstructive sleep apnea in children with malocclusion. Am J Respir Crit Care Med 2002;165:123–7.

38. Carvalho FR, Lentini-Oliveira DA, Machado MA, et al. Oral appliances and functional orthopaedic appliances for obstructive sleep apnoea in children. Cochrane Data Base Systematic Review 2007;(2): CD005520.

39. Mitchell RB. Adenotonsillectomy for obstructive sleep apnea in children: outcome evaluated by pre- and postoperative polysomonography. Laryngoscope 2007;117(10):1844–54.

40. Lipton AL, Gozal D. Treatment of obstructive sleep apnea in children: do we really know how? Sleep Med Rev 2003;7:61–80.

41. Friedman M, Wilson M, Lin HC, et al. Updated systematic review of tonsilectomy and adenoidectomy for treatment of pediatric obstructive sleep apnea/hypopnea syndrome. Otolaryngol Head Neck Surg 2009;140:800–8.

42. Costa DJ, Mitchell R. Adenotonsillectomy for obstructive sleep apnea in obese children: a meta-analysis. Otolaryngol Head Neck Surg 2009;140:455–60.

43. Rieder AA, Ishman SL, Flanary VA. The effect of polysomnography of pediatric adenotonsillectomy postoperative management. In: Friedman M, editor. Sleep apnea and snoring: surgical and non-surgical therapy. China: Elsevier; 2009. p. 420–4.

44. Blum RH, McGowan FX. Chronic upper airway obstruction and cardiac dysfunction: anatomy, pathophysiology and anesthetic implications. Pediatr Anesthes 2004;14:75–83.

45. Brigger MT, Brietzke SE. Outpatient tonsillectomy in children: a systematic review. Otolaryngol Head Neck Surg 2006;135:1–7.

46. Johnson LB, Elluru RG, Myer CM. Complications of adenotonsillectomy. Laryngoscope 2002;112(8 pt 2):35–6.

47. Marioni G, De Filippis C, Tregnanghi A, et al. Cervical emphysema and pneumomediastinum after tonsillectomy: it can happen. Otolaryngol Head Neck Surg 2003;128:298–300.

48. Tomita H, Ohtuka K. Taste disturbance after tonsillectomy Acta Otoalryngol Suppl 2002;546:164–72.

49. Wilson YL, Merer MD, Moscatello AL. Comparison of three common tonsillectomy techniques: a prospective randomized, double-blinded clinical study. Laryngoscope 2009;119(1):162–70.

50. Alexiou VG, Salazar-Salvia MS, Jervis PN, et al. Modern technology assisted vs. conventional tonsillectomy: a meta-analysis of randomized control trials. Arch Otolaryngol Head Neck Surg 2006;137(11): 558–70.

51. Younis RT, Lazar RH. History and current practice of tonsillectomy. Laryngoscope 2002;112(8 pt 2):3–5.

52. Maddern BR. Electrosurgery for tonsillectomy. Laryngoscope 2002;112(8 pt 2):11–13.

53. Temple RH, Timms MS. Paediatric coblation tonsillectomy. Int J Pediatr Otorhinolaryngol 2001;61(3):195–8.

54. Wiatrack BJ, Willging JP. Harmonic scalpel for tonsillectomy. Laryngoscope 2002;112:(8 pt 2):14–16.

55. Grindle CR, Murray RC, Chennupati SK, et al. Revision adenoidectomy. Laryngoscope 2010;121(11):2128–30.

56. Eviatar E, Kessler A, Shlamkovitch N, et al. Tonsillectomy vs. partial tonsillectomy for OSAS in children – 10 years post-surgery follow-up. Int J Pediatr Otorhinolaryngol 2009;73(5):637–40.

57. Koltai PJ, Solares CA, Mascha EJ, et al. Intracapsular partial tonsillectomy for tonsillar hypertrophy in children. Laryngoscope 2002 112 8 pt 2):17–19.

58. Stewart MG, Glaze DF, Friedman EM, et al. Quality of life and sleep study findings after adenotonsillectomy in children with obstructive sleep apnea. Arch Otolaryngol Head Neck Surg 2005;131:308–34.

59. De Serres LM, Derkay C, Sie K, et al. Impact of adenotonsillectomy on quality of life in children with obstructive sleep disorders. Otolaryngol Head Neck Surg 2002;128:489–96.

60. Suen JS, Arnold JE, Brooks LJ. Adenotonsillectomy for treatment of obstructive sleep apnea in children. Arch Otolaryngol Head Neck Surg 1995;121:525–30.

61. Costa DJ, Mitchell R. Adenotonsillectomy for obstructive sleep apnea in children: a meta-analysis. Otolaryngology Head Neck Surg 2009;140(4):455–60.

62. Bhattacharjee R, Kheirandish-Gozal L, Spruyt K, et al. Adenotonsillectomy outcomes in treatment of obstructive sleep apnea in children: a multicenter retrospective study. Am J Resp Crit Care Med 2010; 182:676–83.

63. Mitchell RB, Kelly J. Adenotonsillectomy for obstructive sleep apnea in obese children. Otolaryngol Head Neck Surg 2004;131:104–8.

64. Gozal D, Kheirandish-Gozal L. The multiple challenges of obstructive sleep apnea in children: morbidity and treatment. Curr Opin Pediatr 2008;20:654–8.

65. Mitchel RB, Kelly J. Outcome of adenotonsillectomy for obstructive sleep apnea in obese and normal-weight children. Otolaryngology Head Neck Surg 2007;137:42–8.

66. Marcus CL. Sleep-disordered breathing in children. Am J Respir Crit Care Med 2001;164:16–30.

67. American Academy of Pediatrics. Clinical practice guideline: diagnosis and management of childhood obstructive sleep apnea syndrome. Pediatrics 2002;109(4):704–12.

68. Fujita S, Conway W, Zorick F, et al. Surgical correction of anatomic abnormalities in obstructive sleep apnea syndrome: uvulopalatopharyngoplasty. Otolaryngol Head Neck Surg 1981;89(6):923–34.

69. Wooten CT, Shott SR. Evolving therapies to treat retroglossal and base-of-tongue obstruction in pediatric obstructive sleep apnea. Arch Otolaryngol Head Neck Surg 2010;136(10):983–7.

70. Kuhle S, Urschitz MS, Eitner S, et al. Interventions for obstructive sleep apnea in children: A systematic review. Sleep Med Rev 2009; 13(2):123–31.

71. Prager JD, Hopkins BS, Propst EJ, et al. Oropharyngeal stenosis: a complication of multilevel, single-stage upper airway surgery in children Arch Otolaryngol Head Neck Surg 2010;136:1111–15.

72. Marcus CL, Katz ES, Lutz J, et al. Upper airway dynamic responses in children with the obstructive sleep apnea syndrome. Pediatr Res 2005;57:99–107.
73. Leong SC, Kubba H, White PS. A review of outcomes following inferior turbinate reduction surgery in children for chronic nasal obstruction. Int J Pediatr Otorhinolaryngol 2010;74(1):1–6.
74. Liu CM, Tan CD, Lee FP, et al. Microdebrider-assisted versus radiofrequency-assisted inferior turbinoplasty. Laryngoscope 2009; 119(2):414–18.
75. Kezirian EJ, Powell NB, Riley RW, et al. Incidence of complications in radiofrequency treatment of the upper airway. Laryngoscope 2005; 115(7):1298–304.
76. Guilleminault C, Li K, Quo S, et al. A prospective study on the surgical outcomes of children with sleep-disordered breathing. Sleep 2004; 27:95–100.
77. Merrell JA, Shott SR. OSAS in Down syndrome: T&A versus T&A plus lateral pharyngoplasty. Int J Pediatr Otorhinolaryngology 2007; 71(8):1197–203.
78. Pang KP, Woodson BT. Expansion sphincter pharyngoplasty: a new technique for the treatment of obstructive sleep apnea. Otolaryngol Head Neck Surg 2007;137(1):110–14.
79. Sied AB, Martin PJ, Pransky SM, et al. Surgical therapy of obstructive sleep apnea in children with severe mental insufficiency. Laryngoscope 1990;100(5):507–10.
80. Abdu MH, Feghali JG. Uvulopalatopharyngoplasty in a child with obstructive sleep apnea. J Laryngol Otol 1988;102:5465–8.
81. Carenfelt C, Haradsson PO. Frequency of complications after uvulopalatopharyngoplasty. Lancet1993;341:437.
82. Abdel-Aziz M, Ibrahim N, Ahmed A, et al. Lingual tonsil hypertrophy; a cause of obstructive sleep apnea in children after adenotonsillectomy: operative problems and management. Int J Pediatr Otorhinolaryngol 2011;75(9):1127–31.
83. Lin AD, Koltai PJ. Persistent pediatric obstructive sleep apnea and lingual tonsillectomy. Otolaryngol Head Neck Surg 2009;141(1):81–5.
84. Woodson BT, Fujita S. Clinical experience with ligualplasty as part of the treatment of severe obstructive sleep apnea. Otolaryngol Head Neck Surg 1992;107 40–8.
85. Maturo SC, Mair EA. An effective, novel surgery for pediatric tongue base reduction. Ann Otol Rhinol Laryngol 2006;115(8):624–30.
86. Fernandez-Julian E, Munoz N, Achiques MT, et al. Randomized study comparing two tongue base surgeries for moderate to severe obstructive sleep apnea syndrome. Otolaryngol Head Neck Surg 2009;40(6):917–23.
87. Riley R, Guilleminault C, Powell N, et al. Mandibular osteotomy and hyoid bone advancement for obstructive sleep apnea: a case report. Sleep 1984;7(1):79–82.
88. DeRowe A, Gunther E, Fibbi A, et al. Tongue-base suspension with a soft tissue-to-bone anchor for obstructive sleep apnea: preliminary clinical results of a new minimally invasive technique. Otolaryngol Head Neck Surg 2000;122:100–3.
89. Woodson BT, Steward DL, Mickelson S, et al. Multicenter study of a novel adjustable tongue advancement device for obstructive sleep apnea. Otolaryngol Head Neck Surg 2010;143(4):585–90.
90. Powell NB, Riley RW, Guilleminault C. Radiofrequency tongue base reduction in sleep-disordered breathing: a pilot study. Otolaryngol Head Neck Surg 1999;120(5):656–64.
91. Farrar J, Ryan J, Oliver E, et al. Radiofrequency ablation for the treatment of obstructive sleep apnea: a meta-analysis. Laryngoscope 2008;118(10): 878–83.
92. Chen DK, Truong MT, Koltai PJ. Supraglottoplasty for occult laryngomalacia to improve obstructive sleep apnea syndrome. Arch Otolaryngol Head Neck Surg 2012;138(1):50–4.
93. Bouchard C, Troulis MJ, Kaban LB. Management of obstructive sleep apnea: role of distraction osteogenesis. Oral Maxillofac Surg Clin N Am 2009;21(4):459–75.
94. Ow AT, Cheung LK. Meta-analysis of mandibular distraction osteogenesis: clinical applications and funtional outcomes. Plast Reconstru Surg 2008;121(3):54e–69e.
95. Mandell DL, Yellow RF, Bradley JP, et al. Mandibular distraction for micrognathia and severe upper airway obstruction. Arch Otolaryngol Head Neck Surg 2004;130(3):344–8.
96. Wang X, Wang XX, Liang C, et al. Distraction osteogenesis in correction of micrognathia accompanying obstructive sleep apnea syndrome. Plast Reconstr Surg 2003;112:1549–57.
97. Cistulli PA, Palmisano RG, Poole MD. Treatment of obstructive sleep apnea syndrome by rapid maxiallary expansion. Sleep 1998;21: 831–5.
98. Villa MP, Rizzoli A, Miano S. Efficacy of rapid maxillary expansion in children with obstructive sleep apnea syndrome: 36 months of follow-up. Sleep Breath 2011;159(2):179–84.
99. Guilleminault C, Quo S, Pirelli P, et al. Adenotonsillectomy and maxillary distraction in snoring children. Sleep 2006;29:A97.
100. Guilleminault C, Quo S, Huynh NT, et al. Orthodontic expansion treatment and adenotonsillectomy in the treatment of obstructive sleep apnea in prepubertal children. Sleep 2008;31:953–7.
101. Wetmore RF, Marsh RR, Thompson ME, et al. Pediatric tracheostomy: a changing procedure? Ann Otol Rhinol Laryngol 1999;108(pt 1): 695–9.
102. Conway WA, Victor LD, Magilligan DJ Jr, et al. Adverse effects of tracheostomy for sleep apnea. JAMA 1981;246:347–50.
103. Phillipson EA. Sleep disorders. Philadelphia: W.B. Saunders; 1988.
104. Knill RL, Clement JL. Site of selective action of halothane on the peripheral chemoreflex pathway in humans. Anesthesiology 1984;61:121–6.
105. Sanders JC, King MA. Perioperative complications of adenotonsillectomy in children with obstructive sleep apnea. Anesthes Analges 2006;103(5):1115–21.
106. Galvis AJ. Pulmonary edema compliating relief of upper airway obstruction. Am J Emerg Med 1987;5:294–7.
107. Rosen GM, Muckle RP, Mahowald MW, et al. Post-operative respiratiory compromise in children with obstructive sleep apnea syndrome: can it be anticipated? J Pediatr 1994;93:784–8.
108. Ruboyianes JM, Criuz RM. Pediatric adenotonsillectomy for obstructive sleep apnea. Ear Nose Throat J 1996;75:420–33.
109. Schroeder JW, Anstead AS, Wong H. Complications in children who electively remain intubated after adenotonsillectomy for severe obstructive sleep apnea. Int J Pediatr Otorhinolaryng 2009;73(8):1095–9.
110. Conley SF, Beecher RB, Delaney AL, et al. Outcomes of tonsillectomy in neurologically impaired children. Laryngoscope 2009;119(11):2231–41.
111. Waters KA, Everett FM, Bruderer JW, et al. Obstructive sleep apnea: the use of nasal CPAP in 30 children. Am J Respir Crit Care Med 1995;152:780–5.
112. Marcus CL, Ward SL, Mallory GB, et al. Use of nasal continuous positive airway pressure as treatment of childhood obstructive sleep apnea. J Pediatr 1995;127:88–94.
113. Guilleminault C, Pelayo R, Clerk A, et al. Home nasal continuous positive airway pressure in infants with sleep-disordered breathing. J Pediat 1995;127:905–12.

Sleep Disorder Breathing: A Dental Perspective

Kevin L. Boyd and Stephen H. Sheldon

INTRODUCTION

With their 1981 publication *Western Diseases: Their Emergence and Prevention*,[1] authors Hugh Trowell and Denis Burkitt essentially launched a new paradigm in medical education; many modern diseases are now better understood when viewed from an evolutionary perspective. As healthy circadian sleep cycling during childhood would have been absolutely necessary for our ancestors' survival and reproduction (collectively referred to as *evolutionary fitness*) over the vast time span of human evolutionary history,[2] sleep-related breathing disorders such as obstructive sleep apnea (OSA) were likely not a part of the human experience until fairly recently, and thus can be appropriately categorized as *Western* diseases (WDs).

Evolutionary medicine (EM), also known as Darwinian medicine,[3] is a new approach providing a useful framework for understanding modern diseases from an evolutionary perspective. Evolutionary oral medicine (EOM), or Darwinian dentistry, describes how EM principles can be applied to exploring the evolutionary basis of modern dentofacial maladies such as dental caries, periodontal disease and malocclusion. For example, one proposed explanation by EM/EOM proponents for why humans have only *recently* begun to become vulnerable to many modern diseases such as type 2 diabetes and dental malocclusion, for example, is the *Mismatch* hypothesis,[4] which postulates that current high prevalences of WDs in *industrialized* populations are due, at least in part, to exposure to modern feeding regimens and environmental conditions which are vastly dissimilar, or *mismatched* to, the Paleolithic/pre-agricultural diets and environments to which the human genome has been best adapted.[5]

Pediatric sleep-disordered breathing (SDB) is a pathological condition associated with a wide range of clinical symptoms, historical evidence, dentofacial physical examination findings, environmental components and genetic and/or epigenetic factors. Recently published controlled studies indicate a close association between pediatric SDB/OSA and neurocognitive impairments such as ADD/ADHD and other behavioral disorders.[6,7] Many of the various physical characteristics associated with high prevalences of pediatric SDB/OSA are also strongly associated with a number of pediatric dentofacial abnormalities; the relationship between pediatric SDB/OSA and the developing jaws and facial structures is also well described.[8,9]

Many craniofacial traits are, for the most part, alterable during the early childhood stages of dentofacial growth and thus likely to play a large role in the presence or absence of clinical symptoms associated with pediatric SDB/OSA and its associated clinical morbidities. Consequently, the role of the orthodontist, pediatric dentist and general dentist as an integral member of every child's comprehensive healthcare team has never been more important.[10,11]

ETIOLOGY OF MALOCCLUSION

Anthropological studies confirm that dentofacial malocclusion (poorly aligned jaws and teeth), a known risk indicator of SDB/OSA,[12] was infrequently suffered by our pre-*industrial* ancestors, and seldom occurs with frequency in extant non-*Westernized* aboriginal cultures.[13] In fact, skeletal malocclusion didn't appear appreciably in humans until around the time of the *Industrial Revolution* of the mid-eighteenth century,[14] and wherever occasionally observed before that era, it was usually confined to privileged-class individuals.[15]

In order to most efficiently address the health problems known to be associated with untreated, and/or *inappropriately* treated malocclusion, it would first be helpful to have some idea about why our fairly recent ancestors seldom suffered from these unpleasant dentofacial, dental and skeletal disharmonies. Anthropologists have understood for decades that human craniofacial volume has been steadily diminishing since around the time of the Agricultural Revolution some 10,000–12000 years ago, and most rapidly over the past 350–400 years.[14] While there seems to be a definite observable trend towards increased prevalences of malocclusion over the last three to four centuries, to date there is not yet firm consensus amongst dental anthropologists as to precisely *what happened*, but there does seem to be a growing body of evidence that seems to suggest that feeding behaviors during infancy and early childhood are likely involved.[16] Specifically, *ancestral-type* breastfeeding and weaning are known to be protective against certain forms of malocclusion,[17] likely due to the physical challenges posed to the developing palatal–facial suture complex (P–FSC) during infancy and early childhood; furthermore, the highly processed/soft baby foods and artificial infant formulas/commercial nipples that are in so much use today were simply not readily available to children prior to the *Industrial Revolution*.

With ever-accumulating physical evidence from anthropological studies, combined with advances in the newly emerging scientific disciplines of epigenetics and evolutionary medicine, it can be stated with a reasonable degree of scientific certainty that malocclusion is *not* primarily a *genetically determined* disease entity. Rather, malocclusion is better described as a WD that is primarily mediated through a gene–environment interaction that follows a fairly predictable pattern of pathological progression: initially, most WDs are *preventable* so long as genetically predisposed individuals are identified before early phenotypic expression of the disease is obvious, and where feasible, are allowed to thrive in a nurturing environment; next, WDs can be *reversible*, but only in the very early stages of disease expression, and only when the precipitating environmental pressures (e.g., unhealthy eating, sleep-disordered breathing) have been eliminated; subsequently, in cases where a WD has advanced beyond reversibility, it can still be *treated* with accurate diagnosis and appropriate therapeutic measures (e.g., dietary changes, pharmaceuticals) if the disease state is not too far advanced; and finally, advanced end-stage WDs can be *fatal* if not accurately identified, reversed and/or appropriately controlled.

While a cause-and-effect relationship between malocclusion and the pathophysiology of SDB/OSA is not yet proven,[18] a relationship does indeed appear to exist between the two disease entities. Similar to what is now understood about why diabetes and periodontal disease often coexist in the same host,[19] the underlying mechanism connecting SDB/OSA and malocclusion is more likely to be a *bidirectional* one rather than a unilateral cause-and-effect relationship. Simply stated, measures aimed at preventing the initiation and early progression of one disease entity will aid in preventing the initiation and early progression of the other. Given that many dentofacial physical risk indicators for malocclusion might also identify increased risk for SDB/OSA, it seems fairly obvious that measures aimed at prevention, reversal and/or adequate treatment of malocclusion might also help preclude the negative health outcomes that are often associated with SDB/OSA.

PEDIATRIC ORAL HEALTH AND SLEEP

Dentists who treat children are uniquely positioned to identify patients who might be at increased risk for SDB/OSA. Due in part to the successful implementation of the American Academy of Pediatrics and American Academy of Pediatric Dentistry's (AAPD) joint effort to assure that all children establish a *dental home* by the age of 1 year,[20] pediatric dentists now have a higher frequency of patient encounters than do most other allied health professionals. Additionally, postgraduate specialty training programs in pediatric dentistry and orthodontics purposefully prepare clinicians for identifying patients with interferences to normal dentofacial development, including children with special healthcare needs who might be at even higher risk for developing OSA, such as patients diagnosed with Down syndrome, sickle cell anemia, and Pierre-Robin sequence.

During dental visits, many warning signs that a child might be experiencing sleep disturbances can be ascertained from both a thorough oral–medical health history interview with parents/primary caregivers and a comprehensive clinical dentofacial examination. In order to best assure a comfortable and safe dental visit, questions usually asked during a detailed pediatric oral–medical health history interview are designed not only to obtain information about the child's overall dental/medical health status, but also to acquire information about dietary/feeding history and previous dental and/or medical encounters that might impact a child's possible expectations about the dental appointment. A typical list of questions asked might include, 'Was your child breastfed, and if so, for how long?' and 'What beverage does your child typically drink when thirsty?'

While not necessarily a component of a *typical* pediatric medical–dental health history, it is certainly easy, useful and appropriate for dentists to incorporate into the parent/caregiver interview a short series of questions specifically designed to gain valuable information about a child's possible risks for both malocclusion and/or SDB/OSA; some examples might include, but are not limited to: 'Does your child grind his/her teeth at night?', 'Is your child a noisy open-mouth breather and/or snorer during sleep?', 'Does your child occasionally wet the bed?', 'Does your child ever wake up with either a sore jaw, headache, dry mouth and/or sore legs?', 'Is your child at a healthy weight?', and 'Does your child have night terrors or nightmares?'

In addition to the detailed medical–dental health history interview, a comprehensive dentofacial clinical examination might yield warning signs that a child might be suffering from impaired ability to breathe properly during sleep.

SURGICAL VERSUS NON-SURGICAL TREATMENT OPTIONS FOR PEDIATRIC SDB/OSA

It is well established that surgical removal of the tonsils and/or adenoids is the most common treatment for pediatric OSA. For extremely severe cases of OSA for which adenotonsillar surgery might not be indicated as the best treatment, maxillomandibular advancement surgery (MMA) and/or tracheostomy placement are on occasion considered as better surgical options. According to a recently published guidelines paper by the American Academy of Otolaryngology,[21] craniofacial abnormalities of the maxilla and mandible are definite indications for recommending a PSG sleep study prior to T & A surgery.

Maxillary constriction (MC) is a common craniofacial abnormality that plays an important role in the bi-directional relationship between malocclusion and OSA;[22] MC is typically characterized by narrow/deep-vaulted palate (Figure 34-1), tapered dental arches and retro-position of the mid face relative to the anterior cranial base. Per the various comorbidities associated with various surgical interventions, wherever feasible, collaborative efforts aimed at preventing and treating pediatric OSA non-surgically should be given the highest consideration.

Two commonly implemented *non-surgical* medical interventions include inhaled nasal corticosteroids and usage of CPAP/BPAP devices. While correctly classified as a non-surgical treatment option, long-term usage of CPAP/BPAP facial masks can markedly reduce mid-facial development potential in growing children[23] in much the same manner as adult orthognathic surgical reduction procedures such as mandibular setback and anterior segmental maxillary osteotomy. Other common examples of non-surgical prevention and treatment options for pediatric OSA include, myofunctional training oral appliances (e.g., Infant Trainers, Myo-Munchies, etc.), oral myofunctional therapy (OMT), conjunctive dietary counseling for overweight and obese OSA patients, functional orthodontic mandibular advancement appliances (e.g., Bionator), rapid maxillary expansion (RME) appliances (e.g., bonded Schwartz Plate, Hyrax, etc.) with, or without, reverse pull maxillary protraction appliances (MPA) (e.g., Delaire facemask) and more recently, Biobloc Orthotropic (BBO) postural appliances that are capable of non-surgically increasing posterior airway dimensions through sequential advancement of both the mandible *and* maxilla with a series of removable acrylic mouthpieces.

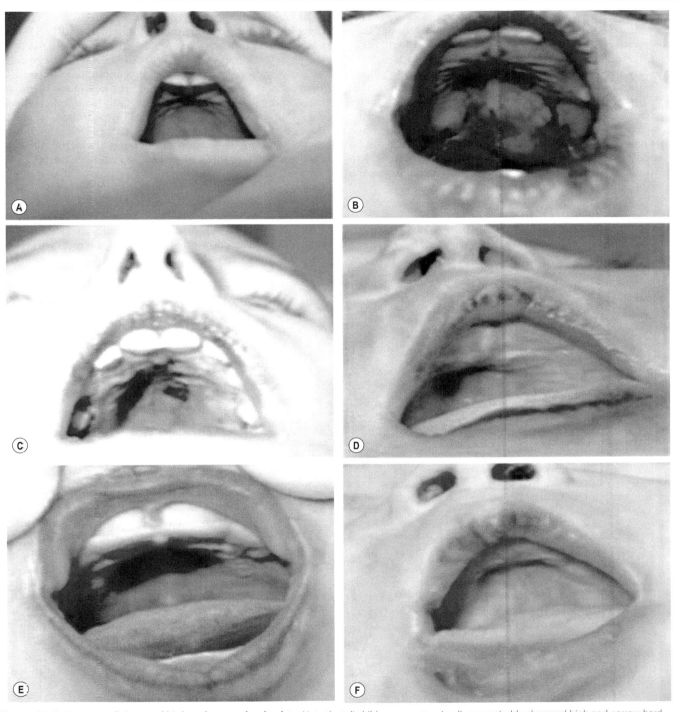

FIGURE 34-1 Montage of abnormal high and narrow hard palate. Note that all children present a visually recognizable abnormal high and narrow hard palate which is related to the development of the naso-maxillary complex during embryonic development considering age of children. On the first row on the left, on the second row in both cases, and on the third row from the top on the right, note the abnormal noses presented by the patients. The asymmetry of the nostril may not be obvious at first investigation; using photographs taken below the nose may help performing better analyses. Asymmetrical opening is often associated with a ymmetrical septum and change in nasal resistance. When associated with high palatal vault, they indicate presence of a higher upper airway resistance and greater risk of abnormal breathing during sleep with addition of infectious or inflammatory reaction. *From Rambaud C, Guilleminault C., Death, nasomaxillary complex, and sleep in young children. Eur J Pediatr. 2012 Sep;171(9):1349–58, with permission of Springer-Verlag 2012.*

Until the recognition of BBO as a non-surgical option for improving posterior airway volume in actively growing children,[24] rapid maxillary expansion (RME) was considered the primary non-surgical orthodontic treatment of choice for treating OSA in children.[25]

Rapid Maxillary Expansion (RME)

Rapid maxillary expansion (RME) is well established as an effective non-surgical treatment option for decreasing upper airway resistance through increasing airway volumes within the nasomaxillary complex.[26,27] Depending on the age of the patient, by exerting orthopedic forces upon the entire maxillary suture complex, primarily with the use of fixed maxillary expansion appliances, RME orthopedic movement will occur when the relatively light forces applied to the teeth and the maxillary alveolar process eventually exceed the forces required for orthodontic tooth movement alone. Following RME, there is an increase in the transverse width of the nasal cavity and hard palate, most notably at the floor of the nose near the mid-palatal suture. In cases where the narrow maxillary arch is also retrognathic (relative to the cranial base), RME can be assisted by reverse-pull headgear (e.g., Delaire facemask) to provide additional nasal airway volume through increasing the anterior dimension of the nasorespiratory space.[28]

Biobloc Orthotropics (BBO) and Oral Myofunctional Therapy (OMT)

As a key participant at the 2012 NESCent Catalysis Conference, Professor Robert Corruccini, a dental anthropologist from Southern Illinois University, was recently cited in *Science*:[29] 'As for malocclusion and jaw disorders, Corruccini noted that a branch of evolutionary dentistry has emerged in which children do mouth exercises and wear devices that put stronger force on their growing jaws.' The branch that Professor Corruccini was referring to is called orthotropics. The orthotropic premise was originally developed in England in the late 1950s by Dr. John Mew, a dual-trained oral surgeon–orthodontist, as an alternative to the then and still commonly held belief that malocclusion is primarily a genetically inherited condition; Mew, also a student of anthropology, studied ancient skulls at the Natural History Museum in London where he was further convinced that malocclusion is an environmentally influenced *disopoly* (*disease of civilization*) which had been brought about by factors related to increased industrialization. Specifically, the orthotropic premise implicitly states that improper tongue and head posture will invariably lead to malocclusion and other associated negative systemic health outcomes.

United by their common focus on assuring optimal dentofacial growth potential and healthy wake–sleep nasorespiratory ability for their young and growing patients, the number of clinicians, mostly orthodontists, pediatric dentists, general dentists, OMTs, sleep medicine physicians and other allied health professionals, who are recommending BBO treatment as a viable non-surgical intervention for SDB/OSA patients is growing rapidly.

The Biobloc appliance system utilizes a series of acrylic intraoral appliances to first develop the upper jaw (maxilla) and mid face to its optimal width and forward position within the cranial base, after which the mandible is *postured* forward with a subsequent appliance to reunite both jaws to a more forward post-treatment position within the cranial base. This maximally forward jaws–facial position provides not only for better esthetics and facial balance, but is also more conducive to development of increased posterior pharyngeal volume and less nasal airway resistance.

There are many other more traditional types of orthodontic appliances such as Twin Blocs, Frankels, Bionators, MARAs, Herbst appliances, class II elastics and others, which all attempt to do the same thing, but most of these appliances are often only begun in the late-mixed to early adult dentition and can exert a backward force, or *headgear effect*, on the growing maxilla that can actually worsen esthetic appearance and/or an already compromised airway.

Biobloc Orthotropics (BBO) differs mainly from conventional orthodontic treatment modalities in that BBO: (1) does not utilize treatment mechanics that place retrusive forces on the jaws, teeth and face; (2) is usually begun in the primary or early mixed dentition when maximum impact upon a child's naso-respiratory competence and neurological, craniofacial and somatic growth is most easily accomplished; and (3) often in conjunction with OMT regimens, is chiefly designed to create a lifelong optimum oral environment for a properly postured and functioning tongue, which is also conducive to lifelong stable and well-aligned adult teeth.

Biobloc as an Alternative to Mandibular Distraction Surgery for Severe OSA: Case Report

The case study described below is a good illustration of how BBO can be utilized as a safe non-surgical alternative to mandibular distraction osteogenesis for severe OSAS. Note the improved cervical spine posture and posterior airway volume seen at the end of BBO Tx (Figure 34-2) and the supportive PSG result. At baseline (Ba) (Figure 34-3), the AHI was elevated at 12.4 events per hour of sleep with the majority of events occurring during REM sleep. Over the course of time, the AHI and REM AHI both decreased steadily, to a degree that at point 1 on the graph the AHI was only 3 events per hour of sleep. Interestingly, as treatment continued from baseline and as the AHI fell, there was a concomitant increase in $EtCO_2$ with a peak when the AHI reached only 3 events per hour. Interpretation of these findings was initially difficult since there was numerical improvement in the frequency of occlusive and partially occlusive respiratory events, but apparent worsening of gas exchange exemplified by increasing obstructive hypoventilation. Etiology of elevation of CO_2 and presence of obstructive hypoventilation related to presumptive development of extremely prolonged partially occlusive respiratory events. For example, if each hypopnea lasted 20 minutes and they were continuously periodic, the AHI will be only 3 events per hour of sleep despite persistence of partial upper airway obstruction. At point 2 at the end of the graph, AHI continued to fall to its nadir of 0.2 events per hour of sleep with concurrent decrease in CO_2 levels to normal and resolution of obstructive hypoventilation. At the same time, there was clear clinical evidence of improvement in symptoms with absence of snoring, resolution of restless sleep, and resolution of daytime sleepiness. At this point, based on both clinical resolution and polysomnographic evidence, sleep-disordered breathing had resolved. Continued follow-up is still warranted and required in order to assure resolution. One final polysomnogram will be conducted to provide objective evidence.

SUMMARY AND FUTURE CONSIDERATIONS

1. OSA is a chronic respiratory disorder that is clearly linked to retrognathic skeletal malocclusions that force the hyoid bone, base of the tongue and its supporting musculature too close to the posterior pharynx. Given what anthropologists have shown with regard to shrinking human craniofacial volume over the past 300 years or so, currently accepted cephalometric normative values are not completely reflective of our true genomic craniofacial growth potential. As a result of this disparity, many clinicians are

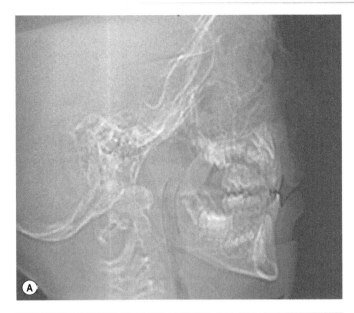

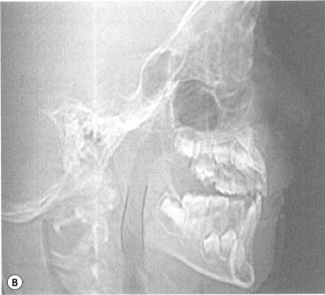

FIGURE 34-2 Note differences in cervical spine erectness and posterior airway area in pre-BBO Tx image (left) vs. post-BBO Tx image (right).

currently being trained to diagnose, treat and evaluate orthodontic treatment progress and final outcomes in accordance with cephalometric norms that are *anthropologically uniformed*, especially with regard to the baseline assessment of maxillary position relative to the anterior cranial base; this is potentially dangerous as this error can sometimes lead to diagnostic and treatment failures which in turn can have negative overall health implications related to inadequate posterior airway volume; e.g., cervical-pull headgear treatment and incisor retraction exacerbating compromised posterior airway volume in class II retrognathic patients.[30,31] Cooperative efforts between anthropologists, dentists and other concerned healthcare professionals should be undertaken to revise currently used cephalometric standards so as to better reflect the true forward growth potential of the human dentofacial complex.

2. Medical and dental educational programs should incorporate more cross-curriculum activities and include evidence-based content into their teaching curriculums within the disciplines of evolutionary medicine, sleep medicine, orofacial myology and nutrition.

3. Overconsumption of sugar and other refined (fermentable) carbohydrates are clearly implicated in recent increases in nationwide prevalences of both early childhood caries (ECC)[32] and childhood obesity.[33,34] Given that childhood obesity[35] and pain associated with untreated caries[36] are both known risk factors associated with fragmented sleep, it seems reasonable to suggest that medical and dental professionals should implement diet counseling as an adjunctive component to their existing preventive and therapeutic treatment protocols.

4. Orthodontists, pediatric dentists and general dentists should collaborate with efforts to raise awareness, amongst themselves and their patients, about the importance of early recognition of pediatric patients who might be at risk for SDB/OSA.

5. Guidelines for identifying SDB/OSA dentofacial risk indicators should be established and disseminated to all members of the allied pediatric health care team.

6. Future well-designed prospective trials will be necessary in order to validate existing scientific and circumstantial evidence that early childhood feeding environments, dentofacial development, naso-respiratory competence, pediatric

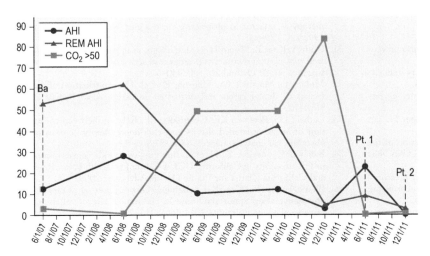

FIGURE 34-3 Longitudinal polysomnograph assessment comparing the patient's AHI, REM AHI, and CO_2 levels as BBO treatment progresses.

sleep hygiene and neuro-cognitive development, are all inter-related.

7. When indicated by the presence of multiple medical and/or dentofacial risk indicators for SDB/OSA, orthodontists, pediatric dentists and general dentists will need to be properly trained to deliver effective non-surgical modes of oral interventions, and be willing and able to intervene or refer for appropriate screening (e.g., PSG) and/or treatment while children are still in their primary dentitions.

8. Pediatric sleep medicine centers should have at least one dentist on their team who is experienced in dentofacial issues related to SDB/OSA.

9. New methods for earlier detection of children at risk for SDB/OSA, such as *in utero* 3-D ultrasonography facial imaging, should continually be explored.

Clinical Pearls

- An increased emphasis on identifying malocclusion as more of a *symptom* rather than as a distinct *disease* entity can help medical and dental clinicians better understand and appreciate the inter-relatedness between malocclusion and SDB/OSA. Evaluating SDB/OSA and malocclusion from an evolutionary perspective helps clarify that, similar to other *Western diseases* such as type 2 diabetes, susceptible individuals need not fully express the disease phenotype if environmental triggers are identified and eliminated early in a child's life.

- The ability to recognize known dentofacial risk indicators of SDB/OSA in early childhood can help dentists, physicians and other allied health professionals better collaborate in providing comprehensive and coordinated care for their mutual patients.

- Both childhood obesity (CO) and pain from untreated early childhood caries (ECC) are known risk factors for SDB/OSA that can negatively impact sleep quality and quantity. As overconsumption of commercially processed fermentable carbohydrates (f-CHOs) in early childhood is a known etiological component of both CO and ECC, dentists and physicians should discourage unhealthy snacking on simple sugars and starches as a component of their CO, ECC and SDB/OSA prevention and treatment protocols.

- As breastfeeding is known to be protective against the development of SDB/OSA, adenotonsillar hypertrophy (ATH) and malocclusion, dentists and physicians should mutually provide consistent and accurate advice to parents regarding options for infant and early childhood feeding regimens.

References

1. Trowell HC, Burkitt DP. Western diseases: their emergence and prevention. Cambridge, MA: Harvard University Press; 1981.
2. Tucci V. Sleep, circadian rhythms, and interval timing: evolutionary strategies to time information. Frontiers Integrat Neurosc 2012;5(92):1–4.
3. Nesse R, Williams GC. The dawn of Darwinian medicine. Q Rev Biol 1991;66(1):1–22.
4. Gluckman P, Hanson M. Mismatch: why our world no longer fits our bodies. Oxford: Oxford University Press; 2006.
5. Cordain L, Eaton SB, Sebastian A, et al. Origins and evolution of the Western diet: health implications for the 21st century. Am J Clin Nutr 2005;81:341–54.
6. Beebe DW, Rausch J, Byars KC, et al. Persistent snoring in preschool children: predictors and behavioral and developmental correlates. Pediatrics 2012;130:382–9.
7. Bonuck K, Freeman K, Chervin RD, et al. Sleep-disordered breathing in a population-based cohort: behavioral outcomes at 4 and 7 years. Pediatrics 2012;129(4):1–9.

8. McNamara J. Influence of respiratory pattern on craniofacial growth. Angle Orthodont 1981;51(4):269–300.
9. Zettergren-Wijk L, Linder-Aronson S, Nordlander B, et al. Longitudinal effect on facial growth after tonsillectomy in children with obstructive sleep apnea. World J Orthodont 2002;3:67–72.
10. Hang W. Obstructive sleep apnea: dentistry's unique role in longevity enhancement. J Am Orthod Assoc 2007;7(2):28–32.
11. Ruoff CM, Guilleminault C. Orthodontics and sleep-disordered breathing. Sleep Breath 2012;16(2):271–3.
12. Flores-Mir C, Korayem M, Heo G, et al. Craniofacial morphological characteristics in children with obstructive sleep apnea syndrome: A systematic review and meta-analysis. JADA 2013;144(3):269–77.
13. Price Weston A. Nutrition and physical degeneration; a comparison of primitive and modern diets and their effects. New York, London: P3. Hoeber; 1945.
14. Gilbert SF. 2001, Ecological developmental biology: developmental biology meets the real world. Dev Biol 2001;233:1–12.
15. Mew John. 2012, personal communication.
16. Boyd KL. Darwinian dentistry part 2: early childhood nutrition, dentofacial development and chronic disease. J Am Orthodont Soc 2012;12(2):28–32.
17. Romero CC, Scavone-Junior H, Garib DG, et al. Breastfeeding and non-nutritive sucking patterns related to the prevalence of anterior open bite in primary dentition. J Appl Oral Sci 2011;19(2):161–8.
18. Darendeliler MA, Cheng LL, Pirelli P, Cistulli PA. Dentofacial Orthopedics. In: Lavigne GJ, Cistulli PA, Smith MT, editors. Sleep medicine for dentists: a practical overview. Chicago: Quentessence Books; p. 88–91.
19. Taylor GW. Bidirectional interrelationships between diabetes and periodontal diseases: an epidemiologic perspective. Ann Periodontol 2001;6(1):99–112.
20. American Academy of Pediatrics Section on Pediatric Dentistry. Oral health risk assessment timing and establishment of the dental home. Pediatrics 2003;111(5):1113–16.
21. Roland PS, Rosenfeld RM, Brooks LJ, et al. Clinical practice guideline: polysomnography for sleep-disordered breathing prior to tonsillectomy in children. Otolaryngol Head Neck Surg 2012;145(1S):S1–15.
22. Seto BH. Maxillary morphology in obstructive sleep apnoea syndrome. Eur J Orthodont 2001;23(6):703–14.
23. Villa MP, Pagani J, Ambrosio R, et al. Mmid-face hypoplasia after long-term nasal ventilation (LTE). Am J Resp Crit Care Med 2002;166:112.
24. Hang W, Singh D. Evaluation of the posterior airway space following biobloc therapy: geometric morphometrics. J Craniomandib Pract 2002; 25(2):84–9.
25. Timms DJ. The effect of rapid maxillary expansion of nasal airway resistance. Br J Orthodont 1986;13:221–8.
26. Pirelli P, Saponara M, Guilleminault C. Rapid maxillary expansion in children with obstructive sleep apnea syndrome. Sleep 2004;27(4): 761–76.
27. Villa MP, Malagola C, Pagani J, et al. Rapid maxillary expansion in children with obstructive sleep apnea syndrome: 12-month follow-up. Sleep Med 2007;8(2):128–34.
28. Yagci A, Uysal T, Usumez S, et al. Nonsurgical treatment of a class III malocclusion with maxillary skeletal retrusion using rapid maxillary expansion and reverse pull headgear. Am J Orthod Dentofac Orthop 2011;140(5):e223–31.
29. Gibbons A. An evolutionary theory of dentistry. Science 2012;336:973–75.
30. Pirilä-Parkkinen K, Pirttiniemi P, Nieminen P, et al. Cervical headgear therapy as a factor in obstructive sleep apnea syndrome. Pediatr Dent 1999;21(1):39–45.
31. Godt A, Koos B, Hagen H, et al. Changes in upper airway width associated with class II treatments (headgear vs activator) and different growth patterns. Angle Orthod 2011;81:440–6.
32. Mobley C, Marshall TA, Milgrom P, et al. The contribution of dietary factors to dental caries and disparities in caries. Acad Pediatr 2009; 9(6):410–14.
33. Ludwig DS, Peterson KE, Gortmaker SL. Relation between consumption of sugar-sweetened drinks and childhood obesity: a prospective, observational analysis. Lancet 2001;357:505–8.
34. Babey SH, Jones M, Yu H, et al. Bubbling over: soda consumption and its link to obesity in California. UCLA Center for Health Policy Research and California Center for Public Health Advocacy; 2009.
35. Bhattacharjee R, Kim J, Kheirandish-Gozal L, et al. Obesity and obstructive sleep apnea syndrome in children: a tale of inflammatory cascades. Pediatr Pulmonol 2011;46(4):313–23.
36. Low W, Tan S, Schwartz S. 1999, The effect of severe caries on the quality of life in young children. Pediatr Dent 1999;21(6):325–6.

Chapter 35

Non-Invasive Positive Airway Pressure Treatment

Yakov Sivan and Guy Gut

INTRODUCTION

Non-invasive positive pressure ventilation (NIPPV) encompasses a variety of noninvasive techniques of ventilatory therapy delivered through an interface, usually a nasal mask and less frequently through a full face mask or nasal prongs. Treatment of obstructive sleep apnea (OSA) by nasal CPAP (nCPAP) was first reported in 1981 in adults.[1] Guilleminault and colleagues reported the first use in children with OSA in 1986.[2] In OSA, CPAP prevents upper airway obstruction by acting as a pneumatic splint, thereby maintaining an open airway. Further advances in non-invasive respiratory support both for sleep-disordered breathing (SDB) and for other pulmonary or neurologic diseases have brought about new NIPPV technologies. In this chapter the term NIPPV refers to and includes all of these techniques including CPAP, automatically titrating CPAP devices, BIPAP techniques, adaptive servo-ventilation (ASV), average volume-assured pressure support (AVAPS) and bi-level positive airway pressure with pressure release technology (Bi-Flex). The new techniques have been used mainly in adults, and have led to changes in pressure titration protocols, allowing for machine-driven pressure titration in the home environment.

CLINICAL INDICATIONS IN SLEEP MEDICINE

Delineation of the specific indications for NIPPV implementation in children has yet to be formally defined in any consensus statement. A recent paper has further emphasized the need for such consensus since it pointed out for the first time that NIPPV leads to amelioration of cognitive deficits in children with SDB.[3] The indications for NIPPV are summarized in Box 35-1.

Use in Obstructive Sleep Apnea Syndrome (OSAS)
Most children with OSAS respond to adenotonsillectomy. A minority who fail surgery and children with other causes of OSAS such as obesity, craniofacial anomalies or hypotonia may require NIPPV.[4] This indication is becoming increasingly relevant due to the secular trends in the prevalence of pediatric obesity around the world.

Use in Central and Peripheral Nocturnal Apnea/Hypoventilation
One of the major applications of NIPPV in children is the treatment of central hypoventilation.[5–7] However, caution must be used when applying NIPPV to very young infants with severe central hypoventilation since such patients might not synchronize the opening of the upper airways and glottis at inspiration.

NIPPV is also extremely useful in severe and progressive forms of neuromuscular, skeletal, lung and airway diseases. In most of these situations, the disease progresses over time, and commonly, the first indication of ventilatory insufficiency is manifested by nocturnal hypoventilation that usually resolves during wakefulness. As the disease progresses, both nocturnal and daytime hypoventilation emerge. Symptoms may include headaches, decreased performance and cardiovascular complications. Although during the first stage, when hypoventilation occurs only during sleep, clinical symptoms may be mild, daytime sleepiness and fatigue are not infrequent. Assisted bi-level positive airway pressure delivered by nasal mask may be used successfully to treat sleep-disordered breathing in these patients. The added value of IPAP techniques that provide support also during the inspiratory phase operates primarily through reduction in the work of breathing.[7] Of note, hypoventilation in these patients may appear first or be more severe during REM sleep. Therefore, the indication to start ventilatory support is based on carbon dioxide and saturation during sleep as observed by polysomnography together with the clinical presentation. The main goal of NIPPV in these situations is to improve arterial blood gases to near normal values without discomfort and in the absence of sleep disruption. It should be noted that specifically in these diseases, isolated low oxygenation during sleep without increased $paCO_2$ might not suggest nocturnal hypoventilation, but rather reflects an underlying pulmonary problem with ventilation/perfusion mismatching that might be adequately treated by supplemental oxygen without NIPPV. Some children may require oxygen supplementation being bled into the ventilator circuit in addition to satisfactory NIPPV due to the concurrent presence of parenchymal lung disease. Since these diseases might progress over time, clinical as well as polysomnographic follow-up should be regularly conducted at a rate that depends on the type of disease, age and progression.

HARDWARE

Interface
The interface is the device positioned on the patient's nose and mouth in order to connect the patient to the ventilator. It includes the device itself and straps that secure the interface to the face. Choosing the correct interface is crucial for patient compliance and effectiveness of treatment. The ideal interface should have minimal leaks, be comfortable and easy to wear.[7] Types of interfaces include: nasal prongs (usually for smaller children), nasal mask (the most popular for sleep disturbances in adults and older children), nasal pillows, oro-nasal mask, full-face mask and helmet. Factors contributing to the selection of the interface include: patient age, neurological status, and

Box 35-1   Indications for Non-Invasive Positive Pressure Ventilation (NIPPV) in Pediatric Sleep Medicine

Obstructive Sleep Apnea
- OSA due to adenotonsillar hypertrophy – 2nd line if adenotonsillectomy has failed
- OSA where obstruction is due to causes other than adenotonsillar hypertrophy
  - obstruction by redundant fat tissue: obesity
  - obstruction by enlarged tongue (macroglossia, Beckwith–Weidemann syndrome, Down syndrome)
  - obstruction by bony and cartilage tissue: craniofacial anomalies (Crouzon, Apert, Pfeiffer syndromes), isolated facial defects (Pierre Robin sequence, Treacher Collins syndrome)
  - obstruction by collapsing UA tissue: hypotonia syndromes and diseases
  - obstruction by collapsing subglottic and lower airway tissue: tracheomalacia

Central Nocturnal Apnea/Hypoventilation
- congenital central hypoventilation
  - congenital central hypoventilation syndrome (Ondine's curse, neonatal and late-onset)
  - secondary to congenital CNS structural anomalies (e.g. Chiari, hydrocephalus, syringomyelia)
  - secondary to congenital CNS (and peripheral) diseases (chromosomal anomalies, e.g. Down syndrome, Noonan syndrome)

- secondary to CNS injury during birth and CP (severe asphyxia, CNS bleeding)
- acquired central hypoventilation
  - CNS damage due to trauma, infection, bleeding, seizures, immune and post-infectious diseases, hypoxia/anoxia, storage diseases, metabolic diseases, obesity

Peripheral Nocturnal Apnea/Hypoventilation
- congenital neuropathies
  - e.g., spinal muscular atrophy
- acquired neuropathies
  - secondary to trauma, infection, immune and post-infectious diseases, metabolic diseases
- congenital myopathies
  - acid maltase deficiency, Duchenne dystrophy, myotonic dystrophy
- acquired myopathies

Skeletal Anomalies
- primary bone and cartilage anomalies and developmental defects
  - severe kyphoscoliosis, Jeune thoracic dystrophy
- Anomalies secondary to neuromuscular diseases (severe kyphoscoliosis)

Lung and Airway Diseases

OSA, obstructive sleep apnea syndrome; UA, upper airway; CNS, central nervous system; CP, cerebral palsy.

---

pulmonary or facial abnormalities. For example, a nasal mask may not be suitable for young and uncooperative children due to mouth air-leaks, and the risk of vomiting and aspiration in disabled patients should be considered when using a full-face mask.[8] Infants and small children might better be treated with masks that have a small dead space. Mask type and size will also need to be adjusted over time as the child grows.

Other features of the interface are: anti-asphyxia valves that allow external air to enter the mask in case of ventilator failure, and ports to connect lines for oxygen supplementation and for capnography. The combination of mask and circuit must have only one exhalation port for venting (producing intentional, calibrated leak). Unfortunately, there are only a few products specifically designed for young children.[8]

Circuit

Simple one-tube (open system) or double-tube (for inhalation and exhalation; closed system) circuits can be used depending on the type of ventilator.

Ventilator

There are two basic types of ventilator, time-cycled-pressure-limited and volume-controlled.[9] The former delivers gas using a preset constant pressure; hence, the volume-delivered, is determined by respiratory mechanics and interface properties. Volume-cycled ventilators provide constant volume and will adjust the driving pressure accordingly until a set-up limit is reached. While the pressure-controlled machines compensate for small to medium air leaks (a pressure drop due to leak will drive the machine to continue delivering gas until the set-up pressure is reached again), the volume-controlled ventilators

do not, since the machine cannot differentiate between inhaled gas and lost gas due to leak resulting in reduced tidal volume and minute ventilation. Although studies in adults comparing these methods did not show clear benefit for one method over the other,[10,11] the pressure mode is usually preferred in children due to the relatively large amount of wasted ventilation in the circuit. Most of the current non-invasive ventilators were designed for adults and, therefore, are often not triggered by very small or weak children with low inspiratory flow rates or with fast breathing rates.[7]

TECHNIQUES OF NON-INVASIVE POSITIVE PRESSURE VENTILATION

Continuous Positive Airway Pressure (CPAP)

This is the simplest and by far the most common NIV mode. Positive pressure is delivered to the patient by continuous airflow and a pressure valve. This method maintains the airways patent throughout the respiratory cycle, improves functional residual capacity (FRC), and decreases the work of breathing. It also results in normalization of the pharyngeal dilator muscle activity during sleep in patients with SDB.[5,12] CPAP requires a spontaneously breathing patient and is unable to support ventilation in the case of apnea.

Pressure requirements will vary among individuals, thus, mandating individual titration in the sleep laboratory.[4] Parameters to program during titration include: expiratory positive airway pressure (EPAP) also named continuous positive airway pressure (CPAP), and FiO_2 in specific ventilators capable of adjusting the concentration of delivered oxygen.

Automatically Titrated Positive Airway Pressure (APAP)

In this method, the ventilator continuously adjusts pressure as needed to eliminate respiratory events during sleep. Usually, it serves for titrating the optimal pressure for CPAP treatment (see titrating section). Its use for long-standing treatment of OSAS was studied in adults. At present, there is no evidence of superiority for APAP over CPAP for the treatment of OSAS.[13]

Bi-Level Positive Airway Pressure Ventilation (BIPAP)

BIPAP is often used for patients who fail a trial of CPAP for OSAS and in the treatment of central apnea/chronic hypoventilation in the pediatric population.[14] Two levels of pressure are then delivered to the patient – a lower pressure during expiration (EPAP) and a higher pressure delivered during inspiration (inspiratory positive airway pressure; IPAP). Hence, this method requires triggering and synchronization with the patient's spontaneous breathing.

Triggering the respiratory cycle is achieved by one of three modes:

Spontaneous (S) (or assist). All breath cycles are triggered by the patient without any background ventilation. The ventilator maintains CPAP and gives the patient pressure support during inspiration. The ventilator is programmed to sense inspiratory effort (by sensing either the negative inspiratory pressure or the inspiratory flow, the latter being more accurate) and to activate IPAP until a drop in the inspiratory flow reaches a threshold that terminates the inhalation phase (expiratory trigger).[15]

Machine settings include: *CPAP* and *IPAP* levels, inspiratory *ramp slope* (regulates the speed of gas flow into the lungs) and in some devices also the *expiratory trigger* level expressed as a percentage of the peak inspiratory flow (usually around 25%; however, in most modern ventilators, this variable is preset by the manufacturer). This may become a problem when a large leakage exists, since the ventilator will compensate with increased flow rates resulting in delayed termination of inspiratory phase. This problem may be avoided by increasing expiratory trigger to 40–70% of peak flow.[15]

Timed (T) or control. All breaths are activated by the ventilator. The ventilator starts and ends inspiration solely according to preset values. This mode is used only in patients who cannot initiate breathing spontaneously (usually not applicable to sleep medicine). Indeed, new NIV ventilators usually have only CPAP S/T modes. Machine parameters that need to be set include, in addition, the delivered breathing rate and the inspiratory time.

Spontaneous/timed (S/T) (or assist-control). These are the same as S mode with a background breathing rate that guarantees a minimum rate and is used in cases of significant bradypnea or apnea (Figure 35-1).[17]

Average Volume Assured Pressure Support (AVAPS)
Combined Modes

This method, designed originally for conventional mechanical ventilation[18] combines volume-controlled and pressure-controlled ventilation. BIPAP with fixed pressure support may not maintain adequate ventilation during the changes in pulmonary mechanics that occur during sleep. Hence, it has been suggested that hybrid modes that target a preset volume by adjustment of the supported pressure may be more effective.[19] These novel modes estimate the expiratory tidal volume and respond by adjusting the inspiratory pressure (IPAP) accordingly to maintain ventilation.

This is achieved by two flow sources that work in parallel, one generating constant flow to achieve desirable volume and the other generating a variable level of flow in order to maintain preset airway pressure. Most studies have been performed in adult patients with obesity hypoventilation syndrome. Dialed parameters include tidal volume, IPAP, EPAP and ramp (slope of flow rise).

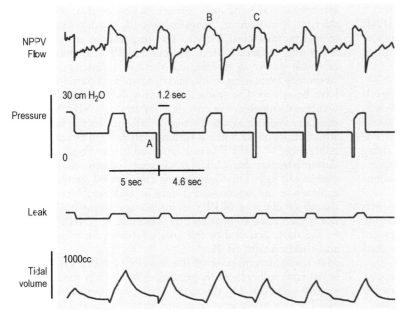

Figure 35-1 Tracing of NIPPV flow, pressure, leak, and tidal volume in a patient receiving BIPAP in the ST mode. Back-up rate is 12/min. When the ventilator did not sense patient's inspiratory effort for 5 seconds, the machine triggered a breath (**A**). Spontaneous (**B**) and ventilator (**C**) triggered breaths have similar peak flows but different duration and tidal volume. *Adapted with permission from ref. 17: Berry RB et al., NPPV Titration Task Force of the American Academy of Sleep Medicine. Best clinical practices for the sleep center adjustment of noninvasive positive pressure ventilation (NPPV) in stable chronic alveolar hypoventilation syndromes. J Clin Sleep Med. 2010; 6:491–509.*

Proportional Assisted Ventilation

By measuring the volume or flow that the patient generates during inspiration (with a pneumotachometer), the ventilator delivers inspiratory flow and pressure proportional to the patient's spontaneous breathing effort.[20] The respiratory pattern is dialed (normal, obstructive, restrictive or mixed) and all other machine variables are then automatically programmed (CPAP, maximum pressure, maximum tidal volume and percent assistance). Manual setting is optional.

Adaptive Servo-Ventilation (ASV)

ASV was developed to treat Cheyne–Stokes central sleep apnea in adult patients with congestive heart failure. It is also approved for use in patients with complex sleep apnea. The subject's ventilation is controlled to equal a target ventilation of 90% of the long-term average ventilation by adjusting IPAP–EPAP difference.[21]

Expiratory Pressure Relief and Flexible Bi-Level Positive Airway Pressure

Exhaling against a positive airway pressure is uncomfortable and believed to be one of the reasons for low compliance to NIPPV treatment in patients with SDB. To address this problem, new ventilators equipped with pressure support algorithms that decrease mask pressure were developed. The main examples are the C-Flex® and the Bi-Flex® technologies (Respironics, Philips). The C-Flex pressure relief technology makes sleep therapy more comfortable by reducing pressure at the beginning of exhalation in order to minimize the back-pressure against which the patient exhales, returning to thera-peutic pressure just before inhalation when upper airway narrowing and collapse are most likely. The level of pressure relief varies, based on the patient's expiratory flow and which of the three C-Flex settings has been selected.[22]

Setting Parameters: EPAP and Gain

The bi-level flexible mode (Bi-Flex) results in pressure decre-ments during both late inspiration and expiration. These adjustments assume to optimize triggering and patient–ventilator synchrony. The magnitude of change of the IPAP and EPAP is proportional to patient effort (as in C-Flex).[23] Parameters to be set are: P_{base} (EPAP), $gain_{ins}$, maximal IPAP, $gain_{exp}$ and minimal PEEP. Experience with these modes of NIV in children with sleep-disordered breathing is emerging.

General Considerations

Leaks. A major issue in NIV is overcoming air leaks that result from mouth breathing and poor interface positioning. Venti-lators compensate for leaks by increasing airflow.[9] Leaks cause a decrease in tidal volume, and problems in triggering. For example, additional flow generated to balance leaks can delay the decrease in inspiratory flow and termination of inspira-tion, resulting in increased asynchrony between the patient and ventilator.

Some of the ventilators include a ramp option which increases pressure gradually to the preset pressure over time allowing the patient to fall asleep on lower inflating pressure that are more comfortable while the desired pressure is reached after the patient is already asleep.

Humidification. High flow of air and unidirectional inspira-tory nasal airflow due to mouth leaks can cause dryness of the nasal mucosa and increase the airway resistance.[24]

Humidification of inspired gas is essential to prevent these complications and also to maintain normal mucociliary func-tion and improve gas delivery. Humidification is especially important in patients with chronic lung disease and in those with a history of chronic rhinitis. Types of humidifiers include: heat-and-moisture exchanger (HME), heated and non-heated pass-overs and pass-through devices. HME is less effective due to the high flows used in NIV. When using pressure-controlled machines only the pass-over humidifier is suitable since the other types may compromise pressure generating and triggering.[9] Most NIPPV devices today have the option for an integrated heated humidifier which is recommended in general, especially for those with nasal symptoms.[14]

Oxygen supplementation. O_2 may be added to NIV after adjustment of other ventilatory parameters (usually increasing CPAP and EPAP) has failed to correct hypoxemia or when the patient does not tolerate higher pressure. Another reason to add oxygen is lung disease.[7] The FiO_2 that is generated and reaches the patient by O_2 supplementation to the ventilator circuit is generally unknown and potentially variable. There are many factors influencing FiO_2 including the IPAP, EPAP, the O_2 flow rate and the site where O_2 is added to the circuit. One study in healthy volunteers found that during NIPPV, the closer the O_2 was connected to the exhalation port (and not the patient) the higher was the FiO_2 achieved.[25] A study in a lung model found conflicting results where the most effective oxygen attachment site was on the mask itself.[25] Due to the uncertainty regarding the FiO_2 actually being delivered to the patient, it is recommended that children who require oxygen supplementation be monitored by pulse oximetry.

RESPONSE TO TREATMENT

Adherence and Compliance

Empiric evidence regarding NIPPV adherence in pediatrics is relatively limited because, compared to adults, NIPPV by CPAP or IPAP modes has only more recently been used in children with OSA. Information from adults clearly shows a positive relationship between the level of adherence to NIPPV treatment and outcomes encompassing health, sleepiness, daytime functioning, neurobehavioral, cardiovascular and mortality measures. Hence, the importance of adherence cannot be underestimated. Although NIPPV use has become relatively common in children, there is a paucity of studies rigorously evaluating its use and outcomes. In particular, there have been very few studies evaluating NIPPV adherence in children using objective criteria.[27,28] Although NIPPV in chil-dren has been shown to be highly effective in the laboratory situation, its use at home is significantly limited by suboptimal adherence.[29,30] NIPPV is not approved by the Food and Drug Administration for children <7 years of age or weighing <40 lb (18 kg). This might have contributed to the limited experience and uncontrolled data in children. Nevertheless, the off-label use of NIPPV in infants and young children has not been shown to bear an increased risk.[27–32] NIPPV might be the most practical or the only treatment for some infants and children with SDB.

A major determinant of the efficacy of NIPPV treatment is patient's adherence. In general, adherence is measured by several variables: (1) the ratio of the number of hours the NIPPV is actually used (machine turned on, mask is applied and fitted and pressures are at required levels) to total sleep time per night; (2) number of nights NIPPV is used for a minimum number of hours a week; and (3) length of time (months/years) NIPPV is used.

Adherence studies are frequently skewed by difficulties in standardization for NIPPV usage and by using populations with average NIPPV application time that is only a little above half of the sleep time. Adult studies, for example, define regular use by at least 4 h of CPAP administered on 70% of the days monitored since only about half of the patients actually use CPAP for equal or greater than these rates.[33–35] Hence, this definition results from practical reasons rather than from medical and outcome considerations. This imposition led to the erroneous assumption that CPAP use of 4 hours/night on 70% of nights is a clinically valid benchmark of CPAP adherence.[36] Recent data show similar findings also in children.[3] It has been shown that even in adherent children and families, the average usage time of NIPPV during sleep is only about 50%.[29,30] The problem with such an approach is that it defines 'outcome' as the *actual patient's usage* in real life and not as a short- and long-term *medical and health consequence*, hence, not representing the potential of NIPPV treatment since the device must be used consistently for all medical benefits to be evaluated and realized. We suggest that patients who do not comply with the treatment should not be considered only as *adherence failure*, but also as *treatment failure*.

Indeed, in many adherence studies, patients who did not use NIPPV or used it during a relatively short time of the total sleep time were excluded and were not included in the outcome analysis. Another problem with adherence is that many studies are based on patients' or parental subjective reports.[37] Objective data from both children and adults show that nCPAP usage is significantly lower compared to reported information.[27,33] Data from adult patients confirm that the reported amount of CPAP use exceeded that recorded electronically.[33,38,39] A recent report in children confirms these findings[40] and highlights the importance of obtaining objective data for adherence in children since previous studies in children reported relatively good rates of subjective adherence on the basis of parental reports.

The application of new generations of NIPPV machines to children that record usage, application time, mode and pressures that are electronically downloaded to a built-in media allows one to objectively evaluate information of compliance and adherence.[27–29] This is important both to allow the clinician to intervene at follow-up visits and for research purposes. Studies in adults have shown that factors that are often thought intuitively by clinicians to be important for NIPPV adherence, such as high pressures or interface issues,[41,42] have not been borne out during scrutiny.[28,43]

CPAP adherence has been linked to multiple factors, such as disease characteristics and severity, patient's characteristics, psychosocial factors, maternal education, titration procedure, mask style, nasal symptoms, pressure discomfort, perceived benefit and the ability to use the therapy. Lower maternal education was associated with lower CPAP use by children in one study.[28] Full-face masks were associated with lower adherence than nasal masks.[30] Conflicting results have been reported for the effect of age.[28–31,37] Yet, most pediatric studies did not include infants and toddlers; hence, less is known about CPAP adherence in younger children. Nevertheless, no differences were found between infants and children who

complied with NIPPV treatment and those who failed regarding gender, underlying diseases, OSAS severity (AHI, oxygen saturation), predisposing factors for OSA and mode of NIPPV delivery.[36,37]

Many children requiring NIPPV treatment have underlying chronic illnesses or developmental delays which further complicate efforts to improve long-term adherence.[27–30,37] NIPPV can be particularly difficult for children with developmental delays, and for those with anxiety or behavioral problems. These children often verbally and physically resist caregivers' efforts to get them to wear the mask, and may develop conditioned anxiety because of poorly fitting equipment and repeated association of the sight, sound, and sensation of NIPPV with discomfort from the mask, physiologic arousal from struggling, or both. They learn that physical and verbal resistance to PAP can cause the caregiver to delay or give up on the use of NIPPV.[44]

Similar findings have been reported from US and Canadian centers. A small cohort including 29 children from four US centers using objective data showed that one-third of children dropped out within 1–6 months of follow-up despite all patients receiving intensive support that included free equipment and continuing assistance.[29] Of the 21 children for whom 6-month adherence data were recorded electronically, the mean nightly use was 5.3±2.5 hours, i.e. only 50% of the sleep which is clinically suboptimal. Of concern is the fact that parental assessment of NIPPV use considerably overestimated actual uses (7.6±2.6 h/night vs. 5.8±2.4 h/night, respectively, $P<0.001$). This may further contribute to failure due to parental false assurance and avoidance of action to improve adherence. In a group of 52 children, the nightly mean use was 170±145 minutes (range: 1–536 minutes).[3] Over the first 60 nights of treatment, children applied NIPPV for only 60±25 nights, i.e., the range of weekly usage was from only a couple of days to an entire week.[3] Another recent small study showed that obese adolescents with OSA adhere poorly to NIPPV.[45] Similar findings were reported in young patients with an average CPAP use of 3.35 h per night.[40] Considering that adherence decreases with treatment time, these data are frustrating and raise concerns on how to significantly improve these unacceptably low adherence rates. More encouraging data from the UK reported that nCPAP was effective and tolerated by 86% of children. A period of acclimatization in the home environment was found to be a useful strategy to achieve success in 26% of patients who initially were intolerant to nCPAP.[37]

It has been suggested that early successful CPAP usage improves subsequent adherence[30,46] with children who were less readily accepting of CPAP (i.e., >90 days to first use after CPAP titration polysomnogram) having also lower CPAP adherence. Probably the most reliable data for children come from a recent prospective study of NIPPV adherence where 56 children and their parents completed a series of psychosocial questionnaires prior to NIPPV initiation.[28] Objective (electronically recorded) adherence data were obtained after 1 and 3 months of NIPPV use. In the first month, NIPPV was worn for an average of 22±8 nights being used by only 78% of children for more than >50% of nights and for only 3±3 hours/night. Adherence rates during the third month were slightly lower: 19±9 nights/month and mean nightly use of 2.8±2.7 hours, corresponding to an average use of only one-third of the sleep time for two-thirds of the nights. Lower maternal education was the strongest predictor of poor NIPPV adherence, implying that intensive training programs might improve adherence. For normally developing children, adherence correlated inversely with age. Adherence did not correlate with severity of apnea, pressure levels, or psychosocial parameters other than a correlation between family social support and nights of NIPPV use. As in adults, severity of baseline polysomnography and nasal symptoms at baseline did not affect adherence.[28,42] Data from adults suggest that short- and long-term adherence are significantly affected by the severity of baseline symptoms, specifically being sleepy at baseline was associated with improved adherence.[33,47–49] This pattern has not been observed in children. Hence, reinforcement from the clinician, regular assessment and motivation sessions are most important.

A major limitation of most studies is that adherence was assessed for only the first 3–6 months of treatment and in some studies children participated in intervention programs with particular efforts being invested to support adherence. Hence, data for long-term adherence in unselected groups cannot be ascertained. Only one recent study looked at adherence beyond the first 6 months of treatment and found an even lower adherence rate with CPAP usage with an average of only 3.5 hours/night.[40] Thus, children demonstrate poor average nightly rates of CPAP use, ranging from 3.5 to 7 h per night. Given that children require between 9 and 12 hours of sleep per night depending on age, it is likely that overall NIPPV adherence in children is very poor.

Adherence – CPAP versus IPAP Modes

It may be reasonable to assume that NIPPV with inspiratory support would be more comfortable than CPAP. Nevertheless, adult data have shown that adherence was similar between CPAP and BIPAP use. Preliminary results show that this is also the case with children.[29] The mean nightly use was 5.6±2.6 hours in the nCPAP group compared with 5.8±2.6 hours for the BIPAP group. The study was not adequately powered to detect a difference between the modes (16 BIPAP and 13 nCPAP cases); nevertheless, the small difference in adherence between the two modes is unlikely to be clinically important.

Conflicting results were found regarding whether the application of auto-bi-level device improves adherence rates.[35,50] Despite the theoretical advantage, the auto-CPAP has not been shown to significantly increase NIPPV usage or succeed in cases where fixed-CPAP failed. A meta-analysis in adults failed to show any differences or even improved hours of usage with auto-CPAP compared to fixed-CPAP despite the fact that the average pressure on auto-CPAP was lower by 2 cmH$_2$O.[51] A randomized, double-blind study compared the use of traditional nCPAP to bi-level positive airway pressure with pressure release technology (Bi-Flex) treatment in children showed no differences in adherence rates.[50] A recent Cochrane database review in adults concluded that device type (auto, bi-level, or CPAP) and pressure contour modification may not play a significant role in influencing adherence to NIPPV therapy.[52]

How to Improve Compliance and Adherence

It should be noted that the American Academy of Sleep Medicine (AASM) standard for management and recommendations and the practice parameters for the use of CPAP and NIPPV refer to adults only.[53,54] These strategies may, however, be applicable to infants and children. For example, educational (reinforced education by prescriber and by homecare provider, one-day education program using video and discussion, demonstration, simple video education), technological (telephone-linked communication, tele-health program, tele-monitoring of CPAP treatment data, internet-based information, support, and feedback system), psychosocial (cognitive behavior therapy), pharmacological (non-benzodiazepine sedative hypnotic agent), and multi-dimensional strategies (intensive support, combination including education, relaxation, and CPAP habituation) can be entertained and adapted to the pediatric age range.[37] Factors that were associated with a successful compliance with NIPPV treatment include: a dedicated staff and an intensive structured program that involved education of families and children and providing ongoing support and follow-up.

Preliminary data on 20 children (aged 1–17 years) with OSAS, referred by physicians for noncompliance with BIPAP, showed that after behavioral intervention 75% of children successfully tolerated BIPAP with increased hours of documented usage versus 0% beforehand.[44] In contrast, no changes occurred in families who declined behavioral therapy.

Initiation of NIPPV Therapy

Since adolescents tend to adhere less than younger children to NIPPV treatment,[28,31] a tailored approach should be undertaken with these patients. Attempts to identify factors that decrease compliance such as the fear of being different from peers, sleeping together with peers at homes or camps, not perceiving potential benefits from therapy and opposing authority should be sought. In addition, it is likely that the older children and adolescents had less parental supervision for NIPPV use. Motivation and self-responsibility seem to be important factors.[28]

A study from Canada of 50 children aged 10±5 years in which almost 50% were using nCPAP for half of the nights for an average of 4.7 hours/night (1.4–7.0 hours/night) showed that by applying a behavior modification program in conjunction with ongoing support and close follow-up, a high implementation rate and a reasonable compliance for using nCPAP could be achieved.[30] A one-on-one educational consultation session of parents and children with a qualified sleep technologist is essential for improved compliance.[30] During this session, families should receive verbal and written information on OSA, the role of nCPAP therapy, the use and care of the nCPAP machine, how to add humidification, how to clean the machine daily using a 1:50 part vinegar:water solution or a mild dish detergent, how to comfortably and appropriately apply the child's mask and how to deal with troubleshooting. Proper mask fit is essential for successful treatment.[55] Hence, during the session, mask fitting is performed. It should be noted that children, especially small ones with tactile aversions such as syndromic children or those with developmental delays or autism and children with minimal nasal airflow (i.e, congenital craniofacial anomalies), may be better treated with a full-face mask.[8] During the session, the effect of changing sleep position on mask and headgear fitting should be evaluated.

For patients in whom the nCPAP trial is unsuccessful or those in whom non-cooperation is suspected from the first consultation, a period of home acclimatization to the NIPPV equipment has been shown to be very effective[37] and is therefore recommended before attempting the NIPPV trial. Children may be given a practice mask and headgear without the NIPPV unit to practice and a gradual application of CPAP therapy is used. This involves letting the child play with the mask and then placement of the mask alone followed by wearing the mask for 2 weeks while awake to help the child habituate to the system. When the child is able to fall asleep with the mask in place, then air is introduced using low pressure and slowly increasing to the prescribed pressure. Once the child accepts NIPPV, overnight laboratory titration study to determine the optimal pressure is performed.

The sudden application of pressure and flow created as the CPAP machine is turned on and applied to the face may significantly affect patient's cooperation, especially in children or when the child is uncooperative and fearful. A gradual progressive approach is, therefore, most important. Some machines have a ramp function, which allows the child to fall asleep on lower pressure levels and then gradually increase the pressure to the required level automatically. When

using BIPAP, the inspiratory and expiratory pressures may be adjusted independently. This lowers the mean airway pressure. It is usually helpful to start with expiratory pressure only, and after the child is cooperative to add and increase the inspiratory pressure by small steps. With BIPAP, cooperative children should be explained that when they inhale, they will feel some air flowing from the machine and that it may take only a few relaxed breaths to synchronize with the machine breaths and then they will feel very comfortable. Hence, the first steps are most important to future compliance and adherence.

Taken together, optimal intervention should be tailored individually according to family and patient characteristics. Effective improvements in adherence may be achieved also by simple, inexpensive efforts, such as weekly phone calls to uncover any problems and encourage use and by written information about sleep apnea and the importance of regular NIPPV use, especially when these are applied at the start of treatment.[56] Suggested protocols for acclimatization to NIPPV are presented in Figure 35-2[36] and Box 35-2. Those dealing with pediatric NIPPV may elect to use all steps and

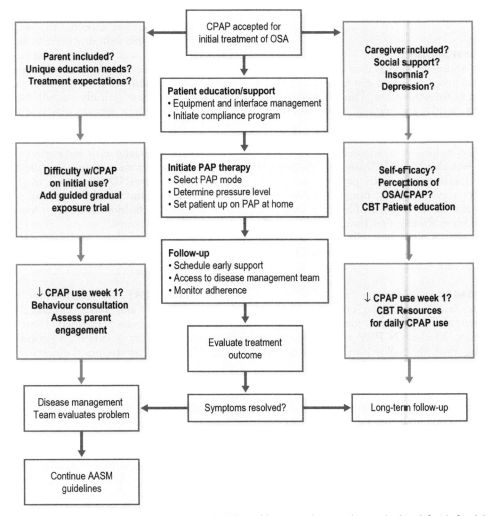

FIGURE 35-2 Intervention to promote CPAP adherence in children and adults. Add-on considerations (green shading, left side for children; right side for older adults and older adults with cognitive impairment) to promote CPAP use. These suggestions extend the American Academy of Sleep Medicine's Adult Obstructive Sleep Apnea Task Force recommendations. AASM, American Academy of Sleep Medicine; CBT, cognitive behavior therapy; CPAP, continuous positive airway pressure; OSA, obstructive sleep apnea; PAP, positive airway pressure. *Flow diagram adapted with permission from ref. 36: Sawyer AM et al. Sleep Med Reviews 2011; 15:343–56.*

Box 35-2 Practical Points for Progressive Initiation of NIPPV to the Child and for Home Acclimatization *(Based on References 8 and 37)*

Some of the steps apply only to small children and depend on child's cooperation.
- Initial exposure to the mask using a nonthreatening and relaxed attitude during an educational consultation session of parents and children with a qualified sleep technologist:
  - Encourage use, discuss importance and benefit.
  - Discuss technical issues, care and maintenance of NIPPV machine, daily cleansing, humidification, prevention of sores.
  - Individualize mask and headgear selection.
  - Appoint a coordinator, provide means of communication.
  - Instruct parents to apply the following steps at home.
- Parents may place the mask in a toy box at home. Encourage the child to play with the mask as a toy during the day.
- Parents should encourage the child to play with the NIPPV

mask which is worn alone (without tubing) until the child is able to wear the open mask without distress.
- Parents should encourage the child to go to sleep wearing the open mask. All ports should be left open without tubing. Parents should remove the mask after the child falls asleep.
- Once the child is able to wear the mask to go to sleep, low CPAP pressure is started (4 cmH$_2$O). Use a heated humidifier from the start of treatment.
- Once the child tolerates the mask and pressure during sleep at home, schedule a titration study in the sleep lab. Avoidance of NIPPV pressures that are too high or too low.
- Use a ramp function, which allows the child to fall asleep on lower pressure levels and then gradually increases the pressure to the required level.

---

measures or adjust the most appropriate ones according to the specific child, the underlying cause and the available facilities.

Ongoing – Long-Term Support

A downward drift in adherence occurs over time.[28,40] Hence, even the best-initiated program might not be efficient if the effect is only assessed in the short term. This is a major challenge since it involves months and years of efforts and intensive follow-up measures to prevent drop-out and to boost participation. Recently, a measure for examining child- and parent-reported barriers to long-term adherence to the CPAP regimen in children was developed.[40] Using this Adherence Barriers to CPAP Questionnaire, both parents and youth detailed many barriers across a diverse range that prevented them from following the CPAP regimen. This brief tool, that was introduced to children for the first time, could be easily administered and scored in a medical clinic by healthcare personnel to determine those obstacles to adherence that are most pertinent to a specific family.

Monitoring Response to Treatment

Electronic monitoring is considered the 'gold standard' for adherence measurement and allows for continuous assessment of long-term adherence. Modern NIPPV machines contain a built-in monitoring card that allows the collection and storage of night-by-night, mask-on CPAP application at effective pressure over each 24-h period. It is important to review the card records for the duration of time when the set pressure was maintained representing actual patient use of the machine (time in use), rather than the duration of time the machine was turned on. This allows obtaining objective compliance data and providing information on the number of days NIPPV was used and the hours of real daily use. NIPPV adherence data can be transmitted to practice sites by several vehicles, including modem, smartcard, or web-portal, depending on the manufacturer. Accordingly, early and routine assessment of CPAP use and treatment response, as recommended by the American Academy of Sleep Medicine, is possible.[36]

Periodic Assessments

Unlike adults, children continue to grow. Pressure requirements can be therefore expected to change over time.[14,57] The mask type and size will also need to be adjusted over time. Hence, a scheduled regular assessment is recommended. Auto-CPAP does not eliminate the need for periodic office visits and evaluations of the clinical course using subjective and objective (electronically stored) data. A study in adults showed that air leak was associated with poor adherence to auto-CPAP therapy.[58] Auto-NIPPV devices may perform suboptimally in the presence of air leak; hence, air leak should be assessed, especially with automated systems, preferentially by objective electronic storage. Specifically, in the presence of air leak, the auto-NIPPV device might fail to detect the events of OSA, and thereby either fail to respond or respond in a suboptimal fashion, leading to lower levels of delivered (therapeutic) pressures.

OUTCOME

CPAP and BIPAP are effective for managing OSAS in both infants[31,57] and older children,[29,32,55] but long-term studies have not been performed. There is a major difference between the ability of NIPPV to correct sleep apnea in the sleep lab (immediate technical outcome) and the clinical benefits of using continuous and lengthy NIPPV treatment in children (short- and long-term clinical outcomes). While studies have shown that neurocognitive and neurobehavioral abnormalities are at least partially reversible with surgical treatment,[59,60] the response to NIPPV has scarcely been studied in children.

There is at present only one study of neurobehavioral outcomes in children with OSA providing some encouraging data showing a significant correlation between the decrease in daytime sleepiness after only 3 months of NIPPV treatment indicating that, despite suboptimal adherence, a significant improvement in neurobehavioral function in children was possible, even in developmentally delayed children.[3] Another recent study in obese adolescents showed that although half of the adolescents prescribed NIPPV for OSA were non-adherent to the treatment and did not use NIPPV at all, Marcus et al. looked also at the effect of NIPPV on quality of life using the Pediatric Quality of Life Inventory (PedsQL)[61] and the OSAS-18.[29] NIPPV was associated with significant improvements in caregiver- and child-reported quality of life for both OSAS-specific and general health-related quality of life.

The time and number of hours/night required for maximal improvements in behavioral function are unknown but might well be longer than 3 months. Unfortunately, no pediatric data are available. Another difficult issue includes the study of the correlation between NIPPV usage and adherence with long-term outcomes including bio-markers. The effect of drop-out and decreased adherence after several months or years of treatment on clinical outcome is also a very complicated topic requiring complex large-scale studies. Another variable that needs further data is the effect of age on clinical response to NIPPV treatment. At present, conflicting results have been reported.[28–31,37] Brain development and plasticity depend on age and it is reasonable to assume that the effects of wearing CPAP for 4 hours a night for 5 nights per week may differ between a teenager, toddler and an infant. Studies that will look at this issue will have to correct also for underlying problems, length and severity of OSA.

TITRATION

The adequate NIPPV setting is one that eliminates all obstructive apneas, other upper airway obstruction episodes, desaturations, and hypercapnia and can still be tolerated by the patient without excessive awakenings. The gold standard for the titration of this optimal pressure is a full PSG in the sleep lab attended by a certified polysomnographic technologist. The pressure is then prescribed for use in the child's home. Direct observation by a trained sleep lab technologist allows for real-time adjustments of mask fitting, eliminating leaks, and helping the patient to adapt to the initial CPAP experience.[62] Any PSG lab should have a written titration protocol to guide the technologist.

Split-night titration. Evidence supporting the use of split-night diagnosis/treatment studies in children younger than 12 years of age is insufficient.[62] Although discouraged, the titration protocol should be identical to that of full-night test. Until recently, only few NIPPV titration protocols were published in the literature, resulting in high variability between centers. In order to standardize diagnosis and NIPPV treatment for SDB, an AASM task force published guidelines for the titration and administration of NIPPV in adults and pediatric population with OSAS and for chronic hypoventilation syndromes.[17,62]

CPAP should be increased by at least 1 cmH$_2$O each time, until obstructive respiratory events (apneas, hypopneas, respiratory effort-related arousal (RERAs), and snoring) are eliminated or the recommended maximum CPAP is reached. In a split-night study one might have to increase pressure at larger increments. Patients uncomfortable or intolerant of high pressures on CPAP and those who continue to have obstructive respiratory events at 15 cmH$_2$O of CPAP during the

titration study should be switched to BIPAP and, again, pressure should be increased by small intervals until respiratory events disappear. A 'down' titration is reasonable due to the 'hysteresis' phenomenon. But the AASM task force recommends that if a down titration is performed, at least one 'up–down' CPAP titration (1 cycle) should be conducted during the night.

The recommended minimum starting IPAP and EPAP are 8 cmH$_2$O and 4 cmH$_2$O, respectively, and the recommended maximum IPAP is 20 cmH$_2$O for patients <12 years and 30 cmH$_2$O for patients ≥12 years. In children who require pressure support (PS), the recommended minimum and maximum levels of PS are 4 and 20 cmH$_2$O, respectively.

Ideally, the patient should be recorded in supine REM sleep for at least 15 minutes. In hypoxemic patients, supplemental O$_2$ should be introduced at 1 L/min and titrated upwards to achieve the target SpO$_2$.[62] Figures 35-3 and 35-4 present titration algorithms.

Auto-adjustable PAP technique (APAP). Manual titration to reach a target pressure could result in higher pressures being prescribed. Auto-adjustable NIPPV techniques (APAP) seem to address this problem, since the machine detects upper airway obstruction by monitoring snoring, airflow reduction (apnea or hypopnea), airflow versus time profile or impedance with the forced oscillation technique and adjusts the pressure in order to eliminate these events. When no such event is recorded, pressure is decreased to the minimum effective pressure.[63] Compared to the fixed airway pressure in conventional CPAP, the variable pressure of auto-CPAP allows for auto-adjustment under different situations such as changing sleeping positions, upper airway infections, and changes in body weight. This technique has been successfully used in adults for almost two decades[64] and is now considered more frequently, including its application to children.[65] A recent review concluded that the use of APAP is sufficient in the majority of adult patients with moderate-to-severe OSAS.[63] One study from Stanford first used auto-CPAP for in-lab pressure titration in children with suspected SDB and has shown that APAP can be used safely for pressure titration in an attended setting.[5]

Of note, APAP is not recommended to diagnose OSA.[66] Patients being treated with fixed CPAP on the basis of APAP titration or being treated with APAP must have close clinical follow-up to determine treatment effectiveness and safety. Appropriate mask fitting to prevent leak is crucial in auto-CPAP since the pressure will unnecessarily increase in the presence of a significant mask leak.

LIMITATIONS, PROBLEMS AND COMPLICATIONS

Several complications have been reported with NIPPV; however, serious complications are rare, and adverse effects have generally been minor.[14] Side effects of NIPPV include patient discomfort, medical side effects and inconveniences. In addition to discomfort, these side effects significantly affect adherence.[36]

Both mask leaks and air leakage through the mouth causing discomfort from nasal and oral mucosal drying are common side effects that are associated with higher NIPPV pressures.

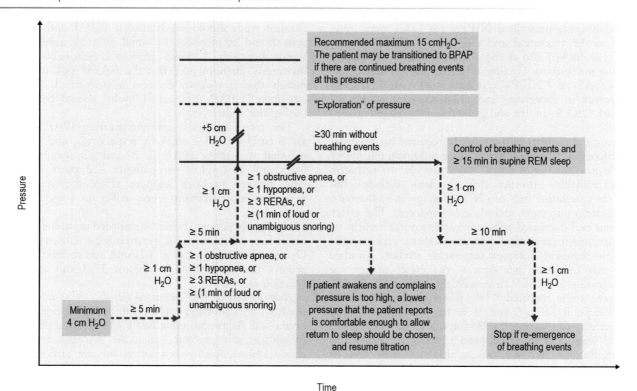

FIGURE 35-3 CPAP titration algorithm for patients <12 years during full- or split-night titration studies. *Adapted with permission from ref. 62: Kushida et al. Clinical guidelines for the manual titration of positive airway pressure in patients with obstructive sleep apnea. J Clin Sleep Med. 2008; 15;4:157–71.*

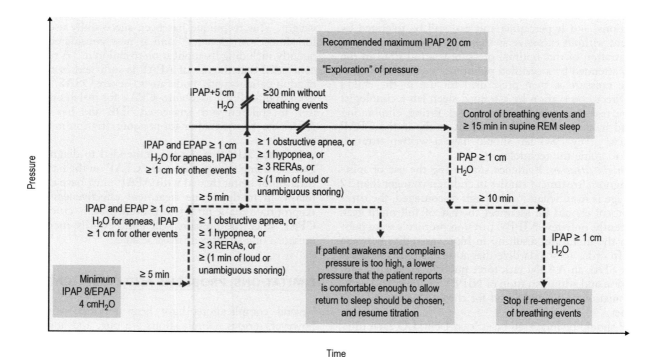

FIGURE 35-4 BIPAP titration algorithm for patients <12 years during full- or split-night titration studies. It is suggested that a higher starting IPAP and EPAP might be selected for patients with an elevated BMI and for re-titration studies. *Adapted with permission from ref. 62: Kushida et al. Clinical guidelines for the manual titration of positive airway pressure in patients with obstructive sleep apnea. J Clin Sleep Med. 2008; 15;4:157–71.*

Mask leak directed to the eyes may cause conjunctival irritation and even conjunctivitis. Skin sores and bruising mainly at the nose bridge are not uncommon and might be prevented by using a well-fitting mask, alternating between different masks and applying colloid dressing to protect the bridge of the nose. Therefore, determination of the minimum pressures required to eliminate apneas and hypopneas is important. In some children who have difficulties or side effects that limit the use of the nasal mask, especially those with nasal side effects, a whole-face (nose and mouth) mask may be successfully used. However, gastric distention and the concern of vomiting into the mask should be taken into consideration, especially in small children. Another option is nasal prongs that may be more adaptable to certain children. Nares irritation is, nevertheless, more common. Pressure on the maxilla from the mask influencing facial development may occur. Facial deformities, malocclusion and mid-facial hypoplasia have been reported as side effects of NIPPV in children, although they are probably rare. Monitoring of facial development and growth is important when using NIPPV masks in young children.

As mentioned, mask size may need to be changed as the child grows. There are relatively few sizes available for children. Experience from the UK shows that children complained of frequent minor discomforts in case of forehead soreness or air leaks, but they responded to simple treatments such as a change of mask size or type, the use of skin cream or protective tape to alleviate skin irritation, and passive humidification in the case of nasal dryness.[37] Particular problems with NIPPV application occur in children with craniofacial anomalies who use NIPPV as a bridging treatment, particularly after they undergo neurosurgery and facial surgeries, since surgical scars and sites may prevent mask and pressure application in the postoperative period.

Nasal congestion might result from the direct pressure applied and from exacerbation of allergic rhinitis which is common in children with SDB. The use of topical steroids has been reported with conflicting results and may be used mainly in atopic children. A 1-month, placebo-controlled adult study failed to show any beneficial effect of nasal steroids.[67] Humidifiers may also improve both mucosal dryness and nasal congestion.

Aspiration has been mentioned as a risk; however, this is rather a theoretical complication. The potential risk is, however, increased in children using a full-face mask. Infectious complication is a concern using humidifiers.[68] The importance of regular cleaning and instructions should be emphasized to parents.

CONCLUSION

The body of evidence regarding treatment of children with SDB with NIPPV is rapidly growing, and parallels the increasing need for this treatment modality. New ventilators and ventilation modalities are being introduced and, therefore, expanded knowledge and practice with these machines and the tailoring of the best modality and settings to the patient will be required from pediatric sleep specialists. To optimize adherence and outcomes, the impact of education, training and continuous support of the patient and family cannot be overemphasized.

Clinical Pearls

- NIPPV is the preferred treatment for SDB when surgery fails or in obese children and those with craniofacial anomalies. However, it provides only a temporary solution rather than a cure.
- CPAP therapy is adequate for most children with OSAS who require NIPPV.
- Poor adherence and compliance are the major barriers to successful treatment.
- Objective measurement of adherence by the new generation of ventilators is recommended.
- Methods to improve compliance and adherence are most important and include education, training and behavioral intervention. However, even with an optimal start, compliance and adherence to treatment decline significantly over time. Hence, long-term follow-up and support using both subjective and objective measures are essential for treatment success.
- There are limited data on long-term outcome of NIPPV in pediatric SDB. Recent data suggest improvement also in neurobehavioral function.
- The gold standard for NIPPV titration for children remains full-night polysomnography. The role of auto-adjustable techniques for titration and for first-line use in children needs further research.

References

1. Sullivan CE, Berthon-Jones M, Issa FG, et al. Reversal of obstructive sleep apnea by continuous positive airway pressure applied through the nares. Lancet 1981;1:862–5.
2. Guilleminault C, Nino-Murcia G, Heldt G, et al. Alternative treatment to tracheostomy in obstructive sleep apnea syndrome: nasal continuous positive airway pressure in young children. Pediatrics 1986;78:797–802.
3. Marcus CL, Radcliffe J, Konstantinopoulou S, et al. Effects of positive airway pressure therapy on neurobehavioral outcomes in children with obstructive sleep apnea. Am J Respir Crit Care Med 2012;185:998–1003.
4. American Academy of Pediatrics. Clinical practice guideline: diagnosis and management of childhood obstructive sleep apnea syndrome. Pediatrics 2002;109:704–12.
5. Villa MP, Dotta A, Castello D, et al. Bi-level positive airway pressure (BiPAP) ventilation in an infant with central hypoventilation syndrome. Pediatr Pulmonol 1997;24:66–9.
6. Guilleminault C, Philip P, Robinson A. Sleep and neuromuscular disease: bilevel positive airway pressure by nasal mask as a treatment for sleep disordered breathing in patients with neuromuscular disease. J Neurol Neurosurg Psychiatry 1998;65:225–32.
7. Robert D, Argaud L. Non-invasive positive ventilation in the treatment of sleep-related breathing disorders. Sleep Med 2007;8:441–52.
8. Kirk V, O'Donnell AR. Continuous positive airway pressure for children: A discussion on how to maximize compliance. Sleep Med Rev 2006;10:119–27.
9. Schonhofer B, Sortor-Leger S. Equipment needs for noninvasive mechanical ventilation. Eur Respir J 2002;20:1029–36.
10. Tuggey JM, Elliott MW. Randomised crossover study of pressure and volume non-invasive ventilation in chest wall deformity. Thorax 2005;60:859–64.
11. Windisch W, Storre JH, Sorichter S, et al. Comparison of volume- and pressure-limited NPPV at night: a prospective randomized cross-over trial. Respir Med 2005;99:52–9.
12. Deegan PC, Nolan P, Carey M, et al. Effects of positive airway pressure on upper airway dilator muscle activity and ventilatory timing. J Appl Physiol 1996;81:470–9.
13. Fleetham J, Ayas N, Bradley D, et al; Canadian Thoracic Society Sleep Disordered Breathing Committee. Canadian Thoracic Society 2011 guideline update: diagnosis and treatment of sleep disordered breathing. Can Respir J 2011;18:25–47.

14. Liner LH, Marcus CL. Ventilatory management of sleep-disordered breathing in children. Curr Opin Pediatr 2006;18:272–6.
15. Medina A, Pons M, Martinon-Torres F. Non-invasive ventilation devices. In: Non-invasive ventilation in pediatrics. 2nd ed. Madrid: Ergon; 2009. p. 41.
16. Medina A, Pons M, Martinon-Torres F. Non-invasive ventilation modes and methods for pediatric patients. In: Non-invasive ventilation in pediatrics. 2nd ed. Madrid: Ergon; 2009. p. 47–58.
17. Berry RB, Chediak A, Brown LK, et al; NPPV Titration Task Force of the American Academy of Sleep Medicine. Best clinical practices for the sleep center adjustment of noninvasive positive pressure ventilation (NPPV) in stable chronic alveolar hypoventilation syndromes. J Clin Sleep Med 2010;6:491–509.
18. Amato MB, Barbas CS, Bonassa J, et al. Volume-assured pressure support ventilation (VAPSV). A new approach for reducing muscle workload during acute respiratory failure. Chest 1992;102:1225–34.
19. Murphy PB, Davidson C, Hind MD, et al. Volume targeted versus pressure support non-invasive ventilation in patients with super obesity and chronic respiratory failure: a randomised controlled trial. Thorax 2012;67(8):727–34.
20. Younes M, Puddy A, Roberts D, et al. Proportional assist ventilation. Results of an initial clinical trial. Am Rev Respir Dis 1992;145:121–9.
21. Teschler H, Döhring J, Wang YM, et al. Adaptive pressure support servo-ventilation: a novel treatment for Cheyne–Stokes respiration in heart failure. Am J Respir Crit Care Med 2001;164:614–19.
22. Aloia MS, Stanchina M, Arnedt JT, et al. Treatment adherence and outcomes in flexible vs standard continuous positive airway pressure therapy. Chest 2005;127:2085–93.
23. Gay PC, Herold DL, Olson EJ. A randomized, double-blind clinical trial comparing continuous positive airway pressure with a novel bilevel pressure system for treatment of obstructive sleep apnea syndrome. Sleep 2003;26:864–9.
24. Richards GN, Cistulli PA, Ungar RG, et al. Mouth leak with nasal continuous positive airway pressure increases nasal airway resistance. Am J Respir Crit Care Med 1996;154:182–6.
25. Thys F, Liistro G, Dozin O, et al. Determinants of Fi,O$_2$ with oxygen supplementation during noninvasive two-level positive pressure ventilation. Eur Respir J 2002;19: 653–7.
26. Schwartz AR, Kacmarek RM, Hess DR. Factors affecting oxygen delivery with bi-level positive airway pressure. Respir Care 2004;9:270–5.
27. Uong EC, Epperson M, Bathon SA, et al. Adherence to nasal positive airway pressure therapy among school-aged children and adolescents with obstructive sleep apnea syndrome. Pediatrics 2007;120:e1203–11.
28. DiFeo N, Meltzer LJ, Beck SE, et al. Predictors of positive airway pressure therapy adherence in children: a prospective study. J Clin Sleep Med 2012;8:279–86.
29. Marcus CL, Rosen G, Ward SL, et al. Adherence to and effectiveness of positive airway pressure therapy in children with obstructive sleep apnea. Pediatrics 2006;117:e442–51.
30. O'Donnell AR, Bjornson CL, Bohn SG, et al. Compliance rates in children using noninvasive continuous positive airway pressure. Sleep 2006;29:651–8.
31. Downey R III, Perkin RM, MacQuarrie J. Nasal continuous positive airway pressure use in children with obstructive sleep apnea younger than 2 years of age. Chest 2000;117:1608–12.
32. Waters KA, Everett FM, Bruderer JW, et al. Obstructive sleep apnea: the use of nasal CPAP in 80 children. Am J Respir Crit Care Med 1995;152:780–5.
33. Kribbs NB, Pack AI, Kline LR, et al. Objective measurement of patterns of nasal CPAP use by patients with obstructive sleep apnea. Am Rev Respir Dis 1993;147:887–95.
34. Stepnowsky C, Moore P. Nasal CPAP treatment for obstructive sleep apnea: developing a new perspective on dosing strategies and compliance. J Psychosom Res 2003;54:599–605.
35. Powell ED, Gay PC, Ojile JM, et al. A pilot study assessing adherence to auto-bilevel following a poor initial encounter with CPAP. J Clin Sleep Med 2012;8:43–7.
36. Sawyer AM, Gooneratne NS, Marcus CL, et al. A systematic review of CPAP adherence across age groups: Clinical and empiric insights for developing CPAP adherence interventions. Sleep Med Rev 2011;15: 343–56.
37. Massa F, Gonsalez S, Laverty A, et al. The use of nasal continuous positive airway pressure to treat obstructive sleep apnoea. Arch Dis Child 2002;87:438–43.
38. Krieger J. Long-term compliance with nasal continuous positive airway pressure (CPAP) in obstructive sleep apnea patients and nonapneic snorers. Sleep 1992;15:S42–6.
39. Rauscher H, Formanek D, Popp W, et al. Subjective versus objective compliance with nasal CPAP therapy for obstructive sleep apnea. Sleep Res 1992;21:252.
40. Simon SL, Duncan CL, Janicke DM, et al. Barriers to treatment of paediatric obstructive sleep apnoea: Development of the adherence barriers to continuous positive airway pressure (CPAP) questionnaire. Sleep Med 2012;13:172–7.
41. Ryan S, Garvey JF, Swan V, et al. Nasal pillows as an alternative interface in patients with obstructive sleep apnoea syndrome initiating continuous positive airway pressure therapy. J Sleep Res 2011;20:367–73.
42. Weaver TE, Grunstein RR. Adherence to continuous positive airway pressure therapy: the challenge to effective treatment. Proc Am Thorac Soc 2008;5:173–8.
43. Aloia MS. Understanding the problem of poor CPAP adherence. Sleep Med Rev 2011;15:341–2.
44. Koontz KL, Slifer KJ, Cataldo MD, et al. Improving pediatric compliance with positive airway pressure therapy: the impact of behavioral intervention. Sleep 2003;26:1010–15.
45. Beebe DW, Byars KC. Adolescents with obstructive sleep apnea adhere poorly to positive airway pressure (PAP), but PAP users show improved attention and school performance. PLoS One 2011;6:e16924.
46. Budhiraja R, Parthasarathy S, Drake CL, et al. Early CPAP use identifies subsequent adherence to CPAP therapy. Sleep 2007;30:320–4.
47. McArdle N, Devereux G, Heidarnejad H, et al. Long-term use of CPAP therapy for sleep apnea/hypopnea syndrome. Am J Respir Crit Care Med 1999;159:1108–14.
48. Barbé F, Mayoralas LR, Duran J, et al. Treatment with continuous positive airway pressure is not effective in patients with sleep apnea but no daytime sleepiness. A randomized, controlled trial. Ann Intern Med 2001;134(11):1015–23.
49. Patel SR, White DP, Malhotra A, et al. Continuous positive airway pressure therapy for treating sleepiness in a diverse population with obstructive sleep apnea: results of a meta-analysis. Arch Intern Med 2003;163(5):565–71.
50. Marcus CL, Beck SE, Traylor J, et al. Randomized, double-blind clinical trial of two different modes of positive airway pressure therapy on adherence and efficacy in children. J Clin Sleep Med 2012;8:37–42.
51. Ayas NT, Patel SR, Malhotra A, et al. Auto-titrating versus standard continuous positive airway pressure for the treatment of obstructive sleep apnea: results of a meta-analysis. Sleep 2004;27:249–53.
52. Smith I, Lasserson TJ. Pressure modification for improving usage of continuous positive airway pressure machines in adults with obstructive sleep apnoea. Cochrane Database Syst Rev 2009:CD003531.
53. Epstein LJ, Kristo D, Strollo PJ, et al; Adult Obstructive Sleep Apnea Task Force of the American Academy of Sleep Medicine. Clinical guideline for the evaluation, management and long-term care of obstructive sleep apnea in adults. J Clin Sleep Med 2009;5:263–76.
54. Kushida C, Littner M, Hirshkowitz M, et al; American Academy of Sleep Medicine. Practice parameters for the use of continuous and bilevel positive airway pressure devices to treat adult patients with sleep-related breathing disorders. Sleep 2006;29:375–80.
55. Palombini L, Pelayo R, Guilleminault C. Efficacy of automated continuous positive airway pressure in children with sleep related breathing disorders in an attended setting. Pediatrics 2004;113:e412–17.
56. Chervin RD, Theut S, Bassetti C, et al. Compliance with nasal CPAP can be improved by simple interventions. Sleep 1997;20:284–9.
57. McNamara F, Sullivan CE. Obstructive sleep apnea in infants and its management with nasal continuous positive airway pressure. Chest 1999;116:10–16.
58. Valentin A, Subramanian S, Quan SF, et al. Air leak is associated with poor adherence to AutoPAP therapy. Sleep 2011;34:801–6.
59. Montgomery-Downs HE, Crabtree VM, Gozal D. Cognition, sleep and respiration in at-risk children treated for obstructive sleep apnoea. Eur Respir J 2005;25:336–42.
60. Li HY, Huang YS, Chen NH, et al. Impact of adenotonsillectomy on behavior in children with sleep-disordered breathing. Laryngoscope 2006;116:1142–7.
61. Franco RA Jr, Rosenfeld RM, Rao M. First place – resident clinical science award 1999. Quality of life for children with obstructive sleep apnea. Otolaryngol Head Neck Surg 2000;123:9–16.
62. Kushida CA, Chediak A, Berry RB, et al; Positive Airway Pressure Titration Task Force; American Academy of Sleep Medicine. Clinical guidelines for the manual titration of positive airway pressure in patients with obstructive sleep apnea. J Clin Sleep Med 2008;4:157–71.
63. Hertegonne K, Bauters F. The value of auto-adjustable CPAP devices in pressure titration and treatment of patients with obstructive sleep apnea syndrome. Sleep Med Rev 2010;14(2):115–19.

64. Teschler H, Berthon-Jones M, Thompson AB, et al. Automated continuous positive airway pressure titration for obstructive sleep apnea syndrome. Am J Respir Crit Care Med 1996;154:734–40.

65. Marcus CL, Ward SL, Mallory GB, et al. Use of nasal continuous positive airway pressure as treatment of childhood obstructive sleep apnea. J Pediatr 1995;127:88–94.

66. Morgenthaler TI, Aurora RN, Brown T, et al; Standards of Practice Committee of the AASM; American Academy of Sleep Medicine. Practice parameters for the use of autotitrating continuous positive airway pressure devices for titrating pressures and treating adult patients with obstructive sleep apnea syndrome: an update for 2007. An American Academy of Sleep Medicine report. Sleep 2008;31(1):141–7.

67. Strobel W, Schlageter M, Andersson M, et al. Topical nasal steroid treatment does not improve CPAP compliance in unselected patients with OSAS. Resp Med 2011;105:310–15.

68. Sanner BM, Fluerenbrock N, Kleiber-Imbeck A, et al. Effect of continuous positive airway pressure therapy on infectious complications in patients with obstructive sleep apnea syndrome. Respiration 2001;68(5):483–7.

Novel Pharmacological Approaches for Treatment of Obstructive Sleep Apnea

Leila Kheirandish-Gozal

INTRODUCTION

Adenotonsillar hypertrophy has been identified as the major pathophysiological factor in the causation of upper airway obstruction in pediatric obstructive sleep apnea (OSA). Over the last few decades, novel immunological techniques have enabled identification of some of the specific tonsillar cells underlying inflammatory immune responses in specific contextual settings; however, the exact mechanisms leading to the adenotonsillar cell proliferation are still not fully understood.[1] It is apparent that a combination of structural and neuromuscular abnormalities contributes to the occurrence of OSA in children.[2] Tonsils and adenoids continue to grow from birth to 12 years of age, with the greatest increase in size during the ages of 2 and 8, a process that is paralleled by the surrounding structures that constitute the upper airway. During this period of time, the gradual growth in the size of the skeletal boundaries of the upper airway and the occurrence of disproportionate growth of adenoids and tonsils relative to the other upper airway structures will result in a relatively narrower upper airway, even if, as mentioned, the growth of all structures during this period is parallel to each other.[3] The relative physiological narrowing of the upper airway space in children is, however, compensated by the activation of the upper airway muscles and through increased central ventilatory drive, preventing the excessive upper airway collapsibility when compared to adults.[4] As such, OSA only occurs when the interaction between the anatomical restriction and the neuromuscular reflexes fails to preserve airway patency, a state-dependent process, since it does not occur during wakefulness.

Nevertheless, the size of the adenoids and tonsils plays a significant role in the severity of OSA.[5,6] This excessive tissue enlargement can be induced by proliferation of specific cellular components and is due to various isolated or recurrent bacterial or viral infections as well as exposure to environmental irritants such as allergens, cigarette smoke and air pollution.[7–11] The location of the adenoids and tonsils at the entrance of the respiratory and alimentary tracts positions them as the first site of contact with a variety of microorganisms and antigenic substances that are present in food and inhaled air, resulting in proliferation and growth in these organs.

Currently, surgical extirpation of these tissues is the first line of treatment for either recurrent infection or pediatric sleep apnea;[12] however, the efficacy of adenotonsillectomy has recently been challenged, with informal assessments of striking reductions in estimated success rates to less than 30% of all cases,[13,14] further intensifying the need for developing non-surgical therapeutic options more than ever.

Inflammation in Pediatric OSA

Since adenotonsillar hypertrophy and hyperplasia are the primary causes of OSA in children, the mechanisms leading to the enlargement of these complex lymphoid structures has been a main focus of investigation among researchers in the field. The earlier studies were primarily focused on assessment of bacterial infections as the underlying cause of recurrent tonsillitis and as contributing factors to recurrent chronic otitis media and their epidemiological links with adenotonsillar hypertrophy.[15–19] Since then, different theories have evolved, particularly in relation to the development of adenotonsillar hypertrophy that underlies OSA in children. Indeed, current opinion surmises that a low-grade systemic inflammation is present in addition to local upper inflammation in pediatric OSA. Multiple studies have investigated the cause and effect of mechanical vibration due to intermittent collapse and occlusion of the upper airway manifested by snoring as a potential primary source of inflammation in children with OSA. In this context, localized inflammation of the upper airway tissue would occur as a result of continuous and periodic mechanical insult due to tissue vibration and intraluminal pharyngeal pressure swings from the repeated upper airway obstructive events.[20,21] Thus, the initiation of mild snoring would promote inflammation that would progressively aggravate the snoring, leading to a vicious cycle of disease progression. Although this theory is definitely attractive, there is no available epidemiological evidence supporting such a temporal trajectory of progressive worsening of OSA in children. Indeed, the time course of disease initiation and progression has yet to be investigated. Some investigators argue that snoring-related mechanical trauma to the soft palate and uvula may not be the sole factor underlying upper airway inflammation considering the fact that both nasal and oropharyngeal mucosal inflammation are also present in patients with OSA, and that the nasal mucosa is not subjected to repeated snoring-induced injury.[22–24] Conversely, the alternations between hypoxia and re-oxygenation could produce excessive free radicals mediated through several intracellular pathways that potentially will lead to both local and systemic inflammation.[25] Another possible mechanism that has been advanced links early life infections with respiratory viruses as eliciting enduring immune cell-mediated amplificatory memory responses that will be triggered upon exposure to inhaled stimuli such as environmental pollution or recurrent viral infections.[26]

Thus, the mechanisms leading to the initiation, generation, and propagation of inflammatory processes within the upper airway among various age groups will definitely require more extensive investigation than simply just the evidence that is presented above.

EVIDENCE OF LOCAL UPPER AIRWAY AND SYSTEMIC INFLAMMATION IN PEDIATRIC OSA

In adults with OSA, increased concentrations of pro-inflammatory markers such as interleukin-6 and 8-isopentane, and oxidative stress markers have been reported in the exhaled upper airway condensate.[27–29] Higher levels of nuclear factor kappaB-dependent genes such as tumor necrosis factor-alpha (TNF-α) and interleukin 6 (IL-6) are also present,[30] and treatment of OSA with continuous positive airway pressure was associated with reductions in serum levels of high-sensitivity C-reactive protein (hsCRP) and IL-6 concentrations,[31] while local airway inflammation was improved, as evidenced by reduced numbers of neutrophils.[32] Thus, adults with OSA present evidence of both local (i.e., upper airway) and systemic low-grade inflammatory changes.

What about children? Since the initial study by Tauman and colleagues, who reported increased plasma hsCRP levels in children with OSA compared to controls, multiple studies have corroborated such findings.[33] Interestingly, improved hsCRP levels and cardiovascular markers after effective treatment of OSA were also demonstrated.[33–36] Recent studies further suggest that variances in the hsCRP levels or in polymorphisms within the NADPH oxidase gene or its functional subunits such as p22phox, both of which reflect systemic inflammatory responses, appear to account for important components of the differences in cognitive function deficits associated with OSA in children.[36–38] Thus, the degree of systemic inflammation and oxidative stress may play a major contributor to the presence of morbidity in children with OSA and, as a result, targeting of such pathways may provide a viable therapeutic strategy towards prevention of end-organ morbidity.[37,38]

Another significant contributor to the pathophysiology of pediatric OSA and the treatment outcomes is obesity, which should be viewed as yet another systemic inflammatory condition. The rather accelerated increase over the last two decades in the prevalence of pediatric obesity has led to substantial changes in the cross-sectional demographic and anthropometric characteristics of the children who are referred for evaluation of suspected OSA.[39,40] Obesity is a proven and definitive risk factor that operates in a synergistic fashion among children at risk for OSA, and such interactions could, in fact, reflect augmented activation of inflammatory pathways.[41–43] Thus, considering the deleterious consequences of OSA in children if left untreated, the use of therapeutic agents towards reduction in inflammation or specific oxidative stress may yield to reverse or palliated morbidities.

The evidence of local inflammatory processes within the upper airway of children with OSA is not as well established and has not been as thoroughly investigated. Here, the author will review the few selected pathways that have thus far gained attention in pediatric OSA, namely leukotriene and glucocorticoid pathways.

LEUKOTRIENE AND LEUKOTRIENE RECEPTORS

Cysteinyl leukotrienes are major mediators of inflammation in both humans and animals, and serve as potent neutrophil chemoattractants and activators.[44] The cysteinyl leukotriene receptors 1 and 2 are expressed on several tissues including the nasal mucosa and the lungs.[45,46] The leukotrienes B4 and the Cys LTs, C4, D4, and E4 can mediate inflammation in both the upper and lower airways by binding to Cys Lt receptors, although LTB4 has 2 cognate receptors that exhibit much higher affinity to this leukotriene. A considerable overlap and interdependency between asthma and OSA[47–49] as well as compelling evidence of the favorable effect of CYS LT1-R antagonists in reducing inflammation in children with inflammatory conditions such as asthma and allergic rhinitis,[50,51] suggested a potential role for leukotriene modifiers in the management of pediatric OSA.

Assessment of the LT1-R and LT2-R expression in tonsils and adenoids of children with OSA compared to children with recurrent infectious tonsillitis without OSA revealed higher protein expression levels of LT1-R and LT2-R, along with a distinct topographical pattern of distribution, suggesting that different mechanisms promoting inflammation are operational in OSA versus infection-induced tonsillitis.[52] In this context, it would appear that leukotrienes may contribute to the higher proliferative pattern of upper airway lymphoid tissues than is present in the generation of adenotonsillar hypertrophy that characterizes the majority of children with OSA. Indeed, immunohistochemical characterization of germinal centers in tonsils of children with OSA showed a peripheral location of LT1 receptor (Figure 36-1), which might be due to either its occurrence during late stages of maturation of lymphoid tissues or, as proposed by others, LT1-R-positive cells might have migrated from the vasculature to occupy sites within the tonsils, where their activation may be of functional importance.[53] The initial characterization of heightened expression of leukotrienes and their receptors in the adenoids and tonsils of OSA patients was subsequently confirmed by Kaditis and colleagues who showed that tonsils of children with OSA display an enhanced expression of cysteinyl leukotriene receptors in T lymphocytes without an associated increase in serum hsCRP concentrations.[54] Of note, an increased preponderance of CD8-positive lymphocytes is present in tonsils of children with OSA (see Figure 37-1). Increased concentrations of either LTB4 or LTC4/D4/E4 in the adenotonsillar tissues of children with OSA could promote upper airway lymphoid hypertrophy/hyperplasia when compared with children with recurrent infectious tonsillitis.[55] Up-regulation of LT1-R and LT2-R expression could potentially promote tonsillar enlargement in children with OSA by promoting the proliferation or the pro-inflammatory activity of T-cell lymphocytes within the tonsillar and adenoidal tissues.[56] Of note, increases in leukotriene concentrations LTB4 and LTC4/LTD4/LTE4 are readily identified in the exhaled breath condensates of children with OSA.[57] Interestingly, and similar to children, LTB4 concentrations were also found to be elevated in the exhaled condensates of adults with OSA and appear to be correlated with the severity of OSA.[58]

To further assess the effects of LTD4 and several LT receptor antagonists on lymphoid tissue proliferation, Gozal and colleagues developed a mixed-cell culture model using freshly dissociated tonsils or adenoids harvested during adenotonsillectomy from children with polysomnographically diagnosed OSA or recurrent tonsillitis. Cellular proliferation and release of inflammatory cytokines were assessed in cell culture supernatants using standard enzyme-linked immunosorbent assays.[59,60] In this *ex vivo* model, LTD4 elicited dose-dependent increases in adenotonsillar cell proliferation that were markedly enhanced in children with OSA.

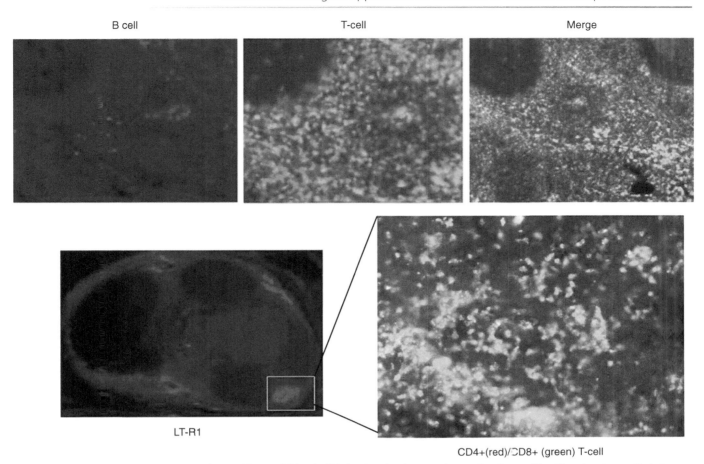

FIGURE 36-1 Immunihistochemical stains of a tonsil from a child with OSA showing the disproportionate abundance of T-cell lymphocytes, particularly CD8-positive lymphocytes, and the high level of expression of leukotriene receptors in the peripheral regions surrounding the germinal centers.

On the other hand, LT antagonists exhibited dose-dependent reductions in adenotonsillar cellular proliferation rates, with montelukast showing superior potency compared to the other antagonists tested, suggesting that LT-dependent pathways underlie components of the intrinsic proliferative and inflammatory signaling pathways and play a significant role in adenotonsillar hypertrophy in children.[61]

Interestingly, the cell substrates mediating the hyperplastic responses of these tissues demonstrate a T-cell preponderance of proliferation of CD3-, CD4-, and CD8-positive lymphocytes in OSA, while B-cell lymphocytes were more likely to be proliferative in RI.[54,60] Circulating levels of LTB4 and Cys LT were also found to be elevated in children with mild and moderate to severe OSA compared to controls, and decreased after treatment.[62]

Therefore, based on the aforementioned studies, it is plausible to conclude that lipoxygenase-dependent pathways are involved in the pathophysiology of OSA in children, and may serve as targets for treatment of this condition, particularly in selected subgroups of children. Improving the severity of residual OSA after adenotonsillectomy with leukotriene antagonists was shown as an effective approach, justifying the use of leukotriene receptor antagonists as potential adjuncts to pre- and to post-T&A in pediatric OSA, in an effort to improve the outcomes associated with this surgery.[63]

Leukotriene modifiers could also be considered as a direct therapeutic option in mild OSA as an alternative to T&A.[10] A recent randomized double-blind, placebo-controlled trial with oral montelukast in children with mild OSA showed significant improvements in apnea index and in adenoid size.[64]

GLUCOCORTICOID RECEPTORS AND CORTICOSTEROIDS IN PEDIATRIC OSA

Corticosteroids (CS) are frequently used by pediatricians for clinical management of conditions such as asthma, allergic rhinitis; however, the favorable response is somewhat uneven in children with asthma, suggesting that some of these children may exhibit differential sensitivity to the activity of CS, a phenomenon that was initially ascribed to differences in glucocorticoid receptor (GCR) subtype expression (i.e., the expression of CS-sensitive GCRα expression was dominant as opposed to the presence of GCRβ expression). Furthermore, reduced ligand binding to corticosteroids, single nucleotide polymorphisms in GCR gene, or defects in GCR translocation to the nucleus and binding to the glucocorticoid-binding response element account for a fraction of corticosteroid-resistant asthma.[65–70] Among other identified mechanisms for resistance to CS, a reduction in histone deacetylase (HDAC)-2 activity and expression, impaired glucocorticoid receptor activity (GCR) and increased pro-inflammatory signaling pathways could all be operational. Both GCRα and GCRβ are expressed in adenotonsillar tissues of children with OSA, are significantly abundant and demonstrate specific topographic patterns within the germinal centers. In addition, the high GCRα:GCRβ ratios found in all tissues analyzed further indicate a favorable therapeutic response profile for topical corticosteroid therapy in snoring children with adenotonsillar hypertrophy.[71] Therefore, there is little if any reason to anticipate that upper airway lymphadenoid tissues exhibit resistance to treatment with CS. In a series of experiments, Gozal and colleagues assessed the cellular proliferation rates and apoptotic rates using the above-mentioned mixed cell model of dissociated tonsils or adenoids harvested intraoperatively from children. *In vitro* treatments were conducted with three selected corticosteroids, namely dexamethasone (DEX), fluticasone (FLU), and budesonide (BUD). All three compounds reduced cellular proliferation rates, and exhibited dose-dependent effects. In addition, increased apoptosis among T-cell lymphocytes and significant reduction in TNF-α, IL-8 and IL-6 concentrations in the supernatants were observed, suggesting the likelihood of successful treatment of pediatric obstructive sleep apnea with CS topical application. Of note, the available cumulative experience with CS use in the treatment of pediatric OSA is quite limited, and will be reviewed below.[72]

In a very early study by Demain and Goetz, a small number of children with chronic obstructive nasal symptoms were randomly assigned to an 8-week, double-blind, placebo-controlled crossover study of standard-dose aqueous nasal beclomethasone followed by a 16-week, open-label intranasal beclomethasone.[73] This trial resulted in significant improvements in obstructive symptom scores as well as in adenoidal hypertrophy, suggesting a favorable outcome for use of topical CS in children with OSA that was primarily due to adenotonsillar hypertrophy.[73] However, the latter study did not include sleep studies, and a pilot open-label study using short-term (5-day) oral prednisone in prepubertal children with OSA yielded no improvements in either clinical symptomatology or in adenotonsillar size.[74]

In a subsequent randomized triple-blind study, the efficacy of topical intranasal steroids in treating 25 children with polysomnographically proven moderately severe OSA who were scheduled for adenotonsillectomy was assessed. Although significant reduction in overall respiratory abnormalities was observed, the indices of adenoidal and tonsillar sizes remained unchanged, suggesting that inflammatory components are important contributors to upper airway collapsibility.[75] In addition, an open-label study of nasal budesonide administered for 4 weeks reported sustained effect of intranasal steroids even months after discontinuation of CS therapy.[76]

Several subsequent studies have reported on the beneficial effect of another topical CS, i.e., mometasone furoate, on adenoid size; however, the authors in this study did not objectively evaluate breathing patterns during sleep.[77-79] In addition, reductions in cytokines were also reported.[80] In a recent randomized, double-blind controlled trial with a crossover design, intranasal budesonide was administered at bedtime for a total of 6 weeks' duration, and was shown to substantially either reduce the severity of mild OSA or normalize sleep

respiratory disturbance, as well as the size of the adenoids relative to the airway, and this beneficial effect persisted for at least 8 weeks after cessation of the therapy.[81] Such findings were substantiated using meta-analytical approaches that ultimately confirmed that long-term safety and efficacy data are unavailable.[82]

Therefore, the use of topical CS appears justified as a viable therapeutic option in otherwise healthy children with mild OSA, but larger and more pointed trials are needed to address issues such as efficacy in younger and older children, the usefulness of CS in obese children, and appropriate and optimal timing of such interventions in the context of other therapies.

Clinical Pearls

- Pediatric obstructive sleep apnea (OSA) is primarily the result of inflammatory processes in the upper airway that involve hyperplasia/hypertrophy of the adenoids and tonsils, and is primarily treated by surgical removal of these tissues (T&A).
- T&A is likely to reduce the severity of OSA in most cases but is rarely curative; furthermore, there is no consensus as to the AHI cut-off value that represents a clear-cut indication for T&A. Therefore, alternative non-surgical therapeutic options in milder cases of OSA should be considered.
- Increased expression of leukotrienes and their receptors is associated with increased proliferation of upper airway lymphoid tissues. Therefore, leukotriene modifiers are emerging as potentially useful agents in the treatment of mild pediatric OSA.
- The glucocorticosteroid receptor expression patterns in adenotonsillar tissues suggest a high likelihood for favorable responses to corticosteroid treatment of pediatric OSA, and this assumption has now been corroborated by a small number of randomized double-blind controlled trials.
- Although the effect of anti-inflammatory therapy in pediatric OSA has only been evaluated in a small group of patients, the encouraging results support the need for randomized, larger-scale prospective and well-controlled trials.

References

1. Heier I, Malmstrom K, Pelkonen AS, et al. Bronchial response pattern of antigen presenting cells and regulatory T cells in children less than 2 years of age. Thorax 2008;63(8):703–9.
2. Marcus CL, McColley SA, Carroll JL, et al. Upper airway collapsibility in children with obstructive sleep apnea syndrome. J Appl Physiol 1994;77(2):918–24.
3. Jeans WD, Fernando DC, Maw AR, et al. A longitudinal study of the growth of the nasopharynx and its contents in normal children. Br J Radiol 1981;54(638):117–21.
4. Marcus CL, Lutz J, Hamer A, et al. Developmental changes in response to subatmospheric pressure loading of the upper airway. J Appl Physiol 1999;87(2):626–33.
5. Brooks LJ, Stephens B, Bacevice AM. Adenoid size is related to severity but not the number of episodes of obstructive apnea in children. J Pediatr 1998;132(4):682–6.
6. Li AM, Wong E, Kew J, et al. Use of tonsil size in the evaluation of obstructive sleep apnoea. Arch Dis Child 2002;87(2):156–9.
7. Ersu R, Arman AR, Save D, et al. Prevalence of snoring and symptoms of sleep-disordered breathing in primary school children in Istanbul. Chest 2004;126(1):19–24.
8. Snow A, Dayyat E, Montgomery-Downs HE, et al. Pediatric obstructive sleep apnea: a potential late consequence of respiratory syncitial virus bronchiolitis. Pediatr Pulmonol 2009;44(12):1186–91.

9. Goldbart AD, Mager E, Veling MC, et al. Neurotrophins and tonsillar hypertrophy in children with obstructive sleep apnea. Pediatr Res 2007;62(4):489–94.

10. Kuhle S, Urschtz MS. Anti-inflammatory medications for obstructive sleep apnea in children. Cochrane Database Syst Rev 2011;(1):CD007074.

11. Siegel G, Linse R, Macheleidt S. Factors of tonsillar involution: age-dependent changes in B-cell activation and Langerhans' cell density. Arch Otorhinolaryngol 1982;236(3):261–9.

12. Schechter MS; American Academy of Pediatrics, Section on Pediatrics Pulmonology, Subcommittee on Obstructive Sleep Apnea Syndrome. Technical report: diagnosis and management of childhood obstructive sleep apnea syndrome. Pediatrics 2002;109(4).

13. Lipton AJ, Gozal D. Treatment of obstructive sleep apnea in children: do we really know how? Sleep Med Rev 2003;7(1):61–80.

14. Bhattacharjee R, Kheirandish-Gozal L, Spruyt K, et al. Adenotonsillectomy outcomes in treatment of obstructive sleep apnea in children: a multicenter retrospective study. Am J Respir Crit Care Med 2010;182(5):676–83.

15. Suzuki M, Watanabe T, Mogi G. Clinical, bacteriological, and histological study of adenoids in children. Am J Otolaryngol 1999;20(2):85–90.

16. Zuliani G, Carlisle M, Duberstein A, et al. Biofilm density in the pediatric nasopharynx: recurrent acute otitis media versus obstructive sleep apnea. Ann Otol Rhinol Laryngol 2009;118(7):519–24.

17. Nistico L, Kreft R, Gieseke A, et al. Adenoid reservoir for pathogenic biofilm bacteria. J Clin Microbiol 2011;49(4):1411–20.

18. Gozal D, Kheirandish-Gozal L, Capdevila OS, et al. Prevalence of recurrent otitis media in habitually snoring school-aged children. Sleep Med 2008;9(5):549–54.

19. Tauman R, Derowe A, Ophir O, et al. Increased risk of snoring and adenotonsillectomy in children referred for tympanostomy tube insertion. Sleep Med 2010;11(2):197–200.

20. Vuono IM, Zanoteli E, de Oliveira AS, et al. Histological analysis of palatopharyngeal muscle from children with snoring and obstructive sleep apnea syndrome. Int J Pediatr Otorhinolaryngol 2007;71(2):283–90.

21. Boyd JH, Petrof BJ, Hamid Q, et al. Upper airway muscle inflammation and denervation changes in obstructive sleep apnea. Am J Respir Crit Care Med 2004;170(5):541–6.

22. Rubinstein I. Nasal inflammation is present in patients with obstructive sleep apnea. Laryngoscope 1995;105:175–7.

23. Müns G, Rubinstein I, Singer P. Phagocytosis and oxidative burst of granulocytes in the upper respiratory tract in chronic and acute inflammation. J Otolaryngol 1995;24:105–10.

24. Sekosan M, Zakkar M, Wenig B, et al. Inflammation in the uvula mucosa of patients with obstructive sleep apnea. Laryngoscope 1996;106:1018–20.

25. Wang Y, Zhang SX, Gozal D. Reactive oxygen species and the brain in sleep apnea. Respir Physiol Neurobiol 2010;174(3):307–16.

26. Goldbart AD, Mager E, Veling MC, et al. Neurotrophins and tonsillar hypertrophy in children with obstructive sleep apnea. Pediatr Res 2007;62(4):489–94.

27. Carpagnano GE, Kharitonov SA, Resta O, et al. 8-Isoprostane, a marker of oxidative stress, is increased in exhaled breath condensate of patients with obstructive sleep apnea after night and is reduced by continuous positive airway pressure therapy. Chest 2003;124(4):1386–92.

28. Li Y, Chongsuvivatwong V, Geater A, et al. Exhaled breath condensate cytokine level as a diagnostic tool for obstructive sleep apnea syndrome. Sleep Med 2009;10(1):95–103.

29. Carpagnano GE, Lacedonia D, Foschino-Barbaro MP. Non-invasive study of airways inflammation in sleep apnea patients. Sleep Med Rev 2011;15(5):317–26.

30. Entzian P, Linnemann K, Schlaak M, et al. Obstructive sleep apnea syndrome and circadian rhythms of hormones and cytokines. Am J Respir Crit Care Med 1996;153(3):1080–6.

31. Yokoe T, Minoguchi K, Matsuo H, et al. Elevated levels of C-reactive protein and interleukin-6 in patients with obstructive sleep apnea syndrome are decreased by nasal continuous positive airway pressure. Circulation 2003;107(8):1129–34.

32. Shadan FF, Jalowayski AA, Fahrenholz J, et al. Nasal cytology: a marker of clinically silent inflammation in patients with obstructive sleep apnea and a predictor of noncompliance with nasal CPAP therapy. J Clin Sleep Med 2005;1(3):266–70.

33. Tauman R, Ivanenko A, O'Brien LM, et al. Plasma C-reactive protein levels among children with sleep-disordered breathing. Pediatrics 2004;113(6):e564–9.

34. Gozal D, Capdevila OS, Kheirandish-Gozal L. Metabolic alterations and systemic inflammation in obstructive sleep apnea among nonobese and obese prepubertal children. Am J Respir Crit Care Med 2008;177(10):1142–9.

35. Kheirandish-Gozal L, Capdevila OS, Tauman R, et al. Plasma C-reactive protein in nonobese children with obstructive sleep apnea before and after adenotonsillectomy. J Clin Sleep Med 2006;2(3):301–4.

36. Goldbart AD, Levitas A, Greenberg-Dotan S, et al. B-type natriuretic peptide and cardiovascular function in young children with obstructive sleep apnea. Chest 2010;138(3):528–35.

37. Gozal D, Khalyfa A, Capdevila OS, et al. Cognitive function in prepubertal children with obstructive sleep apnea: a modifying role for NADPH oxidase p22 subunit gene polymorphisms? Antioxid Redox Signal 2012;16(2):171–7.

38. Gozal D, Crabtree VM, Sans Capdevila O, et al. C-reactive protein, obstructive sleep apnea, and cognitive dysfunction in school-aged children. Am J Respir Crit Care Med 2007;176(2):188–93.

39. Tauman R, Gulliver TE, Krishna J, et al. Persistence of obstructive sleep apnea syndrome in children after adenotonsillectomy. J Pediatr 2006;149(6):803–8.

40. Mitchell RB, Kelly J. Outcome of adenotonsillectomy for obstructive sleep apnea in obese and normal-weight children. Otolaryngol Head Neck Surg 2007;137(1):43–8.

41. Bhattacharjee R, Kim J, Alotaibi WH, et al. Endothelial dysfunction in children without hypertension: potential contributions of obesity and obstructive sleep apnea. Chest 2012;141(3):682–91.

42. Bhattacharjee R, Kim J, Kheirandish-Gozal L, et al. Obesity and obstructive sleep apnea syndrome in children: a tale of inflammatory cascades. Pediatr Pulmonol 2011;46(4):313–23.

43. Spruyt K, Gozal D. A mediation model linking body weight, cognition, and sleep-disordered breathing. Am J Respir Crit Care Med 2012;185(2):199–205.

44. Peters-Golden M, Henderson WR Jr. Leukotrienes. N Engl J Med 2007;357(18):1841–54.

45. Shirasaki H, Kanaizumi E, Watanabe K, et al. Expression and localization of the cysteinyl leukotriene 1 receptor in human nasal mucosa. Clin Exp Allergy 2002;32(7):1007–12.

46. Figueroa DJ, Breyer RM, Defoe SK, et al. Expression of the cysteinyl leukotriene 1 receptor in normal human lung and peripheral blood leukocytes. Am J Respir Crit Care Med 2001;163(1):226–33.

47. Kheirandish-Gozal L, Dayyat EA, Eid NS, et al. Obstructive sleep apnea in poorly controlled asthmatic children: effect of adenotonsillectomy. Pediatr Pulmonol 2011;46(9):913–18.

48. Malakasioti G, Gourgoulianis K, et al. Interactions of obstructive sleep-disordered breathing with recurrent wheezing or asthma and their effects on sleep quality. Pediatr Pulmonol 2011;46(11):1047–54.

49. Ross KR, Storfer-Isser A, Hart MA, et al. Sleep-disordered breathing is associated with asthma severity in children. J Pediatr 2012;160(5):736–42.

50. Bisgaard H, Loland L, Oj JA. NO in exhaled air of asthmatic children is reduced by the leukotriene receptor antagonist montelukast. Am J Respir Crit Care Med 1999;160(4):1227–31.

51. Chauhan BF, Ducharme FM. Anti-leukotriene agents compared to inhaled corticosteroids in the management of recurrent and/or chronic asthma in adults and children. Cochrane Database Syst Rev 2012;(5):CD002314.

52. Goldbart AD, Goldman JL, Li RC, et al. Differential expression of cysteinyl leukotriene receptors 1 and 2 in tonsils of children with obstructive sleep apnea syndrome or recurrent infection. Chest 2004;126(1):13–18.

53. Ebenfelt A, Ivarsson M. Neutrophil migration in tonsils. J Anat 2001;198(Pt 4):497–500.

54. Kaditis AG, Ioannou MG, Chaidas K, et al. Cysteinyl leukotriene receptors are expressed by tonsillar T cells of children with obstructive sleep apnea. Chest 2008;134(2):324–31.

55. Goldbart AD, Goldman JL, Veling MC, et al. Leukotriene modifier therapy for mild sleep-disordered breathing in children. Am J Respir Crit Care Med 2005;172(3):364–70.

56. Tsaoussoglou M, Lianou L, Maragozidis P, et al. Cysteinyl leukotriene receptors in tonsillar B- and T-lymphocytes from children with obstructive sleep apnea. Sleep Med 2012;13(7):879–85.

57. Goldbart AD, Krishna J, Li RC, et al. Inflammatory mediators in exhaled breath condensate of children with obstructive sleep apnea syndrome. Chest 2006;130(1):143–8.

58. Petrosyan M, Perraki E, Simoes D, et al. Exhaled breath markers in patients with obstructive sleep apnoea. Sleep Breath 2008;12(3):207–15.

59. Serpero LD, Kheirandish-Gozal L, Dayyat E, et al. A mixed cell culture model for assessment of proliferation in tonsillar tissues from children with obstructive sleep apnea or recurrent tonsillitis. Laryngoscope 2009;119(5):1005–10.
60. Kim J, Bhattacharjee R, Dayyat E, et al. Increased cellular proliferation and inflammatory cytokines in tonsils derived from children with obstructive sleep apnea. Pediatr Res 2009;66(4):423–8.
61. Dayyat E, Serpero LD, Kheirandish-Gozal L, et al. Leukotriene pathways and in vitro adenotonsillar cell proliferation in children with obstructive sleep apnea. Chest 2009;135(5):1142–9.
62. Abstract [519]: In: Am J Respir Crit Care Med. The American Thoracic Society International Conference. San Francisco, California, USA: 2007;175:A15–1004.
63. Kheirandish L, Goldbart AD, Gozal D. Intranasal steroids and oral leukotriene modifier therapy in residual sleep-disordered breathing after tonsillectomy and adenoidectomy in children. Pediatrics 2006;117(1): e61–6.
64. Goldbart AD, Greenberg-Dotan S, Tal A. Montelukast for children with obstructive sleep apnea: a double-blind, placebo-controlled study. Pediatrics 2012;130(3):e575–80.
65. Adcock IM, Lane SJ. Corticosteroid-insensitive asthma: molecular mechanisms. J Endocrinol 2003;178(3):347–55.
66. Adcock IM, Barnes PJ. Molecular mechanisms of corticosteroid resistance. Chest 2008;134(2):394–401.
67. Barnes PJ, Adcock IM. Glucocorticoid resistance in inflammatory diseases. Lancet 2009;373(9678):1905–17.
68. De Iudicibus S, Franca R, Martelossi S, et al. Molecular mechanism of glucocorticoid resistance in inflammatory bowel disease. World J Gastroenterol 2011;17(9):1095–108.
69. Christodoulopoulos P, Leung DY, Elliott MW, et al. Increased number of glucocorticoid receptor-beta-expressing cells in the airways in fatal asthma. J Allergy Clin Immunol 2000;106(3):479–84.
70. Gagliardo R, Chanez P, Vignola AM, et al. Glucocorticoid receptor alpha and beta in glucocorticoid dependent asthma. Am J Respir Crit Care Med 2000;162(1):7–13.
71. Goldbart AD, Veling MC, Goldman JL, et al. Glucocorticoid receptor subunit expression in adenotonsillar tissue of children with obstructive sleep apnea. Pediatr Res 2005;57(2):232–6.
72. Kheirandish-Gozal L, Serpero LD, Dayyat E, et al. Corticosteroids suppress in vitro tonsillar proliferation in children with obstructive sleep apnoea. Eur Respir J 2009;33(5):1077–84.
73. Demain G, Goetz DW. Pediatric adenoidal hypertrophy and nasal airway obstruction: reduction with aqueous nasal beclomethasone. Pediatrics 1995;95:355–64.
74. Al-Ghamdi SA, Manoukian JJ, Morielli A, et al. Do systemic corticosteroids effectively treat obstructive sleep apnea secondary to adenotonsillar hypertrophy? Laryngoscope 1997;107:1382–7.
75. Brouillette RT, Manoukian JJ, Ducharme FM, et al. Efficacy of fluticasone nasal spray for pediatric obstructive sleep apnea. J Pediatr 2001;138:838–44.
76. Alexopoulos EI, Kaditis AG, Kalampouka E, et al. Nasal corticosteroids for children with snoring. Pediatr Pulmonol 2004;38(2):161–7.
77. Berlucchi M, Valetti L, Parrinello G, et al. Long-term follow-up of children undergoing topical intranasal steroid therapy for adenoidal hypertrophy. Int J Pediatr Otorhinolaryngol 2008;72:1171–5.
78. Berlucchi M, Salsi D, Valetti L, et al. The role of mometasone furoate aqueous nasal spray in the treatment of adenoidal hypertrophy in the pediatric age group: preliminary results of a prospective, randomized study. Pediatrics 2007;119:e1392–7.
79. Rezende RM, Silveira F, Barbosa AP, et al. Objective reduction in adenoid tissue after mometasone furoate treatment. Int J Pediatr Otorhinolaryngol 2012;76:829–31.
80. Esteitie R, Emani J, Sharma S, et al. Effect of fluticasone furoate on interleukin 6 secretion from adenoid tissues in children with obstructive sleep apnea. Arch Otolaryngol Head Neck Surg 2011;137:576–82.
81. Kheirandish-Gozal L, Gozal D. Intranasal budesonide treatment for children with mild obstructive sleep apnea syndrome. Pediatrics 2008;122:e149–55.
82. Kuhle S, Urschitz MS. Anti-inflammatory medications for obstructive sleep apnea in children. Cochrane Database Syst Rev 2011;CD007074.

Chapter 37

Congenital Central Hypoventilation Syndrome

Pallavi P. Patwari

EPIDEMIOLOGY AND HISTORY

In 1970, Dr. Robert Mellins described the first congenital case of primary central alveolar hypoventilation, and reviewed 30 postnatally acquired central hypoventilation reported cases in his seminal publication entitled, *Failure of Automatic Control of Ventilation*.[1] Until then, all reported cases of central hypoventilation were considered as acquired, and were attributed to abnormalities of the central nervous system (e.g., encephalitis or focal medullary abnormality). This now classic case report described a newborn boy of normal birth weight, who cried at birth and demonstrated improved ventilation with crying, but was persistently cyanotic while in the nursery, without identifiable etiology after thorough diagnostic work-up. He improved with negative-pressure ventilation therapy while initially hospitalized, and was subsequently surgically implanted with phrenic nerve electrodes stimulated via radio-frequency transmitter (phrenic nerve diaphragm pacing). Since the pacing was unsuccessful, he succumbed to heart failure and died at 14 months of age. Despite the therapeutic failure,[1] diaphragmatic pacing in congenital central hypoventilation syndrome (CCHS) has become more refined, takes into consideration multiple factors, and is an ideal method of artificial ventilation in the appropriate CCHS candidate.[2] However, the authors provide a compelling description of the physiologic compromise the child suffered during various states, the ventilatory response to exogenous hypercarbic challenge, and also describe some of the sequelae of chronic inadequate ventilatory support.

While many case reports followed, it was not until 1992 that Dr. Weese-Mayer and colleagues described the first relatively large cohort of 32 CCHS cases with description of associated findings (Hirschsprung disease, ophthalmologic abnormalities, growth deficiency) and outcomes.[3] In this cohort, the authors found that about one third died, a third required awake and asleep ventilatory support, and the other third required sleep-only ventilatory support. In 1999, the first American Thoracic Society (ATS) statement on CCHS estimated the existence of at least 160–180 cases worldwide.[4] Further, this publication increased awareness of this rare condition, introduced the concept of autonomic nervous system (ANS) dysregulation (ANSD), and suggested the existence of a genetic basis for CCHS.[4] Subsequently, candidate gene studies focused on the ANS pathways.

A major breakthrough occurred in 2003 with the discovery that *PHOX2B* gene mutations were present among CCHS patients in French,[5] American,[6] and Japanese cohorts.[7] The *PHOX2B* gene is located on chromosome 4, is a transcription factor that plays a key role in embryologic development of the autonomic nervous system,[8,9] and the genetic abnormality is inherited in an autosomal dominant pattern.[6,10] Race and gender are not expected to influence inheritance or severity of illness. The development of clinically available diagnostic testing allowed for earlier and more definitive diagnosis of CCHS with a consequent increase in the number and frequency of identified cases.

In 2010, the second ATS statement on CCHS was published and estimated at least 1000 living children with CCHS worldwide[11] and suggested this number to represent an underestimate since those patients with milder CCHS phenotypes are likely to be missed. The 2010 ATS statement also reiterated the clinical criteria for diagnosis of CCHS and introduced the requirement for identification of *PHOX2B* gene mutations for the definitive diagnosis of CCHS. Over the past decade, mortality and morbidity of CCHS appear to have improved with introduction of genetic testing because of the ability for early, definitive diagnosis that allows for early introduction of chronic artificial ventilatory support, facilitates parental acceptance of diagnosis and provides empowerment in the context of prenatal testing, and allows for anticipatory guidance and insight into prognosis based on specific type of *PHOX2B* mutation. However, specific studies are lacking to conclusively demonstrate the improved outcomes associated with earlier detection and recognition.

PRESENTATION AND DIAGNOSIS

The majority of individuals with CCHS presents in the newborn period with signs of alveolar hypoventilation resulting in hypoxemia and hypercarbia, which are most apparent during sleep, and are usually not accompanied by any associated increases in respiratory rate or arousal.[4] CCHS should be considered if an intubated individual requires minimal pressure (suggesting normal lung compliance) and is unable to tolerate decreases in ventilator rate settings and/or experiences unexpected failed extubations associated with absent cardiorespiratory and behavioral responses to ensuing physiologic compromise. *PHOX2B* genetic testing should be immediately performed while evaluation of other potential etiologies for the alveolar hypoventilation are being pursued – exclusion of pulmonary, cardiac, or neuromuscular disease and brainstem lesions. If feeding intolerance or constipation is present, then evaluation for Hirschsprung's disease should also be considered. Associated pathology and the spectrum of ANSD can include decreased heart rate variability,[12] abrupt sinus pauses,[13] decreased pupillary responses to light,[14] decreased basal body temperature, esophageal dysmotility, constipation, and altered diaphoresis.[4,11,15] These subtle symptoms may be difficult to identify unless specifically sought.

Patients presenting outside of the newborn period are called 'late-onset' CCHS (LO-CCHS). Although the delayed diagnosis may be attributable to subclinical rather than absence of symptoms, alveolar hypoventilation often becomes readily apparent in the context of an instigating event, such as exposure to sedation/substances that decrease the level of consciousness or following an acute pulmonary process such as pneumonia that requires an increase in respiratory drive. With careful, comprehensive review of medical history in these individuals, subtle signs and symptoms of disordered respiratory control from infancy may be uncovered.

At any age, if there is clinical suspicion of alveolar hypoventilation, it behooves the clinician to expedite diagnosis by documenting its presence, and by seeking a more definitive diagnosis through detection of a *PHOX2B* mutation in order to avoid potential devastating events resulting in compromised neurocognitive outcome or even death. Furthermore, delay in diagnosis and institution of artificial ventilatory support can also result in development of cor pulmonale, polycythemia, and seizures.

PAIRED-LIKE HOMEOBOX 2B (PHOX2B) AND GENETIC TESTING

The *PHOX2B* gene consists of three exons; the third exon has two polyalanine repeat regions of which the larger polyalanine repeat region normally has 20 alanines on each allele. Therefore, the *PHOX2B* genotype in a normal individual would be indicated as '20/20.' Ninety percent of CCHS-associated *PHOX2B* mutations are due to heterozygous polyalanine repeat expansion mutations (PARM) with expansions from 24 to 33 alanine repeats on the affected allele (resulting genotypes 20/24 – 20/33).[11] Of these, the most common *PHOX2B* PARMs are genotypes 20/25, 20/26, and 20/27.[16] *PHOX2B* mutations that do not consist of polyalanine expansions are referred to as non-polyalanine expansion repeat mutations (NPARM), and may include frameshift, nonsense, and missense mutations. More recently, whole exon deletions have been identified as causing CCHS in <1% of cases, though these cases may just have components of the full CCHS phenotype in regards to respiratory control deficit and ANSD features.[17]

The variable *PHOX2B* gene mutations result in variable levels of physiologic dysfunction at the cellular level including (1) altered regulation of genes involved with ANS development such as dopamine beta hydroxylase (DBH),[10] (2) altered localization of PHOX2B protein such that it is found in the cytoplasm instead of nucleus of the cell, and (3) altered/absent DNA binding of the PHOX2B protein due to aggregate formation which also interferes with the activity of the normal PHOX2B protein.[10,18] These different mechanisms of cellular dysfunction will ultimately determine the severity of each patient's clinical features, thereby leading to the strong interest in clarifying *PHOX2B*-genotype/CCHS-phenotype associations.

Early MRI studies and autopsies were unremarkable in individuals with CCHS. More recent investigations utilizing functional MRI (fMRI) and diffusion tensor imaging (DTI) in a small cohort with suspected CCHS (*PHOX2B* genetic testing was not performed in all subjects) found brainstem changes in areas known to mediate central chemosensitivity.[19] The neuroanatomic defects in CCHS are likely the result of focal loss of *PHOX2B* expression along with consequences of

recurrent hypoxemia and/or hypercarbia. Based on rodent studies and fMRI in humans, the following regions pertinent to respiratory control show *PHOX2B* expression in the pons and medulla of the brainstem: locus coeruleus, dorsal respiratory group, nucleus ambiguus, and parafacial respiratory group, among other areas. Physiologic evidence suggests that the respiratory failure in these children is mostly based on defects in central mechanisms, but peripheral mechanisms (mainly carotid bodies) also are important.[19]

The majority of *PHOX2B* mutations causing CCHS are *de novo* events with a subset of cases that are inherited in an autosomal dominant manner[6] from an affected parent (typically, genotype 20/25) or parent with somatic mosaicism,[20] even very low-level mosaicism (5%)[21] which may note be identified with commonly available sequencing tests.[20,21] Germline mutation has been described in one case report,[22] emphasizing the importance of genetic counselling and prenatal testing.

Overall, these findings emphasize the importance of requesting *PHOX2B* testing, with particular attention being given to the testing method. Table 37.1 provides indications and limitations of the clinically available genetic testing methods. A three-step process is generally recommended that includes fragment analysis (screening test), sequencing and multiplex ligation-dependent probe amplification (MLPA). Since the most common genotypes are PARMs, the majority of mutations (≈90%) will be identified using fragment analysis. Fragment analysis should be performed using assays that amplify the GC-rich areas in order to detect polyalanine regions expanded to 30–33 repeats.[23] Sequencing is the most commonly available testing method and will identify all NPARMs and the majority of PARMs. With normal results from both the screening and sequencing tests and with continued clinical suspicion of CCHS, MLPA should be performed to identify large deletions or duplications involving exon 3 of the *PHOX2B* gene.

PHOX2B-GENOTYPE/CCHS-PHENOTYPE ASSOCIATION

Since discovery of *PHOX2B* mutations as the mechanism for CCHS, there has been growing evidence of a clear, albeit not absolute, relationship between severity of each of the clinical features and the specific *PHOX2B* mutation. While most evidence available has been in the context of the most common *PHOX2B* genotypes (namely, 20/25, 20/26 and 20/27), in general, findings suggest that the longer PARMs and NPARMs will result in a more severe clinical phenotype. Uncovering these associations has been vital to advancing clinical care through anticipatory guidance and focused screening.

Respiratory Control and Ventilatory Dependence

Individuals with CCHS have monotonous respiratory rates with absent/attenuated increase in minute ventilation in response to hypoxemia and/or to hypercarbia and absent/attenuated asphyxia perception which places them uniquely at risk for adverse and detrimental consequences in the context of otherwise routine activities (swimming, exertion, alcohol intake). Evaluation of respiratory control in individuals with CCHS has been a long-standing curiosity for physicians and scientists, but the number of investigations that include the

TABLE 37.1   Clinically Available *PHOX2B* Testing for Individuals with Suspected Congenital Central Hypoventilation Syndrome (CCHS) and Parents of Affected Children

TESTING METHOD	INDICATION	TYPE OF MUTATION DETECTED	IF RESULTS ARE NORMAL, THEN
Fragment analysis	First step in identifying CCHS in proband	All PARM (24–33 alanines on affected allele)	In proband, consider sequencing
	Parental testing if child has PARM	Large NPARM (35 or 38 base pair deletions)	
	Prenatal testing if sibling has PARM	Somatic mosaicism	
Sequencing test	Second step if there is continued clinical suspicion of CCHS	All NPARM Majority of PARM	Consider fragment analysis if it has not been completed
	If there is a high suspicion for NPARM (such as individuals with Hirschsprung's disease or tumor of neural crest origin)		
Multiplex ligation-dependent probe amplification (MLPA)	Third step if continued clinical suspicion of CCHS	Large deletion of full exon 3 Full exon duplication	No further testing is indicated if fragment analysis and sequencing have already been completed
	Parental testing if child has deletion or duplication		

A three-step process is recommended for identifying PHOX2B mutation in an individual with suspected CCHS.
  PARM, polyalanine expansion repeat mutation; NPARM, non-polyalanine expansion repeat mutation.

PHOX2B genotype is limited.[24] All patients with CCHS demonstrate hypoventilation while asleep and must be provided with artificially supported ventilation. The mildest respiratory phenotype is generally found in individuals with the 20/24 and 20/25 genotype, often requiring sleep-only ventilatory support[11] because of adequate (though potentially not fully normal) awake spontaneous breathing. Accordingly, some individuals with the 20/25 genotype and all those children with the 20/24 genotype will present outside of the newborn period. Individuals with the 20/26 genotype are expected to have variable awake ventilatory requirements and may become more easily compromised with activity. Individuals with 20/27 genotype and NPARMs generally require continuous ventilatory support.[11,23] Because of the few cases with genotypes 20/28 – 20/33, it is not yet clear if the pattern of longer PARM results in incremental severity of respiratory control deficits in this group.

Cardiac Sinus Pause and Pacemakers
Weese-Mayer and colleagues found a clear, linear relationship between the most common PARMs and R-R interval of 3 seconds or greater such that none was found in those children with 20/25 genotype, 19% were present in those patients with 20/26 genotype, and 83% of patients with 20/27 genotype.[24,25] However, it is possible that the prolonged sinus pauses in the individuals with 20/25 genotype will develop later in life during adulthood.[26] Along with increase in the proportion of individuals with prolonged sinus pauses by genotype (for genotypes 20/25, 20/26, and 20/27), there is also an increase in the average R–R interval duration and in the number of patients requiring cardiac pacemaker implantation.[25] There have been no reports of cardiac pacemaker implantation and/or prolonged sinus pauses in CCHS patients with NPARM, but this may be due to the small numbers of individuals with NPARMs and the wide variability of mutations in this group.

Autonomic Nervous System Dysregulation (ANSD)
The spectrum of ANSD that appears to be specific to CCHS includes pupil abnormalities,[27] decreased heart rate variability,[28] altered esophageal and gastrointestinal motility, decreased pain perception, and altered diaphoresis.[15] Of these manifestations, *PHOX2B* genotype has a clear, linear relationship with pupillary diameter and pupillary responses to light such that longer PARMs have increasing miosis and decreasing pupil responses to light.[27]

ANS tissue pathology due to absent development of ganglion cells in the gastrointestinal tract (Hirschsprung's disease; HSCR) or to development of tumors from sympathetic tissue (tumors of neural crest origin) have commonly been described in CCHS cases. HSCR has been reported in 87–100% of individuals with NPARMs in contrast to 13–20% of those with PARMs.[10,11,28] Of those with PARMs, those with the 20/27 genotype have the highest occurrence of HSCR, while no cases of HSCR have been reported in individuals with the 20/25 genotype. Tumors of neural crest origin include neuroblastomas, ganglioneuromas, and ganglioneuroblastomas that are found in the chest and abdomen in paraspinal ganglia or the adrenal glands. In individuals with NPARMs neuroblastoma is the predominant tumor type. Of those with PARMs, ganglioneuromas and ganglioneuroblastomas have been reported in children with the 20/29 – 20/33 genotypes, while the risk for neuroblastoma in PARMs is unknown.[10,29]

Neurocognitive Outcome
Neurocognitive evaluation in children with CCHS has been described in small cohorts, but only one study has been completed since introduction of *PHOX2B* testing.[30] Zelko and colleagues[30] evaluated formal neurocognitive results in 20 genetically confirmed CCHS cases and found mean full-scale intelligence quotient of 84.9 and no apparent relationship between genotype and severity with wide variability in results

(standard deviation, 23.9), but these findings are limited because of multiple factors related to suboptimal medical management that may play a role in neurocognitive outcomes.

MANAGEMENT

Congenital central hypoventilation syndrome is a life-long disorder for which artificial ventilatory support is the mainstay of care and for which there are unique considerations in ventilatory management in the context of disordered respiratory control. Comprehensive, in-patient physiologic evaluations at centers of expertise are recommended every 6 months for children less than 3 years of age, and annually thereafter.[11] These evaluations are intended to facilitate, not replace, care provided by a primary pulmonologist because management of children with CCHS is complex. The comprehensive evaluations should include assessment of ventilatory requirements during varying levels of activity while awake and during all stages of sleep, exogenous ventilatory challenges, 72-hour Holter monitoring, neurocognitive performance, and age-appropriate autonomic testing.[11] With improvements in technology for home monitoring and home ventilation, individuals with CCHS are anticipated to have improved survival and quality of life.

For those <1 year of age, optimal ventilation is provided via tracheostomy with portable home mechanical ventilation. In the older child, non-invasive positive- (or negative-) pressure ventilation or diaphragmatic pacing may be considered, but should be pursued under careful scrutiny and consideration. Non-invasive positive-pressure ventilation (NPPV) is difficult for long-term use and not ideal in children because of risk of development of mid-face hypoplasia. Diaphragmatic pacing is ideal for ambulatory children (>2 years of age) who require daytime ventilatory support, allowing them the freedom to explore their environment without the mechanical ventilator tether. A few of the many important considerations for diaphragm pacing include: inability of the child to undergo MRI once internal components of the pacemaker system are implanted, risk of injury to internal components is highest with the subcutaneously implanted disk-like receiver, decannulation should be implemented with caution after initiating use of diaphragm pacers because of development of upper airway obstruction with each negative-pressure breath.[2] Regardless of mode of ventilatory support, all individuals with CCHS must have home pulse oximetry and end-tidal carbon dioxide monitoring (with home nursing supervision) to allow for tight control of oxygen and carbon dioxide levels via mechanical ventilator adjustments and because outward signs without objective measures can lead to devastating events.[11]

The sinus pauses found in individuals with CCHS are abrupt in onset and can occur while awake. Based on Holter recordings, if R–R intervals of 3 seconds or greater are found, then cardiac pacemaker placement should be considered in order to reduce the risk of neurocognitive delays and sudden death, but formal recommendations for this unique population are not yet covered by the American Heart Association guidelines for pacemaker implantation.[31,32] Hirschsprung's disease should be investigated with rectal biopsy in any individual with clinical signs/symptoms of HSCR and a high level of suspicion should remain in those individuals at risk based on *PHOX2B* genotype.

With early diagnosis and conservative management, individuals with CCHS are not only surviving into adulthood, but now have potential for improved quality of life and excellent neurocognitive outcome.

SUMMARY

Congenital central hypoventilation syndrome is a fascinating disorder of respiratory control and autonomic dysregulation with wide variability in disease severity, elicited by mutations of the *PHOX2B* gene. Over the past decade, increased interest from both basic scientists and clinicians has led to improved understanding of the underlying mechanisms and significance of *PHOX2B* mutations in CCHS. Investigation of genotype–phenotype associations has revealed that, in general, disease severity increases with longer PARMs and with NPARMs. Clinically available *PHOX2B* genetic testing facilitates diagnosis of those with neonatal onset, very mild phenotypes (LO-CCHS), somatic mosaicism, and allows for parents and clinicians to make better-informed decisions.

Clinical Pearls

- Diagnosis of congenital central hypoventilation syndrome (CCHS) is based on the presence of alveolar hypoventilation in the absence of primary neuromuscular, lung, or cardiac disease, or an identifiable brainstem lesion that can account for the full phenotype *and* identification of a *PHOX2B* mutation.
- The most common *PHOX2B* mutations are heterozygous polyalanine expansion repeat mutations (PARM) with genotypes 20/25, 20/26, and 20/27 (normal genotype 20/20). Identification of the type of *PHOX2B* mutation can facilitate anticipatory management in individuals with CCHS.
- Close monitoring of end tidal carbon dioxide and oxygen saturation levels are essential for those with CCHS – because of the intrinsic respiratory control deficit, the patient will not sense or demonstrate signs of ensuing physiologic compromise.
- Individuals with CCHS often develop hypoxemia and/or hypercarbia during routine activities of daily living (eating, drinking, playing, running) and with drowsiness (prior to sleep onset). Therefore, evaluation must include the awake state and can be performed at centers with expertise in disorders of respiratory control.

References

1. Mellins RB, Balfour HH Jr, Turino GM, et al. Failure of automatic control of ventilation (Ondine's curse). Report of an infant born with this syndrome and review of the literature. Medicine (Baltimore) 1970; 49:487–504.
2. Chin A, Shaul DB, Patwari PP, et al. Diaphragmatic pacing in children with congenital central hypoventilation syndrome. In: Gozal D, Gozal LK, editors. Sleep disordered breathing in children: a clinical guide. New York: Springer; 2012. p. 553–73.
3. Weese-Mayer DE, Silvestri JM, Menzies LJ, et al. Congenital central hypoventilation syndrome: diagnosis, management, and long-term outcome in thirty-two children. J Pediatr 1992;120:381–7.
4. Weese-Mayer DE, Shannon DC, Keens TG, et al. Idiopathic congenital central hypoventilation syndrome. diagnosis and management. Am J Resp Crit Care Med 1999;160:368–73.

5. Amiel J, Laudier B, Attie-Bitach T, et al. Polyalanine expansion and frameshift mutations of the paired-like homeobox gene PHOX2B in congenital central hypoventilation syndrome. Nat Genet 2003;33:459–61.

6. Weese-Mayer DE, Berry-Kravis EM, Zhou L, et al. Idiopathic congenital central hypoventilation syndrome: analysis of genes pertinent to early autonomic nervous system embryologic development and identification of mutations in PHOX2B. Am J Med Genet A 2003;123A:267–78.

7. Sasaki A, Kanai M, Kijima K, et al. Molecular analysis of congenital central hypoventilation syndrome. Hum Genet 2003;114:22–6.

8. Pattyn A, Morin X, Cremer H, et al. The homeobox gene PHOX2B is essential for the development of autonomic neural crest derivatives. Nature 1999;399:366–70.

9. Howard MJ. Mechanisms and perspectives on differentiation of autonomic neurons. Dev Biol 2005;277(2):271–86.

10. Trochet D, O'Brien LM, Gozal D, et al. PHOX2B genotype allows for prediction of tumor risk in congenital central hypoventilation syndrome. Am J Hum Genet 2005;76:421–6.

11. Weese-Mayer DE, Berry-Kravis EM, Ceccherini I, et al. An official ATS clinical policy statement: Congenital central hypoventilation syndrome: genetic basis, diagnosis, and management. Am J Respir Crit Care Med 2010;181:626–44.

12. Woo MS, Woo MA, Gozal D, et al. Heart rate variability in congenital central hypoventilation syndrome. Pediatr Res 1992;31:291–6.

13. Gronli JO, Santucci BA, Leurgans SE, et al. Congenital central hypoventilation syndrome: PHOX2B genotype determines risk for sudden death. Pediatr Pulmonol 2008;43:77–86.

14. Patwari PP, Stewart TM, Rand CM, et al. Pupillometry in congenital central hypoventilation syndrome (CCHS): quantitative evidence of autonomic nervous system dysregulation. Pediatr Res 2012;71(3):280–5.

15. Weese-Mayer DE, Silvestri JM, Huffman AD, et al. Case/control family study of autonomic nervous system dysfunction in idiopathic congenital central hypoventilation syndrome. Am J Med Genet 2001;100:237–45.

16. Weese-Mayer DE, Rand CM, Berry-Kravis E, et al. Congenital central hypoventilation syndrome from past to future: model for translational and transitional autonomic medicine. Pediatr Pulmonol 2009;44:521–35.

17. Jennings LJ, Yu M, Rand CM, et al. Variable human phenotype associated with novel deletions of the PHOX2B gene. Pediatr Pulmonol 2012;47:153–61.

18. Parodi S, Bachetti T, Lantieri F, et al. Parental origin and somatic mosaicism of PHOX2B mutations in congenital central hypoventilation syndrome. Hum Mutat 2008;29:206.

19. Patwari PP, Carroll MS, Rand CM, et al. Congenital central hypoventilation syndrome and the PHOX2B gene: a model of respiratory and autonomic dysregulation. Respir Physiol Neurobiol 2010;173(3):322–35.

20. Jennings LJ, Yu M, Zhou L, et al. Comparison of PHOX2B testing methods in the diagnosis of congenital central hypoventilation syndrome and mosaic carriers. Diagn Mol Pathol 2010;19:224–31.

21. Bachetti T, Parodi S, Di Duca M, et al. Low amounts of PHOX2B expanded alleles in asymptomatic parents suggest unsuspected recurrence risk in congenital central hypoventilation syndrome. J Mol Med (Berl) 2011;89:505–13.

22. Rand CM, Yu M, Jennings LJ, et al. Germline mosaicism of PHOX2B mutation accounts for familial recurrence of congenital central hypoventilation syndrome (CCHS). Am J Med Genet 2012;158A(9):2297–301.

23. Matera I, Bachetti T, Puppo F, et al. PHOX2B mutations and polyalanine expansions correlate with the severity of the respiratory phenotype and associated symptoms in both congenital and late onset central hypoventilation syndrome. J Med Genet 2004;41:373–80.

24. Carroll MS, Patwari PP, Weese-Mayer DE. Carbon dioxide chemoreception and hypoventilation syndromes with autonomic dysregulation. J Appl Physiol 2010;108:979–88.

25. Gronli JO, Santucci BA, Leurgans SE, et al. Congenital central hypoventilation syndrome: PHOX2B genotype determines risk for sudden death. Pediatr Pulmonol 2008;43:77–86.

26. Antic NA, Malow BA, Lange N, et al. PHOX2B mutation-confirmed congenital central hypoventilation syndrome: presentation in adulthood. Am J Respir Crit Care Med 2006;174:923–7.

27. Patwari PP, Stewart TH, Rand CM, et al. Pupillometry in congenital central hypoventilation syndrome (CCHS): quantitative evidence of autonomic nervous system dysregulation. Pediatric Research 2012;71(3):280–5.

28. Woo MS, Woo MA, Gozal D, et al. Heart rate variability in congenital central hypoventilation syndrome. Pediatr Res 1992;31(3):291–6.

29. Berry-Kravis EM, Zhou L, Rand CM, et al. Congenital central hypoventilation syndrome: PHOX2B mutations and phenotype. Am J Respir Crit Care Med 2006;174:1139–44.

30. Zelko FA, Nelson MN, Leurgens SE, et al. Congenital central hypoventilation syndrome: neurocognitive functioning in school age children. Pediatr Pulmonol 2010;45:92–8.

31. Epstein AE, DiMarco JP, Ellenbogen KA, et al. ACC/AHA/HRS 2008 Guidelines for Device-Based Therapy of Cardiac Rhythm Abnormalities: a report of the American College of Cardiology/American Heart Association Task Force on Practice Guidelines (Writing Committee to Revise the ACC/AHA/NASPE 2002 Guideline Update for Implantation of Cardiac Pacemakers and Antiarrhythmia Devices) developed in collaboration with the American Association for Thoracic Surgery and Society of Thoracic Surgeons J Am Coll Cardiol 2008;51(21):e1–62.

32. Tsao S, Webster G, Patwari PP, et al. Pacemaker utilization in cohort of 85 children with congenital central hypoventilation syndrome (CCHS) may impact the risk of sudden death. Circulation 2011;124:A17138.

Rapid-Onset Obesity with Hypothalamic Dysfunction, Hypoventilation, and Autonomic Dysregulation (ROHHAD)

Pallavi P. Patwari and Casey M. Rand

EPIDEMIOLOGY AND HISTORY

The first case of rapid-onset obesity with hypothalamic dysfunction, hypoventilation, and autonomic dysregulation (ROHHAD) was described in 1965[1] as a 3.5-year-old boy who developed signs of hypoventilation within 9 months of onset of rapid weight gain. The hypoventilation did not improve with weight loss, suggesting a distinction from Pickwickian syndrome (now known as obesity hypoventilation syndrome). Furthermore, this child developed a transient central diabetes insipidus indicating hypothalamic dysfunction. Accordingly, the case was described as the first patient with alveolar hypoventilation and hypothalamic disease. It was not until 2000 that the possibility of a distinct syndrome was evoked and called late-onset central hypoventilation syndrome with hypothalamic dysfunction (LO-CHS/HD)[2] with description of a new case and review of the 10 existing cases in the literature.

Although children with ROHHAD can present with obstructive sleep apnea after development of obesity, the condition is markedly distinct from obstructive sleep apnea hypoventilation syndrome[3] and obesity hypoventilation syndrome in which chronic obstructive sleep apnea with resulting overnight hypercarbia, hypoxemia, and frequent arousals leads to daytime awake hypoventilation, hypoxemia, and daytime sleepiness. The management of these disorders involves relief of the obstruction, which would be expected to resolve the hypoventilation and daytime sleepiness completely. In contrast, relief of the upper airway obstruction in ROHHAD children often unveils the presence of the underlying primary central alveolar hypoventilation.

Congenital central hypoventilation syndrome (CCHS) is a disorder of the autonomic nervous system (ANS) that is similar to ROHHAD such that respiratory control and ANS dysregulation (ANSD) are key features.[4] In contrast to ROHHAD, CCHS is often diagnosed in the newborn period, but milder cases of CCHS can go undiagnosed even until adulthood. These later-presenting cases of CCHS can potentially lead to some confusion in distinguishing cases of ROHHAD from CCHS. However, within the past decade a genetic basis was identified for CCHS, allowing rapid, objective diagnosis of CCHS, providing a definitive distinction from cases of ROHHAD.

In 2007, a cohort of 23 ROHHAD cases was described and found *not* to have congenital central hypoventilation syndrome (CCHS)-associated *PHOX2B* mutations.[5] With intention to facilitate early diagnosis, the acronym ROHHAD was created at this time. Specifically, the rapid weight gain was most often the presenting sign. In 2008, a new acronym,

ROHHADNET, was introduced because of the finding of neural crest tumors.[6] These authors described six cases, all with ganglioneuromas. The difficulty with this acronym is that only a subset of patients (33–40%)[5,7] with ROHHAD will develop these tumors, which may lead to missed diagnosis. Despite the confusion due to multiple names/acronyms for the same disorder and the high occurrence of cardiorespiratory arrest (50–60%),[5,6,8] there has been a dramatic increase in reported cases since 2007. Currently, it is estimated that there are at least 100 children worldwide affected by ROHHAD. It is not yet clear whether any particular population is at greater risk for developing ROHHAD.

DIAGNOSIS AND PRESENTATION

The diagnosis of ROHHAD is currently based on clinical criteria (Table 38.1): (1) rapid-onset obesity and alveolar hypoventilation starting after the age of 1.5 years, (2) evidence of hypothalamic dysfunction, as defined by ≥1 of the following findings: rapid-onset obesity, hyperprolactinemia, central hypothyroidism, disordered water balance, failed growth hormone stimulation test, corticotropin deficiency, or altered onset of puberty (delayed or precocious), and (3) absence of *PHOX2B* mutation (to genetically distinguish ROHHAD from CCHS). Since a single diagnostic test is not yet available for ROHHAD, it is essential to be attentive to the clinical presentation and course, which should include cooperative consultation by experts in the fields of respiratory, endocrine, and autonomic medicine.

One of the most remarkable features of ROHHAD is that affected children appear to be completely normal prior to the onset of symptoms. Most often, the first sign is a dramatic, unexplained weight gain,[5] which occurs anywhere between 1.5 to 7 years of age. With variable timing, the affected child will then develop further signs of hypothalamic dysfunction. Evidence of hypothalamic dysfunction can potentially be found with laboratory investigation guided by a pediatric endocrinologist. Hypoventilation can also be found soon after presentation of rapid-onset obesity or even years later.[5] Presentation of hypoventilation can include episodes of hypoxemia during sleep, cyanosis while awake (without associated respiratory distress), and most often cardiorespiratory arrest. Features of ANSD may occur early or late in the course, as there appears to be wide variation in age at onset, but tend to be less threatening and more difficult to identify due to limited availability of objective measures of ANSD for use in children.

TABLE 38.1 ROHHAD Phenotypic Spectrum and Diagnostic Criteria

Mandatory for diagnosis	Rapid-onset obesity	20–40 pounds gain over 6–12 months after 1.5 years of age (typically between 3 and 9 years of age)
	Alveolar hypoventilation	Absent or attenuated respiratory and behavioral response to hypercarbia and/or hypoxemia during sleep and wakefulness
≥ 1 of the following	Hypothalamic dysfunction	Rapid weight gain
		Disordered water balance (altered vasopressin secretion) with sodium derangement
		Failed test of growth hormone stimulation
		Hyperprolactinemia
		Precocious or delayed puberty
		Corticotropin deficiency
		Central hypothyroidism
Supportive findings	Autonomic nervous system dysregulation	Mydriasis with decreased pupillary response to light
		Vasomotor dysregulation (cold hands/feet)
		Thermal dysregulation (severe hyper- or hypothermia)
		Bradycardia
		Gastrointestinal dysmotility (constipation or diarrhea)
		Altered diaphoresis
	Other neurologic features	Tumors of neural crest origin (sympathetic tumors)
		Decreased pain perception
		Behavioral or mood problems (flat affect, inability to detect social cues, in severe cases psychosis)
		Altered circadian rhythm; hypersomnolence
		Seizures (potentially due to sodium derangement, hypercarbia, and/or hypoxemia)

COMPREHENSIVE EVALUATION AND MANAGEMENT

As soon as ROHHAD is considered as a potential diagnosis, it is essential that all relevant systems be evaluated to identify the degree to which each is affected. Initial evaluation should include screening endocrinology blood work, overnight polysomnography (PSG) to determine if there are signs of obstructive sleep apnea and/or hypoventilation (with hypoventilation becoming more apparent upon follow-up PSG after the obstruction is resolved), computed tomography (CT) of chest and abdomen to screen for neural crest tumors, MRI of the head to rule out other etiologies of central hypoventilation, and cardiac evaluation (echocardiogram to screen for cor pulmonale, 24-hour Holter recording to screen for bradycardia). Since disease progression varies for each affected child, it is generally recommended to have yearly comprehensive evaluations, but evaluations may need to occur more frequently if there appears to be rapid disease progression (as may occur early in the course).

Since ROHHAD affects multiple systems, successful management involves coordinated multidisciplinary care primarily involving the pediatrician, sleep medicine physician, pulmonologist, and endocrinologist. Over the course of the disease, multiple other subspecialists may be actively involved and can include cardiologists, intensivists, otolaryngologists, surgeons, gastroenterologists, neurologists, ophthalmologists, psychologists, and psychiatrists.[9] As there is no cure for ROHHAD, key to management are close monitoring and symptomatic treatment based on the affected systems.

Obesity and Hypothalamic Dysfunction

The hypothalamic dysfunction seen in ROHHAD patients should be evaluated and treated by a pediatric endocrinologist and care individualized (as there is wide variability of hypothalamic dysfunction in those affected with ROHHAD). Typically between 1.5 and 7 years of life, a child with ROHHAD will demonstrate a dramatic weight gain (20–40 pounds) within 6–12 months and with associated hyperphagia. The

obesity should be controlled with diet and exercise, often requiring very strict calorie restriction. Because of the risk of developing hypoxemia and hypercarbia with exertion, recommendations should start with only mild exertion along with close monitoring. Formal testing should be performed to identify the safe level of exertion and type of support required, based on end-tidal carbon dioxide and pulse oximetry values recorded during exercise. Routine or expected complications of obesity should also be considered and include development of non-alcoholic steatohepatitis, hyperlipidemia, and diabetes mellitus.

Evaluation for other hypothalamic abnormalities can include prolactin level (hyperprolactinemia), cortisol levels (rule out Cushing's disease), thyroid panel (central hypothyroidism), growth factors, fasting arginine vasopressin levels (partial diabetes insipidus or SIADH), and other focused testing relating to altered onset of puberty and corticotropin deficiency. These can develop soon after onset of obesity or even years later. Therefore, repeated testing is required. Accordingly, treatments may include a strict fluid intake regimen and/or DDAVP, hormone replacement, and more.

Hypoventilation

Hypoventilation is the most insidious and life-threatening feature, requiring proactive and repeated investigation, ideally including awake and asleep endogenous and exogenous ventilatory challenges. Specifically, evaluation should include response to endogenous challenges while asleep and spontaneously breathing in various conditions (sitting up, supine, sleep onset, and within sleep). Since awake ventilatory needs will vary, respiratory evaluation should also include endogenous ventilatory challenges (assessment of spontaneous breathing during typical activities of daily living such as playing, running, and eating, among others) and exogenous ventilatory challenges (response based on exposure to hyperoxia, hyperoxia/hypercarbia, hypoxemia/hypercarbia, and hypoxemia). Despite multiple case reports that clearly demonstrate abnormal chemoreception, systematic evaluation of carbon dioxide chemoreception in ROHHAD cohorts has yet to be formally evaluated and published.[10]

All children with ROHHAD develop alveolar hypoventilation as demonstrated by inability to increase rate and/or depth of breathing in response to hypoxemia and/or hypercarbia. Therefore, artificial ventilatory support is mandatory at some point in the course of the disease for those with ROHHAD. From one of the largest cohorts with detailed physiologic evaluation, it appears that about half (7 of 15 cases) required tracheostomy and 24-hour/day ventilatory support and that the remaining half (8 of 15 cases) were supported with overnight mask ventilation.[5] It is important to note that the severity of respiratory control deficit may evolve over time and is often exacerbated by the mechanical effects of obesity (decrease in functional residual capacity, restrictive lung disease). Other methods of artificial ventilatory support such as phrenic nerve diaphragm pacing may have limited success due to the associated morbid obesity.

Home monitoring for children with respiratory control deficits is distinctly more conservative than other chronically ventilated children because of the absent or attenuated physiologic, behavioral, and arousal responses to hypoxemia and hypercarbia. With development of physiologic compromise, there would be an absence of outward signs and the only means of determining adequate ventilation and oxygenation would be with objective measures from a pulse oximeter and end-tidal carbon dioxide monitor. Ideally, children with ROHHAD should have both awake and asleep home monitoring since they will not be able to sense or adequately respond to a developing respiratory challenge (acute respiratory illness, increased activity, or even with eating).

Autonomic Nervous System Dysregulation

At some point, all patients with ROHHAD develop signs of ANSD. These include ophthalmologic abnormalities such as mydriasis and attenuated pupil response to light, strabismus, altered gastrointestinal motility (commonly leading to chronic constipation), altered thermoregulation (leading to extreme hypothermia <92° Fahrenheit and/or hyperthermia >104° Fahrenheit), decreased pain sensation (increasing risk of self injury), bradycardia (even <40 bpm necessitating cardiac pacemaker), altered diaphoresis, and altered peripheral perfusion (suggesting vasomotor dysregulation). ANSD requires symptomatic treatment. For example, the altered thermoregulation requires careful monitoring of body temperature and adjustment of ambient temperature. Chronic constipation can be easily controlled with stool softeners.

ANS testing is limited in children and may only include a comprehensive review of ANS symptoms. Depending on the child's ability to cooperate, the ANS testing may also include pupillometry, heart-rate-deep-breathing, Valsalva maneuver, tilt test, orthostatic response, quantitative sudomotor evaluation, and pulse wave velocity analysis.

A subset of cases with ROHHAD (33–39%)[5,7] develops tumors of neural crest origin such as ganglioneuromas or ganglioneuroblastomas. These can be found in the paraspinal area along the sympathetic chain or in the adrenal gland, and most often require only surgical removal, but should be managed in consultation with an oncologist. If initial CT or MRI of chest and abdomen has been performed, yearly screening can include chest radiograph, ultrasound of adrenals, and urine catecholamines.

Other Neurologic Features

Other features that can develop in children with ROHHAD include behavioral problems (blunt affect, emotional lability, or even psychosis), developmental delay which may be secondary to recurrent episodes of hypoxemia or cardiorespiratory arrest, and seizures (which may also be secondary to hypoxemia). Annual neurocognitive testing is recommended as an early and objective marker of effectiveness (or compliance) with ventilatory management or development of progressive neurologic decline. Concomitant mood and behavior problems may prevent completion of formal neurocognitive testing and may even be so severe that medical care, including initiating ventilator support, can be compromised.

SUSPECTED ETIOLOGY

Since ROHHAD affects seemingly normal children, etiologic investigations may provide insight into maturational mechanisms of the hypothalamus, ANS, and respiratory control. More promising is that the clinical course is variable between and within each affected child, suggesting a plasticity, which if identified, can potentially lead to substantive treatments. Currently, there are several hypothesis and lines of investigation into the etiology of ROHHAD.

Genetic/Epigenetic

The similarities between the ROHHAD phenotype and CCHS suggest that the etiology of the ROHHAD syndrome may involve mutations in genes known to be important to the development or regulation of the ANS. Furthermore, since ROHHAD demonstrates a wider spectrum of systems involved than CCHS, an alternate pathway involved in ANS and hypothalamic development is likely to be involved. However, to date, candidate gene analyses by Sanger sequencing in several studies (Table 38.2) have failed to identify any disease-causing or disease-associated mutations.[5,7,11] The etiologies of several diseases have now been shown to be based on, related to, or associated with aberrant epigenetic patterning including atherosclerosis, Prader–Willi syndrome, Angelman syndrome, schizophrenia, bipolar disorder, and several forms of cancer.[12–16] The existence in some of these diseases of relatively late age of onset and peaks of susceptibility, discordance of monozygotic twins and major fluctuations on the course of disease severity can be at least partially explained by epigenetic phenomena. Since all of these epigenetically suggestive features are seen in ROHHAD, interest in the epigenetics of ROHHAD has increased. Current investigation into possible genetic and epigenetic mechanisms in ROHHAD is underway.

TABLE 38.2   Candidate Genes Previously Tested in ROHHAD Cohorts

GENES	ASSOCIATED SYSTEM	REFERENCE
HTR_{1A}, OTP, PACAP	Hypothalamic	11
NECDIN		7
ASCL1	Neuroendocrine	7
PHOX2B	Autonomic	5
TRKB, BDNF	Neuronal development	5

Paraneoplastic/Autoimmune

Several investigators have hypothesized that a secondary phenomenon, such as an autoimmune process or paraneoplastic syndrome, may be responsible for ROHHAD.[7,9,17–21] Paraneoplastic conditions result from secondary autoimmune responses to the presence of a tumor in the body and can be successfully treated with immunosuppressive therapy and/or tumor removal. Tumors of neural crest origin are known to lead to paraneoplastic conditions, and are found in a subset of ROHHAD patients. Additionally, broad clinical improvement was observed in a recent reported ROHHAD case treated with an immunosuppressive drug.[19] However, as this case did not present with the hypoventilation as normally seen in ROHHAD, it is unclear whether this treatment will prove effective in typical cases of ROHHAD, and how the treatment could affect long-term prognosis. Additionally, tumors are only identified in a subset of ROHHAD cases, and therefore a paraneoplastic phenomenon is not likely to explain the majority of ROHHAD cases. Further, tumor removal has not been found to dramatically alter the phenotype of these cases, as would be expected in a strictly paraneoplastic condition. Therefore, the development of ROHHAD may involve a 'two-hit' phenomenon, i.e., genetic predisposition coupled with development of a paraneoplastic process.

CONCLUSION

Previously known as late-onset central hypoventilation syndrome with hypothalamic dysfunction (LO-CHS/HD), ROHHAD is an acronym intended to facilitate early diagnosis and describe the evolving clinical course. Considering the multi-system involvement, these children are best served with coordinated, multi-subspecialist care. With early initiation of treatment and conservative management, outcome in these children can be optimized, including excellent neurocognitive function, quality of life, and potentially normal life span.

Clinical Pearls

- Diagnosis of ROHHAD is based on development of rapid weight gain (20–40 pounds within 6–12 months) and alveolar hypoventilation (with absence of *PHOX2B* mutation) after 1.5 years of age in addition to evidence of hypothalamic dysfunction.
- Considering the multi-system involvement, these children are best served with coordinated, multi-subspecialist care.
- Individuals with ROHHAD often have an evolving clinical course and benefit from repeated evaluations at centers with expertise in disorders of respiratory control.
- Since the etiology of ROHHAD is still elusive, there is no cure for ROHHAD. Therefore, management of ROHHAD cases is based on careful monitoring and symptomatic treatment.

References

1. Fishman LS, Samson JH, Sperling DR. Primary alveolar hypoventilation syndrome (Ondine's curse). Am J Dis Child 1965;110:155–61.
2. Katz ES, McGrath S, Marcus CL. Late-onset central hypoventilation with hypothalamic dysfunction: a distinct clinical syndrome. Pediatr Pulmonol 2000;29(1):62–8.
3. Rosen CL. Clinical features of obstructive sleep apnea hypoventilation syndrome in otherwise healthy children. Pediatr Pulmonol 1999;27(6):403–9.
4. Weese-Mayer DE, Berry-Kravis EM, Ceccherin I, et al. An official ATS clinical policy statement: Congenital central hypoventilation syndrome: genetic basis, diagnosis, and management. Am J Respir Crit Care Med 2010;181(6):626–44.
5. Ize-Ludlow D, Gray JA, Sperling MA, et al. Rapid-onset obesity with hypothalamic dysfunction, hypoventilation, and autonomic dysregulation presenting in childhood. Pediatrics 2007;120(1):e179–88.
6. Bougneres P, Pantalone L, Linglart A, et al. Endocrine manifestations of the rapid-onset obesity with hypoventilation, hypothalamic, autonomic dysregulation and neural tumor (ROHHADNET) syndrome in early childhood. J Clin Endocrinol Metab 2008;93(10):3971–80.
7. De Pontual L, Trochet D, Caillat-Zucman S, et al. Delineation of late onset hypoventilation associated with hypothalamic dysfunction syndrome. Pediatr Res 2008;64(6):689–94.
8. Chew HB, Ngu LH, Keng WT. Rapid-onset obesity with hypothalamic dysfunction, hypoventilation and autonomic dysregulation (ROHHAD): a case with additional features and review of the literature. BMJ Case Rep 2011;March 1.
9. Patwari PP, Rand CM, Berry-Kravis EM, et al. Monozygotic twins discordant for ROHHAD phenotype. Pediatrics 2011;128(3):e711–15.
10. Carroll MS, Patwari PP, Weese-Mayer DE. Carbon dioxide chemoreception and hypoventilation syndromes with autonomic dysregulation. J Appl Physiol 2010;108(4):979–88.
11. Rand C, Patwari PP, Rodikova EA, et al. Rapid-onset obesity with hypothalamic dysfunction, hypoventilation, and autonomic dysregulation: analysis of hypothalamic and autonomic candidate genes. Pediatr Res 2011;70(4):375–8.
12. Zaina S, Lindholm MW, Lund G. Nutrition and aberrant DNA methylation patterns in atherosclerosis: more than just hyperhomocysteinemia? J Nutr 2005;135(1):5–8.
13. Esteller M, Corn PG, Baylin SB, et al. A gene hypermethylation profile of human cancer. Cancer Res 2001;61(8):3225–9.
14. Petronis A. Epigenetics and bipolar disorder: new opportunities and challenges. Am J Med Genet C Semin Med Genet 2003;123C(1): 65–75.
15. Costa E, Chen Y, Davis J, et al. REELIN and schizophrenia: a disease at the interface of the genome and the epigenome. Mol Interv 2002; 2(1):47–57.
16. Nicholls RD, Knepper JL. Genome organization, function, and imprinting in Prader-Willi and Angelman syndromes. Annu Rev Genomics Hum Genet 2001;2:153–75.
17. Abaci A, Catli G, Bayram E, et al. A case of rapid-onset obesity with hypothalamic dysfunction, hypoventilation, autonomic dysregulation, and neural crest tumor: ROHHADNET syndrome. Endocr Pract 2012:1–19.
18. Ouvrier R, Nunn K, Sprague T, et al. Idiopathic hypothalamic dysfunction: a paraneoplastic syndrome? Lancet 1995;346(8985):1298.
19. Paz-Priel I, Cooke DW, Chen AR. Cyclophosphamide for rapid-onset obesity, hypothalamic dysfunction, and autonomic dysregulation syndrome. J Pediatr 2011;158(2):337–9.
20. Sirvent N, Berard E, Chastagner P, et al. Hypothalamic dysfunction associated with neuroblastoma: evidence for a new paraneoplastic syndrome? Med Pediatr Oncol 2003;40(5):326–8.
21. Armangue T, Petit-Pedrol M, Dalmau J. Autoimmune encephalitis in children. J Child Neurol 2012;27(11):1460–9.

PARASOMNIAS

Chapter **39** **Disorders of Arousal**
Gerald M. Rosen
Disorders of arousal constitute a clinical spectrum of behaviors that occur during incomplete wakings from sleep. They vary from mild (a child who quietly sits up in bed, mumbles briefly, and then lies back down and returns to sleep) to major (the adolescent who has a sudden arousal that begins with a bloodcurdling scream followed by headlong flight, with no concern regarding safety). All of the disorders of arousal share a common pathophysiology and have many similarities in family history, genetic predisposition, timing during the sleep cycle, and clinical features. This group of disorders comprises some of the most common and (for parents) disturbing sleep problems seen in children.

Chapter **40** **REM Behavior Disorder**
Stephen H. Sheldon and Darius A. Loughmanee
REM behavior disorder, or REM motor parasomnia (RMP), is rare in children. This disorder is typified by abnormal behaviors occurring during REM sleep that may cause injury to the child or others. Symptoms can include talking, laughing, shouting, gesturing, flailing, punching, kicking, sitting up, leaping from the bed, crawling, or running. This chapter reviews the presentation, comorbid states, and treatment of RMP, and discusses the means of differentiating it from NREM parasomnias.

Chapter **41** **Other Parasomnias**
Harsha Kumar and Sindhuja Vardhan
Parasomnias can be seen in children. It is very important to obtain a good history and, when required, obtain sleep studies and other tests to rule out disease conditions that can be seen along with parasomnias. Good sleep hygiene is important for management of many parasomnias. Patients should be advised to allow at least 7–8 hours of sleep and maintain a consistent sleep–wake cycle. Creating a safe sleep environment is very important and should include secure windows and doors, sleeping on a low bed to minimize injury from falls and electronic alarm devices to alarm the family members if the patient is leaving the room. Bed alarms for patients with incontinence are beneficial. Resist awakening sleepwalkers as it can worsen the situation; instead, take them back to bed. It is most crucial to identify the underlying disorders and triggers for the parasomnia, which need to be addressed appropriately.

Disorders of Arousal

Gerald M. Rosen

INTRODUCTION

Parasomnias represent a broad group of sleep disorders that are defined as undesirable phenomena occurring predominantly during sleep, first described by Broughton.[1] These sleep disorders are of great interest to sleep specialists, primary care providers, and patients (and their parents) because this group comprises some of the most common and bizarre sleep problems seen in children. Disorders of arousal are the most common of the parasomnias seen in children. Disorders of arousal are defined similarly by the Diagnostic and Statistical Manual of Mental Disorders, 5th edition (DSM-V)[2] and the International Classification of Sleep Disorders, 3rd edition (ICSD-3).[3] Both classification schema define subtypes: sleepwalking, confusional arousals and sleep terrors.

CLINICAL DESCRIPTION

The clinical features common to most children experiencing any of the disorders of arousal include the timing during the nighttime sleep cycle, misperception of and unresponsiveness to the environment, automatic behavior, a high arousal threshold, varying levels of autonomic arousal, and (on waking after an event or in the morning) variable retrograde amnesia. The disorders of arousal typically begin abruptly at the transition from the first period of the deepest phase of non-REM (NREM) sleep (slow-wave sleep, stage N3) of the night (Figures 39.1 and 39.2), which accounts for the typical timing 60 to 90 minutes after sleep onset at the end of the first sleep cycle. The duration of each event can vary from less than 1 minute to over 30 minutes. In most cases, the arousal terminates with the child returning to sleep without ever fully awakening. Although only a single event usually occurs on a given night, some children may have multiple ones. When there are multiple events, they often will recur at 60- to 90-minute intervals during the night, corresponding to subsequent transitions out of slow-wave sleep at the end of each subsequent ultradian sleep cycle, though the arousals may occur at any time during the night. Successive events on the same night tend to be progressively milder.

Although the clinical manifestations of the disorders of arousal occur along a spectrum, for ease of description and to establish a common nomenclature, the DSM-V and ICSD-3 have divided the spectrum of arousal disorders into three distinct entities: sleepwalking, confusional arousals, and sleep terrors; however, in the pediatric literature, no clear distinction is generally made between confusional arousals and sleep terrors. Confusional arousals are much more common in children, especially in young children. Sleep terrors occur much less frequently, are more violent, and typically occur in older children and adolescents. At the mildest end of the clinical spectrum, a child will simply awaken from sleep, sit up in bed, look around briefly, lie back down, and return to sleep. These arousals are rarely noticed unless the child sleeps with a parent. This type of arousal is usually not characterized as a problem by parents and is seldom brought to the attention of the child's physician. These arousals may be noted as an incidental finding in children who are studied by overnight polysomnography for other reasons. At the other end of the spectrum are sleep terrors, which are the most dramatic and least common of the disorders of arousal. They are seen more often in older children and young adults. The events usually begin precipitously with the child bolting upright with a scream. There is generally a high level of autonomic arousal. The eyes are usually open, the heart is racing, and often there is diaphoresis and mydriasis. The facial expression is one of intense fear. A youngster may jump out of bed and run blindly as if to frantically avoid some unseen threat.

Sleepwalking

The presentation of sleepwalking is similar at all ages. At a minimum, there is a partial arousal from sleep with some ambulation. The young child may simply awaken and crawl about in the crib before returning to sleep; such events may go unnoticed unless the child sleeps with another family member. An older child may get up and walk to the parents' room, or he may simply be found asleep at a location different from where he went to bed, with no recollection of having left his bed. Some inappropriate behavior, such as urinating in the closet or next to the toilet, is common. A sleepwalking child may be easily led back to bed, with little evidence of a complete awakening and no recall of the event the next day. Sleepwalking can be triggered in most children by simply standing them up within the first few hours of sleep onset. Because the child is unaware of their environment during a sleepwalking episode, they may be injured or put themselves into dangerous situations during a quiet sleepwalking episode.

Sleepwalking is common in children, as documented in two large, population-based studies by Klackenberg[4] in Sweden, and Laberge and Petit[5,6] in Quebec. Klackenberg studied a group of 212 randomly selected children in Stockholm, longitudinally from ages 6 to 16 years. The prevalence of quiet sleepwalking (occurring at least once during the 10-year data collection period in this group) was 40%. The yearly incidence varied from 6% to 17%, although only 3% had more than one episode per month. In Klackenberg's study, the sleepwalking persisted for 5 years in 33% of children and for over 10 years in 12%.

Laberge[5] and Petit et al.[6] studied 2675 randomly selected children in Quebec who were part of the Québec Longitudinal Study of Child Development conducted by the Québec Institute of Statistics. The parents completed a yearly sleep questionnaire regarding the presence of parasomnias in their children from 2.5 to 13 years of age. Occasional or frequent sleepwalking was present in 14% of the children at some time during that period. The yearly incidence of sleepwalking, as shown in Table 39.1, varied from 2.5% to 7.5%. Table 39.2 describes the ages of onset and offset of sleepwalking and confusional arousals/night terrors. In the majority of these children, the sleepwalking began and ended between the ages of 3 and 13 years. At 13 years of age 3% of the children were still sleepwalking. There was no gender difference in sleepwalking prevalence. In the studies of Laberge, Petit and

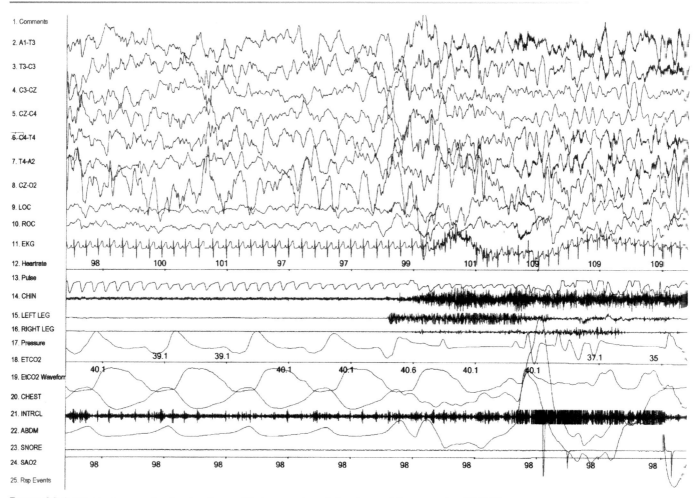

FIGURE 39-1 Polysomnogram of a disorder of arousal that occurred precipitously out of slow-wave sleep(NREM 3).

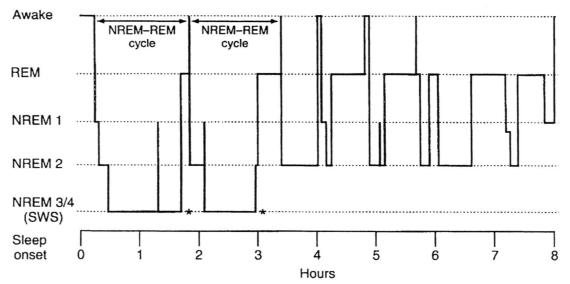

FIGURE 39-2 Idealized sleep hypnogram showing ultradian rhythm through the night. NREM–REM cycles are approximately 90 minutes; the majority of SWS occurs early in the sleep period, and the majority of REM sleep occurs late in the sleep period. Disorders of arousal generally occur during the transition out of SWS (asterisks). NREM, non-REM; REM, rapid eye movement; SWS, short-wave sleep. *Rosen GM, Ferber R, Mahowald MW: Evaluation of parasomnias in children. Child Adolesc Psychiatr Clin North Am 1996;5:601–616.*

TABLE 39.1   Prevalence of Parasomnias at Various Ages in the Same Children

AGE	SLEEPWALKING (%)	CA&NT (%)
2 5	3.3	19.9
3 5	2.5	20.8
4 0	4.1	17.4
5 0	4.8	11.8
6 0	7.8	11.3
11	7.0	3.8
12	6.8	2.3
13	3.3	1.2
Overall	13.8	39.8

CA&NT, confusional arousals and night terrors.

Modified with permission from Laberge L, Tremblay RE, Vitaro F, Montplasir J: Development of parasomnias from childhood to early adolescence. Pediatrics 2000 106:67–74; Petit D, Touchette E, Tremblay R, Boivin M, Montplaisir J: Dysomnias and parasomnias in early childhood. Pediatrics 2007;119:e1016–1025.

TABLE 39.2   Age of Onset and Disappearance of Parasomnias at Various Ages in the Same Children

AGE	SLEEPWALKING (%)	CA&NT (%)
2.5		
Onset	22.7	50.1
3.5		
Onset	13.3	25.8
Disappearance	12.7	15
4.0		
Onset	15.3	12.5
Disappearance	5.3	19
5.0		
Onset	20.7	6.3
Disappearance	13.3	20.2
6.0		
Onset	28.0	5.3
Disappearance	14.7	17.4
11		
Onset	17.2	9.4
Disappearance	18.1	14.8
12		
Onset	12.9	4.0
Disappearance	34.5	11.4
13		
Onset	3.5	2.0
Persisting	24.1	6.7

CA&NT, confusional arousals and night terrors.

Modified with permission from Laberge L, Tremblay RE, Vitaro F, Montplasir J: Development of parasomnias from childhood to early adolescence. Pediatrics 2000 106:67–74; Petit D, Touchette E, Tremblay R, Boivin M, Montplaisir J: Dysomnias and parasomnias in early childhood. Pediatrics 2007;119:e1016–1025.

Klackenburg, sleepwalking was frequently seen in those children who had confusional arousals at a younger age.

Confusional Arousals/Sleep Terrors

The Confusional arousal/sleep terrors seem bizarre and are frightening for parents. The arousal usually starts with some movements and moaning, progressing to crying, often in association with intense thrashing about in the bed or crib. An infant may be described simply as crying inconsolably. These arousals are common in infants and toddlers. The child is typically described as appearing confused, with the eyes open or closed. These events can last anywhere from a few minutes to over 1 hour, with 5 to 15 minutes being typical. Even if the child calls for the parents, the child often does not recognize them. Even vigorous attempts to wake the child are often unsuccessful. Holding and cuddling usually do not provide reassurance; instead, the child often resists, twists, and pushes away and may become more agitated. It is the parents' inability to comfort their child, who appears to be in great distress, that is often of the greatest concern to them.

In the studies of Laberge[3] and Petit,[6] there was no distinction between confusional arousals, sleep terrors, and night terrors. However, from the age distribution and the description of the events, the current nomenclature would characterize these as confusional arousals. In the Laberge and Petit studies, the prevalence of confusional arousals between the ages of 2.5 and 6 years was 39.8% (see Table 39.1). The yearly incidence was 19.9% at age 2.5 years , 11.3% at age 6 years, 3.8% at 11 years of age, and 1.2% at 13 years of age . In 85% of the children the confusional arousals first appeared between the ages of 3 and 10 years, and in the majority of these children, they disappeared before the age of 10 years (see Table 39.2). The confusional arousals persisted beyond 13 years of age in 6.7% of the children.

In the studies of Laberge, Petit, and Klackenberg, sleepwalking and confusional arousals were often seen in the same child at different ages Thirty-six percent of the children with sleepwalking in the study of Laberge had confusional arousals as preschoolers, and all of the children with confusional arousals in Klackenburg's study had at least one episode of sleepwalking when they were older.

PATHOPHYSIOLOGY OF DISORDERS OF AROUSAL

Disorders of arousal are best understood as a dissociated state during which elements of wakefulness, and NREM sleep occur simultaneously resulting in behavior that is neither fully awake or fully asleep. This concept, first put forward by Mahowald[7,8] is consistent with the current understanding of sleep neurophysiology. During the disorders of arousal, some facets of wakefulness appear during the transition out of slow-wave sleep. This usually occurs at the end of the first sleep cycle. As a consequence, the transition out of slow-wave sleep, which is usually behaviorally inapparent, can be dramatic. The child appears caught between deep NREM sleep and wakefulness. The child's behavior at this time has elements that we associate with wakefulness (walking, talking, crying, running) complex motor behaviors) and sleeping (misperception of and unresponsiveness to the environment, high arousal threshold, amnesia, automatic behavior) occurring simultaneously. The EEG during these arousals from sleep is typically characterized by a mixture of waking and sleeping rhythms with the simultaneous occurrence of alpha, theta, and delta frequencies, and suggests that different areas of the brain are in different states simultaneously. This dissociated state is inherently unstable, and eventually one state is fully declared. In most cases, the child appears to simply return to quiet sleep. Alternatively, the child may awaken totally but will have no recall of the arousal and will usually rapidly return to sleep.

The causes of the disorders of arousal are multifactorial. Genetic predisposition, homeostatic drive, sleep–wake cycling and synchronization, and behavioral and emotional states all seem to play some role in the clinical appearance of the disorders of arousal. Of these factors, genetic predisposition is probably the most important, though the mechanism is unknown. Sleep–wake cycling and synchronization are affected by age, homeostatic factors, circadian factors, hormones, and drugs. Affective disorders, anxiety, and environmental stress have all been identified as important factors in the appearance of the disorders of arousal in clinical studies,[9,10] although the mechanisms by which these factors lead to the arousal is not known.

GENETICS OF DISORDERS OF AROUSAL

A familial predisposition toward the disorders of arousal has been recognized since these disorders were first described. The genetics of the disorders of arousal has been explored by Hublin et al.[11,12] and Nguyen et al.[13] (in population-based twin studies) and also by Lecendreux.[14] In Hublin's retrospective study of adults the phenotypic variance of sleepwalking was attributable to genetic factors at 65%, which he believed was the result of many genes, each with minor effects. In Nguyen's study, environmental information was gathered in an attempt to understand the relative contribution of genetic, shared environmental, and non-shared environmental factors leading to confusional arousals in children. They concluded that the best explanation was a two-component model with 44% of the variance explained by genetic factors and 56% of the variance explained by non-shared environmental factors. These results are consistent with the results of Lecendreux, who looked at human leukocyte antigens and sleepwalking. The familial predisposition to disorders of arousal may be secondary to the familial aggregation of restless leg syndrome or sleep-disordered breathing, which are recognized as triggers for disorders of arousal.[18] A positive family history of a first-degree relative with a disorder of arousal is present in 60% of the children with a disorder of arousal compared with 30% in children without disorders of arousal.

SLEEP HOMEOSTASIS AND DISORDERS OF AROUSAL

There is good theoretical support and some experimental evidence that the familial predisposition toward the disorders of arousal is mediated by the genetic control of the of the sleep homeostatic process. This process has been shown to be under strong genetic control in animal studies.[16] Studies in mice have demonstrated that sleep loss leads to an increase in homeostatic drive, with a change in slow-wave sleep activity as measured by delta power, in a dose–response fashion that varies with the duration of prior wakefulness and is different in different genotypes. A quantitative trait–loci analysis revealed that this trait is the product of multiple genes. Human EEG studies have also shown that slow-wave sleep and EEG slow-wave activity are markers for measuring homeostatic drive.[17–19] Increases in slow-wave sleep and slow-wave activity occur after sleep deprivation and decline after sleep. The synchronization of the homeostatic and circadian processes optimizes the quality of sleep and wakefulness. This

interaction is described in a comprehensive article by Dijk and Lockley.[18] Adequate sleep duration occurs only when the circadian and homeostatic systems are fully synchronized. The clinical implication of this observation is that a child with an irregular and/or chaotic sleep–wake schedule will simply not be able to have optimum synchronization of the homeostatic and circadian systems; this inevitably leads to sleep disruption and sleep deprivation, which may lead to a clinical event in a child who may be predisposed to the disorders of arousal.

POLYSOMNOGRAPHY IN DISORDERS OF AROUSAL

Polysomnographic studies have shown that individuals with the disorders of arousal, when compared with normal control subjects, have no consistent differences in sleep efficiency or sleep stage distribution.[20] However, there are subtle differences in the cyclic alternating patterns and arousal rates,[21,22] arousals from slow-wave sleep,[22] and slow-wave sleep activity delta counts between the sleep of patients with the disorders of arousal and that of control subjects.[20] These differences are the most prominent during the first sleep cycle, which is when the disorders of arousal usually occur. There were increased numbers of brief EEG arousals from slow-wave sleep, decreases in slow-wave sleep activity delta counts at the end of the first ultradian cycle, and increases in arousals from the cyclic alternating patterns compared with control subjects. The subjects for these research studies were carefully screened for the presence of sleep-disordered breathing, sleep deprivation, and restless legs syndrome.

Sleep-disordered breathing and restless legs syndrome with periodic limb movements have both been identified as triggers for disorders of arousal.[18,23] In children with these comorbid sleep disorders, the disorders of arousal disappeared after adenotonsillectomy in the children with sleep-disordered breathing and after drug treatment in the children with restless legs syndrome, suggesting that these clinical causes of sleep disruption can unmask a disorder of arousal.

Several lines of evidence suggest that the fundamental abnormality that underpins the disorders of arousal is the instability of slow-wave sleep. This conclusion is supported by the clinical observation and experimental evidence that in individuals predisposed to the disorders of arousal, an event is much more likely to occur after a night of sleep deprivation[24] or after sleep fragmentation from sleep apnea or periodic movements of sleep that increases the homeostatic drive and would be expected to make an unstable homeostatic system more unstable.

CLINICAL EVALUATION OF CHILDREN WITH DISORDERS OF AROUSAL

The children described in this chapter will generally present with the complaint of unusual nocturnal awakenings. It is important to recognize that there are many causes of unusual nocturnal awakenings in children. The most important tool for evaluating children with unusual nocturnal awakenings is a complete sleep and medical history. The sleep history will usually allow the clinician to distinguish between the different causes of unusual nocturnal arousals and to formulate an appropriate evaluation and treatment plan. The facets of the

Box 39-1   Sleep History

- Circadian
  - Sleep log for 2 weeks (time in bed, sleep onset, awakening time) (weekdays/weekends)
  - Vacation sleep schedule
  - 24-hour daily schedule of activities (school, work, meals, play)
  - Amount of light in room
  - Seasonal variations
  - Preferred sleep time and duration
- Sleep Environment
  - Describe bedroom (What is in it? Who is there? How much natural light is there? Is there a television or radio?)
- Sleep Onset
  - How does the child fall asleep?
  - Who is present at sleep onset and what do they do?
  - Are there curtain calls, fears, hypnagogic hallucinations, sleep-onset paralysis, restless legs, head banging, body rocking?
- Arousals
  - Time of night, frequency
  - Triggers, association with injury
  - Description of the way in which the arousal terminates
  - Level of agitation/manner in which the ambulation child returns to sleep?
  - Association with eating and drinking, recall the next day
  - Level of consciousness, age of onset
  - Duration
- Other Sleep Behavior
  - Seizures, enuresis, diaphoresis, restlessness, snoring, cough, choking, apnea, periodic movements of sleep, vomiting, nightmares, bruxism
- Waking Behavior
  - Hypnopompic hallucinations, paralysis, headaches
- Daytime Sleep
  - Naps, cataplexy, excessive daytime sleepiness, settings where sleep occurs
- Medical
  - Neurologic: Migraine headaches, attention-deficit disorder, seizures, tics, mental retardation, narcolepsy, neuromuscular disease
  - Psychiatric: Depression, anxiety, dissociative disorders, conduct disorder, panic disorder, physical/sexual abuse, post-traumatic stress disorder
  - Ear, Nose, Throat: Ear infections, ear effusions, nasal airway obstruction, sinusitis, streptococci infections
  - Cardiorespiratory: Asthma, cough, heart disease, pneumonia
  - Gastrointestinal: Vomiting, diarrhea, constipation, swallowing problems
  - Growth: Failure to thrive
  - Allergies: Milk, seasonal, asthma, eczema
  - Drug: Legal/illegal, prescription
  - School/behavior: School/developmental problems, behavioral problems
  - Acute medical illness
- Family History
  - Sleep apnea/snoring
  - Arousals (sleepwalking, confusional arousals, night terrors, restless legs/periodic movements)
  - Psychiatric condition (depression, anxiety)
  - Social issues (stress at home, divorce, family violence, drug/ethyl alcohol use)
  - Narcolepsy, hypersomnolence
  - Restless legs syndrome
  - Delayed/advanced sleep phase

sleep history that are the most important in the evaluation of the disorders of arousal are listed in Box 39.1. Any problem that causes sleep disruption, which results in awakenings, or affects sleep duration or synchronization can lead to the appearance of the disorders of arousal in a child.

There are a number of distinguishing clinical characteristics in the histories of children with the disorders of arousal. The salient features are listed and discussed below.
- *Timing*: The first event generally though not always occurs about 60–90 minutes after sleep onset. If a second event occurs during the night, it typically occurs 90 minutes after the first, at the time of the transition out of slow-wave sleep. Arousals occurring within 30 minutes of sleep onset, or awakening from sleep in the morning, are more likely to represent unusual sleep-related seizures.
- *Description of the event*: The onset can be gradual, with sleepwalking and confusional arousals, or sudden, with sleep terrors. The behavior during an event is often bizarre and may be complex but is not stereotypical. The child is not normally responsive to the environment, although he or she may be partially responsive. A child will not typically recognize parents and often cannot be comforted by them. The events generally terminate with a return to sleep and without a complete awakening.
- *Frequency*: The frequency of occurrence is highly variable, from several times a night to once in a lifetime; multiple episodes in a single night may occur but are uncommon.

- *Level of consciousness*: This child is generally not arousable.
- *Memory of event*: Most children will have no recall the day after the event.
- *Daytime sleepiness*: Most children have no evidence of daytime sleepiness the next day.
- *Family history*: The family history is often positive in parents and siblings for any of the disorders of arousal.

Box 39.2 lists those conditions that mimic the disorders of arousal and those that may trigger them. The conditions that may mimic the disorders of arousal include seizures, particularly nocturnal frontal lobe seizures;[25,26] cluster headaches; psychiatric disorders such as nocturnal panic attacks, post-traumatic stress disorder, and nocturnal dissociative disorder; nightmares; REM sleep behavior disorder; and rhythmic movements of sleep. The conditions that may trigger disorders of arousal in a child include obstructive sleep apnea, the periodic movements of sleep, gastroesophageal reflux, behavioral or psychiatric disorders, sleep deprivation, and an irregular sleep–wake schedule. The last two of these are the most common and most easily corrected triggers for the disorders of arousal.

The distinction between disorders of arousal and sleep related seizures is often difficult to make. The most consistent clinical difference between seizures and disorders of arousal are that seizures are usually stereotypical events, which can occur at any time throughout the night. Seizures occur exclusively during sleep 30% of the time, and may not always have abnormal EEG correlates recorded from routine surface

Box 39-2 Conditions That Mimic or Trigger Disorders of Arousal

- Neurologic
  *Seizures
  *Cluster headaches
- Medical
  †Obstructive sleep apnea
  †Gastroesophageal reflux
- Behavioral/Psychiatric
  *Conditioned arousals
  *Post-traumatic stress disorder
  *Nocturnal dissociative state
  *Nocturnal panic
- Sleep
  *Nightmares
  *Rhythmic movements of sleep
  *Rapid eye movement sleep behavior disorders
  †Periodic movements of sleep
  †Sleep deprivation
  †Irregular sleep–wake schedule

*Conditions that mimic disorders of arousal.
†Conditions that trigger disorders of arousal.

TABLE 39.3 Comparison of Disorders of Arousal and Seizures

CLINICAL CHARACTERISTICS	DISORDER OF AROUSAL	SEIZURES
Age of onset (typical)	2–10 years	Any age
Timing of event	60–90 minutes after sleep onset	Any time of night, often multiple times during night, often at sleep onset or upon awakening
Sleep stage	Arises at end of stage N3	Arises out of stage N1,N2
Duration	2–60 minutes	1–2 minutes
Description of event	Variable, quiet-agitated	Stereotypical, repetitive
Family history	Positive	Positive for NFLE
EEG/PSG	Sudden arousal from stage N3, mixed alpha, theta, delta, OSA/PLMS	Normal, spikes may be present, focal or generalized
Triggering events	OSA, PLMS, fever, sleep deprivation, irregular sleep	None
Amnesia	Yes	Yes
Daytime behavior	Normal, no EDS	Often EDS

electrodes , especially in children with nocturnal frontal lobe epilepsy.[25,26] Evaluation in specialized centers is often necessary to establish the correct diagnosis and to develop an appropriate treatment. See Table 39.3 for comparison between disorders of arousal and seizures.

POLYSOMNOGRAPHY

The American Academy of Sleep Medicine has published a review of the non-repiratory indications for PSG in children.[27,28] Polysomnography using an expanded EEG montage was indicated in children to confirm the diagnosis of an atypical or potentially injurious parasomnias, to differeentiate a parasomnia from sleep related epilepsy, or to identify when sleep-disordered breathing or PLMD is believed to be contributing to frequent parasomnias or control of seizures. Polysomnography was not indicated for the evaluation of children with typical parasomnias or confirmed sleep related epilepsy.[27,28] The routine use of polysomnography in the evaluation of the disorders of arousal is limited because the sleep macroarchitecture in children with these disorders is generally normal. The primary role of polysomnography in the evaluation of children with suspected disorders of arousal is to rule out other sleep disorders and nocturnal seizures, which may either trigger or mimic the disorders of arousal.

If nocturnal seizures are suspected, based on the history of the stereotypical nature or the timing of the arousals throughout the sleep period or if there is an increased likelihood of seizures because of a concomitant neurologic problem, further diagnostic studies should be obtained. In most clinical settings, sleep-related seizures can be best evaluated with sleep-deprived EEG or an overnight study in an EEG telemetry unit. These children should be evaluated in a sleep lab only if the lab staff are experienced in the diagnosis and treatment of sleep-related seizures.

TREATMENT OF CHILDREN WITH DISORDERS OF AROUSAL

The most appropriate treatment for the child with a disorder of arousal will depend on the diagnosis. Before considering a treatment strategy, one must have completed a comprehensive medical, neurologic, and sleep evaluation such as the one described in this chapter. If the disorders of arousal are thought to be the most likely cause of the awakenings, the treatment may include some or all of the following recommendations, but one should start with the first five items listed, which represent essential components in any effective treatment plan for children with the disorders of arousal.

- *Education* of the parents and their children about the benign, self-limiting nature of the disorders of arousal. Discuss the pathophysiology of these disorders in a manner that is comprehensible to both the child and parents. *Child safety* is of paramount concern in managing children with the disorders of arousal. During an event, children can put themselves in danger such as by walking out of the house or by running into a glass door. In most cases, these concerns can be addressed using a simple, commonsense approach. The child should not sleep on the upper level of a bunk bed, obstructions should be removed from the room, double-cylinder locks may need to be installed on the doors of the house, or a security system (alerting the parents that a door or window has been opened) may need to be installed.
- *Demystification* of the disorders of arousal. The parents often misunderstand the problem and fear that the intensity of the arousal reflects severe psychological distress.
- *Sleep extension and schedule regularization* should always be considered. Sleep deprivation and an irregular sleep–wake schedule are very common problems for children and are often causally related to the appearance of these disorders
- *Elimination of caffeine* if its use is identified.

- *Institution of a bedtime routine that is pleasant for both the parent and the child,* ideally one ending within 15 minutes of the transition to sleep. If there is conflict at bedtime, if sleep onset latency is prolonged, or if the child is fearful or requires close contact with a parent, these issues may need to be addressed.
- *Medication* may be a good short-term strategy, in a child with frequent, disruptive, or potentially dangerous arousals, while other nonpharmacologic modalities are initiated. Medication has been described as an effective treatment for the disorders of arousal in several series of case reports, although it has not been the subject of well-controlled studies , and no medications are FDA approved for the treatment of disorders of arousal. Clonazepam[29,30] has been the most widely used off-label medication for the treatment of disorders of arousal. Clinicians should be cautious when begining pharmacotherapy for these disorders in children because in most cases the events are benign and self-limiting and have no direct, adverse impact on the child. If medication is used, it should be given 1–1.5 hours before the anticipated sleep onset to ensure that there are adequate drug levels in the brain at the beginning of the night, when these disorders are most likely to occur. The beginning dose of clonazepam is generally 0.125 mg, increasing until the arousals are eliminated, or the appearance of side effects. Once the arousals are eliminated, continuation of medication for 4–6 weeks, during which time the family can work on sleep extension and regularization of the schedule. This allows everyone in the family to recover from the effects of the previous sleep disruption. Thereafter, the medication can be gradually tapered to ascertain if the arousals recur. If there is a recurrence of the arousals there needs to be a discussion of the risks and benefits of longer-term use of medication. If medications are used long term, an attempt at a medication taper , and a reassesment of possible triggers and mimics, should be done every 3–6 months.
- In adolescents, one should discuss the potential risks posed by the disorders of arousal when the teen moves out of the home, and the impact of alcohol use, sleep restriction, and an irregular sleep schedule.
- *Scheduled* awakening is a behavioral treatments for confusional arousals that has been described anecdotally in the literature first by Lask.[31] Although it is not clear why this intervention is helpful, several case reports have described its efficacy.[31,32] The recommended treatment is simple enough: the child is awakened 15 to 30 minutes before the usual time of the arousal and needs to open his or her eyes and at least mumble a response before being allowed to return to sleep. The parents continue this intervention nightly for 1 month. In some cases this simple intervention has been effective. However, it should be noted that in some cases these scheduled awakenings actually trigger an arousal or cause one that usually occurs early in the night to occur later.
- *Relaxation and/or mental imagery and biofeedback* are behavioral approaches that have been described in case reports as being useful treatments for the disorders of arousal in school-aged children.[34]
- *Psychotherapy and counseling* are important interventions for any child who has evidence of significant psychological distress. However, a disorder of arousal is not a symptom of a psychological problem.

SUMMARY

To the casual observer, the disorders of arousal represent a paradox during which an individual appears to engage in waking behavior while still asleep. With the understanding that sleep and wakefulness are not always mutually exclusive states of being, the paradox disappears. The concept of state dissociation provides an explanation for these events that is founded in the current understanding of the neurophysiology of sleep. The disorders of arousal are common problems, especially in young children, and can usually be fully evaluated and treated by a knowledgeable sleep clinician without the use of high technology.

Clinical Pearls

- The timing of all of the disorders of arousal is most often 1–1.5 hours after sleep onset. This can be one of the most useful clinical signs for differentiating disorders of arousal from other causes of sudden arousals from sleep.
- Disorders of arousal rarely have a stereotypical character.
- Regularization and extension of nocturnal sleep are important interventions.
- During any of the disorders of arousal children can put themselves in harm's way, making a discussion of safety with the children (especially adolescents) and their parents a necessary part of the treatment plan.

References

1. Broughton RJ. Sleep disorders: Disorders of arousal? Science 1968; 159:1070–8.
2. American Psychiatric Association. Diagnostic and statistical manual of mental disorders. 5th ed. Arlington, VA: APA; 2013.
3. American academy of sleep medicine. International classification of sleep disorders. Diagnostic and coding manual. 3rd ed. Westchester, Illinois: American Academy of Sleep Medicine; 2014.
4. Klackenberg G. Somnambulism in childhood – prevalence, course and behavioral correlates: A prospective longitudinal study (6-16 years). Acta Paediatr Scand 1982;71:495–9.
5. Laberge L, Tremblay RE, Vitaro F, et al. Development of parasomnias from childhood to early adolescence. Pediatrics 2000;106:67–74.
6. Petit D, Touchette E, Tremblay R, et al. Dyssomnias and parasomnias in early childhood. Pediatrics 2007;119:e1016–25.
7. Mahowald MW, Schenck CH. Dissociated states of wakefulness and sleep. Neurology 1992;42:44–52.
8. Mahowald M, Cramer Bornemin C, Schenck C. State dissociation, human behavior, and consciousness. Curr Topics Med Chem 2011;11: 2392–402.
9. Simonds JF, Parago H. Sleep behavior and disorders in children and adolescents evaluated at psychiatry clinics. Dev Behav Pediatr 1984; 6:6–10.
10. Dahl RE, Puig-Antich J. Sleep disturbance in children and adolescent psychiatric disorders. Pediatrician 1990;167:32–7.
11. Hublin C, Kaprio J, Partinen M, et al. Prevalence and genetics of sleep-walking: A population-based twin study. Neurology 1997;48:177–81.
12. Hublin C, Kaprio J, Partinen M, et al. Parasomnias: Co-occurrence and genetics. Psychiatr Gen 2001;11:65–70.
13. Nguyen B, Perusse D, Paquet J, et al. Sleep terrors in children: A prospective study of twins. Pediatrics 2008;122:e1164–7.
14. Lecendreux M, Bassetti C, Dauvilliers Y, et al. HLA and genetic susceptibility to sleepwalking. Mcl Psychiatry 2003;8:114–17.
15. Cao M, Guilleminault C. Families with sleepwalking. Sleep Med 2010;11:726–34.
16. Franken P, Chollet D, Tafti M. The homeostatic regulation of sleep need is under genetic control. J Neurosci 2001;21:2610–21.
17. Dijk DJ, Czeisler CA. Contribution of the circadian pacemaker and the sleep homeostat to sleep propensity, sleep structure, electroencephalographic slow waves, and sleep spindle activity in humans. J Neurosci 1995;15:3526–38.

18. Dijk DJ, Lockley SW. Functional genomics of sleep and circadian rhythm: Integration of human sleep-wake regulation and circadian rhythmicity (invited lecture). J Appl Physiol 2002;92:852–62.

19. Gaudreau H, Joncas S, Zadra A, et al. Dynamics of slow-wave activity during the NREM sleep of sleepwalkers and control subjects. Sleep 2000;23:755–60.

20. Guilleminault C, Poyares D, Aftab FA, et al. Sleep and wakefulness in somnambulism: A spectral analysis study. J Psychosom Res 2001;51:411–16.

21. Zuconi M, Oldani A. Arousal fluctuation in non-rapid eye movement parasomnias: The role of cyclic alternating pattern as a measure of sleep instability. J Clin Neurophysiol 1995;12:147–54.

22. Smirne S, Ferini-Strambi L. Clinical applications of cyclic alternating pattern. In: Comi G, Lucking C, Kimura J, et al, editors. Clinical neurophysiology: from receptors to perception. Philadelphia: Elsevier Science; 1999. p. 109–12.

23. Guilleminault C, Palombini L, Pelayo R, et al. Sleepwalking and sleep terrors in prepubertal children: What triggers them? Pediatrics 2003;111:e17–25.

24. Joncas S, Zadra A, Paquet J, et al. The value of sleep deprivation as a diagnostic tool in adult sleepwalkers. Neurology 2002;58:936–40.

25. Tinuper P, Provini F, Bisulli F, et al. Movement disorders in sleep: guidelines for differentiating epileptic from non-epileptic motor phenomena arising from sleep. Sleep Med Rev 2007;11:255–67.

26. Mallow BA. Paroxysmal events in sleep. J Clin Neurophysiol 2002;19:522–34.

27. Kotagal S, Nichols C, Grigg-Danberger M, et al. Non-respiratory indications for polysomnography and related procedures in children: an evidenced-based review. Sleep 2012;35:1451–66.

28. Aurora R, Lamm C, Zak R, et al. Practice parameters for the non-respiratory indications for polysomnography and multiple sleep latency testing for children. Sleep 2012;35:1467–73.

29. Mahowald M, Schenck C. NREM parasomnias. Neurol Clin N Am 1996;14:675–96.

30. Dahl R. The pharmacologic treatment of sleep disorders. Psych Clin North Am 1992;15:161–78.

31. Lask B. Novel and non-toxic treatment for night terrors. Br Med J 1988;297:592.

32. Tobin J. Treatment of somnambulism with anticipatory awakening. J Pediatr 1993;122:426–7.

33. Frank C, Spirito A. The use of scheduled awakenings to eliminate childhood sleepwalking. J Pediatr Psychol 1997;22:345–53.

34. Kohen DP, Mahowald MW, Rosen GM. Sleep-terror disorder in children: The role of self hypnosis in management. Am J Clin Hypnosis 1991;4:233–44.

REM Behavior Disorder

Stephen H. Sheldon and Darius A. Loughmanee

REM sleep behavior disorder (RBD) is classified as a parasomnia usually associated with REM sleep. It has been defined as abnormal behaviors occurring during REM sleep that may cause injury to self or others or may result in sleep disruption.[1] Alternate names include *onirism*; stage 1 REM sleep, REM sleep without atonia, paradoxical sleep without atonia, and REM sleep motor parasomnia (RMP). As RBD has been noted only sporadically in the pediatric sleep medicine literature and consists mostly of case reports, the latter terminology (RMP) appears more appropriate when referring to this symptom complex in children and adolescents. It is unclear whether this complex and polysomnographic findings have similar implications in the pediatric population when compared to adults.

In 1975, a disorganized relation of tonic and phasic events during REM sleep was described in a patient with a tumor located in the brainstem.[2] RBD as a clinical entity was described by Schenck and colleagues in 1986 as a parasomnia that typically occurred in older male patients[3] and was associated with synucleinopathic degenerative disorders (for example Parkinson disease, Lewy body dementia, and multiple system atrophy).[4,5] Certain medications have also been associated with RBD in adults including serotonin reuptake inhibitors.[6] Although symptoms of RBD in childhood and adolescence were thought to be rare, there is increasing information that RBD, or a disorder that may fulfill criteria for this diagnosis, exists in the pediatric population.[7-9]

Dream reports and nightmares are common in childhood.[10] NREM sleep partial arousal disorders are also common. Differentiation of REM dream reports and mentation during partial arousals from NREM sleep is at times problematic since children will often report a story line when asked if they were having a 'nightmare' regardless of dream content, making diagnosis using adult criteria difficult. Similarly, since there are no systematic studies of RBD/RMP in children and adolescents and literature consists mainly of case reports, it is difficult to conclude RBD in adults and RBD/RMP in children are manifestations of the same disorder. Putative pathophysiological etiologies are speculative and complex.[11]

Symptoms of RBD/RMP in children and adolescents are based on clinical history of movement and apparent dream enactment. Nonetheless, this may often be difficult to clinically differentiate from confusional arousals where there may be a report of a dream of being chased or attacked, agitation, and unusual and/or aggressive movements during a spell. Time of night and a history of NREM parasomnia may be helpful in differentiation. Symptoms of RBD in adults include talking, laughing, shouting, gesturing, and reaching, grabbing, arm flailing, punching, kicking, sitting up, leaping from bed, crawling, and running. Quiet walking is uncommon. These symptoms can be similar to symptoms classically associated with NREM partial arousal disorders including but not limited to sleep terrors, agitated sleepwalking, and confusional arousals. They may also be seen in patients with paroxysmal hypnogenic dystonia.

An essential feature of RBD/RMP is dream enactment.[1] This appears to be due to absence of normal REM sleep skeletal muscle atonia. Paradoxical muscle activity results in gross complex body movements allowing for 'acting out' dreams. Adults can typically report vivid dream recall following a spell. Dream recall may be more difficult to elicit and content may not be as clear in the pediatric patient.

Abnormalities of REM sleep that appear during polysomnographic recording include augmentation of chin muscle tone, increased chin or limb phasic twitching, excessive episodic limb movements, gross body jerking, somewhat purposeful movements and/or vocalizations, and occasional violent behavior.

Assessment of symptoms suggesting RBD/RMP can be problematic in children. This is particularly true of the dream report. Pediatric patients communicate perceptions differently than adults, tend to be more concrete in descriptions, and there may be impairment in the ability to adequately verbalize symptoms and/or dream content. Additionally, there may be considerable 'programming' of the child's report by parents/caretakers. When clinical history is difficult to interpret, the child's behavior at the time of the dream might be helpful.[8]

Medical and scientific literature regarding RBD/RMP in children consists mainly of case reports. In 1975, Barros-Ferreira et al. described an 8-year-old female with an infiltrating pontine tumor.[2] The patient presented with symptoms of agitation at night along with mouth movements, somniloquy, and laughing during sleep. These clinical findings were associated with reported disorganized relationships of phasic and tonic REM sleep. Subsequently, Schenck and colleagues[12] described a syndrome of excessive restlessness and complex stereotypic movements during sleep in a 10-year-old following the removal of a midline cerebellar astrocytoma. These were associated with intermittent loss of REM atonia associated with some of these complex movements and frequent episodic limb movements in REM and NREM sleep. Interestingly, the patient's 8-year-old brother had similar polysomnographic findings, without clinical symptoms.

In 1998, five patients who were evaluated for unusual behaviors during sleep associated with unusual nightmares, displacement from the bed, and sleep-related motor activity were reported.[7] Dissociated state of REM sleep was suspected because limb movements and/or body movements were associated with vivid dream recall, nightmares associated with dream enactment, or injurious motor activity during sleep. Five matched comparison subjects who had been referred for evaluation of pediatric obstructive sleep apnea were chosen since movement and electrocortical arousals were common following occlusive and/or partially occlusive respiratory events, particularly during REM sleep. There were more reports of nightmares, excessive muscle tone during REM sleep, more frequent gross body movements, and increased phasic chin muscle activity (without increased eye movement activity) during REM sleep in subjects with RMP.

REM sleep motor abnormalities have also been reported in patients with autistic spectrum disorder,[13] seizures,[14] post-traumatic stress disorder,[15] hereditary quivering chin with tongue biting,[16] and Tourette's syndrome.[17]

Nevsimalova and colleagues have reported RMP as the presenting symptom of narcolepsy–cataplexy in two children.[18] Presenting symptoms included excessive daytime sleepiness and sporadic cataplectic attacks. Diagnosis of narcolepsy–cataplexy was established based on short sleep latency on standard MSLT testing, multiple sleep onset REM periods, low cerebrospinal fluid hypocretin levels, and the presence of human leukocyte antigen (HLA)-*DQB1*0602*. Along with the onset of EDS and cataplexy, the patients exhibited restless sleep, nightmares, and movements during sleep, somniloquy, and harmful behaviors. RBD has been reported in about one-third of adults with narcolepsy-cataplexy.[19]

Lloyd and colleagues[9] retrospectively evaluated 15 patients with symptoms of RMP and REM sleep without atonia. Mean age at diagnosis was 9.5 years with a range of 3–17 years. Nightmares were reported in 13 of the patients. Excessive daytime sleepiness was noted in about half. Other comorbid states included anxiety, attention deficit disorder, developmental delay, Smith–Magenis syndrome, pervasive developmental disorder, narcolepsy, idiopathic hypersomnia, and Moebius syndrome. Reviewing both presentations and response to therapy (including benzodiazepine, melatonin) and response to discontinuing a tricyclic medication, it was concluded that RMP may be associated with neurological abnormalities, narcolepsy, or medication. It seems to be distinct from NREM partial-arousal disorders and adult RBD. Although Rye and colleagues[23] reported REM sleep without atonia, dream enactment, and excessive daytime sleepiness in a patient with juvenile Parkinson's disease, neurodevelopmental disorders, narcolepsy, and medication effect occur in some patients, but specific neurodegenerative disorder appears to be quite uncommon.

Limited evidence exists regarding appropriate treatment for RMP in children. Treatments have typically been guided by those that have been successful in adults. About 90% of adult patients with RBD clinically respond well to clonazepam at doses from 0.5 to 2.0 mg.[20] Use of clonazepam may be limited in children due to its long half-life and duration of action. A shorter-acting benzodiazepine (for example, lorazepam) may be better tolerated by children and anecdotally has been as effective as clonazepam without a residual daytime 'hangover' effect noted to be associated with long-acting benzodiazepines. In adults, there has been little, if any, tendency for the development of tolerance, dependency, abuse, or sleep disruption with clonazepam for long-term treatment of RBD.

In summary, RMP appears to represent state dissociation during REM sleep associated with paradoxical motor activity and vivid dream recall that can result in injury in children and adolescents. This motor dyscontrol may be a final common pathway for a variety of disorders ranging from narcolepsy–cataplexy, to post-traumatic stress disorder,[7,16,17] and autistic spectrum disorder.[8,21] Interestingly, early in development, motor activity during REM sleep is common and normal, resulting in the term 'active sleep.' Therefore, RMP may also occur in otherwise normal children and represent dysfunction of maturation, particularly in the pontine tegmental region.[21,22] By clinical history alone, other more commonly recognized childhood parasomnias, such as confusional arousals, sleepwalking, and sleep terrors, might be considered. However, these NREM partial-arousal disorders are characteristically associated with amnesia for the event, absence of vivid dream recall, and occur during the first third to first half of the sleep period. Nonetheless, diagnosis can be difficult and requires a high index of suspicion. When symptoms suggestive of RMP occur in children or adolescents, underlying etiologies and/or comorbidities require comprehensive evaluation. RMP requires further research and longitudinal studies aimed at epidemiology, pathophysiology, and predictive significance of REM sleep motor dyscontrol during childhood.

CHAPTER SUMMARY

REM behavior disorder, or REM motor parasomnia (RMP), is rare in children. This disorder is typified by abnormal behaviors occurring during REM sleep that may cause injury to the child or others. Symptoms can include talking, laughing, shouting, gesturing, flailing, punching, kicking, sitting up, leaping from the bed, crawling, or running. This chapter reviews the presentation, comorbid states, and treatment of RMP, and discusses the means of differentiating it from NREM parasomnias.

Clinical Pearls

- RMP represents state dissociation during REM sleep associated with motor activity and vivid dream recall.
- RMP can be differentiated from NREM parasomnias by the presence of vivid dream recall, memory of the episode, and the occurrence of the episode in the last half to two thirds of the night.
- If RMP is noted in a patient with no other known comorbidities further evaluation for narcolepsy or post-traumatic stress disorder should be considered.

References

1. American Academy of Sleep Medicine. International classification of sleep disorders, 2nd edn. Diagnostic and coding manual. Westchester, Illinois: American Academy of Sleep Medicine; 2005.
2. Barros-Ferreira M, Chodkiewicz J-P, Lairy GC, et al. Disorganized relations of tonic and diphasic events of REM sleep in a case of brain-stem tumour. Electroencephalogr Clin Neurophysiol 1975;38:203–7.
3. Schenck CH, Bundlie SR, Ettinger MG, et al. Chronic behavioral disorders of human REM sleep: A new category of parasomnia. Sleep 1986;9:293–308.
4. Boeve BF, Silber MH, Parisi JE, et al. Synucleinopathy pathology and REM sleep behavior disorder plus dementia or Parkinsonism. Neurology 2003;61:40–5.
5. Postuma RB, Gagnon, JF, Vendette M, et al. Quantifying the risk of neurodegenerative disease in idiopathic REM sleep behavior disorder. Neurology 2009;72:1296–300.
6. Schenck CH, Mahowald MW, Kim SW, et al. Prominent eye movements during NREM sleep and REM sleep behavior disorder associated with fluoxetine treatment of depression and obsessive-compulsive disorder. Sleep 1992;15:226–35.

7. Sheldon SH, Jacobsen J. REM-sleep motor disorder in children. J Child Neurol 1998;13:257–60.

8. Stores G. Rapid eye movement sleep behaviour disorder in children and adolescents. Dev Med Child Neurol 2008;50:728–32.

9. Lloyd R, Tippmann-Peikert M, Slocumb N, et al. Characteristics of REM sleep behavior disorder in childhood. J Clin Sleep Med 2012; 8:127–31.

10. Sheldon SH. The parasomnias. In: Sheldon SH, Ferber R, Kryger MH, editors. Principles and practice of pediatric sleep medicine. Philadelphia: Elsevier/Saunders; 2005. p. 305–15.

11. Boeve BF, Silber MH, Saper CB, et al. Pathophysiology of REM sleep behavior disorder and relevance to neurodegenerative disease. Brain 2007;130:2770–88.

12. Schenck CH, Bundlie SR, Smith SA, et al. REM behavior disorder in a 10-year-old girl and aperiodic REM and NREM sleep movements in an 8-year-old brother. Sleep Res 1986;15:162.

13. Thirumalai SS, Shubin RA, Robinson R. Rapid eye movement sleep behavior disorder in children with autism. J Child Neurol 2002;17: 173–8.

14. Cipolli C, Bonanni E, Maestri M, et al. Dream experience during REM and NREM sleep of patients with complex partial seizures. Brain Res Bull 2004;63:407–13.

15. Ross RJ, Ball WA, Dinges DF, et al. Motor dysfunction during sleep in post-traumatic stress disorder. Sleep 1994;17:723–32.

16. Blaw ME, Leroy RF, Steinberg JB, et al. Hereditary quivering chin and REM behavioral disorder. Ann Neurol 1989;26:471.

17. Trajanovic NN, Voloh I, Shapiro CM, et al. REM sleep behavior disorder in a child with Tourette's syndrome. Can J Neurol Sci 2004;31:572–5.

18. Nevsimalova S, Prihodova I, Kemlink D, et al. REM behavior disorder (RBD) can be one of the first symptoms of childhood narcolepsy. Sleep Med 2007;8:784–6.

19. Nightingale S, Orgill JC, Ebrahim IO, et al. The association between narcolepsy and REM behavior disorder (RBD). Sleep Med 2005;6: 253–8.

20. Arora RN, Zak RS, Maganti RK, et al. Standards of Practice Committee; American Academy of Sleep Medicine. Best practice guide for the treatment of REM sleep behavior disorder (RBD). J Clin Sleep Med 2010;6:85–95.

21. Green RA, Gillin JC, Wyatt RJ. The inhibitory effect of intraventricular administration of serotonin on spontaneous motor activity of rats. Psychopharmacology 1976;198:12–22.

22. Chadwick D, Hallet M, Harris, R, et al. Clinical, biochemical, and physiological features distinguishing myoclonus responsive to 5-hydroxytryptophan, tryptophan with monoamine oxidase inhibitor and clonazepam. Brain1977;100:455–87.

23. Rye DB, Johston LH, Watts RL, Bliwise, DL. Juvenile Parkinson's disease with REM sleep behavior disorder, sleepiness, and daytime REM onset. Neurology1999;53:1868–70.

Other Parasomnias

Harsha Kumar and Sindhuja Vardhan

INTRODUCTION

Parasomnias are undesirable events or experiences that occur during sleep. Parasomnia is derived from 'para' meaning 'beside or alongside of' in Greek and 'somnus' meaning 'sleep' in Latin. The word parasomnia was coined by the French researcher Henri Roger in 1932.

Parasomnias typically occur when falling asleep (hypnogogic), during sleep, or when waking up (hypnopompic) from sleep. Parasomnias are thought to be a result of activation of the central nervous system and transmission of impulses to skeletal muscles and the autonomic nervous system. Parasomnias also include abnormal behaviors, perceptions and abnormal sleep-related movements.

The latest International Classification of Sleep Disorders (ICSD-2) divides parasomnias into three categories:
1. Disorders of arousal (from NREM sleep)
2. Parasomnias usually associated with REM sleep
3. Other parasomnias.

Other parasomnias will be discussed in this chapter.

Other parasomnias as per ICSD-2 include:
1. Sleep-related dissociative disorders
2. Sleep enuresis
3. Sleep-related groaning (catathrenia)
4. Exploding head syndrome
5. Sleep-related hallucinations
6. Sleep-related eating disorder
7. Unspecified parasomnia
8. Parasomnia due to a drug or substance
9. Parasomnia due to a medical condition.

Here we review the more common disorders in this group. Epidemiological data on this group of parasomnias are scant. General prevalence at the population level is not known for most of the above parasomnias. The occurrence of parasomnias in children is thought by some researchers as physiologic and part of normal development, whereas in adults it is sometimes associated with psychological disorders.[1–3]

SLEEP-RELATED DISSOCIATIVE DISORDERS

Definition

Sleep-related dissociative disorders are parasomnias that can emerge from any stage of sleep, either at transition from wakefulness or within several minutes after awakening from non-rapid eye movement (NREM) sleep or rapid eye movement (REM) sleep.[1]

Sleep-related dissociative disorders are also known as nocturnal (psychogenic) dissociative disorders, hysterical somnambulistic trance, and dissociative pseudoparasomnia. Dissociative identity disorder, dissociative fugue and dissociative disorder NOS (not otherwise specified) have been identified with sleep-related dissociative disorders.[1,4,5]

Etiology

Dissociation is a defense mechanism when other mature adaptive defenses fail. It is a primitive psychological defense wherein the distressing experience is kept apart from typical consciousness, resisting integration with the individual's daily activities. These experiences may emerge as activity when environmental conditions are conducive or prompt them.[6] The pathophysiology of dissociation is not clear. It is proposed that it is a functional disconnection among various brain regions. Sleep periods are vulnerable to a wide range of dissociative phenomena across all sleep stages and after arousals and full awakenings from all sleep stages.

Epidemiology

Women are more often affected than men. Onset ranges from childhood to adulthood. The course often remains chronic and severe. Events can occur several times weekly to multiple times nightly.[1]

Signs and Symptoms

Most sleep-related dissociative disorders have corresponding daytime episodes of disturbed behavior, confusion, and associated amnesia. Additionally, patients with sleep-related dissociative disorder have often experienced[7] combat,[8] adult interpersonal violence[9] or natural disasters.[10] Dissociation is often associated with post-traumatic stress and is considered to be mainly a post-traumatic response.[8,10] Complications include injuries to the patient and/or bed partner, including ecchymoses, lacerations, fractures, and burns.[1]

Diagnostic Criteria

A. Meets the criteria for dissociative disorder as per Diagnostic and Statistical Manual of Mental Disorders, Fourth edition, and emerges in close association with the main sleep period.
B. One of the following is present:
   1. Polysomnography demonstrates a dissociative episode, or episodes that emerge during sustained EEG wakefulness, either in the transition from wakefulness to sleep or after an awakening from NREM or REM sleep.
   2. In the absence of a polysomnographically recorded episode of dissociation, the history provided by observers is compelling for a sleep-related dissociative disorder, particularly if the sleep-related behaviors are similar to observed daytime dissociative behaviors.
C. The sleep disturbance is not better explained by another sleep disorder, medical or neurologic disorder, medication use, or substance use disorder.

Differential Diagnosis

1. Parasomnias such as sleepwalking, sleep terrors and REM sleep behavior disorder (RBD).

2. Disorders of arousal like confusional arousals, sleepwalking, and sleep terrors.
3. Abnormal toxic metabolic states or medical disorders that can cause altered states of consciousness may mimic a dissociative disorder and must be excluded.

PSG Findings
EEG wakefulness before, during and after the episodes. The alpha EEG rhythm with disorders of arousals and sleep-related dissociative disorders can be distinguished by looking at the lag time between EEG arousal and behavioral arousal. There is a lag time of 15 to 60 seconds in sleep-related dissociative disorder. There is no lag time in disorders of arousals.[11]

Management
Comprehensive approach that includes cognitive-behavioral therapy, supportive psychotherapy, and post-traumatic disorder treatment.[5]

Early identification and intensive therapeutic interventions for dissociative symptoms in children appear to be particularly efficacious. A psychiatric treatment plan is helpful for supporting cognitive/emotional processing of trauma-related material in order to develop greater affect regulation capacities.[10]

Prognosis/Clinical Course
The course often remains chronic and severe.

SLEEP ENURESIS (see also Chapter 13)

Definition
Sleep enuresis is defined as recurrent involuntary voiding of urine occurring during sleep at least twice a week, for at least 3 consecutive months, in a child who is at least 5 years of age.[1] Sleep enuresis is considered primary in a child who has never been consistently dry for 6 consecutive months. It is considered secondary in a child who had previously been dry for 6 consecutive months and then began wetting at least twice a week for a period of at least 3 months.[1]

Etiology
The exact etiology of primary sleep enuresis is unknown. Factors thought to contribute to persistent nocturnal incontinence after 5 years of age include:
1. Disorders of arousal from sleep causing children to continue to sleep during a full and contracting urinary bladder, leading to incontinence
2. Nocturnal polyuria
3. Reduced bladder capacity (anatomical and/or functional capacity)
4. Anatomical abnormalities usually present as both daytime and night-time enuresis.

Secondary sleep enuresis is more commonly associated with:
1. Urinary tract infections
2. Genitourinary tract malformations
3. Extrinsic pressure on the bladder (chronic constipation)
4. Polyuria secondary to excessive fluid intake, diuretics, caffeine ingestion, diabetes mellitus or diabetes insipidus
5. Neurologic conditions, leading to neurologic bladder
6. Sleep-disordered breathing (obstructive sleep apnea)
7. Seizure disorder

8. Psychological stressors such as parental divorce, neglect, physical abuse, sexual abuse, and institutionalization can cause secondary sleep enuresis.[12]

Epidemiology
Primary sleep enuresis is seen in approximately 30% of 4-year-olds, 10% of 6-year-olds, 7% of 7-year-olds and 5% of 10-year-olds. Primary sleep enuresis is more common in boys than in girls in the ratio of 3:2. The spontaneous cure rate for primary sleep enuresis is about 15% per year.[1]

There is a high prevalence of enuresis among the parents, siblings, and other relatives of the child with primary enuresis. If both parents were enuretic as children, the prevalence in their child is 77%. If one parent was enuretic, the prevalence is 44%. Studies indicate putative linkage of sleep enuresis to a region on chromosomes 22q, 13q, and 12q across different families.[1]

Signs and Symptoms
Signs and symptoms are determined by the etiology of sleep enuresis. In many patients, there may be no finding other than the enuresis. In patients with secondary sleep enuresis, it is more likely to have other signs and symptoms from the underlying condition.

Diagnosis
It is important to diagnose whether the etiology of enuresis is primary or secondary, as it is essential for the success of treatment. History should include familial predisposition, emotional state, sleep habits, dietary habits (including daytime and fluid intake in the evenings).[13] Physical examination should be performed with attention to adenotonsillar hypertrophy, urinary bladder distension, constipation, genital abnormalities, and spinal cord anomalies.

Laboratory investigation can include urine analysis and culture, depending on the history,[14] ultrasonography and bladder sphincter electromyography. Cystoscopy may be considered if organic etiology is suspected. Nocturnal polysomnography is rarely required for the diagnosis of sleep enuresis and should only be performed when other underlying sleep-related disorders are suspected.

Diagnostic Criteria
Primary Sleep Enuresis
1. The patient is older than 5 years of age.
2. The patient exhibits recurrent involuntary voiding during sleep, occurring at least twice weekly.
3. The patient has never been consistently dry during the night.

Secondary Sleep Enuresis
1. The patient is older than 5 years of age.
2. The patient exhibits recurrent involuntary voiding during sleep, occurring at least twice weekly.
3. The patient has previously been consistently dry during sleep for at least 6 months.

Differential Diagnosis
It is crucial to distinguish between primary and secondary sleep enuresis. Other diseases, such as diabetes mellitus, nocturnal seizures, spina bifida, urinary tract infection, and sleep-disordered breathing, must be excluded.

PSG Findings

Polysomnographic study is indicated in the evaluation of secondary sleep enuresis only when another sleep disorder, such as OSA or sleep-related seizure disorder, is suspected. Enuretic episodes, in both primary and secondary enuresis, can occur in all sleep stages.

Management

It is important to identify if the sleep enuresis is primary or secondary, as treatment strategies are very different.

Primary Enuresis

No treatment is recommended until an affected individual reaches 5–6 years of age. Clinical monitoring may be sufficient in children greater than 6 years, if the episodes are intermittent and improving. Treatment strategies include sleep hygiene, evening fluid restriction, supportive therapy, motivational therapy and pharmacotherapy. Punishing children may contribute to the existing problem, rather than to the treatment.

Depending on the age of the child, enuresis alarm, bladder control training, psychotherapy, hypnosis and biofeedback[15] can be beneficial. Desmopressin, Imipramine, and oxybutynin are drugs commonly used when non-pharmacologic measures are insufficient.

Secondary Sleep Enuresis

Management of secondary enuresis depends on the underlying cause. Occasionally, primary and secondary enuresis may coexist. In such cases, techniques used in the treatment of primary enuresis may be used along with the treatment of underlying pathology. Children with recurrent urinary tract infections often benefit from hygiene efforts and prophylactic antibiotics. Treatment of sleep-disordered breathing with adenotonsillectomy and non-invasive positive-pressure ventilation might be required, as pediatric obstructive sleep apnea is a common cause for secondary enuresis. Studies have shown that sleep enuresis is more common in children with pediatric obstructive sleep apnea and habitual snoring, than in non-snoring children.[16]

Prognosis/Clinical Course

The spontaneous cure rate for primary sleep enuresis is about 15% per year.[1]

SLEEP-RELATED GROANING (CATATHRENIA)

Definition

Sleep-related groaning is defined as a deep inspiration followed by a prolonged expiration, accompanied by a monotonous sound that resembles groaning. This happens most commonly during REM sleep.

Other names for sleep-related groaning include expiratory groaning during sleep, sleep-related respiratory dysrhythmia with bradypnea and vocalization, and REM-sleep-associated long, inarticulate expiratory phonation.

Etiology

The pathophysiology for sleep-related groaning is unclear. Sleep-related groaning is a complex respiratory event that involves the closure of glottis and withheld breath, followed by expiration. It is hypothesized that central respiratory generators in the brainstem are involved in this action. Children exhibiting sleep-related groaning do not have anatomical abnormalities in the larynx.

Epidemiology

Sleep-related groaning is common in adolescence and early adulthood.

Signs and Symptoms

In most cases, the patient is not affected by groaning. Rather, it is the partner or family who are disturbed, leading them to evaluation.

Groaning is asymptomatic and is not associated with dreaming, sleep talking, sleep-related disorders, respiratory disorders, psychologic or psychiatric disorders. Sleep-related groaning does improve with change in position, but usually resumes again.

Usually, these patients are asymptomatic and may occasionally complain of restless sleep, hoarseness, and mild daytime fatigue. No association with respiratory disorders, psychological problems or psychiatric disorders has been found.

Diagnosis

Sleep-related groaning is a clinical diagnosis. Neurological, psychiatric, otorhinolaryngological and pulmonary investigations in the majority of cases are normal. Polysomnography may be beneficial when the history is atypical.

Differential Diagnosis

Differential diagnosis for sleep-related groaning includes obstructive sleep apnea, upper airway anomalies, central sleep apnea, sleep talking, sleep-related laryngospasm and nocturnal asthma. A good history, physical examination, and polysomnogram should be able to differentiate these disorders from sleep-related groaning.

PSG Findings

Sleep-related groaning is a clinical diagnosis. PSG findings include decreased respiratory rate, prolonged expiratory phase with vocal sounds resembling groaning, preceded by inspiration. These events happen mostly in REM sleep. The rest of the sleep tracings are normal. No gas exchange abnormalities are noted during the groaning periods.

Management

There is no treatment available for sleep-related groaning. Reassurance is helpful for patients and patients' families. Pharmacologic agents such as trazodone, clonazepam, gabapentin and carbamazapine have been tried with very limited success.[11] Non-invasive positive-pressure ventilation is an option for patients who also have coexisting sleep-disordered breathing.[17–19]

Prognosis/Clinical Course

The course of sleep-related groaning is chronic and it usually occurs every night. Catathrenia is not known to progress clinically. The long-term prognosis and health consequences are unknown and prospective studies are much needed.

Onset of catathrenia is usually seen during adolescence and early adulthood. No predisposing or precipitating factors have been identified. The course and long-term prognosis of catathrenia are chronic. The available follow-up data are still incomplete, but seem to exclude a clinical progression or complication of catathrenia.[20,21]

SLEEP-RELATED EATING DISORDER

Definition
Sleep-related eating disorder (SRED) is defined as repeated episodes of drinking and eating done without conscious control during arousals from various stages of sleep. These disorders often lead to untoward consequences.

Etiology
As with most parasomnias, the etiology is unclear. There seems to be an abnormal relationship between sleep and eating, the two basic drive states. SRED can be idiopathic, iatrogenic, or secondarily associated with primary sleep disorders.

Common sleep disorders associated with SRED include obstructive sleep apnea, sleepwalking, periodic limb movement disorder, narcolepsy, bulimia nervosa, and circadian rhythm disorder. SRED has been reported with use of medications such as zolpidem and lithium, and secondary to cessation of alcohol, tobacco and other substance abuse.

Epidemiology
Sleep-related eating disorder is more common in women. It has also been reported that it is more common in patients who have been diagnosed with eating disorders such as anorexia nervosa and bulimia nervosa.

Signs and Symptoms
Episodes of eating commonly occur during partial arousals with variable recall of the event. The number of these episodes is variable and can occur a few times a week to many times in a night. Food consumed is usually high in calories and not preferred during the day. Alcohol is not usually consumed during these episodes. Consumption of ready-to-eat foods and preparation of entire hot or cold meals have been reported. Clumsy handling of food and related injuries are common. Disturbance of a patient during an episode can lead to agitation.

Diagnostic Criteria
A. Recurrent episodes of involuntary eating and drinking during the main period of sleep.
B. One or more of the following must be present with the recurrent episodes of involuntary eating and drinking:
   1. Consumption of peculiar forms or combinations of food or inedible or toxic substances (such as frozen pizzas, raw bacon, buttered cigarettes, cat food, salt sandwiches, coffee grounds, ammonia cleaning solutions)
   2. Insomnia related to sleep disruption from repeated episodes of eating, with a complaint of non-restorative sleep, daytime fatigue, or somnolence
   3. Sleep-related injury
   4. Dangerous behaviors performed while in pursuit of food or while cooking food
   5. Morning anorexia
   6. Adverse health consequences from recurrent binge eating of highly calorific foods.
C. The disturbance is not better explained by another sleep disorder, medical or neurological disorder, mental disorder, medication use, or substance use disorder.

Complications
Injuries such as burns and lacerations are seen secondary to clumsy food preparation, handling and ingestion of food.

Obesity, hypercholesterolemia, uncontrolled diabetes from high-calorie foods and anaphylactic reactions from consuming food to which the patient is allergic are possibilities.

Differential Diagnosis
Nocturnal eating syndrome, bulimia nervosa, Kleine–Levin syndrome, and Kluver–Bucy syndrome need to be differentiated from sleep-related disordered breathing.

PSG Findings
Multiple arousals can arise from any stage of sleep, but most commonly from slow-wave sleep. These arousals may or may not be associated with eating episodes. In the majority of these patients, polysomnogram have helped in diagnosis of a primary sleep disorder.

Management
Medications such as benzodiazapenes, sertraline, topiramate, melatonin, oxazepam, and sibutramine have been used with varying results, depending on the patient's underlying medical conditions. Some medications showed improvement but have significant adverse effects and had to be discontinued.

Further controlled clinical trials of pharmacological agents for the treatment of SRED are warranted.

Non-pharmacologic approaches, such as having a meal before sleep, limiting the amount of food available at home, and locking the food cabinets and refrigerators made no difference.[22]

Clinical Pearls

- NREM parasomnias are common, while REM and other parasomnias are rare.
- It is important to understand that obstructive sleep apnea, periodic limb movement disorder, restless leg syndrome and sleep deprivation can trigger parasomnias. Appropriate management of these conditions can improve, or even resolve, parasomnias in children.
- Parasomnias in children are most commonly diagnosed based on clinical history from the parents or caregivers who may observe the patient sleep or share the sleep place with them.
- Most often polysomnograms are not necessary for the diagnosis of parasomnias. Polysomnograms are important in children when other sleep disorders are suspected, which may be aggravating the parasomnia. These sleep disorders include obstructive sleep apnea, periodic limb movement disorder, and restless leg syndrome.
- Management of parasomnias includes good sleep hygiene, reassurance, modification of the sleep environment, treatment of the underlying disorder and avoidance of substances such as caffeine, alcohol and other substances of abuse. In certain parasomnias, pharmacologic agents may be beneficial in treating the parasomnia or the underlying condition. Underlying conditions may be triggers for parasomnia.
- It is very important to create a safe sleep environment. This should include secure windows and doors, sleeping on a low bed or the ground to minimize injury from falls, and electronic alarm devices to warn the family members if the patient is leaving the room.

References

1. The International Classification of Sleep Disorders-2. Westbrook, IL: American Academy of Sleep Medicine; 2005.
2. Mahowald MW, Bornemann MC, Schenck CH. Parasomnias. Semin Neurol 2004;24(3):283–92.
3. Stores G. Parasomnias of childhood and adolescence. Sleep Med Clin 2007;2:405–17.
4. Schenck CH, Milner DM, Hurwitz TD, et al. A polysomnographic and clinical report on sleep-related injury in 100 adult patients. Am J Psychiatry 1989;146(9):1166–73.
5. Mason TB 2nd, Pack AI. Pediatric parasomnias. Sleep 2007;30(2):141–51.
6. Hartman D, Crisp AH, Sedgwick P, et al. Is there a dissociative process in sleepwalking and night terrors? Postgrad Med J 2001;7(906):244–9.
7. Chu JA, DDill DL. Dissociative symptoms in relation to childhood physical and sexual abuse. Am J Psychiatry 1990;147(7):887–92.
8. Bremner JD, Southwick SM, Brett E, et al. Dissociation and posttraumatic stress disorder in Vietnam combat veterans. Am J Psychiatry 1992;149(3):328–32.
9. Feeny NC, Zoellner LA, Fitzgibbons LA, et al. Exploring the roles of emotional numbing, depression, and dissociation in PTSD. J Trauma Stress 2000;13(3):489–98.
10. Briere J. Dissociative symptoms and trauma exposure: specificity, affect dysregulation, and posttraumatic stress. J Nerv Ment Dis 2006;194(2):78–82.
11. Thorpy M, Plazzi G. The parasomnias and other sleep-related movement disorders. New York: Cambridge University Press; 2010; 163–74.
12. Sheldon SH. Sleep-related enuresis. Child Adolesc Psychiatr Clin North Am 1996;5:661–72.
13. Hjalmas K, Arnold T, Bower W, et al. Nocturnal enuresis: an international evidence based management strategy. J Urol 2004;71(6 Pt 2):2545–61.
14. Kotagal S. Parasomnias in childhood. Sleep Med Rev 2009;13(2):157–68.
15. Mattelaer P, Mersdorf A, Rohrmann D, et al. Biofeedback in the treatment of voiding disorders in childhood. Acta Urol Belg 1995;63(4):5–7.
16. Alexopoulos EI, Kostadima E, Pagonari I, et al. Association between primary nocturnal enuresis and habitual snoring in children. Urology 2006;68(2):406–9.
17. Iriarte J, Alegre M, Urrestarazu E, et al. Continuous positive airway pressure as treatment for catathrenia (nocturnal groaning). Neurology 2006;66(4):609–10.
18. Guilleminault C, Hagen CC, Khaja AM. Catathrenia: parasomnia or uncommon feature of sleep disordered breathing? Sleep 2008;31(1):132–9.
19. Songu M, Yilmaz H, Yucetuk AV, et al. Effect of CPAP therapy on catathrenia and OSA: a case report and review of the literature. Sleep Breath 2008;12(4):401–5.
20. Oldani A, Manconi M, Zucconi M, et al. 'Nocturnal groaning': just a sound or parasomnia? J Sleep Res 2005;14(3):305–10.
21. Vetrugno R, Lugaresi E, Plazzi G, et al. Catathrenia (nocturnal groaning): an abnormal respiratory pattern during sleep. Eur J Neurol 2007;14(11):1236–43.
22. Provini F, Albani F, Vetrugno R, et al. A pilot double-blind placebo-controlled trial of low-dose pramipexole in sleep-related eating disorder. Eur J Neurol 2005;12(6):432–5.

MOVEMENT DISORDERS

Sleep-Related Movement Disorders

Jonathan D. Cogen and Darius A. Loghmanee

INTRODUCTION

Sleep-related movement disorders (SRMD) present a unique challenge to practitioners caring for children, as they can cause significant distress in parents and families. This class of clinical conditions is characterized by relatively simple, non-purposeful, and usually stereotyped movements that occur in sleep, primarily during sleep–wake transitions. These generally benign movements can represent self-soothing mechanisms, but at times are associated with physical injury, interfere with the sleep of the child and family, and cause excessive daytime sleepiness. Typically, these movement disorders resolve spontaneously and do not have significant long-term consequences. Although the International Classification of Sleep Disorders (ICSD-2) lists restless legs syndrome (RLS) and periodic limb movements of sleep (PLMS) as sleep-related movement disorders,[1] these conditions will only be covered briefly, as they are described elsewhere in this book.

ASSESSMENT OF RHYTHMIC MOVEMENTS SURROUNDING THE SLEEP PERIOD

When considering the diagnosis of a sleep-related movement disorder, it is essential to have a systematic and thorough approach (Box 42-1). In order to differentiate SRMD from neurologic conditions with variable persistence during sleep such as a seizure disorder, dystonia, or Tourette's syndrome, one must first determine if the movement disorder occurs only during sleep or if it also occurs during periods of wakefulness. If the movements occur only during sleep–wake transitions, then one must next decide if the movements are simple or complex. Complex, purposeful, and goal-directed movements, such as those represented by sleepwalking or confusional arousals, are considered parasomnias and are not included in this category. If the movement occurs only during wake–sleep transitions and appears to be relatively simple and stereotypic, the SRMD diagnosis can be initially assessed by comprehensive history, physical examination, neurological examination, and if necessary, a polysomnogram (PSG). If a PSG is required, an expanded EEG electrode array is usually needed to rule out seizure. A dedicated sleep-deprived EEG may be warranted if clearly indicated by clinical signs or symptoms or if abnormal findings are noted on the EEG montage performed with the PSG.

SLEEP-RELATED MOVEMENT DISORDERS

Rhythmic Movement Disorder

Rhythmic movement disorder (RMD) is defined as a group of stereotyped, repetitive movements most often involving large muscles that typically begins prior to sleep onset and may be sustained into transitional sleep. The most frequent forms of RMD are head banging (often referred to as *jactatio capitis nocturna*), body rocking, and body rolling, while leg rolling and leg banging are less common (Table 42.1).[2] These movements can range in intensity from subtle to violent, and treatment is not usually required unless daytime consequences related to sleep quality are present, sleep-related injury occurs, or there are significant life-threatening issues for other family members.[1] The duration of these movements can last from several minutes to several hours. The movement frequency can vary, but the rate is usually between 0.5 and 2 per second, with duration of the individual cluster of movements generally less than 15 minutes.[1] In contrast to sleep-related epilepsy, children with RMD usually can voluntarily stop the movements upon request. Movements can be manifest at sleep onset, after nocturnal arousals, or in combination. Patients in whom frequent episodes of RMD are noted during the night should be clinically evaluated for causes of sleep fragmentation such as obstructive sleep apnea or periodic limb movements of sleep. In patients with head banging, physical examination can demonstrate bruising, callus formation, or discrete patches of hair loss at the point of contact with the object they are striking with their head. Patients with leg rolling or body rolling may demonstrate bruising at sites of impact with furniture or the wall. Polysomnography is rarely needed to make the diagnosis, but will generally demonstrate rhythmic movements during wakefulness and extending into transitional sleep.[3]

Rhythmic head banging, body rocking, and head rolling are very common in childhood, with up to 60% of infants displaying the characteristic signs and symptoms by 9 months of age. RMD prevalence decreases with age, and is only seen in 5% of 5-year-olds. This disorder is more common in males, with a 4:1 male to female ratio.[1] Though less common, RMD can continue into adolescence or adulthood.[4-6] Although initially thought to be suggestive of autism and mental retardation, RMD is common in neurodevelopmentally normal patients, even when it persists into adulthood.[5] An association between attention deficit hyperactivity disorder (ADHD) and RMD has been demonstrated in one small study,[7] but more research is required.

Various management and treatment strategies have been suggested. The key aspect of rhythmic movement disorder management is helping prevent injury to the child and providing parental education about the nature of this condition. In a typical child with RMD who has no apparent daytime behavioral or social issues, parents should be reassured that the condition is common and almost always self-limiting. Parents should be instructed to place the child in an environment where injury from these repetitive and sometimes violent movements can be avoided. Cribs and beds should be in good repair and inspected regularly. If falling off the bed is a concern, safe bedrails might be considered. Parents can also move the bed away from the wall or have the child sleep on a mattress on the floor to ensure his or her safety.

Interventions to control the movements generally seek to provide the child with alternative means of self-soothing. The establishment of a bedtime routine made up of consistent and progressively less stimulating activities focused on helping the

Box 42-1   Diagnostic Criteria for Sleep-Related Rhythmic Movement Disorder (ICSD-2, 2005)

A. The patient exhibits repetitive, stereotyped, and rhythmic motor behaviors.

B. The movements involve large muscle groups.

C. The movements are predominantly sleep-related, occurring near nap or bedtime, or when the individual appears drowsy or asleep.

D. The behavior results in a significant complaint as manifest by at least one of the following:
   i. interference with normal sleep
   ii. significant impairment in daytime function
   iii. self-inflicted bodily injury that requires medical treatment (or would result in injury if preventable measures were not used).

E. The rhythmic movements are not better explained by another current sleep disorder, medical or neurological disorder, mental disorder, medication use, or substance use disorder.

TABLE 42.1   Clinical and Pathophysiological Subtypes of SRMD (ICSD-2, 2005)

Body rocking type	The whole body is rocked while on the hands and knees
Head banging type (*jactatio capitis nocturna*)	The head is forcibly moved, striking an object
Head rolling type	The head is moved laterally, typically while in the supine position
Other type	Includes body rolling, leg rolling, and leg banging
Combined type	Includes two or more of the individual types

child decelerate can be a sufficient intervention to help the child fall asleep without needing to engage in rhythmic movements. Fixing a wake-up time and manipulating naps can also be effective in helping the child fall asleep without relying on repetitive motions to relax. A more comprehensive review of these behavioral approaches is included in Chapter 9, Promoting Healthy Sleep Practices for Children and Adolescents.

Other behavioral and psychological approaches have given attention to replacing the rhythmic movements with alternate means of soothing. The use of a metronome as a stimulus substitution demonstrated some success in one study,[4] as has holding the child while patting or rocking the child at the same rate as their rhythmic movements. Etzioni and colleagues used a 3-week controlled sleep restriction regimen, and found that the combination of mild sleep deprivation along with usage of hypnotics at treatment initiation abolished rhythmic movements and treat the disorder.[8] This study suggests that RMD may represent a learned behavior that the child uses to help transition from wakefulness to sleep. In severe cases, or in cases in which the patient's rhythmic movements are a threat to the child's safety, pharmacologic treatment can be considered. A small dose of clonazepam has been

shown to be effective in up to 50% of cases.[4] Antidepressants have also been tried with limited success.

Benign Sleep Myoclonus of Infancy

This sleep-related movement disorder occurs solely in infants, and consists of repetitive myoclonic jerks involving the whole body, limbs, or trunk. These movements usually disappear by 6 months of age, and occur only during sleep. As soon as the child is aroused or awakened from sleep, the movements abruptly and consistently stop. This disorder can sometimes be difficult to distinguish from sleep-related epilepsy and infantile spasms. If focal findings are present on examination, developmental issues are present, or clinical concern is heightened for a seizure disorder, an EEG may be ordered. The prevalence and etiology of this sleep-related condition are unknown. Rare, occasional myoclonic jerks often greatly worry the infant's parents, who may quickly seek out their pediatrician for a consultation. Parents can be reassured that this condition is benign without sequelae, and that symptoms will disappear after a few months of life.

Sleep Starts

Sleep starts, known also as hypnic or hypnagogic jerks, are sudden, single, brief contractions of the legs and occasionally the arms or head that occur at sleep onset. This disorder is a transition problem from wakefulness; it is extremely common and has been experienced by almost everyone at one time or another. Often, these movements are associated with a subjective impression of falling or a visual hypnagogic dream or hallucination. It has been hypothesized that sleep starts represent aberrant muscle contractions triggered as a result of instability of the brainstem reticular formation at the transition between wakefulness and sleep.[9] These movements can be frightening for parents, especially when they are accompanied by vocalization or crying. Parents should be reassured that sleep starts are a normal phenomenon and have no sequelae for the growing child. No treatment is necessary unless the movements result in injuries from kicking hard surfaces such as the crib railings, wall or a bedpost. In these cases, treatment modalities similar to those used in RMD could be considered.

Hypnagogic Foot Tremor/Alternating Leg Muscle Activation (ALMA)

Hypnagogic foot tremors occur at the transition between wake and sleep or during light sleep, and consist of rhythmic foot movements occurring every second or so for several minutes. This sleep-related movement disorder may represent a variant of rhythmic movement disorder (RMD); polysomnographic monitoring typically demonstrates recurrent EMG potentials or foot movements at the 0.5–3-hertz range in one or both feet as well as burst potential longer than the myoclonic range (greater than 250 ms).[1] The prevalence in childhood is unknown, but one study estimated the adult prevalence at 7.5%.[10] Hypnagogic foot tremors are considered a benign entity with no known sequelae, and no treatment has been found to be effective.

Alternating leg muscle activation (ALMA) is a term used to describe brief contractions of the lower leg alternating with activation of the muscle in the other leg. This sleep-related condition may represent the same disorder as hypnagogic foot tremor, except for the alternating nature seen clinically.

Polysomnography shows the characteristic anterior tibialis activation in one leg alternating with similar activation in the other leg. Both hypnagogic foot tremor and ALMA have been seen in one series in patients who were taking antidepressants,[11] and many patients with ALMA have been found concurrently to have obstructive sleep apnea syndrome or periodic limb movement disorder.[12] While no treatment has been successful in reducing symptoms associated with hypnagogic foot tremor, dopamine agonists have been shown to be of benefit in patients with ALMA who report disrupted sleep.[13]

Sleep-Related Bruxism

Sleep-related bruxism (SB) is a stereotyped movement disorder characterized by grinding or clenching of the teeth during sleep. These rhythmic movements are the result of involuntary, repetitive contractions of the masseter, temporalis, and pterygoid muscles.[3] The child or adolescent may report jaw muscle discomfort, jaw lock, or headaches upon awakening in the morning. According to the International Classification of Sleep Disorders (2005), a diagnosis of sleep-related bruxism requires that one or more of the following must be present: (1) abnormal wear of the teeth; (2) jaw muscle discomfort, fatigue, or pain and jaw lock upon awakening; or (3) masseter muscle hypertrophy upon voluntary forceful clenching. Poor sleep can also be seen in severe cases. The exact prevalence of this condition is unclear, although several epidemiological studies have shown that 14–20% of children are affected by sleep-related bruxism.[14] There appears to be an equal sex distribution, a familial pattern without clear genetic transmission has been observed, and the condition decreases with age.

While SB can be a sign of an underlying sleep disorder (e.g. OSA or periodic limb movement disorder) or dental disorders (e.g. malocclusion, poor oral habits, or temporomandibular disorders, it can also represent emotional conditions such as high stress or anxiety.[16] SB can occur during all stages of sleep, but is most common in non-REM stages 1 and 2.[1] In children, bruxism can be associated with obstructive sleep apnea. This is thought to represent an attempt to open the airway during obstructive events by advancing the mandible, and is usually noted during arousals at the termination of respiratory events. Khoury et al. demonstrated that sleep-related bruxism is linked to transient sleep arousal, higher sleep-time sympathetic-cardiac activity, and a rise in respiration prior to and during the rhythmic masticatory muscle activity that typifies bruxism.[15] While the relevance of these findings is still unclear, these physiologic changes during sleep may contribute to the morning orofacial pain and headaches seen in patients with this movement disorder.

While SB can be a sign of an underlying sleep disorder (e.g. OSA or periodic limb movement disorder) or dental disorders (e.g. malocclusion, poor oral habits, or temporomandibular disorders), it can also represent emotional conditions such as high stress or anxiety.[16] Dental treatment focuses on preventing tooth destruction, reducing pain, and improving overall sleep quality. In many cases these goals can be achieved through the use of a mouth guard. Treatment strategies focused on addressing emotional concerns rely primarily on behavioral approaches designed to teach the child about relaxation[17] and establishing a consistent and relaxing bedtime routine in order to reduce stress or anxiety. Benzodiazepines and muscle relaxants have been shown to improve

	SLEEP-RELATED BRUXISM	FACIOMANDIBULAR MYOCLONUS
Tooth destruction	Yes	No
Temporomandibular dysfunction	Yes	No
Masseter muscle hypertrophy	Yes	No

TABLE 42.2 Sleep-Related Bruxism versus Faciomandibular Myoclonus

sleep-related bruxism, and other medications (e.g. propranolol, clonidine, levodopa) are currently being looked at in an attempt to decrease SB events. Given the complex nature of treatment plans for SB, consultation between sleep medicine physicians, dentists, psychologists, and psychiatrists is often required.

Faciomandibular myoclonus is similar to sleep-related bruxism, but is considered to be more benign (Table 42.2). Compared to the more sustained jaw closure seen in SB, faciomandibular myoclonus is associated with rapid jaw jerks or twitches. Children and adolescents with this movement disorder, in contrast to SB, show no tooth wear, temporomandibular dysfunction, or masseter muscle hypertrophy. While rarely required clinically, a polysomnogram can differentiate between these two disorders.

Restless Legs Syndrome

Restless legs syndrome (RLS) is a sleep-related movement disorder with several cardinal features, including an urge to move the legs, typically accompanied by an uncomfortable sensation in the lower extremities. These urges usually begin or worsen on lying down to go to sleep, and can interfere with the onset of sleep. Patients describe the sensations as 'aches,' 'creeping,' 'tingling,' 'prickling' or 'itching,'[1] which are partially or completely relieved with leg movement. Younger children may report these symptoms as pain due to their limited vocabulary. In severe cases, other parts of the body, including the arms, can also be affected.[9] These symptoms may last from a few minutes to several hours, but even the most severely affected patients can still sleep for several hours each night. Diagnosis generally can be made based on clinical features; however, polysomnography and actigraphy can be performed if diagnosis is in doubt. Both of these diagnostic modalities are very sensitive and specific in detecting and diagnosing RLS by monitoring the activity of the anterior tibialis muscle.[14]

Periodic Limb Movement Disorder

Periodic limb movement disorder (PLMD) is characterized by periodic episodes of stereotyped, repetitive limb movements that manifest during sleep. In contrast to restless leg syndrome, PLMD does not occur prior to sleep onset, but only when the child or adolescent is asleep. Polysomnographic monitoring demonstrates repetitive episodes of muscle contraction and intermittent arousals or awakenings. However, recent studies have questioned the correlation between severity of PLMD and excessive daytime sleepiness, including one in which several surveys investigating this link did not show any association between PLMD and sleep–wake complaints.[17]

Box 42-2   Diagnostic Criteria for Sleep-Related Leg Cramps (ICSD-2, 2005)

A. A painful sensation in the leg or foot is associated with sudden muscle hardness or tightness indicating a strong muscle contraction.

B. The painful muscle contractions in the legs or feet occur during the sleep period, although they may arise from either wakefulness or sleep.

C. The pain is relieved by forceful stretching of the affected muscles, releasing the contraction.

D. The sleep-related leg cramps are not better explained by another current sleep disorder, medical or neurological disorder, medication use, or substance abuse disorder.

Clinical Pearls

- A detailed history and physical examination are necessary to distinguish sleep-related movement disorders from neurological conditions such as seizures or dystonia, as well as to differentiate from complex sleep-related movements as seen in parasomnias.

- As sleep-related movement disorders are largely behavioral in nature, it is essential to reassure and educate families that these simple, non-purposeful, and usually stereotyped movements are benign and generally self-limited.

- Treatment should also focus on ensuring the safety of the child and easing the transition between wakefulness and sleep, often achieved by establishing consistent bedtime routines consisting of progressively more relaxing activities and strengthening positive associations between the sleep environment and relaxation.

Sleep-Related Leg Cramps

Sleep-related or nocturnal leg cramps are painful sensations of muscular hardness, tightness, or tension that occur in the calf or foot during sleep (Box 42-2). These leg cramps can last for a few seconds and remit spontaneously, or in some cases persist for up to 15–30 minutes. These painful sensations can result in arousals or awakenings from sleep, and may occur many times each night and up to several times a week. Polysomnographic monitoring reveals increased electromyographic activity in the affected leg with associated arousal or awakening. The exact prevalence of this condition is unknown, but sleep-related leg cramps can occur at any age, with the highest frequency found in the elderly. Patients affected by neurological conditions (e.g. peripheral neuropathies) and metabolic disturbances (e.g., hypokalemia, hypothyroidism, or dehydration) may be at increased risk for sleep-related leg cramps. If these illnesses are contributing to this movement disorder, first-line treatment should clearly be to effectively manage the underlying condition. Otherwise, nocturnal leg cramps can usually be relieved by local massage, application of heat, stretching, or movement of the affected limb. Treatment with vitamin E or quinine can sometimes be effective,[9] but no one pharmacologic approach has been shown to be effective in every case.

Excessive Fragmentary Myoclonus

Excessive fragmentary myoclonus (EFM) is characterized by brief, involuntary 'twitch-like' local contractions involving various areas of both sides of the body. These contractions are asymmetric and asynchronous, and occur during sleep. In many cases, this movement disorder is diagnosed strictly as an incidental finding of polysomnography. Involved areas may include muscles from the face, arms, legs, fingers, or toes. The EMG findings in EFM are similar to REM twitches that are a normal finding in REM sleep, except that these twitches also occur in other, non-REM stages of sleep.[9] Awareness of the twitch-like movements is usually not present. When severe, patients can complain of excessive daytime sleepiness, although the vast majority of cases are benign and self-limiting. There is no know treatment, and this disorder is rare in childhood and adolescence, occurring more frequently in older men.[9]

References

1. American Academy of Sleep Medicine. International classification of sleep disorders, revised: Diagnostic and coding manual. Chicago, Illinois: American Academy of Sleep Medicine; 2005.
2. Merlino G, Serafini A, Dolso P, et al. Association of body rolling, leg rolling, and rhythmic feet movements in a young adult: a video-polysomnographic study performed before and after one night of clonazepam. Move Disorder 2008;23(4):602–7.
3. Sheldon SH, Ferber R, Kryger MH. Principles and practice of pediatric sleep medicine. Philadelphia: Elsevier Saunders; 2005. p. 312.
4. Haywood PM, Hill CM. Rhythmic movement disorder: managing the child who head-bangs to get to sleep. Pediatr Child Health 2012;22(5):207–11.
5. Attarian H, Ward N, Schuman C. A multigenerational family with persistent sleep related rhythmic movement disorder (RMD) and insomnia. J Clin Sleep Med 2009;5(6):571–2.
6. Su C, Miao J, Lin Y, et al. Multiple forms of rhythmic movements in an adolescent boy with rhythmic movement disorder. Neurology 2009;63: 2272–9.
7. Walters AS, Silvestri R, Zucconi M, et al. Review of the possible relationship and hypothetical links between attention deficit hyperactivity disorder (ADHD) and the simple sleep related movement disorders, parasomias, hypersomnias, and circadian rhythm disorders. J Clin Sleep Med 2008;4(6):591–600.
8. Etzioni T, Katz N, Hering E, et al. Controlled sleep restriction for rhythmic movement disorder. J Pediatr 2005;147:393–5.
9. Walters AS. Clinical identification of the simple sleep-related movement disorders. Chest 2007;131:1260–6.
10. Wichniak A, Tracik F, Geisler P, et al. Rhythmic feet movements while falling asleep. Movet Disord 2001;16:1164–70.
11. American Academy of Sleep Medicine. Hypnagogic foot tremor and alternating leg muscle activation. In: Sateia MJ, editor. The International Classification of Sleep Disorders: Diagnostic and Coding Manual. 2nd ed. Westchester, IL: American Academy of Sleep Medicine; 2005. p. 213–15.
12. Chervin RD, Consens FB, Kutluay E. Alternating leg muscle activation during sleep and arousals: a new sleep-related motor phenomenon? Movem Disord 2003;18:551–9.
13. Cosentino FI, Iero I, Lanuzza B, et al. The neurophysiology of the alternating leg muscle activation (ALMA) during sleep: study of one patient before and after treatment with pramipexole. Sleep Med 2006;7:63–71.
14. Merlino G, Gigli GL. Sleep-related movement disorders. Neurolog Sci 2012;33:491–513.
15. Khoury S, Rouleau GA, Rompre PH, et al. A significant increase in breathing amplitude precedes sleep bruxism. Chest 2008;143:332–7.
16. Hornyak M, Feige B, Riemann D, et al. Periodic leg movements in sleep and periodic limb movement disorder: prevalence, clinical significance and treatment. Sleep Med Rev 2006;10:169–77.
17. Monaca A, Ciammella NM, Marci MC, Pirro R, Giannoni M. The anxiety in bruxer child. A case-control study. Minerva Somatol 2002;51(6):247–50.
18. Restrepo CC, Alvarez E, Jaramillo C, Velez C, Valencia I. Effects of psychological techniques on bruxism in children with primary teeth. Journal of Oral Rehabilitation 2001;28:354–60.

Restless Legs Syndrome, Periodic Leg Movements and Periodic Limb Movement Disorder

Jeffrey S. Durmer

Chapter 43

INTRODUCTION

A feeling of restlessness can describe both a physical and a psychological sensation that prompts movement or the urge to move. This ubiquitous human experience is at once recognizable as normal yet, in genetically susceptible individuals, an exaggeration of these (sometimes painful) sensations results in intrusive compensatory movements and the degradation of rest, sleep, performance and health. It is in these instances – when feelings of internal restlessness and the urge to move interfere with routine activities – that we use the term restless legs syndrome (RLS) or Willis–Ekbom disease. The characteristic symptoms of RLS have been known for hundreds of years and were first reported in medicine in the 1600s. The Swedish neurologist Karl Ekbom formally described the clinical, epidemiologic and pathophysiologic correlates of the condition in 1945.[1]

The syndrome has four well-known clinical criteria: (1) an uncomfortable sensation or unexplainable urge to move the legs or other affected body part; (2) increasing symptoms with rest or inactivity; (3) a reduction of symptoms with movement; and (4) a circadian enhancement of symptoms in the evening or night. Ekbom reported all aspects of RLS occurring in children, but it was not until the mid 1990s that the first case reports of children with RLS were published and research began to focus on the potential genetic causes for this familial disorder.[2,3]

Much has been discovered with regards to the genetics, potential pathophysiology, and epidemiology of RLS in the past 20 years, but advances have included very little specific information about children. The recognition of significant correlations between RLS and select pediatric conditions – such as attention-deficit hyperactivity disorder (ADHD) and iron deficiency – has helped generate new perspectives with regards to pathophysiology. Because pediatric-specific information concerning RLS is limited, age-adjusted adult criteria have been adopted for the diagnosis of this condition in children. Although additional criteria were included to increase the selectivity for children, having to rely on verbal descriptions in a linguistically developing population to diagnose a largely subjective disorder increases the clinical complexity. Still, an accurate diagnosis of RLS is the single most important aspect of treating children with this condition. Clinicians must consider potential mimics as well as comorbid and associated conditions. More objective findings, such as of periodic leg movements in sleep (PLMS) and of a family history of RLS, can increase diagnostic certainty.

Periodic limb movement disorder (PLMD), which is clinically defined as a disorder distinct from RLS, is noted in children as well as adults. The diagnostic criteria for PLMD include increased PLMS for age (>5 per hour) and a clinical

sleep disturbance that is not accounted for by another sleep disorder, including RLS. Clinical case studies suggest that children may manifest PLMD before developing RLS later in childhood.[4] Observations such as these help our understanding of the biological relationships between the sensory and motor components of these seemingly distinct but related disorders. Due to the limited available pediatric research, this chapter provides consensus opinion-based – as well as current evidence-based – information on the subject of childhood RLS and PLMD. Prevalence, pathophysiology, diagnosis, treatment and clinical associations of these conditions are also discussed.

SYMPTOMS AND PREVALENCE OF RLS AND PLMD IN CHILDREN

Restless legs syndrome and PLMD are very common in northern European populations and are believed to be among the most common inherited conditions known. Surveys show that between 4% and 15% of adults in the US and Western Europe have symptoms consistent with RLS.[5-7] In addition, there is evidence that up to 40% of adult RLS sufferers may have had the onset of symptoms in childhood or adolescence.[8,9] Prevalence rates vary from population to population due to genetic heterogeneity as well as to differences in survey tools used.

Validated RLS inventories, such as the *International Restless Legs Syndrome Study Group Rating Scale (IRLS)*,[10] have allowed investigators to utilize common tools in adult studies. The occurrence of RLS is increased in women compared to men (3:2 female:male). In younger populations the female:male ratio is closer to 2:1. Studies of adults over the age of 65 years show RLS prevalence increasing up to 10–20%.[11]

Approximately 8% to 20% of adults fulfill standard RLS criteria,[12,13] but only 2.7–3.9% of adults meet criteria for moderate to severe RLS (episodes twice or more per week with moderate to severe distress).[12,14] Not all people with RLS symptoms require medical attention.

Picchietti and colleagues – using the NIH consensus criteria for the diagnosis of *definite* RLS in children – performed the most comprehensive prevalence survey to date of RLS in children from the US and UK.[15] They demonstrated that 1.9% of 8–11-year-olds and 2% of 12–17-year-olds fulfilled these criteria. The prevalence of moderately severe RLS was 0.5% and 1% in 8–11-year-olds and 12–17-year-olds, respectively. There was no gender preference noted, unlike in adult RLS. In addition, the data showed a potentially strong genetic predisposition for RLS with 71–80% of children having at least one affected parent.[15] In 2010, an RLS symptom severity scale for children and adolescents was developed,[16] although large-scale validation studies have yet to be performed.

PERIODIC LIMB MOVEMENT DISORDER AND PERIODIC LEG MOVEMENTS

PLMD is delineated as a separate sleep-related movement disorder,[17] although many experts in the field consider PLMD to exist on a continuum with RLS. Both disorders are associated with low ferritin levels, respond to dopaminergic medications, share similar genetics, and are more common in Caucasian children than in other racial groups (OR=9.5).[18] The supposition of a continuum from PLMD to RLS is further bolstered by clinical evidence that some children manifest PLMD or PLMS years before the symptoms of RLS develop.[4] In a retrospective longitudinal study, Picchietti and Stevens identified PLMD or probable/possible RLS in 18 children (mean age=10.3 years) and subsequently diagnosed these children with definite RLS an average of 11.6 years later. In addition, these children had many of the comorbidities commonly associated with RLS such as ADHD, parasomnias, and a low serum ferritin level.[4] Thus, despite the differentiation of RLS from PLMD on clinical grounds, this evidence illustrates their potentially common pathophysiology and treatment.

With the recent discovery of a dose-dependent association between the BTBD9 gene (on chromosome 6p) and the findings in RLS of both PLMS and low serum ferritin, there remains no doubt that the motor and sensory features of RLS are related.[19] In addition, given that the vast majority of RLS sufferers have PLMS on polysomnography (PSG) testing (reports vary from 80% to 100%), the presence of a common neural mechanism for both sensory and motor symptoms is suggested. In contrast, PLMS are noted in a number of other disorders (such as Parkinson's disease and Tourette's syndrome), in association with certain medical conditions (such as pregnancy), in association with other sleep disorders (such as narcolepsy, sleep deprivation, and obstructive sleep apnea (OSA)), as a result of OSA treatment with continuous positive airway pressure),[20] and as a result of certain medications (such as selective serotonin reuptake inhibitors (SSRIs) and tricyclic antidepressants (TCAs)).[21-27]

Since PLMS are not disease-specific, some authorities question whether or not PLMS (and thus PLMD) should be considered abnormal. They also increase with age and occur in up to 30% of adults over the age of 50 years,[8] suggesting neurological deterioration that is part of normal aging.

Counter to the argument – that PLMS represent normal motor activity – are data that demonstrate the impact of PLMS and RLS on both health and psychological well-being. Sympathetic over-activation may explain the association between PLMS and chronic cardiovascular conditions in adults;[28] and, in RLS sufferers, this relationship is thought to elevate the risk for stroke and even the risk for insulin resistance and type II diabetes.[29] The natural state of sympathetic *hyperactivity* associated with youth may actually place children and younger adults at an even higher risk.[30] A number of adult and pediatric studies demonstrate a strong relationship with ADHD, behavioral disorders, and cognitive deficits as well as with depression and anxiety in RLS populations.[31-34] Adults with RLS carry a 4–5-fold increased risk for depression and a 13-fold increased risk for panic disorder.[35-38] Patient-reported outcome measures demonstrate a significant impact of RLS in adults.[12,39-42] Studies demonstrating that RLS causes clinical morbidity in pediatric populations, however, are lacking (Figure 43-1).

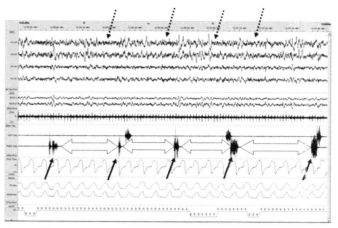

FIGURE 43-1 Periodic leg movements during sleep (PLMS) depicted on 2-minute PSG recording page. Each solid arrow demonstrates an individual PLM in a sequence of PLMS recorded with right and left anterior tibialis EMG. Block arrows denote the inter-movement interval, which is very consistent as noted in RLS. Also, note cortical arousals (dashed arrows) associated with PLMS that are thought to confer excessive autonomic activity and sleep fragmentation. *From: Durmer JS and Quraishi GH. Restless legs syndrome, periodic leg movements and periodic leg movement disorder in children. Pediatric Clinics of North America 2011;58:591–620.*

Measuring Periodic Leg Movements in Sleep

PLMS in children are not uncommon, especially in children with RLS; and, studies suggest that between 8.4% and 11.9% of children may have PLMD.[43] Normative pediatric data from studies that record PLMS via PSG and/or accelerometry (also referred to as actigraphy and actometry) demonstrate that most children and adolescents exhibit a periodic leg movement index (PLMi) no greater than 5/hour.[43-47] By contrast, up to 74% of children with definite RLS have a PLMi in excess of 5/hour.[48] When a PLMi are noted in children, clinicians should consider further investigation into the possibility of RLS.

Standardized criteria commonly utilized to score PLMS recorded via bilateral anterior tibialis electromyography (EMG)[49] have been modified in the past 5 years. Specifically, four movements must be scored in a row to qualify as periodic leg movements, and each of these movements must have an EMG amplitude greater than 8 microvolts, the movements must be separated by between 5 and 90 seconds, and individual movements must last between 0.5 seconds and 10 seconds.[50] These criteria allow for significant variability in the expression and periodicity of PLMS. Investigation based on rhythmic firing characteristics of neural systems provides a less variable measure of PLMS and provides a more scientific assessment for the potential generation of PLMS. Using the technique of a Markov-based stochastic mathematical process to measure inter-movement intervals and characterize the periodicity of PLMS,[51] researchers have demonstrated that subjects with RLS-related PLMS (and likely PLMD) have less inter-movement interval variability (with intervals clustering between 24 and 28 seconds) than is seen in PLMS due to other conditions (such as narcolepsy and ADHD).[52-54] There has been speculation that this particular frequency range is caused by neural pattern generators in the spinal cord and/or diencephalon.

PLMS demonstrate marked night-to-night variability, in children as well as in adults, and multiple nights of testing may be required to accurately quantify and diagnose PLMS.[55] Ambulatory or home-based PLMS measurements made using accelerometry in adults correlate with PLMS measured by PSG, and the same technique may be useful in the clinical evaluation of a child.[56,57]

PATHOPHYSIOLOGY OF RLS/PLMD

The neurobiological mechanisms leading to the motor and sensory symptoms of RLS/PLMD remain the topic of scientific inquiry. Clinical observations demonstrate that most primary cases of RLS respond to dopaminergic treatments such as levodopa/carbidopa, ropinirole and pramipexole. These observations suggest that monoaminergic neurotransmitter systems within the central nervous system play a pivotal role in the expression of RLS/PLMD symptoms. Neuroanatomic and physiologic models of diencephalic and spinal cord dopaminergic systems support an intriguing hypothesis related to the sole source of dopamine innervation in the spinal cord, namely the bilateral A-11 hypothalamic cell groups. These cells project to all levels of the spinal cord and provide dorsal (sensory), ventral (motor) and mediolateral (sympathetic) dopaminergic activity. This important neuroanatomic property suggests that the A-11 dopaminergic cell groups may be major contributors to the development of RLS.[58] Animal models using dopamine receptor (D2-like) knock-out mice suggest that the loss of spinal cord gating via D2-like receptors may precipitate the sensory and motor symptoms of RLS/PLMD (Figure 43-2).[59]

An association between iron deficiency and RLS was first noted by Nordlander in 1954.[60] Impairment of brain iron availability is hypothesized to play a role in the pathogenesis of RLS and PLMD, based on several studies in animals and humans. Serum iron indices, such as total iron, hemoglobin levels, and hematocrit, are usually within the normal ranges in RLS patients. Nevertheless, brain iron deficiency has been implicated in humans from investigations using cerebrospinal fluid analysis of iron and ferritin,[61,62] magnetic resonance imaging and ultrasound of the substantia nigra,[63–65] and autopsy examination of brain tissue from RLS subjects.[66,67] The link between iron deficiency and dysfunction of central dopaminergic systems is based on evidence that iron is a cofactor for the rate-limiting enzyme in dopamine synthesis, tyrosine hydroxylase, and is required for postsynaptic D2 receptor function. Iron deficiency results in down-regulation of striatum and nucleus accumbens dopamine receptors as well as dysregulation of dopamine vesicular release.[68–70] Correlations between peripheral serum ferritin levels and cerebrospinal ferritin levels in RLS patients demonstrate that serum ferritin levels below 50 ng/mL correlate with relative body iron storage deficiency.[61,62]

Recent evidence suggests that lower ferritin status in RLS may not only correlate with alterations in dopamine metabolism and neural transmission but may also be associated with an inability to retain intracellular ferritin.[71] In a study comparing 24 women with early-onset RLS with a control group of 25 women without RLS, Earley et al. demonstrated there were marked differences in proteins associated with iron trafficking into cells (soluble transferrin receptor (TfR) and

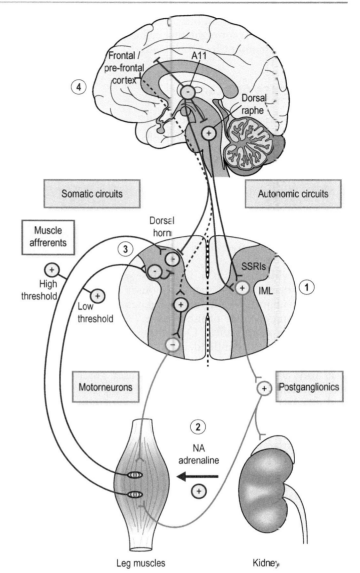

FIGURE 43-2 The proposed role of the diencephalic dopaminergic cell group A-11 in the pathophysiology of RLS. A11 neurons project caudally to inhibit the dorsal raphae nucleus. This results in less sympathetic excitation via the spinal cord intermediolateral cell column (IML). A-11 neurons also project to all levels of the spinal cord and inhibit dorsal horn sensory transmission as well as the afferent projections of the IML (#1) As proposed in RLS, a loss of A-11 dopaminergic inhibition results in increased sensory input to cortex (uncomfortable sensations or urge to move), increased sensory activation of the spinal cord reflex arc (#3) (causing PLMS), and increased sympathetic activity (#2) (accentuating PLMS and associated medical conditions such as hypertension and pro-inflammatory states). The loss of rostral A11 projections would also enhance cortically mediated sensory discomfort associated with RLS (#4). *From: Clemens S, Rye D, Hochman S. RLS revisiting the dopamine hypothesis from the spinal cord perspective. Neurology. 2006;67:125-130.*

divalent metal transporter 1 protein (DMT-1) and out of cells (ferroportin protein). RLS patients had higher TfR and DMT-1 levels consistent with an increased cellular need for iron. Paradoxically, they also had higher ferroportin protein levels, which would normally signify high intracellular iron levels since this protein regulates iron efflux. Thus, patients with RLS seem to have an intracellular need for iron; yet, the proteins responsible for regulating cellular iron content create a situation tantamount to a *leaky bucket*.

THE GENETICS OF RLS/PLMD

Genetic investigations over the past 12 years using twin concordance, family association, familial linkage, and genomic association methods have created a more complex picture. Twin studies suggest a heritability of approximately 54% for RLS.[72] Additional genomic and linkage studies suggest that different sensorimotor phenotypes may be linked to different genetic loci. Ten different genetic loci for RLS have been identified (on multiple chromosomes) using familial linkage analysis, and these findings suggest that RLS/PLMD is a complex genetic trait that interacts with environmental factors.[73–86]

Initial evidence from a familial segregation analysis in Germany demonstrated that early-onset RLS (patients <30 years old) supported a single major gene model with an autosomal dominant mode of inheritance.[87] Late-onset RLS did not demonstrate this effect. On further analysis, two distributions of RLS were identified, based on age of onset (with the dividing point at 26.3 years). These data suggest that RLS is primarily genetic in younger age-of-onset groups but that environmental components influence the expression of RLS and may be more relevant in the later age-of-onset groups.[88] Many studies of familial RLS demonstrate genetic anticipation where subsequent generations show a progressively earlier ages of symptom onset.[89–92] Thus far, there is no evidence to support a trinucleotide repeat mechanism for RLS (as is the case in certain other disorders that also demonstrate genetic anticipation, such as spinocerebellar ataxia and Huntington's disease).[93,94]

To understand if there are more common RLS alleles with particular phenotypes, genomic association studies using single nucleotide polymorphisms (SNPs) have been performed since 2007. An Icelandic investigation of 306 RLS cases and 15,664 controls identified three genes (BTBD9, GLO1, and DNAH8) on chromosome 6p that were associated with RLS patients with PLMS as a major component of their phenotype.[19] This study demonstrated dose-dependent associations among the BTBD9 allele, PLMS, and serum ferritin levels. Heterozygous individuals for this allele showed twice the risk for RLS with PLMS, while those homozygous for this variant had four times the risk. Serum ferritin levels were also lower in those with the additional BTBD9 allele. In a second genomic study performed in a German cohort of 401 familial RLS sufferers and 1644 controls, four genes (MEIS1 – ch 2p, BTBD9 – ch 6p, MAP2K5 – ch15q, and LBXCOR1 – ch 15q) were found in association with RLS.[95] In both the German and Icelandic investigations, the BTBD9 allele, which is widely distributed in the brain and body, was found to be associated with RLS.

Replication studies of the familial and genomic findings from adult studies have proven inconclusive in children. One study assessed gene variants in 23 children and found an 87% positive family history of RLS and a trend toward association with MEIS1 and MAP2K/LBX-COR1 variants, but no association was found with BTBD9.[96] Another study of 386 children with ADHD and RLS did not find a genetic association.[97]

THE DIAGNOSIS OF RLS/PLMD IN CHILDREN

As stated above, the diagnosis of PLMD in children and adolescents formally requires: (1) PLMS documented by polysomnography and exceeding a PLMi of 5 per hour, (2) clinical sleep disturbance, and (3) the absence of another primary sleep disorder or reason for the PLMS (including RLS). In 1995, the *International Restless Legs Syndrome Study Group* developed standardized criteria for the diagnosis of RLS in adults.[98] In addition to the four essential features (noted above), five additional clinical features of RLS were included: (1) sleep disturbance, or daytime results of sleep disturbance, (2) involuntary movements during sleep (PLMS) and during wake (periodic leg movements during wakefulness (PLMW)), (3) neurological examination findings consistent with RLS, (4) typical clinical course and exacerbating factors, and (5) positive family history. Idiopathic or primary RLS was also distinguished from reactive or secondary RLS (which may be caused by conditions such as uremia, neuropathy, medications, and anemia).

In 2003, an NIH workshop produced expert consensus criteria for the diagnosis of RLS in children and special populations.[99] Categories of diagnostic certainty for RLS in children aged 2–12 years old were established based on varying levels of clinical evidence (see Box 43-1). The essential four adult criteria were retained for the diagnosis of *definite* RLS in adolescents (13–18 years old). In addition, categories of *possible* and *probable* RLS were established, suggesting that individuals with incomplete RLS should be followed for progression of symptoms.

The 2003 NIH expert panel consensus criteria for the diagnosis of pediatric RLS included a requirement that children be able to state in their own words their experience of the symptoms. These criteria not only reduce potential misdiagnoses but also raise a diagnostic challenge (due to the developmental nature of verbal fluency). Up to 40% of adults first experience RLS symptoms in childhood or adolescence, and PLMS and PLMD precede the diagnosis of RLS in children by an average of 11–12 years.

In 2010, a multi-dimensional, self-administered, patient-reported outcome questionnaire (the *Pediatric Restless Legs Syndrome Severity Scale* (P-RLS-SS)) was published to assess pediatric RLS symptom severity and impact.[16] In addition to establishing a metric, this study demonstrated that children experience RLS symptoms during both daytime and nighttime. They experience pain in association with RLS and often utilize countermeasures such as rubbing or moving. Many children provided non-verbal descriptions of their symptoms using a visual analog scale and free-hand drawings of their experiences.[100] Despite variations of interpretation, such visual approaches may be more appropriate for diagnosing RLS in younger or less fluent children, especially when one is searching for a starting point in the diagnostic process (Figure 43-3).

In the diagnostic interview for RLS it is important to provide a non-leading introduction in order to allow the child to express his or her own experience. Adult family members should be questioned as well since they may have similar symptoms or even have an RLS diagnosis themselves. However, clinicians should direct their inquiry toward the child to help them recreate the last time they experienced something that made it hard 'to fall asleep' or 'to lie still in bed.' Often, the presenting complaint from the child or

Box 43-1 Definite RLS Criteria for Pediatrics

NIH Workshop Diagnostic Criteria for RLS in Children and Adolescents

For definite RLS, children (ages 2–12 years) must meet ALL of the following adult criteria:

- An urge to move the legs, usually accompanied or caused by uncomfortable and unpleasant sensations in the legs. (Sometimes the urge to move is present without the uncomfortable sensations and sometimes the arms or other body parts are involved in addition to the legs.)
- The urge to move or unpleasant sensations begin or worsen during periods of rest or inactivity such as lying or sitting.
- The urge to move or unpleasant sensations are partially or totally relieved by movement, such as walking or stretching, at least as long as the activity continues.
- The urge to move or unpleasant sensations are worse in the evening or night than during the day or only occur in the evening or night. (When symptoms are very severe, the worsening at night may not be noticeable but must have been previously present.)

AND

- A description of the leg discomfort in the child's own words using terms that are age-appropriate

OR

- Demonstrate at least 2 of 3 following supportive criteria
- Sleep disturbance for age (e.g.; sleep onset/maintenance insomnia)
- A biologic parent or sibling with definite RLS
- The child has documented PLMS index of ≥ 5/hour.

For definite RLS, adolescents (ages 13–18 years) must meet ALL of the 4 adult criteria above.

Adapted from: Allen RP, Picchietti DL, Henning WA, Trenkwalder C, Walters AS, Montplaisir J. Restless legs syndrome: diagnositic criteria, special considerations, and epidemiology. A report from the RLS diagnosis and epidemiology workshop at the NIH. Sleep Med 2003;4:101–119

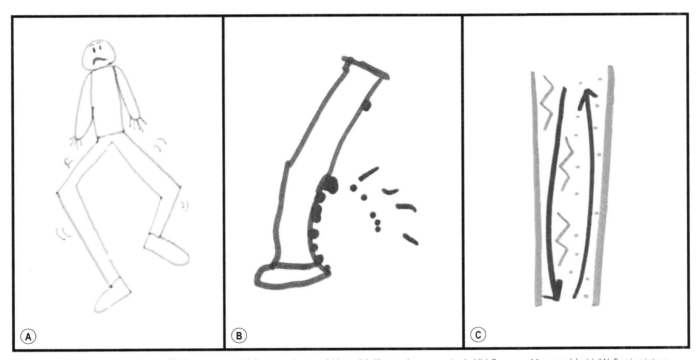

FIGURE 43-3 Children's drawings of RLS symptoms: (a) From an 8-year-old boy: 'It's like my legs are wiggly;' (b) From an 11-year-old girl: 'Well his picture shows like, see like it's ant bites that's kind of showing you that it's really hurting me like in those areas;' (c) From a 14-year-old girl: 'I feel stuff going up and down my legs where it just tingles. And that's more when it starts feeling like a little numb and then these represent my tingles. And then the red would be just when it hurts.' *Adapted from: Picchietti DL, Arbuckle RA, Abetz L, Durmer JS, Ivanchenko A, Owens J, Croenlein J, Allen RP, Walters AS. Pediatric restless legs syndrome: analysis of symptom descriptions and drawings. Journal of Child Neurology 2011;26(11):1365–76.*

parent may not appear to be related to 'restlessness' or 'kicking.' Common complaints in pediatric RLS are difficulty falling asleep, not wanting to go to sleep, and (occasionally) difficulty remaining asleep. By directing the conversation to a description of the bedtime routine, a young or forgetful child can start by reporting the bedroom surroundings to contextualize the sleep-onset experience. Since this is the most common time for symptoms to emerge, the child may then recall the last time he or she had a problem falling asleep. The clinician can use similar techniques to help the child remember symptoms that occur at other times of the day, such as sitting in class at a desk, attempting to nap, or while doing homework after school. Children provide imaginative descriptions of RLS symptoms – e.g., 'soda bubbles in my legs,' 'ants biting my leg,' 'just want to move,' or 'got to kick.'[4,15,101] It is not common for children to use the term 'urge to move' in relationship to their description of RLS symptoms, but it is helpful to allow them to physically demonstrate compensatory maneuvers such as wiggling, rubbing, kicking, hitting and even constantly moving 'to find the cool spot.' After exhausting one's direct inquiry with a child it is sometimes helpful to incorporate the parent into the discussion to remind the child of bedtime rituals and activities that may provide some recall.

Additional diagnostic criteria, including timing of the symptoms, exacerbating conditions, and compensatory maneuvers, can be elicited by focusing on the *bad feeling* that the child describes. During the day, it is common to note some degree of classroom difficulty, and the child's teacher or parent may be helpful in this regard. Difficulty sitting quietly at a desk and paying attention, irritability, and hyperactivity may be notable symptoms of children with RLS. The overlap with ADHD-like symptoms is often brought up in this context. To distinguish between these two sets of *restlessness* symptoms it is helpful to remember that in RLS the hyperactivity is caused by an *internal* sensory discomfort while in ADHD it is related to an interaction with the *external* environment.

Clinicians must be aware of causes of secondary or reactive RLS in children since their treatment may be quite different from that of primary RLS. Age-associated causes of secondary RLS include joint pain and arthritis, Osgood–Schlatter disease, dysasthesias related to peripheral neuropathy or radiculopathy, akathesia related to anti-dopaminergic medications, and cutaneous pain related to dermatitis or rashes (see Box 43-2). Identification of one of these entities or RLS should prompt clinicians to ask for symptoms of the other. Another condition commonly associated with, and often possibly identical to, RLS is that of *growing pains*. Children diagnosed with growing pains unrelated to any other identifiable disorder commonly demonstrate a strong family history of RLS and, in many cases, fulfill the diagnostic criteria for RLS.[102] The prevalence of growing pains in children ages 4–6 years measured with validated instruments is as high as 37%.[103] And, the presence of typical growing pains in children with either a family history of growing pains or RLS should prompt clinicians to consider a diagnosis of RLS.

It is helpful to note that, in children, symptoms commonly associated with RLS may also be seen with other sleep or medical/psychiatric disorders. Irritability, depression, anxiety, and hyperactivity may occur secondary to sleep deprivation; they may also be symptoms of comorbid conditions such as panic disorder, generalized anxiety disorder, ADHD, ODD and depression. Parasomnias, sleep-related movement disorders, and the insomnias also may be the presenting symptoms in some cases of childhood RLS.[4,101,104] It is important to note mood and behavioral symptoms since these secondary symptoms of RLS may be most prominent.

Although RLS is a clinical diagnosis that does not require testing, it is not possible to determine the presence or effect of PLMS on a child's sleep without a test. Parental reports and even clinical evaluation by trained sleep clinicians are not adequate predictors of PLMS.[105,106] Sleep testing is also required when symptoms suggest other sleep disorders. Traditionally, PSG is employed to detect PLMS; however, accelerometry may also be considered.

Box 43-2 Conditions that may Result in Secondary (or Reactive) RLS in Children

- Endocrine
  - Diabetes
  - Thyroid disease
- Musculoskeletal
  - Osgood–Schlatter
  - Muscle soreness
  - Injury (e.g. sprain, bruise, strain)
  - Cramps
  - Arthritis
  - Connective tissue disorders (e.g. plantar fasciitis)
  - Myopathy (congenital or acquired)
- Neurovascular
  - Positional discomfort (e.g. 'pins-and-needles')
  - Peripheral neuropathy
  - Radiculopathy
  - Myelopathy
  - Sickle cell disease
  - Multiple sclerosis
- Neoplasm
- Skin
  - Dermatitis
  - Dry skin substances
- Anti-dopaminergic medications
  - SSRI medications
  - Tricyclic medications
  - Caffeine
- Other
  - ADHD
  - Iron deficiency
  - Oppositional defiant disorder
  - Pregnancy
  - Celiac disease
  - Uremia

RLS AND ADHD

From the mid 1990s to the present, an increased prevalence of RLS and PLMD has been noted in children with symptoms consistent with ADHD.[31,107] Despite limited sample sizes (between 19 and 98 individuals/study), estimates for RLS in the ADHD pediatric population range between 10.5% and 44%, and the estimated prevalence of ADHD in the RLS population is similarly increased (18–30%).[15,108–112] The epidemiological survey study by Picchietti and colleagues also demonstrates a strong relationship between ADHD and RLS with 23.9% of 8–11-year-olds and 28.6% of 12–17-year-olds demonstrating both definite RLS and attentional deficit disorder (ADD)/ADHD.[113] The relationship between RLS and ADD/ADHD is complex since sleep deprivation in children may mimic the hyperactivity and inattention noted in ADD and ADHD. In addition, physiologic and genetic investigations suggest that these two conditions may share similar features such as iron deficiency and dopamine dysfunction.

Objective sleep measures demonstrate increased sleep disruption in children with ADHD (with findings of PLMS, sleep-disordered breathing (SDB), increased sleep onset latency, and increased number of stage shifts per hour of sleep).[114,115] Theories concerning the high correlation between RLS/PLMD and ADHD often focus on sleep deprivation as a cause for the symptoms of hyperactivity and inattention in ADHD. Sleep deprivation may even help explain the higher incidence of other sleep disorders (such as SDB) also seen in ADHD. Although sleep deprivation may help explain some of the general overlap between RLS and ADHD, converging areas of genetic evidence support a more specific dopaminergic connection between these conditions. ADHD, like RLS, is a complex neurodevelopmental disorder with multiple subtypes that likely represent dysfunction within several neural systems. ADHD candidate genes are notably related to the dopamine system. The dopamine relationship is supported by additional evidence, namely that the most effective treatments for ADHD are stimulants (which block dopamine transport), that neural imaging findings in ADHD demonstrate neuroanatomical and physiological dysfunction of the frontostriatal system, and that the executive function deficits noted in ADHD are secondary to dopaminergic transmission abnormalities. Genes associated with ADHD include the D4 (DRD4), D5 (DRD5), and D1 (DRD1) dopamine receptor genes, and the dopamine transporter gene (DAT1).[116–122] Additional genetic associations are also noted within dopamine metabolic pathways including the DDC gene (which catalyzes the conversion of DOPA to dopamine), the DβH gene (which regulates an enzyme responsible for the conversion of dopamine to norepinephrine), a polymorphism of the catechol-O-methyl transferase (COMT) gene, and the monoamine oxidase A (MAOA) gene.[123] There are also associations between ADHD and other monoaminergic genes responsible for noradrenergic and serotonergic activity. Initial investigations using several of the previously identified RLS-linked SNPs (MEIS1, BTBD9 and MAP2K5) demonstrated no significant associations with ADHD. Although BTBD9 SNPs show nominal significance, however, when one controls for multiple testing, this association is seen to be at best a trend.[124] Additional investigations utilizing various RLS and ADHD phenotypes in genetic linkage and genomic association studies are needed to understand the relationship of these co-occurring and perhaps comorbid conditions.

Both RLS and ADHD demonstrate an association with iron deficiency. Studies of children with RLS, ADHD, or both show a relationship with relatively low serum ferritin measures when compared to age- and gender-matched controls.[115,125–127] Treatment for relative iron deficiency using oral iron repletion in children with ADHD has been studied in a small randomized, double-blind, placebo-controlled trial.[128] Iron treatment demonstrated benefits in both Clinical Global Impression scales and ADHD rating scales.

For additional discussion, also see Chapter 15.

TREATMENT AND MANAGEMENT OF RLS/PLMD

The Behavioral Approach

Children with RLS or PLMD (or their parents) often report symptoms of behavioral sleep disorders that have become ingrained in a family's approach to sleep. Sleep-onset association and limit-setting behavioral sleep disorders, inadequate sleep hygiene, and insufficient sleep can all result in symptomatic worsening and render even the best medical therapies ineffective (see Chapters 8 and 14). The initial approach to RLS/PLMD treatment is education, for example to establish proper bedtime behaviors, ensure a non-stimulating environment, avoid exercise and excitement before bed, and control access to food and drink during the night. The use of cognitive and physical countermeasures for RLS symptoms – such as physical relaxation techniques, warm baths, and cognitive restructuring – may be helpful during the sleep-onset routine in children suffering from RLS. It is also critical to consider activators of RLS symptoms such as sleep deprivation and certain drugs and medications (caffeine, nicotine, SSRIs, TCAs, anti-emetics and antihistamines).

The Pharmacologic Approach
Iron Supplementation
In a study by Konofal et al. children with RLS and ADHD had lower ferritin levels than children with ADHD alone, and they also had more severe symptoms of ADHD.[127] More recently, a retrospective analysis of 30 consecutive Japanese children with RLS treated with oral iron therapy showed a clear benefit that was noted on average 3 months after starting therapy.[129] Symptom resolution occurred in 57% of children, and improvement in 33%; only 10% were non-responders.

Given the evidence of relative iron body storage deficits in children with RLS, it is now common practice to obtain serum levels before embarking on any particular therapy. Studies of familial RLS demonstrate that, aside from an earlier age of onset, patients typically have lower serum ferritin levels (which also predict future therapeutic challenges such as augmentation to dopaminergic therapies).[130,131] At a minimum, the serum ferritin and a complete blood count (CBC) should be obtained, although total iron binding capacities, transferrin, and TfR are often included. It is important to remember that infection, liver disease, cancer, or significant stress can elevate ferritin levels and lead to inaccurate conclusions about iron status. Serum ferritin levels (and iron stores) may also be decreased without overt iron deficiency anemia (i.e., without low hemoglobin or hematocrit levels). It is particularly important to understand the physiology of body iron compartmentalization when testing RLS patients (see Figure 43-4). Functional iron constituents such as hemoglobin, generally used as surrogates for body iron levels, are preserved at the expense of stored iron. Thus, just knowing that hemoglobin levels are normal is incomplete information; it is important to also note the relative ferritin and transferrin levels to complete the iron metabolism picture.

Current recommendations for iron supplementation in children with RLS symptoms suggest treatment when the serum ferritin falls below 50 ng/mL.[132] This recommendation is partially based on the finding that in adult RLS patients a serum ferritin below 50 ng/mL is associated with increased symptoms.[133,134] Also, subjects with ferritin levels below that level are significantly more responsive to iron repletion therapy. The goal of therapy is to achieve a ferritin level of 80–100 ng/mL since saturation of peripheral iron stores typically occurs in this range.

Deficits in serum ferritin often go unrecognized, even with testing, since the lower end of the normal reference ranges typically are listed as being well below the 50 ng/mL level, i.e., below the level where RLS and PLMD symptoms may emerge.

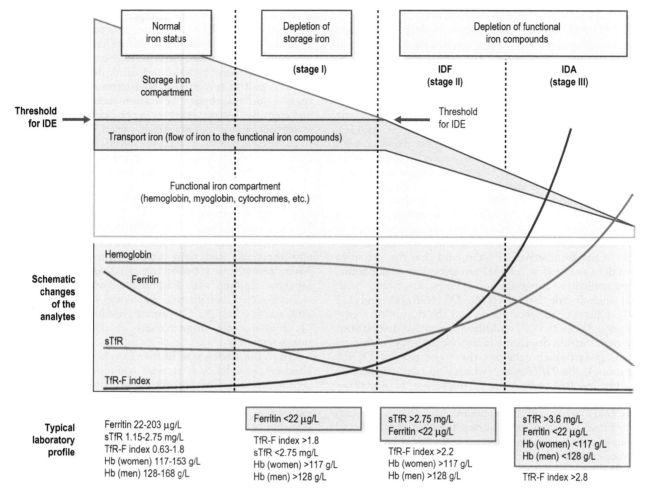

FIGURE 43-4 Stages of iron deficiency (ID) in the body correlated with typical laboratory values. From left to right, as body iron stores become depleted, storage becomes increasingly reduced as reflected by falling serum ferritin levels. As the stages of ID progress (defined by laboratory values within the boxes at the bottom of the figure), transport and functional iron compartments become impacted resulting in iron-deficient erythropoiesis (IDE) and iron deficiency anemia (IDA). Of note, hemoglobin values do not reflect iron depletion until the last stages of iron deficiency. *From: Suominen P, Punnonen K, Rajamaki A, Irjala K. Serum transferrin receptor and transferrin receptor-ferritin index identify healthy subjects with subclinical iron deficits. Blood 1998;92(8):2934–39*

The literature supports the use of iron repletion therapy to treat both RLS and PLMS symptoms in children.[104,129,135,136] Although extensive clinical data are lacking with regards to this therapy, both oral and intravenous (IV) iron repletion methods for RLS are available. Oral supplementation may take 3 months or more to achieve adequate ferritin elevations, and clinical evidence suggests a similar response time for symptoms.[129] Oral dosing is usually 3–6 mg/kg/day and supplements should be taken on an empty stomach with vitamin C for improved absorption. Liquids and tablet preparations are available. The most common side effects are gastrointestinal. To help reduce side effects and maximize absorption, supplements should be taken without calcium-containing foods or drinks. Repeat testing is recommended within 2–3 months to confirm a change in iron levels and also to assure that levels do not exceed the therapeutic range. Once serum ferritin levels reach 80–100 ng/mL, iron therapy may be discontinued or tapered. Some clinicians prefer to continue a low-maintenance iron supplementation with vitamins, but no data regarding the effectiveness of this strategy are available.

In adults, trials of IV iron therapy have demonstrated significant effects on serum ferritin levels and, in some cases, complete amelioration of RLS symptoms.[137–139] There are no similar studies using IV iron in children. When iron infusions are given serially, there is a reliable increase in ferritin levels with each infusion followed by a gradual fall, and the rate of fall decreases progressively over successive treatments.[137] In fact, a return to previously low ferritin levels may follow the initial courses of any form of iron therapy. Serum ferritin retesting should be considered if a child reports a return of RLS symptoms or to ensure that ferritin levels remain above 50 ng/mL. Clinically, the use of low-molecular-weight IV iron dextran compounds is noted to result in a superior outcome without the previously noted hypersensitivity and allergic reactions related to higher-molecular-weight formulations.[140,141]

Other Forms of Pharmacotherapy

In addition to iron repletion, other forms of pharmacotherapy may be required if symptoms impact sleep or daytime activities on a regular basis, although no current FDA-approved options are available for children. The utility of medication depends on the symptom frequency and intensity. Occasional symptoms, occurring less than once a week, may be treated on an as-needed basis rather than with daily prophylactic treatment. When moderately severe RLS symptoms are present in adults (symptoms 2 days/week or more), daily drug therapy is suggested. Painful, intrusive nighttime symptoms, or those that cause daytime dysfunction, are more likely to engender a medical response. Clinicians must understand the array of medical interventions available to adults and help parents and children make an informed decision.

The five general categories of medications most commonly used to treat RLS symptoms are dopaminergic agents, anti-adrenergics, opioids, anticonvulsants, and benzodiazepines.

Dopaminergics

The most widely used and most successful medical therapies for RLS are those that produce their effect through the dopaminergic system. This class of therapies is so helpful that the diagnostic criterion for adult RLS even includes a response to dopaminergic medication as a supportive feature. Treatment with dopamine therapy may control both sensory and motor symptoms. Dopaminergic medications have also proven successful in case reports and small open-label studies of children with RLS with and without ADHD;[4,142-150] but, to date, there have been no large-scale, double-blind, placebo-controlled trials using dopaminergic medications in children with RLS or PLMD. The effect of L-dopa on symptoms of ADHD and RLS in children was investigated in a 2011 small randomized, double-blind study. Twenty-nine children diagnosed with ADHD and RLS, and 29 with ADHD and no RLS, were either treated with L-dopa or a placebo and assessed pre- and post-intervention. Despite a significant impact on RLS and PLMS, there were no effects on objective neuropsychiatric measures of ADHD.[151] Although ADHD and RLS share a significant clinical overlap, multiple therapies may be required to control symptoms.

L-dopa was the first dopamine agent shown to be effective for both the sensory and motor symptoms of RLS.[152] Due to its short half-life (1.5–2 hours), it is usually reserved as an abortive or diagnostic agent and is not routinely used for prophylaxis.[21] In addition, L-dopa has a high reported rate of augmentation (up to 60–73% of adult users).[153,154] The rate of augmentation in children has not been studied; however, unpublished anecdotal evidence suggests very little augmentation is observed in children. A more common cause for cessation of dopaminergic therapy in children is related to side effects including gastrointestinal upset, nausea, disturbed dreams and sedation.

Augmentation, as defined by the Max Planck Institute Criteria, includes three basic features: (1) increased symptoms in 5 of the previous 7 days, (2) no other identifiable cause for the symptom change, and (3) a prior positive response to dopamine therapy. Two additional features of augmentation are: (1) persistence or paradoxical response to additional dopaminergic therapy, and (2) an earlier return of symptoms.[155] Augmentation causes a shift of RLS symptoms to earlier in the day, it leads to an increase in body parts involved, and it may be associated with change in severity or quality of discomfort during pharmacologic therapy. All these effects are reversible by withdrawal of the therapy. Also, augmentation is increased when serum ferritin levels are low and when dopaminergic medications have been used for extended time periods.[154] It is important to distinguish augmentation from tolerance, early morning rebound, neuroleptic-induced akathesia, and RLS disease progression.[154] Progression of RLS symptoms may also appear similar to augmentation, but generally this occurs on a timescale of years rather than weeks or months.

Tolerance is a reduction in medication effectiveness over time, often necessitating an increase in dose. It is unclear if this is related to the development of augmentation, but it has been reported to precede some cases of augmentation in adults.

Neuroleptic-induced akathesia is distinguished from augmentation by its non-circacian pattern as well as the inner *sense* of overall body restlessness rather than discrete limb restlessness.

If augmentation is noted, the first course of action is to test serum ferritin levels and treat the patient accordingly. Following this, an immediate reduction of dopaminergic therapy to the lowest tolerated dose should both result in symptomatic improvement and serve to confirm the diagnosis of augmentation. Other causes for RLS exacerbation should be identified and eliminated. If augmentation persists, the dopaminergic agent should be discontinued and alternative medical therapy (such as described below) may be instituted.[154]

Dopaminergic agents that are FDA-approved to treat moderate to severe RLS in adults include the non-ergot selective D2, D3, D4 agonists ropinirole, pramipexole and rotigotine. The longer half-lives of the first two of these (oral) agents (6–8 hours for ropinirole and 8–10 hours for pramipexole) and the lower total daily dose and lower augmentation rate (3.5–30%) favors them for prophylactic therapy in moderate to severe RLS.[156] In 2012, a transdermal dopamine agonist delivery system with rotigotine was approved by the FDA for moderate to severe RLS. Initial studies conducted with this delivery system demonstrate significant benefit for adult RLS patients with less augmentation and side effects when compared to oral treatments.[157] The most common side effect with transdermal therapy is local skin irritation, but it seems that very few patients discontinue due to this effect, even after 5 years of treatment.[158] The risk/benefit of dopamine agonist therapies in children should be addressed on a case-by-case basis. With oral, and now transdermal alternatives, clinicians are better equipped than ever to provide alternatives for children and their parents seeking an effective medical therapy.

The common side effects of dopamine agonists in adults include nausea, vomiting, nasal congestion, headaches, insomnia, hypersomnia, fluid retention and augmentation. The neurodevelopmental effects of dopamine agonists on humans are not known. Given the plasticity of the central nervous system's dopaminergic pathways, it is difficult to predict the rates of side effects, augmentation, and any potential detrimental effects in children. In some cases, particularly with co-occurring ADHD or obsessive–compulsive disorder (OCD), children may manifest increased impulsive behaviors and even obsessive thinking with dopaminergic therapy. The long-term effects of childhood dopamine agonist therapy on the symptomatic progression of RLS are also unknown, and longitudinal research is required to understand the complex interaction between therapy and the course of disease progression from childhood into adulthood.

Anti-Adrenergics

Clonidine is sometimes employed in the treatment of RLS and comorbid ADHD-related insomnia, although it is generally used as an anti-hypertensive or anxiolytic (due to its alpha-2-receptor agonist properties).[159,160] In a small randomized, double-blind, placebo-controlled trial, clonidine was shown to effectively treat RLS sensory symptoms in adults without significant side effects.[161] Clonidine is commonly used as a pediatric sleep aid[162] (even though not FDA approved for this purpose) and has pharmacological attributes which make it particularly useful for treating hyperactivity-related symptoms in children. For RLS sufferers, it may also aid in reducing overactive sympathetic nervous system outflow that is theorized to contribute to PLMS and the exacerbation of associated medical conditions such as hypertension and cardiovascular disease. The most common side effects are sedation and hypotension.

Opioids

Opioids are not often prescribed as prophylactic therapy but usually are reserved for treatment of painful refractory RLS or cases of dopaminergic augmentation. In adults with RLS, the efficacy of oral and intrathecal opioids – such as methadone, morphine and oxycodone – has been demonstrated in double-blind, placebo-controlled trials and case reports.[163–167] The pharmacologic action of opioids with regards to RLS is thought to be mediated through interactions with the dopamine system.[168] In 2011, a 10-year retrospective analysis compared adults who were treated for moderate to severe RLS with dopamine agonists (pergolide and pramipexole) with those treated with methadone and demonstrated some important outcomes favoring opioid therapy.[169] Treatment with low-dose methadone (median of 10 mg), for example, demonstrated none of the discontinuation or augmentation that is seen with dopamine agonists. In addition, the successful use of opioids as a bridging agent after withdrawal from dopaminergic therapy (partly due to an indirect dopaminergic mechanism) suggests that opioids may be safely implemented in specific RLS populations. The effective control of refractory pain-related symptoms (that can occur in severe RLS or as a result of augmentation) is a primary reason to consider opioid therapy. Polysomnographic studies also demonstrate that opioids do not consistently reduce PLMS but do reduce associated arousals.[164]

The centrally acting, non-narcotic analgesic, tramadol, is an alternative to opioid use in children, given its lower abuse potential and fewer adverse side effects. Small open-label studies have demonstrated the effectiveness of this medication in treating the subjective complaints associated with RLS in adults;[170] however, similar studies have not been conducted in children.

Anticonvulsants

In adults, studies demonstrate the acute and long-term benefits of the alpha 2-delta agonist gabapentin[171–173] and the pro-drug gabapentin enacarbilin[174–176] in the management of RLS-related symptoms. Data suggest that the major effect of this class of agents in the treatment of RLS is amelioration of sensory symptoms; however, a significant reduction in PLMS has been noted as well.[171,172] Gabapentin is often considered a first choice for children experiencing sleep onset difficulty and RLS symptoms since this drug is known to enhance slow-wave sleep. There are few adverse side effects (emotional lability and edema are most notable). Since there is no appreciable metabolism of gabapentin in humans, resulting in circulatory renal excretion, it is safe to use in combination with many other medications. In 2011, gabapentin enacarbil was approved by the FDA for the treatment of moderate to severe RLS in adults.[177] A single dose of 600 mg was suggested. However, there is no evidence to support this treatment in children. Gabapentin is excreted in human breast milk and both gabapentin and gabapentin enacarbil are classified as pregnancy category C, which means they should only be used in pregnancy if the potential benefits justify the potential risks to the fetus.

Benzodiazepines

In the years prior to FDA approval of dopamine agonists and gabapentin enacarbil for the treatment of RLS in adults, clonazepam was the most commonly used medication for this condition. This was largely due to its noted effects in controlling myoclonic jerks and myoclonus following anoxia. The first published uses of clonazepam for RLS were case reports in 1979 and 1980.[178,179] Subsequent double-blind, placebo-controlled trials demonstrated significant benefits in objective sleep efficiency and subjective sleep quality despite an absence of effects on PLMS.[180] Clonazepam has a very long half-life of 18–50 hours, which may be useful in children due to prolonged sleeping times. Clonazepam is approved by the FDA for use in children with epilepsy and adults with panic attacks. The side effects include mental confusion, muscle relaxation, and depression. When it has been used to treat children with RLS and ADHD, hyperactivity has been aggravated in some children. In adults with RLS, the benefits of other benzodiazepines, such as temazepam, and non-benzodiazepine sedative hypnotics in the imidazopyridine class, such as zolpidem, are documented in the literature.[181,182]

Other Agents

Pharmacotherapies that alter dopaminergic and/or other monoaminergic pathways have demonstrated benefits for RLS sufferers. Bupropion inhibits dopamine and noradrenaline reuptake and is typically used as an antidepressant. A number of small studies in the adult literature demonstrate the beneficial effects of bupropion use for RLS sensory symptoms and sleep quality outcomes.[183,184] Research in adults also supports the use of bupropion for treating PLMS and PLMD.[183,185] Of note, bupropion is often a treatment of choice for cases of co-occurring RLS and depression. It may be especially useful when antidepressant-induced RLS exacerbation occurs and as an alternative to traditional SSRI and TCA treatments. The side effects of bupropion include potentiating seizures (in epilepsy patients) and hypomania (in genetically susceptible individuals) due to heightened dopaminergic function. In children and adolescents, an increased risk for suicide has also been reported with the use of some antidepressants. For these reasons, clinicians should discuss the potential risks with parents prior to prescription.

Clinical Pearls

- Childhood RLS is usually familial.
- Periodic leg/limb movement disorder may be present before sensory symptoms of RLS appear.
- RLS incidence is increased in children with ADHD, depression, iron deficiency, or central nervous system disorders; it is also increased in those taking medications that impact dopamine function.
- Low iron stores – and iron-dependent dopamine impairment – are common in RLS.
- Low iron stores are detected by measurement of ferritin (not iron, hemoglobin, or hematocrit).
- Patients with low iron stores, as determined by findings of ferritin levels below 50 ng/mL, may benefit from iron therapy.
- Although there are no FDA-approved medications for childhood RLS, there are several medical and behavioral therapies available that provide symptomatic relief with limited side effects.

References

1. Ekbom KA. Restless legs; a clinical study. Acta Med Scand Supp 1945;158:1–122
2. Walters AS, Picchietti DL, Ehrenberg BL, et al. Restless legs syndrome in childhood and adolescence. Ped Neurol 1994;11(3):241–5.
3. Picchietti DL, Walters AS. Restless legs syndrome and periodic limb movement disorder in children and adolescents comorbidity with attention-deficit hyperactivity disorder. Child Adoles Psych Clinics North Amer 1996;5:729–40.
4. Picchietti DL, Stevens HE. Early manifestations of restless legs syndrome in childhood and adolescence. Sleep Med 2008;9(7):770–81.
5. Lavigne GJ, Montplaisir JY. Restless legs syndrome and sleep bruxism: prevalence and association among Canadians. Sleep 1994;17:739–43.
6. Berger K, Luedemann J, Trenkwalder C, et al. Sex and the risk of restless legs syndrome in the general population. Arch Intern Med 2004;164:196–202.
7. Ulfberg J, Nystrom B, Carter N, et al. Prevalence of restless legs syndrome among men aged 18 to 64 years: an association with somatic disease and neuropsychiatric symptoms. Mov Disord 2001;16:1159–63.
8. Montplaisir J, Boucher S, Poirier G, et al. Clinical, polysomnographic, and genetic characteristics of restless legs syndrome: a study of 133 patients diagnosed with new standard criteria. Mov Disord 1997;12:61–5.
9. Walters AS, Hickey K, Maltzman J, et al. A questionnaire study of 138 patients with restless legs syndrome: the 'Night-Walkers' survey. Neurology 1996;46(1):92–5.
10. The International RLS Study Group. Validation of the International Restless Legs Syndrome Study Group rating scale for restless legs syndrome. Sleep Med 2003;4:121–32.
11. Zucconi M, Ferni-Strambi L. Epidemiology and clinical findings of restless legs syndrome. Sleep Med 2004;5:293–9.
12. Allen RP, Walters AS, Montplaisir J, et al. Restless legs syndrome prevalence and impact: REST general population study. Arch Intern Med 2005;165(11):1286–92.
13. Juuti AK, Laara E, Rajala U, et al. Prevalence and associated factors of restless legs in a 57-year-old urban population in northern Finland. Acta Neurol Scand DOI. 2009;10.1111.
14. Henning W, Walters AS, Allen RP, et al. Impact, diagnosis and treatment of restless legs syndrome (RLS) in a primary care population: the REST (RLS epidemiology, symptoms and treatment) primary care study. Sleep Med 2004;5(3):237–46.
15. Picchietti D, Allen RP, Walters AS, et al. Restless legs syndrome: prevalence and impact in children and adolescents – the Peds REST study. Pediatrics 2007;120(2):253–66.
16. Arbuckle R, Abetz L, Durmer JS, et al. Development of the pediatric restless legs syndrome severity scale (P-RLS-SS): a patient-reported outcome measure of pediatric RLS symptoms and impact. Sleep Med 2010;11:897–90.

17. American Academy of Sleep Medicine. International classification of sleep disorders. 2nd ed. Diagnostic and coding manual. Westchester, Illinois: American Academy of Sleep Medicine; 2005
18. O'Brien LM, Holbrook CR, Jones F, et al. Ethnic difference in periodic limb movements in children. Sleep Med 2007;8(3):240–6.
19. Stefansson H, Rye DB, Hicks A, et al. A genetic risk factor for periodic limb movements in sleep. N Eng J Med 2007;357(7):639–47.
20. Walters AS, Lavigne G, Hening, et al. The scoring of movements in sleep. J Clin Sleep Med 2007;3(2):155–67.
21. Gamaldo CE, Earley CJ. Restless legs syndrome: a clinical update. Chest 2006;130(5):1596–604.
22. Benes H, Walters AS, Allen RP, et al. Definition of restless legs syndrome, how to diagnose it, and how to differentiate it from RLS mimics. Mov Disord 2007;22(Suppl. 18):S401–8. Review. Erratum in: Mov Disord 2008;23(8):1200.
23. Yang C, White DP, Winkelman JW. Antidepressants and periodic leg movements of sleep. Biol Psychiatry 2005;58:510–514.
24. Hoque R, Chesson AL. Pharmacologically induced/exacerbated restless legs syndrome, periodic limb movements of sleep, and REM behavior disorder/REM sleep without atonia: literature review, qualitative scoring, and comparative analysis. J Clin Sleep Med 2010;6(1):79–83.
25. Shraf SM, Tubman A, Smale P. Prevalence of concomitant sleep disorders in patients with obstructive sleep apnea. Sleep Breath 2005;(9):50–6.
26. Al-Alawi A, Mulgrew A, Tench E, et al. Prevalence, risk factors and impact on daytime sleepiness and hypertension of periodic leg movements with arousals in patients with obstructive sleep apnea. J Clin Sleep Med 2006;2(3):281–7.
27. Baran AS, Richert AC, Douglass AB, et al. Change in periodic limb movement index during treatment of obstructive sleep apnea with continuous positive airway pressure. Sleep 2003;26(6):717–20.
28. Sforza E, Pichot V, Barthelemy JC, et al. Cardiovascular variability during periodic leg movements: a spectral analysis approach. Clin Neurophysiol 2005;116:1096–104.
29. Walters AS, ad Rye DB. Review of the relationship of restless legs syndrome and periodic limb movements in sleep to hypertension, heart disease and stroke. Sleep 2009;32(5):589–97.
30. Gosselin N, Lanfranchi P, Michaud M, et al. Age and gender effects on heart rate activation associated with periodic leg movements in patients with restless legs syndrome. Clin Neurophysiol 2003;114:2188–95.
31. Picchietti DL, England SJ, Walters AS, et al. Periodic limb movement disorder and restless legs syndrome in children with attention-deficit hyperactivity disorder. J Child Neuol 1998;13(12):588–94.
32. Chervin RD, Archbold KH, Dillon JE, et al. Associations between symptoms of inattention, hyperactivity, restless legs and periodic leg movements. Sleep 2002;25(2):213–18.
33. Chervin RD, Dillon JE, Archbald KH, et al. Conduct problems and symptoms of sleep disorders in children. J Am Acad Child Adolesc Psychiatry 2003;42(2):201–8.
34. Pearson VE, Allen RP, Dean T, et al. Cognitive deficits associated with restless legs syndrome (RLS). Sleep Med 2006;7:25–30.
35. Sevim S, Dogu O, Kaleagasi H, et al. Correlation of anxiety and depression symptoms in patients with restless legs syndrome: a population based survey. J Neurol Neurosurg Psychiatry 2004;75(2):226–30.
36. Picchietti D, Winkelman JW. Restless legs syndrome, periodic limb movements in sleep, and depression. Sleep 2005;28(7):891–8.
37. Winkelmann J, Prager M, Lieb R, et al. 'Anxietas Tibiarum' depression and anxiety disorders in patients with restless legs syndrome. J Neurol 2005;252(1):67–71.
38. Lee HB, Hening WA, Allen RP, et al. Restless legs syndrome is associated with DSM-IV major depressive disorder and panic disorder in the community. J Neuropsychiatr Clin Neurosci 2008;20(1):101–5.
39. Winkelman JW, Redline S, Baldwin CM, et al. Polysomnographic and health-related quality of life correlates of restless legs syndrome in the sleep heart health study. Sleep 2009;32(6):772–8.
40. Happe S, Reese JP, Stiasny-Kolster K, et al. Assessing health-related quality of life in patients with restless legs syndrome. Sleep Med 2009;10(3):295–305.
41. Allen RP, Burchell BJ, MacDonald B, et al. Validation of the self-completed Cambridge–Hopkins questionnaire (CH-RLSq) for ascertainment of restless legs syndrome (RLS) in a population survey. Sleep Med 2009;10(10):1097–100.
42. Rothdach AJ, Trenkwalder C, Haberstock J, et al. Prevalence and risk factors of RLS in an elderly population: the MEMC study. Memory and morbidity in Augsburg elderly. Neurology 2000;54(5):1064–8.

43. Crabtree VM, Ivanenko A, O'Brien LM, et al. Periodic limb movement disorder of sleep in children. J Sleep Res 2003;12:73–81.

44. O'Brien LM, Holbrook CR, Faye Jones V, et al. Ethnic difference in periodic limb movements in children. Sleep Med 2007;8:240–6.

45. Montgomery-Downs HE, O'Brien LM, Gulliver TE, et al. Polysomnographic characteristics in normal preschool and early school-aged children. Pediatrics 2006;117(3):741–53.

46. Pennestri MH, Whittom S, Adam B, et al. PLMS and PLMW in healthy subjects as a function of age: prevalence and interval distribution. Sleep 2006;29(9):1183–7.

47. Traeger N, Schultz B, Pollock AN, et al. Polysomnographic values in children 2–9 years old: additional data and review of the literature. Pediatr Pulmonol 2005;40(1):22–30.

48. Picchietti DL, Picchietti MA. Pediatric restless legs syndrome and periodic limb movement disorder: parent–child pairs. Sleep Med 2009;10:925–31.

49. Walters AS, Lavigne G, Hening W, et al. The scoring of movements in sleep. J Clin Sleep Med 2007;3(2):155–67.

50. Iber C, Ancoli-Israel A, Chesson AI, et al. for the AASM. The AASM manual for the scoring of sleep and associated events; rules, terminology and technical specifications. Westchester, IL: 1 Westbrook Corporate Center, Suite 920; 2007.

51. Ferri R, Zucconi M, Manconi M, et al. New approaches to the study of periodic leg movements during sleep in restless legs syndrome. Sleep 2006;29(6):759–69.

52. Ferri R, Manconi M, Lanuzza B, et al. Age-related changes in periodic leg movements during sleep in patients with restless legs syndrome. Sleep Med 2008;9(7):790–8.

53. Ferri R, Franceschini C, Zucconi M, et al. Sleep polygraphic study of children and adolescents with narcolepsy/cataplexy. Dev Neuropsychol 2009;34(5):523–38.

54. Bruni O, Ferri R, Verrillo E, et al. New approaches to the study of leg movements during sleep in ADHD children. In: Proceedings of the 20th meeting of the Associated Sleep Societies. Sleep 2006;29(Suppl. 2006):259.

55. Trotti LM, Bliwise DL, Greer SA, et al. Correlates of PLMs variability over multiple nights and impact upon RLS diagnosis. Sleep Med 2009;10:668–71.

56. Sforza E, Johannes M, Bassetti C. The PAM-RL ambulatory device for detection of periodic leg movements: a validation study. Sleep Med 2005;6:407–13.

57. Morrish E, King MA, Pilsworth SN, et al. Periodic limb movement in a community population detected by a new actigraphy technique. Sleep Med 2002;3:489–95.

58. Rye DB. Parkinson's disease and RLS: the dopaminergic bridge. Sleep Med 2004;5:317–28.

59. Clemens S, Rye D, Hochman S. RLS revisiting the dopamine hypothesis from the spinal cord perspective. Neurology 2006;67:125–30.

60. Nordlander NB. Restless legs. Brit J Phys Med 1954;17:160–2.

61. Earley CJ, Connor JR, Beard JL, et al. Abnormalities in CSF concentrations of ferritin and transferrin in restless legs syndrome. Neurology 2000;54(8):1698–1700.

62. Mizuno S, Mihara T, Miyaoka T, et al. CSF iron, ferritin and transferrin levels in restless legs syndrome. J Sleep Res 2005;14(1):43–7.

63. Earley CJ, Barker PB, Horska A, et al. MRI-determined regional brain iron concentrations in early- and late-onset restless legs syndrome. Sleep Med 2006;7:459–61.

64. Allen RP, Barker PB, Wehrl F, et al. MRI measurement of brain iron in patients with restless legs syndrome. Neurology 2001;56(2):263–5.

65. Schmidauer C, Sojer M, Seppi K, et al. Transcranial ultrasound shows nigral hypoechogenicity in restless legs syndrome. Ann Neurol 2005;58(4):630–4.

66. Connor JR, Boyer PJ, Menzies SL, et al. Neuropathological examination suggests impaired brain iron acquisition in restless legs syndrome. Neurology 2003;61(3):304–9.

67. Connor JR, Wang XS, Patton SM, et al. Decreased transferrin receptor expression by neuromelanin cells in restless legs syndrome. Neurology 2004;62(9):1563–7.

68. Erikson KM, Jones BC, Beard JL. Iron deficiency alters dopamine transporter functioning in rat striatum. J Nutr 2000;130:831–7.

69. Erikson KM, Jones BC, Hess EJ, et al. Iron deficiency decreases dopamine D1 and D2 receptors in rat brain. Pharmacol Biochem Behav 2001;69:409–18.

70. Wang X, Wiesinger J, Beard J, et al. Thy1 expression in the brain is affected by iron and is decreased in restless legs syndrome. J Neurol Sci 2004;220(1–2):59–66.

71. Earley CJ, Ponnuru P, Wang X, et al. Altered iron metabolism in lymphocytes from subjects with restless legs syndrome. Sleep 2008;31(6): 847–52.

72. Desai AV, Cherkas LF, Spector TD, et al. Genetic influences in self-reported symptoms of obstructive sleep apnoea and restless legs: a twin study. Twin Res 2004;7(6):589–95.

73. Desautels A, Turecki G, Montplaisir J, et al. Identification of a major susceptibility locus for restless legs syndrome on chromosome 12q. Am J Hum Genet 2001;69(6):1266–70.

74. Desautels A, Turecki G, Montplaisir, J, et al. Restless legs syndrome: confirmation of linkage to chromosome 12q, genetic heterogeneity, and evidence of complexity. Arch Neurol 2005;62(4):591–6.

75. Bonati MT, Ferini-Strambi L, Aridon P, et al. Autosomal dominant restless legs syndrome maps on chromosome 14q. Brain 2003;126(Pt 6):1485–92.

76. Chen S, Ondo WG, Rao S, et al. Genomewide linkage scan identifies a novel susceptibility locus for restless legs syndrome on chromosome 9p. Am J Hum Genet 2004;74(5):876–85.

77. Winkelmann J, Lichtner P, Putz B, et al. Evidence for further genetic locus heterogeneity and confirmation of RLS-1 in restless legs syndrome. Mov Disord 2006;21(1):28–33.

78. Pichler I, Marroni F, Volpato CB, et al. Linkage analysis identifies a novel locus for restless legs syndrome on chromosome 2q in a South Tyrolean population isolate. Am J Hum Genet 2006;79(4):716–23.

79. Levchenko A, Provost S, Montplaisir J, et al. A novel autosomal dominant restless legs syndrome locus maps to chromosome 20p13. Neurology 2006;67(5):900–1.

80. Levchenko A, Montplaisir JY, Asselin G, et al. Autosomal dominant locus for restless legs syndrome in French-Canadians on chromosome 16p.12.1. Mov Disord 2009;24(1):40–50.

81. Kemlink D, Plazzi G, Vetrugno R, et al. Suggestive evidence for linkage for restless legs syndrome on chromosome 19p13. Neurogenetics 2008;9:75–82.

82. Winkelmann J, Czamara D, Schormair B, et al. Genome-wide association study identifies novel restless legs syndrome susceptibility loci on 2p14 and 16q12.1. PLos Genetics 2011;7(7):e1002171.

83. Desautles A, Turecki G, Montplaisir J, et al. Dopaminergic neurotransmission and restless legs syndrome: a genetic association analysis. Neurology 2001;57:1304–6.

84. Schormair B, Kemlink D, Roeske D, et al. PTPRD (protein tyrosine phosphatase receptor type delta) is associated with restless legs syndrome. Nature Genetics 2008;40:946–8.

85. Winkelmann J, Lichtner P, Schormair B, et al. Variants in the neuronal nitric oxide synthase (nNOS, NOS1) gene are associated with restless legs syndrome. Mov Disord 2008;23:350–8.

86. Oexle K, Schormair B, Ried JS, et al. Dilution of candidates: the case of iron-related genes in restless legs syndrome. Eur J Hum Genet 2012 [Epub ahead of print]

87. Winkelmann J, Muller-Myhsok B, Wittchen HU, et al. Complex segregation analysis of restless legs syndrome provides evidence for an autosomal dominant mode of inheritance in early age at onset families. Ann Neurol 2002;52(3):297–302.

88. Mathias RA, Hening W, Washburn M, et al. Segregation analysis of restless legs syndrome: possible evidence for a major gene in a family study using blinded diagnosis. Hum Heredity 2006;62(3):157–64.

89. Lazzarini A, Walters AS, Hickey K, et al. Studies of penetrance and anticipation in five autosomal-dominant restless legs syndrome pedigrees. Mov Disord 1999;14(1):111–16.

90. Trenkwalder C, Seidel VC, Gasser T, et al. Clinical symptoms and possible anticipation in a large kindred of familial restless legs syndrome. Mov Disord 1996;11(4):389–94.

91. Esteves AM, Pedrazzoli M, Bagnato M, et al. Two pedigrees with restless legs syndrome in Brazil. Braz J Med Biol Res 2008;41(2): 106–9.

92. Babacan-Yildiz G, Gursoy E, Kolukisa F, et al. Clinical and polysomnographic features of a large Turkish pedigree with restless legs syndrome and periodic limb movements. Sleep Breath 2012; Aug 2 [Epub ahead of print]

93. Roos RA. Huntington's disease; a clinical review. Orphanet J Rare Dis 2010;5(1):40.

94. Schols L, Bauer P, Schmidt T, et al. Autosomal dominant cerebellar ataxias : clinical features, genetics and pathogenesis. Lancet Neurol 2004;3(5):291–304.

95. Winkelmann J, Schormair B, Lichtner P, et al. Genome-wide association study of restless legs syndrome identifies common variants in three genomic regions. Nat Genetics 2007;39(8):1000–6.

96. Muhle H, Neumann A, Lohmann-Hedrich K, et al. Childhood-onset restless legs syndrome: clinical and genetic features of 22 families. Mov Disord 2008;23(8):1113–21.

97. Young JE, Vilariño-Güell C, Lin SC, et al. Clinical and genetic description of a family with a high prevalence of autosomal dominant restless legs syndrome. Mayo Clin Proc 2009;84(2):134–8.

98. The International Restless Legs Syndrome Study Group. Toward a better definition of the restless legs syndrome. Mov Disord 1995;10: 634–42.

99. Allen RP, Picchietti DL, Henning WA, et al. Restless legs syndrome: diagnositic criteria, special considerations, and epidemiology. A report from the RLS diagnosis and epidemiology workshop at the NIH. Sleep Med 2003;4:101–19.

100. Picchietti DL, Arbuckle RA, Abetz L, et al. Pediatric restless legs syndrome: analysis of symptom descriptions and drawings. J Child Neurol 2011;26(11):1365–76.

101. Mohri I, Kato-Nishimura K, Tachibana N, et al. RLS: an unrecognized cause for bedtime problems and insomnia in children. Sleep Med 2008;9:701–2.

102. Rajaram A, Walters AS, England SJ, et al. Some children with growing pains may actually have restless legs syndrome. Sleep 2004;27(4): 767–73.

103. Evans AM, Scutter SD. Prevalence of growing pains in young children. J Pediatrics 2004;145:255–8.

104. Kryger MH, Otake K, Foerster J. Low body stores of iron and restless legs syndrome: a correctable cause of insomnia in adolescents and teenagers. Sleep Med 2002;3:127–32.

105. Martin BT, Williamson BD, Edwards N, et al. Parental symptom report and periodic limb movements of sleep in children. J Clin Sleep Med 2008;4(1):57–61.

106. Chervin RD, Hedger KM. Clinical prediction of periodic leg movements during sleep in children. Sleep Med 2001;2:501–10.

107. Picchietti DL, Walters AS. Restless legs syndrome and periodic limb movement disorder in children and adolescents comorbidity with attention-deficit hyperactivity disorder. Child Adoles Psych Clinics North Amer 1996;5:729–40.

108. Cortese S, Konofal E, Lecendreux M, et al. Restless legs syndrome and attention-deficit/hyperactivity disorder: a review of the literature. Sleep 2005;28(8):1007–13.

109. Oner P, Dirik EB, Taner Y, et al. Association between low serum ferritin and restless legs syndrome in patients with attention deficit hyperactivity disorder. Tohoku J Exp Med 2007;213(3):269–76.

110. Silvestri R, Gagliano A, Arico I, et al. Sleep disorders in children with attention-deficit/hyperactivity disorder (ADHD) recorded overnight by video-polysomnography. Sleep Med 2009;10(10):1132–8.

111. Wagner ML, Walters AS, Fisher BC. Symptoms of attention-deficit/hyperactivity disorder in adults with restless legs syndrome. Sleep 2004;27(8):1499–504.

112. Wiggs L, Montgomery P, Stores G. Actigraphic and parent reports of sleep patterns and sleep disorders in children with subtypes of attention-deficit hyperactivity disorder. Sleep 2005;28(11):1437–45.

113. Picchietti D, Allen RP, Walters AS, et al. Restless legs syndrome: prevalence and impact in children and adolescents – the Peds REST study. Pediatrics 2007;120(2):253–66.

114. Silvestri R, Gagliano A, Arico I, et al. Sleep disorders in children with ADHD recorded overnight by video-polysomnography. Sleep Med 2009;10:1132–8.

115. Konofal E, Lecendreux M, Cortese S. Sleep and ADHD. Sleep Med 2010;11:652–8.

116. Faraone SV, Doyle AE, Mick E, et al. Meta-analysis of the association between the 7-repeat allele of the dopamine D(4) receptor gene and attention deficit hyperactivity disorder. Am J Psychiatry 2001;158(7): 1052–7.

117. Li D, Sham PC, Owen MJ, et al. Meta-analysis shows significant association between dopamine system genes and attention deficit hyperactivity disorder (ADHD). Hum Mol Genet 2006;15(14):2276–84.

118. Lowe N, Kirley A, Hawi Z, et al. Joint analysis of the DRD5 marker concludes association with attention deficit/hyperactivity disorder confined to the predominately inattentive and combined subtypes. Am J Hum Genet 2004;74(2):348–56.

119. Misener VL, Luca P, Azeke O, et al. Linkage of the dopamine receptor D1 gene to attention-deficit/hyperactivity disorder. Mol Psychiatry 2004;9(5):500–9.

120. VanNess SH, Owens MJ, Kilts CD. The variable number of tandem repeats element in DAT1 regulates in vitro dopamine transporter density. BMC Genet 2005;6:55.

121. Cook EH, Stein MA, Krasowski MD, et al. Association of attention-deficit disorder and the dopamine transporter gene. American J Hum Genet 1995;56:993–8.

122. LaHoste GJ, Swanson JM, Wigal SB, et al. Dopamine D4 receptor gene polymorphism is associated with attention deficit hyperactivity disorder. Molec Psychiatry 1996;1:21–124.

123. Coghill D, Banaschewski T. The genetics of ADHD. Expert Rev. Neurother 2009;9(10):1547–55.

124. Schimmelmann BG, Friedel S, Nquyen TT, et al. Exploring the genetic link between RLS and ADHD. J Psychiatr Res 2009 43(10):941–5.

125. Oner P, Dirik EB, Taner Y, et al. Association between low serum ferritin and restless legs syndrome in patients with attention deficit hyperactivity disorder. Tohoku J Exp Med 2007;213:269–76.

126. Konofal E, Lecendreux M, Arnulf I, et al. Iron deficiency in children with attention-deficit/hyperactivity disorder. Arch Pediatr Adolesc Med 2004;158:1113–15.

127. Konofal E, Cortese S, Marchand M, et al. Impact of restless legs syndrome and iron deficiency on attention-deficit/hyperactivity disorder in children. Sleep Med 2007;8:711–15.

128. Konofal E, Lecendreux M, Deron J, et al. Effects of iron supplementation on attention deficit hyperactivity disorder in children. Ped Neurol 2008;38:20–6.

129. Mohri I, Kato-Nishimura K, Kagitani-Shimono K, et al. Evaluation of oral iron treatment in pediatric restless legs syndrome (RLS). Sleep Med 2012;13(4):429–32.

130. Frauscher B, Gschliesser V, Brandauer E, et al. The severity of RLS and augmentation in a prospective patient cohort: association with ferritin levels. Sleep Med 2009; doi:10.1016/j.sleep.2008.09.007.

131. Whittom S, Dauvilliers Y, Pennestri MH, et al. Age-at-onset in restless legs syndrome: a clinical and polysomnographic study. Sleep Med 2007;9(1):54–9.

132. Earley CJ. Restless legs syndrome. N Engl J Med 2003;348(21): 2103–9.

133. Sun ER, Chen CA, Ho G, et al. Iron and the restless legs syndrome. Sleep 1998;21:371–7.

134. O'Keeffe ST, Gavin K, Lavan JN. Iron status and restless legs syndrome in the elderly. Age Ageing 1994;23(3):200–3.

135. Simakajornboon N, Gozal D, Vlasic V, et al. PLMS and iron status in children. Sleep 2006;26(6):735–8.

136. Davis BJ, Rajput A, Rajput ML, et al. A randomized double-blind placebo-controlled trail of iron in restless legs syndrome. Eur Neurol 2000;43:70–5.

137. Early CJ, Heckler D, Allen RP. Repeated IV doses of iron provide effective supplemental treatment of restless legs syndrome. Sleep Med 2005;6(4):301–5.

138. Ondo WG. IV iron dextran for severe refractory RLS. Sleep Med 2010;11:494–6.

139. Grote L, Leissner L, Hedner J, et al. A randomized, double-blind, placebo controlled, multi-center study of intravenous iron sucrose and placebo in the treatment of restless legs syndrome. Mov Disord 2009;24(10):1445–52.

140. Vaage-Nilsen O. Acute, severe and anaphylactoid reactions are very rare with low-molecular-weight iron dextran, CosmoFer. Nephrol Dial Transplant 2008;23(10):3372; author reply 3372.

141. Auerbach M, Al Talib K. Low-molecular weight iron dextran and iron sucrose have similar comparative safety profiles in chronic kidney disease. Kidney Int 2008;73(5):528–30.

142. Walters AS, Mandelbaum DE, Lewin DS, et al. and the Dopaminergic Study Group. Dopaminergic therapy in children with restless legs/periodic limb movements in sleep and ADHD. Pediatric Neurol 2000;22:182–6.

143. Konofal E, Arnulf I, Lecendreux M, et al. Ropinirole in a child with ADHD and RLS. Pediatric Neurol 2005;32:350–1.

144. Kotagal S, Silber MH. Childhood-onset restless legs syndrome. Ann Neurol 2004;56(6):803–7.

145. Muhle H, Neumann A, Lohmann-Hedrich K, et al. Childhood-onset restless legs syndrome: clinical and genetic features of 22 families. Mov Disord 2008;23(8):1113–21.

146. Starn AL, Udall JN Jr. Iron deficiency anemia, pica, and restless legs syndrome in a teenage girl. Clin Pediatr (Phila) 2008-47(1):83–5.

147. Cortese S, Konofal E, Lecendreux M. Effectiveness of ropinirole for RLS and depressive symptoms in an 11-year-old girl. Sleep Med 2009;10(2):259–61.

148. Picchietti DL, Walters AS. Moderate to severe periodic limb movement disorder in childhood and adolescence. Sleep 1999;22(3):297–300.

149. Guilleminault C, Palombini L, Pelayo R, et al. Sleepwalking and sleep terrors in prepubertal children: what triggers them? Pediatrics 2003;111(1):e17–25.

150. Martinez S, Guilleminault C. Periodic leg movements in prepubertal children with sleep disturbance. Dev Med Child Neurol 2004;46(11): 765–70.

151. England SJ, Picchietti DL, Couvadelli BV, et al. L-Dopa improves restless legs syndrome and periodic limb movements in sleep but not attention-deficit–hyperactivity disorder in a double-blind trail in children. Sleep Med 2011;12(5):471–7.

152. Conti CF, de Oliveira MM, Andriolo RB, et al. Levodopa for idiopathic restless legs syndrome: evidence-based review. Mov Disord 2007;22(13): 1943–51.

153. Allen RP, Earley CJ. Augmentation of the restless legs syndrome with carbidopa/levodopa. Sleep 1996;19:205–13.

154. Garcia-Borreguero D, Williams A. Dopamine augmentation of restless legs syndrome. Sleep Med Rev 2010;14:339–46.

155. Paulus W, Trenkwalder C. Less is more: pathophysiology of dopaminergic related augmentation in restless legs syndrome. Lancet Neurol 2006;5:878–86.

156. Garcia-Borrequerro D, Hogl B, Ferini-Strambi L, et al. Systemic evaluation of augmentation during treatment with ropinirole in restless legs syndrome (Willis–Ekbom disease): results from a prospective, multicenter study over 66 weeks. Mov Disord 2012;27(2):277–83.

157. Trenkwalder C, Benes H, Poewe W and the SP790 study group. Efficacy of rotigotine for treatment of moderate to severe restless legs syndrome; a randomized, double-blind, placebo-controlled trial. Lancet Neurol 2008;7:595–604.

158. Oertel W, Trenkwalder C, Benes H, et al. and the SP710 study group. Long-term safety and efficacy of rotigitine transdermal patch for moderate-to-severe idiopathic restless legs syndrome: a 5-year open label extension study. Lancet Neurol 2011;10:710–20.

159. Newcorn JH, Schulz K, Harrison M, et al. Alpha 2 adrenergic agonists. Neurochemistry, efficacy, and clinical guidelines for use in children. Pediatr Clin North Am 1998;45(5):1022–99 [viii].

160. Prince JB, Wilens TE, Biederman J, et al. Clonidine for sleep disturbances associated with attention-deficit hyperactivity disorder: a systematic chart review of 62 cases. J Am Acad Child Adolesc Psychiatry 1996;35(5):599–605.

161. Wager ML, Walters AS, Coleman RG, et al. Randomized double-blind placebo-controlled study of clonidine in restless legs syndrome. Sleep 1996;19(1):52–8.

162. Owens JA, Rosen CL, Mindell JA. Medication use in the treatment of pediatric insomnia: results of a survey of community-based pediatricians. Pediatrics 2003;111(5 Pt 1):e628–35.

163. Walters AS, Wagner ML, Hening WA, et al. Successful treatment of the idiopathic restless legs syndrome in a randomized double-blind trial of oxycodone versus placebo. Sleep 1993;16:327–32.

164. Kaplan PW, Allen RP, Buchholz DW, et al. A double-blind, placebo-controlled study of the treatment of periodic limb movements in sleep using carbidopa/levodopa and propoxyphene. Sleep 1993;16:717–23.

165. Ross DA, Narus MS, Nutt JG. Control of medically refractory RLS with intrathecal morphine:case report. Neurosurgery 2008;62(1):e263.

166. Jakobsson B, Ruuth K. Successful treatment of RLS with an implanted pump for intrathecal drug delivery. Acta Anaesthsiol Scand 2002;46: 114–17.

167. Ondo WG. Methadone for refractory RLS. Mov Disord 2005;20(3): 345–8.

168. Walters AS. Review of receptor agonist and antagonist studies relevant to the opiate system in restless legs syndrome. Sleep Med 2002;3:301–30.

169. Silver N, Allen RP, Senerth J, et al. A 10-year longitudinal assessment of dopamine agonists and methadone in the treatment of restless legs syndrome. Sleep Med 2011;12:440–4.

170. Laurma H, Markkula J. Treatment of restless legs syndrome with tramadol: an open study. J Clin Psychiatr 1999;60:241–4.

171. Garcia-Borreguero D, Larrosa O, de la Llave Y, et al. Treatment of restless legs syndrome with gabapentin: a double-blind, cross-over study. Neurology 2002;59(10):1573–9.

172. Happe S, Klosch G, Saletu B, et al. Treatment of idiopathic restless legs syndrome (RLS) with gabapentin. Neurology 2001;57(9):1717–19.

173. Happe S, Sauter C, Klosch G, et al. Gabapentin versus ropinirole in the treatment of idiopathic restless legs syndrome. Neuropsychobiology 2003;48(2):82–6.

174. Cundy KC, Sastry S, Luo W, et al. Clinical pharmacokinetics of XP13512, a novel transported prodrug of gabapentin. J Clin Pharmacol 2008;48(12):1378–88.

175. Kushida CA, Becker PM, Ellenbogan AL, et al; XP052 Study Group. A randomized, double-blind, placebo-controlled trial of XP13512/GSK1838262 in patients with RLS. Neurology 2009;72(5):439–46.

176. Bogan R, Bornemann MA, Kushida CA, et al; XP060 Study Group. Long-term maintenance treatment of RLS with gabapentin enacarbil: a randomized control study. Mayo Clinic Proc 2010;85(7):693–4.

177. Lee DO, Zinman RB, Perkins AT, et al; and XP053 Study Group. A randomized, double-blind, placebo-controlled study to assess the efficacy and tolerability of gabapentin enacarbil in subjects with restless legs syndrome. J Clin Sleep Med 2011;7(3):282–92.

178. Matthews WB. Treatment of restless legs syndrome with clonazepam. BMJ 1979;1:751.

179. Oshtory MA, Vijayan N. Clonazepam treatment of insomnia due to sleep myoclonus. Arch Neurol 1980;37:119–20.

180. Saletu M, Ander P, Prause W, et al. RLS and PLMD acute placebo-controlled sleep laboratory studies with clonazepam. Eur Neuropsychopharm 2001;11:153–61.

181. Silber MH, Ehrenberg BL, Allen RP, et al. Henisequent references and text citations.ng WA, Rye DB, and the medical advisory board of the restless legs syndrome foundation. An algorithm for the management of restless legs syndrome. Mayo Clin Proc 2004;79(7):916–22.

182. Hening W, Allen R, Earley C, et al. The treatment of restless legs syndrome and periodic limb movement disorder. An American academy of sleep medicine review. Sleep 1999;22(7):970–99.

183. Kim SW, Shin IS, Kim JM, et al. Bupropion may improve restless legs syndrome. A report of three cases. Clin Neuropharmacol 2005;28: 298–301.

184. Lee JJ, Erdos J, Wilkosz MF, et al. Bupropion as a possible treatment option for restless legs syndrome. Ann Pharmacother 2009;43:370–4.

185. Nofzinger EA, Fasiczka A, Berman S, et al. Bupropion SR reduces periodic limb movements associated with arousals from sleep in depressed patients with periodic limb movement disorder. J Clin Psychiatry 2000;61:858–62.

SLEEP IN MEDICAL DISORDERS AND SPECIAL POPULATIONS

Chapter **48** **Sleep and School Start Times**

Amy R. Wolfson and Michaela Johnson

Sleep problems in children and adolescents are often observed in school settings. Features of sleepiness and degraded school performance are usually the first clues that a sleep problem is present. The sleep problems are generally related to disorders (e.g., narcolepsy or sleep apnea) or due to an incompatibility between the student's circadian biology and the school start time. Over 30 years of research clearly suggests that delaying middle and high school start times allows adolescents to obtain at least an adequate amount of sleep, which translates to positive implications for health behaviors and academic performance. In demonstrating the importance of delaying school start times for adolescents, this chapter reviews adolescents' sleep–wake needs and developmental changes in sleep–wake regulatory systems, accounting for a biological delay and environmental constraints and life style decisions. Studies demonstrating delaying start times as an effective countermeasure to adolescents' chronic insufficient sleep are reviewed along with the barriers to change and creative solutions. The chapter concludes with a discussion of the latest global-level forms of advocacy supporting the benefits of delaying school start times. Finally, future directions of research in this area and recommendations for healthcare professionals are outlined, most especially stressing the importance of sleep education for adolescents, parents, and school administrators.

Sleep and Sleep Disorders in Epilepsy

Madeleine M. Grigg-Damberger

INTRODUCTION

Sleep problems and primary sleep disorders are far more likely to be found in children with epilepsy (CWE) than the general pediatric population.[1-14] The etiology of sleep disruption in children with epilepsy may be multifactorial including: epilepsy *per se*, frequent nocturnal seizures disrupting nocturnal sleep organization, effects of antiepileptic medications on daytime alertness and nighttime sleep, and treatable primary sleep disorders. Comorbidities such as physical disability,[8] intellectual disability,[2,15,16] neurodevelopmental syndromes,[17,18] autism spectrum disorder,[19] and behavioral disorders[1,7-9,20] may add to the likelihood of sleep disorders in a child with epilepsy. In CWE, they are associated with negative effects on daytime behavior and academic performance.[21-23] Recognizing this has led to increasing numbers of children or adolescents referred to sleep specialists to evaluate whether undiagnosed sleep disorders are contributing to their seizures.

QUESTIONNAIRE-BASED STUDIES ON THE PREVALENCE OF SLEEP DISORDERS IN CHILDREN WITH EPILEPSY

Children with epilepsy (CWE) are much more likely to have sleep problems than the general pediatric population.[1-10,24] Sleep problems in CWE may be due to varying combinations of: epilepsy *per se*, nocturnal seizures disrupting nocturnal sleep organization, effects of antiepileptic medications on daytime alertness and nighttime sleep, and treatable primary sleep disorders. Worse yet, comorbidities such as physical disability,[8] intellectual disability,[2,15,16] neurodevelopmental syndromes,[17,18] autism spectrum disorder,[19] and behavioral disorders[1,7-9,20] often increase the likelihood of sleep disorders in CWE.

A recently published study prospectively explored the relationships between the effect of pediatric epilepsy on child sleep, parental sleep and fatigue, and household sleeping arrangements in 105 households with a child with epilepsy and 79 controls.[25] Using multiple different validated pediatric sleep questionnaires, the authors found: (1) increased rates of both parent–child room sharing and cosleeping compared to controls; (2) CWE had significantly more sleep disturbances, especially for parasomnias, nocturnal awakenings, sleep duration, daytime sleepiness, sleep onset delay and bedtime resistance than controls. Parents of CWE were more likely to report fatigue and sleep dysfunction. Severity of a child's epilepsy correlated positively with the degree of child and parent sleep dysfunction and parental fatigue. Antiepileptic drug polytherapy predicted that greater childhood sleep disturbances would be reported. Child sleep problems were associated with room sharing and cosleeping. Sixty-two percent of parents described decreased quantity and/or quality of sleep when cosleeping. Forty-four percent of parents reported rarely or never feeling rested because they were concerned about their children having seizures during sleep.

An earlier prospective study found 89 children with idiopathic partial or generalized epilepsy (in whom seizures were more often well controlled and not associated with comorbidities) were significantly more likely to have more sleep problems than their 49 siblings or 321 age-matched healthy controls.[1] Post-hoc comparisons found the CWE had significantly more excessive daytime sleepiness (EDS), bedtime difficulties, sleep fragmentation, and parasomnias than their siblings or controls. Multiple regression analysis showed that sleep complaints, longer sleep latencies, and shorter sleep times were much more likely to be found in the children whose seizures were poorly controlled. Furthermore, daytime seizures and high nighttime interictal epileptiform discharge (IED) rates predicted daytime drowsiness, and explained 15% of its variance. Sleep problems in these CWE greatly increased the likelihood they would have far more behavior problems (inattention, hyperactivity, impulsivity, oppositional defiant disorder) than their siblings or controls. Three variables (age, higher rates of IEDs during sleep, and length of freedom from seizures) accounted for 24% of the variance of which CWE were at greatest risk.

Juvenile myoclonic epilepsy (JME) is one of the most common adolescent-onset epilepsies. Patients with JME typically have generalized convulsive motor seizures heralded by myoclonic jerks which typically occur soon after awakening. Seizures are often triggered by sleep deprivation with or without alcohol ('activation by celebration'). Krishnan et al. prospectively studied the effect of epilepsy on sleep in patients with JME, comparing them with age- and gender-matched controls using detailed clinical assessment, EEG, neuroimaging and multiple different sleep questionnaires.[26] They found that patients with JME had significant sleep disturbances characterized by EDS and disturbed nocturnal sleep despite adequate AED therapy and good seizure control.

Another case-control study found sleep problems were twofold higher (mean 4 ± 3 vs. 2 ± 2) in 79 CWE (mean age 10 ± 3 years) compared with 73 age- and gender-matched controls. Other questionnaire-based studies have demonstrated: (1) symptoms of OSA were 15 times more likely to be reported by the parents of 26 children with epilepsy (mean age 15 years) than a similar number of healthy controls (65% vs. 4%); ((2) children with epilepsy compared with control subjects had more daytime sleepiness, less on-task behavior, and less attention;[16] and (3) children with benign rolandic epilepsy had significantly shorter sleep duration, more frequent parasomnias, and daytime sleepiness than a reference sample of children.[5,24]

Poor sleep hygiene may contribute to sleep problems in CWE. A prospective case-control study found 121 CWE needed to be put to bed by their parents, take an afternoon nap, awaken during the night, take >30 minutes to fall asleep, express fear of the dark, awake complaining of a distressing dream or worry, call for parent(s) during the night and/or visit the parental bed.[2] These studies have further found that: (1) CWE whose seizures are poorly controlled are more likely to have poor sleep habits compared to those whose seizures are controlled; and (2) CWE whose seizures occur primarily during sleep are significantly more likely to have difficulty falling asleep, afternoon napping, nocturnal awakenings, awakening with fear or a dream, calling out for their parents at night, or visiting the parental bed when compared to CWE whose seizures occur primary when awake.

IS SLEEP ARCHITECTURE ABNORMAL IN CHILDREN WITH EPILEPSY?

Pereira et al. recorded a single night of polysomnography (PSG) in 31 CWE who had drug-resistant epilepsies comparing sleep architecture in them with a group of normal age-matched healthy controls and a group of children with benign rolandic epilepsy.[27] Compared to normal controls, the children with drug-resistant epilepsy showed a significant reduction of time in bed, total sleep time, rapid eye movement (REM) sleep, sleep stage NREM 3, and sleep efficiency, and a significant increase in wake after sleep onset. Compared to children with benign rolandic epilepsy, those with drug-resistant epilepsy had greater reduction in NREM 3, REM sleep and sleep efficiency.

Other small case-control studies[28–32] recording in-laboratory PSG have shown that abnormalities in sleep architecture are significantly more likely to be found in CWE compared to healthy age-matched controls. Findings among the case-control studies were: (1) children who had partial seizure(s) during a comprehensive in-laboratory overnight PSG with 24-channel EEG had significantly less time in bed and sleep time compared to CWE who did not have seizures during the study or normal controls;[31] (2) children with primary generalized epilepsy whose seizures were well controlled still had significantly more NREM 1 and longer REM sleep latency than normal controls;[32] (3) compared to controls, children with Lennox–Gastaut syndrome (a severe childhood-onset epileptic encephalopathy with medically refractory seizures) had reduced percentages of REM, NREM 2 and NREM 3 sleep;[33] (4) children with benign rolandic epilepsy (who often have few or no seizures) still had reduced total sleep time, sleep efficiency, and percent REM sleep compared to controls;[30] (5) compared to controls, children with intellectual disability and epilepsy (mean age 13±4 years) had longer sleep latency, higher percentage of wake after sleep onset and NREM 3 sleep, lower sleep efficiency, more awakenings and stage shifts, a higher CAP rate, increased A1 index, long and less numerous CAP sequences;[34] and (6) abnormalities in the density and frequency of sleep spindles were observed in children with untreated epilepsy compared to CWE whose seizures were treated or healthy controls.[35] However, two studies found normal sleep architecture in overnight PSG in children with absence epilepsy (and whose petit mal seizures typically occur when awake).[36,37]

Another small case-control study compared PSG findings in 10 children (mean age 11) with tuberous sclerosis complex (TSC) and 10 healthy controls.[38] They found the children with TSC more often had lower sleep efficiency (ranging from 60% to 88%), increased WASO (>10%), more nocturnal awakenings and stage shifts, poorly organized sleep cycles, increased NREM 1, and decreased REM sleep compared with controls. Furthermore, sleep architecture was significantly more disrupted in the three children who had at least one seizure recorded during their PSG (sleep efficiency 69%, WASO 24%, mean awakenings 16/h) compared to the TS children who did not (sleep efficiency 88%, WASO 5%, and mean awakenings 3/h).

PREVALENCE OF SLEEP APNEA ON SLEEP STUDIES IN CHILDREN WITH EPILEPSY

A retrospective case-control study compared PSG findings in 40 CWE referred for suspected obstructive sleep apnea (OSA) with 11 children who had moderate pediatric OSA (pediatric obstructive apnea–hypopnea indexes (PAOHI)) of 5–10/h of sleep.[28] Twenty percent of the CWE had OSA (PAOHI >1/h), 33% obstructive hypoventilation, 8% upper airway resistance syndrome, 18% primary snoring, and 10% periodic limb movements (>5/h). These findings are not particularly revelatory, given the children were symptomatic. The CWE and OSA compared with those with uncomplicated moderate OSA had a higher body mass index (BMI), were more likely to be obese (BMI >95th percentile in 62% vs. 18%), had longer sleep latencies (51 vs. 16 min), higher arousal indexes, and lower nadir SpO_2 (86% vs. 90%) even though their mean PAOHI was only 3/h compared to 7/h in the children with uncomplicated moderate OSA. The investigators further found CWE whose seizures were poorly controlled had significantly lower sleep efficiency, a higher arousal index, and a higher percentage of REM sleep compared with children who were seizure-free or exhibited good seizure control.

A recently published small prospective study found OSA was more likely to be found in CWE who were on multiple antiepileptic medications and whose seizures were poorly controlled.[39] Uncontrolled epilepsy was a risk factor for OSA (80%) compared with primary snoring (47%, $P=0.02$). The obstructive apnea–hypopnea index increased with increasing number of AEDs. Based on these findings, the investigators argue that children with uncontrolled seizures on multiple AEDs should be routinely screened for obstructive sleep apnea.

IMPACT OF TREATING OBSTRUCTIVE SLEEP APNEA IN CHILDREN WITH EPILEPSY

Few studies have examined the effects of treating OSA in children with epilepsy. A recent retrospective analysis by Segal et al. evaluated the effects of adenotonsillectomy on seizure frequency in 27 CWE (median age 5 years).[40] Three months after surgery they found median reduction in seizure frequency for the group was 53%; 10 (37%) patients became seizure-free, 3 (11%) had a >50% reduction in the frequency of their seizures, 6 (22%) showed lesser degrees of improvement. Seizure frequency was unchanged in 2 (7%) and worse in 6 (22%). Multivariate analysis demonstrated a trend toward seizure freedom with each percentile increase in BMI and early age of surgery. A 45% or greater reduction in seizure frequency was found in three of six adults with epilepsy who used CPAP and ≥60% in one of three children who tolerated it.[41]

SLEEP–WAKE AND CIRCADIAN PATTERNS AND TYPES OF SEIZURES IN CHILDREN

Three retrospective studies from the same research group have recently been published investigating sleep–wake, day/night and 24-h periodicity of different types of seizures in children with epilepsy.[42–4] Among these papers, the investigators reported that: (1) tonic seizures were more frequently seen in sleep; (2) clonic seizures awake between 6 to 9 a.m. and 12 to 3 p.m.; (3) absence seizures 9 a.m. to 12 p.m. and 6 p.m. to 12 a.m. primarily awake; (4) atonic seizures between 12 to 6 p.m.; (5) myoclonic seizures occurred in wakefulness (6 a.m. to noon);[42] (6) primarily generalized tonic–clonic seizures 9 a.m. and 12 p.m.; (7) focal-onset generalized convulsions emanating from the temporal lobe were more likely to occur when awake, extratemporal during sleep;[43] and (8) infantile (epileptic) spasms in children less than age 3 between 9 a.m. and 12 p.m. and 3 to 6 p.m., 6 a.m. to 9 a.m. in children older than age 3.[44]

NREM PARASOMNIAS ARE MORE COMMON IN PATIENTS WITH NOCTURNAL FRONTAL LOBE EPILEPSY

Nocturnal frontal lobe seizures in children are often initially misdiagnosed as sleepwalking, sleep terrors, nightmares or even a psychiatric problem.[45,46] A case series found frontal lobe seizures in 22 children occurred almost exclusively during sleep in 77%, were brief (30 seconds to 2 minutes), frequent (3–22 per night) and characterized by a sudden arousal from NREM 2 sleep accompanied by screaming, agitation, dystonic posturing, kicking or bicycling of the legs, and/or urinary incontinence.[45] Interictal EEGs were normal in 86% of the children, although frontal or bifrontal electrographic seizure activity accompanying some of the frontal lobe seizures was seen in 95%. Given these clinical and EEG features, it is understandable why they are often initially misdiagnosed as sleepwalking, sleep terrors, nightmares or even a psychiatric problem.[45,46] Adding to the diagnostic challenge, NREM arousal disorders and sleep bruxism are significantly more common in patients and their relatives with NFLE.

A prospective case-control study found a higher incidence of parasomnias among 89 children with idiopathic epilepsy compared with 49 siblings and 321 healthy control children using parental sleep questionnaires. A recent retrospective study found the lifetime risk for NREM arousal disorders was sixfold greater in individuals with NFLE and fivefold higher for sleep bruxism compared to controls.[47] Among relatives of those with NFLE, the lifetime prevalence of a NREM arousal disorder was 4.7 times greater and nightmares 2.6 times higher compared to the relatives of control subject. NREM arousal disorders which are frequent (≥2–3 per week) warrant overnight PSG, which often identify another primary sleep

disorder (most often OSA, less often RLS or PLMD). If OSA is found with PSG, tonsillectomy often eliminates both sleep disorders.[48]

INDICATIONS FOR VIDEO-POLYSOMNOGRAPHY IN CHILDREN WITH SUSPECTED OR KNOWN EPILEPSY

Comprehensive video-PSG is most often done in CWE for suspected OSA or to identify primary sleep disorders contributing to complaints of sleepiness, fragmented sleep and/or poorly controlled seizures. When symptoms suggest this, a PSG is warranted.[49] Sometimes, we are asked to confirm whether paroxysmal nocturnal behaviors are epileptic or not in children with or without known epilepsy. The majority of children referred for parasomnias have NREM sleep disorders of arousal. This is not surprising since a recently published longitudinal study of child development reported an overall prevalence of 39.8% for sleep terrors and 14.5% for sleepwalking in children 6 years or younger.[50]

The American Academy of Sleep Medicine (AASM) practice parameters for PSG suggest a PSG is unnecessary if the nocturnal behavior events are typical, non-injurious, infrequent, and not disruptive to the child or family.[51] Common, uncomplicated, non-injurious parasomnias (such as typical disorders of arousal, nightmares, enuresis, sleeptalking and bruxism) can usually be diagnosed by a clinical history. One caveat, though: unusually frequent sleep terrors or sleepwalking events (more than 2–3 times per week) warrant PSG to identify another sleep disorder precipitating them (most often OSA, occasionally PLMD). OSA was found on overnight PSG in 58% of 84 prepubertal children who had sleep terrors and/or sleepwalking.[48] OSA and parasomnias were eliminated in 43 who had tonsillectomy. Two had restless legs syndrome and treatment of it with pramipexole eliminated the confusional arousals, restless legs and PLMS.

A PSG is indicated if the paroxysmal nocturnal events are atypical, frequent, potentially injurious, and/or disruptive to patient or family.[51] The AASM recently published practice parameters[52] for non-respiratory indications for PSG in children, accompanied by an evidence-based review justifying these.[53] These recommend a PSG may help differentiate atypical paroxysmal nocturnal behaviors from nocturnal seizures or to identify when sleep-disordered breathing or other sleep disorders contribute to frequent parasomnias, enuresis or affect control of seizures. Box 44.1 summarizes the differential diagnosis of nocturnal behavioral events in children. Box 44.2 provides a summary of the clinical features which are typical for a NREM arousal disorder. Box 44.3 summarizes red flags for atypical parasomnias which warrant consideration of video-PSG.

DIAGNOSTIC ALGORITHM FOR EVALUATING SEIZURES IN CHILDREN WITH SUSPECTED SLEEP-RELATED SEIZURES

Clinical features which warrant concern for sleep–related epileptic seizures are: (1) events occur any time in the night, just after falling asleep, or shortly before awakening in the morning; (2) multiple events a night; (3) occasional occurrence of these events awake or during a brief nap. If one suspects the

Box 44-1 Differential Diagnosis of Nocturnal Behavioral Events in a Child

- NREM partial arousal disorder (confusional arousal; sleep walking; sleep terror)
- Sleep-related epilepsy
- REM sleep-behavior disorder (RBD)
- Nightmare disorder
- Sleep-related dissociative disorder
- Sleep-related panic disorder
- Sleep-related choking, laryngospasm or gastroesophageal reflux
- Sleep-related rhythmic movement disorder with vocalization
- Sleep-related expiratory groaning (catathrenia)

Box 44-2 'Typical' NREM Arousal Disorders Usually Do Not Need a Sleep Study

- Occur first third of night when NREM 3 sleep predominates
- Appear confused and disoriented
- Usually cannot be fully aroused from event
- If aroused, dream imagery recalled only fragmentary
- Exhibit automatic motor behaviors and autonomic disturbances suggest sympathetic activation
- Cannot console; may resist intervention
- Little or no responsiveness to external environment
- Positive family history
- Moderate to high likelihood of injury in agitated sleepwalking or sleep terrors

Box 44-3 Red Flags for Atypical Parasomnias

- Spells are stereotyped
- Spells occur just after sleep onset
- Spells frequently occur second half of the night
- Behaviors potentially injurious or have caused injury to child or others
- Multiple episodes per night, not just ≤3 hours after sleep onset
- More than 2–3 spells per week
- Excessive daytime sleepiness
- Impaired daytime functioning
- Symptoms suggestive of sleep apnea or periodic limb movements
- Failure of conventional therapy

parasomnia may be sleep-related seizures and the child has not had an EEG with sleep, request one first. A prospective study of EEG done on 534 children referred for possible epilepsy reported epileptiform activity in 37% of the children with definite epilepsy, and 13% of clinically suspected cases.[54] However, the initial routine EEG will be normal in approximately one-half of children with clinically diagnosed epilepsy.[55,56]

Order the EEG without (or only partial) sleep deprivation because a recent prospective study of 820 EEGs specifically examining the diagnostic utility of sleep or varying degrees of sleep deprivation for finding IEDs in a child's EEG showed:

(1) NREM sleep was observed in 57% of sleep-deprived, 44% of partially sleep-deprived, and 21% of non-sleep-deprived pediatric EEGs; (2) a sixfold increased yield of recording NREM 2 sleep with sleep deprivation, 2.8-fold increase with partial sleep deprivation; (3) the odds ratio that IEDs would be found was *not* increased by the presence of sleep, nor the use of total or partial sleep deprivation; and (4) the *only* significant effect of sleep deprivation was to increase the odds sleep would occur.[57] Sleep is likely to occur with only partial sleep deprivation and more stringent sleep deprivation will not increase the yield.[58] The better mix of sleep yield and cost containment is to order an EEG with partial sleep deprivation, asking that a child >2 years of age stays awake 2 hours later than usual the night before the EEG and performing sleep-deprived EEGs in the morning, and no naps the day of the EEG for those <2 years.

Do request video be recorded during *routine* or sleep-deprived outpatient pediatric EEGs. Adding video when recording routine EEGs for an average duration of only 26 minutes helped confirm the diagnosis in 45% of children referred for frequent paroxysmal events, and in 55% of the children with cognitive impairment.[59] Using videos, it was possible to confirm the nature of many non-epileptic events including staring spells, tics, stereotypies, tremor, paroxysmal eye movements, breath holding or cyanotic spells.

If the child's paroxysmal events are daily (and only in sleep), a day of recording in the laboratory (with partial sleep deprivation or sleep deprivation the night before) can be diagnostic.[60,61] A retrospective study of prolonged v-EEG monitoring in 230 children found outpatient in-laboratory daytime recordings (4–8 hours) captured and confirmed the nature of the paroxysmal events in 80% of children whose events occurred on a daily basis.[60] Ordering 1 day of v-EEG done outpatient in-laboratory is best reserved for children whose events occur daily.[60,61]

If the first (or second) routine EEG with sleep is normal and clinical suspicion for a sleep-related epilepsy remains, request continuous inpatient video-EEG monitoring (LTM) for 2–5 days: (1) when the nocturnal behaviors do not occur nightly or every other night; (2) a primary sleep disorder (e.g., OSA or childhood RLS) is unlikely; (3) a history exists of post-ictal agitation or wandering; and/or (4) cooperation of the patient is questionable. Typical spells will be recorded in prolonged LTM in 45% to 80% of patients who have one or more event per week.[60,62,63] Characteristic events were captured in 53% of 444 children with suspected epileptic seizures by recording 1–5 days of inpatient video-EEG, confirming the diagnosis of epilepsy in 34%.[63] The likelihood of capturing an event was greater if a patient had an event frequency of at least 1 per week.

LTM can help confirm other non-epileptic paroxysmal behavior. One study of the diagnostic yield of LTM in 666 children (ages 2 weeks to 17 years) found they were able to confirm events in 96% of cases: staring in 34%, sleep-related arousals in 13%, benign infant sleep myoclonus in 15%, motor tics 11%, and shuddering in 7%.[62]

If a patient's spells occur only at night and are frequent, consider ordering a video-PSG with expanded EEG before prolonged inpatient video-EEG monitoring, especially if concomitant OSA or RBD is suspected. If the typical events are not captured on a single night of video-PSG, consider recording a second or order LTM. Prolonged inpatient video-EEG monitoring from the beginning is often a better choice in patients with undiagnosed paroxysmal nocturnal events when: (1) the nocturnal behaviors do not occur nightly or every other night; (2) a primary sleep disorder (e.g., OSA) is unlikely; (3) a history exists of postictal agitation or wandering; and/or (4) cooperation of the patient is questionable.

TECHNICAL CONSIDERATIONS WHEN RECORDING VIDEO-POLYSOMNOGRAPHY IN CHILDREN WITH EPILEPSY

The AASM practice parameters recommend that video-PSGs done to diagnose parasomnias need: (1) 'additional EEG derivations in an expanded bilateral montage' to diagnose paroxysmal arousals or other sleep disruptions thought to be seizure-related when the initial clinical evaluation and results of a standard EEG are inconclusive; (2) recording surface EMG activity from the left and right anterior tibialis and extensor digitorum muscles; (3) obtaining good audio-visual recording; (4) having a sleep technologist present throughout the study to observe and document events; and (5) sleep specialists who are not experienced or trained in recognizing and interpreting both PSG and EEG abnormalities should seek appropriate consultation or should refer patients to a center where this expertise is available.[51]

Regarding how many additional EEG derivations should be recorded in a PSG in a person with epilepsy, a study by Foldvary-Schaefer et al. found that recording 18 channels of EEG during video-PSG did not improve the ability to recognize frontal lobe seizures.[64] The ability to recognize frontal lobe seizures by EEG alone was not helped by either more EEG channels, slower screen times or midline electrodes. When seizures are suspected or known, recording 18 channels of EEG during a video-PSG is warrented, particularly if seizures, electrographic seizure activity or IEDs are thought to contribute to the sleep–wake complaints.

Unfortunately, the habitual nocturnal event may not be captured by one night of in-laboratory video-PSG (unless the child has NFLE). One to two consecutive nights of video-PSG provided valuable diagnostic information in 69% of 41 patients whose paroxysmal motor behaviors were 'prominent,' 41% of 11 patients referred for minor motor activity in sleep, and 78% of 36 patients with known epilepsy.[65] Another study found video-PSG was diagnostic in 65% and 'helpful' in another 26% of 100 consecutive adults referred for frequent sleep-related injuries; video-PSG identified DoA in 54, RBD in 36, sleep-related dissociative disorders in seven, nocturnal seizures in two, and OSA in one.[66] Unfortunately, only one-third of patients with paroxysmal nocturnal events will have a typical spell on a single night of video-PSG.[65,67]

Sleep researchers have found they were able to increase the diagnostic yield of one night of video-PSG for recording NREM arousal disorders by recording in-laboratory PSG after 25 hours of total sleep deprivation then ringing loud auditory stimuli. Patients arrived at their customary bedtime, remained awake the entire night, then were permitted to fall asleep 1 hour later than their usual wake time (i.e., 25 hours of prior wakefulness). To further provoke DoA events, patients are subjected to auditory stimuli delivered via earphones inserted in both ears. The auditory stimulus was a pure sound lasting 3 seconds. Most often 40–90 dB was needed to arouse both sleepwalkers and healthy controls from NREM 3. Using this technique, the investigators found they could trigger 1–3 sleepwalking events in 30% of 10 patients with DoA by sounding a 40–70 dB buzzer during NREM 3 sleep. After 25 hours of total sleep deprivation, the buzzer technique provoked NREM arousal disorder behaviors in 100% of their subjects (and none of their controls). Sleep deprivation nearly tripled the percentage of auditory stimulus trials that induced a behavioral event (57% vs. 20%).

Scoring sleep studies in patients with epilepsy can be difficult, especially when IEDs are frequent, even more difficult when their sleep spindles are dysmorphic or low in amplitude, or they have inappropriate alpha intrusions in their sleep EEG.[68] Almost continuous generalized spike-wave discharges first appearing during NREM sleep in a child warrant consideration of continuous electrographic status epilepticus in NREM sleep.[69,70] Figure 44.1 shows an example of this, and how the discharges are easier to identify in a 15-second epoch compared to 30 seconds. Electrographic seizures and IEDs in video-PSG are best identified by increasing the high-frequency filter of the EEG derivations to 70 Hz, re-mapping the frontal, central, and occipital channels to the ipsilateral mastoid to more easily recognize laterality of the discharges, and reviewing portions of the recording using vertical screen times (epochs) of 10 or 15 seconds.[53,71] Figure 44.2 shows focal spike-wave discharges emanating from the midline central (Cz)–left central (C3) region. These were activated by NREM sleep. Note how these are least frequent during REM sleep. Seizures and IEDs are least likely to be seen during REM sleep, perhaps because the EEG is desynchronized during REM sleep and skeletal atonia present then. Figures 44.3 and 44.4 show electrographic seizures which occurred from NREM 2 sleep in two different patients; both had nocturnal frontal lobe epilepsy, one whose seizures were primarily hypermotor, the other tonic.

EFFECTS OF VAGAL NERVE STIMULATION ON RESPIRATION DURING SLEEP

Vagal nerve stimulation (VNS, a treatment for medically refractory epilepsy) often alters the rate and amplitude of breathing when it 'activates' during sleep.[72-77] Most often, the respiratory change is an increase in the respiratory rate and fall in respiratory amplitude when the device fires, which usually does not cause an arousal or desaturation. Frank obstructive events with significant desaturation when the VNS activates are uncommon. When observed, consider reducing the VNS stimulation current from 1 to 2 milliamps. This often suppresses the effect of VNS on respiration. The effects of VNS on breathing in sleep do *not* usually warrant its removal.

USE OF MELATONIN TO TREAT SLEEP DISORDERS IN CHILDREN WITH EPILEPSY

Alterations in the circadian rhythm secretion of melatonin and lower nocturnal melatonin levels have been reported in CWE, especially those with medically intractable epilepsy.[78,79] Melatonin may have anticonvulsant effects, demonstrated in several different animal models of epilepsy.[4,80-84] Mechanisms

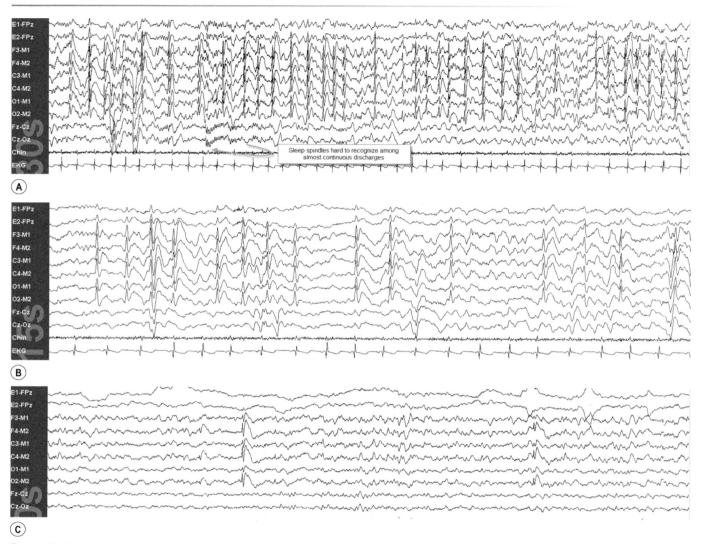

FIGURE 44-1 (A) Staging sleep challenging when interictal epileptiform discharges almost continuous. (B) Discharges easier to recognize if reviewed in 15-second epochs. (C) Note how much fewer discharges are seen in REM sleep.

by which melatonin may improve seizure control include its ability to reduce the electrical activity of neurons secreting glutamate (the primary central nervous system excitatory neurotransmitter) while enhancing neuronal release of neurons which secrete γ-aminobutyric acid (GABA, the primary CNS inhibitory neurotransmitter). Moreover, melatonin is metabolized to kynurenic acid (an endogenous anticonvulsant). Lastly, melatonin and its metabolites may have neuroprotective effects in that they can act as a free radical scavenger and antioxidant. However, relatively high doses of melatonin are needed to inhibit experimental seizures and such doses are much more likely to have undesirable adverse effects of decreased body temperature, and even cognitive and motor impairment.

Four randomized, double-blind, placebo-controlled studies of bedtime oral melatonin in children with epilepsy have shown positive effects on sleep.[4,82,85,86] These studies found: (1) oral melatonin improved sleep latency and quality and reduced parasomnias by a mean of 60% in 31 children with epilepsy (ages 3–12);[85] (2) nightly oral melatonin in 23 children with medically refractory epilepsy resulted in significant improvements in bedtime resistance, sleep duration, sleep latency, nocturnal arousals, sleepwalking, nocturnal enuresis, daytime sleepiness, and even seizure frequency;[4] (3) nightly use of oral melatonin (3 mg increased weekly to 9 mg as needed) in 25 children with epilepsy, mental retardation, and sleep–wake disorders (mean age 10.5 years) resulted in significant subjective improvements in sleep;[86] and (4) significantly fewer nocturnal awakenings and better control of convulsions in 10 children with severe medically intractable epilepsy given 3 mg of oral melatonin before bed nightly for 3 months followed by placebo for 3 months.[82] In humans, melatonin has relatively low toxicity, rare reports of nightmares, hypotension, and daytime sleepiness. A recently published Cochrane Database Review found there were too few studies and of poor methodological quality to draw any

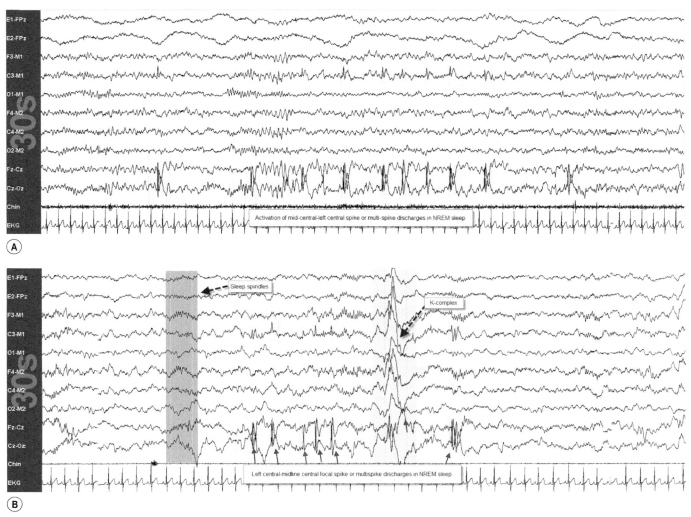

FIGURE 44-2 (A) Activation of focal spike or multi-spike discharges midline central–left central in NREM 1 sleep in 3-year-old girl. (B) Midline central–left central spike-wave discharges during NREM 2.

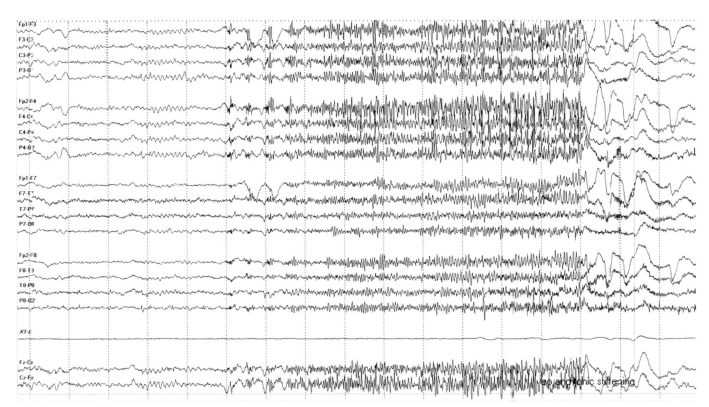

FIGURE 44-3 Brief Frontal Lobe Seizure from NREM 2 Sleep

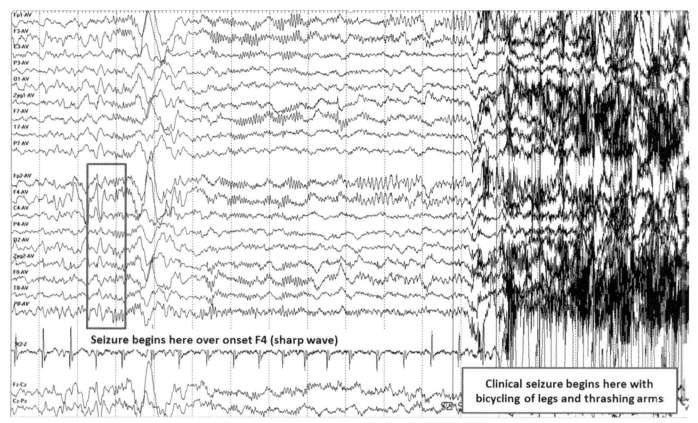

Seizure begins here over onset F4 (sharp wave)

Clinical seizure begins here with bicycling of legs and thrashing arms

FIGURE 44-4 Nocturnal Frontal Lobe Hypermotor Seizure

conclusions about the role of melatonin in reducing seizure frequency or improving quality of life in patients with epilepsy.[87]

SUMMARY

The relationship between sleep and epilepsy is a fruitful and rewarding area for research. Much more research and knowledge is needed to better understand: (1) why sleep macro- and microarchitecture is altered in patients with epilepsy; (2) whether treating OSA in patients with epilepsy improves seizure control; (3) the influence of circadian rhythms and chronotypes on different epilepsy syndromes, and (4) whether frequent IEDs during sleep with few or no seizures should be treated. Better understanding of the link between particular epilepsies, non-epileptic parasomnias, sleep fragmentation, and arousal to understand how to best improve overall function and that a multidisciplinary model will best serve patients with these disorders.

Clinical Pearls

- Children with epilepsy are much more likely to have parasomnias, nocturnal awakenings, shorter sleep duration, daytime sleepiness, sleep onset delay, and bedtime resistance than controls.
- Even children with epilepsy whose seizures were controlled were more likely to have sleep problems than their siblings or controls.
- Sleep problems in children with epilepsy increase the likelihood of inattention, hyperactivity, impulsivity and oppositional defiant disorder than in their siblings or controls.
- Poor sleep hygiene may contribute to sleep problems in children with epilepsy, especially in those whose

seizures occur primarily during sleep and/or are poorly controlled.
- Abnormalities in sleep architecture seen in some children with epilepsy include reduced sleep efficiency, decreased sleep time, increased NREM 1, increased arousals and awakenings, and reduced REM sleep time.
- Obstructive sleep apnea is more likely to be found in children with epilepsy who are on multiple antiepileptic medications and whose seizures are poorly controlled; children with uncontrolled seizures on multiple antiepileptics should be screened for obstructive sleep apnea.

Clinical Pearls

- Tonic and hypermotor seizures more often occur during sleep; clonic and absence seizures while awake.
- Nocturnal frontal lobe seizures are often initially misdiagnosed as sleepwalking, sleep terrors, nightmares or a psychiatric problem.
- The life-time risk of NREM arousal disorders is sixfold higher in individuals with nocturnal frontal lobe epilepsy.
- Video-PSG with expanded EEG is indicated in children with epilepsy for suspected obstructive sleep apnea, to identify primary sleep disorders contributing to complaints of sleepiness, fragmented sleep and/or poorly controlled seizures, and/or to confirm whether nocturnal events are epileptic or not.

- Sleep deprivation the night before a sleep study may increase the likelihood a NREM arousal disorder occurs during a single night of in-laboratory video-PSG.
- When a vagal nerve stimulator fires for 30 seconds during sleep, it most often causes an increase in respiratory rate and fall in respiratory amplitude for the time the stimulator fires. This usually does not cause an arousal or desaturation. On occasion, obstructive apneas occur during and when the vagal nerve stimulator fires; reducing the stimulator current from 1 to 2 milliamps often lessens this effect.
- Melatonin may have anticonvulsive effects and can have positive effects on sleep in children with epilepsy, especially those with other neurological comorbidities.

References

1. Cortesi F, Giannotti F, Ottaviano S. Sleep problems and daytime behavior in childhood idiopathic epilepsy. Epilepsia 1999;40(11):1557–65.
2. Batista BH, Nunes ML. Evaluation of sleep habits in children with epilepsy. Epilepsy Behav 2007;11(1):60–4.
3. Ong LC, Yang WW, Wong SW, et al. Sleep habits and disturbances in Malaysian children with epilepsy. J Paediatr Child Health 2010;46(3):80–4.
4. Elkhayat HA, Hassanein SM, Tomoum HY, et al. Melatonin and sleep-related problems in children with intractable epilepsy. Pediatr Neurol 2010;42(4):249–54.
5. Tang SS, Clarke T, Owens J, et al. Sleep behaviour disturbances in rolandic epilepsy. J Child Neurol 2010.
6. Maganti R, Hausman N, Koehn M, et al. Excessive daytime sleepiness and sleep complaints among children with epilepsy. Epilepsy Behav 2006;8(1):272–7.
7. Stores G, Wiggs L, Campling G. Sleep disorders and their relationship to psychological disturbance in children with epilepsy. Child Care Health Dev 1998;24(1):5–19.
8. Wirrell E, Blackman M, Barlow K, et al. Sleep disturbances in children with epilepsy compared with their nearest-aged siblings. Dev Med Child Neurol 2005;47(11):754–9.
9. Byars AW, Byars KC, Johnson CS, et al. The relationship between sleep problems and neuropsychological functioning in children with first recognized seizures. Epilepsy Behav 2008;13(4):607–13.
10. Williams J, Lange B, Sharp G, et al. Altered sleeping arrangements in pediatric patients with epilepsy. Clin Pediatr (Phila) 2000;39(11):635–42.
11. de Weerd A, de Haas S, Otte A, et al. Subjective sleep disturbance in patients with partial epilepsy: a questionnaire-based study on prevalence and impact on quality of life. Epilepsia 2004;45(11):1397–404.
12. Khatami R, Zutter D, Siegel A, et al. Sleep-wake habits and disorders in a series of 100 adult epilepsy patients – a prospective study. Seizure 2006;15(5):299–306.
13. Piperidou C, Karlovasitou A, Triantafyllou N, et al. Influence of sleep disturbance on quality of life of patients with epilepsy. Seizure 2008;17(7):588–94.
14. Jenssen S, Gracely E, Mahmood T, et al. Subjective somnolence relates mainly to depression among patients in a tertiary care epilepsy center. Epilepsy Behav 2006;9(4):632–5.
15. Didden R, Korzilius H, van Aperlo B, et al. Sleep problems and daytime problem behaviours in children with intellectual disability. J Intellect Disabil Res 2002;46(Pt 7):537–47.
16. Didden R, de Moor JM, Korzilius H. Sleepiness, on-task behavior and attention in children with epilepsy who visited a school for special education: a comparative study. Res Dev Disabil 2009;30(6):1428–34.
17. Conant KD, Thibert RL, Thiele EA. Epilepsy and the sleep–wake patterns found in Angelman syndrome. Epilepsia 2009;50(11):2497–500.
18. Segawa M, Nomura Y. Polysomnography in the Rett syndrome. Brain Dev 1992;14(Suppl):S46–54.
19. Liu X, Hubbard JA, Fabes RA, et al. Sleep disturbances and correlates of children with autism spectrum disorders. Child Psychiatry Hum Dev 2006;37(2):179–91.
20. Becker DA, Fennell EB, Carney PR. Daytime behavior and sleep disturbance in childhood epilepsy. Epilepsy Behav 2004;5(5):708–15.
21. Chan S, Baldeweg T, Cross JH. A role for sleep disruption in cognitive impairment in children with epilepsy. Epilepsy Behav 2011;20(3):435–40.
22. Parisi P, Bruni O, Pia Villa M, et al. The relationship between sleep and epilepsy: the effect on cognitive functioning in children. Dev Med Child Neurol 2010;52(9):805–10.
23. Manni R, Terzaghi M. Comorbidity between epilepsy and sleep disorders. Epilepsy Res 2010;90(3):171–7.
24. Tang SS, Clarke T, Owens J, et al. Sleep behavior disturbances in rolandic epilepsy. J Child Neurol 2011;26(2):239–43.
25. Larson AM, Ryther RC, Jennesson M, et al. Impact of pediatric epilepsy on sleep patterns and behaviors in children and parents. Epilepsia 2012;53(7):1162–9.
26. Krishnan P, Sinha S, Taly AB, et al. Sleep disturbances in juvenile myoclonic epilepsy: a sleep questionnaire-based study. Epilepsy Behav 2012;23(3):305–9.
27. Pereira AM, Bruni O, Ferri R, et al. The impact of epilepsy on sleep architecture during childhood. Epilepsia 2012;53(9):1519–25.
28. Kaleyias J, Cruz M, Goraya JS, et al. Spectrum of polysomnographic abnormalities in children with epilepsy. Pediatr Neurol 2008;39(3):170–6.
29. Miano S, Bruni O, Arico D, et al. Polysomnographic assessment of sleep disturbances in children with developmental disabilities and seizures. Neurol Sci 2010.
30. Bruni O, Novelli L, Luchetti A, et al. Reduced NREM sleep instability in benign childhood epilepsy with centro-temporal spikes. Clin Neurophysiol 2010;121(5):665–71.
31. Nunes ML, Ferri R, Arzimanoglou A, et al. Sleep organization in children with partial refractory epilepsy. J Child Neurol 2003;18(11):763–6.
32. Maganti R, Sheth RD, Hermann BP, et al. Sleep architecture in children with idiopathic generalized epilepsy. Epilepsia 2005;46(1):104–9.
33. Eisensehr I, Parrino L, Noachtar S, et al. Sleep in Lennox–Gastaut syndrome: the role of the cyclic alternating pattern (CAP) in the gate control of clinical seizures and generalized polyspikes. Epilepsy Res 2001;46(3):241–50.
34. Miano S, Bruni O, Arico D, et al. Polysomnographic assessment of sleep disturbances in children with developmental disabilities and seizures. Neurol Sci 2010;31(5):575–83.
35. Myatchin I, Lagae L. Sleep spindle abnormalities in children with generalized spike-wave discharges. Pediatr Neurol 2007;36(2):106–11.
36. Sato S, Dreifuss FE, Penry JK. The effect of sleep on spike-wave discharges in absence seizures. Neurology 1973;23(12):1335–45.
37. Terzano MG, Parrino L, Anelli S, et al. Effects of generalized interictal EEG discharges on sleep stability: assessment by means of cyclic alternating pattern. Epilepsia 1992;33(2):317–26.
38. Bruni O, Cortesi F, Giannotti F, et al. Sleep disorders in tuberous sclerosis: a polysomnographic study. Brain Dev 1995;17(1):52–6.
39. Jain SV, Horn PS, Simakajornboon N, et al. Obstructive sleep apnea and primary snoring in children with epilepsy. J Child Neurol 2012.
40. Segal E, Vendrame M, Gregas M, et al. Effect of treatment of obstructive sleep apnea on seizure outcomes in children with epilepsy. Pediatr Neurol 2012;46(6):359–62.
41. Malow BA, Weatherwax KJ, Chervin RD, et al. Identification and treatment of obstructive sleep apnea in adults and children with epilepsy: a prospective pilot study. Sleep Med 2003;4(6):509–15.

42. Zarowski M, Loddenkemper T, Vendrame M, et al. Circadian distribution and sleep/wake patterns of generalized seizures in children. Epilepsia 2011;52(6):1076–83.

43. Ramgopal S, Vendrame M, Shah A, et al. Circadian patterns of generalized tonic-clonic evolutions in pediatric epilepsy patients. Seizure 2012;21(7):535–9.

44. Ramgopal S, Shah A, Zarowski M, et al. Diurnal and sleep/wake patterns of epileptic spasms in different age groups. Epilepsia 2012;53(7):1170–7.

45. Sinclair DB, Wheatley M, Snyder T. Frontal lobe epilepsy in childhood. Pediatr Neurol 2004;30(3):169–76.

46. Oldani A, Zucconi M, Asselta R, et al. Autosomal dominant nocturnal frontal lobe epilepsy. A video-polysomnographic and genetic appraisal of 40 patients and delineation of the epileptic syndrome. Brain 1998;121(Pt 2):205–23.

47. Bisulli F, Vignatelli L, Naldi I, et al. Increased frequency of arousal parasomnias in families with nocturnal frontal lobe epilepsy: A common mechanism? Epilepsia 2010.

48. Guilleminault C, Palombini L, Pelayo R, et al. Sleepwalking and sleep terrors in prepubertal children: what triggers them? Pediatrics 2003;111(1):e17–25.

49. Aurora RN, Zak RS, Karippot A, et al. Practice parameters for the respiratory indications for polysomnography in children. Sleep 2011;34(3):379–88.

50. Petit D, Touchette E, Tremblay RE, et al. Dyssomnias and parasomnias in early childhood. Pediatrics 2007;119(5):e1016–25.

51. Kushida CA, Littner MR, Morgenthaler T, et al. Practice parameters for the indications for polysomnography and related procedures: an update for 2005. Sleep 2005;28(4):499–521.

52. Aurora RN, Lamm CI, Zak RS, et al. Practice parameters for the non-respiratory indications for polysomnography and multiple sleep latency testing for children. Sleep 2012;35(11):in press.

53. Kotagal NC, Grigg-Damberger MM, et al. Non-respiratory indications for polysomnography and related procedures in children: an evidence-based review. Sleep 2012;35(11):in press.

54. Aydin K, Okuyaz C, Serdaroglu A, et al. Utility of electroencephalography in the evaluation of common neurologic conditions in children. J Child Neurol 2003;18(6):394–6.

55. Camfield P, Gordon K, Camfield C, et al. EEG results are rarely the same if repeated within six months in childhood epilepsy. Can J Neurol Sci 1995;22(4):297–300.

56. Gilbert DL, Gartside PS. Factors affecting the yield of pediatric EEGs in clinical practice. Clin Pediatr (Phila) 2002;41(1):25–32.

57. Gilbert DL. Interobserver reliability of visual interpretation of electroencephalograms in children with newly diagnosed seizures. Dev Med Child Neurol 2006;48(12):1009–10; author reply 1010–11.

58. Gilbert DL, DeRoos S, Bare MA. Does sleep or sleep deprivation increase epileptiform discharges in pediatric electroencephalograms? Pediatrics 2004;114(3):658–62.

59. Watemberg N, Tziperman B, Dabby R, et al. Adding video recording increases the diagnostic yield of routine electroencephalograms in children with frequent paroxysmal events. Epilepsia 2005;46(5):716–19.

60. Chen LS, Mitchell WG, Horton EJ, et al. Clinical utility of video-EEG monitoring. Pediatr Neurol 1995;12(3):220–4.

61. Valente KD, Freitas A, Fiore LA, et al. The diagnostic role of short duration outpatient V-EEG monitoring in children. Pediatr Neurol 2003;28(4):285–91.

62. Bye AM, Kok DJ, Ferenschild FT, et al. Paroxysmal non-epileptic events in children: a retrospective study over a period of 10 years. J Paediatr Child Health 2000;36(3):244–8.

63. Mohan KK, Markand ON, Salanova V. Diagnostic utility of video EEG monitoring in paroxysmal events. Acta Neurol Scand 1996;94(5):320–5.

64. Foldvary-Schaefer N, De Ocampo J, Mascha E, et al. Accuracy of seizure detection using abbreviated EEG during polysomnography. J Clin Neurophysiol 2006;23(1):68–71.

65. Aldrich MS, Jahnke B. Diagnostic value of video-EEG polysomnography. Neurology 1991;41(7):1060–6.

66. Schenck CH, Milner DM, Hurwitz TD, et al. A polysomnographic and clinical report on sleep-related injury in 100 adult patients. Am J Psychiatry 1989;146(9):1166–73.

67. Blatt I, Peled R, Gadoth N, et al. The value of sleep recording in evaluating somnambulism in young adults. Electroencephalogr Clin Neurophysiol 1991;78(6):407–12.

68. Marzec ML, Malow BA. Approaches to staging sleep in polysomnographic studies with epileptic activity. Sleep Med 2003;4(5):409–17.

69. Brazzo D, Pera MC, Fasce M, et al. Epileptic encephalopathies with status epilepticus during sleep: new techniques for understanding pathophysiology and therapeutic options. Epilepsy Res Treat 2012 2012:642–725.

70. Loddenkemper T, Fernandez IS, Peters JM. Continuous spike and waves during sleep and electrical status epilepticus in sleep. J Clin Neurophysiol 2011;28(2):154–64.

71. Grigg-Damberger M, Ralls F. Primary sleep disorders and paroxysmal nocturnal nonepileptic events in adults with epilepsy from the perspective of sleep specialists. J Clin Neurophysiol 2011;28(2):120–40.

72. Nagarajan L, Walsh P, Gregory P, et al. Respiratory pattern changes in sleep in children on vagal nerve stimulation for refractory epilepsy. Can J Neurol Sci 2003;30(3):224–7.

73. Hsieh T, Chen M, McAfee A, et al. Sleep-related breathing disorder in children with vagal nerve stimulators. Pediatr Neurol 2008;38(2):99–103.

74. Pruvost M, Zaaimi B, Grebe R, et al. Cardiorespiratory effects induced by vagus nerve stimulation in epileptic children. Med Biol Eng Comput 2006;44(4):338–47.

75. Zaaimi B, Heberle C, Berquin P, et al. Vagus nerve stimulation induces concomitant respiratory alterations and a decrease in SaO_2 in children. Epilepsia 2005;46(11):1802–9.

76. Khurana DS, Reumann M, Hobdell EF, et al. Vagus nerve stimulation in children with refractory epilepsy: unusual complications and relationship to sleep-disordered breathing. Childs Nerv Syst 2007;23(11):1309–12.

77. Zaaimi B, Grebe R, Berquin P, et al. Vagus nerve stimulation induces changes in respiratory sinus arrhythmia of epileptic children during sleep. Epilepsia 2009;50(11):2473–80.

78. Paprocka J, Dec R, Jamroz E, et al. Melatonin and childhood refractory epilepsy – a pilot study. Med Sci Monit 2010;16(9):CR389–96.

79. Ardura J, Andres J, Garmendia JR, et al. Melatonin in epilepsy and febrile seizures. J Child Neurol 2010;25(7):888–91.

80. Scorza FA, Colugnati DB, Arida RM, et al. Cardiovascular protective effect of melatonin in sudden unexpected death in epilepsy: a hypothesis. Med Hypotheses 2008;70(3):605–9.

81. Sanchez-Forte M, Moreno-Madrid F, Munoz-Hoyos A, et al. [The effect of melatonin as anti-convulsant and neuron protector]. Rev Neurol 1997;25(144):1229–34.

82. Uberos J, Augustin-Morales MC, Molina Carballo A, et al. Normalization of the sleep–wake pattern and melatonin and 6-sulphatoxymelatonin levels after a therapeutic trial with melatonin in children with severe epilepsy. J Pineal Res 2010.

83. Fenoglio-Simeone K, Mazarati A, Sefidvash-Hockley S, et al. Anticonvulsant effects of the selective melatonin receptor agonist ramelteon. Epilepsy Behav 2009;16(1):52–7.

84. Molina-Carballo A, Munoz-Hoyos A, Sanchez-Forte M, et al. Melatonin increases following convulsive seizures may be related to its anticonvulsant properties at physiological concentrations. Neuropediatrics 2007;38(3):122–5.

85. Gupta M, Aneja S, Kohli K. Add-on melatonin improves sleep behavior in children with epilepsy: randomized, double-blind, placebo-controlled trial. J Child Neurol 2005;20(2):112–15.

86. Coppola G, Iervolino G, Mastrosimone M, et al. Melatonin in wake-sleep disorders in children, adolescents and young adults with mental retardation with or without epilepsy: a double-blind, cross-over, placebo-controlled trial. Brain Dev 2004;26(6):373–6.

87. Brigo F, Del Felice A. Melatonin as add-on treatment for epilepsy. Cochrane Database Syst Rev 2012;(6):CD006967.

Neoplasms and Sleep: Impact and Implications

Valerie McLaughlin Crabtree and Chasity Brimeyer

INTRODUCTION

Each year more than 61,000 children and adolescents under the age of 20 are diagnosed with a malignancy.[1] Significant advances in treatment including surgery, intensive chemotherapy, and targeted radiation therapy have led to substantial increases in survival, with survival rates of 83% by 2009.[1] As survival rates have increased over the past several years, both researchers and clinicians have increased focus on quality of life, including sleep and fatigue, in pediatric oncology patients and survivors.

Fatigue and sleep disturbances have consistently been found to be among the most frequently reported symptoms experienced by both adult and pediatric oncology patients undergoing cancer-directed therapy.[2-4] Both fatigue and sleep disturbance have been reported in these patients, and it is important to distinguish between these two complaints. Fatigue, which is reported to be one of the most distressing symptoms in pediatric oncology patients, is defined as the subjective feeling of physical, emotional, or cognitive tiredness that interferes with the ability to participate in physical or social activities.[5] In pediatric oncology patients, this may be directly caused by treatments including chemotherapy and/or radiation therapy, a side effect of specific medications, such as corticosteroids, and/or secondary to treatment-related effects such as anemia. Sleep disturbances are also observed in oncology patients and can be the direct cause of the fatigue identified by these patients. Sleep disturbances and fatigue are of particular concern for children and adolescents with cancer because they may negatively impact immune functioning and healing, daily functioning, social activities, depressive symptoms, behavior problems, and overall quality of life.[2,6-9]

COMMON SLEEP COMPLAINTS

Sleep complaints are commonly associated with pediatric cancer, and include restless sleep, excessive daytime sleepiness (EDS), obstructive sleep apnea symptoms, and difficulty initiating and maintaining sleep.[5,10] Zupanec and colleagues[11] observed a detrimental impact on sleep habits in children following a diagnosis of acute lymphocytic leukemia (ALL), the most common childhood cancer. Sixty-seven percent of parents reported sleep problems, increased restlessness, nighttime awakenings, bedtime resistance, frequency of nightmares, and more changes in sleep location during the night. Parents attributed their children's poorer sleep habits and subsequent decreased sleep quality to medication schedules and side effects, among other psychological factors related to their diagnosis and treatment.[11] Hinds and colleagues[12] reported that children on ALL maintenance therapy slept longer while receiving dexamethasone treatment (a backbone of leukemia treatment) but demonstrated poorer sleep quality with more nighttime awakenings, more restless sleep, and more daytime napping as documented by actigraphic recording.

Sleep complaints are frequently reported not only when children are undergoing treatment for cancer, but also in the survivorship period. One study of childhood cancer survivors referred to a sleep center revealed that 60% of children presented with EDS, 40% with sleep-disordered breathing, 24% with insomnia, 4% with circadian rhythm dysfunction, and 9% demonstrated parasomnias.[13] Furthermore, sleep disruptions in pediatric brain tumor survivors may be enduring. While sleep complaints have been found to resolve following treatment in child survivors of leukemias, brain tumor survivors continue to experience sleep disruptions even 1 year post treatment[14] and report excessive daytime sleepiness more than 5 years post treatment.[15] In addition to excessive daytime sleepiness, adolescents with cancer have continued to report significant fatigue up to 5 years after treatment and even into adulthood.[16,17]

Excessive Daytime Sleepiness

Excessive daytime sleepiness (EDS) is the most commonly reported sleep problem in children and adolescents with cancer with rates higher than those observed in otherwise healthy obese adolescents.[13,13,15,18-20] EDS is characterized by increased total duration of sleep, recommencement of daytime naps, inability to easily awaken in the morning, and/or difficulty staying awake during daytime activities.[10,19] It is especially prevalent and more severe in children with brain tumors; 50–60% of all pediatric oncology patients report fatigue and EDS, while 80% of children with brain tumors involving the hypothalamus, thalamus, and brainstem experience these symptoms.[19,21] In survivors of pediatric brain tumors, up to one-third self-reported significant EDS that was not well recognized by their parents.[15] Not surprisingly, children and adolescents with brain tumors report EDS-related impairments in their functioning at home and school.[5]

Insomnia

Sleep onset or maintenance insomnia is characterized by difficulty initiating or maintaining sleep; in children, it may be the result of inadvertent, behavioral conditioning from their parents.[13] Given the demands of treatment and the physiological symptoms experienced by children with cancer, it is not uncommon for parents to become overly involved in their child's bedtime routine. This sometimes results in conditioning the child to require parental presence to initiate and/or maintain sleep. Insomnia has also been linked to uncontrolled pain[13] (see Chapter 12) and/or high-dose corticosteroid treatments, which frequently accompany oncological therapy.

CONTRIBUTORS TO SLEEP DISTURBANCE

Many factors contribute to sleep disturbances in children and adolescents who are receiving cancer-directed therapy, including disease process, treatment modality,[6] frequent nocturnal awakenings in hospitalized patients,[3] nighttime caretaking needs, and poor sleep quality.[22]

Disease-related variables are likely to account for the significant fatigue in pediatric oncology patients both during and after treatment. Several studies have investigated children's sleep and fatigue while receiving treatment, typically for ALL, and have found that use of steroids, a backbone of leukemia treatment, may contribute to fatigue. Both actigraphic recording and parent report have indicated that children with ALL have poor sleep while receiving treatment. This poor sleep has been characterized by decreased total sleep time at night, increased daytime napping, increased nighttime awakenings, and more restless sleep, particularly while children are receiving steroid treatment in comparison to days when they are not receiving steroids.[12,23]

Excessive daytime sleepiness can result from the cumulative effect of insufficient sleep, fragmented sleep, irregular sleep–wake schedules, and circadian rhythm disruption.[10] In pediatric patients with centrally located brain tumors, the mechanism of EDS is likely twofold because the hypothalamus regulates both neurological sleep control and weight. First, EDS may result from hypothalamic injury following tumor resection and/or from the tumor itself, resulting in the child's inability to effectively maintain sleep and wakefulness. Second, increased risk for obesity due to hypothalamic dysfunction or injury may result in obstructive sleep apnea.[10,13,18,24,25] In this way, tumor location, rather than type, is more of a determinant of EDS symptoms. One study of children referred to a sleep center who were currently receiving cancer treatment or had completed treatment found that children with brain tumors, particulary tumors of the hypothalamus, thalamus, and brainstem, accounted for over two-thirds of all referrals.[13] In pediatric brain tumor survivors evaluated during their survivorship clinic visits who had not been referred to a sleep clinic, however, tumor location was not as consistently related to levels of excessive daytime sleepiness.[15] Thus, while survivors of CNS tumors have increased likelihood of sleep disturbances, the etiology of these sleep disruptions is complex and likely multifactorial.

DEMOGRAPHIC VARIABLES RELATED TO DIFFERENCES IN SLEEP PROBLEMS

Demographic variables that may relate to differences in sleep and fatigue in pediatric oncology patients have received limited attention; however, there is some evidence to suggest that gender and age may contribute to sleep disturbance and fatigue. For example, in a study examining sleep disruption in pediatric ALL patients in the maintenance phase of treatment, girls were found to nap more and had more consolidated nighttime sleep than did boys. This finding was consistent even after controlling for differences in age, treatment, and risk group.[26] Another study examining changes in fatigue over the course of cancer treatment also found that girls reported more fatigue than boys.[27] However, this is an equivocal finding, as other studies of pediatric oncology

patients have found no gender differences.[28] Research related to age differences has also yielded mixed results. One study compared children with ALL to their healthy same-age peers and found that only younger children with ALL exhibited significantly longer sleep duration.[8] Conversely, a study of children successfully treated for CNS tumors found that patients aged 8–12 exhibited significantly more sleep disturbances, while patients aged 4–8 and 12–18 did not exhibit greater sleep difficulties than their same-age peers.[29] On the other hand, children aged 6–12 have been reported to experience a decrease in fatigue over the course of treatment while adolescents aged 13–18 experienced no change.[28]

IMPACT OF SLEEP DISTURBANCE

Sleep disturbances have been associated with poorer health, mood, behavior regulation, academic performance, neurocognitive function, immune function, and overall quality of life.[30–32] The consequences of sleep disturbances are of particular concern to pediatric oncology patients because sleep is critical for neural recovery and tissue renewal; disrupted sleep may hinder the child's recovery.[17,30] Similarly, the consequences of sleep disruption on the child's psychological well-being should be considered. More specifically, reduced adaptive functioning, limited engagement in social activities, behavioral and mood problems, and/or negative impact on treatment adherence have been associated with nocturia, fatigue, and disturbance of sleep–wake cycles.[2,6,7,27]

Academic Functioning

Poor and insufficient sleep has been found to negatively impact academic functioning in children with obesity.[33,34] While the relationship between sleep, cancer, and school performance has not been explicitly studied, the impact of sleep disturbances on school performance has been researched in otherwise healthy children. For example, treatment of obstructive sleep apnea has been linked with significantly improved academic performance.[35] Moreover, a 'learning debt' has been hypothesized whereby sleep-disordered breathing in early childhood may impair future school performance.[36] Children with pediatric cancers are already at risk for poor school performance due to extended school absences and neurocognitive late effects of cancer treatments;[37–39] problematic sleep may only compound this risk, and warrants further investigation.

Mood and Behavior

A growing body of research suggests that sleep deprivation has its greatest impact on an adolescent's ability to regulate behavior, emotions, and attention.[40] Studies investigating the link between sleep regulation and emotional/behavioral regulation in healthy adolescents have revealed an interactive relationship, wherein emotional disorders influence sleep quality, regulation, and duration, and sleep quality and duration influence an adolescent's ability to regulate emotions and behavior.[40,41] Similarly, in a study of 67 children and adolescents undergoing chemotherapy, sleep disturbances (e.g., nighttime awakenings, poor sleep duration) *and* fatigue negatively influenced interpersonal relations, anxiety, and depressive symptoms in adolescents, whereas fatigue alone was associated with depressive symptoms and behavioral changes in children.[7]

Anxiety may have a similar effect. In addition to nausea, vomiting, and frequent bathroom use, nightmares and fear were among the most commonly reported reasons for nighttime awakenings in a study on sleep quality in children with cancer.[11] The authors surmised that anxiety may play more of a role in sleep disruption than previously understood, suggesting that the child's or adolescent's ability to self-soothe may have been negatively impacted by their illness and treatment experiences. Treatment-related anxiety and disease-related cognitive rumination may also contribute to difficulty with sleep onset.[42-46]

Environmental stressors such as family stress or hospital-related sleep interruptions (e.g., entry and exit from the patient's room), have also been shown to impact sleep quality.[3,47] While undergoing cancer treatment certainly qualifies as a stressful event, most children with cancer do not meet diagnostic criteria for depression or anxiety but remain at risk for these difficulties.[48-50] Given the neurocognitive sequelae associated with their disease, children and adolescents with brain tumors continue to be at risk for anxiety and depression in the survivorship period.[51] Increased risk for both emotional difficulties and sleep disruptions may create compounding sleep-related problems in this population.

Quality of Life

Quality of life is defined as an individual's functional independence within physical, emotional, social, and cognitive domains[52] and emphasis on improving quality of life has increased with improved childhood cancer survival rates.[53] Adolescents undergoing cancer therapy have reported lower quality of life when compared to healthy peers, particularly with regard to physical functioning and mood.[54] Cancer diagnoses and therapy have also have been shown to impact quality of life, with higher-risk disease and extended, aggressive treatment related to lower quality of life.[55]

One important contributor to overall quality of life that has received more recent attention is sleep. Sleep disturbances have the potential to interfere with functional domains independently or in combination with other factors, therein negatively impacting quality of life.[56] For example, adolescents with cancer have endorsed EDS and difficulty with sleep onset, insufficient sleep duration, and multiple nighttime awakenings that interfere with their daily functioning.[8] Moreover, symptoms of nausea, pain, worry, and anxiety have also been reported,[42-45] which also decrease opportunities to engage in developmentally typical activities, resulting in poorer quality of life.[56] Combining symptoms of disrupted sleep, EDS, and the physical and social/emotional consequences of pediatric cancer may result in greater detriment to quality of life than any of these symptoms alone.[42] Dissatisfaction with functional independence has been found to affect psychosocial functioning both during and after treatment.[57,58] As a result, interventions targeted toward improving sleep and fatigue have the potential to improve quality of life in pediatric oncology patients.

INTERVENTIONS

Interventions that facilitate efficient sleep and developmentally appropriate maintenance of daily activities should be explored.[56] Research in the efficacy of interventions to improve sleep quality in children and adolescents with pediatric cancer is lacking, potentially because no formalized interventions have been developed specifically for this population at this time. However, interventions for facilitating sleep that have been used to address the antecedents to sleep disruptions, such as bedtime refusal, anxiety, and problematic sleep-wake cycles, may be effective. Because sleep involves both biological and psychological components,[10] a variety of potential interventions are offered. Similarly, the cause of the child's sleep disruption, such as cancer treatment, hospitalization, or behavioral disruptions, should be identified to better tailor sleep interventions.[56]

Behavioral Sleep Medicine Interventions

Behavioral strategies may facilitate and maintain development of healthy sleep habits in children with cancer. Establishing and maintaining effective sleep hygiene is a mainstay in sleep intervention. Families of children with cancer may be tempted to disregard a sleep routine, given the child's health status, parental distress, overprotectiveness, or disrupted routines as a result of medication schedules or hospitalizations.[11] Thus, establishing a daily schedule with specific periods of rest and activity may be beneficial.[11,56] Enforcing a consistent bedtime and wake time, developing a bedtime routine, eliminating stimulating activities before sleep, decreasing caffeine intake, and providing a cool and quiet sleep environment are recommended.[11,59,60] Nurses may assist parents in maintaining these limits while the child is on the inpatient unit in an effort to reduce parental distress.[61] Graduated extinction methods have also demonstrated effectiveness in case reports for children with sleep onset difficulties who also have medical complications.[62] Gradually reducing parental attention to sleep disturbances, rather than traditional extinction methods, may facilitate parental adherence to the intervention by reducing aversive extinction bursts in which the negative behavior temporarily worsens prior to extinguishing.[63] Moreover, stimulus control (or minimizing negative associations of frustration with the child's bed) with consideration for the child's current medical presentation has demonstrated benefit.[5,11]

Interventions that target mood-related antecedents to sleep disturbances are also recommended. For example, cognitive-behavioral therapy to reduce anxiety, as well as interventions that promote self-soothing behaviors after nighttime awakenings, may be beneficial.[11] Guiding the child in cognitive restructuring may be helpful in reducing maladaptive sleep cognitions. Furthermore, relaxation training, including diaphragmatic breathing, progressive muscle relaxation, autogenic training, and imagery techniques, may facilitate a child's sleep onset and ability to return to sleep after nighttime awakenings (see Chapter 12). Finally, improving illness management, such as decreasing pain or managing obesity, may indirectly benefit a child's sleep.[64]

Hospital-Based Interventions

Environmental restructuring of the hospital environment may serve to protect children's sleep while they are admitted for cancer-directed treatment. During an inpatient stay, children were found to have an average of 11 room entries/exits by staff during the nighttime period with a mean of 12–16 nighttime awakenings each night of the admission. Not surprisingly, over the course of the hospital admission, children's reported fatigue steadily increased, which was associated with the number of nighttime awakenings.[3] Changes in nursing practices such as 'bundling care' whereby all necessary, scheduled care occurs simultaneously during the night with the remainder of room entries confined to unexpected needs that arise may help protect children's sleep while an inpatient. Furthermore, nursing-led interventions to facilitate improved sleep in oncology patients admitted for high-dose chemotherapy have been shown to be feasible. Feasible changes to the inpatient unit included having the child and parent determine a bedtime and wake time, use of white noise machines and light-blocking blinds, pre-bedtime routines, bundled care, and out-of-bed activity during the day.[65]

Pharmacological Interventions

Pharmacological intervention that is used conjointly with behavioral strategies, such as administration of melatonin,[66] may facilitate sleep onset in those patients with difficulty initiating sleep. Similarly, sedative hypnotics have been used to address steroid-induced insomnia.[13] Tricyclic antidepressants have also been prescribed for use at bedtime to assist in sleep consolidation (see Chapter 12). Stimulant medications, such as methylphenidate, amphetamines, and modafinil, have demonstrated promise in treating EDS in children with brain tumors.[10] Relatedly, assisted breathing devices, such as continuous positive airway pressure (CPAP) or bilevel positive airway pressure (BIPAP), may improve symptoms of sleep-disordered breathing in those patients with hypothalamic obesity.[10,13]

Both pharmacologic and non-pharmacologic interventions that show evidence for effective symptom management of sleep disturbances in the pediatric cancer population are needed. Continuing to enhance our understanding of the contributors to common sleep complaints will help guide future research in developing successful treatment strategies.

SUMMARY

As research into the impact of cancer, its treatment, and the survivorship period is a relatively new area of study, many more questions than answers exist. It is becoming increasingly clear that children and adolescents receiving cancer-directed treatment are at increased risk for a number of sleep disturbances that likely contribute to fatigue, which is one of the more burdensome symptoms of pediatric oncology patients. These sleep disturbances are multifactorial and include difficulty initiating and maintaining sleep and restless sleep, likely caused by a combination of direct physiological effects of cancer and medications (particularly corticosteroids), changes in routine, stress and anxiety, and environmental disruptions on the inpatient unit. Resulting fatigue may be related not only to sleep disruptions but also to the physiological effects of cancer-directed therapy such as pain and anemia. After completion of cancer-directed therapy, pediatric survivors of brain tumors are at risk for hypothalamic obesity, which can lead to symptoms of obstructive sleep apnea above and beyond otherwise healthy children, and to excessive daytime sleepiness. Interventions are needed to target symptoms during both the treatment and the survivorship periods and should include a combination of both behavioral and pharmacologic interventions targeted to the specific symptoms of the child. Although much research is necessary, targeted interventions should demonstrate a positive impact on patients' quality of life.

Clinical Pearls

- Fatigue is one of the most commonly reported symptoms in children and adolescents undergoing treatment for cancer.
- Restless sleep, excessive daytime sleepiness (EDS), obstructive sleep apnea symptoms, and difficulty initiating and maintaining sleep are common sleep disturbances observed in pediatric oncology patients and survivors.
- Disease process, treatment modality, frequent nocturnal awakenings in hospitalized patients, nighttime caretaking needs, and poor sleep quality may individually or in combination affect sleep quality in pediatric patients undergoing cancer-directed therapy.
- Poor sleep in pediatric oncology patients is associated with reduced adaptive functioning, limited engagement in social activities, behavioral and mood problems, and/or negative impact on treatment adherence.
- Both behavioral sleep medicine and pharmacological interventions should be considered in this patient population.

References

1. National Cancer Institute. Surveillance Epidemiology and End Results. 2013; www.seer.cancer.gov. Accessed February 26, 2013.
2. Ancoli-Israel S, Rissling M, Neikrug A, et al. Light treatment prevents fatigue in women undergoing chemotherapy for breast cancer. Support Care Cancer 2012;20(6):1211–19.
3. Hinds P, Hockenberry M, Rai S, et al. Nocturnal awakenings, sleep environment. Interruptions, and fatigue in hospitalized children with cancer. Oncol Nurs Forum 2007;34(2):393–402.
4. Kim B, Chun M, Han E, et al. Fatigue assessment and rehabilitation outcomes in patients with brain tumors. Support Care Cancer 2012;20(4):805–12.
5. Crabtree VM. Sleep in children with cancer and other chronic diseases. In: Kushida CA, editor. The encyclopedia of sleep, vol. 2. Waltham, MA: Academic Press; 2013. p. 632–3.
6. Erickson J, Beck S, Christian B, et al. Patterns of fatigue in adolescents receiving chemotherapy. Oncol Nurs Forum 2010;37(4):444–55.
7. Hockenberry M, Hooke M, Gregurich M, et al. Symptom clusters in children and adolescents receiving cisplatin, doxorubicin, or ifosfamide. Oncol Nurs Forum 2010;37(1):E16–27.
8. van Litsenburg R, Huisman J, Hoogerbrugge P, et al. Impaired sleep affects quality of life in children during maintenance treatment for acute lymphoblastic leukemia: an exploratory study. Health Quality Life Outcomes 2011;9(1):25.
9. Corser NC. Sleep of 1- and 2-year-old children in intensive care. Issues Comprehens Pediatr Nursing 1996;19(1):17–31.
10. Rosen GM, Shor AC, Geller TJ. Sleep in children with cancer. Curr Opin Pediatr 2008;20(6):676–81.
11. Zupanec S, Jones H, Stremler R. Sleep habits and fatigue of children receiving maintenance chemotherapy for ALL and their parents. J Pediatr Oncol Nurs 2010;27(4):217–28.
12. Hinds PS, Hockenberry MJ, Gattuso JS, et al. Dexamethasone alters sleep and fatigue in pediatric patients with acute lymphoblastic leukemia. Cancer 2007;110(10):2321–30.
13. Rosen G, Brand SR. Sleep in children with cancer: case review of 70 children evaluated in a comprehensive pediatric sleep center. Support Care Cancer 2011;19(7):985–94.
14. Meeske K, Katz ER, Palmer SN, et al. Parent proxy-reported health-related quality of life and fatigue in pediatric patients diagnosed with brain tumors and acute lymphoblastic leukemia. Cancer 2004;101(9):2116–25.
15. Crabtree VM, Brimeyer C, Zhu L, et al. Sleep complaints in child survivors of CNS tumors. Sleep Abstract Supplement 2013 in press;36.
16. Ream E, Gibson F, Edwards J, et al. Experience of fatigue in adolescents living with cancer. Cancer Nursing 2006;29(4):317–26.
17. Clanton NR, Klosky JL, Li C, et al. Fatigue, vitality, sleep, and neurocognitive functioning in adult survivors of childhood Cancer: A report from the childhood cancer survivor study. Cancer 2011;117(1):2559–68.

18. O'Gorman CS, Simoneau-Roy J, Pencharz P, et al. Sleep-disordered breathing is increased in obese adolescents with craniopharyngioma compared with obese controls. J Clin Endocrinol Metab 2010;95(5): 2211–18.
19. Rosen GM, Bendel AE, Neglia JP, et al. Sleep in children with neoplasms of the central nervous system: case review of 14 children. Pediatrics 2003;112(1 Pt 1):e46–54.
20. Poder U, Ljungman G, von Essen L. Parents' perceptions of their children's cancer-related symptoms during treatment: a prospective, longitudinal study. J Pain Symptom Manage 2010;40(5):661–70.
21. Kaleyias J, Manley P, Kothare SV. Sleep disorders in children with cancer. Sem Pediatr Neurol 2012;19(1):25–34.
22. Zupanec S, Jones H, Stremler R. Sleep habits and fatigue in children receiving maintenance chemotherapy for ALL and their parents. J Pediatr Oncol Nursing J 2010;27(4):217–28.
23. Hinds PS, Hockenberry-Eaton M, Gilger E, et al. Comparing patient, parent, and staff descriptions of fatigue in pediatric oncology patients. Cancer Nursing 1999;22(4):277–88; quiz 288–9.
24. Marcus CL, Trescher WH, Halbower AC, et al. Secondary narcolepsy in children with brain tumors. Sleep 2002;25(4):435–9.
25. Lipton J, Megerian JT, Kothare SV, et al. Melatonin deficiency and disrupted circadian rhythms in pediatric survivors of craniopharyngioma. Neurology 2009;73(4):323–5.
26. Sanford SD, Okuma JO, Pan J, et al. Gender differences in sleep, fatigue, and daytime activity in a pediatric oncology sample receiving dexamethasone. J Pediatr Psychol 2008;33(3):298–306.
27. Perdikaris P, Merkouris A, Patiraki E, et al. Changes in children's fatigue during the course of treatment for paediatric cancer. Int Nurs Rev 2008;55(4):412–19.
28. Hooke MC, Garwick AW, Gross CR. Fatigue and physical performance in children and adolescents receiving chemotherapy. Oncol Nurs Forum 2011;38(6):649–57.
29. Greenfeld M, Constantini S, Tauman R, et al. Sleep disturbances in children recovered from central nervous system neoplasms. J Pediatr 2011;159(2):268–72 e261.
30. Mandrell BN, Wise M, Schoumacher RA, et al. Excessive daytime sleepiness and sleep-disordered breathing disturbances in survivors of childhood central nervous system tumors. Pediatr Blood Cancer 2012;58(5):746–51.
31. Beebe DW. Neural and neurobehavioral dysfunction in children with obstructive sleep apnea. PLoS med 2006;3(8):e323.
32. Donaldson DL, Owens J. Sleep and sleep problems. In: Bear GG, Minke KM, editors. Children's needs III: development, prevention, and intervention. Washington, D.C.: National Association of School Psychologists; 2006. p. 1025–39.
33. Beebe DW, Lewin D, Zeller M, et al. Sleep in overweight adolescents: shorter sleep, poorer sleep quality, sleepiness, and sleep-disordered breathing. J Pediatr Psychol 2007;32(1):69–79.
34. Chaput JP, Brunet M, Tremblay A. Relationship between short sleeping hours and childhood overweight/obesity: results from the 'Quebec en Forme' Project. Int J Obes (Lond) 2006;30(7):1080–5.
35. Gozal D. Sleep-disordered breathing and school performance in children. Pediatrics 1998;102(3 Pt 1):616–20.
36. Gozal D, Pope DW Jr. Snoring during early childhood and academic performance at ages thirteen to fourteen years. Pediatrics 2001;107(6): 1394–9.
37. Moore BD 3rd. Neurocognitive outcomes in survivors of childhood cancer. J Pediatr Psychol 2005;30(1):51–63.
38. Daly BP, Brown RT. Scholarly literature review: management of neurocognitive late effects with stimulant medication. J Pediatr Psychol 2007;32(9):1111–26.
39. Spencer J. The role of cognitive remediation in childhood cancer survivors experiencing neurocognitive late effects. J Pediatr Oncol Nurs 2006;23(6):321–5.
40. Dahl RE, Lewin DS. Pathways to adolescent health sleep regulation and behavior. J Adolesc Health 2002;31(Suppl. 6):175–84.
41. Chorney DB, Detweiler MF, Morris TL, et al. The interplay of sleep disturbance, anxiety, and depression in children. J Pediatr Psychol 2008;33(4):339–48.
42. Berger AM, Parker KP, Young-McCaughan S, et al. Sleep wake disturbances in people with cancer and their caregivers: state of the science. Oncol Nurs Forum 2005;32(6):E98–126.
43. Dodd MJ, Miaskowski C, Lee KA. Occurrence of symptom clusters. J Nat Cancer Instit Monographs 2004;(32):76–8.
44. Hockenberry M, Hooke MC. Symptom clusters in children with cancer. Semin Onc Nurs 2007;23(2):152–7.
45. Roscoe JA, Kaufman ME, Matteson-Rusby SE, et al. Cancer-related fatigue and sleep disorders. Oncologist 2007;12 (Suppl. 1):35–42.
46. Barsevick AM. The elusive concept of the symptom cluster. Oncol Nurs Forum 2007;34(5):971–80.
47. Sadeh A, Raviv A, Gruber R. Sleep patterns and sleep disruptions in school-age children. Develop Psychol 2000;36(3):291–301.
48. Kashani J, Hakami N. Depression in children and adolescents with malignancy. Can J Psychiatry Revue canadienne de psychiatrie 1982; 27(6):474–7.
49. Allen L, Zigler E. Psychological adjustment of seriously ill children. J Am Acad Child Psychiatry 1986;25(5):708–12.
50. Patenaude AF, Kupst MJ. Psychosocial functioning in pediatric cancer. J Pediatr Psychol 2005;30(1):9–27.
51. Zeltzer LK, Recklitis C, Buchbinder D, et al. Psychological status in childhood cancer survivors: a report from the Childhood Cancer Survivor Study. J Clin Oncol 2009;27(14):2396–404.
52. Brown R, DuPaul G. Promoting school success in children with chronic medical conditions. School Psychol Rev 1999;28(2):175–81.
53. Jemal A, Siegel R, Xu J, et al. Cancer statistics, 2010. CA: a cancer journal for clinicians 2010;60(5):277–300.
54. Landolt MA, Vollrath M, Niggli FK, et al. Health-related quality of life in children with newly diagnosed cancer: a one year follow-up study. Health Qual Llife Outcomes 2006;4:63.
55. Bhat SR, Goodwin TL, Burwinkle TM, et al. Profile of daily life in children with brain tumors: an assessment of health-related quality of life. J Clin Oncol 2005;23(24):5493–500.
56. Erickson JM, Beck SL, Christian BR, et al. Fatigue, sleep-wake disturbances, and quality of life in adolescents receiving chemotherapy. J Pediatr Hematol/Oncol 2011;33(1):e17–25.
57. Varni JW, Limbers CA, Burwinkle TM. Impaired health-related quality of life in children and adolescents with chronic conditions: a comparative analysis of 10 disease clusters and 33 disease categories/severities utilizing the PedsQL 4.0 Generic Core Scales. Health Qual Life Outcomes 2007;5:43.
58. Zebrack BJ, Chesler MA. Quality of life in childhood cancer survivors. Psycho-oncology 2002;11(2):132–41.
59. Ward TM, Rankin S, Lee KA. Caring for children with sleep problems. J Pediatr Nurs 2007;22(4):283–96.
60. Stepanski EJ, Wyatt JK. Use of sleep hygiene in the treatment of insomnia. Sleep Med Rev 2003;7(3):215–25.
61. Mindell JA, Kuhn B, Lewin DS, et al. Behavioral treatment of bedtime problems and night wakings in infants and young children. Sleep 2006;29(10):1263–76.
62. Wiggs L, France K. Behavioural treatments for sleep problems in children and adolescents with physical illness, psychological problems or intellectual disabilities. Sleep Med Rev 2000;4(3):299–314.
63. Lawton C, France K, Blampied NM. Treatment of infant sleep disturbance by graduated extinction. Child Family Behavior Ther 1991; 13(1):39–56.
64. Meltzer LJ, Moore M. Sleep disruptions in parents of children and adolescents with chronic illnesses: prevalence, causes, and consequences. J Pediatr Psychol 2008;33(3):279–91.
65. Mandrell B, Pritchard M, Coan A, et al. A pilot study to examine sleep in pediatric brain tumor patients hospitalized for high dose chemotherapy. Sleep Abstract Supplement 2013 in press;36.
66. Owens JA, Babcock D, Blumer J, et al. The use of pharmacotherapy in the treatment of pediatric insomnia in primary care: rational approaches. A consensus meeting summary. J Clin Sleep Med 2005;1(1):49–59.

Sleep in Psychiatric Disorders

Anna Ivanenko, Jonathan Kushnir, and Candice A. Alfano

INTRODUCTION

Behavioral and emotional development in children and adolescents is closely linked to the maturation of sleep–wake regulatory systems. Early disruptions in the organization of sleep states may contribute to dysregulation of affect and behavior and subsequently lead to the development of psychopathology. Alternatively, psychiatric disorders can contribute to the development of sleep disturbances that are long-lasting and require specific interventions to prevent further deterioration of the neurobehavioral functions.

Sleep problems are commonly reported among children and adolescents with psychiatric disorders. Growing numbers of epidemiological studies in patients attending child psychiatric clinics have described a high prevalence of sleep-related disorders that include: bedtime refusal, fear of the dark, nightmares, night terrors, and restless sleep.[1] Long sleep latencies, short sleep durations, frequent nocturnal awakenings, and restless sleep have all been shown to correlate with the severity of psychiatric symptoms in a diverse cohort of children with psychiatric disorders.[2]

Numerous surveys have indicated a strong association between sleep complaints and symptoms of emotional distress, depression, and anxiety in children.[3–6] In a large community-based prospective study of 6-year-old children, 13% of those with trouble sleeping were found to have clinically elevated anxiety and depressive scores compared to just 3% of children without problems sleeping; at age 11, the percentage of children with anxiety or depressive symptoms increased to 29% and 4%, respectively.[7]

Adolescents with sleep problems have significantly elevated rates of depression, anxiety, low self-esteem, excessive worry, and irritability, as well as an increased likelihood of using alcohol, nicotine, and caffeine.[8–12] A recent cross-sectional and prospective study of 12–18-year-olds found that 54% of adolescents with insomnia reported depressive symptoms, 26% had suicidal ideation, and 10% indicated a history of suicide attempts, with all frequencies higher than those found in a non-insomnia group (which were 32%, 12%, and 3%, respectively).[13]

SLEEP IN EARLY-ONSET MAJOR DEPRESSION

Major depressive disorder (MDD) is a severe and debilitating clinical condition that is often recurrent and associated with poor psychosocial, academic, and occupational outcomes. Approximately 2% of children and 8% of adolescents are affected by MDD with a male-to-female ratio of 1:1 in children and 1:2 in adolescents.[14] Suicide is the most dramatic outcome of MDD and the third leading cause of death for people aged 15 to 24.[15]

Subjective sleep complaints are characteristic of MDD in adults and include: sleep initiation and sleep maintenance insomnia, early morning awakenings, non-refreshed sleep, disturbed dreams, and decreased total sleep time. A subset of adult patients with MDD present with hypersomnia and daytime fatigue. Objective polysomnographic (PSG) studies of adults with MDD yielded consistent findings with prolonged sleep onset latency, short rapid eye movement (REM) sleep onset latency, reduced slow-wave sleep, and increased sleep fragmentation.[16] Furthermore, research data suggest that insomnia predicts relapse of depression in previously remitted patients,[17] and that objectively measured prolonged sleep onset latency and short sleep duration, with or without complaints of insomnia, are risk factors for poor depression treatment outcome.[18]

Subjective Sleep Complaints in Early-Onset Major Depression

Early studies of sleep complaints in clinically depressed preadolescent children revealed that two-thirds of children with depression reported sleep onset and sleep maintenance problems and half suffered from terminal insomnia. Furthermore, their sleep complaints continued throughout the depressive episode with 10% of children experiencing insomnia after remission.[19,20] In a large community sample of 1507 adolescents, 88.6% of those who met diagnostic criteria for major depression reported sleep disturbances.[21] Interestingly, the 75.7% of adolescents who went on to develop a major depressive episode over a 12-month period had insomnia as an initial complaint. A more recent study assessed sleep-related symptoms among children and adolescents ages 7.3 to 14.9 years diagnosed with major depression using a structured diagnostic interview.[22] Sleep complaints were present in 72.7% of the patients. Children and adolescents with sleep disturbances had more severe depression with higher rates of anxiety symptoms. In that same clinical sample, 53.5% of those with sleep complaints reported insomnia, 9% experienced hypersomnia alone, and 10.1% had both insomnia and hypersomnia (with that combination of symptoms seemingly associated with the most severe forms of depression).[22]

Sleep Complaints and Adolescent Suicide

Sleep disturbances, especially insomnia and nightmares, have been associated with increased rates of reported suicidal ideation and suicide attempts in youngsters.[23–25] In the only known study that examined sleep disturbances in 15 to 19-year-old suicide completers, insomnia was 10 times more likely to have been reported in that group than it was in community controls. Furthermore, adolescents who completed suicide were five times more likely than controls to have exhibited insomnia in the week preceding death.[26]

An association between suicidality and sleep duration was examined using the Youth Risk Behavior Surveys from 2007 and 2009, which consist of school-based, nationally representative samples ($n=12154$ for 2007, $n=14782$ for 2009). Adolescents who reported sleeping ≤5 or ≥10 hours had a significantly higher risk for suicidality compared to those with a total sleep time (TST) of 8 hours. The largest odds ratios were found among the most severe forms of suicide attempt behaviors (such as those requiring treatment) with an odds ratio of 5.9 for a TST ≤4 hours and 4.7 for a TST ≥10 hours.[27]

In a 2011 prospective study of high-risk adolescents, Wong et al. compared 392 children (280 boys and 112 girls, 12–14 years old) from high-risk alcoholic families to controls.[28] They found that having sleep problems at 12 to 14 years significantly predicted suicidal thoughts and self-harm behaviors at 15 to 17 years, even when controlling for other variables such as gender, parental alcoholism or prior suicidal thoughts. Interestingly enough, variables such as depression and substance-related problems at age 12 to 14 were not significant predictors. This study emphasized the importance of sleep assessment when screening for risk factors for suicidal behaviors in adolescents.

Objective Sleep Measures in Early-Onset Major Depression: PSG/EEG Studies

PSG characteristics of sleep have been examined in prepubertal children with major depression and have yielded inconsistent results. The early work by Puig-Antich and colleagues (1982) failed to reveal significant differences in any sleep variables between children with major depression and normal controls.[19] Their findings were later supported by other studies that demonstrated no differences in PSG characteristics between children with MDD and healthy controls.[29,30] However, when depressed children were recruited from inpatient facilities, reduced REM onset latencies, increased REM time, and increased sleep onset latencies were found in a subset of prepubertal children with MDD[30,31] Based on such PSG characteristics, it was suggested that inpatient status, severity of MDD, and presence of other psychiatric comorbidities may influence sleep characteristics in pre-adolescent depressives. Over the years of PSG research, a prolonged latency to sleep onset has emerged as one of the more stable characteristics of sleep dysregulation associated with early-onset MDD.[32]

PSG characteristics have been examined much more extensively in adolescents with MDD. The first such study, which compared 13 depressed adolescents with 13 age-matched normal controls, revealed shorter REM onset latencies and greater REM densities in the depressed patients.[33] At least one subsequent study found PSG abnormalities in early-onset MDD to be similar to those found in depressed adults.[34] However, a few other studies failed to differentiate adolescents with MDD from normal controls based on REM sleep characteristics.[35–37]

In a more recent mixed-age group sample of children aged 7 to 17 years with either MDD or an anxiety disorder, subjective and objective sleep characteristics were similar in the MDD group and normal controls.[38] When electroencephalographic (EEG) sleep measures during an episode were compared to those during recovery, 15–17-year-old adolescents with MDD demonstrated lower sleep efficiencies and REM latencies than controls, a reduction that remained unchanged even in remission, suggesting that EEG sleep changes are state-independent and represent a biological trait of MDD.[39]

The discrepancies between studies may be explained by the subtypes of depression, severity of clinical state, gender, age

range of participants, and presence of anxiety, attention deficit hyperactivity disorder (ADHD), or other psychiatric symptoms.[40,41]

Based on the available research data, there seems to be a stronger association between subjective sleep complaints and depression than there is to objective instrumental measures of sleep and MDD. When both subjective and EEG sleep characteristics were examined in youngsters with MDD, there was no evidence of EEG sleep disruptions in children with depression compared to healthy controls, even in the presence of significant sleep-related complaints. What is even more interesting is that children with the highest rating of insomnias showed the highest sleep efficiencies according to PSG reports.[42] Perception of sleep thus seems to be different in depressed individuals than in normal controls.

In summary, increased sleep onset latency emerged as the most consistent finding across all studies of sleep and early depression, with some subgroups of children and adolescents with MDD also having reduced REM latency.

Objective Sleep Measures in Early-Onset Major Depression: Actigraphic Studies

Actigraphy has been used to assess sleep characteristics, such as sleep onset latency, sleep efficiency, the frequency and duration of nocturnal awakenings, nocturnal and diurnal activity levels, and circadian rhythmicity in patients with MDD.

Abnormal circadian rhythms were described in children and adolescents with depression compared to controls; these were characterized by blunted activity level with diurnal variations that did not peak until early evening.[43,44] Armitage et al. found that among children (as opposed to adolescents) with MDD, there were sex differences noted, with damped circadian amplitudes seen only in girls.[44]

When children with depression were compared, by actigraphic study, both with normal children and ones with a history of abuse, the children who had been abused showed both the highest levels of nocturnal activity and the longest sleep onset latencies.[45] The authors concluded that abuse has a more profound effect on sleep regulation than does depression alone.

SLEEP IN EARLY-ONSET BIPOLAR DISORDER

Bipolar disorder is a chronic severe psychiatric illness with a prevalence rate in the pediatric population of 1.8%.[46] There are four types of bipolar disorder currently defined in the DSM-IV: bipolar-I disorder, bipolar-II disorder, bipolar disorder-not otherwise specified (NOS), and cyclothymia. Research studies in adults with bipolar disorder showed sleep problems to be associated with every phase of bipolar illness and usually include insomnia with reduced need for sleep during the manic phase, and insomnia with hypersomnia during depressed phase.[47–50]

Circadian and social rhythm dysfunction has been proposed as one of the pathophysiological mechanisms of bipolar disorder in adults.[51] Although research on circadian rhythms in pediatric bipolar disorder is limited, some evidence exists that interpersonal and social rhythm therapy is beneficial to adolescents with bipolar illness.[52,53] Interpersonal and social rhythm therapy is based on the belief that sleep deprivation, and disruptions of our circadian rhythms, may provoke or exacerbate symptoms commonly associated with bipolar disorder. This form of therapy uses methods from both interpersonal psychotherapy and cognitive-behavioral therapy to teach patients the importance of, and help them maintain in a regular fashion their daily circadian rhythms and activity routines such as of eating and sleeping.

Sleep Complaints in Early-Onset Bipolar Disorder

Examinations of sleep complaints among different samples of children and adolescents with bipolar disorder-I, bipolar disorder-II, and cyclothymia revealed a weighted average of 72% of patients reporting a decreased need for sleep with symptoms of mania.[54] Geller et al. compared the clinical characteristics of 7–16-year-old children and adolescents with bipolar disorder, ADHD, and healthy controls and found a reduced need for sleep in 40% of children with mania compared to only 6.2% of those with ADHD and 1.1% of normal controls.[55] Thus, decreased need for sleep is one of the core symptoms of pediatric mania along with hypersexuality, elated mood, racing thoughts, and grandiosity.

When both parent and child reports of sleep problems were analyzed in patients with early-onset bipolar disorder, Lofthouse et al. found that 96.2% of children suffered from sleep disturbances related to manic, depressive, or comorbid symptoms during different phases of their illness.[56] In their more recent web-based survey completed by parents of children with bipolar disorder, the following sleep problems were frequently reported: insomnia, daytime sleepiness, parasomnias, night wakings, bedtime resistance, anxiety, and sleep-disordered breathing.[57] Nearly all children whose parents completed the web-based survey (96.9%) were affected by sleep disturbances that required either pharmacological or non-pharmacological sleep interventions.[57,58]

Diurnal variations of mood have been described in youth with bipolar disorder, with findings of evening acceleration of mood and energy and of delayed sleep onset with difficulty waking up in the morning. Nearly 30% of children exhibited elevated mood during the day switching into depression overnight.[59]

In their 2012 study, Baroni et al. evaluated sleep complaints in youth with bipolar-I and bipolar-NOS using a structured diagnostic interview (K-SADS-PL) during both manic and depressive episodes.[60] At least one sleep symptom was reported by 84.3% of subjects: 71.4% of patients had insomnia during depressive episodes, 51.4% experienced decreased need for sleep during hypomania/mania, 22% of subjects reported circadian reversal, and 27% reported nocturnal enuresis. Decreased need for sleep correlated significantly with measures of global functioning, which suggests that manic symptoms, perhaps, have a more profound impact on global functioning in youth. There were no significant differences found in sleep characteristics between bipolar-I and bipolar-NOS, according to this study.

Objective Sleep Measures in Early-Onset Bipolar Disorder

There are only a few studies that have used PSG or actigraphic assessment of sleep in bipolar youth. In the first such study, published by Rao et al. in 2002, EEG characteristics of sleep were compared among three groups: adolescents with unipolar depression, those with bipolar disorder, and normal healthy controls.[51] There were no differences in REM sleep

found among the groups; however, those with bipolar disorder demonstrated increased amounts of stage 1 sleep and reduced percentages of stage 4 sleep.

In a study by Mehl et al., PSGs of children, whose results on the Child Behavior Checklist (CBCL) were suggestive of bipolar disorder, were compared with normal controls.[62] Sleep measures of children with *bipolar profile* revealed reduced sleep efficiencies, reduced amounts of REM sleep, and increased numbers of nocturnal awakenings. On sleep questionnaires, parents of children with bipolar profile reported that their children had more problems with sleep onset, more restlessness, and more frequent nightmares and morning headaches than did controls. This study, however, was limited by the lack of validated clinical assessment of bipolar disorder in children participating in the study.

In a 2011 study, sleep was assessed in a small sample of adolescents with bipolar disorder, who were between mood episodes, and compared both to children with ADHD and to normal controls.[63] Patients with bipolar disorder experienced their sleep as more fragmented and less restorative than their peers. However, actigraphy indicated the reverse, namely longer periods of sleep and fewer interruptions compared to their peers. Further research is needed to understand the discrepancy between self-perception of sleep and actigraphic sleep measures in this population.

SLEEP IN CHILDHOOD ANXIETY DISORDERS

The presence and frequency of sleep disruption in children with anxiety disorders is among the highest seen in any form of child psychopathology. For example, in addition to rates of sleep problems above 90% in samples of anxious youth,[64–66] group-based comparisons found that anxious youth experienced more frequent and more varied types of sleep problems than did their counterparts with ADHD.[67] Conversely, children presenting with insomnia complaints were also most likely to have co-occurring anxiety disorders.[2,68] Problems with sleep initiation, nighttime awakenings, nightmares, and bedtime resistance are among the problems most commonly reported.[65,66]

Retrospective reports of sleep are nonetheless subject to a range of potential limitations including reporter and recall biases. Far fewer studies have investigated the sleep of anxious youth prospectively. In one of the few studies to examine at-home sleep patterns, anxiety-disordered and healthy control children completed prospective 1-week sleep diaries. Later bedtimes, less sleep on weekdays, and more variable weekend sleep patterns were found among those with anxiety.[69]

Reports of sleep also have been found to vary based on informant. In particular, and in contrast to community samples where parents tend to underestimate child sleep problems,[70,71] anxious youth reported fewer sleep problems than did their parents.[66,72] Differential findings may be explained by greater parental awareness of, or sensitivity to, sleep problems in clinically anxious youth due to these problems commonly being covert or of an embarrassing nature (e.g., nighttime fears, requests to co-sleep, night terrors). It is also possible that anxious youth possess distorted perceptions about their sleep. Children with anxiety disorders have been found to underreport sleep disruption compared to objective sleep measures.[73]

In one of the few studies to examine PSG sleep patterns in these children, Forbes et al. used two nights of laboratory-based PSG to compare the EEG sleep patterns of three groups of children, all aged 7–17 years: those with anxiety disorders (including generalized anxiety disorder, panic disorder, separation anxiety disorder, or social phobia), those with depression, and those comprising a group of healthy controls.[73] On both nights the anxiety group had more awakenings than the depressed group and less slow-wave (deep) sleep than depressed and control children. On the second PSG night anxious youth exhibited a prolonged sleep onset latency, whereas the latency to REM sleep decreased in both other groups. A greater percentage of missing data from night two was also reported in the anxious group. Thus, in addition to alterations in sleep architecture, results suggest that anxious children experience greater difficulty adapting to the sleep lab environment. Such data underscore a need for research examining objective sleep patterns in the home environment.

There is also evidence to suggest that rates and types of sleep problems differ among the various forms of anxiety. The following sections provide a review of available findings across specific anxiety diagnoses most closely associated with sleep disruption.

Generalized Anxiety Disorder

Diagnostic criteria and empirical data indicate that sleep plays an important role in pediatric generalized anxiety disorder (GAD). First, in addition to excessive and uncontrollable worry, DSM-IV criteria specifically include 'difficulty falling or staying asleep' as one of six possible physiological symptoms.[74] Similar to rates in adults with GAD,[75] a majority of youth experience difficulty sleeping, with rates as high as 94%.[64–66] Other common sleep-related problems include nightmares and daytime sleepiness. Although a majority of research is based on parent report, one study found 87% of youth with a primary GAD diagnosis self-report difficulty sleeping and difficulty awakening in the morning, a greater proportion than seen in children with other primary anxiety disorders.[66]

In a study of EEG-based sleep patterns, Alfano and colleagues examined the sleep of prepubescent children (7 to 11 years) with GAD in comparison to a matched healthy control group based on one night of PSG.[76] Anxious children studied were not depressed or taking any psychotropic medications at the time of the study. Children with GAD exhibited significantly longer sleep onset latency and reduced latency to REM sleep than controls. A marginally significant increase in REM sleep, and a decrease in sleep efficiency, also was found in the GAD group. Thus, although anxious children did not meet criteria for comorbid depressive diagnoses, objective sleep findings correspond in part with the trait-like sleep alterations found in clinically depressed and at-risk samples of adults.[77–79] A shared genetic basis for GAD and depression, with overlapping of clinical features (i.e., negative affectivity) and/or of other neurobiological markers of risk, may serve to explain a similar overlap in sleep parameters.[80]

Separation Anxiety Disorder

Separation anxiety disorder (SAD) is characterized by developmentally inappropriate and excessive anxiety surrounding separation from major attachment figures.[74] Two possible diagnostic symptoms of SAD are specific to sleep: persistent reluctance or refusal to sleep alone, and repeated nightmares involving themes of separation. Refusing to sleep alone is among the most common reasons for referral to an anxiety specialty clinic.[81] Although empirical studies examining sleep problems in children with SAD specifically are limited, one study, based on parent and clinician reports, found that 97% of children with SAD had at least one sleep problem, which was more than that seen in children with social anxiety disorder (but not more than seen in children with GAD).[65] Based on child reports, 60% of children with SAD reported difficulty sleeping.[66] The most frequently listed sleep problems were insomnia, reluctance or refusal to sleep alone, and nightmares.[65] Parents of children with primary SAD also reported that their children exhibited more parasomnias (including sleepwalking, bedwetting, and night terrors) than did parents of youth with social anxiety disorder.[66] This last finding agrees with results, reported by Verduin and Kendall, that parasomnias commonly occur in the presence of SAD diagnosis.[82]

Obsessive–Compulsive Disorder

Although sleep-related difficulties are not DSM-IV diagnostic criteria for pediatric obsessive–compulsive disorder (OCD), youth with OCD commonly do experience sleep-related problems. One study found 92% of pediatric OCD patients experienced at least one type of sleep problem.[72] Less sleep also was associated with greater OCD severity. Two other studies have reported lower (56% and 54%), albeit still clinically meaningful, rates of sleep problems in this population of youth.[66,83] Sleep may be especially problematic for young children and females with OCD.[72]

In the only published OCD study to utilize PSG, Rapaport and colleagues compared the sleep of nine adolescents with OCD to a matched healthy control group.[84] Adolescents with OCD exhibited less total sleep, longer sleep onset latency, and shortened latency to REM sleep than did controls. However, because a majority of subjects had a current or previous depressive disorder, the extent to which these sleep patterns were reflective of other forms of psychopathology is unclear.

In a small, non-depressed sample of 7 to 11-year-old children, Alfano and Kim used subjective reports as well as seven nights of actigraphy to examine the sleep patterns of children with OCD and compare them to those from a matched healthy control group.[85] In line with parental reports indicating clinically significant sleep problems, actigraphy data revealed significantly fragmented sleep in children with OCD as well as less total sleep and longer nighttime awakenings. A significant negative association between total sleep time and severity of compulsive behaviors was also found, potentially reflecting the negative impact of insufficient sleep on ability to monitor and inhibit behavior.[85]

Post-Traumatic Stress Disorder and Trauma

Post-traumatic stress disorder (PTSD) is characterized by distressing symptoms including re-experiencing of a traumatic event, avoidance of situations, places, or people that are reminders of the trauma, and hyperarousal.[74] Sleep disturbances, including trauma-related nightmares and difficulty initiating or maintaining sleep, are core features of PTSD. In lieu of a wealth of investigations focused on the relationship between trauma exposure and sleep disruption in adults, research in pediatric samples is limited. Nightmares, bedwetting, and night terrors nonetheless appear to be common in the aftermath of trauma.[86] In a study of children and adolescents exposed to Hurricane Hugo, bad dreams showed strong diagnostic correlation to a subsequent PTSD diagnosis.[87] In a longitudinal study of children exposed to Hurricane Katrina, the presence of sleep problems 2 years after the hurricane predicted the maintenance of existing PTSD symptoms, as well as the emergence of new ones, 6 months later.[88]

In an actigraphy-based study of a sample of trauma-exposed children, Glod and colleagues reported that abused children demonstrated significantly longer sleep onset latency than did both a sample of depressed youth and a group of controls.[45] A lower sleep efficiency was also seen in the abused group compared to controls, and also in those with a history of physical as opposed to sexual abuse. Differences in sleep patterns as a function of a PTSD diagnosis were not found.

Other research, too, suggests that the negative impact of early trauma on sleep may persist into the adult years. For example, Bader and colleagues found childhood trauma to be the strongest predictor of values of sleep onset latency, sleep efficiency, and nocturnal activity in adulthood, even after controlling for levels of stress and depression.[89] Similarly, females who experienced sexual abuse as children were more likely to experience sleep problems as adults irrespective of depressive symptoms.[90] Overall, available research suggests that trauma exposure, more so than a PTSD diagnosis *per se*, is closely associated with persistent sleep disruption.

SHARED FACTORS AND MECHANISMS OF INTEREST

At a basic level an increased state of arousal, which is a central feature of all anxiety disorders, is incompatible with quiescence and sleep.[91] Similarly, insufficient sleep produces increases in arousal systems, mood disturbance, anxiety, and tension.[92–95] At a more complex level, the pervasive overlap between symptoms of sleep and anxiety disorders appears rooted in a variety of potentially mediating and synergistic factors including genetics, cognitive style, and environmental influences. For example, genetic factors alone have been found to account for 74% of the covariance in the association between early sleep and anxiety symptoms.[96] Certain circadian clock-related genes, specifically *BCL2*, *DRD2*, and *PAWR*, are also associated with anxiety disorders.[97] The latter set of genes belongs to the signaling pathway connecting circadian rhythmicity and anxiety-related behavior, thus suggesting a possible shared genetic predisposition for problems in both domains. However, a specific link with anxiety, as opposed to a broader range of psychiatric symptoms and disorders, has not been established. For example, results from a large study of 8-year-old twin pairs reported that the genes influencing sleep problems are more closely associated with depression than anxiety.[98] Also, the serotonin transporter gene (*5-HTTLPR*) has been implicated in sleep disturbance[99] and depression[100] as well as in anxiety.[101,102]

Problems sleeping are also consistently associated with a range of cognitive factors and styles shared by anxious individuals. *Catastrophizing*, which is a negative, iterative thought process similar to rumination or worry, is hypothesized to play a critical role in the development and maintenance of insomnia.[103] In support of this theory, Barclay and Gregory found that poor sleepers are more likely than good sleepers to catastrophize about the consequences of sleeplessness as well as other topics, though findings were largely mediated by anxiety and worry.[104]

Using an experimental paradigm among both adolescent and adult participants, Talbot and colleagues did not find that sleep restriction resulted in increased worries or longer catastrophizing sequences, but they did find that catastrophizing following sleep restriction produced more anxiety and increased estimation of the likelihood that 'catastrophes' might occur.[94] Furthermore, an early adolescent subgroup (aged 10–13 years) rated their most threatening worry as significantly more threatening when they were sleep deprived than when rested.

Other studies highlight significant associations between a negative attributional style and dysfunctional cognitions in connection with sleep disruption, depression, and anxiety in youth.[105–107] One study found a significant association between cognitive errors (such as catastrophizing, overgeneralization, personalizing, and selective abstraction errors) and sleep problems, specifically during adolescence.[105] Additionally, an association between decreased total sleep duration and greater levels of pre-sleep cognitive arousal has been documented in children with various anxiety disorders.[66]

In addition to evolving interest in genetic and cognitive factors, the sleep environment in which problems develop remains a critically important area of investigation. In the large twin study conducted by Gregory and colleagues, longitudinal associations between sleep problems at age 3–4 years and anxiety at age 7 were largely mediated by shared environmental factors.[108] Research examining specific familial characteristics of, and parenting behaviors within, the early sleep environment interestingly revealed that both under- or over-involvement in behaviors related to sleep impacted sleep in a negative manner. For example (in a manner consistent with findings that the regularity of children's sleep schedules is essential for optimal daytime functioning[109,110]) familial disorganization (e.g., lacking structure and routines in the home) was found to account for a significant portion of the variance in childhood sleep problems and anxiety.[108] Although the precise pathways through which *familial disorganization* impacts children's sleep remain to be delineated, it is known that lack of parental rules with respect to sleep is associated with shorter sleep duration in school-aged children.[111]

On the other hand, parental over-involvement in their children's sleep may be problematic, particularly for at-risk and anxious children. Warren and colleagues found mothers with anxiety disorders were overly involved in infant and toddler bedtime sleep routines (e.g., co-sleeping or putting children to bed when already asleep), and these behaviors were associated with higher rates of child sleep problems.[112] Such parental behaviors might function as moderators of both sleep and anxiety-based outcomes in this population of children. More specifically, at-risk children who do not adequately learn how to negotiate sleep onset independently may similarly struggle with, and feel ineffective in their ability to manage, anxiety-producing daytime situations. Sleep disruption that results from prolonged sleep onset or nighttime awakenings related to a need for parental support could further exacerbate daytime anxiety.[113] Overall, the broad range of intra- and inter-individual factors impacting both sleep and anxiety dictate a need for investigations aimed at understanding how multiple levels of factors interact to create these commonly co-occurring problems.

PSYCHOSOCIAL TREATMENT

Although sleep disturbances commonly co-occur with psychiatric disorders (particularly those of mood and anxiety) in both children and adults,[22,114-116] understanding of optimal methods for, and ideal timing of, treatment targeting sleep problems in this context is limited.[65,116] Lack of understanding is directly linked to the fact that empirically supported treatments for anxiety and mood disorders do not typically address sleep problems directly, and behavioral interventions for childhood sleep problems do not specifically measure changes in anxiety or mood.[117] Thus, current understanding in children has largely evolved from theoretical models, adult-based studies, and case reports. A growing body of evidence nonetheless suggests that addressing sleep in anxious and depressed youth might be critical for positive long-term outcomes.

A meta-analysis of research in adults shows that cognitive behavioral treatments (CBT) for anxiety reduce co-occurring sleep difficulties.[118] CBT for insomnia (CBT-I) also appears to reduce anxiety and depressive symptoms in adults with primary insomnia.[117] In one study, patients receiving combined CBT-I and treatment for depression reported improvements in sleep and depressive symptoms.[119] Although far less is known about treatment in children, research highlighting a bidirectional relationship between sleep and emotional functioning in youth underscores the potential importance of addressing functioning in both domains.[113]

As in anxious and depressed adults, the most common sleep problems in youth relate to difficulty initiating and/or maintaining sleep.[65,113,116] Also, as with adult-based interventions, effective child-focused treatments consider the behavioral, somatic, and cognitive symptoms present, as each may have relevance for sleep disruption. Behavioral aspects of treatment target maladaptive sleep-related behaviors such as bedtime avoidance, inconsistent sleep schedules and routines, interfering sleep-onset associations (e.g., parental presence), and poor sleep hygiene.[120,121] However, since sleep problems may be more disruptive to parents than to children, a lack of motivation for change on the part of the child can be a significant barrier to treatment success. For youth who are initially hesitant or unwilling to address maladaptive sleep behaviors, intangible and tangible rewards may be used with success. In other cases, setting firmer parental limits surrounding sleep may be necessary.[122-124]

Worrisome thoughts, rumination and catastrophizing among anxious and depressed youth, which often prolong sleep onset, can be particularly problematic during the pre-sleep period due to the absence of environmental distracters.[66,125] Reduction of problematic nighttime cognitive activity through provision of corrective information about sleep and the effects of sleep loss, use of positive imagery techniques, and scheduled *worry periods* during afternoon hours can be effective.[126] Pre-sleep cognitive activity also may result in increased somatic arousal at night for which progressive muscle relaxation techniques are commonly used. Importantly, increased levels of arousal and wakefulness at bedtime can also contribute to feelings of frustration at bedtime, thereby undermining development of positive sleep-onset

associations. Temporarily delaying a child's bedtime can serve to increase the homeostatic sleep drive and better align the sleep–wake schedule.

At present, it is not fully understood whether or how sleep is impacted by interventions that do not specifically target sleep problems co-occurring with anxiety or depressive disorders.[65,72] Results from the *Treatment for Adolescents With Depression Study* (TADS)[127] indicate sleep problems were the most common residual symptoms in depressed youth who responded to mood-focused treatment (either CBT, fluoxetine, or their combination) but had not yet progressed to full remission.[128] Emslie and colleagues found that among adolescents successfully treated for depression, those with a longer sleep onset latency were significantly more likely to relapse within 12 months.[129] Thus, similar to experience with adult populations,[130] joint treatment of sleep and mood disorders (i.e., based on the use of strategies targeting both problems) may improve outcomes in younger populations[116] or even prevent initial onset of depression.[131]

Finally, several case reports and controlled studies have reported significant reductions in nighttime fears and associated sleep difficulties following the use of behavioral sleep interventions.[132] The development of these interventions has followed the general direction of effective treatments for fears, phobias, and anxiety in children[133] and are based on standard CBT techniques.[132] Efficacy of treatments for severe nighttime fears has been demonstrated in case studies and in a limited number of controlled studies.[132,134-136] In 2011, Kushnir and Sadeh reported the effectiveness of two brief interventions for nighttime fearful preschool-aged children. Both interventions provided children a puppy doll along with either directions to take care of the doll or, alternatively, reassurance that the doll would protect them.[137] Both interventions significantly reduced children's nighttime fears and sleep problems. Furthermore, they both also significantly reduced parental fear management behaviors, and results were maintained at 6 months post treatment.

PHARMACOLOGICAL TREATMENT

There is very limited evidence-based research for the pharmacological treatment of depression-related sleep problems in children and adolescents. Some antidepressants may cause changes in sleep characteristics when used in pediatric population. For example, imipramine can increase stage 2 sleep and wakefulness and decrease stage 4 sleep, and it also appears to decrease sleep efficiency and cause REM suppression.[138,139] Similarly, fluoxetine was found to increase stage 1 sleep and REM density. However, REM suppression was not evident in this sample of children. Fluoxetine may also cause oculomotor abnormalities, increased myoclonic activity, and subjectively reported lower-quality sleep and more awakenings.[140] Trazodone has been shown to be therapeutic in alleviating insomnia in a small sample of children with depression.[141] However, it should be used with caution as it has the potential for significant side effects due to its interactions with fluoxetine.[142,143]

Concurrent treatment of insomnia and depression or anxiety should be considered in youth, with careful selection of sedative–hypnotic agents based on knowledge of the drugs' pharmacological properties and individual patient characteristics.

Clinical Pearls

- Sleep assessment is an essential part of the comprehensive evaluation of children and adolescents with mood and anxiety disorders.
- Increased sleep onset latency is the most consistent finding in the sleep of children and adolescents with early depression.
- Some subgroups with major depression also have reduced REM latency.
- In adolescents, there is an apparent relationship between the presence of sleep disturbances and an increased risk for suicide.
- Children presenting with insomnia complaints also have an increased likelihood of currently or subsequently meeting criteria for a disorder of anxiety.
- Childhood sleep and anxiety disorders are linked by a range of genetic, behavioral, cognitive, and environmental influences.
- Effective psychosocial interventions target child behaviors and cognitions, physiologic tensions, and parenting and environmental influences that maintain hyperarousal at night.

References

1. Simonds JF, Parraga H. Sleep behaviors and disorders in children and adolescents evaluated at psychiatric clinics. J Dev Behav Pediatr 1984;5:6–10.
2. Ivanenko A, Crabtree VM, O'Brien LM, et al. Sleep complaints and psychiatric symptoms in children evaluated at a pediatric mental heath clinic. J Clin Sleep Med 2006;2(1):42–8.
3. Blader JC, Koplewicz HS, Abikoff H, et al. Sleep problems of elementary school children: A community survey. Arch Pediatr Adolesc Med 1997;151:473–80.
4. Smedje H, Broman JE, Hetta J. Parents' reports of disturbed sleep in 5–7-year-old Swedish children. Acta Pædiatr 1999;88:858–65.
5. Paavonen EJ, Aronen ET, Moilanen I, et al. Sleep problems of school-aged children: a complementary view. Acta Pædiatrics 2000;89:223–8.
6. Stein MA, Mendelson J, Obermeyer WH, et al. Sleep and behavior problems in school-aged children. Pediatrics 2001;107(4):e60.
7. Johnson EO, Chilcoat HD, Breslau N. Trouble sleeping and anxiety/depression in childhood. Psychiatry Res 2000;94:93–102.
8. Price VA, Coates TJ, Thoresen CE, et al. Prevalence and correlates of poor sleep among adolescents. Am J Dis Child 1978;132:583–6.
9. Kirmil-Gray K, Eagleston JR, Gibson E, et al. Sleep disturbance in adolescents: sleep quality, sleep habits, beliefs about sleep, and daytime functioning. J Youth Adol 1984;13:375–84.
10. Morrison DN, McGee R, Stanton WR. Sleep problems in adolescence. J Am Acad Child Adolesc Psychiatry 1992;31:94–9.
11. Manni R, Ratti MT, Marchioni E, et al. Poor sleep in adolescents: a study of 869 17-year-old Italian secondary school students. J Sleep Res 1997;6:44–9.
12. Saarenpää-Heikkilä O, Laippala P, Koivikko M. Subjective daytime sleepiness and its predictors in Finnish adolescents in an interview study. Acta Pædiatr 2001;90:552–7.
13. Roane BM, Taylor DJ. Adolescent insomnia as a risk factor for early adult depression and substance abuse. Sleep 2008;31(10):1351–6.
14. American Academy of Child and Adolescent Psychiatry. Practice parameter for the assessment and treatment of children and adolescents with depressive disorders. J Am Acad Child Adolesc Psychiatry 2007;46:1503–26.
15. Centers for Disease Control. Suicide Factsheet. 2009. www.cdc.gov/violenceprevention/pdf/suicide-datasheet-a.pdf.
16. Benca RM. Mood disorders. In: Kryger MH, Roth T, Dement WC, editors. Principles and practice of sleep medicine. 3rd ed. Philadelphia: WB Saunders; 2000. p. 1140–57.
17. Perlis ML, Smith LJ, Lyness JM, et al. Insomnia as a risk factor for onset of depression in the elderly. Behav Sleep Med 2006;4(2):104–13.
18. Troxel WM, Kupfer DJ, Reynolds CF III, et al. Insomnia and objectively measured sleep disturbances predict treatment outcome in depressed patients treated with psychotherapy or psychotherapy–pharmacotherapy combinations. J Clin Psychiatry 2012;73(4):478–85.
19. Puig-Antich J, Goetz R, Hanlon C, et al. Sleep architecture and REM sleep measures in prepubertal children with major depression. A controlled study. Arch Gen Psychiatry 1982;39:932–9.
20. Puig-Antich J, Goetz R, Hanlon C, et al. Sleep architecture and REM sleep measures in prepubertal major depressives. Studies during recovery from the depressive episode in a drug-free state. Arch Gen Psychiatry 1983;40:187–92.
21. Roberts RE, Lewinsohn PM, Seeley JR. Symptoms of DSM-III-R major depression in adolescence: evidence from an epidemiological survey. J Am Acad Child Adolesc Psychiatry 1995;34 1608–17.
22. Liu X, Buysse DJ, Gentzler AL, et al. Insomnia and hypersomnia associated with depressive phenomenology and comorbidity in childhood depression. Sleep 2007;30:83–90.
23. Bailly D, Bailly-Lambin I, Querleu D et al. Sleep in adolescents and its disorders. A survey in schools. L'encéphale 2004;30(4):352–9.
24. Liu X. Sleep and adolescent suicidal behavior. Sleep 2004;27:1351–8.
25. Barbe RP, Williamson DE, Bridge JA, et al. Clinical differences between suicidal and nonsuicidal depressed children and adolescents. J Clin Psychiatry 2005;66 (4):492–8.
26. Goldstein TR, Bridge JA, Brent DA. Sleep disturbance preceding completed suicide in adolescents. J Consult Clin Psychol 2008;76(1):84–91.
27. Fitzgerald CT, Messias E, Buysse DJ. Teen sleep and suicidality: results from the youth risk behavior surveys of 2007 and 2009. J Clin Sleep Med 2011;7(4):351–6.
28. Wong MM, Brower KJ, Zucker RA. Sleep problems, suicidal ideation, and self-harm behaviors in adolescence. J Psychiatr Res 2011;45:505–11.
29. Young W, Knowles JB, MacLean AW, et al. The sleep of childhood depressives: comparison with age-matched controls. Biol Psychiatry 1982;17:1163–8.
30. Dahl RE, Ryan ND, Birmaher B, et al. Electroencephalographic sleep measures in prepubertal depression. Psych Res 1991;38:201–14.
31. Emslie GJ, Rush AJ, Weinberg WA, et al. Children with major depression show reduced rapid eye movement latencies. Arch Gen Psychiatry 1990;47:119–24.
32. Dahl RE, Ryan ND, Matty MK, et al. Sleep onset abnormalities in depressed adolescents. Biol Psychiatry 1996;39:400–10.
33. Lahmeyer HW, Poznanski EO, Bellu SN. EEG sleep in depressed adolescents. Am J Psychiatry 1983;40:1150–3.
34. Emslie GJ, Roffwarg HP, Rush AJ, et al. Sleep EEG findings in depressed children and adolescents. Am J Psychiatry 1987;144:668–70.
35. Goetz RR, Puig-Antich J, Ryan N, et al. Electroencephalographic sleep of adolescents with major depression and normal controls. Arch Gen Psychiatry 1987;44:61–8.
36. Appelboom-Fondu J, Kerkhofs M, Mendlewicz J. Depression in adolescents and young adults – polysomnographic and neuroendocrine aspects. J Affect Disord 1988;14:35–40.
37. Khan AU, Todd S. Polysomnographic findings in adolescents with major depression. Psychiatry Res 1990;33:313–20.
38. Forbes EE, Bertocci MA, Gregory AM, et al. Objective sleep in pediatric anxiety disorders and major depressive disorder. J Am Acad Child Adolesc Psychiatry 2008;47(2):148–55.
39. Rao U, Poland RE. Electroencephalographic sleep and hypothalamic–pituitary–adrenal changes from episode to recovery in depressed adolescents. J Child Adolesc Psychopharmacol 2008;18(5):607–13.
40. Ivanenko A, Crabtree VM, Gozal D. Sleep and depression in children and adolescents. Sleep Rev 2005;9(2):115–29.
41. Lofthouse N, Gilchrist R, Splingard M. Mood-related sleep problems in children and adolescents. Child Adolesc Psychiatric Clin N Am 2009;18(4):893–916.
42. Bertocci MA, Dahl RE, Williamson DE, et al. Subjective sleep complaints in pediatric depression: a controlled study and comparison with EEG measures of sleep and waking. J Am Acad Child Adolesc Psychiatry 2005;44:158–66.
43. Teicher MH, Glod CA, Harper D, et al. Locomotor activity in depressed children and adolescents: I. Circadian dysregulation. J Am Acad Child Adolesc Psychiatry 1993;32:760–9.
44. Armitage R, Hoffman R, Emslie G, et al. Rest–activity cycles in childhood and adolescent depression. J Am Acad Child Adolesc Psychiatry 2004;43:761–9.
45. Glod CA, Teicher MH, Hartman CR, et al. Increased nocturnal activity and impaired sleep maintenance in abused children. J Am Acad Child Adolesc Psychiatry 1997;36:1236–43.

46. Van Meter AR, Moreira AL, Youngstrom EA. Meta-analysis of epidemiological studies of pediatric bipolar disorder. J Clin Psychiatry 2011;72:1250–6.

47. Wehr TA, Sack DA, Rosenthal NE. Sleep reduction as a final common pathway in the genesis of mania. Am J Psychiatry 1987;144(2): 201–4.

48. Barbini B, Bertelli S, Colombo C, et al. Sleep loss, a possible factor in augmenting manic episode. Psychiatry Res 1996;65(2):121–5.

49. Leibenluft E, Albert PS, Rosenthal NE, et al. Relationship between sleep and mood in patients with rapid-cycling bipolar disorder. Psychiatry Res 1996;63(2–3):161–8.

50. Harvey AG, Schmidt DA, Scarna A, et al. Sleep-related functioning in euthymic patients with bipolar disorder, patients with insomnia, and subjects without sleep problems. Am J Psychiatry 2005;162(1):50–7.

51. Goodwin FK, Jamison KR. Manic-depressive illness: Bipolar disorder and recurrent depression. 2nd ed. Oxford, UK: Oxford University Press; 2007.

52. Harvey AG, Mullin BC, Hinshaw SP. Sleep and circadian rhythms in children and adolescents with bipolar disorder. Dev Psychopathol 2006;18(4):1147–68.

53. Hlastala SA, Frank E. Adapting interpersonal and social rhythm therapy to the developmental needs of adolescents with bipolar disorder. Dev Psychopathol 2006;18(4):1267–88.

54. Kowatch RA, Youngstrom EA, Danielyan A, et al. Review and meta-analysis of the phenomenology and clinical characteristics of mania in children and adolescents. Bipolar Disord 2005;7(6):483–96.

55. Geller B, Zimerman B, et al. DSM-IV mania symptoms in a prepubertal and early adolescent bipolar phenotype compared to attention-deficit/hyperactive and normal controls. J Child Adolesc Psychopharmacol 2002;12:11–25.

56. Lofthouse N, Fristad M, Splaingard M, et al. Parent and child reports of sleep problems associated with early-onset bipolar spectrum disorders. J Fam Psychol 2007;21(1):114–23.

57. Lofthouse N, Fristad M, Splaingard M, et al. Web survey of sleep problems associated with early-onset bipolar spectrum disorders. J Pediatr Psychol 2008;33(4):349–57.

58. Lofthouse N, Fristad M, Splaingard M, et al. Web-survey of pharmacological and non-pharmacological sleep interventions for children with early-onset bipolar spectrum disorders. J Affect Disord 2010;120:267–71.

59. Staton D, Volness LJ, Beatty WW. Diagnosis and classification of pediatric bipolar disorder. J Affect Disord 2008;105(1–3):205–12.

60. Baroni A, Hernandez M, Grant MC, et al. Sleep disturbances in pediatric bipolar disorder: a comparison between bipolar I and bipolar NOS. Front Psychiatry 2012;3:article 22.

61. Rao U, Dahl RE, Ryan ND, et al. Heterogeneity in EEG sleep findings in adolescent depression: unipolar versus bipolar clinical course. J Affect Disord 2002;70(3):273–80.

62. Mehl RC, O'Brien LM, Jones JH, et al. Correlates of sleep and pediatric bipolar disorder. Sleep 2006;29(2):193–7.

63. Mullin BC, Harvey AG, Hinshaw SP. A preliminary study of sleep in adolescents with bipolar disorder, ADHD, and non-patient controls. Bipolar Disord 2011;13(4):425–32.

64. Alfano CA, Beidel DC, Turner SM, et al. Preliminary evidence for sleep complaints among children referred for anxiety. Sleep Med 2006;7(6):467–73.

65. Alfano CA, Ginsburg GA, Kingery JN. Sleep-related problems among children and adolescents with anxiety disorders. J Am Acad Child Adolesc Psychiatry 2007;46:224–32.

66. Alfano CA, Pina AA, Zerr AA, et al. Pre-sleep arousal and sleep problems of anxiety-disordered youth. Child Psychiatry Hum Dev 2010;41(2):156–67.

67. Hansen BH, Skirbekk B, Oerbeck B, et al. Comparison of sleep problems in children with anxiety and attention deficit/hyperactivity disorders. Eur Child Adolesc Psychiatry 2011;20(6):321–30.

68. Chase RM, Pincus DB. Sleep-related problems in children and adolescents with anxiety disorders. Behav Sleep Med 2011;9(4):224–36.

69. Hudson JL, Gradisar M, Gamble A, et al. The sleep patterns and problems of clinically anxious children. Behav Res Ther 2009;47(4):339–44.

70. Gregory AM, Rijsdijk FV, Eley TC. A twin-study of sleep difficulties in school-aged children. Child Dev 2006;77(6):1668–79.

71. Schreck KA, Mulick JA, Johannes R. Parent perception of elementary school aged children's sleep problems. J Child Fam Stud 2005;14(1): 101–9.

72. Storch EA, Murphy TK, Lack CW, et al. Sleep-related problems in pediatric obsessive-compulsive disorder. J Anxiety Disord 2008;22(5): 877–85.

73. Forbes EE, Bertocci MA, Gregory AM, et al. Objective sleep in pediatric anxiety disorders and major depressive disorder. J Am Acad Child Adolesc Psychiatry 2008;47(2):148–55.

74. American Psychiatric Association. Diagnostic and Statistical Manual of Mental Disorders. 4th ed-TR. Washington, DC: American Psychiatric Association; 2000.

75. Monti JM, Monti D. Sleep disturbance in generalized anxiety disorder and its treatment. Sleep Med Rev 2000;4(3):263–76.

76. Alfano CA, Reynolds KC, Scott N, et al. Polysomnographic sleep pattern of non-medicated, non-depressed children with generalized anxiety disorder. J Affect Disord in press.

77. Giles DE, Kupfer DJ, Roffwarg HP, et al. Polysomnographic parameters in first-degree relatives of unipolar probands. Psy Res 1989; 27:127–36.

78. Giles DE, Kupfer DJ, Rush AJ, et al. Controlled comparison of electrophysiological sleep in families of probands with unipolar depression. Am J Psychiatr 1998;155:192–9.

79. Reynolds CF 3rd, Kupfer DJ. Sleep research in affective illness: state of the art circa 1987. Sleep 1987;10(3):199–215.

80. Kendler KS. Major depression and generalised anxiety disorder Same genes, (partly) different environments – revisited. Br J Psychiatry Suppl 1996;(30):68–75.

81. Eisen AR, Schaefer CE. Separation anxiety in children and adolescents: An individualized approach to assessment and treatment. New York: The Guilford Press; 2005.

82. Verduin TL, Kendall PC. Differential occurrence of comorbidity within childhood anxiety disorders. J Clin Child Adolesc Psychol 2003;32(2): 290–5.

83. Piacentini J, Bergman RL, Keller M, et al. Functional impairment in children and adolescents with obsessive–compulsive disorder. J Child Adolesc Psychopharmacol 2003;13(Suppl 1):S61–9.

84. Rapoport J, Elkins R, Langer DH, et al. Childhood obsessive–compulsive disorder. Am J Psychiatr 1981;138(12):1545–54.

85. Alfano CA, Kim KL. Objective sleep patterns and severity of symptoms in pediatric obsessive compulsive disorder: A pilot investigation. J Anx Disord 2011;25(6):835–9.

86. Pynoos RS, Frederick C, Nader K, et al. Life threat and posttraumatic stress in school-age children. Arch Gen Psychiatry 1987;44(12): 1057–63.

87. Lonigan CJ, Phillips BM, Richey JA. Posttraumatic stress disorder in children: diagnosis, assessment, and associated features. Child Adolesc Psychiatr Clin N Am 2003;12(2):171–94.

88. Brown TH, Mellman TA, Alfano CA, et al. Sleep fears, sleep disturbance, and PTSD symptoms in minority youth exposed to Hurricane Katrina. J Trauma Stress 2011;24(5):575–80.

89. Bader K, Schafer V, Schenkel M, et al. Adverse childhood experiences associated with sleep in primary insomnia. J Sleep Res 2007;16(3): 285–96.

90. Noll JG, Trickett PK, Susman EJ, et al. Sleep disturbances and childhood sexual abuse. J Pediatr Psychol 2006;31(5):469–80.

91. Dahl RE. The regulation of sleep and arousal: Development and psychopathology. Dev Psychopathol 1996;8(1):3–27.

92. Dinges DF, Pack F, Williams K, et al. Cumulative sleepiness, mood disturbance, and psychomotor vigilance performance decrements during a week of sleep restricted to 4–5 hours per night. Sleep 1997;20(4): 267–77.

93. Pilcher JJ, Huffcutt AI. Effects of sleep deprivation on performance: a meta-analysis. Sleep 1996;19(4):318–26.

94. Talbot LS, McGlinchey EL, Kaplan KA, et al. Sleep deprivation in adolescents and adults: changes in affect. Emotion 2010;10(6):831–41.

95. Yoo SS, Gujar N, Hu P, et al. The human emotional brain without sleep – a prefrontal amygdala disconnect. Curr Biol 2007;17(20):R877–8.

96. Gregory AM, Buysse DJ, Willis TA, et al. Associations between sleep quality and anxiety and depression symptoms in a sample of young adult twins and siblings. J Psychosomat Res 2011;71(4):250–5.

97. Sipila T, Kananen L, Greco D, et al. An association analysis of circadian genes in anxiety disorders. Biol Psychiatry 2010;67(12):1163–70.

98. Gregory AM, Rijsdijk FV, Dahl RE, et al. Associations between sleep problems, anxiety, and depression in twins at 8 years of age. Pediatrics 2006;118(3):1124–32.

99. Barclay NL, Eley TC, Mill J, et al. Sleep quality and diurnal preference in a sample of young adults: associations with 5HTTLPR, PER3, and CLOCK 3111. Am J Med Genet B Neuropsychiatr Gene 2011; 156B(6):681–90.

100. Stockmeier CA. Involvement of serotonin in depression: evidence from postmortem and imaging studies of serotonin receptors and the serotonin transporter. J Psychiatr Res 2003;37(5):357–73.

101. Gunthert KC, Conner TS, Armeli S, et al. Serotonin transporter gene polymorphism (5-HTTLPR) and anxiety reactivity in daily life: a daily process approach to gene–environment interaction. Psychosom Med 2007;69(8):762-8.

102. Jorm AF, Prior M, Sanson A, et al. Association of a functional polymorphism of the serotonin transporter gene with anxiety-related temperament and behavior problems in children: a longitudinal study from infancy to the mid-teens. Mol Psychiatry 2000;5(5):542–7.

103. Harvey AG, Greenall E. Catastrophic worry in primary insomnia. J Behav Ther Exp Psychiatry 2003;34(1):11–23.

104. Barclay NL, Gregory AM. The presence of a perseverative iterative style in poor vs. good sleepers. J Behav Ther Exp Psychiatry 2010;41(1): 18–23.

105. Alfano CA, Zakem AH, Costa NM, et al. Sleep problems and their relation to cognitive factors, anxiety, and depressive symptoms in children and adolescents. Depress Anxiety 2009;26(6):503–12.

106. Gregory AM, Cox J, Crawford MR, et al. Dysfunctional beliefs and attitudes about sleep in children. J Sleep Res 2009;18(4):422–6.

107. Gregory AM, Eley TC. Sleep problems, anxiety and cognitive style in school-aged children. Infant Child Dev 2005;14(5):435–44.

108. Gregory AM, Eley TC, O'Connor TG, et al. Etiologies of associations between childhood sleep and behavioral problems in a large twin sample. J Am Acad Child Adolesc Psychiatry 2004;43(6):744–51.

109. Bates JE, Viken RJ, Alexander DB, et al. Sleep and adjustment in preschool children: sleep diary reports by mothers relate to behavior reports by teachers. Child Dev 2002;73(1):62–75.

110. Lavigne JV, Arend R, Rosenbaum D, et al. Sleep and behavior problems among preschoolers. J Dev Behav Pediatr 1999;20(3):164–9.

111. Meijer AM, Habekothe RT, van den Wittenboer GL. Mental health, parental rules and sleep in pre-adolescents. J Sleep Res 2001;10(4): 297–302.

112. Warren SL, Gunnar MR, Kagan J, et al. Maternal panic disorder: Infant temperament, neurophysiology, and parenting behaviors. J Am Acad Child Adolesc Psychiatry 2003;42(7):814–25.

113. Cousins JC, Whalen DJ, Dahl RE, et al. The bidirectional association between daytime affect and nighttime sleep in youth with anxiety and depression. J Pediatr Psychol 2011;36(9):969–79.

114. Benca RM, Obermeyer WH, Thisted RA, et al. Sleep and psychiatric disorders – a metaanalysis. Arch Gen Psychiatry 1992;49(8):651–68.

115. Harvey AG. A transdiagnostic approach to treating sleep disturbance in psychiatric disorders. Cogn Behav Therap 2009;38:35–42.

116. Clarke G, Harvey AG. The complex role of sleep in adolescent depression. Child Adolesc Psychiatr Clin N Am 2012;21(2):385–400.

117. Belleville G, Cousineau H, Levrier K, et al. Meta-analytic review of the impact of cognitive-behavior therapy for insomnia on concomitant anxiety. Clin Psychol Rev 2011;31(4):638–52.

118. Belleville G, Cousineau H, Levrier K, et al. The impact of cognitive-behavior therapy for anxiety disorders on concomitant sleep disturbances: A meta-analysis. J Anx Disord 2010;24(4):379–86.

119. Manber R, Edinger JD, Gress JL, et al. Cognitive behavioral therapy for insomnia enhances depression outcome in patients with comorbid major depressive disorder and insomnia. Sleep 2008;31(4):489–95.

120. Tikotzky L, Sadeh A. The role of cognitive-behavioral therapy in behavioral childhood insomnia. Sleep Med 2010;11:686–91.

121. Sadeh A. Cognitive-behavioral treatment for childhood sleep disorders. Clin Psychol Rev 2005;25(5):612–28.

122. Alfano CA, Lewin D. Sleep in children with anxiety disorders. In: Ivanenko A, editor. Sleep and psychiatric disorders in children and adolescents. New York, USA: Informa Healthcare; 2008. p. 315–27.

123. Mindell JA, Owens JA, Carskadon MA. Developmental features of sleep. Child Adolesc Psychiatr Clin N Am 1999;8(4):695–725.

124. Kuhn BR, Elliott AJ. Treatment efficacy in behavioral pediatric sleep medicine. J Psychosomat Res 2003;54(6):587–97.

125. Harvey AG, Schmidt DA, Scarna A, et al. Sleep-related functioning in euthymic patients with bipolar disorder, patients with insomnia, and subjects without sleep problems. Am J Psychiatry 2005;162(1):50–7.

126. Harvey AG, Payne S. The management of unwanted pre-sleep thoughts in insomnia: distraction with imagery versus general distraction. Behav Res Ther 2002;40(3):267–77

127. March J, Silva S, Petrycki S, et al. Fluoxetine, cognitive-behavioral therapy, and their combination for adolescents with depression – treatment for adolescents with depression study (TADS) randomized controlled trial. JAMA 2004;292(7):807–20.

128. Kennard B, Silva S, Vitiello B, et al. Remission and residual symptoms after short-term treatment in the Treatment of Adolescents with Depression Study (TADS). J Am Acad Child Adolesc Psychiatry 2006;45(12):1404–11.

129. Emslie GJ, Armitage R, Weinberg WA, et al. Sleep polysomnography as a predictor of recurrence in children and adolescents with major depressive disorder. Int J Neuropsychopharmacol 2001;4(2):159–68.

130. Perlis ML, Smith LJ, Lyness JM, et al. Insomnia as a risk factor for onset of depression in the elderly. Behav Sleep Med 2006;4(2): 104–13.

131. Smith MT, Huang MI, Manber R. Cognitive behavior therapy for chronic insomnia occurring within the context of medical and psychiatric disorders. Clin Psychol Rev 2005;25(5):559–92.

132. Gordon J, King NJ, Gullone E, et al. Treatment of children's nighttime fears: The need for a modern randomised controlled trial. Clin Psychol Rev 2007;27(1):98–113.

133. Compton SN, Burns BJ, Helen LE, et al. Review of the evidence base for treatment of childhood psychopathology: internalizing disorders. J Consult Clin Psychol 2002;70(6):1240–66.

134. Graziano AM, Mooney KC Family self-control instruction for children's nighttime fear reduction. J Consult Clin Psychol 1980;48(2): 206–13.

135. Graziano AM, Mooney KC. Behavioral treatment of nightfears in children – maintenance of improvement at 2 1/2-year to 3-year follow-up. J Consult Clin Psychol 1982;50(4):598–9.

136. King N, Ollendick TH, Tonge BJ. Children's nighttime fears. Clin Psychol Rev 1997;17(4):431–43.

137. Kushnir J, Sadeh A. Assessment of brief interventions for nighttime fears in preschool children. Eur J Pediatr 2012;171:67–75.

138. Kupfer DJ, Coble P, Kane J, et al. Imipramine and EEG sleep in children with depressive symptoms. Psychopharmacology 1979;60:117–23.

139. Shain BN, Naylor M, Shipley JE, et al. Imipramine effects on sleep in depressed adolescents: A preliminary report. Biol Psychiatry 1990; 28:459–62.

140. Armitage R, Emslie G, Rintelmann J. The effect of fluoxetine on sleep EEG in childhood depression: a preliminary report. Neuropharmacology 1997;17:241–5.

141. Kallepalli BR, Bhatara VS, Fogas BS, et al. Trazodone is only slightly faster than fluoxetine in relieving insomnia in adolescents with depressive disorders. J Child Adolesc Psychopharmacol 1997;7:97–107.

142. Metz A, Shader RI. Adverse interactions encountered when using trazodone to treat insomnia associated with fluoxetine. Int Clin Psychopharmacol 1990;5(3):191–4.

143. Nierenberg AA, Cole JO, Glass L. Possible trazodone potentiation of fluoxetine: a case series. J Clin Psychiatry 1992;53(3):83–5.

Evaluation of Sleep in Cancer

Gerald Rosen and Sarah R. Brand

INTRODUCTION

Caring for children with cancer presents a sleep clinician with unique challenges and opportunities. Children with cancer face a life-threatening illness which may require painful and toxic therapies. The opportunities to positively impact the child and family rests in identifying sleep-related issues that are generally similar to sleep problems seen in children without cancer. These sleep disorders are likely to be familiar to sleep clinicians, are easy to recognize, and typically respond well to appropriate therapy. Managing sleep-related disorders in children with cancer can provide much-needed respite from the rigors of required therapeutic interventions.

OVERVIEW OF CANCER IN CHILDREN

Prevalence of cancer is 15 per 100000 children.[1] Neoplasia occurs due to a breakdown of the existing biological balance of cellular renewal and cellular apoptosis/elimination within the body. This disruption is the result of an imbalance of the signaling pathways that control essential cellular functions including cell growth, differentiation and survival.[2,3] The majority of cancers are caused by random mutations or alternations to molecular pathways, which increase cancer susceptibility, though some may be the result of hereditary and/or environmental factors. Childhood cancers comprise a wide spectrum of markedly different malignancies, which vary by histology, gender, age, site of origin and race. The most commonly diagnosed childhood cancers are acute lymphocytic leukemia (ALL) and central nervous system (CNS) malignancies, which comprise 27% and 22% of all childhood cancers, respectively.[1] CNS tumors are the most commonly diagnosed solid tumors in children.

The 5-year survival rate for childhood cancer has dramatically improved over the past 10 years. The overall survival rate averaged across all types of cancers, is about 75%. To achieve this high cure rate, however, children must often endure several years of intensive treatment, which may involve, chemotherapy, radiation therapy, and surgery. Cancer treatment is often a traumatic process requiring frequent and painful procedures or therapies. Morbidity from cancer may be the direct result of the destructive effect of the cancer, or may be from collateral injury to normal tissues caused by toxic treatments. Morbidity in cancer may occur immediately, as a result of acute toxic side effects of treatment, or may develop as the child grows older.[4] Some morbidities may not become apparent until well after the cancer has been cured. With respect to sleep-related comorbidity, when investigated, sleep problems have been recognized in children during and after treatment for leukemia[5-10] and brain tumors,[11,12] the two most common malignancies in children (Table 47.1).

SLEEP IN CHILDREN WITH CANCER

The sleep problems in children with cancer can be understood as the result of four distinct processes:
1. Children with cancer are expected to have the same background prevalence of sleep problems seen in all children.
2. Sleep problems that are the result of the stress on the child and family from the child having a life-threatening disease.
3. Sleep problems that are the direct result of brain injury from brain tumors and CNS-directed therapies including cranioradiotherapy (CRT) for children with brain tumors and leukemia.
4. Sleep problems that are the indirect result of chemotherapy and the many medical complications of cancer including: cancer-related fatigue (CRF), pain, seizures, obesity, endocrinopathies, heart failure, blindness, medication.

There have been no prospective studies of sleep in children with cancer, so the prevalence of sleep problems in this group of children is not known. However, there have been published case series reviews of children with CNS tumors followed in the neurosurgery clinic after surgery,[13] children with CNS tumors and other non-CNS malignancies followed in oncology clinics,[12] and of children with cancer who were referred for a sleep evaluation because of a sleep complaint identified by their oncologist or primary care doctor.[11] Together, these studies provide some insights into the types and frequency of sleep problems in children with cancer.

Sleep problems seen in a study of 70 children with cancer, 48 with CNS tumors, 18 with leukemia or lymphoma, and 4 with solid tumors who were referred for an evaluation and seen over a 15-year period in a single institution, are described in Box 47-1. Sleep problems identified were: excessive daytime sleepiness (EDS), present in 60% of the children; apnea, present in 40%; insomnia, present in 24%; parasomnias present in 9% and circadian rhythm disorders present in 4% of the children. More than one sleep problem was identified for many of the children. Excessive daytime sleepiness was the most common sleep problem identified. Parents did not describe EDS as present at the time of diagnosis, but rather developing after the treatment with CNS-directed therapies were instituted. Insomnia was present in 24% of the children, but in most cases was not of great concern to the parents, who viewed it as an inevitable consequence of cancer treatment. Noteworthy in this case series was the distribution of sleep problems seen in children with cancer. This distribution varied significantly from the expected prevalence of sleep problems in children. The type of sleep problem was related to both the type of cancer, and more specifically the location of the cancer, particularly in the case of brain tumors. Although accounting for only 25% of cancers in children, those with brain tumors were the most commonly referred group of children seen in this study, accounting for almost 70% of the

TABLE 47.1 Sleep Problems in Children with Cancer Referred for a Sleep Evaluation[11]

CHILDREN WITH CANCER SEEN IN SLEEP CLINIC 1994–2009	TOTAL # OF PATIENTS	EDS/LONG SLEEPERS	APNEA	INSOMNIA	CIRCADIAN	PARASOMNIA
Total	70	42/70 (60%)	28/70 (40%)	17/70 (24%)	3/70 (4%)	6/70 (9%)
Tumors of CNS	48					
Hypothalamus/brainstem	35	28/35 (80%)	16/35 (46%)	5/35 (14%)	2/35 (6%)	2/35 (6%)
Posterior fossa	7	6	2	2	0	1
Cortex	6	4	2	1	0	2
Leukemia/other blood	18	4/18 (22%)	6/18 (33%)	7/18 (39%)	1/18 (6%)	1/18 (6%)
Other solid tumors	4					
Upper airway	3	0	2	1	0	0
Kidney	1	0	0	1	0	0

Box 47-1 Sleep History in Children with Cancer

Chief complaint – insomnia, EDS, unusual awakenings from sleep, snoring/OSA (often more than one complaint)

History of Present Illness
Cancer
- Leukemia:
  - Age of diagnosis, presenting symptoms
  - CNS radiation
  - Corticosteroid treatment
  - Chemotherapy protocol
- Brain tumor:
  - Type, location (if solid tumor), age of diagnosis, presenting symptoms of cancer, initial treatment
  - Surgeries – dates, type (biopsy, partial resection, gross total research, shunt)
  - Cranial radiation – dose _____ cGray
  - Field _____
  - Chemotherapy – protocol_____
  - Corticosteroids

Sleep History
- Sleep before cancer diagnosis
  - Bedtime, wake time, naps
  - Problems with sleep – sleep onset, snore/OSA, awakenings, circadian – regularity, timing
  - Number of hours of sleep child averaged/night
- Current sleep history
  - Sleep log – 2 weeks
  - Bedtime – weekday/weekend
  - Wake time – weekday/weekend
  - Preferred vacation sleep schedule – timing, duration
  - Sleep onset – restless legs, fears, pain, parents present or not, hypnagogic hallucinations, sleep onset paralysis. How and where does the child fall asleep, who else is present at sleep onset, is there any inadvertent reinforcement of problem behaviors
  - Sleep – snore/OSA, CSA, choke, vomit, seizures, enuresis, sleepwalking, confusional arousals, night terrors, nightmares, sleep eating

- Awakenings – frequency, response to awakenings by parents, any inadvertent reinforcement of awakenings by parents (allowing child to co-sleep, if so how often does it occur and by which parent)
- Daytime cataplexy

Past Medical History
- Current medications
  - Corticosteroids?
  - What medications have been used for sleep? With what success?
  - Caffeine use – type (pop, coffee, tea, energy drinks), amount
  - Recreational drugs – nicotine, alcohol, marijuana, other – use/abuse
- Hospitalizations
- Allergies
- HEENT – eye: visual impairment, blindness
- ENT – ear infections, enlarged tonsils and adenoids, strep infections, sinusitis, chronic mouth breathing, difficulty swallowing, aspiration/choking on food
- Cardiopulmonary – asthma, pneumonia, heart disease, cardio-toxic chemotherapy
- GI – reflux, vomiting, abdominal pain, constipation, diarrhea
- Neuro – headaches, seizures, hypotonia, hypertonia, developmental/cognitive/behavioral problems, pain, ADD
- School – grade, academic performance, behavior
- Endocrine – deficiencies/replacement hormones – thyroid, growth hormone, cortisol, sex hormones, diabetes insipitus, diabetes, obesity

Family History
- Identified sleep problems in parents and other family members – OSA, RLS, circadian chronotypes of parents
- Parents' parenting style; parents' belief around sleep and their child's illness
- Parental concern about child's illness (including prognosis, course of treatment, psychological impact on child and family)

referrals. Excessive daytime sleepiness was the most common problem in children with brain tumors, presenting in almost 80% of these children. In contrast, only 22% of the children with leukemia/lymphoma present with EDS as their predominant complaint. In one-third of children with brain tumors and EDS which began after their brain tumor

diagnosis, the mean sleep latency on a multiple sleep latency test (MSLT) was greater than 15 minutes. This objective measure of daytime sleepiness would not meet criteria for hypersomnolence as defined by the International Classification of Sleep Disorders, 2nd Edition. Nonetheless, these children had a history of an increase in total 24-hour sleep duration, resumption of daytime napping, inability to awaken at the desired morning rise time, and/or an inability to remain awake during daytime activities, all of which began after their cancer diagnosis. When these children were treated with stimulant medication, their symptoms of EDS improved, allowing them to fully participate in the activities of their day.

Sleep-disordered breathing was present in 40% of the children. The majority of these children had obstructive sleep apnea (OSA), though clinically significant central sleep apnea (CSA) was present in 10% of the children. All of the children with CSA had brain tumors and/or CNS-directed therapies affecting the respiratory control center of the medulla. In two children with sleep apnea, the event that led to their referral was a respiratory arrest during conscious sedation for an elective procedure. In one other child, the CSA was a manifestation of a seizure disorder and was effectively treated with anticonvulsants. Three children with CSA required nocturnal ventilation.

All of the children diagnosed with EDS were provided with education regarding sleep hygiene to regularize and extend their sleep duration, but in most cases this alone did not correct their EDS. In all of the children, stimulant medications were prescribed, methylphenidate (10–56 mg/day), modafinil (200–400 mg/day), or amphetamine salts (20–40 mg/day) and were all effective in correcting the EDS. The medication was titrated clinically with the primary goal to help the children remain awake during the school day and allowing them to participate in after-school activities. Once an effective dose was established, hypersomnia remained well controlled without the need for significant escalation in dose. Side effects of medications were uncommon but did included headaches and anorexia. In children with EDS, the symptoms persisted long term, recurring whenever the stimulant medication was discontinued over a 15-year follow-up. Though insomnia was identified in 24% of the children referred to the sleep clinic for an evaluation, it was rarely the reason for the referral. Insomnia was considered an incidental problem in a child who was referred for either EDS or OSA, and for most of the parents treatment of insomnia was not a priority.

Sleep in children with cancer is often made worse during hospitalization because of frequent interruptions of the child's sleep by caregivers. This was described in a study of 29 children with cancer hospitalized for 2–3 days. The children were awakened 0–40 times/night, mean 14. The longest duration of uninterrupted sleep for 70% of the children was 1 hour.[14]

NEUROANATOMY OF SLEEP AND WAKEFULNESS

Sleep and wake are complex neurologic processes which are actively generated by coordinated, overlapping mechanisms controlled by nuclei in the hypothalamus, thalamus, basal forebrain and brainstem.[15] Each of these systems controls a different facet of sleep and/or wake, and each has different roles, so the loss of any one system may be partially compensated by other systems. CNS-directed therapies for cancer may impact sleep by direct damage to the brain centers that are responsible for the regulation of sleep–wake by a brain tumor or neurosurgery, or by the neurotoxic effects of CRT and chemotherapy. The relationship between injury to the brain and the development of sleep problems was first described by Von Economo,[16] based on his observations of patients with encephalitis. Since Von Economo's original clinical observations, many other types of injuries to this critical area of the brain have been recognized as causing problems with sleep. The most commonly reported sleep problem after a CNS injury is EDS. Brain injuries that have resulted in EDS have been summarized in a comprehensive review of symptomatic narcolepsy by Nishino and Kanbayashi.[17] The 116 cases of symptomatic narcolepsy which have been reported in the literature were associated with: inherited disorders (34%), brain tumors (29%), head trauma (16%), demyelinating disorders (9%), stroke (5%), infection (3%), and degenerative disorders (3%). In Nishino's series, many different types of brain tumors were associated with EDS. Seventy percent of the tumors involved the hypothalamus or adjacent structures including pituitary, supracellar, or optic chiasm, and 10% involved the brainstem. Some tumors involved multiple sites, but in only 12% were areas of the brain other than the brainstem or hypothalamus involved, and in many of these cases CRT was one of the treatments. In 10 of the patients with brain tumors in Nishino's review, cerebrospinal fluid (CSF) hypocretin was measured. Hypocretin was found to be low in 3/10, and normal in 7/10; suggesting that in the majority of cases EDS in patients with brain tumors is not simply caused by the destruction of the hypocretin-secreting cells in the lateral hypothalamus.

CRANIAL RADIATION THERAPY (CRT)

Cranial radiation is a common treatment modality for pediatric brain tumors, and for the treatment of CNS leukemia. CRT has substantial morbidity, which is related to the radiation dose and field, and is especially toxic to children under age 3 years. Though no systematic survey has been done of sleep in children receiving radiotherapy, sleep problems do appear to be common in case reports of children with brain tumors and leukemia treated with CRT. The most common sleep problem reported is EDS. The increase in daytime sleepiness after treatment with CRT can be transient or permanent. Radiation hypersomnia is a constellation of symptoms including EDS, increased total sleep time, irritability, anorexia, low-grade fever, nausea, vomiting, dysphagia, and headaches, which can be seen in up to 60% of children treated with 2400 cGy cranial radiation.[18–20] The syndrome typically appears 3–12 weeks post radiation, and lasts for 3–14 days. Affected children become sleepier, increasing the amount of sleep they require on a daily basis and often, in spite of an increased total sleep time, experience significant fatigue and EDS making it difficult for them to participate in normal activities of daily living. These findings were described in a long-term follow-up study of sleep in adult brain tumor survivors, who were treated as children with cranial radiation 5–15 years earlier.[21] Actigraphy was used to compare the sleep of the survivors to that of normal controls. The radiation-treated group showed an increase in sleep duration, decreased sleep fragmentation, and decreased tolerance for alterations in the timing of sleep. There was a clear dose–effect relationship with higher doses of cranial radiation associated with longer sleep bouts and decreased tolerance for alterations in the timing of sleep. The underlying mechanism responsible for these changes is not understood.

CANCER-RELATED FATIGUE

Cancer-related fatigue (CRF) is described as a near universal experience of individuals with cancer, present in over 70% of patients.[22–29] Fatigue is clinically different from sleepiness, a distinction that is often not made by parents and/or oncologists. Fatigue is a subjective complaint quantified by using standardized questionnaires. However, all standardized questionnaires utilized to measure fatigue include questions regarding sleep. Therefore, distinction between fatigue and sleepiness is often blurred. Children and their parents characterize CRF as multidimensional, with physical, emotional, and mental facets. The multidimensional fatigue scale is a validated questionnaire which distinguishes general fatigue, sleep/rest fatigue, and cognitive fatigue. This scale has demonstrated an increasing level of fatigue in children with brain tumors, after they have completed therapy, and have been 'cured' of their cancer.[27] Children with brain tumors had more fatigue than children with leukemia, and two-thirds of children with brain tumors were >1 SD below the norms of fatigue of healthy control children (greater fatigue). Numerous causes and comorbidities for CRF have been proposed, including: pain, depression, anxiety, anemia, poor nutrition, sleep disorders, physical deconditioning, infection and organ system failure.[24] It has been suggested that sleepiness and fatigue may share some common biologic pathways mediating both symptoms, which would explain the great deal of overlap between fatigue and sleepiness. Inflammatory cytokines, tumor necrosis factor alpha and interleukin-6, both seem to be important mediators of both fatigue and sleep.[25] Fatigue from whatever cause often results in an increased time in bed, with an earlier bedtime and a later rise time. These schedule modifications are often accompanied by a decrease in daytime activity, which in turn may result in a decrease in morning light exposure. The net result of all of these changes, many of which seem to make intuitive sense and are often recommended by physicians who encourage their patients to get more 'rest,' is a loss of the normal synchronization between circadian rhythmicity and homeostatic sleep drive. This inevitably leads to a poorer-quality sleep, with decreased sleep efficiency, a poorer quality of wakefulness as well as contributing to physical deconditioning, all of which leads to worsening fatigue. In surveys, children with cancer describe feeling impaired by fatigue and rate it as one of the most distressing treatment-related symptoms they experience.[28]

SLEEP-DISORDERED BREATHING IN CHILDREN WITH CANCER

Snoring is a common pediatric symptom, present in 12% of all children, and OSA in about 2%, so either may be present before a child develops cancer.[30] Obstructive sleep apnea is always a multifactorial problem, the cumulative result of craniofacial, neuromuscular and soft tissue factors. In children with brain tumors, the neurologic contributors to OSA may be secondary to: (1) state-dependent change in pharyngeal tone during sleep, (2) hypotonia, (3) hypertonia, (4) injury to the medulla resulting in a loss of the synchronization of the pharyngeal dilators with the diaphragmatic contractions, and (5) peripherally mediated injury to the vagus, glossopharyngeal or hypoglossal nerves, which control the pharyngeal dilators. Two important non-respiratory, non-neurologic contributors to OSA seen in children with cancer are obesity and hypothyroidism. In most children with OSA, the sleep-disordered breathing is present whenever the child is asleep, but in some children the OSA is only present or is much worse when the child is asleep, sedated with drugs such as benzodiazepines, chloral hydrate, or when treated for pain with narcotic analgesics. These dangers are especially important in children with cancer because these children frequently undergo conscious sedation for diagnostic procedures and are commonly treated with narcotics for pain control. Both conscious sedation and good pain control can be achieved in children with OSA, but it is important that the appropriate precautions are taken.

CENTRAL SLEEP APNEA

Clinically significant central sleep apnea is uncommon in children older than 1 year, unless they have a brainstem malformation such as an Arnold–Chiari malformation, or have sustained a severe brain injury from a tumor, infection, trauma or stroke. Central nervous system injury may result in CSA or centrally mediated OSA. Central sleep apnea in children with cancer is most commonly caused by: (1) an injury to the respiratory control center of the brain located in the medulla oblongata, (2) an unusual manifestation of a seizure, or (3) damage to the phrenic nerve. The symptom of a child with central sleep apnea typically is non-obstructive hypoventilation during sleep; which leads to sleep-related hypoxemia and/or hypercarbia, and, if severe, may cause waking hypercapnia, and/or cor pulmonale.

PSYCHOLOGICAL/BEHAVIORAL INFLUENCES

When parents are specifically asked about sleep problems in their children using standardized questionnaires, 60% of parents of children with cancer rate their children as problem sleepers[31] and acknowledge that the sleep problems have a negative impact on both their lives and their children's lives. However, the majority of these parents view insomnia as an inevitable consequence of either cancer or the chemotherapy, and rarely seek treatment for the insomnia.

Sleep is an arena where many of the forces that control a child's life play out. The predominant forces are biological, circadian, neurodevelopmental and behavioral/psychological/environmental. The sleep–wake system is dynamic, and can be thought of as functioning like a mobile hanging from a ceiling. Counterbalancing forces can lead to either a delicate stable balance or chaotic movement. When the system is balanced, a child will fall asleep independently at a consistent bedtime without difficulty, sleeps through the night without behavioral awakenings, spontaneously awakens in the morning feeling refreshed, and maintains a high level of daytime alertness the following day except for well-defined nap times. When balance is not achieved, the child has difficulty falling asleep. Sleep will occur at variable times and the child may need a parent's presence for transition. Numerous behavioral awakenings during the night may also occur, often requiring parental assistance for the child to return to sleep. The child may not wake spontaneously at a desired time in the morning, is fatigued during the day, and often naps at irregular times.

Because of the importance of sleep for both a child with cancer, and the parents of children with cancer, keeping the system balanced should be a high priority.

For any child, the periods of transition from wakefulness to sleep, which occur at sleep onset and again at numerous times throughout the night after normal spontaneous awakenings, are vulnerable to the influences of behavioral, psychological, and environmental factors. In children with cancer, the amount of potentially influencing factors across all three domains increases exponentially, thereby increasing the likelihood of problems during this transition. Parents of children with cancer are typically much more vigilant and often have justifiable fears for their child's safety and health. This often results in changes in parental behavior including increased parental monitoring at night and alterations in sleeping arrangements such as co-sleeping. While this has not been empirically examined in pediatric cancer, research investigating alterations in sleeping arrangements of epilepsy patients found that 22% of children experienced a change towards less independent sleeping arrangements after diagnosis. Parents of these children were more likely to endorse worry about seizure activity as the reason for the change in sleeping arrangements.[32]

As a result of heightened parental vigilance and fears, it is not uncommon for parents of cancer patients to be involved in the child's falling asleep. This may inadvertently set the stage for the development of a conditioned sleep-onset association disorder. The hallmark symptom of this problem is the parental presence as the child transitions to sleep at bedtime; and the necessity of parental involvement after the child has a nighttime awakening. The symptom arises because the transition to sleep may be difficult for the child because of anxiety, or as a result of parents wanting to be present with the child at bedtime for the reasons described above. When the parent is present at the beginning of the night at sleep onset, this often does help the child transition to sleep at bedtime more quickly, but it may also inadvertently create a learned association, resulting in the child's wanting and/or needing to have the parents present to facilitate the return to sleep after normal awakenings, which might occur 5–6 times throughout the night. When the parent responds to these awakenings by again helping the child return to sleep during the night, they are inadvertently re-enforcing the sleep onset association and perpetuating the arousals. This pattern often results in adequate sleep for the child, but very disrupted sleep for the parents. For parents already dealing with other stressors related to their child's medical illness, this can significantly impact their daytime functioning.

PAIN

Pain is common in children with cancer, particularly at the time of diagnosis, and when pain is present sleep is often disrupted. In a study of pain in children with cancer,[33] at the time of their diagnosis 78% experienced significant pain and in almost three-quarters of them the pain led to sleep disruption, causing multiple awakenings from sleep. Nine percent had severe sleep disruption and were unable to return to sleep, even with analgesic medication, 32% had a moderate degree of sleep disruption and were able to return to sleep only after medication, and 20% had mild sleep disruption, returning to sleep without medication. In many clinical settings, acute and chronic pain leads to sleep fragmentation, which in turn has

been associated with increased pain sensitivity,[34] establishing a vicious spiral. In adults, pain has also been shown to play a mediating role in the development of CRF.[35] Medications used to treat pain, particularly the narcotic analgesics, can also cause sleep problems, including the development or exacerbation of sleep-disordered breathing, and daytime sedation. These reactions to medication may lead to daytime napping, and in turn may impact circadian rhythmicity and synchronization with the homeostatic sleep drive.

OTHER MEDICAL PROBLEMS

Sleep disruption may occur in many other medical problems which may be present in a child with cancer including: obesity, asthma, endocrinopathies, gastroesophageal reflux, heart failure, abdominal pain, arthritis, seizures and atopic dermatitis. These medical problems may cause sleep fragmentation which may contribute to the symptoms of insomnia, increase in pain sensitivity and/or daytime sleepiness.

MEDICATIONS

Sedation and/or insomnia are listed as a side effect of over 500 prescription and over-the-counter drugs in the side effect index of the physicians desk reference.[36] These drugs may affect sleep–wake directly by leading to either an increased level of arousal (causing insomnia) or a decreased level of arousal (causing sedation), or indirectly by causing sleep fragmentation. In many of the medications that affect the CNS neurotransmitters the drugs may have a primary effect (often sedation or increased arousal), or the opposite effect, which may be secondary to withdrawal or to an idiosyncratic reaction to the drug. This has most commonly been described with diphenhydramine (H1 antagonist), which usually results in sedation; but may cause hyperactivity in some children. Opioid analgesics are an important part of the pain management of children with cancer. Good pain control is essential for good sleep in children. However, opioids may also be a factor that can negatively impact on sleep in a number of ways. Opioids may cause daytime sedation and fatigue, raise the arousal threshold for sleep apnea, and lead to respiratory depression. High-dose corticosteroids have become a mainstay in the treatment of many types of cancer. Most chemotherapy protocols for standard-risk and high-risk acute lymphoblastic leukemia include 30–60 mg/m^2 of dexamethasone for 2 to 3 years given monthly. Sleep disruption is a commonly reported adverse side effect of dexamethasone amongst affected children, present in 30–50% of the children.[7,8] Insomnia and hypersomnia are both commonly reported. Insomnia is more common among adolescents and hypersomnia in children less than 10 years of age.

SLEEP DURING THE TERMINAL PHASE OF CHILDHOOD CANCER

Two studies have detailed sleep during the terminal phase of cancer treatment from the perspective of palliative care providers[37] and parents.[38] In the last month of the child's life, parents and the doctors reported fatigue in 92%, daytime sleepiness in 60%, and insomnia in 16–40% of children.

Treatment of sleep problems may need to be addressed within the context of palliative care in these children.

LATE EFFECTS OF CANCER

As a result of advances in treatment, 75% of children and adolescents who are diagnosed with cancer as a child are long-term survivors. The cancer survivors often suffer from a variety of late effects, which were documented in a recent study of long-term survivors of childhood cancer.[4] Severe or life-threatening medical problems occurred in 27.5%. Chemotherapy and radiation therapy but not surgery were most commonly associated with the late effects, suggesting that the treatments more than the cancer itself are responsible for the late effects. In a study of acute lymphoblastic leukemia survivors ages 18 to 41 who were off treatment for an average of 14 years, sleep problems (not specified) were the most common late effect, present in 49% of the adults surveyed.[10] Neurocognitive impairment is among the most common late effects experienced by long-term survivors of pediatric cancer, with 20–40% of patients exhibiting deficits. In a study of 1426 survivors from the Childhood Cancer Survivors Study, using sibling controls, 20% of cancer survivors had neurocognitive deficits. Multivariate regression models revealed daytime sleepiness and poor sleep quality as two of the most important factors contributing to the neurocognitive deficits. The relative risk of neurocognitive deficits associated with fatigue and sleep disturbance was equivalent to that of high-dose cranial radiation.[39]

EVALUATION AND TREATMENT OF SLEEP PROBLEMS

Sleep is the result of the interaction and synchronization of a number of different physiologic processes. The sleep process matrix (Figure 47-1) is a tool for organizing and analyzing the processes that regulate sleep and is particularly helpful when evaluating children with complex medical problems such as cancer. The sleep history is the primary tool for evaluating sleep problems in children (see Box 47-1). The history can be organized into the different domains important to sleep regulation: circadian, ultradian, homeostatic, developmental, radiation, cardio-respiratory, neurologic, behavioral-psychiatric, drugs/alcohol, other medical. The hypotheses, which are developed within each domain, are confirmed or refuted as the history unfolds to best explain the sleep problems. This process leads to an analysis/synthesis which may require a diagnostic test such as a PSG, actigraphy or MSLT to confirm a diagnosis. Though the causes of sleep-disordered breathing and excessive daytime sleepiness in children with cancer are often related to their cancer; the evaluation and treatment for these conditions is not substantially different in children with or without cancer.

However, treating insomnia in child cancer patients differs significantly. Behavioral management strategies to treat insomnia in healthy infants, toddlers, and preschoolers have been well-studied and validated. The standard treatments include unmodified extinction and graduated extinction. In an unmodified extinction treatment paradigm, the parents put the child to bed at a designated bedtime and then ignore the child until morning, with the objective of reducing the undesirable behavior (e.g., crying) by eliminating the reinforcer (parental attention). In a graduated extinction paradigm, parents are instructed to ignore bedtime crying for a predetermined period before briefly checking on the child. A progressive/graduated checking schedule or fixed checking schedule can be used, depending on parental preference. Similar to the unmodified extinction, the goal is to remove the reinforcer of parental attention and enable the child to develop self-soothing skills, allowing them to fall asleep independently.[40]

Sleep process	Circadian	Homeostatic	Ultradian	Develop-mental	Cardiopulm	Neuro	Radiation	Psychiatric/behavior	Drugs/chemo	Other/medical problems
Hypothesis										
Data to gather										
Analysis synthesis										
Treatment										

FIGURE 47-1 Sleep process matrix is a tool for organizing and analyzing how the fundamental processes that regulate sleep interact with each other and lead to sleep symptoms. Generally, the sleep history provides the information necessary to develop hypotheses within each pathophysiologic domain. As the patient's history unfolds, the data gathered either confirm or refute these hypotheses. Diagnostic sleep studies may be necessary to establish the diagnosis.

These standard treatment recommendations are often not practical, nor successful, when treating insomnia in pediatric cancer patients for a number of reasons. First and foremost, parents of a medically ill child have justifiable fears about their child's safety and health, and therefore they will be extremely reluctant to 'ignore' cries of distress from their child, as these cries could indicate a medical distress. While extinction paradigms allow for parents to monitor for these issues, it is often difficult to distinguish between crying as an attention-seeking behavior and crying due to physical distress, especially in young children. Even a modified extinction program, such as that with parental presence, is often difficult for parents to implement, for the same reasons identified above.

Because the standard behavioral therapies can often not be used with this population, an alternative treatment plan that harnesses the power of the combined forces of the homeostatic and circadian drives has been developed by the authors.

Prior to implementing the treatment plan one must:

1. Form an alliance with the family so the parents believe and trust the recommendations given to them.
2. Educate the parents regarding normal sleep physiology so they understand that children learn how to transition to sleep at bedtime, and often do it the same way after they have a normal awakening during the night. If the parent is part of the child transitioning to sleep at bedtime, they often need to be part of the return to sleep after normal awakenings during the night.
3. Understand the child's circadian chronotype and typical sleep need.
4. Establish with the parents that the goal is to teach the child to fall asleep by themselves at bedtime and after normal spontaneous awakenings which occur throughout the night.
5. Obtain a careful sleep history and 2 weeks of sleep logs prior to beginning treatment.

Developing the Individual Treatment Plan:

1. Based on the sleep log (Figure 47-2), determine how many hours the child is sleeping (not time in bed) during the night at present.
2. Based on the scheduling demands of the child and parent, determine at what time the child needs to awaken. This will be wake time 7 days/week.
3. Schedule bedtime so that the number of hours of sleep the child averages equals the number of hours of time in bed. For children with significant sleep-onset and sleep-maintenance insomnia this calculation leads to a much later bedtime than their current bedtime. Parents need to be reminded that this calculation is based on the number of hours of sleep the child is currently getting so that the later bedtime does not mean less sleep, just less time in bed awake.
4. Develop with the parents a pleasant bedtime routine in a neutral family space, not in the child's or the parents' bedroom, preceding the designated bedtime. The parents' job becomes keeping their child awake until the designated bedtime, instead of struggling to get the child to sleep, even if the child is tired and wants to fall asleep earlier some nights.
5. Limit electronics – television, cell phones, computers, video games – and high-energy activities for the several hours before bedtime.
6. If the child is not ready to go to bed at the designated bedtime; this is not a problem. The parent should allow the child to go to bed as late as they wish. Prior to bedtime the child can play quietly until he or she is clearly ready to fall asleep. However, no matter when the child goes to sleep, wake time remains the same.
7. Before bedtime, parents should anticipate all of the typical stalling tactics their child will use – one more drink, one more hug, etc. – so they are not responding to the child's demands at bedtime.
8. Once the child is in bed, parents check on the child regularly (intervals depending on the child and parent) until the child is asleep. If the child leaves the bed, gently take the child back to bed. If the child does not fall asleep within 15 minutes, the parents are permitted to take the child out of bed and allow the child to play until the child becomes sleepy, at which point the child is placed back into bed.
9. Parents continue this until they win no matter how long it takes. The goal is for the child to fall asleep in their own bed by themselves, without a parent present, which is what the child will need to do to return to sleep after a normal nighttime awakening.
10. If the child awakens during the night parents adopt the same routine as at bedtime.
11. Parents never lie with the child in the child's bed nor do they allow the child to sleep in the parents' bed. If the parents are not willing to accept this, this strategy may not be feasible.
12. Wake time in the morning stays the same regardless of how late the child went to sleep, how many times it awakened during the night, and how long the child was awake during the night. Upon awakening, the child should be exposed to bright natural light (30 min of phototherapy may be necessary if this is before sunrise).
13. Daytime naps are limited to a predefined nap windows, to be decided with the parents based on the child's typical schedule. The child is not allowed to fall asleep before nap time and is awakened at the end of the nap window regardless of how long the child has been asleep. The timing and duration of the nap window may be modified based on the child's response to the treatment. The child may choose to skip naps but should not be allowed to nap outside of the designated nap window.

This approach is simply a variation of good sleep hygiene, it maintains the child's circadian rhythm by fixing the wake time and exposing the child to bright light upon awakening in the morning, gradually builds an increasing amount of homeostatic drive through sleep restriction, and limits the inadvertent reinforcement by the parents. The homeostatic drive is a very powerful one, especially in young children and, if harnessed, can overpower almost any other problem leading to insomnia except severe anxiety.

Once the child has consolidated the nighttime sleep and is falling asleep independently and not having behavioral awakenings during the night, the bedtime is gradually moved earlier (in about 15-min increments) until the sleep restriction is eliminated. When the sleep–wake pattern is reset, most children are able to maintain it.

Using this approach, parents are exerting leverage on the child's sleep where they have control – in keeping the child awake, and awakening them in the morning – and not attempting to exert control where they have none – getting the child to fall asleep.

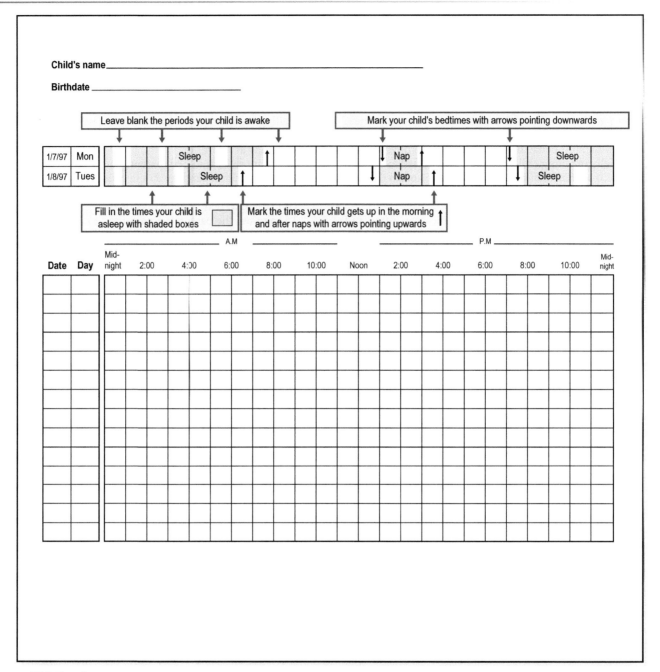

FIGURE 47-2 Sleep log.

Clinical Pearls

- Fatigue is an almost universal and generally multifactorial symptom in children with cancer that overlaps with but needs to be distinguished from sleepiness.
- Corticosteroids are commonly used as chemotherapy for cancer and can lead to either sleepiness and insomnia.
- Excessive daytime sleepiness is most commonly seen in children with tumors or treatment involving the hypothalamus.

- Excessive daytime sleepiness and sleep-disordered breathing in children with cancer respond well to treatment.
- For the treatment of insomnia in children with cancer, standard behavioral treatments may not be appropriate. Utilizing treatment methods that harness the combined forces of the circadian and homeostatic drives is key to success in treating insomnia in this population.

References

1. Reis LM, Kosary C, et al. SEER cancer statistics review, 1975–2002. Bethesda (Eisner MD: National Cancer Institute; 2005.
2. Song Y, Smaulsk T, Van Dyke T. Cancer: a conceptual framework. In: DeVita V, Lawrence T, Rosenberg S, editors. Cancer principles and practices of oncology. 8th ed. Philadelphia: Lippincott Williams & Wilkins; 2008. p. 3–12.
3. Weinberg RA. The nature of cancer. In: The biology of cancer. New York: Garland Science, Taylor & Francis Group, LLC.; 2007. p. 25–56.
4. Oeffinger K, Mertens A, Sklar C, et al. Chronic health conditions in adult survivors of childhood cancer. N Engl J Med 2006;355(15): 1572–82.
5. Hockenberry-Eaton M, Hinds P. Fatigue in children and adolescents with cancer: evolution of a program of study. Semin Oncol Nurs 2000;16:261–72.
6. Van Litsenburg RR, Huisman J, Hoogerbrugge P, et al. Impaired sleep affects quality of life in children during maintenance treatment for acute lymphoblastic leukemia: an exploratory study. Health Qual Life Outcomes 2011;9:25–32.
7. Hinds P, Hockenberry M, Gattuso J, et al. Dexamethasone alters sleep and fatigue in pediatric patients with acute lymphoblastic leukemia. Cancer 2007;110:2321–30.
8. Harris J, Carel C, Rosenberg L, et al. Intermittent high dose corticosteroid treatment in childhood cancer: behavioral and emotional consequences. J Am Acad Child Psychiatry 1986;25(1):120–4.
9. Drigan R, Spirito A, Gelber R. Behavioral effects of corticosteroids with acute lymphoblastic leukemia. Med Pediatr Oncol 1992;20:13–21.
10. Meeske K, Siegel S, Globe D, et al. Prevalence and correlates of fatigue in long-term survivors of childhood leukemia. Clin Oncol 2005;23(24):5501–10.
11. Rosen GM, Brand SR. Sleep in children with cancer: case review of 70 children evaluated in a comprehensive pediatric sleep center. Supportive Care Cancer 2011;19:985–94.
12. Verberne L, Maurice-Stam H, Grootenhuis M, et al. Sleep disorders after treatment for a CNS tumor. J Sleep Res 2012;21:461–9.
13. Greenfeld M, Constanti S, Taumann R, et al. Sleep disturbance in children recovered from central nervous system neoplasms. J Peds 2011;159: 268–72.
14. Hinds PS, Hockenberry M, Rai SN, et al. Nocturnal awakenings, sleep environment interruptions, and fatigue in hospitalized children with cancer. Oncol Nurs Forum 2007;34:393–402.
15. Fuller P, Lu J. Neubiology of sleep. In: Amlaner E, Uller P, editors. Basics of sleep guide. 2nd ed. Westchester, Ill: Sleep Resesrach Society; 2009.
16. Von Economo C. Sleep as a problem of localization. J Nerv Ment Dis 1930;71:249–59
17. Nishino S, Kanbayashi T. Symptomatic narcolepsy, cataplexy and hypersomnia, and their implications in the hypothalamic hypocretin/orexin system. Sleep Med Rev 2005;9:269–310.
18. Ryan J. Radiation somnolence syndrome. J Pediatr Oncol Nurs 2000; 17:50–3.
19. Faithful S, Brada M. Somnolence syndrome in adults following cranial irradiation for primary brain tumors. Clin Oncol 1998;10:250–4.
20. Jereczek-Fossa E, Marsiglia H, Orecchia R. Radiotherapy-related fatigue. Crit Rev Oncol Hematol 2002;41:317–25.
21. Someren E, Swart-Heikens J, Endert E, et al. Long term effect of cranial irradiation for childhood malignancy on sleep in adulthood. Eur J Endocrinol 2004;150:503–10.
22. National Comprehensive Cancer Network Practice Guidelines. Cancer-Related Fatigue Panel 2004 Guidelines. 2004.
23. Kline N, DeSwarte J. Consensus statements, research on fatigue in children with cancer. Semin Oncol Nurs 2000;16:277–8.
24. Cella D, Davis K, Breibart W, et al. Cancer related fatigue: prevalence of proposed diagnostic criteria in a United States sample of cancer survivors. J Clin Oncol 2001;19:3385–91.
25. Kim H, Barsevick A, Fang C, et al. Common biological pathways underlying the psychoneurological symptom cluster in cancer patients. Cancer Nurs 2012;35:E1–20.
26. Hockenberry MJ, Hinds PS, Barrera P, et al. Three instruments to assess fatigue in children with cancer: the child, parent, and staff perspective. J Pain Symptom Manage 2003;25:319–28.
27. Varni JW, Burwinkle TM, Katz ER, et al. The peds ql in pediatric cancer. Cancer 2002;94:2090–106.
28. Meeske K, Katz ER, Burwinkle T, et al. Parent proxy-reported health related quality of life and fatigue in pediatric patients diagnosed with brain tumors and acute lymphoblastic leukemia. Cancer 2004;101: 2116–25.
29. Morrow G, Shelke A, Roscoe J, et al. Management of cancer related fatigue. Cancer Invest 2005;23:229–39.
30. Brooks L. Obstructive sleep apnea syndrome in infants and children: clinical features and pathophysiology. In: Sheldon S, Ferber R, Kryger M, editors. Principles and practice of pediatric sleep medicine. Philadelphia: Elsevier; 2005. p. 223–31.
31. Rosen G, Harrris A, Lui M, et al. The effects of dexamethasone on sleep in young children with acute lymphoblastic leukemia. Supp Cancer Care; Under review.
32. Williams J, Lange B, Sharp G, et al. Altered sleeping arrangements in pediatric patients with epilepsy. Clin Pediatr 2000;39(11):635–42.
33. Miser A, McCalla J, Dothage J, et al. Pain as a presenting symptom in children and young adults with newly diagnosed malignancy. Pain 1987;29:85–90.
34. Ljungman G, Gordh T, Sorensen S, et al. Pain variations during cancer treatment in children: a descriptive study. Pediatr Hematol Oncol 2000;17:211–21.
35. Smith M, Haythornthwaite J. How do sleep disturbance and chronic pain inter-relate? Insight's from the longitudinal and cognitive-behavioral clinical trials literature. Sleep Med Rev 2004;8:119–32.
36. Thompson Healthcare. Physicians desk reference. 57th ed. Montvale (NJ): Medical Economics Company; 2003.
37. Goldman A, Hewitt M, Collins G, et al. Symptoms in children/young people with progressive malignant disease: United Kingdom children's cancer study group/pediatric oncology nurses forum study. Pediatrics 2006;117(6):e1179–86.
38. Jalmsell L, Kreicbergs U, Onelov E, et al. Symptoms affecting children with malignancies during the last month of life: a nationwide followup. Pediatrics 2006;117(4):1314–20.
39. Clanton N, Klosky J, Chenghong L, et al. Fatigue, vitality, sleep and neurocognitive functioning in adult survivors of childhood cancers. Cancer 2011;117:2559–68.
40. Mindell J, Kuhn B, Lewin D, et al. Behavioral treatment of bedtime problems and night wakings in infants and young children. Sleep 2006;29(10):1263.

Sleep and School Start Times

Amy R. Wolfson and Michaela Johnson

INTRODUCTION

One important feature of sleep problems in children and adolescents is that academic performance degrades or they fall asleep in class or are inattentive. This is often (and sometimes erroneously) attributed to attention deficit hyperactivity disorder. In some instances the problem is due to sleep pathology (such as sleep apnea or narcolepsy, which is covered elsewhere in this volume) and in other instances is due to a lack of synchrony between a child's circadian rhythm and the school schedule. To help an individual student succeed, schools might have a role by physical accommodation (e.g., making nap rooms available for children with narcolepsy) or by changing a student's class and activity schedule (as might be the case in a child or adolescent with a disorder of circadian rhythm). In this chapter we focus on the adolescent without sleep pathology whose circadian rhythm is not compatible with his or her school start time. Sleep in adolescents is impacted not just by their biology, but their lifestyles and often irregular sleep–wake schedules.

Over the last three decades, an accumulation of studies have clearly demonstrated that delaying school start times works as an effective countermeasure to adolescents' chronic insufficient sleep while also enhancing students' health, safety, and academic success.[1–5] Inadequate sleep is one of the most common, significant, and potentially reparable health challenges that adolescents struggle with over the middle through high school years. From a biological perspective, at about the time of puberty, the majority of adolescents begin to experience later sleep onset and offset times (i.e., a circadian phase delay).[6–10] This shift can be as long as 2 hours in comparison to elementary schoolers' sleep–wake schedules. For more than two decades, studies have demonstrated that three key changes in sleep regulation are probably responsible for this phenomenon: (1) adolescents experience a delay of the evening onset of melatonin secretion, expressed as a shift in circadian phase preference from *lark* to *owl* type, resulting in difficulty falling asleep at an earlier bedtime; (2) adolescents undergo a change in regulatory homeostatic 'sleep drive' whereby the accumulation of sleep propensity while awake slows relative to younger children, making it easier for them to stay up later; (3) adolescents' sleep *needs* do not decline from pre-adolescent levels with optimal sleep amounts ranging from 8.5 to 9.5 hours per night.[8,7,10–13] On a practical level, this means that the average adolescent has difficulty falling asleep before about 11 p.m., and is unlikely to wake up before 8 a.m. In addition to these three significant developmental changes, environmental and lifestyle factors interfere with adolescents getting sufficient and regular sleep. There is clear and compelling evidence that delaying middle and high school start times gives adolescents the opportunity to obtain an adequate amount of sleep with implications for academic performance and health. In the chapter that follows, we review over 30 years of research on adolescent sleep–wake patterns and the countermeasures and interventions where schools delayed their school start times.

ADOLESCENTS' SLEEP–WAKE NEEDS AND PATTERNS

It is not surprising that adolescents often ignore their need for sleep to accommodate social, technology, academic, and escalating extracurricular demands.[8,14–16] Teenagers' ability to function throughout the school day, however, is influenced by the quantity, regularity, and quality of their sleep. As observed in many countries, self-reported sleep patterns show marked changes over the adolescent years.[17–20] Beginning as early as sixth or seventh grade (approximately age 12), the majority of adolescents report increasingly later bedtimes, especially on weekend and vacation nights.[20–23] School-night bedtimes range from 9:30 p.m. to midnight with high school-aged adolescents (ages 14–19 years), reporting significantly later bedtimes than their early adolescent peers (ages 10–13 years).[3,24] Rise times on school days remain relatively stable across this developmental stage largely due to school schedules.[3,7,22,24] Many schools in the USA, Great Britain, Canada, and elsewhere, however, start significantly earlier than 8 a.m., leading to wake times that range from about 6:00 a.m. to 7:00 a.m. (Figure 48-1).[25–27]

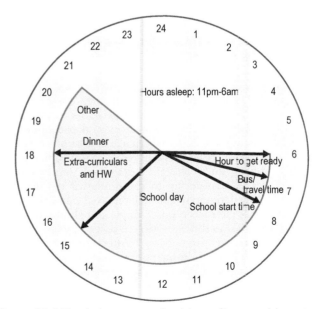

FIGURE 48-1 This clock represents a breakdown of how an adolescent may spend the 24 hours of his or her day. The orange pie shape represents the hours spent awake, while the blue signifies hours spent asleep, compared with the recommended 9.2 hours. The overlap shows the difference in hours of sleep lost when school start time is earlier than recommended by research.

Due largely to early wake times and delayed bedtimes on school days, adolescents tend to report increasingly less sleep during the week over the middle and high school years. Time in bed ranges from as little as 5 to closer to 8 hours, with older adolescents reporting less time in bed than younger adolescents.[3,24,28,29] In striking contrast to self-report studies, laboratory-based research reveals that older adolescents may need the same amount or even more sleep in comparison to their younger early adolescent peers.[8,12,30,31]

In Carskadon and colleagues' landmark research, now known as the *Stanford Sleep Camp* study, pre- and early adolescents, ages 10 to 12, were assessed during three consecutive summers.[31] Participants were given the opportunity to sleep for a maximum of 10 hours (10 p.m.–8 a.m.) while in the laboratory for three consecutive nights. Using polysomnographic (PSG) recordings, Carskadon and colleagues found that the amount of time spent asleep during these 10 hours remained constant across puberty stages (Tanner stages 1–5), and averaged 9.2 hours.[31] In fact, if anything, it was the older and more mature adolescents who needed to be awakened after 10 hours, suggesting that they may have slept longer if given the opportunity.

Research suggests that many adolescents attempt to make up for insufficient school-night sleep by oversleeping on the weekend. Time in bed averages about 0.5 to 2.5 hours more on weekend compared to school nights, and this disparity increases from ages 14 to 18.[3,24,32,33] Likewise, most adolescents typically delay going to sleep about 1 to 2 hours on weekends in comparison to school nights, and extend their sleep period by waking 1 to 4 hours later on weekends. Self-reported bedtimes characteristically range from about 10:30 p.m. to midnight or later on weekend nights, and weekend wake times typically range between 9 and 10 a.m. or later on weekend mornings, with older adolescents reporting later sleep–wake schedules than their younger siblings and friends.[3,22,32,33]

DEVELOPMENTAL CHANGES TO SLEEP/WAKE REGULATORY SYSTEMS

The adolescent's circadian system also undergoes significant developmental changes.[11,34] In self-report, questionnaire-based studies, more advanced pubertal status is associated with owl-like preferences, and laboratory studies demonstrate that more mature adolescents experience later onset and offset melatonin secretion or what is referred to as a circadian phase delay.[7,11,35] Sadeh and colleagues examined developmental sleep changes in relationship to the timing of the onset of puberty.[36] Using actigraphy and self-reported pubertal status, they found that later sleep onset times and shortened sleep times emerge prior to the expression of secondary sexual characteristics associated with puberty.[36] Alterations to the sleep–wake regulatory systems during puberty seem to allow mature adolescents to stay awake later at night to finish their favorite You-Tube or Netflix video or to text message a few more friends, while their younger and less mature peers are more likely to fall asleep more easily. As a result, it is more difficult for adolescents to fall asleep and awaken early compared to their elementary school or pre-adolescent-aged friends and siblings. Parents might experience this as the 'sleep-over' problem. In other words, it is easier for older adolescents to

act like they can remain alert after a late night sleepover, whereas younger, middle school-aged adolescents cannot function following a sleepover. This pronounced sleep debt leads to school absenteeism and tardiness, daytime sleepiness, emotion regulation difficulties, and academic struggles.[3,5,28,37] Moreover, adolescents perhaps compensating for sleep loss with increased caffeine and stimulant use or drug use and abuse.[38–41] There is little doubt that adolescents are getting insufficient and inconsistent sleep, with clear negative implications for physical and emotional well-being, academic performance, and other daytime behaviors and activities.

Environmental constraints and lifestyle decisions including family socioeconomic status, substance use, after-school employment hours, and high-tech use further exacerbate and interfere with many adolescents' ability to obtain sufficient sleep or to maintain a regular sleep–wake schedule.[3,14,22,40,42–44] Undoubtedly, the biological delay in sleep onset and the social pressures of the teen years in combination with the need to arise early in the morning for school easily creates a situation in which the adolescent chronically obtains inadequate sleep. Extracurricular activities and technology use may be more or less under an adolescent's control; however, the determination of high school and middle school start times is not in their hands.

MEETING ADOLESCENTS' SLEEP NEEDS: DELAYING SCHOOL START TIMES

Minimal research exists to explain why high schools historically start earliest, followed by middle schools, and why elementary schools traditionally start the latest.[25] High school start times across the United States have been informally and formally surveyed. One pilot study compared data over the period of 1975–1996 for 59 early-starting (before 8:00 a.m.) and late-starting (8:00 a.m. and later) high schools. Early-starting schools maintained their early schedules over the 20-year time period.[45] A sampling of 1996–1997 school year schedules posted on the Internet from 40 high schools throughout the United States found that 48% had start times of 7:30 a.m. or earlier, with only 12% starting between 8:15 and 8:55 a.m.[44] Another assessment of 50 high schools from around the country for the 2001–2002 school year found 35% of schools posted start times before 7:30 a.m. and 16% between 8:15 and 8:55 a.m.[46] Ten years later, in a 2012 web-based sampling of 50 high schools' school year bell schedules, 40% of the high schools still listed start times for before 7:30 a.m., with 10% of the high schools listing 8:15–9:00 a.m. as their 2012–2013 school start times. In comparison, a sampling of 50 middle schools' 2012–2013 schedules revealed that 14% set start times for 7:30 a.m. or earlier, with 20% starting between 8:15 and 8:55 a.m. Previously, Wolfson and Carskadon conducted a comprehensive analysis of factors that contributed significantly to the determination of high school start times and whether these times changed across the decades.[25] Over 4000 public high schools, representing 10% of public high schools in the United States, were randomly selected from the National Center for Education Statistics' online database and asked to complete a brief survey regarding the pattern of school schedules and student demographics. Additionally, schools were asked about whether or not they had considered changing the school start times and perceived barriers to making the change. Results indicated that, on average, school start and end times did not change across the 15-year span from 1986–1987 to 2001–2002 (mean=7:55 a.m.); however, early-starting schools reported increasingly earlier starting times over this period, whereas late-starting schools reported increasingly delayed bell schedules.[25] Factors associated with earlier start times were higher socioeconomic status, urban environment, and larger student populations with busing systems that operate multiple routes at different times each day.[25]

Research on the impact of delaying the start time of middle and high schools for adolescents' sleep and daytime functioning is discussed below.

In a now hallmark school transition study, Carskadon and colleagues assessed the impact of a 65-minute school start time advance across the transition from 9th grade (8:25 a.m.) to 10th grade (7:20 a.m.) for 40 14–16-year-olds attending a suburban, public school in the northeastern part of the US.[7] In the spring of 9th and fall of 10th grades, assessments involved 2 weeks of actigraphy and sleep–wake diaries and an overnight laboratory evaluation that included dim light salivary melatonin and the Multiple Sleep Latency Test (MSLT). Actigraphic sleep records demonstrated that just over 60% of the 9th-graders and fewer than 50% of the 10th-graders obtained an average of 7 hours or more of sleep on school nights, and they awakened significantly earlier on school mornings, obtained less sleep, yet they did not go to sleep earlier in 10th than in 9th grade. In 10th grade, students' DLSMO phase was significantly later and they also displayed atypical sleep patterns on the MSLT. For example, they fell asleep faster in 10th versus 9th grade, and about 50% of the 10th-graders experienced at least one REM sleep episode on the MSLT. Transitioning to an earlier school start time from 9th to 10th grade was associated with insufficient sleep and daytime sleepiness that is ordinarily seen in narcolepsy.[47]

Since the 1990s, researchers have examined the effects of school start times on adolescents' sleep patterns and daytime functioning. Allen demonstrated that students from early- compared to late–starting schools reported shorter sleep times and a longer sleep phase delay.[48] His own follow-up study indicated that students at an earlier-starting school (7:40 a.m.) slept less on school nights and woke up later on weekends than students at a later-starting school (8:30 a.m.).[49] Moreover, later weekend bedtimes were associated with poorer grades in all students, with a higher percentage of students with 'average grades' reporting bedtimes after 2:30 a.m. in comparison to students who reported the highest grades. Another study that examined early-starting schools (7:20 a.m.) versus late (9:30 a.m.) found that students at both schools reported similar bedtimes, but students at the earlier-starting schools had shorter total sleep times and more irregular sleep schedules, which were also associated with poorer grades.[50]

Struck by Carskadon and colleagues' laboratory school transition study, Wahlstrom and colleagues conducted a large-scale, convenience study in Minneapolis, Minnesota.[5,7] Over 18 000 high school students in the Minneapolis School District were evaluated before and after the district delayed its high school start times from 7:15 a.m. to 8:40 a.m. beginning with the 1997–1998 school year.[5,27] Wahlstrom and colleagues found the following: (1) attendance rates for students in grades 9 through 11 improved; (2) the percentage of high

school students continuously enrolled in the district or the same school increased; (3) grades showed a slight but not statistically significant improvement; and (4) high school students, themselves, reported bedtimes similar to students in schools that did not change start times, obtaining nearly 1 hour more of sleep on school nights during the 1999–2000 school year.[5,27] Similarly, Dexter and colleagues compared 10th- and 11th-graders attending late versus early-starting public high schools in the Midwest and found that adolescents at the late-starting high school reported more sleep and less daytime sleepiness as measured by the Epworth Sleepiness Scale.[51] Htwe and colleagues surveyed high school students before and after their New England public school district delayed school start times from 7:35 to 8:15 a.m.[52] As in previous studies, students reported sleeping, on average, 35 additional minutes and experienced less daytime sleepiness with the delayed high school start time.[52]

In a more recent study of 9th through 12th-graders at a private high school that instituted a 30-minute delay (from 8 to 8:30am), mean self-reported school night sleep duration increased by 45 minutes and mean bedtimes advanced by 18 minutes.[4] The percentage of students getting less than 7 hours of sleep decreased by nearly 80% and those reporting at least 8 hours of sleep increased from 16% to 55%. Owens and colleagues also found that students reported significantly more satisfaction with their sleep, improved motivation as well as less daytime sleepiness, fatigue, and depressed mood following the delayed school start time.[4] Health-related variables such as health center visits for fatigue-related complaints and class attendance also improved.[4]

Research on the impact of early versus delayed school start times for early adolescents has demonstrated strikingly similar findings. Specifically, 7th and 8th-graders at a later-starting urban middle school (8:37 a.m.) reported less tardiness, less daytime sleepiness, better academic performance (especially the 8th-graders), more school-night total sleep, and later rise times in comparison to middle school students at an earlier-starting school (7:15 a.m.) in the same district.[26] A pilot study of 116 5th and 6th-graders attending early (7:45 a.m.) versus late (8:25 a.m.) starting elementary schools from the same large, urban New England district mentioned above found that students at the later-starting school reported later rise times, more sleep, and less daytime sleepiness than their pre- and early adolescent peers at the earlier-starting school.[21] Likewise, Epstein and colleagues' study of 811 10–12-year-olds from 18 Israeli schools with starting times that ranged from 7:10 to 8:30 a.m. demonstrated the importance of delaying school start times for pre- and early adolescents.[53] Nearly 15 years ago, they compared schools that started at least 2 days per week at 7:15 a.m. or earlier with schools that started regularly at 8:00 a.m. Based on self-report, the pre- and early adolescents attending the early-starting schools obtained significantly less sleep (8.7 vs. 9.1 hours), complained more of daytime sleepiness, dozed off in class more often, and reported more attention and concentration difficulties than the students at the later-starting schools.[53] Using an experimental design, Lufi and colleagues examined the impact of delaying middle school start time by 1 hour on sleep duration and attention in two groups of 14-year-olds.[2] The experimental group was on a delayed schedule for 1 week and back on the original schedule for the second week of the study, while the control group kept their regular schedule for the 2 weeks.[2]

Participants' sleep was estimated using actigraphy and attention was measured with two different measures of attention. In keeping with previous studies, during the delayed condition, the experimental group of middle schoolers slept nearly an hour longer and they performed better than the comparison group on tests requiring attention beyond practice effects.[2] Undoubtedly, delaying the start of middle school allows early adolescents to obtain sufficient sleep and to perform better in school, similar to their older, high-school-aged peers.

COMPLEMENTARY BENEFITS OF LATER HIGH SCHOOL START TIMES

With adolescents and emerging adults at particular risk for sleepy driver and *fall asleep at the wheel* motor vehicle accidents, researchers have also assessed the effects of delayed high school start times on sleep patterns and automobile accidents.[54–56] Danner and Phillips queried middle school and high-school-aged students in a school district that delayed high school start times by 1 hour (7:30 to 8:30 a.m.) from one school year to the next, keeping middle school start times the same.[53] Similar to the studies discussed above, after delaying high school start times by 1 hour, students averaged from 12 minutes (grade 9) to 30 minutes (grade 12) more self-reported nightly sleep. Students who got at least 8 hours of sleep prior to the start time change increased from 37% to 50% and those who got 9 hours increased from 6.3% to 10.8%.[53] Moreover, average additional weekend sleep decreased from nearly 2 hours to 1 hour when start times were delayed, suggesting that the adolescents were getting insufficient sleep and needed to catch up on sleep under the earlier school start time schedule.[54] These researchers also examined the automobile accident records for the 17–18-year-olds. Separate accident rates were computed for the county that changed high school start times and for the state as a whole with crash rates computed for the 2 years prior to the school start change through 2 years following the school start change. Analyses revealed a decrease of 16.5% in the 2 years following the school start time delay; however, there was a significant increase of 7.8% across the same time period for the rest of the state. Similarly, Vorona and colleagues compared neighboring cities' teen driver crash rates where one school district's high school start times were 75 to 80 minutes earlier.[56] The city with the earlier high school start times reported significantly higher teen crash rates with teen drivers' accident peaks occurring 1 hour earlier in the morning in the city with earlier high school start times.[55] Taken together, these studies document a troubling consequence of early school start times and insufficient sleep – drowsy driving.[54,56] However, these studies didn't utilize individual-level data, making it difficult to draw reliable conclusions. Future studies should clarify which aspects of adolescents' insufficient sleep and/or circadian timing contribute to drowsy driving and fall-asleep motor vehicle accidents.

Clinkinbeard and colleagues examined sleep deprivation and crime rates in adolescents.[57] Sleep deprivation was positively associated with the amount of violent and property crime in the sample of adolescents.[57] Sleeping just 1 hour less (7 hours) than the recommended reference group (8–10 hours of sleep) contributed to an increased likelihood of property delinquency, and the effect increased for each hour of sleep

loss. The hours immediately after school release times had the highest rates of juvenile crime, suggesting that delayed school end times may lead to some reduction in crime.[58]

Furthermore, economic and education policy researchers have recently examined data surrounding school start times and academic achievement in an effort to construct a cost-benefit ratio for later start times.[59–61] In the Hamilton Report,[59] economists calculated a 9:1 benefit-to-cost ratio for later start times. They utilized studies conducted by Carrell and colleagues and Edwards to show that delaying start times by 1 hour might increase test scores by an average of 0.175 standard deviations.[60,61] In particular, Carrell and colleagues examined first-year Air Force Academy students who keep varying regimented schedules and complete standardized assessment examinations and found that students beginning classes before 8:00 a.m. performed the poorest in all of their courses.[60] A 1-hour delay corresponded to a 0.5 standard deviation increase in performance.[60] Edwards found that Wake County, North Carolina, middle school students who started school 1 hour later experienced a 2.2 percentile increase in their standardized math test scores and a 1.5 percentile increase in reading, on average, with increased benefits for disadvantaged students.[61] Starting school 1 hour later had further benefits, including less television viewing per day, more time devoted to homework per week, and fewer absences.[61] At the district level, transportation costs for changing school start times were estimated based on recent research to range from $0 to $1950 per student over their entire school career, putting the benefit to cost ratio at a minimum of 9:1.[59–61]

In addition, delaying middle and high school start times might have particular benefits for adolescents from lower socioeconomic status (SES) backgrounds. In Marco and colleagues' study of seventh-graders in an urban school district where middle schools started at 8:37 a.m., the timing and consistency of actigraphically estimated school- and weekend-night sleep were associated with demographic, behavioral, and neighborhood aspects of SES.[22] In other words, early adolescents from lower SES backgrounds obtained less sleep and had more erratic sleep–wake schedules than their peers from higher SES families. As noted, the adolescents in this study attended schools with relatively late school start times (8:37 a.m.) in comparison to middle schools throughout the United States.[25] As Marco and colleagues discuss, if these seventh-graders had to get to an early-starting middle school, it is likely that their sleep would be further disadvantaged, as suggested by a study by Wolfson et al. in the same school district.[22,26] Because insufficient and inconsistent sleep patterns place young adolescents at greater risk for behavioral disorders, academic difficulties, and physical illness, the findings of this study strengthen the concern regarding the negative ramifications of early-starting schools for adolescents, especially those from lower SES households.[20,22,23]

All together, it is clear that when schools designed for adolescents carefully consider the start time of school, middle- and high-school-aged students obtain more sleep and behavioral well-being and academic performance improves. Contrary to earlier questions and concerns, students obtain more sleep due to later school morning rise times and bedtimes remain fairly consistent. Overall, adolescents at later-starting schools also report less daytime sleepiness, decreased tardiness, better academic performance, improvement on other daytime functioning factors.

TRIALS AND TRIBULATIONS WITH CHANGING POLICIES TO DELAY SCHOOL START TIMES

The numerous studies discussed throughout in this chapter document how school-night sleep time is drastically reduced because of early school start times.[3,5,7,8] Additionally, the problem has intensified as schools' start times have drifted to earlier times over at least the past 25 years.[25] Despite the substantial evidence that delaying school start time is beneficial for adolescents, a seemingly simple quick fix actually presents a complicated and sometimes controversial situation for many communities.[62] School districts and communities are faced with a number of opportunities and challenges when working to delay school start times for middle- and high-school-aged adolescents. Because schools and school districts usually make policy decisions based on historical precedent, and districts typically have the natural tendency to resist change, it makes it that much more difficult for the logical, research-based argument to prevail.[63,64] Individual communities must assess their priorities because, without parental and school cooperation, changes are very difficult to implement, even when clear, positive outcomes have been demonstrated.[62,65]

The barriers to changing school start times largely stem from the diverse groups within a community affected by school scheduling. From teachers, administrators, and staff to custodial, transportation, and food service employees, before and after school childcare staff, and local businesses that employ students, school districts and the schools, themselves, need to consider a range of constituents and stakeholders when making system-wide decisions.[4,63] As stated in Wolfson and Carskadon's analysis of the factors significantly contributing to the determination of high school start times, earlier start times were associated with higher socioeconomic status, urban environment, and larger student populations with a greater number of bus tiers in the transportation systems.[25] For example, a three-tier transportation system means that the elementary-, middle-, and high-school-level buses are staggered to start and end at different times, coordinating so that one bus can run three separate routes instead of three buses running one each.[66] One large school district in Fort Worth, Texas, created a committee of transportation partners and school officials to gather information about transportation tiers, including routes, schedules, and school start times, to best meet the needs of the entire district.[66] They arranged that the high school buses run on the latest fleet of buses to accommodate this student body's sleep patterns and have tried to accommodate after-school sports and work schedules as well.[66]

The long-standing belief that high schools should start the earliest has become engrained in many school districts; despite what the research clearly demonstrates.[63] Public opinion remains divided over whether or not different types of tiered scheduling are efficient and necessary.[63] However, Wahlstrom found that both suburban and urban school districts are able to implement delayed high school start times without impacting transportation budgets.[64] Nevertheless, one of the primary parental concerns is before and after school childcare costs and questions about elementary school-aged children's sleep needs and schedules if middle and high school start times are delayed.[4,63] Also, for those working parents who rely on high-school students for childcare, an alternative may be needed with later schedules.

Some coaches and athletic directors argue that delayed high school start times make it difficult to accommodate some after-school sports.[5] A variety of creative solutions to this problem have been proposed previously, such as exempting athletes from physical education requirements and adjusting class schedules so that late dismissal times are minimized.[4,63] If study halls or free periods could be scheduled at the end of the day, it would allow for less delayed participation in a variety of different after-school extracurricular activities. To address certain concerns such as delayed playtime on athletic fields, lights could be installed and transportation schedules could be shifted for the older students.[62,63]

Despite these political and logistical barriers to change, delaying school start times ultimately comes down to school districts appreciating the impact of sufficient sleep on learning, feasibility, and openness to change within a community. Previously, research on the impact of delaying school start times was not systematic; however, as discussed throughout this chapter, a significant number of studies demonstrate the clear, positive impact on adolescents' sleep and daytime functioning.[4,26,64]

On a national level in the United States, a small number of politicians have taken on school start times. For example, California's US Representative Zoe Lofgren recently reintroduced a bill in Congress called the 'Zs to As' Act (H.Con. Res. 176–111th Congress Zzz's to A's Resolution, 2009).[67] As an incentive, this bill would allow school districts considering later school times to apply to the federal government for grants of up to $25 000.[67] At a national, community-organizing level, a petition was brought to Congress during the 2012 National Sleep Awareness Week arguing that US public schools should not start before 8 a.m. *Start School Later* is a group of health professionals, educators, and researchers committed to raising public awareness about ensuring health and safety through proper sleep and school hours.[68] Their mission is to advocate for what the data clearly show about the benefits of later start times, and one of the goals is to support school communities striving to implement these changes.[68]

Undoubtedly, local, national, and international-level advocacy is required to bring about creative school start time solutions. To stress the urgency of the problem, community stakeholders need to be fully informed of the scientific rationale that supports the benefits of delaying school start times. Education on the merits of delaying school start times and about adolescents' sleep needs is key to working with school districts on changing school start times.[64] For example, sleep-smart techniques need to be added to health and science curriculums in order to teach adolescents about sleep and healthy sleep hygiene practices.[22] Sleep needs to be valued as much as diet and exercise for maintaining good health. Studies have demonstrated that insufficient sleep may be a screening indicator for poor overall health.[69] For example, appropriate caffeine and high-tech use in relationship to sleep may not be obvious.[14,40] Adolescents need to be taught how caffeinated drinks in the hours before bedtime further delay sleep onset and, in particular, to stay away from the dangers associated with excessive energy drink usage, such as caffeine dependence and using caffeine to get through the day.[14,40] Healthcare providers including pediatricians, family medicine physicians, nurses, physicians assistants, psychologists, and social workers can begin to play a significant role in advocating and working with educators so that schools start at times that are best for adolescents' health and academic endeavors.

FUTURE DIRECTIONS AND RECOMMENDATIONS

1. Pediatricians should educate adolescents and parents regarding the optimal amount of sleep teens need to match physiologic sleep needs (8.5 to 9.5 hours). While napping, extending sleep on weekends and caffeine consumption can temporarily counteract sleepiness, these actions are not a substitute for consistent sufficient sleep.
2. Healthcare professionals should educate themselves on adolescent sleep needs and educate parents, teens, teachers, education administrators, athletic coaches, and others about the biological and environmental factors, including early school start times, which contribute insufficient sleep for adolescents.
3. Pediatricians and other healthcare providers should educate school administrators, PTAs, and school boards about the benefits of delaying school start times as a cost-effective countermeasure to adolescent sleep deprivation.
4. Pediatricians and other healthcare professionals should provide research, evidence-based rationales, guidance, and support in their communities to school districts contemplating delaying school start times in schools that educate adolescents.
5. Researchers, partnering with communities and school districts, need to continue to collect data on the impact of delayed school start times and other countermeasures on adolescents' sleep and overall well-being in order to insure that developing adolescents obtain adequate sleep and, in turn, do their best academically and in other facets of their lives.

SUMMARY

In conclusion, insufficient sleep in children and adolescents should be treated as a public health concern. With school start times being the main determinant of wake times and, therefore, significantly contributing to adolescents' average sleep duration, school districts, educators, healthcare providers, parents, and adolescents, themselves, should advocate for delaying school start times as a countermeasure, along with interventions at the individual level such as improving sleep hygiene.[4,26] Administrators considering a shift to a later school start time are advised to initiate a district-wide assessment on start times, varying scheduling options, decreasing nightly homework hours, and instituting sleep education into the curriculum.[26] Schools are systems of highly choreographed activities and therefore many different fiscal, financial, psychological, and logistical factors must be taken into account, as one solution does not fit all.[63,64] As discussed in this chapter, however, research clearly demonstrates that later school start times allow adolescents to obtain sufficient sleep and, in so doing, do better in school and in their daily lives.[1,2,21]

Healthcare providers can initiate positive behavior changes by educating adolescents and their parents about sleep needs, and by serving as ambassadors in their communities.[63] Pediatricians and other healthcare providers who work closely with children and adolescents can reinforce what is known from the research by passing the information along to families, and encouraging parents and teens, themselves, to be advocates for change in their communities. Sleep medicine professionals can help adolescents and their parents assess the etiology of

problems such as excessive daytime sleepiness and whether their sleep concerns are due to a sleep disorder versus inadequate sleep due to early middle and high school start times.

Clinical Pearls

- The assessment of the child or adolescent with sleep problems should include a review of how the child is doing at school.
- Accommodations such as the availability of nap rooms, or changing a child's schedule can help a child or teen who has sleep problems to succeed in school.
- Delaying the start time of middle and high schools allows adolescents to obtain adequate sleep throughout the week, along with evidence of improved academic performance and behavior, and are associated with improved health and mental health outcomes.
- Pediatricians, school and child psychologists, other healthcare professionals, and researchers have the tools and information to educate adolescents, parents, and education administrators concerning evidence-based rationales, guidance, and support for adolescent sleep needs and delaying school start times.

References

1. O'Malley EB, O'Malley MB. School start time and its impact on learning and behavior. In: Ivanenko A, editor. Sleep and psychiatric disorders in children and adolescents. New York: Informa Healthcare; 2008. p. 79–94.
2. Lufi D, Tzischinsky O, Hadar S. Delaying school starting time by one hour: Some effects on attention levels in adolescents. J Clin Sleep Med 2011;7(2):137–43.
3. Wolfson AR, Carskadon MA. Sleep schedules and daytime functioning in adolescents. Soc Res Child Dev 1998;69(4):875–87.
4. Owens JA, Belon K, Moss P. Impact of delaying school start time on adolescent sleep, mood, and behavior. Arch Pediatr Adolescent Med 2010;164(7):608–14.
5. Wahlstrom K. Changing times: findings from the first longitudinal study of later high school start times. NASSP Bulletin 2002;86(633):3–21.
6. Carskadon MA. Evaluation of excessive daytime sleepiness. Clin Neurophysiol 1993;23:91–100.
7. Carskadon MA, Wolfson AR, Acebo C, et al. Adolescent sleep patterns, circadian timing, and sleepiness at a transition to early school days. Sleep 1998;21(8):871–81.
8. Carskadon MA, Acebo C. Regulation of sleepiness in adolescence: Update, insights, and speculation. Sleep 2002;25:606–16.
9. Crowley SJ, Acebo C, Fallone G, et al. Estimating dim light melatonin onset (DLMO) phase in adolescents using summer or school year sleep/wake schedules. Sleep 2006;29(12):1632–41.
10. Carskadon MA, Acebo C, Richardson GS, et al. An approach to studying circadian rhythms of adolescent humans. J Biolog Rhythms 1997;12(3):278–9.
11. Crowley SJ, Acebo C, Carskadon MA. Sleep, circadian rhythms, and delayed phase in adolescence. Sleep Med 2007;8:602–12.
12. Jenni O, Achermann P, Carskadon MA. Homeostatic sleep regulation in adolescents. Sleep 2005;28:1446–54.
13. Taylor DJ, Jenni OG, Acebo C, et al. Sleep tendency during extended wakefulness: insights into adolescent sleep regulation and behavior. J Sleep Res 2005;14:239–44.
14. Calamaro CJ, Mason TBA, Ratcliffe SJ. Adolescents living the 24/7 lifestyle: Effects of caffeine and technology on sleep duration and daytime functioning. Pediatrics 2009;123(6):e1005–10.
15. Dahl RE, Lewin DS. Pathways to adolescent health sleep regulation and behavior. J Adolesc Health 2002;31:175–84.
16. Wolfson AR, Acebo C, Fallone G, et al. Actigraphically-estimated sleep patterns of middle school students. Sleep (Abstract Supplement) 2003;26:313–15.
17. Dohnt HK, Gradisar MS, Short M. Insomnia and its symptoms in adolescents: Comparing DSM-IV and ICSD-II diagnostic criteria. J Clin Sleep Med 2012;(3):295–99.

18. Iglowstein I, Jenni OG, Molinari L, et al. Sleep duration from infancy to adolescence: reference values and generational trends. Pediatrics 2003;111(2):302–7.

19. Thorleifsdottir I, Bjornsson J.K, Benediktsdottir B, et al. Sleep and sleep habits from childhood to young adulthood over a 10-year period. J Psychosomatic Res 2002;53:529–37.

20. Fredriksen K, Rhodes J, Reddy R, et al. Sleepless in Chicago: tracking the effects of adolescent sleep loss during the middle school years. Child Dev 2004;75(1):84–95.

21. Spaulding N, Butler E, Daigle A, et al. Sleep habits and daytime sleepiness in students attending early versus late starting elementary schools. Sleep (Supplement) 2005;28:A78.

22. Marco CA, Wolfson AR, Sparling M, et al. Family socioeconomic status and sleep patterns of young adolescents. Behav Sleep Med 2012;10(1): 70–80.

23. Wolfson AR, Richards M. Young adolescents struggles with insufficient sleep. Sleep and development: familial and socio-cultural considerations. Oxford: Oxford University Press; 2011.

24. National Sleep Foundation. Sleep in America Poll. Teens and Sleep. National Sleep Foundation website; 2006. Available at http://www. sleepfoundation.org/article/sleep-america-polls/2006-teens-and-sleep/ html.

25. Wolfson AR, Carskadon MA. A survey of factors influencing high school start times. NASSP Bulletin 2005;89:47–66.

26. Wolfson AR. Adolescent sleep update: Narrowing the gap between research and practice; 2007. On-line publication: March/April 2007, www.sleepreview-mag.com.

27. Wahlstrom K. Accommodating the sleep patterns of adolescents within current educational structures: An uncharted path. In: Carskadon M, editor. Adolescent sleep patterns: biological, social, and psychological influences. Cambridge, UK: Cambridge University Press; 2002.

28. Carskadon MA. Patterns of sleep and sleepiness in adolescents. Pediatrician 1990;17:5–12.

29. Carskadon MA, Labyak SE, Acebo C, et al. Intrinsic circadian period of adolescent humans measured in conditions of forced desynchrony. Neurosci Lett 2009;260:129–32.

30. Carskadon MA, Harvey K, Duke P, et al. Pubertal changes in daytime sleepiness. Sleep 1980;19:453–60.

31. Carskadon MA, Dement WC. Cumulative effects of sleep restriction on daytime sleepiness. Psychophysiology 1981;18:107–13.

32. Strauch I, Meier B. Sleep need in adolescents: A longitudinal approach. Sleep 1988;11(4):378–86.

33. Szymczak JT, Jasinska M, Pawlak E, et al. Annual and weekly changes in the sleep–wake rhythm of school children. Sleep 1993;16(5): 433–35.

34. Giannotti F, Cortesi F, Sebastiani T, et al. Circadian preference, sleep and daytime behavior in adolescence. J Sleep Res 2002;11:191–9.

35. Yoon C, May CP, Hasher L. Aging, circadian arousal patterns, and cognition. In: Schwarz N, Park D, Knauper B, et al, editors. Aging, cognition and self reports. Washington, DC: Psychological Press; 1999. p. 117–43.

36. Sadeh A, Dahl RE, Shahar G, et al. Sleep and the transition to adolescence: a longitudinal study. Sleep 2009;32(12):1602–9.

37. Wolfson AR, Carskadon MA. Understanding adolescents' sleep patterns and school performance: a critical appraisal. Sleep Med Rev 2003;7(6): 491–506.

38. Cohen-Zion M, Drummond SP, Padula CB, et al. Sleep architecture in adolescent marijuana and alcohol users during acute and extended abstinence. Addict Behav 2009;34(11):976–9.

39. Orbeta RL, Overpeck MD, Ramcharran D, et al. High caffeine intake in adolescents: associations with difficulty sleeping and feeling tired in the morning. J Adolesc Health 2006;38(4):451–3.

40. Ludden AB, Wolfson AR. Understanding adolescent caffeine use: connecting use patterns with expectancies, reasons, and sleep. Health Educ Behav 2010;37(3):330–42.

41. Pollack CP, Bright D. Caffeine consumption and weekly sleep patterns in US seventh, eighth, and ninth graders. Pediatrics 2003;111(1):42–6.

42. Singleton RA Jr, Wolfson AR. Alcohol consumption, sleep, and academic performance among college students. J Stud Alcohol Drugs 2009;0(3): 355–63.

43. Pieters S, Van Der Vorst H, Burk WJ, et al. Puberty-dependent sleep regulation and alcohol use in early-adolescents. Alcohol Clin Exp Res 2010 in press.

44. Wolfson A. Bridging the gap between research and practice: What will adolescents' sleep/wake patterns look like in the 21st century. In: Carskadon MA, editor. Adolescent sleep patterns: Biological, social and psychological influences. New York: Cambridge University Press; 2002. p. 198–219.

45. Carskadon MA, Acebo C. Historical view of high school start time: preliminary results. Sleep 1997;26:184.

46. Acebo C, Wolfson AR. Inadequate sleep in children and adolescents. In: Kushida CA, editor. Sleep deprivation: clinical issues, pharmacology, and sleep loss effects. New York: Marcel Dekker; 2004.

47. Guilleminault C, Anagnos A. Narcolepsy. In: Kryger MH, Roth T, Dement WC, editors. Principles and practice of sleep medicine. 3rd ed. Philadelphia: Saunders; 2000. p. 676–86.

48. Allen RP. School-week sleep lag: Sleep problems with earlier starting of senior high schools. Sleep Res 1991;20:198.

49. Allen R. Social factors associated with the amount of school week sleep lag for seniors in an early starting suburban high school. Sleep Res1992;21:114.

50. Kowalski NA, Allen RP. School sleep lag is less but persists with very late starting high school. Sleep Res 1995;24:124.

51. Dexter D, Bijwardia J, Shilling D, et al. Sleep, sleepiness and school start times: a preliminary study. Wisconsin Med J 2003;102(1):44–6.

52. O'Malley EB, O'Malley MB. School start time and its impact on learning and behavior. In: Ivanenko A, editor. Sleep and psychiatric disorders in children and adolescents. New York, NY: Informa Healthcare; 2008. p. 79–94.

53. Epstein R, Chillag N, Lavie P. Starting times of school: Effects of daytime functioning of fifth-grade children in Israel. Sleep 1998;21(3):250–6.

54. Danner F, Phillips B. Adolescent sleep, school start times, and teen motor vehicle crashes. J Clin Sleep Med 2009;4:533–5.

55. Pack AI, Pack AM, Rodgman D, et al. Characteristics of crashes attributed to the driver having fallen asleep. Accident Anal Prevent 1995;27:769–75.

56. Vorona RD, Szklo-Coxe M, Wu A, et al. Dissimilar teen crash rates in two neighboring southeastern Virginia cities with different high school start times. J Clin Sleep Med 2011;7(2):145–51.

57. Clinkinbeard SS, Simi P, Evans MK, et al. Sleep and delinquency: Does the amount of sleep matter? J Youth Adolesc 2011;40(7):916–30.

58. National Archive of Criminal Justice Data, 2008.

59. Jacob BA, Rockoff JE. Organizing schools to improve student achievement: start times, grade configurations, and teacher assignments . Washington, D.C.: Brookings Institution; 2011.

60. Carrell SE, Maghakian T, West JE. A's from ZZZZ's? The causal effect of school start time on the academic achievement of adolescents. Am Econ J 2011;3(3):62–71.

61. Edwards F. Early to rise: The effect of daily start times on academic performance. Working paper, University of Illinois at Urbana-Champaign. 2011.

62. National Sleep Foundation. Backgrounder: Later School Start Times.' (2011).(http://www.sleepfoundation.org/article/hot-topics/backgrounder-later-school-start-times)

63. Davison CM, Newton L, Brown RS, et al. Systematic review protocol: later school start times for supporting the education, health, and well-being of high school students. The Campbell Collaboration 2011.

64. Wahlstrom K. School start time and sleepy teens. Arch Pediatr Adolesc Med 2010;164(7):676–7.

65. Wolfson AR, O'Malley EB. Sleep-related problems in adolescence and emerging adulthood. In: Morin CE, Espie CA, editors. The Oxford handbook of sleep and sleep disorders. Oxford: Oxford University Press; 2010.

66. 'Eagle Mountain-Saginaw. New School Hours Facts'. http://www. emsisd.com/domain/4

67. H.Con.Res. 176–111th Congress: Zzz's to A's Resolution. 2009. In: GovTrack.us (database of federal legislation) from http://www.govtrack.us/congress/bills/111/hconres176).

68. 'Start School Later – Health, Safety, and Equity in Education'. www .startschoollater.net. Accessed November 1, 2013.

69. Moore M, Kirchner HL, Drotar D, et al. Relationships among sleepiness, sleep time, and psychological functioning in adolescents. J Pediatr Psychol 2009;34(10):1175–83.

SCORING AND ASSESSMENT OF SLEEP AND RELATED PHYSIOLOGICAL EVENTS

Chapter 49 **Polysomnography and MSLT**

Jyoti Krishna

While clinical evaluation alone suffices to make many diagnoses in sleep medicine, it frequently falls upon the sleep laboratory to lend support to clinical suspicions. Studying children in the sleep laboratory poses unique challenges stemming from their smaller size, changing developmental needs and any associated special clinical conditions. These warrant appropriately sized equipment, as well as creativity and diligence in running the test successfully. Moreover, the rules of scoring and interpreting sleep studies are significantly different from those in adults. Further, the pediatric population is a 'moving target,' as it were, since many physiological parameters change even within the pediatric age group as the baby transitions into adulthood. This requires expertise at all levels of care, beginning with technologists and ending with the sleep specialist. This chapter discusses the polysomnogram and multiple sleep latency tests in the context of the child-friendly sleep laboratory.

Polysomnography and MSLT

Jyoti Krishna

INTRODUCTION

Cliched as it may be the wisdom in the art of medical evaluation of the sick lies primarily in a thorough history and clinical examination. The preceding chapters have aptly illustrated the complexities of evaluating the child with sleep disorders in this regard. Thus, the reader will have appreciated that several medical and non-medical conditions can lead to, or, even masquerade as, a sleep disorder. The reverse is certainly true as well. For instance, excessive daytime sleepiness (EDS) may present with depressive symptoms and obstructive sleep apnea syndrome (OSAS) as attention deficit disorder. As in all other branches of medicine, recourse to diagnostic testing is helpful to clarify clinical suspicions and confirm diagnoses. It is now clearly established by several studies that no combination of clinical history and physical examination will reliably distinguish the presence or absence of OSAS in a snoring child.[1-3] This observation illustrates the need for confirmatory diagnostic testing, specifically polysomnography (PSG). Similarly, PSG is required for the diagnosis of rapid eye movement (REM) sleep behavior disorder where the absence of the skeletal muscle atonia normally present during REM sleep is useful to confirm clinical suspicion. Furthermore, the multiple sleep latency test (MSLT) is a standard tool to objectively ascertain the propensity of daytime sleepiness in patients with symptoms suggestive of EDS.

Alternate tools for the evaluation of the child with a sleep disorder do exist. For instance, with respect to the child with suspected OSAS (the commonest indication for PSG), it has been felt that due to a shortage of pediatric sleep testing centers in the United States or for financial reasons, substitute diagnostic tests such as home video monitoring, daytime nap testing, abbreviated sleep studies (such as overnight oximetry and portable home recordings) may be tried.[4] However, the relatively lower predictive values of these tests make them less desirable when compared to the 'gold standard' PSG.[3] Other tools often used in sleep clinics include a variety of sleep logs and questionnaires for sleep habit screening and to evaluate daytime sleepiness or circadian preferences.[5] Actigraphs, which are wrist-watch-sized devices housing accelerometers, sense motion or lack thereof as a measure of rest and activity levels. These activity-reporting data are then useful as surrogate indicators of wake and sleep. Less commonly, HLA-markers as well as cerebrospinal fluid hypocretin levels are used in the evaluation of patients with EDS who are suspected to have narcolepsy.[6,7]

In this chapter, we will discuss the indications and techniques pertaining to PSG and MSLT, with special emphasis on infants and children. Technical details relative to the standards of clinical practice and laboratory space, laboratory protocols, instrumentation, and specific scoring rules are not discussed in detail in this chapter. The reader is directed to the official guidelines set forth in publications by the American Academy of Sleep Medicine (AASM).[8-10] Excellent information on the requirements for maintaining accreditation of sleep diagnostic facilities is also available at the AASM's website (http://www.aasm.net.org/accred_centerstandards.aspx). Furthermore, while the merits and standards of studying childhood sleep disorders in integrated adult and pediatric laboratories versus pediatric specific accredited laboratories is being hotly debated,[11,12] this chapter will simply describe the traditional 'attended in-lab' types of sleep studies in a child-friendly setting.

INDICATIONS FOR POLYSOMNOGRAPHY

By far, the commonest reason for ordering a sleep study is to confirm the suspected diagnosis of OSAS and other types of sleep-related breathing disorders (SRBD) prior to any therapeutic intervention. In recent statements, the American Academy of Pediatrics and the AASM have outlined their positions on the diagnosis and management of OSAS and emphasized that follow-up PSG should be additionally performed after an intervention such as tonsilloadenoidectomy (T&A) in children with persisting symptoms as well as those at high risk for incomplete resolution of OSAS with T&A. Such children include those with severe preoperative OSAS, obesity, craniofacial anomalies impacting the upper airway, certain neurological conditions (e.g., meningomyelocele) and genetic disorders (e.g., Down syndrome). These children may require additional interventions for persisting SRBD such as positive airway pressure (PAP) therapy.[3,13] Evidence is less robust for the use of PSG for suspected SRBD accompanying chronic lower airway diseases such as asthma, cystic fibrosis, pulmonary hypertension, bronchopulmonary dysplasia, or chest wall abnormality such as kyphoscoliosis.[13] Non-respiratory indications for PSG include apparent life-threatening events (ALTE), periodic limb movement disorder (PLMD), REM sleep behavior disorder (RBD) and selected cases of childhood restless legs syndrome (RLS)[14] (Table 49.1).

ORGANIZATION OF SLEEP SERVICES IN THE CONTEXT OF THE SLEEP STUDY

Equipment and Study Timing

While the pediatric sleep study is broadly very similar to its adult counterpart in the scope of the sleep disorders tested,[15] several key differences are worthy of emphasis. Pediatric populations are diverse in age, and any sleep laboratory catering

TABLE 49.1	Respiratory and Non-Respiratory Indications for and against PSG in Children	
	RESPIRATORY	**NON-RESPIRATORY**
Standard indications	To confirm clinically suspected OSAS After T&A in children with mild OSAS pre-operatively only if suspicion of non-resolution remains on clinical follow-up To confirm resolution of OSAS after T&A in children with high pre-operative risk of non-resolution of OSAS following T&A For PAP titration studies for treatment of OSAS	To confirm clinical suspicion of PLMD For evaluation of narcolepsy (in conjunction with MSLT)
Guideline indications	For suspected hypoventilation due to congenital central hypoventilation, neuromuscular, or chest wall disease For selected cases of primary sleep apnea of infancy or ALTE In children being considered for T&A for suspected OSA To monitor for changes in PAP support requirement in growing children, in those with recurrence of symptoms, or those treated with other methods for OSAS	For evaluation of nocturnal phenomena such as non-REM parasomnia, epilepsy or enuresis when there is clinical suspicion of comorbid OSAS or PLMD
Optional indications	To assess response of OSAS to rapid maxillary expansion or oral appliance To titrate non-invasive positive pressure ventilation in breathing disorders other than OSAS To adjust mechanical ventilator settings To assess readiness for decannulation of tracheostomy for sleep related breathing disorder To assess suspected sleep related breathing disorder in certain chronic pulmonary airway, parenchymal, vascular or chest wall conditions	In conjunction with MSLT for hypersomnia other than narcolepsy Utilizing an expanded montage EEG to investigate atypical or dangerous parasomnia behaviors (including RBD) or to distinguish these from suspected seizures To support clinical suspicion of RLS
PSG not recommended	For diagnosis of OSAS using abbreviated duration PSG (Nap study) For titration of oxygen therapy	Sleep related bruxism

Standard, guideline and optional categories reflect patient-care strategy with high, moderate, and conflicting degrees of clinical certainty based on expert opinion or available evidence.
Abbreviations: OSAS, obstructive sleep apnea syndrome; T&A, tonsilloadenoidectomy; PAP, positive airway pressure; ALTE, apparent life-threatening events; PLMD, periodic limb movement disorder; RBD, REM sleep behavior disorder; RLS, restless legs syndrome.

Adapted from Aurora RN, Zak RS, Karippot A, et al; American Academy of Sleep Medicine. Practice parameters for the respiratory indications for polysomnography in children. Sleep. 2011; 34(3):379–88 and Aurora RN, Lamm CI, Zak RS, et al. Practice parameters for the non-respiratory indications for polysomnography and multiple sleep latency testing for children. Sleep. 2012; 35(11):1467–73.

to childhood sleep disorders needs to be equally adept in monitoring a newborn infant as well as an older teenager. It is therefore essential to maintain the equipment to cater to these age groups in the inventory. This applies to the sensors (e.g., nasal cannula) as well as therapy (e.g., interfaces to deliver positive airway pressure).

The study may need to be timed to match the variable sleep times of children at different levels of maturity. Newborns will sleep for substantial periods in the day and planning of daytime PSGs may free up beds at night for the laboratory. Conversely, a delayed testing schedule may be needed to match the teenager apt to present with a circadian phase delay.[16]

Location

While the physical location of the sleep laboratory is typically in an outpatient setting for adults, many pediatric centers do cater to medically complex children within the hospital setting. For example, 'ventilator checks' and tracheotomy decannulation protocols may be safer to run in an inpatient setting. As a result, many exclusively pediatric sleep laboratories are located within the floor space of a pediatric ward. In other instances, mobile equipment capable of running a complete attended sleep study is utilized at bedside within the hospital, while the bulk of the sleep studies are run in an outpatient laboratory setting. Although the clear advantage of in-hospital PSG is the availability of trained on-call staff to respond to emergencies, should such a need arise for the complex medically unstable child, the latter scenario has the distinct potential disadvantage of poor sound and electrical insulation from the ambient hospital environment. Nonetheless, creative ways of

assuring an uninterrupted night (e.g., private room) may be utilized since safety and reassurance of trained back-up is the priority driving a bedside study in such cases.

Friendliness Factor

Perhaps the single most important factor that makes a sleep laboratory worthy of qualifying as a pediatric sleep laboratory is its 'child friendliness factor.' This applies not only to the physical space itself, but also extends most vitally to the friendliness of the technical and non-technical staff. Zaremba and colleagues have described the ingredients of such a setting very well.[17] As soon as they enter the door, the child's experience often begins to shape the likelihood of cooperation. The decor, the friendliness of the reception area and reassuring words, all go a long way in setting the stage. While teens should not be talked down to or patronized, the younger children may need repeated reassurance and gentle handling. Simple language should be used to describe the plan for the night. A 'show and tell' attitude for equipment needs to be borne in mind before the hook-up. The child should understand that the hook-up will be painless ('no ouchies,' 'no needle sticks') and the technologist must not neglect to assure the young patient that all equipment will come off painlessly next morning. A quick little demonstration with an EEG sticker application on a parent (with the child's permission!) may be very reassuring to reinforce this fact as well as to enlist the child's active participation in the process. Younger girls may be excited about wearing 'shiny hair jewelry,' whereas boys may like to hear they will look 'like a space cadet' once they are all hooked up with the EEG electrodes. Asking families to bring their cameras along to take 'cool looking pictures adds to the excitement of 'camping out at the sleep center!'; TV, DVD and other diversions help. The child may need reassurance that their parent will be in the room and that their favorite teddy bear can accompany them to bed (Figure 49-1).

The beds used in the pediatric sleep laboratory have to be configurable to allow for a parent to room-in with the child in their own separate bed. Ability to bring in a crib or toddler bed for the younger patient or substitute these with a full-size bed for the teenager requires adequate planning for storage space for extra beds. Furthermore, beds have to have safety rails for the appropriate cases, and other safety cautions may have to be modified for the child.[18] Finally, easy access to restroom facilities, odor-sealing diaper disposals, and accommodations for wheelchairs or special equipment for the medically challenged child all need to be considered while planning and designing the sleep center.

Pre-Planning the Logistics of the Study

Given the foregoing description, the reader will have appreciated the complexity of the task involved in running a sleep laboratory smoothly. Both equipment and personnel must work together in a situation where the patient may be fearful, anxious or simply unwilling for the procedure. It is perhaps

safe to say that every pediatric sleep laboratory will have a few 'failed studies' for one reason or another from time to time. Barring illness on the day of study which can rarely be predicted, there are many things that can be preempted to increase the likelihood of an optimal outcome.

First, the clinical encounter must clarify if a study is needed at all and articulate the exact clinical question to be answered during the study. This becomes especially important if the laboratory accepts direct referrals from non-sleep physicians. Tailoring the study to the child is highly desirable to prevent or minimize chance of failure. To this effect, information on the child's age, baseline state of health, and nature of sleep issues must be available to the testing laboratory. Usually, accredited laboratories have standardized sleep order sets that ask the appropriate screening questions from ordering physicians.

All orders ideally should be carefully scrutinized by a knowledgeable person in the laboratory to ascertain that the study can be run as directed. For instance, usually one PSG technologist runs two studies at night in most adult settings. This is commonly referred to as 1:2 staffing. In the pediatric setting, however, due to the laborious nature of the task, especially in children with special needs or the younger child, a ratio of 1:1 is often required. Timing of the start of the

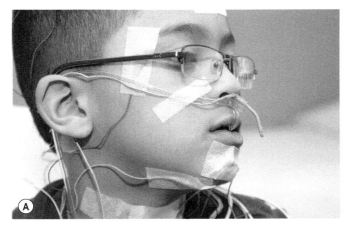

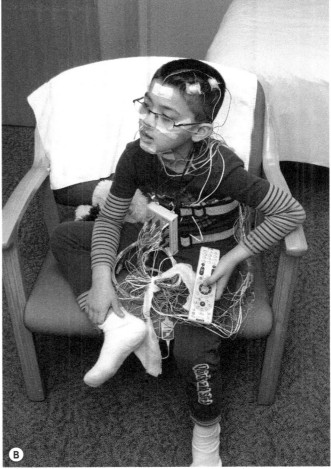

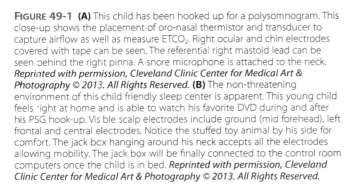

FIGURE 49-1 (A) This child has been hooked up for a polysomnogram. This close-up shows the placement of oro-nasal thermistor and transducer to capture airflow as well as measure ETCO$_2$. Right ocular and chin electrodes covered with tape can be seen. The referential right mastoid lead can be seen behind the right pinna. A snore microphone is attached to the neck. *Reprinted with permission, Cleveland Clinic Center for Medical Art & Photography © 2013. All Rights Reserved.* **(B)** The non-threatening environment of this child friendly sleep center is apparent. This young child feels right at home and is able to watch his favorite DVD during and after his PSG hook-up. Visible scalp electrodes include ground (mid forehead), left frontal and central electrodes. Notice the stuffed toy animal by his side for comfort. The jack box hanging around his neck accepts all the electrodes allowing mobility. The jack box will be finally connected to the control room computers once the child is in bed. *Reprinted with permission, Cleveland Clinic Center for Medical Art & Photography © 2013. All Rights Reserved.*

PSG ('lights out') will be very different for a toddler versus a teenager who sleeps late, or a patient who is traveling multiple time zones to a referral center. Furthermore, sleep technologists often come with prior training in other fields. The supervising technologist will use this knowledge to ensure that the sleep technologist assigned to run any particular study is matched to the clinical need. Thus, a technologist with a respiratory therapy background may be more suited to run a 'ventilator check' while the child with complex parasomnia with suspected seizure disorder may be the forte of the EEG-trained technologist. For 1:2 staffing, the anticipated 'easy hook-up' may be paired with a 'tough hook-up,' or the early 'lights out' study be matched with a late sleeper to allow the technologist time to accomplish the studies on both patients more comfortably.

Preparing the Family for the Sleep Study

Any visit to the doctor is an anxiety-provoking experience for the child and the family. For most, the sleep study is a novel experience. Therefore, seeds for a successful study are best planted during the clinical visit. Careful explanation of the reason for the study and the types of sensors and their importance are crucial to enlist patient and parental cooperation during the PSG. For instance, while most children dislike the nasal cannula, a partnership with the parents helps provide reassurance to the child and transmits the expectation to keep the device on. Similar considerations apply to the other sensors as well. An informed parent is the technologist's best ally when struggling with an uncooperative child at night. The use of sedation to accomplish the PSG is not recommended, and adverse events have been reported in children with OSA.[19] Accordingly, the family may benefit from touring the laboratory a few days prior to the test night. This approach not only reduces anxiety, but also helps the parents and child to plan what clothing, personal effects, or entertainment items to bring along in their overnight bags to make the child comfortable at night. Besides, they get an opportunity to see the sleeping options for the accompanying parent.

The importance of maintaining a sleep schedule leading up to the sleep study should be discussed to avoid, for instance, that late-night party on Friday and consequently a non-representative study night on Saturday. Similarly, a late afternoon nap may delay sleep onset at night significantly. Parents should also be advised to reschedule the PSG if the child is sick. An acute upper airway infection may compromise the accuracy of OSAS diagnosis. Medications that may affect the sleep study should be discussed and an adequate wash-out period should be allocated prior to the sleep study. This is especially true if an MSLT study is to follow the next day, since several medications are known to compromise the quality of the MSLT by direct or withdrawal–rebound effect on the sleep architecture.[9]

RUNNING THE POLYSOMNOGRAM

The PSG Montage

The standard overnight PSG measures sleep parameters utilizing limited electroencephalogram (EEG), electrooculogram (EOG), chin and leg electromyogram (EMG), electrocardiogram (EKG), respiratory effort at the chest and abdomen via respiratory inductance plethysmographic (RIP)

belts, pulse oximetry, capnometry via end-tidal or transcutaneous measurement ($ETCO_2$, $TcpCO_2$), and oro-nasal airflow via pressure transducer and thermistor (see Figure 49-1A and B).

The EEG electrode placement is based on an imaginary grid on the head measured in a standard fashion using the widely accepted 10–20 system.[20] While specialized sleep centers may occasionally utilize the more extensive EEG montage essential for seizure diagnosis, only frontal (F), central (C), occipital (O) and eye (E) exploring electrodes are used to capture EEG and EOG data during the standard PSG. These are referenced to the contralateral mastoid (M) electrode on either side. Standardized numbering of these electrodes is based on location (e.g., C3, C4) with odd numbers represented on the left side by convention (Figure 49-2). EOG leads help monitor rapid eye movements (REM) of dream sleep (Figure 49-3). When combined with EMG

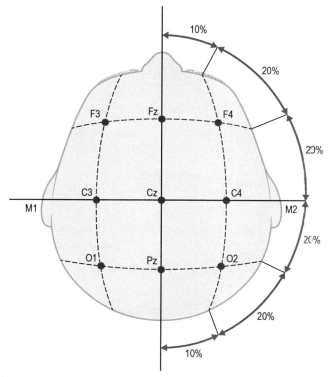

FIGURE 49-2 The International 10–20 system of electrode placement utilizes bony landmarks on the skull to delineate an imaginary grid which is numbered using standard nomenclature as shown. Measurements are made as a fraction of the total head circumference. See text for details. *Reprinted with permission, Cleveland Clinic Center for Medical Art & Photography © 2013. All Rights Reserved.*

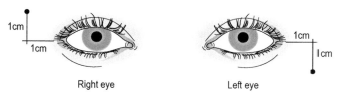

FIGURE 49-3 Recommended placement of ocular leads. The distances may be halved for younger children. *Reprinted with permission, Cleveland Clinic Center for Medical Art & Photography © 2013. All Rights Reserved.*

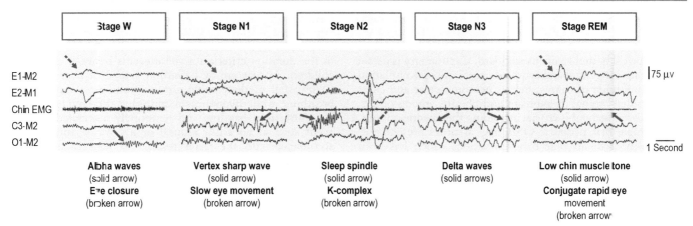

Stage W	Stage N1	Stage N2	Stage N3	Stage REM

E1-M2
E2-M1
Chin EMG
C3-M2
O1-M2

75 µv

1 Second

Alpha waves
(solid arrow)
Eye closure
(broken arrow)

Vertex sharp wave
(solid arrow)
Slow eye movement
(broken arrow)

Sleep spindle
(solid arrow)
K-complex
(broken arrow)

Delta waves
(solid arrows)

Low chin muscle tone
(solid arrow)
Conjugate rapid eye movement
(broken arrow)

FIGURE 49-4 This composite illustrates key features of various sleep stages using standard PSG electrodes. See text for details. *Taken from Krishna J, Foldvary-Schaefer N, Budur K. Introduction to the sleep laboratory. In Foldvary-Schaefer N, Krishna J, Budur K, eds. A Case A Week – Sleep disorders from the Cleveland Clinic; pp. 19; fig. 12.4. By permission of Oxford University Press; 2010.*

data from chin leads, these channels allow for the scoring of sleep and wake into several stages (Figure 49-4). Each stage has several key characteristics that are well described elsewhere.[8] Briefly, stage Wake shows some eye movements, persistent EMG tone in the chin, and age-appropriate dominant posterior rhythm in the occipital leads when the eyes are closed. Stage N1 is characterized by slow rolling eye movements and vertex sharp waves in the central leads. This gives way to sleep spindles and K-complexes characteristic of stage N2 as sleep progresses. Stage N3 is the deepest stage of sleep and comprises abundant delta waves which are 0.5–2 Hz in frequency and 75 µV in amplitude. Stage REM is scored when rapid eye movements are seen alongside mixed-frequency low-voltage EEG and importantly, a low EMG tone. Saw-tooth waves are characteristic as well. Thus, Wake, N1, N2, N3, and REM sleep stages can be scored throughout the sleep record. The EEG and EMG are also used to score arousals which are defined as 3 second long EEG frequency shifts in any sleep stage. There needs to be an accompanying EMG increase in REM stage, however. Arousals in turn are also of importance in the scoring of hypopneas.[21]

A special case is made for stage scoring of very young infants. Here, due to the normal maturational delay of several months in the evolution of sleep spindles and K complexes, the scoring is simplified to comprise Active (equivalent of REM sleep), Quiet (equivalent of NREM sleep), and Indeterminate sleep.[22]

Measuring Breathing

Sensors useful for measurement of respiratory status during PSG include the chest and abdominal effort belts, nasal pressure transducer and thermistor (which both measure oro-nasal airflow), as well as instruments to measure gas exchange. Reliability and validity of respiratory event measurement and scoring has been recently reviewed and forms the basis for the current recommendations by the AASM.[23]

Respiratory effort implies that there is a signal from the central neuronal control centers to the motor neurons targeting muscles of respiration to fire. In the normal circumstance, this results in abdominal and thoracic excursion and alternating ingress and egress of air from the upper airway. The absence of airflow from the nose or mouth over a specified duration is termed apnea. It is 'central' in nature if there are no respiratory efforts associated with absent airflow; it is 'obstructive' if there is lack of airflow in the face of continuing efforts to respire.

Respiratory inductance plethysmography (RIP) belts are now the instrument of choice for measuring respiratory effort. Mercury strain gauges and piezoelectric sensor-equipped belts are no longer used. The RIP belts are essentially elastic belts that go around the patient's chest and abdomen. They have a wire woven into the fabric which reliably measures the cross-sectional expansion and contraction of the thorax and abdomen due to the change in self-inductance that the instrument creates. While RIP belts may be calibrated against a known measure of pulmonary volume such as a pneumotachometer, uncalibrated RIP belts are most commonly used in pediatric settings. The direction of these signals can be used to distinguish respiratory paradox which may be a sign of increased respiratory effort, particularly beyond the age of 3 years.[24] Another technology for measuring effort is the esophageal pressure (Pes) catheter. This is considered the most reliable of all in recognizing respiratory effort by detecting intrathoracic respiratory pressure swings. Pes values become negative with inspiration and increasing negativity is expectedly seen with increased upper airway resistance.[25] However, the invasive nature of Pes limits its popularity. Intercostal EMG applied to the lower intercostal region may also be used by some laboratories to capture diaphragmatic and intercostal muscle firing.[26] Airflow is measured by the nasal pressure cannula and the thermistor. The advent of the nasal pressure transducer has provided a reasonable alternative to Pes as well. The nasal pressure cannula is essentially hollow plastic tubing that captures airflow at the nose and mouth. It looks very much like the ubiquitous oxygen cannula used in hospitals. It is connected to a pressure transducer at the other end to generate a signal that is unique in two respects. First, the amplitude of the signal correlates with the size of the breath. Second, the flattened shape of the waveform correlates with airflow resistance.[23] It is the recommended sensor for hypopnea detection while the thermistor is the recommended sensor for apnea detection.

Most cannulae are able to sample $ETCO_2$ as well from one of the nasal ports. $TcpCO_2$ is an alternative. The author's laboratory utilizes both in most studies. Both instruments need to be calibrated against a standard. Capnometry is useful in assessing congenital and acquired causes of hypoventilation from a multitude of causes such as neuromuscular and chest wall disorders, spinal dysraphism and obesity, among others. Thus, this assessment is crucial in guiding therapeutic options. It is notable that pediatric OSA may at times present predominantly with alveolar hypoventilation, which has been termed obstructive hypoventilation.[27,28] In general, alveolar hypoventilation is deemed to be present if more than 25% of the total sleep time is spent with $ETCO_2$ above 50 mmHg.[8,10]

The pulse oximeter is a vital part of the PSG. Finger, toe, and pinna in the older child or the lateral aspect of the young baby's foot are useful sites for application of the sensor. It is essential that the averaging time of the instrument be relatively short (e.g., 3 seconds) to improve responsiveness to changes in oxygenation with each breath.[29] Accuracy of readings may be compromised by a loosely applied sensor, interference from ambient light, motion of the finger or toes, nail polish, artificial nails, hemoglobinopathies such as sickle cell, and peripheral vasoconstriction.[23]

Thus, using the above respiratory sensors, hypopneas, apneas and hypoventilation may be scored (Figure 49-5).

Criteria for scoring are set forth and recently updated.[8,10] Although a detailed discussion is not within the scope of this chapter, it should be noted that there is a critical difference in the duration criteria for these events between adults and children. Apneas are by definition a total or near complete ($\geq$90%) fall of discernable airflow from pre-event baseline breathing, while hypopneas require that the flow be reduced by $\geq$30% from baseline and temporally associated with an event such as an EEG arousal or a $\geq$3% desaturation. In accordance with the faster respiratory rates in childhood, apneas and hypopneas need to be only the equivalent of 'two breaths' in duration before being counted (unlike the 10-second duration for adults). This duration criteria increases to 20 seconds in the case of central apneas unless accompanied by EEG arousals and/or $\geq$3% desaturations (and/or bradycardia in infants), in which case the 'two breaths' rule holds.

Ancillary Channels

Snoring, limb EMG, EKG, video, body position, vagal nerve channel, and pH probe are additional channels utilized in the PSG. Of these, the last two are only used in special circumstances.

Snoring is the hallmark of OSA and its presence implies at least some increased upper airway resistance. It is usually recorded via a microphone attached to the patient's neck and

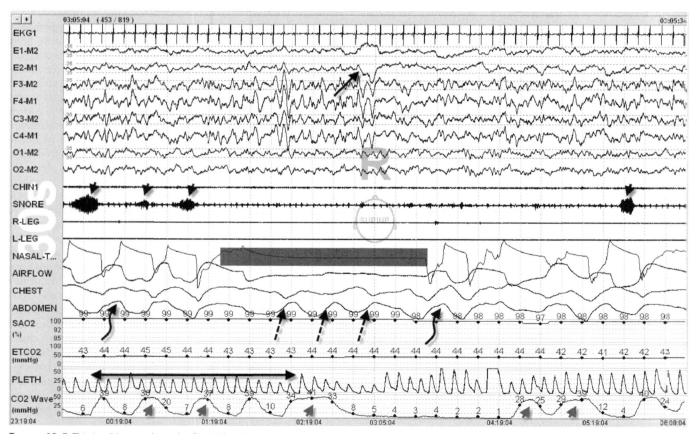

FIGURE 49-5 This is a 30-second epoch of a child in REM sleep showing an obstructive apnea (red bar) with absent flow in both the nasal transducer (Nasal-T) and thermistor (Airflow) channels. Snoring disappears with the onset of the apnea and reappears a few breaths after offset of apnea (black arrowheads). A rapid eye movement (black arrow) is seen in the eye channels. The chest and abdominal RIP belts show paradoxical out-of-phase respirations (broken black arrows) during the apnea indicating distress. Before and after the apnea the belts are in phase (curved arrows). Of note, unlike hypopneas, apnea scoring does not require the presence of arousals or desaturations. The oximeter shows a good plethysmographic signal (double headed arrow), and there is a good plateau in the $ETCO_2$ wave channel (red arrowheads). Both of these features provide reassurance of reliable readings.

displayed as a separate channel in the PSG (see Figure 49-1). Piezoelectric sensors to detect snore vibration in the neck have been used as well.[10] As such, snoring often serves to differentiate central from obstructive events, especially when the efforts channels may be compromised or equivocal. It is also a criterion used to score respiratory effort-related arousals (RERAs), where the fall in airflow is accompanied by an EEG arousal but falls short of meeting the criteria for scoring an apnea or hypopnea.[10]

Leg EMG is useful to score a host of abnormalities of leg movements of sleep including periodic leg movements, hypnagogic foot tremor, and alternating leg muscle activation.[30] Periodic limb movements (PLM), for instance, are scored in a very specific fashion. Each component limb movement begins with an initial EMG amplitude rise of at least 8 µV above the resting baseline. The limb movement is deemed to start at the point where such an increase occurs and ends at a point where the EMG is less than 2 µV above resting baseline. The duration between the start and end points must be at least 0.5 seconds but no more than 10 seconds to be counted as a limb movement. To be counted as a PLM series, there need to be four such movements in succession with 5–90 seconds between each individual limb movement. Such PLM scoring may be supportive of the diagnosis of PLMD or corroborate a clinical suspicion of pediatric RLS.[31] Typically, the anterior tibialis muscle is used to obtain the leg EMG. Rarely, in children, if there is clinical suspicion of absence of the normal REM sleep-related atonia in disorders of dream enactment (RBD), extra limb leads may be useful in the upper limb as well.[32,33]

The EKG is a standard single-channel recording (lead II). It is useful to correlate cardiac dysrhythmia with respiratory events. Sleep-related normative data are available.[34,35] Since EKG artifact can sometimes contaminate the EEG trace, an EKG channel is useful to distinguish this EEG artifact with certainty from true EEG abnormalities such as spikes.

Body position is best scored using real-time video although body position sensors are available as well. Most laboratories have low-light or infra-red cameras which is additionally useful in observing motor phenomena such as parasomnia, bruxing, rhythmic movements of sleep, restless legs, or seizures. OSA is often positional (e.g., worse when supine) and this may be useful knowledge to plan intervention in certain cases.[36] Indeed, occasional insights into sleep-related behaviors such as sleep-onset association disorder, or the use of television or cell phone during the sleep period may be apparent. In the case of neonates where eye closure is important in differentiating sleep from quiet wakefulness, a camera with zoom-in capability is very useful.[22]

Vagal nerve stimulators (VNS) are commonly seen in the pediatric sleep setting in tertiary care centers. It has been noted that their discharge can cause changes in respirations and heart rate and may result in OSA (Figure 49-6). These changes are distinguished by their repetitive nature and a prior knowledge of the setting (firing interval and duration) of the VNS device is useful when interpreting the study.[37]

Esophageal pH probes are used in some centers to test for gastroesophageal reflux (GER) associated with SRBD.[26] In general, the pH probe is not commonly utilized due to its invasive nature, and it is to be further noted that a temporal relationship has not been proven between SRBD and GER episodes.[38] Thus, the AASM does not consider it an essential part of the standard PSG set-up.

Positive airway pressure titration study

Since T&A does not cure OSA in a significant number of cases, an alternative therapeutic recourse often used is PAP therapy.[3,39] Continuous or bi-level PAP (CPAP, BPAP) is the most common mode of delivering this therapy. Before titration can be attempted, however, the child and the family ought to have been educated and prepared to accept the treatment. This implies that, unlike adult studies, PAP titration in children is generally not initiated during a 'split-night' protocol (which refers to initial part-night PSG and subsequent part-night PAP titration). Instead, low pressure, say 5 cmH_2O PAP, is initially empirically chosen after careful mask fitting to habituate the child to the device for several nights at home. Finally, the PAP study is run in a laboratory setting where the goal is to titrate the pressure in various sleep stages and body positions to optimally control the respiratory events.[40] A final prescription pressure is thus obtained.

The montage for PAP titration is very similar to the standard PSG, with the flow measurements obtained from the mask interface rather than nasal cannula or thermistor, and transcutaneous CO_2 measured in lieu of $ETCO_2$.[10] Variations to the use of PSG studies include testing for readiness of tracheotomy decannulation and checking for adequacy of ventilator management.[13,41,42] (see Table 49.1).

THE MSLT

Excessive sleepiness is a common presenting complaint in the pediatric sleep center. Generally speaking, abnormal daytime sleepiness implies the inability to stay alert during the expected waking period and may be accompanied by unanticipated or unintentional periods of sleep.[15] Various disorders may lead to this complaint. Although screening instruments may raise the index of suspicion,[43,44] an accurate history and detailed physical examination are the cornerstone of such diagnoses. The MSLT is frequently employed to confirm clinical suspicion by objectively quantifying and characterizing daytime sleepiness.[45]

The MSLT is mainly indicated for the diagnosis of narcolepsy/idiopathic hypersomnia. It essentially comprises a series of daytime nap tests that is used in conjunction with the PSG. Strict guidelines of conduct including restrictions on stimulants such as caffeine, smoking and exercise need to be followed to maintain the validity of the test. Specific rules are also described for the environment of the study, light exposure, and timing of meals. Furthermore, it is prescribed that certain REM-suppressing medications and stimulants be stopped at least 2 weeks prior to the test to avoid REM rebound or REM suppression. Careful planning is required to avoid sleep deprivation in the several days leading up to the test. Many sleep laboratories require drug screening on the day of the test to ensure substance abuse is not a potential confounder. The AASM has put forth detailed practice parameters describing the indications for this test and its format.[9]

The MSLT typically comprises five nap opportunities given 2 hours apart during the day. The first nap begins 2 hours after the patient rises in the morning following the overnight PSG. Following this awakening, most of the sensors that were used during the PSG are discontinued barring those essential for scoring sleep stages including EEG, EOG, chin

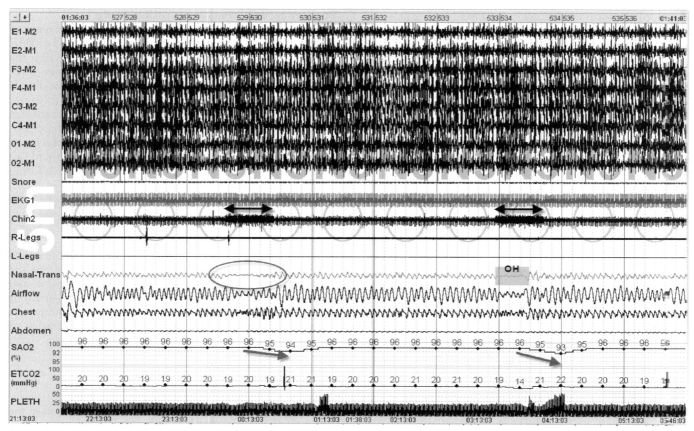

FIGURE 49-6 This child had difficult-to-control epilepsy and had a vagal nerve stimulator (VNS) in place. A PSG was done to screen for breathing disorder associated with her condition. This 5-minute epoch shows VNS discharges occurring every 2 minutes for about 20 seconds each. These are captured on the chin electrode (double-head arrows). Concomitant reduction in oro-nasal airflow is seen (red oval). The chest belt shows continued respiratory efforts. The abdominal belt is not working. The second event (green bar) meets scoring criteria for obstructive hypopnea (OH) due to an associated 3% fall in oxygen saturation (compare red arrows). The end tidal CO_2 reading is unreliable but the plethysmographic signal from the pulse oximeter is robust. The EEG showed florid spikes which are not apparent in this view.

EMG, and EKG. These sensors are kept on for the rest of the day until all five naps are done. Each nap opportunity usually lasts for 20 minutes. However, multiple pediatric laboratories have recommended the use of 30-minute nap opportunities due to the longer normative sleep latency in young prepubertal children.[46,47] At the start of each nap the patient is asked to lie quietly in a comfortable position with eyes closed and instructed to try and fall sleep. The underlying premise is that the sleepier the person, the more likely they are to fall asleep given the chance and conditions to do so. If sleep onset occurs within the assigned 20 minutes, the nap opportunity is extended for an additional 15 minutes to allow other stages of sleep to emerge. Of special interest is the emergence of REM sleep during daytime nap testing. Narcoleptics classically show two or more REM episodes during the five-nap test. Such REM episodes occurring soon after sleep onset are termed sleep-onset REM periods (SOREMPs). If no sleep occurs within the assigned 20 or 30 minutes, the test is terminated. The mean sleep latency is calculated as an arithmetic average of the sleep onset latencies of five naps. SOREMPs are reported as well.

It should be readily evident to the reader that this test has a high likelihood of being confounded by sleep debt, use of medications and drugs, or any disruption of the protocol including extraneous noise in the sleep-testing environment. Motivation may also impact the mean sleep latency.[48] At the risk of being repetitious, it cannot be overemphasized that strict protocol needs to be followed. Given appropriate testing conditions, the MSLT is known to have high test–retest reliability (0.97). Uncertainties arise in using this test in children below the age of 8 years or outside of the standard 8 a.m. to 6 p.m. hours.[15] Challenges may arise in the case of children (especially teenagers) who may have abnormal circadian rhythms in conjunction with a suspicion for an additional intrinsic hypersomnia disorder. Further, compromises are often needed when discontinuation of certain medications is contraindicated or medically problematic.

There are varying opinions about the normative values of the mean sleep latency. There is evidence that mean sleep latency is longer in prepubertal children and reduces by several minutes with advancing Tanner stages.[49] Sometimes, serial MSLT studies may be required in evolving childhood narcolepsy for establishing a definitive diagnosis.[50] Nevertheless, a mean sleep latency of less than 8 minutes and the presence of two SOREMPs support a diagnosis of narcolepsy.[15]

A cautionary note in the interpretation of the adequately run MSLT remains the fact that the mean sleep latency by itself does not distinguish well between clinical and control populations but rather lends support to clinical suspicion. Up to 30% of normal populations may have a mean sleep latency of less than 8 minutes but fewer than 2% of normal controls exhibit SOREMPs.[15] Extensive data for children are lacking.

SCORING AND INTERPRETING THE DATA

Once the sleep study has been accomplished, typically a trained technologist will be assigned to analyze the raw data in 30-second intervals (epochs) using standard AASM criteria for scoring of sleep and associated events.[8–10] It is then the

sleep specialist's task to examine the study in its entirety in order to accurately and judiciously interpret the data presented. In order to do this skillfully, the physician has to be knowledgeable in several areas. To begin with, it is very important to understand the clinical context within which the study was ordered. This will allow the final report to be tailored to the question at hand. Next, attention needs to be turned to any changes in the child's clinical status, including changes in medications or sleep habits, since the time of ordering the study until its execution. For example, an inadvertently taken nap or caffeinated beverage just prior to the sleep study may skew the findings of the test. Similarly, the

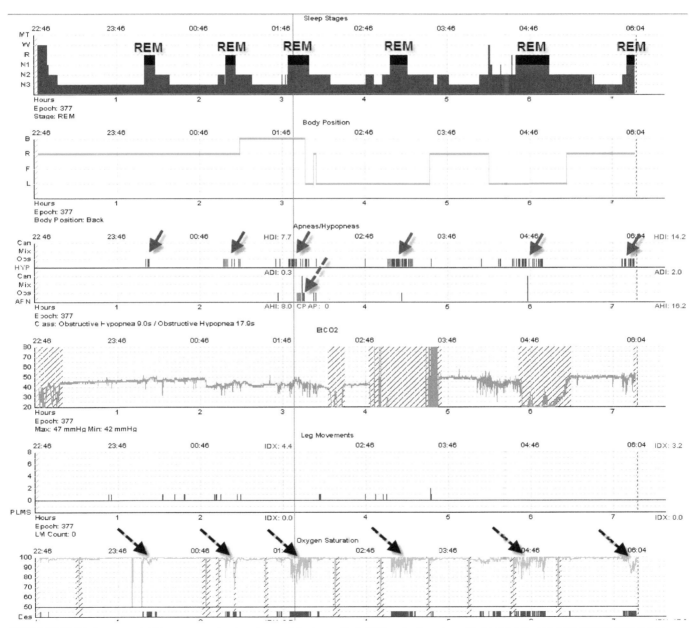

FIGURE 49-7 This is an overnight hypnogram showing sleep architecture with six REM cycles (top channel) separated by non-REM periods. From top to bottom, the remaining channels are body position (B, back or supine; R, right; L, left; F, front or prone), apneas and hypopneas, ETCO₂, leg movements, and oxygen saturation. Notice the clustering of hypopneas (solid red arrows) and apneas (broken red arrow) in temporal conjunction with desaturations (broken black arrows) and REM. For the sake of accuracy in generating cumulative data for the final report, 'bad data' in the ETCO₂ and oxygen channels has been manually 'artifacted out' (crosshatches).

start and stop of certain medications may alter sleep architecture by suppressing REM or other sleep stages or conversely causing a rebound of certain sleep stages.[51] It is useful also to know if the parents thought the recorded sleep period represented a typical night for the child or not. In order to help with this, most sleep centers use pre-study and post-study questionnaires which not only record pertinent clinical status immediately prior to the study, but also allow the patient and/or the parent to feed back on the conditions of the study itself.

Much information is also gathered from the attending technologist's log and this needs to be reviewed by the interpreting sleep expert as well. Problematic environmental and technical conditions that may have interfered with the study are noted. As an example, such notes may be useful in distinguishing whether the noise on the microphone is patient-related snoring, wheezing, stertor, or parental snoring artifact. Similarly, semiology of nocturnal events such as parasomnia or seizures may be crucial, as can notes such as 'head cold, thick nasal discharge' while interpreting sleep data.

Having acquired this background information, the sleep expert needs to bring to bear knowledge of developmental neurology and respiratory physiology while reviewing the data. A fair depth of knowledge is required to be able to interpret the rapidly evolving EEG in the growing infant, for example. The pediatric expert will need to keep in mind that periodic breathing may be normal in infants and that babies may regularly exhibit paradoxical respiration, the frequency of which reduces over the first few years of life, as mentioned previously. A frequent problem in the interpretation of pediatric sleep studies is the presence of artifact from parental intervention such as feeding, holding, patting or rocking, or from technologist intervention to replace sensors. The use of pacifiers is a common cause for dislodgment of nasal or oral airflow sensors. Occasionally, the parent may need to co-sleep with the anxious child and this itself may induce either movement or snore artifact into the child's recording. It is therefore important to have a plethysmographic signal to lend support to the reliability of pulse oximetry. Similarly, visualization of a plateau in the $ETCO_2$ waveform is reassuring that *end-tidal* CO_2 is indeed being measured (see Figure 49-5). Accordingly, capnometry, and pulse oximetry trends need to be reviewed carefully lest such artifact be erroneously used to score events in the night.

Review of the video in real time is additionally very helpful in these circumstances. The video is also vital to confirm rhythmic movement disorder and characterize parasomnias or seizures. Often, reviewing portions of the record at 10, 60, or 120-second epoch lengths is useful to clarify certain observations.

While attention to minute details during epoch-by-epoch review of the study is critical, a careful perusal of the hypnogram is essential prior to formulating a report. This bird's-eye view of the full study period is very useful for analyzing sleep architecture and discerning patterns that may not be evident during event scoring (Figure 49-7). Based upon a detailed review of the sleep study, a report is generated which not only contains a descriptive summary of the numeric data from the PSG/MSLT, but also attempts to correlate this data to the clinical question at hand.

In the end, it is the interpretive portion of the report that is most crucial for further therapeutic interventions. Therefore, despite the fact that normative PSG data have been published[52–54] and diagnostic criteria have been refined over time,[15] the final analysis and interpretation of complex data from the sleep study remains as much art as it is science.

SUMMARY

The study of children in the sleep laboratory poses unique challenges which many adult laboratories may not be well equipped to handle. The requirements and the rules of scoring and interpreting sleep studies are significantly different from those in adults. Indeed, many physiological parameters change even within the pediatric age group as the infant matures into a teenager. The pediatric sleep laboratory should therefore be able to cater for children from birth through adulthood with equal ease. This requires expertise at all levels, beginning with technologists and ending with the sleep specialist.

Clinical Pearls

- A thorough clinical evaluation and formulation of a testing hypothesis is essential before ordering a sleep study in order that a well-defined clinical query may be addressed.
- The utility of adequate pre-test education cannot be overstated. This serves to reduce patient and parent anxiety and enlist their cooperation.
- Essential pre-planning for the sleep study also includes attention to behavioral and developmental needs, age-appropriate sleep requirements, unique sleep habits (including circadian timing), comorbid conditions (including acute illnesses), and medication effects (both at time of initiation and withdrawal).
- The pediatric-friendly sleep lab lives up to its name less because of its ambient decor and toys, but more importantly by the patience, kindness, knowledge and skills exhibited by its technological personnel and medical providers.

References

1. Carroll JL, McColley SA, Marcus CL, et al. Inability of clinical history to distinguish primary snoring from obstructive sleep apnea syndrome in children. Chest 1995;108(3):610–18.
2. Wang RC, Elkins TP, Keech D, et al. Accuracy of clinical evaluation in pediatric obstructive sleep apnea. Otolaryngol Head Neck Surg 1998; 118(1):69–73.
3. Marcus CL, Brooks LJ, Draper KA, et al. Diagnosis and management of childhood obstructive sleep apnea syndrome. American Academy of Pediatrics. Pediatrics 2012;130(3):576–84.
4. American Academy of Pediatrics, Section on Pediatric Pulmonology. Subcommittee on obstructive sleep apnea syndrome. Clinical practice guidelines: Diagnosis and management of childhood obstructive sleep apnea syndrome. Pediatrics 2002;109:704–12.
5. Spruyt K, Gozal D. Pediatric sleep questionnaires as diagnostic or epidemiological tools: a review of currently available instruments. Sleep Med Rev 2011;15(1):19–32.
6. Mignot E, Young T, Lin L, et al. Nocturnal sleep and daytime sleepiness in normal subjects with HLA-DQB1*0602. Sleep 1999;22(3):347–52.
7. Nishino S, Ripley B, Overeem S, et al. Hypocretin (orexin) deficiency in human narcolepsy. Lancet 2000;355(9197):39–40.
8. Iber C, Ancoli-Israel S, Chesson A, et al. for the American Academy of Sleep Medicine. The AASM manual for the scoring of sleep and associated events: Rules, terminology and technical specifications. 1st ed Westchester, Il: American Academy of Sleep Medicine; 2007.
9. Littner MR, Kushida C, Wise M, et al. Practice parameters for clinical use of the multiple sleep latency test and the maintenance of wakefulness test. Sleep 2005;28(1):113–21.

10. Berry RB, Budharaja R, Gottlieb DJ, et al. Rules for scoring respiratory events in sleep: Update of the 2007 AASM Manual for the Scoring of Sleep and Associated Events. Deliberations of the Sleep Apnea Definitions Task Force of the American Academy of Sleep Medicine. J Clin Sleep Med 2012;8(5):597–619.

11. Owens J, Kothare S, Sheldon S. PRO: 'Not just little adults': AASM should require pediatric accreditation for integrated sleep medicine programs serving both children (0–16 years) and adults. J Clin Sleep Med 2012;8(5):473–6.

12. Gozal D. CON: Specific pediatric accreditation is not critical for integrated pediatric and adult sleep medicine programs. J Clin Sleep Med 2012;8(5):477–9.

13. Aurora RN, Zak RS, Karippot A, et al.; American Academy of Sleep Medicine. Practice parameters for the respiratory indications for polysomnography in children. Sleep 2011;34(3):379–88.

14. Aurora RN, Lamm CI, Zak RS, et al. Practice parameters for the non-respiratory indications for polysomnography and multiple sleep latency testing for children. Sleep 2012;35(11):1467–73.

15. American Academy of Sleep Medicine. International classification of sleep disorders. 2nd ed. Diagnostic and coding manual. Westchester, Il: American Academy of Sleep Medicine; 2005.

16. Wolfson AR, Carskadon MA. Sleep schedules and daytime functioning in adolescents. Child Dev 1998;69:875–87.

17. Zaremba EK, Barkey ME, Mesa C, et al. Making polysomnography more child friendly: A family-centered care approach. J Clin Sleep Med 2005;1:189–98.

18. Kothare SV, Vendrame M, Sant JL, et al. Fall-prevention policies in pediatric sleep laboratories. J Clin Sleep Med 2011;7(1):9–10.

19. Biban P, Baraldi E, Pettennazzo A, et al. Adverse effect of chloral hydrate in two young children with obstructive sleep apnea. Pediatrics 1993;92:461–3.

20. Jasper HH. The ten-twenty electrode system of the International Federation. Electroencephalogr Clin Neurophysiol 1958;10:371–5.

21. Grigg-Damberger M, Gozal D, Marcus CL, et al. The visual scoring of sleep and arousals in infants and children: development of polygraphic features, reliability, validity, and alternative methods. J Clin Sleep Med 2007;3:201–40.

22. Anders T, Emde R, Parmelee A, editors. A manual of standardized terminology, techniques and criteria for scoring of states of sleep and wakefulness in newborn infants. Los Angeles: UCLA Brain Information Service: NINDS Neurological Information Network; 1971.

23. Redline S, Budhiraja R, Kapur V, et al. Reliability and validity of respiratory event measurement and scoring. J Clin Sleep Med 2007;3:169–200.

24. Glautier C, Praud JP, Canet E, et al. Paradoxical inward ribcage motion during rapid eye movement sleep in infants and young children. J Dev Physiol 1987;9 391–7.

25. Guilleminault C, Stoohs R, Clerk A, et al. A cause of excessive daytime sleepiness. The upper airway resistance syndrome. Chest 1993;104:781–7.

26. Spriggs WH. Instrumentation. In: Spriggs WH, editor. Principles of polysomnography. 1st ed. Salt Lake City, UT: Sleep Ed, LLC; 2002. p. 50–121.

27. American Thoracic Society. Standards and indications for cardiopulmonary sleep studies in children. Am J Resp Crit Care Med 1996;153:866–78.

28. Brouillette RT, Fernbach SK, Hunt CE. Obstructive sleep apnea in infants and children. J Pediatr 1982;100:31–40.

29. Farre R, Monserrat JM, Ballester E, et al. Importance of the pulse oximeter averaging time when measuring oxygen desaturation in sleep apnea. Sleep 1998;21:386–90.

30. American Academy of Sleep Medicine. International classification of sleep disorders. 2nd ed. Diagnostic and coding manual. Westchester, Il: American Academy of Sleep Medicine; 2005.

31. Simakajornboon N, Kheirandish-Gozal L, Gozal D. Diagnosis and management of restless legs syndrome in children. Sleep Med Rev 2009;13(2):149–56.

32. Stores G. Rapid eye movement sleep behaviour disorder in children and adolescents. Dev Med Child Neur 2008;50:728–32.

33. Boeve BF. REM sleep behavior disorder: updated review of the core features, the rbd-neurodegenerative disease association, evolving concepts, controversies, and future directions. Ann NY Acad Sci 2010;1184:15–54.

34. Caples SM, Rosen CL, Sher WK, et al. The scoring of cardiac events during sleep. J Clin Sleep Med 2007;3:147–54.

35. Archbold KH, Johnson NL, Goodwin JL, et al. Normative heart rate parameters during sleep for children aged 6 to 11 years. J Clin Sleep Med 2010;6:47–50.

36. Pereira KD, Roebuck JC, Howell L. The effect of body position on sleep apnea in children younger than 3 years. Arch Otolaryngol Head Neck Surg 2005;131(11):1014–16.

37. Hsieh T, Chen M, McAfee A, et al. Sleep-related breathing disorder in children with vagal nerve stimulators. Pediatr Neurol 2008;38:99–103.

38. Noronha AC, de Bruin VM, Nobre e Souza MA, et al. Gastroesophageal reflux and obstructive sleep apnea in childhood. Int J Pediatr Otorhinolaryngol 2009;73(3):383–9.

39. Bhattacharjee R, Kheirandish-Gozal L, Spruyt K, et al. a multicenter retrospective study. Am J Respir Crit Care Med 2010;182(5):676–83.

40. Kushida CA, Chediak A, Berry RB, et al. Positive airway pressure titration task force of the American Academy of Sleep Medicine. Clinical guidelines for the manual titration of positive airway pressure in patients with obstructive sleep apnea. J Clin Sleep Med 2008;4:157–71.

41. Tunkel DE, McColley SA, Baroody FM, et al. Polysomnography in the evaluation of readiness for decannulation in children. Arch Otolaryngol Head Neck Surg 1996;122(7):721–4.

42. Mukherjee B, Bais AS, Bajaj Y. Role of polysomnography in tracheostomy decannulation in the paediatric patient. J Laryngol Otol 1999;113(5):442–5.

43. Drake C, Nickel C, Burduvali E, et al. The pediatric daytime sleepiness scale (PDSS): sleep habits and school outcomes in middle-school children. Sleep 2003;26:455–8.

44. Spilsbury JC, Drotar D, Rosen CL, et al. The Cleveland adolescent sleepiness questionnaire: a new measure to assess excessive daytime sleepiness in adolescents. J Clin Sleep Med 2007;3:603–12.

45. Carskadon MA, Dement WC, Mitler MM, et al. Guidelines for the multiple sleep latency test (MSLT): A standard measure of sleepiness. Sleep 1986;9:519–24.

46. Gozal D, Wang M, Pope DW Jr. Objective sleepiness measures in pediatric obstructive sleep apnea. Pediatrics 2001;108(3):693–7.

47. Gozal D, Kheirandish-Gozal L. Obesity and excessive daytime sleepiness in prepubertal children with obstructive sleep apnea. Pediatrics 2009;123(1):13–18.

48. Bonnet MH, Arand DL. Impact of motivation on multiple sleep latency test and maintenance of wakefulness test measurements. J Clin Sleep Med 2005;1(4):386–90.

49. Carskadon MA, Dement WC. Sleepiness in the normal adolescent. In: Guilleminault C, editor. Sleep and its disorders in children. New York: Raven Press; 1987. p. 53–66

50. Kotagal S, Goulding PM. The laboratory assessment of daytime sleepiness in children. J Clin Neurophysiol 1996;13:208–13.

51. Schweitzer PK. Effects of drugs on sleep. In: Barkoukis TJ, Avidan AY, editors. Review of sleep medicine. 2nd ed. Philadelphia: Butterworth-Heinemann; 2007. p. 169–84.

52. Montgomery-Downs HE, O'Brien LM, Gulliver TE, et al. Polysomnographic characteristics in normal preschool and early school-aged children. Pediatrics 2006;117:741–53.

53. Uliel S, Tauman R, Greenfield M, et al. Normal polysomnographic respiratory values in children and adolescents. Chest 2004;125:872–8.

54. Traeger N, Schultz B, Pollock AN, et al. Polysomnographic values in children 2–9 years old: additional data and review of the literature. Pediatr Pulmonol 2005;40:22–30.

Index

Page numbers followed by 'f' indicate figures, 't' indicate tables, and 'b' indicate boxes.

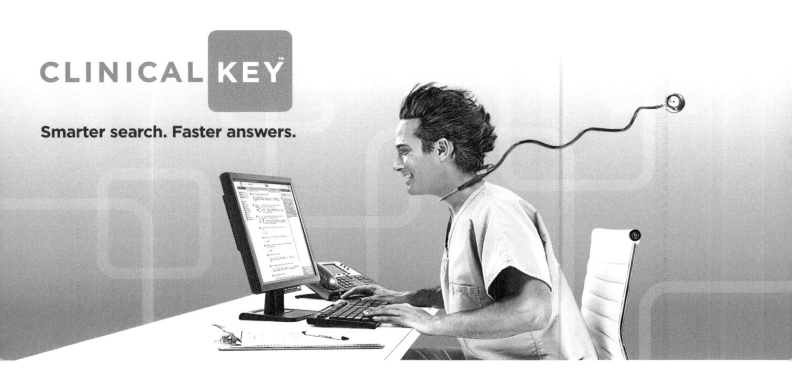

Printed and bound by CPI Group (UK) Ltd, Croydon, CR0 4YY

03/10/2024

01040303-0007